MEDICAL-SURGICAL NURSING

KATHLEEN NEWTON SHAFER
R.N., M.A.

Formerly Associate Professor in Out-Patient Nursing, the Cornell University-New York Hospital School of Nursing, New York, N. Y.; formerly Assistant Consultant in Orthopedic Nursing, the National League for Nursing Education; formerly Instructor in Medical Nursing and Instructor in Surgical Nursing, the Cornell University-New York Hospital School of Nursing, New York, N. Y.

JANET R. SAWYER
R.N., A.M.

Instructor, School of Education, Department of Nurse Education, New York University, New York, N. Y.; formerly Instructor in Surgical Nursing, the Cornell University-New York Hospital School of Nursing, New York, N. Y.; formerly Instructor in Surgical Nursing, Hartford Hospital, Hartford, Conn.

AUDREY M. McCLUSKEY
R.N., M.A.

Associate Professor in Nursing, the Cornell University-New York Hospital School of Nursing, New York, N. Y.; formerly Coordinator of Nursing Instruction in Chronic Illness and Rehabilitation and Instructor in Medical Nursing, the Cornell University-New York Hospital School of Nursing, New York, N. Y.; formerly staff member, Visiting Nurse Service of New York.

EDNA LIFGREN BECK
R.N., M.A.

Associate Director of Nursing Education, Muhlenberg Hospital School of Nursing, Plainfield, N. J.; formerly Assistant Professor in Fundamentals of Nursing and Instructor in Surgical Nursing, the Cornell University-New York Hospital School of Nursing, New York, N. Y.; formerly Clinical Instructor in Surgical Nursing, Roosevelt Hospital School of Nursing, New York, N. Y.

MEDICAL-SURGICAL NURSING

KATHLEEN NEWTON SHAFER, R.N., M.A.

JANET R. SAWYER, R.N., A.M.

AUDREY M. McCLUSKEY, R.N., M.A.

EDNA LIFGREN BECK, R.N., M.A.

SECOND EDITION

with 141 *illustrations*

St. Louis

THE C. V. MOSBY COMPANY

1961

Previous edition copyrighted 1958

Printed in the United States of America

Library of Congress Catalog Card Number 61-5952

Distributed in Great Britain by Henry Kimpton, London

Preface to the second edition

In this edition of *Medical-Surgical Nursing* new material has been incorporated, current references have been added, and sections have been clarified by rearrangement and by the inclusion of more subheadings. As in the first edition, emphasis remains on nursing care of the *patient* who is ill and on nursing and medical care as it relates to major health problems in the United States. However, references have been included for those interested in conditions that occur less frequently or regionally.

We are particularly grateful to the many instructors throughout the United States and in Canada who thoughtfully reviewed the first edition and offered extremely helpful suggestions. Effort has been made to correct all errors called to our attention and, within the limits of the book's size, to include new material suggested.

Again we wish to state our belief that a textbook in nursing should contain primarily *nursing*—not medical content. It is not our intention that this book be turned to for medical information about each of the many diseases which the student will encounter while receiving practice in medical and surgical nursing. The primary purpose of the book is to provide the student with *nursing* knowledge. It is our firm conviction that only when the profession of nursing has at its command a definite body of knowledge, adequately recorded and not handed down by word of mouth as in an apprenticeship system, can it lay firmer claim to being a true profession.

We acknowledge with gratitude the help given by Miss Margaret R. Bonnell, librarian at the Muhlenberg Hospital, Plainfield, N. J.

Kathleen Newton Shafer
Janet R. Sawyer
Audrey M. McCluskey
Edna Lifgren Beck

Preface to the first edition

Much has been written in recent years about total patient care or comprehensive nursing care. Yet few nurses have sufficient opportunity to practice this concept. The very nature of much hospital nursing service organization and nursing education limits opportunity to care for the "whole person." In hospital practice, boundaries—artificial, but all too well established—are often set up to separate the "medical" patient from the "surgical" patient. Few patients, however, are purely "medical" or purely "surgical" by strict definition. Basic principles of nursing used in caring for the patient as a person are the same regardless of his definitive treatment.

The idea of teaching nursing of patients needing both surgical and medical care as one course is not new. The *Curriculum Guide,* published by the National League of Nursing Education in 1937, made this recommendation. Increase in chronic illness, multiplicity of diagnoses in an aging population, and the newer emphasis on rehabilitation have increased the need to review methods of teaching nursing. The material in this book, however, has been so arranged that it can be used in teaching medical nursing, surgical nursing, or any of the specialties separately.

It is the purpose of this book to give a broad general background in the nursing of patients who require medical and surgical treatment. Details of physical care for some common conditions are included as a guide for the nurse in making adaptations for individual patients. To equip the nurse to give comprehensive care, the cause, prevention, medical care, principles of nursing care, and the significance of the disease to the patient, his family, the community, and the nation are considered. The nurse's appreciation of the feelings of individual patients who go through a sequence of events in illness—diagnostic, medical, surgical, rehabilitative—is judged equally important as knowledge of pathologic changes taking place and physical nursing needs that must be met.

Each year it becomes more apparent that the nurse as a professional team member must know the why and wherefore of her nursing acts and take legal responsibility for them. A better informed patient is demanding more specific information from doctors and nurses. While the nurse needs refined judgment in what she tells the patient, she can no longer hide behind the covering statement, "Your doctor will tell you." She must learn to work with the patient in the common undertaking of his recovery, teaching him and his family the care during illness and the prevention of future illness. Because of this newer concept in nursing, attention has been given in this book to some simple everyday conditions about which the nurse may be asked and to teaching the patient and his family both in the home and in the hospital.

The problem of what to include in a book such as this is very real. To give intelligent care, the nurse must know what is the matter with the patient, what the doctor is attempting to accomplish, and what the signs of success or failure may be. She must know the reasons why she is doing what she does for the patient. A book of this kind, however, if it includes nursing detail, cannot give too much space to medical care. For more detailed information we refer the nurse to medical texts, periodicals, and lectures. No attempt has been made to duplicate details of basic nursing procedures that are part of the course in fundamentals of nursing and included in texts on that subject.

The book is divided into two sections. The first deals with general subjects and trends. It is intended to focus thinking on the *nursing needs* of patients and to prevent endless repetition. The second section considers nursing care for patients having specific medical and surgical treatment. Study questions at the beginning of each chapter have been prepared to assist the student to review basic preclinical subject matter not repeated in the text. The references preceded by an asterisk indicate material particularly well suited for student reading.

This book could never have been completed without the help of many people. Miss Virginia M. Dunbar, Dean of the Cornell University-New York Hospital School of Nursing, gave us constant encouragement. Nurses with special knowledge and experience gave generously of their time in reading chapters and offering helpful suggestions. They include Frances L. Boyle, R.N., Carmen Brescia, R.N., Elizabeth Brooks, R.N., Julia Dennehy, R.N., Virginia Dericks, R.N., Alberta Evans, R.N., Mary J. Foster, R.N., Ena Stevens Fisher, R.N., Elizabeth C. Madore, R.N., Frances McVey, R.N., Margery T. Overholser, R.N., Henderika J. Rynbergen, M.S., Doris R. Schwartz, R.N., Margaret H. Terry, R. N., Ethel M. Tschida, R.N., Edna Tuffley, R.N., Carolyn Wagner, R.N., and Margie Warren, R.N., most of whom are on the faculty of the Cornell University-New York Hospital School of Nursing. All the manuscript has been reviewed by members of the teaching staff of the Cornell Medical College. Special gratitude is due John M. Beal, M.D., Peter Dineen, M.D., and S. Frank Redo, M.D., of the Department of Surgery, Frederic T. Kirkham, Jr., M.D., and George G. Reader, M.D., of the Department of Medicine, and James R. McCarroll, M.D., of the Department of Preventive Medicine, who, in spite of other important work, reviewed each chapter and gave us their suggestions. For any misrepresentation of the suggestions of our reviewers, we take full responsibility.

We acknowledge with gratitude the help of Miss M. J. Munroe and Mrs. A. S. Miller, librarians in the School of Nursing; Mr. Milton L. Zisowitz, who edited most of the manuscript; and Mrs. Ethel M. Young, who also helped with editing. Thanks are due Miss Shirley Baty, who did the drawings; Mr. Percy S. Brooks, who took many of the photographs; and Mrs. Doris Baldwin, Mrs. Zetta Murray, and Mrs. Margaret MacGuire, who helped with the typing. Special thanks are also due to relatives and friends for their understanding and encouragement during this undertaking.

Kathleen Newton Shafer
Janet R. Sawyer
Audrey M. McCluskey
Edna E. Lifgren

Contents

MEDICAL-SURGICAL NURSING

Section I

General considerations

Trends and problems influencing patient care

Study questions for review

1. Keep a record for a week of each patient for whom you care. Include the patient's age, his nationality, his place of birth, the language spoken in his home, his education, his place in his family, his religion, and his age. Consider whether or not any of these influenced the nursing care you gave.
2. How has knowledge of the patient's background, as listed above, influenced your teaching of a patient during his preparation for leaving the hospital?
3. What are some of the ways you believe anxiety may be expressed? List some questions that patients and members of their families have asked you that indicate anxiety.

The nurse's understanding of herself and the patient

Chapter 1

THE NURSE'S CONCEPT OF THE PATIENT

The nurse-patient relationship is a term commonly used to identify the complex interaction between the patient and the nurse. Every nurse needs to understand this relationship, for upon it will rest her success in helping the patient and in achieving personal satisfaction.

Each one of us is an individual—the nurse, other hospital personnel, the patient, members of his family, and his friends. Each one is reacting in a particular manner to a specific situation based upon his own social and cultural background, his total life experience, his learned reactions, and his individual make-up. Thus, each will react differently to illness. The nurse needs to learn to distinguish between her own goals and standards of value and conduct and those of her patient. She should be alert to the patient's behavior, try to interpret this wisely, and use his behavior as a guide to his care. A nurse should show sincere interest, sensitivity, and understanding, be friendly and helpful, and recognize that it is important for the patient to maintain his identity and dignity as a person. She should be aware of her own prejudices and work toward meeting each person with an open mind.

In caring for patients with medical and surgical conditions, the nurse encounters many situations which require acceptance of things that cannot be changed. She cares for patients with incurable illnesses which may result in immediate death or chronicity and eventual death. Some patients may require disfiguring surgery. Some may have deformities or communicable diseases with attendant social stigmas. The nurse needs to develop a genuine ability to accept things that cannot be changed and to respect the opinions of others in the determination of what can or should be changed.

The nurse might well ask herself whether she really likes people and is interested in working with them. Does she try to understand what the situation means to a particular patient in the light of his own personality? Does she have a genuine acceptance of others as they are, without judgment and without censure? For example, does she look away from an amputee? This may be because she rejects the deformity, or it may be because she has underestimated the indomitable drive of the human spirit under trying circumstances. These reactions will greatly decrease her effectiveness in caring for the patient. There will be situations that the nurse cannot accept and in which she may herself need help.

Since attitudes speak louder than words, the nurse must be sincere in all her responses and try to become aware of them. There can be no set rules to guide her in her responses to patients. Each response must be spontaneous. A few suggestions follow:

1. Be yourself, for nothing draws more genuine response from others than this.
2. Continue to grow intellectually, emotionally, and socially by developing broad interests both within and outside nursing.
3. Let others respond in their own way rather than trying to make them respond the way you would.
4. In situations that appear unsatisfactory and frustrating, ask yourself, "What am *I* doing?" "Am I really appreciating the values of the patient?"

THE PATIENT'S CONCEPT OF THE NURSE

The patient's concept of the nurse is influenced by his cultural background, his previous knowledge and experience, his social and economic status, his sex, and his emotional make-up. The nurse should be aware that each patient has a stereotype of nurse in mind and that wide variations of this exist. These stereotypes need to be considered as she gives care to each patient.

The patient may have come from a cultural background in which women are considered inferior to men, one in which women unquestionably wait upon the men. For example, a man who had recently come to this country antagonized all the members of a nursing staff by ordering them about and by refusing to help himself at all. His convalescence was being delayed by his firm conviction that the women about him, the nurses, must "do for him" on all occasions. Only when an alert nurse noticed that he ordered his wife about during visiting hours and that she accepted this in a satisfied fashion did the nurses realize the meaning of his behavior. In this particular instance the situation was remedied by working through the doctor, whose opinions, suggestions, and judgments were accepted readily by the patient as those of the nurses were not. There was no need for resentment on the part of the nurses. There was need only for an understanding of the patient and for appropriate action with this in mind.

The patient's concept of the nurse is frequently based on the general public's idea, particularly if the patient has had no previous contact with nurses. The nurse is commonly held in a position of respect by the public. She is often thought of as a person who is good, immaculately groomed, efficient, and kind. She is less often considered a teacher, though the public frequently turns to her for answers to questions regarding health. She is thought of as one who "does for the sick." The new philosophy of rehabilitation and of letting the patient "do for himself" may place the nurse in a position in which her motives may be misunderstood and her actions questioned. This can happen easily unless she takes the time to explain to the patient why he may be asked to do things for himself and finds out if he objects to this, and unless she takes time to teach, to give encouragement, and to help him see his own progress. Her attitude as she does these things conveys to the patient her interest in his comfort and his welfare.

Some patients may have traumatic experiences which lead them to distrust and reject the nurse. Others have listened to harrowing experiences of their friends and assume that their association with nurses will not be pleasant. The nurse should try to help the patient correct this distortion by encouraging him to relate to her as an individual.

Psychologic factors may affect the patient's response to the nurse. When any person becomes ill and dependent upon others, he regresses to some extent. Some patients unconsciously respond to the nurse as they did to their mothers during childhood. This may be demonstrated by docile obedience, eagerness for approval, playing childish tricks to see if they can "get away with anything," or by a number of other ways. Others may identify the nurse with a domineering mother from whom they may be seeking emancipation or with an unwanted mother-in-law. They may respond with stubborn and contradictory behavior which the nurse must try to understand.

Interpretation of all we see is based on our own experiences and learning. Therefore, it is not strange that the nurse is seen in a different light by each person she encounters. Accepting this, she needs to work toward responding to each patient individually, respecting his differences, and placing her emphasis on common elements. In this way she will give the most effective care.

EMOTIONAL RESPONSES TO ILLNESS

Anxiety and *fear* are part of the natural reaction of every normal human being when threats to his health appear. Anxiety has been defined as a feeling of uncertainty and helplessness in the face of danger. It is caused to some extent by the nature of the human organism but can be intensified by lack of knowledge, by lack of faith, and by social, economic, and cultural forces bearing directly upon the affected individual. Fear of cancer, for instance, is becoming almost universal in our society. This fear can be transferred from one person to another in such a way that it has been defined recently as one of the most common "communicable diseases" of man. It is imperative that the nurse have some understanding of the anxieties and fears of her patients. A large part of her work is to encourage the patient in most instances to express his anxieties, to help him see the universality of fear in his situation, and to help him seek outlets for these fears and tensions and to allay them whenever possible.

The signs of anxiety, fear, and tension are variable. An indifference to his symptoms and to the tests being made may mean that the patient has not accepted the possibility that anything may be wrong. He may not be able to face reality and still maintain stability and integrity of his personality. The patient who is noisy and demanding, perhaps declaring that he is not worried, is one who, if closely observed, may reveal what he dares not verbalize. The patient who "forgets" the clinic appointment at which he is to learn the results of a test is probably fearful of these results. Other patients manifest their anxiety, consciously or unconsciously, by repeatedly asking the same question, making many complaints, or being preoccupied with bodily functions. Still others will "battle it out alone," leaving the nurse unaware of their problems. Insomnia, anorexia, frequent urination, and irritability are often signs of anxiety. Sometimes marked physical signs such as perspiring hands, increased pulse and respiratory rates, and dilated pupils denote anxiety and fear. Perhaps the best way a nurse can estimate her helpfulness is by the patient's progress. If he gets more tense or repeats the same question over and over, she should seek expert assistance.

One's cultural background may influence attitudes toward certain diseases. These may have implications that are not culturally acceptable to the patient or his family. In some societies it is a disgrace to become ill at all. In our culture venereal disease often is associated with uncleanliness, and diseases such as epilepsy and mental illness may be carefully guarded secrets within families. Various parts of the body may have significant meaning in certain cultures. Some patients may refuse to permit amputation of a limb because physical fitness and the "body beautiful" are valued highly. The modern woman in the United States may have an almost intolerable emotional reaction to a mastectomy because of the emphasis placed upon women's breasts in our culture.

Illness may be a new experience for the patient. He may be unsure of the reactions expected of him by others, or he may be censured for displaying behavior acceptable in his own cultural group. For instance, in one culture "the picture of health contains a normal amount of disease."[27] For this reason, early medical care or a program of prevention may meet resistance. In another culture the family usually prefers to care for the patient at home, but if hospitalization is necessary many relatives and friends cluster around lest the patient feel rejected in his time of need. In still another culture it is proper to go to bed with much moaning and groaning if one is ill, so that the relatives may fulfill their rightful role of beneficence. Hospital personnel frequently consider these patients "problems" rather than recognizing that such behavior is culturally determined and trying to work out acceptable adjustments. Explanation to the patient and his family of hospital policies such as visiting hours and isolation requirements may prevent undue anxiety in both the patient and his relatives.

Anxiety may be caused by the patient's inability to participate in his usual religious experiences. It is important for the patient to retain religious medals and perform religious rites. If this is not possible, an interpretation of the reasons by a religious adviser is usually helpful in decreasing anxiety.

During illness the patient may be denied certain foods considered necessary in his culture. This may produce anxiety. For example, after two weeks in the respirator, one young patient became anxious over his first meal because the food was not sanctioned by his church law. His family and religious leader had to be called to reassure him before he would eat. Some people believe that one should fast when ill; imagine the anxiety and uncertainty produced when a nourishing diet is served and these patients are told by the doctors and nurses that they must eat.

Economic problems may add to the patient's anxiety. Economic effects of illness are a threat not only to the patient but also to those he loves. This may be particularly so if he is head of the household. Most patients respond to this threat with negative behavior, and the nurse may be the recipient of some of this hostility. She must learn to be a good listener and to accept this as a normal and necessary release of tension. Often the social service worker can help the patient resolve some of his problems, for she will know of available community resources such as funds, housekeepers, child-placement facilities, nursing homes, equipment for home care, and job-placement agencies. To help meet the financial problem common to illness, many organizations have hospital insurance for their employees and many people invest in individual health plans. Hospitals are establishing home-care programs to facilitate the care of chronically and terminally ill patients in their own homes. These can ease many anxieties inherent in institutional care, obviate many problems of readjustment to the patient's own life situation, diminish the economic pressure, and keep hospital beds available for the acutely ill.

THE NURSE'S CONTRIBUTION TO PREVENTION AND RELEASE OF ANXIETY

The nurse cannot possibly know all the factors contributing to anxiety or their particular application for each patient. However, by recognizing anxiety and understanding that all behavior has meaning, the nurse may be guided by some rules. She must remember that it is the patient, his family, and his friends who are primarily concerned with his welfare, and she must try to keep them informed.

Each new experience should be explained to the patient and, if possible, related to familiar experiences. Orienting the newly admitted patient and his family to the hospital routine tends to minimize anxiety. It is helpful to inform the patient how he may call the nurse, when he will see his doctor, the hours the religious adviser is available, and how he may contact his family. In addition, the family should be told how to obtain information concerning the patient, when they may visit, and any immediate plans for the patient.

If a patient is to have a treatment or test, he must be given some idea of what will be done, the preparation involved, and the reasons why the procedure is necessary. To remove the water pitcher and inform a patient that he cannot have any more water until after his x-ray examination can leave him with many anxious thoughts: "What x-ray examination?" "I wonder when it is?" "What will it be like?" "It must be something special if I can't have any water." Lack of knowledge as a cause of anxiety reflects the nurse's lack of consideration for the patient's rights as an individual.

Explanations should be given in the patient's own terms at appropriate times and repeated as necessary. If the patient is very anxious, he may need repeated explanation, since extreme anxiety reduces intellectual function. Detailed explanations should not be given to a patient under sedation, with high temperature, or in severe pain because he will not remember them. Repetition is often required for older persons and children because they may have a short memory span.

Time spent in giving explanations to relatives is not wasted. Not only does it relieve their anxieties which may be transmitted to the patient, but it also saves having to untangle misinformation. Often the family is helpful in interpreting necessary instructions to the patient in such a manner that he understands and accepts them.

The nurse should provide opportunities for the patient to talk, but she should not probe. Without seemingly unduly curious, one can usually find some topic of personal interest to the patient that will provide an opening. A picture on the bedside table may create such an opening. Then, if the nurse will listen with sincere interest and without making judgments about the patient's character, she may gain insight into the patient as a person. More important, the patient may begin to verbalize his fears. At this point the nurse who feels inadequate herself may cut off the conversation. For instance, if a patient says, "You know, I don't think I'll ever get to see my little boy again," a common response is, "Oh, don't say that, certainly you will; you're going to be all right." The patient may very well not be all right. Would it not be better to respond, "Not see your little boy again? What makes you feel this way?" or whatever similar rejoinder is comfortable for the nurse and helps the patient explore the subject. This leaves opportunity for the patient to answer and to examine this fear himself. It also gives the nurse a chance to find out what the patient fears. The nurse should give only factual reassurance and explore the implications with the patient who must solve his own problems. The nurse who is willing to listen to patients, to be guided by their reactions, and to work with them rather than to make decisions for them will find it easier to give needed emotional support, because she is giving them real help.

Even if we could solve patients' problems for them, this is not the aim of nursing. The nurse is prepared only to help the patient look at those problems which he himself is able to bring into awareness. Underlying problems should be handled by a psychotherapist. A nurse needs to be able to recognize normal anxiety reactions and to report exaggerated reactions that may indicate the need for psychiatric referral. Stuttering and blocking of words may indicate increasing tension. Depression and sadness are normal reactions to illness and particularly to surgery, but feelings of guilt and worthlessness should make the nurse aware of the possibility of suicide. Apathy may indicate that the patient has given up not only fear but also hope. Fortunately, most of these states are selflimiting and improve with a cheerful and encouraging attitude on the part of the staff, renewed activity for the patient, and a chance to talk. Independence should be allowed and encouraged as soon as possible, since for most people nothing is so demoralizing as complete dependence upon others. Independence cannot be forced; it results from the patient's own motivation. This motivation may be established by allowing the patient to be dependent. The desired goal is interdependence—the result of collaboration of the health team and the patient to help the patient regain and maintain normal health.

The nurse has a responsibility to her patient for maintaining channels of communication with others who may be better prepared to meet his needs. The patient should feel free to communicate with others such as the doctor, his family, spiritual advisers, and social workers. At times the nurse may need to be a "go-between" because some patients are uneasy as to whether their questions are appropriate. A statement by the nurse such as "Mr. Jones asked about how long he would be hospitalized, and I believe you have some other questions, don't you, Mr. Jones?" may provide the necessary opening.

Throughout the patient's illness, the nurse must be aware that he is a member of a family and of a community to which he will return. This must be considered in planning for home care, or there will be anxiety. This is often the problem confronting the patient who is said to have "hospitalitis." It is important for the nurse to ascertain with whom the family authority lies, since such a person is usually the one who should be brought into planning. She also needs to gain insight into reactions to such things as disability, infectious diseases, and care of the aged, which may be culturally determined. Also, a patient may find it difficult for others to accept him; in such a case the nurse should try to prepare him for this adjustment.

The aged patient is not always readily taken back into the home of his children. In some cultures this is rarely a problem, since the older person is highly respected as the head of the family. In others it may be expected that the aged person who is widowed will go to a home for the aged when he is no longer able to live by himself. Awareness of any such possibilities should make the nurse alert to early planning with the patient and his family for his discharge, whether it be for convalescent, rehabilitative, chronic, or terminal care. Here again, the plans must stem from the patient and his family.

Planning is also necessary in carrying out any patient-teaching program. The nurse suggests needed materials, routines, and techniques. The patient, with his family, should be encouraged to work out the details, such as the equipment available, the best time of day, the best place, and the easiest technique. They must plan, for example, how a special diet can be worked in with the family meals. The nurse should be available to give guidance as needed. In teaching patients, the following principles are helpful:

1. Learn about the patient and his family's circumstances of living.

2. Explain to the patient the desired results, suggesting possible means to these ends.

3. Explore with the patient and his family the possibilities of carrying out instructions. Listen carefully for factors which might interfere with carrying out instructions and try to make adjustments which will make the treatment acceptable and practical to the patient and his family.

4. Have the patient practice the procedure as it is to be carried out in the home.

5. Provide for some channel of assistance if the patient should meet with difficulty.

As she gives physical care to her patient, the nurse should always be using her abilities to provide for comprehensive care. Not every problem will be solved during one patient contact. Some may never be solved or at least not in the manner which seems, in the nurse's judgment, to be for the best interest of the patient.

In this chapter great stress has been placed on the nurse's understanding of human behavior, her acceptance of different patterns of living, and her skill in working with people. Most important is the emotional overtone in the "way" things are done, conveying to the patient inherent warmth, responsiveness, sensitivity, and understanding. Good nurse-patient relationships develop from *genuine feelings* and *appropriate techniques.*

REFERENCES AND SELECTED READINGS*

1 Alfano, Genrose J.: What Rapport Means to Me, Nursing Outlook **3**:326-327, June 1955.

2 *Arnstein, Margaret: Balance in Nursing, Am. J. Nursing **58**:1690-1692, Dec. 1958.

3 *Ashbrook, James B.: Not By Bread Alone, Am. J. Nursing **55**:164-168, Feb. 1955.

4 Averill, Lawrence A., and Kempf, Florence C.: Psychology Applied to Nursing, ed. 4, Philadelphia, 1951, W. B. Saunders Co.

5 Berengarten, Sidney: The Significance of Interpersonal Relationships, Am. J. Nursing **52**:1219-1222, Oct. 1952.

6 *Bird, Brian: Psychological Aspects of Preoperative and Post-operative Care, Am. J. Nursing **55**:685-687, June 1955.

7 *Bogardus, Emory S., and Brethorst, Alice B.: Sociology Applied to Nursing, ed. 3, Philadelphia, 1954, W. B. Saunders Co.

8 Brown, Francis J., and Rouček, Joseph S.: One America, ed. 3, New York, 1952, Prentice-Hall, Inc.

9 *Church, Gertrude M.: Understanding Each Other to Achieve a Common Goal, Am. J. Nursing **56**:201-204, Feb. 1956.

10 Cooley, Carol H.: Social Aspects of Illness, Philadelphia, 1951, W. B. Saunders Co.

11 *Dicks, Russell L.: Who Is My Patient? New York, 1943, The Macmillan Co.

12 *Frake, Carolyn M.: What Kind of Help Is Best for My Patient? Am. J. Nursing **54**:997-998, Aug. 1954.

13 *Freeman, Ruth: Nurses, Patients and Progress, Nursing Outlook **7**:16-18, Jan. 1959.

14 *Frey, Vera S.: The Creative Approach to Nursing, Am. J. Nursing **53**:301-302, March 1953.

15 *Gilbertson, Evelyn: Mental Health Aspects, Am. J. Nursing **54**:1358-1359, Nov. 1954.

16 Gorer, Geoffrey: The American People, New York, 1948, W. W. Norton & Co., Inc.

*References preceded by an asterisk indicate material particularly well suited for student reading.

17 *Greenville, Maurice H.: Interviewing With a Purpose, Am. J. Nursing **56**:1259-1262, Oct. 1956.

18 *Gregg, Dorothy: Reassurance, Am. J. Nursing **55**:171-174, Feb. 1955.

19 *Gregg, Dorothy E.: Anxiety—A Factor in Nursing Care, Am. J. Nursing **52**:1363-1365, Nov. 1952.

20 *Hart, Betty, and Rohweder, Anne W.: Support in Nursing, Am. J. Nursing **59**:1398-1401, Oct. 1959.

21 Hayes, Wayland J., and Gazaway, Reva: Human Relations in Nursing, Philadelphia, 1959, W. B. Saunders Co.

22 *Ingles, Thelma, and Campbell, Emily: The Patient With a Colostomy, Am. J. Nursing **58**:1544-1546, Nov. 1958.

23 *Jourard, Sidney M.: How Well Do You Know Your Patients? Am. J. Nursing **59**:1568-1571, Nov. 1959.

24 *Jourard, Sidney M.: The Bedside Manner, Am. J. Nursing **60**:63-66, Jan. 1960.

25 *Knowles, Lois N.: How Can We Reassure Patients? Am. J. Nursing **59**:834-835, June 1959.

26 *Koos, Earl L.: The Sociology of the Patient, New York, 1954, McGraw-Hill Book Co., Inc.

27 Mead, Margaret: Cultural Patterns and Technical Change, Paris, 1954, UNESCO Manual.

28 Murphy, Gardner: Professional Progress Through Personal Growth, Am. J. Nursing **54**:1464-1467, Dec. 1954.

29 *Norris, Catherine: The Nurse and the Crying Patient, Am. J. Nursing **57**:323-327, March 1957.

30 Peplau, Hildegarde E.: Interpersonal Relations in Nursing, New York, 1952, G. P. Putnam's Sons.

31 *Perry, George S.: Families of America, New York, 1949, Whittlesey House, McGraw-Hill Book Co., Inc.

32 Roberts, Dorothy I.: A Psychiatrist Helps Them Understand Their Patients, Am. J. Nursing **56**:1302-1303, Oct. 1956.

33 Saunders, Lyle: Cultural Difference and Medical Care, New York, 1954, Russell Sage Foundation.

34 *Simmons, Leo W.: The Manipulation of Human Resources in Nursing Care, Am. J. Nursing **51**:452-456, July 1951.

35 *Troy, Crescentia: Let's Start With the Patient, Am. J. Nursing **51**:699-700, Dec. 1951.

36 *Wolff, Ilse S.: Should the Patient Know the Truth? Am. J. Nursing **55**:546-548, May 1955.

Our aging population

Chapter 2

Study questions for review

1 Review the conspicuous physical differences between a young adult and a very old person.
2 From what you have read in newspapers and current magazines, what would you select as major problems of old people in our society?
3 From what you have learned in fundamentals of nursing, what are some practical measures you can take to prevent accidents involving elderly patients in the hospital environment and in their own homes?
4 Review the eating patterns of an elderly person of your acquaintance; compare their food intake with your understanding of an adequate diet.

Many patients on medical and surgical wards of general hospitals are 65 years of age and over. Also, many elderly persons with medical and surgical conditions are cared for in their homes by public health nurses. In the future proportionately more and more nursing time will be spent with such patients. While the care of older patients is not a specialty, such patients do have special problems and special nursing needs. The nurse should know the general economic, social, emotional, and physical differences between older patients and younger ones and should understand how these differences affect the elderly patient, his family, the community, and society as a whole. It must be remembered, however, that each patient is an individual and that generalizations do not necessarily apply to all elderly patients.

A tremendous change in the age distribution of our population has taken place in the last fifty years. Social adjustments to meet the many challenges presented by an aging population have not kept pace with the increasing proportion of older people in the United States. At present over 8.6 per cent of the population of our country are 65 years of age or over; in 1900 only 4.1 per cent were of that age and in 1850 only 2.6 per cent. There are now over 15 million elderly persons in the United States, and it is estimated that by 1970, 9.4 per cent (or over 19½ million) will be 65 years of age or over.[12] These changes have come about largely through the control of communicable disease in the young which has enabled many children to survive to old age. Other reasons for this marked increase include the discovery of the sulfonamides and the antibiotics, the high fertility of our population, and the influx, at the beginning of the century, of many young vigorous persons who are now old.

It has been demonstrated repeatedly that there is no specific age at which the characteristics of old age appear in all people. Tremendous individual variations exist, and age is really physiologic rather than chronologic, although 65 years of age is usually considered the beginning of late maturity or old age. This is because some arbitrary age must be used for many purposes; for example, a person can begin to receive Social Security benefits at the age of 65 years (62 years for women since 1956) and compulsory retirement and many pension plans usually take effect at this age. At present, those persons 75 years of age and over are increasing proportionately faster than the total age group who are 65 years and over. This is leading to new terminology, and the terms "young old" and "old old" or "really old" are being used to refer to those 65 to

75 years and those 75 years and older, respectively. The problems and the needs of these two groups are quite different.

Special study and interest in older persons has brought new terminology into common use. Geriatrics is a term meaning care of the elderly; it is derived from the Greek *geras,* meaning old age, and *iatrikos,* the service or care of. Gerontology means the study of aging. The term "elderly" is preferred to "old." The word "old" has unfortunate connotations in our culture and is seldom used by the person 65 years of age or older in referring to himself. Senile, another word meaning old, has undesirable connotations; it should never be used in speaking of the aged person who is normal or the physically ill but should be reserved for those elderly persons who have severe mental deterioration.

Since 1950 much progress has been made in social planning to meet the needs of older persons. In 1950 the first National Conference on Aging was held in Washington, D. C., and the Committee on Aging and Geriatrics was formed in the Department of Health, Education, and Welfare of the federal government. In 1956 the President created a Federal Council on Aging to coordinate present programs in various departments of the federal government and to broaden the range of federal activities, and in January of 1961 the first White House Conference on aging will be held. The year 1956 was also the one in which the Center for Aging Research in the National Institutes of Health was established. Many state and local committees have been formed and have a broad area of interest. In several states, joint legislative committees have been formed to guide lawmaking bodies in passing legislation concerning the welfare of older people. Voluntary groups have also been particularly active since 1950. For example, the Committee on Aging of the National Social Welfare Assembly* was formed in that year and has worked intensively on a variety of matters affecting the aged, such as standards for sheltered care, economic status, and retirement regulations. This Committee is a valuable source for literature on all activities relating to older persons. Some cities have mayors' committees on aging, and many church and other local groups have set up special committees to study what their contribution can be to housing, recreation, and other community planning for the aging. An interesting development to observe is the close cooperation of federal, state, and voluntary groups as they work for the benefit of our senior population.

Many county medical societies now have geriatric sections, and there are two national scientific societies devoted exclusively to the aging and the aged. The Gerontological Society, Inc., founded in 1940, is concerned with the study of aging. Membership includes scientists from a wide variety of disciplines and is open to nurses. The American Geriatrics Society, founded in 1942, is primarily concerned with the medical care of aged people; those in allied disciplines such as nursing can become associate members.

PSYCHOSOCIAL, ECONOMIC, AND CULTURAL ASPECTS OF CARE OF THE AGED

When the older person becomes ill, he is particularly apprehensive and worried. Probably this is because his security is more profoundly affected by illness than that of younger persons. Life in our society is lacking in security for older persons. Our scientific achievements in controlling the diseases of the young, and thereby enabling so many to become old, has produced a curious paradox. While life has become more secure, living has become less secure. The white infant born today has a life expectancy of 68.6 years. However, this infant has little assurance that his additional years will be either happy or productive. Urbanization, with its crowded housing, industrialization, and centralization of production, often makes

*Headquarters, 345 East Forty-sixth Street, New York, N.Y.

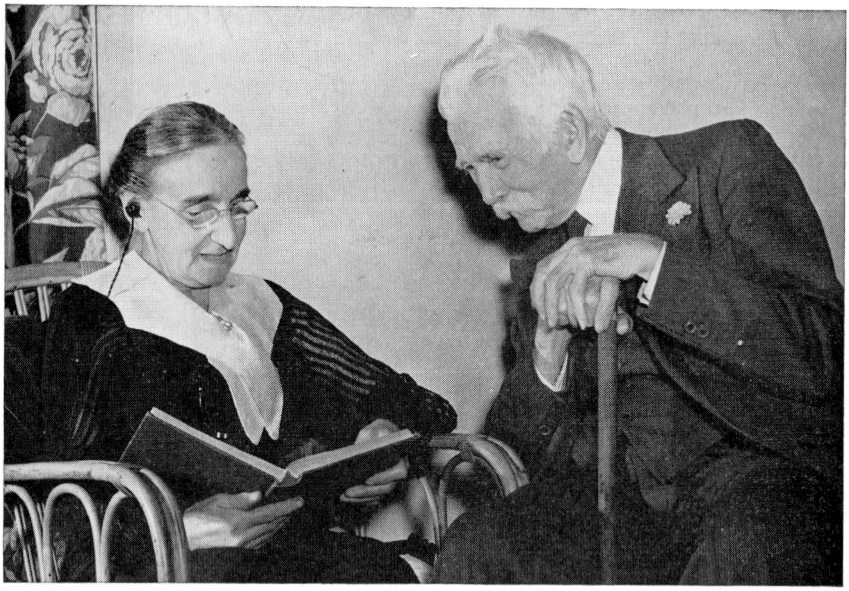

Figure 1

Adjustment is difficult when death of a spouse brings loss of the companionship developed over many years. (Courtesy New York League for the Hard of Hearing, New York, N.Y.)

it impossible for younger family members to care for their elders in the old accepted pattern, and this seriously jeopardizes the older person's chances for security and happiness in his declining years.

In one survey[6] elderly persons were asked what they considered essential for their happiness. They mentioned good health, a place to live and enough money to live comfortably, recognition by others and participation with others, and opportunity for a variety of experiences. These needs are really no different from those of any normal person. We all wish to live as long as possible without being a burden to others, to maintain our independence, to have an opportunity to participate with others in common experiences, to be recognized and accepted, to love and to be loved.

The aged face many adjustments which make it difficult and sometimes impossible for their basic emotional needs to be met. Often they must adjust to the death of a husband or wife as well as friends (see Figure 1). They may have to adjust to lowered income, housing difficulties, retirement, decreased participation in affairs about them, depleted physical energy, and chronic illness.

Ideally, it would be best that one never know that he is through with active life. He should never feel superfluous or unwanted, never be without love or purpose in his life, and never be without outlets for his creative urges.[5] It is a major challenge of our civilization to find some means of meeting the physical and emotional needs of the many whose lives have been prolonged through scientific advancement.

Economic situation. The older patient is almost always at a financial disadvantage. Enforced retirement at 65 years of age means that many workers will spend about eleven years in retirement even though they may not wish to retire and may still be capable of productive work. High costs of living, high taxes, and family responsibilities make it impossible for many persons to accumulate adequate savings to live on when they reach 65 years of age. Most elderly people now have a small income from Old Age and Survivors Insurance, private or government pensions, and other sources. Average income per family unit, however, is substantially below that of families the heads of which are 45 to 64 years of age. In addition, only one third of all those over 65 and one fifth of those who are retired have insurance to cover medical care or hospitalization in the event of illness.[15]

Over one half of our population is now covered by Old Age and Survivors Insurance under the Social Security Act, and in 1959 over 10 million persons 65 years of age and over received income from this source.[10] As of January 1959 new provisions of the law permit persons 65 and over to receive benefits for any month in which they earn no more than $100 regardless of earnings for other months. Old Age and Survivors Insurance, however, was never intended to provide complete support. Average payments in 1959 were $67.50 per month for the retired worker without dependents and $119.50 for the retired couple.[3] In 1959 between 2 and 4 million elderly persons received financial help from (Old Age Assistance), a state-administered program which receives substantial federal support. There is overlapping of benefits; for example, in 1959, 6 million elderly persons received some financial support from both sources.[3]

Private pension plans provide some needed financial security, and individual savings give further help. An additional solution to the problem of financial security may be to permit older persons to earn their support for as long as they wish to and are able to do so. Each year, more union contracts are drawn up with statements to assure the employment of some older workers.

When financial resources are cut, social life becomes curtailed. Clubs may be given up, annual vacations may not be possible, and less money is available for community participation of all kinds. Even if financial support is adequate social outlets for the aged may become limited. Friends die and children marry and move away. Because physical resources decline, it becomes more and more difficult for elderly persons to participate actively in groups and thus make new friends. A social outlet, whether it be an expensive club, an evening of poker at home with friends, or a church gathering, meets an important need, and its loss is sorely felt. Recreational centers for the aged are becoming numerous (see Figure 2). These are a help in many communities, but it must not be assumed that they are a complete answer to loneliness, or that they are necessarily good for everyone. They can never replace regular, recognized, remunerative work which has become an essential part of many people's lives.

Housing. Most elderly persons live in some kind of family unit. Only about 6 per cent of those over 65 years of age live in a communal housing facility, which includes homes for the aged. Many aged persons live in private homes that are too large, in poor neighborhoods, in isolated rural areas, in the top floor of walk-up tenements, and in housing that is otherwise unsuitable. They live in these dwellings for financial reasons and because they may wish to remain in familiar surroundings. Many live with children, and disturbing problems have occurred from crowding, economic pressures, and dissimilarity in cultural backgrounds of various members of the family. Some elderly persons live with distant relatives or friends, and sometimes they are happier than those who live with sons and daughters.

It is believed that the aged need a variety of kinds of housing; what one older person may prefer, another may not. While homes for the aged are good for those who fear to be alone and who need the security and protection of group living, they are not the answer for everyone. Even if they are small and homelike and close to familiar neighbors, many elderly persons do not wish to live in them. Every effort should be made to enable the aged person to live in his own

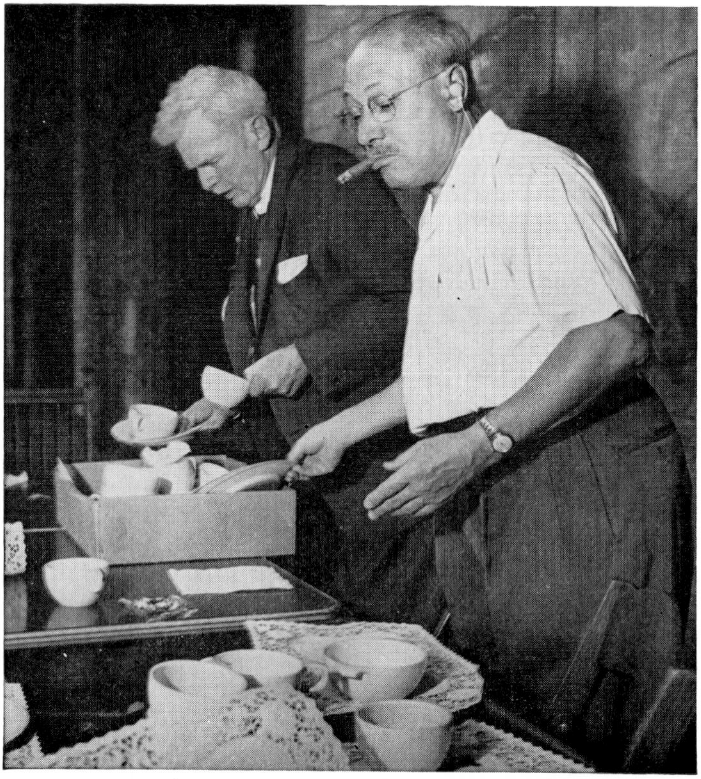

Figure 2

Community recreational programs fill in many empty hours. (Courtesy New York League for the Hard of Hearing, New York, N. Y.)

home and in his customary setting if he so wishes. This is sometimes made possible by providing such services as housekeeping for the frail and visiting nursing for the ailing. In some communities one hot meal each day served in the neighborhood school cafeteria may be all that is necessary to enable a feeble elderly couple to carry on together. Arrangements for the person to enter a home for the aged whenever he may need to have made it possible for many elderly persons to continue on their own with less apprehension. Group housing which provides an overseer, a shopper, a nurse, and a housekeeper is the answer to housing problems for some older persons, whereas others prefer to live with a cross section of all ages. Progress has been made recently in setting aside a portion (recommended 10 per cent or more) of low-cost housing for elderly persons. These housing units, erected with the help of state aid, are available to elderly couples and single aged persons in some states. They are located on ground floors of buildings with special heating and safety features such as electric instead of gas stoves, good lighting, and doorways without sills to minimize the danger of the person with locomotor disability stumbling and falling.

Health care. Health is precious to all, since it represents an assurance of the ability to move about freely, to be with loved ones, to be physically independent, and to compete favorably with others for recognition. Physical freedom or good health is even more precious to the older person, because the threat that he may have to give up his freedom at any moment is ever present. The implications of illness are more important to the aged person than is the actual pain or physical disability itself. Perhaps he cannot afford to be ill, and he may be uncertain of who wants to care for him during illness. General hospitals often admit the aged patient with reluctance, and he may find himself in a poorly equipped hospital for the chronically ill, or in a poorly staffed nursing home.

It is difficult and often impossible for the older person to get hospitalization insurance. Hospital costs are a source of real worry to him, and he often hesitates to have a public health nurse come into his home because he does not understand the plan for charges. He may refuse to spend his savings for fear that his money will be exhausted before his life ends. He may put off medical care, delay the purchase of medications, and sometimes not buy sufficient food. When medical care becomes imperative, he may become panicky about costs, and this may interfere with his cooperation in undergoing tests and in following a prescribed course of treatment.

Illness may break down the barriers to overt aggression that have been built up over a long period of time, and the aged patient may appear irritable out of all proportion to his circumstances. He may use his illness as an occasion for revolt and aggression against years of neglect to his self-esteem and to almost overwhelming economic and emotional problems. The trivial event precipitating the irritability during illness may be purely incidental. Similarities between childhood and old age should not be assumed because they are not valid. Even in the matter of helplessness there is no similarity. The child is in ascendance; he is developing new power daily and marking up achievements over his environment. The aged person's helplessness is infinitely more frustrating because it is increasing rather than decreasing.

ANATOMIC AND PHYSIOLOGIC CHANGES IN AGING

Certain anatomic and physiologic changes take place with age. These influence the development of disease, its progress when established, and the ultimate outcome for the patient. The aim of geriatric medical and nursing care is to keep the patient completely well for his age; it is not to make him like the younger person in health or during illness.

Age changes are due to heredity and to the strains and accidents of living; they are different for each person. Because of these changes, the aged person's margin of safety may be less than that of a younger person who is ill with the same disease. With age there is general tissue desiccation and a slowing of cell division. This means that healing will take place more slowly and that the body response to infection will be less rapid and, perhaps, less effective. It has been estimated that for each five years of life approximately one additional day will be needed to accomplish healing after an operation or to recover from an illness.[13] There is a gradual loss of elasticity of connective tissue. This leads to decreased speed of response and decreased strength. It also causes some increased rigidity of body structures; for example, diminishing elasticity in the rib cage, which may in turn decrease chest expansion and predispose to lung congestion. This may cause problems following anesthesia or during a disease such as pneumonia. Bones become rarefied and fractures occur easily. This is true particularly of the neck of the femur and the vertebral bodies.

In old age there is fatty infiltration of cells and lessened elasticity of the blood vessels. The patient's circulation may not tolerate changes in position such as lowering of the head for postural drainage or long intervals in lithotomy position in the operating room. With prolonged standing, blood may accumulate in the lower extremities so that not enough is provided for the brain, and dizziness and accidents may follow. Since hardened arteries provide less blood to vital structures such as the brain, shortages of essential nutrients in the blood may be quickly felt. Thus faintness and even shock can follow long periods without food. In Europe during World War II it was found that elderly persons withstood starvation even less well than children. Hardened arteries may reflect hemorrhage and signs of shock less quickly, and therefore smaller changes in blood pressure may be of great significance in judging the patient's progress.

There is gradual degeneration and atrophy of the nervous system in old age, which leads to lessened nerve acuity and to impaired sensation. This means, for example, that the aged person's gag reflex may be less acute than that of the younger person, and aspiration of mucus or other foreign material may occur easily following a bronchoscopy or surgical anesthesia or even during a relatively simple procedure such as feeding the patient.

The liver, heart, kidneys, and other vital organs of many elderly patients are working so hard to maintain normal function that there is little margin of safety. The additional burden of anesthesia and operation, or infection, may be enough to tip the balance unfavorably for the patient unless particular care is given. It can be expected that many tests such as kidney function tests, liver function tests, and electrocardiograms may be ordered for older patients. Blood pressure and other vital signs, as well as fluid intake and output, must be watched carefully after surgery and during acute episodes of medical illness. The mechanisms that maintain a fairly constant internal environment for the patient, such as electrolyte balance and temperature, are less efficient in the aged. Evidences of slight changes are therefore of greater significance.

Some evidence exists that mental faculties decline gradually after the age of approximately 22 years.[14] It has been estimated that the average loss is about three points in the intelligence quotient for each decade of life, but individual differences and interest in learning are much more important than changes in intelligence quotient in determining whether or not the older person can learn easily. The learning capacity of the aged needs further study. Interests change with age, and this has not been considered sufficiently in the content of material used for tests of learning ability. It is never wise to assume that because a person is elderly his ability to learn is lessened.

NURSING CARE OF THE ELDERLY PATIENT

The nurse must remember that each aged patient is an individual. He brings to his situation, in illness or in health, his own particular personality which has been developed from inheritance and from his complex environment, his own sense of values, and his own reactions to stresses in his environment. Each elderly patient will react differently to his social, economic, emotional, cultural, and physical problems as he becomes old. On the whole, he will react essentially the same way he has reacted to other stresses throughout his life.

When giving nursing care to elderly patients, it is necessary to build up and protect their sense of worth and their feelings of adequacy. Remembering the names of patients and calling them by name instead of using such terms as "grandma" or "grandpa" will help in this. The patient will appreciate clear explanations so that he is spared the embarrassment of mistakes caused by misunderstanding. His sense of dignity and self-respect can be preserved by facing him when speaking so that he may lip-read inconspicuously if this is necessary and by placing equipment conveniently so that assistance need not be requested.

Necessary nursing care depends upon the physiologic and anatomic changes that have taken place, the disease from which the patient is suffering, and his own emotional make-up and apparent adjustment to his particular situation. Most diseases from which the aged suffer are chronic, and many patients have several chronic ailments. Some of these are not particularly troublesome; most have developed slowly and usually take time to alleviate or cure. Heart disease, cancer, nephritis, vascular disease such as cerebrovascular accident, chronic lung disease such as emphysema, and accidents are the most common problems that bring older patients to the hospital. Other chronic ailments such as arthritis, skin disorders, and mild neuromuscular conditions are very common but are usually cared for while the patient is ambulatory.

Bathing and skin care. The skin of older patients is thin, delicate, and sensitive to trauma and pressure. The tiny arterioles near the skin surface atrophy and harden, causing the skin to lose the rosy bloom of youth and become sallow. Loss of subcutaneous fat leads to wrinkles and sagging. Sweat glands atrophy, and the excretory function of the skin is lessened. Bathing is less necessary and, in fact, may be harmful if too frequent. Usually one or two baths per week are sufficient, although the incontinent patient needs local sponging at frequent intervals and tub baths daily if he can be placed in a tub. The old-style tub with a curved rim is best, since it provides a firm surface which can be easily grasped by the patient. Two nurses or assistants can easily move the patient up the sloping end to a stool or chair provided that the tub is so placed that assistants may approach it from both sides.

Mild superfatted soaps or detergent solutions should be used because regular soaps can be irritating. Some elderly persons suffer from so-called bath itch caused by too frequent bathing. This is a troublesome condition which produces itching and desquamation along the shin bone and may extend to other parts of the body. Bathing should be followed by gentle massage over bony prominences and by the light application of lanolin or emollient creams. Alcohol is drying and should not be used. Bony prominences and weight-bearing areas should be massaged each hour if the patient is confined to bed. An alternating positive-pressure and negative-pressure mattress is excellent in preventing decubiti from developing. Pieces of sponge rubber and soft chamois skin seem to be unusually effective in relieving pressure and preventing irritation of the skin.

Feet. The feet usually show the results of limitation in peripheral circulation before any other part of the body. The nails become hard and thick and the skin dry, cold, and peeling. Well-fitting shoes, daily massage of the feet, toe exercises (curling and extension), and periodic elevation of the lower limbs help to ensure adequate circulation. Hard, thickened toenails should not be cut until they have been softened; warm oil may be used for this and may be left on the nails for a day or two. Foot soaks in warm water also soften the skin and nails and make cutting of the nails and care of the cuticles easier. It must be remembered, however, that even plain water, if used too often, is drying to the skin and nails, and soaks should be followed by massage with a lotion containing lanolin. Daily foot hygiene should include powdering between the toes, because it is almost impossible for the fungus infection of epidermophytosis to thrive on a dry skin surface. Epidermophytosis develops quickly on the skin of elderly persons probably because of the poor circulation and lowered resistance to infection. This infection has been found to be a forerunner of arteriosclerotic gangrene of the toes. Since many elderly patients have toenails that are too difficult for the nurse to manage, the services of a podiatrist are needed.

Hair. The hair becomes thin, dry, and colorless as the tissues age and the blood vessels diminish in activity. Massage of the scalp and daily brushing with a soft bristled brush help to preserve the beauty of the hair. Lanolin cream in small amounts may be used for massage, and oil treatments may be given before shampoos. Too frequent shampooing should be avoided; every two to four weeks is sufficient for most aged patients, although some people who have washed their hair more frequently throughout their lives may wish to continue to do so. A mild soap dissolved in water is the best shampoo for general use. The older person should not experiment with new shampoos because many preparations contain alcohol and other agents which may have a drying effect. In the hospital it is not advisable to use tincture of green soap for elderly patients because it, too, contains alcohol.

Care of the hair during health or illness contributes immeasurably to morale, and patients should be encouraged to care for their own hair. The nurse should ask what is needed and arrange equipment so that this part of the daily routine can be carried out by each patient. If the patient cannot care for her own hair, this must be done for her; hair should be arranged in the manner that is preferred by the patient and is becoming to her. It is a deplorable practice to arrange the hair of all women patients in one certain way, a braid for example, simply because this may be quick, routine, and easy for the nurse.

The distribution and quality of hair change with age. Hair in the axillary and pubic areas becomes finer and scanty, while that of the eyebrows becomes coarse and bristly. To many women hair on the face is a most annoying feature of growing old. If the patient is ill for a long time and is unable to care for herself, the nurse may have to assist in the removal of superfluous hair on the face. Shaving or using a pumice stone, followed by the application of cream to prevent drying, usually suffices. Plucking stray hairs from the face is often necessary. Hairs should not be plucked from moles but may be snipped close to the surface of the skin with small scissors; care must be taken not to cut or otherwise traumatize the mole. Stray hairs on the face may be made less conspicuous by bleaching them daily with a weak solution of hydrogen peroxide and ammonia if this can be done without irritating the skin. Moles and other flaky, scaly, or pigmented areas of the skin should be watched carefully for sudden growth or other changes since they may develop into malignant lesions.

Eyes. Most people over 60 years of age need glasses, at least for reading. Care of glasses, making certain that they are not lost or broken, is important in the nursing care of the elderly patient. Glasses should be kept clean; smudged glasses rather than failing vision may be the cause of difficulty in sight. The patient should have his glasses available at all times since confusion and inability to deal with situations in an adequate fashion may result if they become misplaced. Light should be adjusted over the patient's bed so that reading can be done without eyestrain.

Eye discomfort can be the result of poor lighting and many other causes. Irritation and tearing may follow a decrease in conjunctival secretions. Sometimes the lower lid droops (ectropion) and the moistening fluid of the eye is lost. An accumulation of secretions at the inner canthus of the eye may be present in aged patients, particularly upon awakening. This may be uncomfortable and unsightly. A sterile cotton sponge moistened with boric acid solution or physiologic solution of sodium chloride can be used to cleanse the eyes. Great care must be taken not to press upon the eyeballs or to irritate any exposed conjunctiva. Smoke is sometimes more irritating to the elderly patient's eyes than to the eyes of younger persons.

Teeth. Elderly patients should be encouraged to give good care to their teeth and mouth. Free hydrochloric acid in the stomach may be decreased, thus predisposing to impaired digestion and poor oral health. Gum tissues become less elastic and less vascular and the gums may recede from any remaining teeth, exposing areas of a tooth not covered with enamel. Such areas are sensitive to injury from brushes and coarse dentifrices. Many elderly persons have decayed, broken, or missing teeth. This leads them to avoid foods that are difficult to eat but which may be necessary for health. The effect of mouth health upon nutrition is very real; surprising improvement in appetite has followed correction of unhealthy conditions in the mouth.

Approximately 80 per cent of women and 70 per cent of men have lost their teeth by the time they are 70 years of age and therefore wear dentures. Consequently, care of dentures and their protection from loss are part of the general nursing care of most elderly patients. Patients are usually encouraged by their dentists to keep dentures in place while they sleep as well as when they are awake since this helps to preserve the normal contours of the face. Dentures should be cleansed following each meal. Because dental plates may be conductors of heat, and since the mouths of aged patients are often not too sensitive to excessive heat, care must be taken in feeding elderly patients to prevent serious burns.

Clothing and ventilation. More and more hospitals are permitting patients to wear their own clothing. The elderly patient should wear the clothing that is comfortable for him. In the hospital he might wear socks, woolen underwear, a bed jacket, a cap, or other items of clothing to which he is accustomed. Some provision must be made for the care of this clothing; sometimes members of the family are glad to care for special clothing that the patient needs. The hospitalized patient should always have his shoes at his bedside since they are needed when he is out of bed. Firm shoes with good support are necessary to prevent damage to the arches of the feet when muscles have become weakened from even a few days in bed, and the elderly person is less likely to stumble, fall, or slip when he wears footwear to which he is accustomed.

Fresh air is necessary for the elderly patient. The diminished chest expansion of most aged persons makes it necessary that the air breathed have a normal amount of oxygen. Some, however, do not like windows wide open because of drafts, and their beds should be placed so that they are protected from drafts. The aged are susceptible to drafts not even noticed by younger persons; many suffer from mild arthritis and fibrositis which produce vague muscle and joint pains, and these conditions are aggravated by chilling, dampness, drafts, and changes in barometric pressure. Adipose protective tissue under the skin disappears with age, and the volume of circulating blood, particularly to the small outer arteries, may be diminished, thus affecting the ability to withstand chilling without discomfort. Decreased activity also lessens circulatory function, resulting in lowering of skin temperature and susceptibility to chilling from drafts and from sudden changes of external temperature.

Rest, relaxation, and sleep. Elderly patients should never be rushed. Geriatricians instruct their patients to take twice the usual time to shave, to dress slowly, and to avoid hurry of any kind, particularly during the morning hours. The morning routine of the average busy hospital makes it difficult to achieve a slower pace; laboratory specimens must be collected, examinations must be made, roentgenograms must be taken. Some of the routines and some of the pressure are necessary and cannot be avoided; others can be adjusted to the geriatric patient, and usually some changes can be made to meet individual patient needs. Because of the increased number of elderly patients and the trend to have most patients out of bed for at least part of the day, most general hospitals find that their bathroom facilities are woefully inadequate. The resourceful nurse can often alleviate this situation somewhat by encouraging some patients who have been used to having a bath or shower in the evening to continue to do so rather than insisting that this be part of the morning program for everyone.

In the home, members of the family may need an understanding of the aged person's need for a leisurely pace. For example, allowing time for the performance of simple household chores such as washing dishes without appearing impatient with slow progress does a great deal to improve the morale of the elderly person who lives in the home of others.

Noise is disturbing to the elderly ill person; this is particularly true when he has a hearing loss. Partial deafness may set the person "on edge" and alert him to catch every sound. This interferes with the capacity to relax. Even though ability to hear conversation may be limited, the sound of a distant radio, shrill voices, or rattling equipment may be most disturbing.

Elderly patients usually sleep lightly and intermittently, with frequent waking. At home the aged person may get out of bed, read, wander about the house, and even prepare something to eat at odd hours. In the hospital, although some wakefulness should be anticipated, the nurse must be alert for wakefulness that is not intermittent but constant. Little reliance should be placed on medications for sleep. The elderly person may respond to sedation in an untoward fashion and be greatly upset by it. The time-tested aids such as a warm drink, a back massage, and quiet surroundings may help to get the night of sleep off to a good start. Interesting activities to keep patients awake during the day may result in better sleep at night. Most important, however, are the patient's peace of mind and feeling of well-being. These may be achieved by giving individual attention to the elderly patient, making him feel at home and secure and that he is in safe surroundings. A kind word and a wish for a good night of sleep and an unobstrusive inquiry into some mentioned fear or uncertainty may alleviate worries and will do much to help the patient sleep. Confusion upon awakening is much more common among elderly patients than among younger ones and should be watched for carefully by nursing personnel. This is much more likely to occur during night hours than after naps taken during the day.

Rest is essential for the aged; however, too much rest can be dangerous. It is important for the nurse caring for a patient in the home to instruct the family about this. Since the nurse is seldom in the home long enough to see that the patient is out of bed as much as is desirable, she must depend upon the understanding and cooperation of the patient and his family. The family should know that oversolicitous care and too much waiting on may do physical and psychologic damage to the aged patient. The patient who is confused often benefits a great deal from being out of bed part of the time, since this improves his circulation and seems to contribute to better rest during the time spent in bed.

Most elderly patients are anxious to be out of bed, since this represents to them the assurance that they are progressing favorably. They look forward to and value very highly each small step toward their increased independence following acute illness. The value of early mobilization to circulation, respiration, and other physiologic processes is undisputed for all patients and particularly for elderly ones. Sitting in a chair each day adds to the patient's interest in his surroundings. The environment can be altered; he may be taken in a wheel chair to visit other patients or to a porch. He is much happier doing these things, and often this will avoid the apprehension that so easily occurs in elderly patients.

Posture and exercise. In old age, muscular activity becomes less adequate, and slumped posture may result in many changes. The abdomen may sag, the spine becomes rounded, and the chest and shoulders droop forward. Lessened elasticity of tissue tends to make these changes fixed. Attention to preventive posture is, therefore, essential. Corrective postural exercises and general exercise must, however, be carefully prescribed by a physician, but teaching good posture and encouraging deep breathing are part of the daily nursing care of all elderly patients. Any improvement in posture will enable the elderly patient to use his diminishing resources to better advantage. Breathing exercises are often helpful. Improvement of posture and muscle tone has been shown to decrease states of fatigue associated with low blood pressure. Marked increase of blood pressure and mitigation of symptoms have followed strengthening of the abdominal musculature to provide better support of the viscera.

Good body alignment adds to the comfort of the patient confined to bed. A firm mattress is usually preferable and helps to make use of pillows more effective. If greater stability is needed, a fracture board can be placed under the mattress. Bedcovers should be light and warm and should be tucked loosely, giving sufficient room for the patient to move about in bed. Cradles are not usually satisfactory because they tend to hamper free movement in the bed, but a block or board placed at the foot of the bed helps in keeping covers off the toes and provides something firm against which the patient may press his feet and thereby get some exercise. A pillow placed lengthwise under the head and shoulders helps to bring the chest forward, thereby permitting good chest expansion. Pillows placed under the arms support the muscles of the shoulder girdle and provide comfort for the patient who must have the head of the bed raised for long periods of time. Overbed trapeze fixtures with cross bars designed for use by patients in traction may be helpful for elderly persons, enabling them to move about in bed independently and to release the pressure of weight on the lower spine for brief intervals. Side rails often serve the same purpose. Their use should be explained since they may be interpreted as an indication of lack of faith in the patient's reliability. Side rails are extremely useful to the elderly person with some limitation of motion. They enable him to grasp the rail with the good hand and thereby change his position and move about more than would otherwise be possible. A rope tied to the foot of the bed and on which the patient may pull often helps him to assume a sitting position.

Unless there is some particular contraindication, exercises for the arms and legs, exercises to keep abdominal and gluteal muscles in good tone, and exercises to strengthen the extensor muscles of the spine should be performed several times each day by every bed patient. These exercises should be taught to the patient by the nurse, and their daily supervision is her responsibility. The regular performance of exercises will help to prevent the loss of muscle tone which occurs in all bed patients unless activity is continued. (For details of routine bed exercise see Chapter 4.)

Diet. Nutritional needs of older patients differ little from those of other adults. Because activity is decreased, fewer calories are needed, and usually carbohydrates and fats should be reduced. Protein and mineral requirements are about the same except that larger amounts of calcium are needed because of decreased absorption of this mineral. Older patients need a generous intake of vitamins, but caloric needs are determined by the individual's weight and the amount of his activity. Caloric demands of the aged are roughly estimated as between 30 and 40 calories per kilogram of body weight per day.

Many elderly patients are undernourished, and for this reason a great deal of emphasis is placed on nutrition for the aged. There appear to be several causes of malnutrition. Other than acute and chronic illness, possible causes are limited financial resources, psychologic factors such as boredom and lack of companionship in eating, edentia, lifelong faulty eating patterns, fads and notions regarding certain foods, lack of energy to prepare foods, and lack of sufficient knowledge of the essentials in a well-balanced diet. Many elderly persons, particularly those living alone, subsist on a diet high in carbohydrates and low in vitamins, minerals, and protein. Often they think that because they are elderly they do not need much food and that a diet largely composed of tea and toast seems sufficient.

Appetitie can be improved in a number of ways. A slow unhurried period for eating is necessary. Attention to how an elderly person likes a certain dish prepared will yield good results in improvement of the appetite. For example, many persons like a cup of hot coffee before eating breakfast and do not appreciate a pot of lukewarm coffee served with their main breakfast.

The nurse should instruct the patient and those responsible for his care in the essentials of a well-balanced diet. Dietary patterns should not be changed too quickly, and it is useless to attempt to change many established food patterns. Simply prepared and easily digested foods are best, and meals should be distributed throughout the day. Elderly persons usually do not tolerate too much fried food. Large amounts of roughage should also be avoided, but bulk is necessary. Fluid intake is important, yet many do not drink much water; tea, coffee, and other beverages are usually preferred. Drinks prepared with dry skimmed milk supply essential protein and are useful in helping to meet the protein needs of older patients without supplying too many calories.

Some elderly persons are obese even though they are undernourished. Excess weight burdens the heart, liver, kidneys, and musculoskeletal system and should be avoided throughout life. Weight reduction for the aged person, however, should be gradual and must be supervised by a physician. Sudden loss of weight is poorly tolerated by many elderly persons whose vascular system has become adjusted to their overweight condition. It may lead to serious consequences, including confusion associated with lowered blood pressure, exhaustion, and vasomotor collapse.

Elimination. Elderly patients may worry about their bowel function. They tend to forget that less food and less activity will result in reduced bowel function. Any marked change in bowel habits, however, and any unusual reactions to normal doses of laxatives should be reported, since malignancies of the large bowel are fairly common.

Regularity in going to the toilet is important, since it provides stimulus to evacuate the bowel. Motor activity of the intestinal musculature may be decreased with age, and supportive structures in the intestinal walls become weakened. Sense perception is less acute so that the signal for bowel elimination may be missed and constipation may occur and in turn lead to impactions. The very elderly patient should be reminded to go to the bathroom following meals. In caring for the helpless patient, a commode helps in noting whether or not a bowel movement has occurred. Daily attention must be given to elimination, and sometimes small enemas may be needed every two or three days. Occasional inspection with a gloved finger is sometimes necessary to be certain that impaction has not occurred. Small daily doses of a mild laxative may be ordered. The mild bulk laxatives such as psyllium seed and agar-agar combined with mineral oil are usually preferred to the saline cathartics which may cause dehydration.

Frequency of micturition is common in old age and becomes a problem during illness. One of the first signs of diminishing or failing kidney function is night frequency. The ability of the kidneys to concentrate urine during sleeping hours is usually gradually lost with age. In addition, decreased muscle tone in the bladder with resultant impairment of emptying capacity may result in residual urine in the bladder and subsequent mild infection. Frequency and slight burning on urination are symptoms of mild bladder infection. Elderly women have relaxation of perineal structures which may also interfere with complete emptying of the bladder and further predispose to the development of bladder infection. Some elderly patients have decreased sensation and do not realize when the bladder must be emptied. The nurse should observe the patient for distention until she gets to know her patient; by palpating the lower abdomen it is usually possible to know whether or not the bladder is distended. If the nurse has any doubt about this, she should ask a more experienced nurse or a doctor to check her findings. Unless there is a definite contraindication to high fluid intake, the elderly patient should be urged to take sufficient fluids to dilute urine and decrease its irritating properties. Fluids may be limited in the evening if nocturia is troublesome and is interfering with sleep. If the patient is likely to be up and about at night, the nurse should be certain that a light is convenient at the bedside and that surroundings are such that danger of accidents is minimal. If the patient is quite feeble, it is well to suggest that a urinal or bedpan be used during the night. Urinals may be kept at the side of the bed on a metal hook; bedpans can be kept either at the foot of the bed or on a chair within the patient's easy reach.

Elderly women patients are often annoyed by relatively benign but troublesome conditions associated with the reproductive system. Involutional changes in the lining of the vagina lead to lessened resistance to invasion of organisms; mild infections with troublesome discharge are not unusual. Such a condition should be reported to the doctor. Frequent local bathing is often helpful in allaying itching and skin irritation from the discharge; a douche of mild vinegar solution (2 tablespoonfuls to 1 quart of water) is often ordered by the doctor.

Almost all elderly men have hypertrophy of the prostate, which makes urination more difficult. The nurse must report, or urge her patient to report, such complaints to his doctor because specific treatment is often necessary and can be safely administered even when the patient is far advanced in years.

Drugs. The nurse needs to be familiar with the expected action of the medication she administers and certain that the correct dose is given. Reactions of aged persons to drugs may be bizarre and entirely out of proportion to that expected from the usual dosage of the drug. Older patients, like the very young, usually need smaller doses of drugs such as sedatives. On the other hand, as age advances, larger doses of stimulating drugs are required for therapeutic effect. Differences in rate of absorption and in rate of excretion of drugs may occur. When circulation is slowed down, the effect of medications given hypodermically or intramuscularly may be delayed. Kidney or liver function may be impaired, normal excretory rate may be decreased, and cumulative effects of drugs may appear. For example, careful supervision of the patient receiving digitalis is necessary since storage of the drug within the body may lead to fatal heart block. Bromides may accumulate in the tissues of the older person who has limited excretory function, and toxic signs of overdose of the drug may appear. Barbiturates are likely to have a cumulative effect and may, in some instances, produce the opposite reaction from that desired. Restlessness and even maniacal states may accompany cumulative or secondary effects of the drug. In treating sleeplessness, entirely too much reliance is placed on barbiturates in general hospitals and in nursing homes. Chloral hydrate is one of the best sedatives for the aged because the cumulative and toxic effects are minimal. Many geriatricians recommend small amounts of wine as a sedative for relaxation and sleep provided that this is psychologically acceptable to the patient.

The ataractic or "tranquilizing" drugs have been widely used in treating restlessness and anxiety in aged persons. Use of these drugs, however, is still in the experimental stage and possible ill effects have not yet been fully appraised.

REFERENCES AND SELECTED READINGS*

1 *Age: Selected Papers From University of Michigan Conference, July 1956, Pub. Health Rep. **71**:1167-1208, Dec. 1956.

2 *Austin, Catherine L.: The Basic Six Needs of the Aging, Nursing Outlook **7**:138-141, March 1959.

3 Bruel, Frank R.: Social Insurance. In Kurtz, Russell H. (editor): Social Work Year Book 1960, Issue 14, New York, 1960, National Association of Social Workers.

4 Buckley, Bonita: Feeding the Aged Person, Am. J. Nursing **59**:1591-1593, Nov. 1959.

5 Gitelson, Maxwell: The Emotional Problems of Elderly People, Geriatrics **3**:135-150, May-June 1948.

6 Havighurst, Robert J., and others: Psychology of Aging, Bethesda Conference, Pub. Health Rep. **70**:837-856, Sept. 1955.

*References preceded by an asterisk indicate material particularly well suited for student reading.

7 Kutner, Bernard, and others: Five Hundred Over Sixty, New York, 1956, Russell Sage Foundation.

8 Lemkau, Paul V.: Mental Hygiene of Aging, Pub. Health Rep. **67**:237-241, March 1952.

9 Litin, Edward M.: Mental Reaction to Trauma and Hospitalization in the Aged, J.A.M.A. **162**:1522-1524, Dec. 22, 1956.

10 Mathiasen, Geneva: The Aging. In Kurtz, Russell H. (editor): Social Work Year Book 1960, Issue 14, New York, 1960, National Association of Social Workers.

11 *Newton, Kathleen: Geriatric Nursing, ed. 3, St. Louis, 1960, The C. V. Mosby Co.

12 Population Outlook for 1970; Statistical Bulletin, June 1959, Metropolitan Life Insurance Co.

13 *Randall, Ollie A., and others: The Problems of Extended Illness and Old Age, Am. J. Nursing **54**:1220-1225, Oct. 1954.

14 Stieglitz, Edward J. (editor): Geriatric Medicine, ed. 2, Philadelphia, 1949, W. B. Saunders Co.

15 Tibbitts, Clark: The Aging. In Kurtz, Russell H. (editor): Social Work Year Book 1957, Issue 13, New York, 1958, National Association of Social Workers.

Increase in chronic illness

Chapter 3

Study questions for review

1 Review the case histories of patients on a medical or surgical ward in your hospital. What proportion has a chronic illness as either primary or secondary diagnosis? What proportion has more than one chronic condition? What age group is affected most by multiple diseases?

2 Consult your notes on social and community health aspects of nursing, and review what you learned about the facilities for care of the chronically ill patient in your immediate community. What is the total patient capacity of these facilities, and what percentage of the total population of the city or town could hope to receive care from them if necessary? How are these facilities supported financially?

Prevention and control of chronic illness is the major health problem today. In 1959 the United States Public Health Service reported that on a basis of interviews conducted in the National Health Survey, 10 per cent of the population of the United States was limited in normal activities by some chronic condition. About 4,855,000 persons, or 3 per cent of the entire population, have difficulty "moving about"; approximately 1 million of these are confined to their homes.[4]

In the National Health Survey the list of chronic diseases included asthma, allergy, tuberculosis, severe bronchitis, sinusitis, rheumatic fever, arteriosclerosis, hypertension, heart disease, cerebral vascular accident and other vascular conditions, hemorrhoids, gallbladder or liver disease, gastric ulcers, kidney stones, arthritis, prostrate disease, diabetes mellitus, thyroid disease, epilepsy or convulsions, spinal disease, cancer, chronic dermatosis, and hernia.

DIFFERENCES BETWEEN ACUTE ILLNESS AND CHRONIC ILLNESS

An acute illness is one caused by a disease which produces symptoms and signs within a short period of time, which runs a short course, and from which there is usually a full recovery or an abrupt termination in death. Acute illnesses may become chronic. For example, a common cold may become chronic sinusitis. A chronic illness is one caused by disease which produces symptoms and signs within a variable period of time, which runs a long course, and from which there is only partial recovery. The symptoms and general reactions caused by chronic disease may subside with proper treatment and care. This period during which the disease is controlled and symptoms are not obvious is known as a *remission*. However, at a future time the disease becomes active again with recurrence of symptoms. This period is known as an *exacerbation*. A chronic disease is characterized by remissions and exacerbations and slowly progressive physical changes. Mention of many emotional, social, and economic implications of chronic illness will be made later in this chapter.

Acute exacerbations of chronic disease often cause the patient to seek medical attention, and this may lead to hospitalization. Distinction must be made between acute illness and an acute phase of a chronic illness. The needs of a patient with an acute illness may be very different from those of one with an acute exacerbation of a chronic illness. For example, a young person may enter the hospital with complaints of fever, chest pain, shortness of breath, easy fatigue, and a productive cough. If the diagnosis is pneumonia, the patient usually can be assured of recovery after a period of rest and a course of antibiotic treatment. However, if the diagnosis is rheumatic heart disease and if this is the patient's third, fourth, or fifth admission, the reassurance needed will not be so definite, clear cut, or easy to give. In this instance it will be necessary for the nurse to begin planning care which extends beyond the period of hospitalization, taking into consideration many aspects of the patient's total life situation. The concerns of the patient who has had repeated attacks of illness will be much different than those of the one who has a short-term illness.

The nurse needs to be aware of patients who are admitted to the hospital with an acute illness but who also have an underlying chronic condition. For example, the elderly patient who enters the general hospital with pneumonia may receive treatment for the pneumonia and recover from his illness. However, he may still be hampered by the arteriosclerotic heart disease and arthritis which he has had for years. These two chronic conditions may have been aggravated by the acute infection, or the patient's return to his former activity may be hindered by joint stiffness resulting from enforced bed rest and inactivity. The nurse who considers the patient's several diagnoses can help in preventing new problems associated with his chronic illness.

EXTENT OF CHRONIC ILLNESS

Medical advances in the prevention of disease and in the control and treatment of acute illness have reduced mortality and have led to longer life expectancy. Chronic illness has not been controlled in the same way. For example, children may be victims of such chronic conditions as cerebral palsy, epilepsy, rheumatic fever, and blood dyscrasias. Young people in the productive years of life develop arthritis, tuberculosis, diabetes, and cardiovascular disease. The older person is most likely to have a chronic disease; many have several.

Of the people who were reported chronically ill in 1955, 45 per cent were under 45 years of age, 34 per cent were between 45 and 65 years of age, and 21 per cent were over 65 years of age.[11] Approximately 5 million had been disabled for three months or longer.[11] Of the 5 million who were disabled, 27 per cent were under 45 years of age, 34 per cent were 45 to 65 years of age, and 41 per cent were 65 years of age or over.[11]

The problems of chronic illness and old age are often confused. Many people think of chronic illness as being synonymous with old age. It is true that a large percentage of elderly persons are chronically ill and that the average age of those admitted to hospitals is constantly increasing,[3] but the figures presented in the preceding paragraph show that the majority of those with chronic illness are middle-aged or younger. According to these same figures, it is clear that of those severely disabled the older age group stands out, but considering the total number of people with chronic illness, the older age group at this time is not so involved as are the younger age groups. With the population of the United States shifting toward old age, however, an increase in chronic illness with resultant disability can be expected.

A study done in four hospitals in Boston in 1953-1954, showed that although only about 6 per cent of all patients were hospitalized 30 days or longer, these 6 per cent accounted for one third of the total patient days per year. Of these long-term patients, 42 per cent did not need continued hospital care, but they did need some type of sheltered care.[12]

CONTROL OF CHRONIC ILLNESS

In the control of chronic disease the health team must make the maximum application of existing knowledge and resources to reduce the impact of the disease on the patient, his family, and society. To accomplish this, five areas need to be considered: health promotion, specific prevention, early recognition and prompt treatment of disease, limiting the extent of disability, and rehabilitation.[6]

Health promotion is an area in which the nurse plays a major role. Positive health teaching concerning proper diet, adequate rest, appropriate recreation, safe living, and personal hygiene should be considered in every patient contact. Health practices need to be evaluated and a planned program of teaching and follow-up instituted. The nurse should also be aware of her community's resources for health and illness, encourage their use, and speak out as a citizen concerning the need for additional resources. Improving the general health of the people will decrease the incidence of disabling chronic illness now and in later life. An excellent example of how nurses may contribute in this area is the program recently (1959) begun by the Nursing Services of the American National Red Cross. This course entitled "Fitness After Forty" is available to anyone of that age in the community and stresses positive health practice as a means to prevention of chronic illness in the later years of life.

Much research is being done to gain knowledge of ways to provide *specific* protection. For example, studies are being made concerning accidents in industry and in automobile travel since crippling injuries account for a large number of chronically disabled people. Industry is being studied to determine if carcinogenic substances are being used, and it is being helped to find ways to decrease the danger of these both to employees and the public. Study also is underway concerning the causes of cancer and heart disease. The nurse needs to be informed about the most recent advancements in these fields of investigation so that she can interpret this to the public and help them to profit by preventive measures that are available.

Many facilities are already available to ensure *early recognition and prompt treatment* of chronic illness. A few of these are multiphasic screening programs, mass screening tests for diabetes mellitus, special eye health weeks, tuberculosis case-finding programs, well-baby and well-child clinics, and well-oldster conferences where counseling, guidance, health appraisal, and appropriate referral is done. The nurse should know the diagnostic facilities available in her community and should encourage the public to use them. Also, she should encourage persons to have periodic physical examinations and be alert herself to case finding. Since earlier medical treatment is sought by families who carry medical and hospitalization insurances, plans which give as broad health insurance coverage as possible are advisable.

The nurse who is working with patients who have chronic diseases whether she is in the hospital, outpatient clinic, doctor's office, school, industrial plant, public health nursing agency, or special nursing home has a responsibility to see that *disability from disease* is limited in so far as possible and that a *rehabilitation program* is planned and implemented. She should be alert to the prevention of complications, to the early recognition of symptoms of exacerbations or complications, and to the prevention of deformity. These areas are more specifically discussed under appropriate sections throughout this book. The nurse also, should help to teach the patient, his family, and his employer if necessary, about his limitations and the rehabilitative expectations.

EFFECT OF CHRONIC ILLNESS ON THE PATIENT AND HIS FAMILY

Chronic illness is not always apparent to others, and the chronically ill patient and his family are often misjudged by neighbors, friends, and the public. This is particularly true if the illness is not an obvious one. The person with a chronic ailment may appear healthy, and only his living patterns may reveal signs of his limitations. For example, a man with a heart ailment may meet his wife carrying many bundles and packages at the end of a long day of shopping, but he may take only a light package leaving her to carry the rest. He may be observed riding only three blocks on a bus day after day and this may be questioned as being different from normal. In our culture it is customary for the man to carry the woman's packages and most people walk a distance of three blocks rather than ride. Most onlookers are quick to jump to conclusions and to pass judgment. The onlooker's judgment is based on his own standard of appropriate conduct.

Obvious physical ailments may also cause problems. If an onlooker were to observe someone with a cane and a marked limp carrying packages or riding a short distance by bus, no doubt he would feel sympathetic toward that person and would want to assist him. The more obvious the disability, the more sympathy and help may be extended to him. However, if the disability is disfiguring or unpleasant to see, the observer may feel revulsion and may avoid the handicapped person.

The chronically ill patient is very often misjudged by even the closest members of his family because of lack of understanding. The nurse needs to help the patient's family to understand his limitations and his necessary restrictions. Both the patient and his family may benefit from association with others who have had similar experiences. Patients and their families often meet together in organized groups to share experiences; for example, the organizations for patients who have ileostomies and the organizations for patients who have multiple sclerosis. There has been a recent growth of such groups because of the increase in chronic illness and because people are reluctant to accept the isolation which chronic illness has imposed.

Marked changes often taken place in family living as a result of chronic illness. Families often find themselves drawn closer together and new relationships develop. For example, when it is suddenly learned that the mother has a "heart condition," the husband and teen-age children may rally to assist in household chores. All seem to work together with a special purpose in mind. On the other hand many families may drift apart and be incapable of helping one another. Chronic illness may threaten an individual's basic emotional stability, and the whole situation may be unbearable to others. Sometimes the patient's emotional needs may not have been apparent to the family early in the illness, but, as such needs develop and grow obvious, relatives feel inadequate in the situation. The length of the illness, periodic hospitalization, increased financial burdens, and emotional and social burdens are sometimes more than families can withstand. Public assistance is accepted by many families, whereas others find this degrading. Many persons struggle on their own to assume the full financial burden and consequently expose other members of the family to lower standards of nutrition, housing, and care. Many times relatives move in with one another, arguments develop, and family ties are strained or broken. Some accept public and other assistance without reservation and make little attempt to help themselves.

The effects upon patient and family are numerous and varied. Usually the patient and the family as a whole will respond in a manner similar to that in which they have reacted to problems in the past. However, the first impact of the disability may practically immobilize both the patient and his family. For example, a person who is almost totally helpless as a result of a crippling disease such as poliomyelitis at first may seem to have no interest in learning ways to help himself. His family may react in the same way and be of little help to him. At this time both the patient and his family need interest and support from professional persons. With this reassurance the patient may learn that he can do just one small activity such as turning pages in a book and this small success may be stimulus enough to strengthen his motivation so that he and his family may make amazing strides in thinking through and working out future problems themselves.

NURSING CARE OF THE CHRONICALLY ILL PATIENT

In contrast to the acutely ill patient, the chronically ill patient may receive few specific therapeutic treatments. Whereas the care of the acutely ill patient usually is exciting and momentarily dramatic, the care of the chronically ill patient may seem tedious, repetitive, and unrewarding. The nurse needs to develop a long-range point of view and can derive immediate satisfactions from observing small day-to-day improvements. Many days may pass before even a very small improvement can be recognized by the patient and the nurse. Great and permanent satisfactions, however, are gained by the nurse from experiences such as seeing a chronically ill person who has been bedridden for months and months walking after persistent effort.

Since medical diagnoses do not accurately reflect the physical capacity of the chronically ill person, the use of a *physical profile system* may be instituted as a guide for those working with the patient.[8] The patient is graded from 1 to 4 in six categories. The categories are (1) physical condition such as cardiovascular, pulmonary, gastrointestinal, genitourinary, endocrine, or cerebrovascular disorders, (2) upper extremities including shoulder girdle, cervical and upper dorsal spine, (3) lower extremities including pelvis, lower dorsal and lumbar sacral spine, (4) sensory components relating to speech, vision and hearing, (5) excretory function including bowels and bladder, and (6) mental and emotional status. Grade 1 indicates no unexpected difficulty; grade 2 indicates a minor difficulty which does not preclude normal life activity but which may require occasional medical supervision; grade 3 indicates a difficulty which requires medical and/or nursing supervision but which does not prevent limited activity; grade 4 indicates severe impairment requiring constant and complete care.

The nurse should assist in making the evaluation of each patient and in interpreting it to others who may care for him or who may be making plans with him. Limitations which place a patient in grades 3 or 4 should be specifically outlined as well as the amount and kind of necessary care included. The nurse can use the guide in planning for nursing care, both immediate and long-term, and will find it useful in assisting the family to make realistic plans for the patient's care. Since the condition is not static, reassessment should be made at regular intervals to indicate improvement or regression.

Nursing care of chronically ill patients requires alertness of feeling, seeing, and hearing. Continued warmth and interest are necessary to the well-being of a chronically ill person. Very often it is the nurse who helps the patient change and become highly motivated. It may be taxing to listen to the same person and to say the same things day after day, yet the nature of chronic illness may require this, and the way in which the nurse listens must convey warmth and interest. The world of a chronically ill person, whether in the hospital or elsewhere, becomes narrowed and circumscribed. He treasures and is interested in those things and those people close about him. His conversations may be largely about himself, his immediate environment, a few close objects, and those persons close to him. Although he is confined to bed and to room, others can keep him up to date with outside news. Many patients welcome hearing about outside events, but others may not be able to think beyond themselves. Newspapers, magazines, radio, and television help patients to keep up their interest in others and in outside world events.

Public libraries in many communities provide facilities for disabled persons. Ceiling projectors for books, books of current interest printed in large type, and recordings of books and music are often available on loan. Volunteer workers may act as readers both in hospitals and in homes. Many libraries have elevators and ramps that make library facilities available to the person who is unable to climb stairs and may make taking a person to the library in a wheel chair possible. The publication *Books for Tired Eyes** should be of interest to nurses.

Some communities have organized "Friendly Visiting Programs" in which volunteer workers come to the hospital or the home to provide companionship and to do errands for patients. The nurse should evaluate the advisability of such a plan, and sometimes the physician should be consulted. "Visitors" are not advisable for all patients and should be carefully selected. If the visitor is not prepared to meet the patient's needs, he may upset the patient. Often the nurse can help the visitor to give appropriate help to the patient.

Much has been said in Chapter 1 about the nurse knowing and understanding herself as a person as well as understanding her patient. This is particularly important in caring for the chronically ill patient. Before a nurse can help a patient help himself, she needs to distinguish between her values, standards, and goals and those of the patient. In day-to-day contact with a patient who is making little or no progress, the nurse may be tempted to make plans for his future because of a sincere interest in helping him. This is particularly true when the patient is about the same age as the nurse. She may feel that something must be done to speed progress. She may become frustrated by the feeling of wanting to do something or wanting to see some marked change. However, she needs to recognize that care of the chronically ill patient requires a slow-moving, persistent pace with possibly little or no change for a long time. The patient must be maintained at his present level and effort must be made to further his progress, his prognosis, and his and his family's acceptance of his condition. His eagerness and readiness to progress will be determining factors of his future. The "doing" in the care of the chronically ill patient is not always an active, physical "doing" with the hands. Many times it is maintenance of continuity in approach and attitude and demonstration of real interest which helps the patient most.

Recognizing what is meaningful to the patient is one of the first steps toward helping him to help himself. Personal needs become of paramount importance to the chronically ill patient. Meeting these physical needs provides a way for the nurse to convey to the patient her interest in his progress and welfare. By helping the patient to take his own bath, to attend to toilet needs, and to groom himself, the nurse can give him some sense of accomplishment and maintain his self-esteem. Helping him to be dressed appropriately is important. Patients who are in their homes or in substitute homes should be encouraged to dress in regular, comfortable street clothing rather than in pajamas or gowns. Visitors coming into the home or members of the family who constantly see them dressed for bed think of them as sick and are reminded of the illness. Seeing them dressed as they ordinarily would be helps to maintain normal attitudes, relationships, and expectations. An appropriately dressed housewife seated in a wheel chair paring vegetables is much more conducive to ordinary cheerful conversation with neighbors than one who is sitting in a gown, robe, and slippers with her hands idle.

Activity with a purpose, no matter how small this activity may be, is desirable for the chronically ill person. One may hear the patient say to friends that he does not have time to visit because he has to take care of the plants, do personal laundry, or perform some other task that may seem unimportant to the casual observer. Actually to the patient these jobs may appear to be the most important in the world.

Keeping the patient's body in good alignment, maintaining muscle tone, and

*Published by the American Public Library Association.

preventing contractures are physical measures which every nurse must bear in mind constantly as she works with a patient. A careful plan of rest and activity helps to preserve physical resources and to make the day purposeful. If assistance is needed, the nurse or trained aid can help the patient with the activity.

The nurse should think of each chronically ill person as someone who must live his life although his problems may seem insurmountable to her. She should recognize that many times life has meaning for the patient even though this may not be apparent to her. Nurses with this understanding can help make the patient's life more satisfying and can alter the attitudes of the family, her co-workers, and the public.

FACILITIES FOR THE CHRONICALLY ILL PATIENT

Most patients with a chronic or long-term illness can be cared for at home and actually prefer to be at home where family and friends are close by and where they can still contribute something to family life. They all require medical supervision. The arrangements which can be made vary greatly, depending upon the patient's needs and the facilities available. Many patients are ambulatory and during remissions are able to visit their local clinic. Others manage with visits from their personal physicians with periodic diagnostic work-up done in the office or with the assistance of a technician who goes into the home. For many years public health nurses from voluntary and official agencies have extended help to the sick in their homes. Visits to chronically ill patients (see Figure 3) now occupy a large percentages of their daily case loads.

The development of homemaker service programs is fairly new in many communities and is proving to be most helpful to many families in the care of a chronically ill member. These services are described in a bulletin* published by the American Medical Association Council on Medical Service in cooperation with the Executive Committee of the National Conference on Homemaker Services.

Home-care programs. More and more chronically ill persons are being offered services provided by an organized home-care program extending from a voluntary hospital, medical center, or city institution. These programs allow the patient to receive many hospital services in the home. In addition to physicians' services, some home-care programs provide arrangements for nursing, dental care, services of social workers, instruction in nutrition, homemaking, and housekeeping, and occupational therapy and other rehabilitative services. However, most programs provide only nursing and services of social workers in addition to the physicians' service. Provisions are made for drug and medical supplies as well as hospital equipment to be brought into the home when needed.

Most patients have been in the hospital before referral to home care and often have periodic short hospital stays for acute exacerbations or complicated treatments interspersed with home care. As a result of home-care programs, more beds in the hospital are available for acutely ill patients. In addition this service provides care which could not easily be equaled in institutional care. Not only does the patient have the security of knowing that he is counted as a part of the hospital census and will receive continuing care, but he also has the satisfaction of being cared for in his own environment by a group of professional people who know him, his family, and his total situation.

The philosophy of home care can be traced as far back as 1796 when the Boston Dispensary provided medical care to the sick poor. One of the first institutions to study and demonstrate the advantages of continuous medical care for patients at home was the University Hospital in Syracuse, New York, in 1940. The Montefiore Hospital Home-Care Program in New York City is a more recent example of provision of adequate health services in the home. Their services started in 1947, and

*First issue, January, 1960.

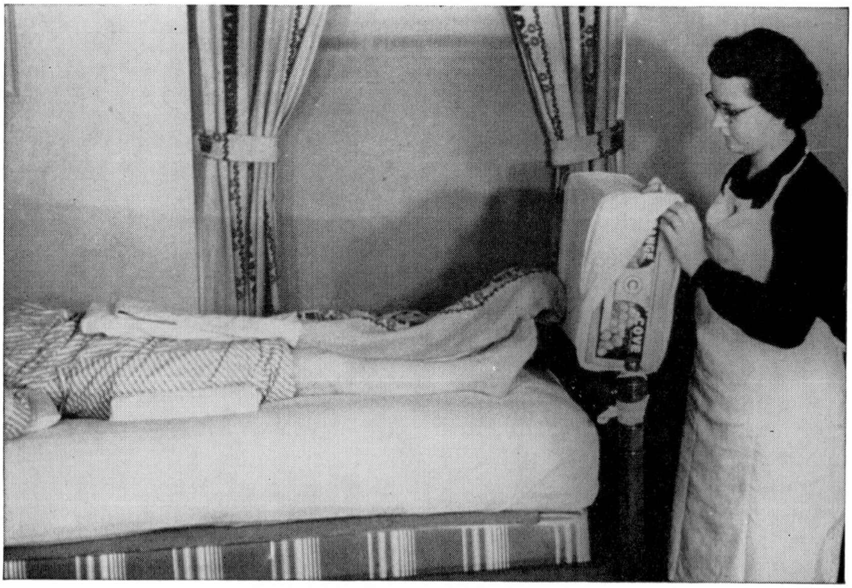

Figure 3

Caring for the chronically ill patient at home. Note improvised foot block and trochanter rolls used to prevent deformity. (Courtesy Visiting Nurse Association of Brooklyn, Inc., Brooklyn, N. Y., and Clay-Adams, Inc., New York, N.Y.)

within a year the New York City Department of Hospitals initiated similar programs in five city hospitals. By 1950 eleven additional New York City hospitals offered this service. Many communities in the United States now have some plan for home care.

Home care is not the solution for all patients. The present social trend is toward smaller dwellings, and adequate space for the patient and other members of the family may be at a premium. The choice of home care or institutional care will depend largely on the desires of the patient and his family. Despite many inconveniences, some families wish to have the patient with them. The family's understanding of the patient and his situation and their ability to support one another will make a great difference. Not only may space be inadequate, but many times it is impossible to have a member of the family in attendance with the patient during the day. Members of the family who work cannot afford to sacrifice jobs to stay with the patient. However, many families find it easier financially to have the patient at home and are able to make satisfactory arrangements even though the facilities are meager.

Some communities now provide "Meals on Wheels" for home-bound chronically ill and feeble aged patients. Most programs provide one hot meal daily and unheated food for at least one other meal. The cost differs widely (from a few cents to $2 per day) depending on the services offered, such as special diets, and on the sponsorship of the plan. Volunteer groups frequently act as delivery messengers. The local public health nursing service usually participates actively in the plan by selecting suitable patients and by being a resource for the workers who encounter health problems on their "rounds." This service alone often makes it possible for a chronically ill person to remain at home.

Institutional resources. Many patients and families have to resort to institutional care for the patient because their own facilities are not suitable, no member of the family can be in attendance during the day, or the kind of care needed by the patient requires close professional supervision. A vast or limited selection of outside facilities may be available, depending on the community. The types of homes include chronic disease hospitals, convalescent homes, rest homes, homes for the aged, and nursing homes.

A national inventory of nursing homes was made in 1954 by the Division of Hospital Facilities of the United States Public Health Service. It was found that there are approximately 25,000 "homes" in the United States. These accommodate about 450,000 people. For the purpose of inventory, homes were classified as follows: skilled nursing homes; personal care homes with skilled nursing; personal care homes without skilled nursing; and sheltered homes. The number of homes found in each group varied. The average-sized "skilled nursing home" has an average bed capacity of about 25 and provides 180,000 beds, or an average of 1.1 beds per 1,000 population. The "personal care homes with skilled nursing" have an average bed capacity of about 40 and provide 80,000 beds. The "personal care homes without skilled nursing" have an average bed capacity of about 15 and provide approximately 110,000 beds. The "sheltered homes" average 10 beds and provide approximately 80,000 beds. The availability of these facilities varies widely over the states, with some states having more of the "skilled nursing homes" and only few of the "sheltered home" type and vice versa. Whether these facilities are suitable in terms of public needs is still to be determined. The Commission on Chronic Illness, in its study of such institutions, found that the standards of medicine, nursing, and personal care in many of these are not acceptable. The licensing and standard-setting authorities for these institutions have been urged to exercise their jurisdiction to bring about improvement in physical facilities and care. Educational programs for the personnel of these homes would also improve care. Better financing for these institutions is imperative. If they are provided with better financial support, licensing authorities and nursing home operators can succeed in applying knowledge and in raising the standards, particularly in those institutions which do not have professional management.

Foster homes. Care in foster homes is a relatively new service which is now being widely used in many communities. Carefully selected families volunteer to take chronically ill persons into their own homes and provide the nonprofessional care that is needed. The family is paid either by the patient or his family, from public funds, or by some social agency. This plan is primarily for those patients who have no family and who cannot live alone, but who neither desire nor need institutional care.

REFERENCES AND SELECTED READINGS*

1 A Joint Project of the Public Health Service and the Commission on Chronic Illness: A Study of Selected Home Care Programs, Public Health Monograph No. 35, U. S. Department of Health, Education, and Welfare, 1955, Public Health Service.
2 *Brown, Francis Gold: Therapeutic Group Discussions, Am. J. Nursing **58**:836-839, June 1958.
3 Chapman, A. L.: Considering the Aged, Pub. Health Rep. **74**:333-337, April 1959.
4 Commission on Chronic Illness: Chronic Illness in the United States—Care of the Long Term Patient, Cambridge, Mass., 1956, Commonwealth Fund by Harvard University Press.
5 *Hill, Thelma M.: Twenty-Nine Men, Am. J. Nursing **59**:1718-1719, Dec. 1959.
6 Leavell, Hugh Rodman, and Clark, E. Gurney: Preventive Medicine for the Doctor in His Community, ed 2, New York, 1958, Blakiston Division, McGraw-Hill Book Co., Inc.
7 Manheimer, Robert H., and Delagi, Edward F.: A Home Care Rehabilitation Program for Ex-Urban Communities, J. Chron. Dis. **6**:589-594, Dec. 1957.

*References preceded by an asterisk indicate material particularly well suited for student reading.

8 *Moskowitz, Eugene, and McCann, Cairbre B.: Classification of Disability in the Chronically Ill and Aging, J. Chron. Dis. **5**:342-346, March 1957.

9 *Priest, Prudence I., and McCann, Virginia H.: Home Care for Mrs. Murphy, Am. J. Nursing **57**:1578-1580, Dec. 1957.

10 Reid, Mabel: Nursing in New York City's Home Care Programs, Nursing Outlook **2**:530-532, Oct. 1954; **2**:591-593, Nov. 1954; **2**:647-649, Dec. 1954; **3**:26-27, Jan. 1955.

11 Roberts, Dean W.: The Over-All Picture of Long-Term Illness, J. Chron. Dis. **1**:149-159, Feb. 1955.

12 Rosenfeld, Leonard, Goldman, Franz, and Kaprio, Leo A.: Reasons for Prolonged Hospital Stay, J. Chron. Dis. **6**:141-151, Aug. 1957.

13 Waterman, Theda L., and Lang, Valonis F.: Chronic Illness, Today's Major Health Problem; a Challenge to Every Community, St. Louis, 1955, The C. V. Mosby Co.

14 *Williams, James R.: Major Medical: A New Frontier in Health Insurance, Nursing Outlook **7**:26-28, Jan. 1959.

Study questions for review

1 Define rehabilitation in your own words. What kinds of patients do you think are most in need of rehabilitation? What professional people are able to contribute to a patient's rehabilitation? Select a patient from one of the hospital wards to illustrate rehabilitation needs.
2 From what you have learned in anatomy and fundamentals of nursing, outline in detail the physical movements necessary for one to rise from a sitting position in a chair to a standing position. Describe how you would assist a patient to a standing position while allowing him opportunity to help himself.

The patient needing rehabilitation

Chapter 4

Rehabilitation has been defined by many persons, and each definition seems to express the particular viewpoint of the person or organization offering it. One simple definition is "Rehabilitation is an adjustment to living."[11] An expanded definition is "Rehabilitation is the process of assisting the individual with a handicap to realize his particular goals, physically, mentally, socially, and economically."[11] The purpose or extent of rehabilitation ranges from employment or reemployment for the handicapped person to the more limited result of his achieving the ability to give his own daily care. This latter accomplishment can be just as important to the individual as earning money and other activities and may represent his greatest life achievement. This might be true, for example, for a person who was born with a severe physical handicap such as cerebral palsy.

For centuries disabled persons have received help, but never before have so many people been interested in this endeavor. In speaking of rehabilitation, Kessler states "It evolved from the idea of isolated and fragmentary activity on behalf of the crippled and the disabled to the modern concept of integrated and continued service."[4] World War II probably increased interest in rehabilitation more than any other force in modern times. Newer techniques have been developed to help persons with specific types of disability. Special equipment and facilities have become increasingly available. Rehabilitation centers and services have been established. There has been mounting national and community interest in the crippled child and the injured worker. The Social Security Act passed in 1935 included children as persons eligible for services for the handicapped, and passage of the Vocational Rehabilitation Act in 1954 expanded the program to enable even more people in the United States to be rehabilitated each year. Disabled veterans have received tremendous benefits from planned, coordinated programs of rehabilitation, and chronically disabled persons are beginning to receive more attention.

A public program for vocational rehabilitation has been serving the nation since 1920 as a partnership between the states and the federal government. Services for disabled persons are provided by state divisions of vocational rehabilitation (DVR). The federal government, through the Office of Vocation Rehabilitation (OVR), administers grants-in-aid and provides technical assistance and national leadership for the program. Opportunities and services are available in each of the 50 states, the District of Columbia, and Puerto Rico. The purpose of this service is to preserve, develop, or restore the ability of disabled persons to earn their own living. The individual services offered are medical care, counseling and guidance, training, and job finding. Thirty-six states have separate rehabilitation programs for the blind. Application for such services can be made to the Division of Vocational Rehabilitation or to the agency serving the blind. All persons of working age with a substantial job handicap resulting from either physical or mental impairment are eligible for these services.

Despite these growing interests and efforts, many persons are still in need of rehabilitation. In 1953 it was estimated that approximately 2 million disabled persons could be rehabilitated and could possibly return to work.[3] The number of persons becoming disabled annually was estimated to be 250,000, and under the existing rehabilitation programs about 60,000 of these were being returned to full and productive lives each year.[3] Goals were set to expand rehabilitation resources progressively so that by 1959 at least 200,000 of the 250,000 persons disabled each year could be rehabilitated. In response to these appeals the Vocational Rehabilitation Act was designed to expand rehabilitation facilities, to authorize training programs to meet the shortage of professionally qualified rehabilitation workers, and to make it possible for the states to bring better rehabilitation services to more disabled persons.

REHABILITATION PLANNING

How is one to know if a patient needs rehabilitation? Does the patient want to be rehabilitated? Does every patient need rehabilitation or only those who have an obvious physical disability such as loss of a part of the body or loss of function of a part of the body? These are a few of the questions nurses might ask. Those with neuromuscular-skeletal conditions have long been the group on whom major interest has been focused and to whom help has been extended. Special attention has been given those patients who have an obvious physical disability such as an amputation, paraplegia, or hemiplegia. Something which can be seen and touched is usually easier to cope with than something unseen and out of reach. For example, it is easier to remember to help the amputee exercise his stump than it is to remember to help the person with chronic pulmonary emphysema to do his breathing exercises.

Evaluation by the rehabilitation team. It is well to assume that each patient may need rehabilitation. However, one cannot know what is needed until a thorough evaluation is made. This includes consideration of the patient's past, present, and future. Observations and data concerning the patient's physical, emotional, social, and economic status are required before a valid evaluation can be made. If the particular disease or illness is known to be acute, of short duration, and without common sequelae, the patient's possible needs for rehabilitation may be few or nonexistent. For example, a normally healthy individual who has a bout of pneumonia may recover and resume all previous activities with little help aside from proper chemotherapy. However, when an alcoholic has a bout of pneumonia, he needs much more than chemotherapy.

Few or numerous professional personnel may be needed to obtain all of the information necessary for patient evaluation. The *rehabilitation team* usually consists of a patient, a doctor, a nurse, and a social worker (see Figure 4). Depending on the needs of the patient being considered, services of other personnel such as a psychiatrist, a physical therapist, an occupational therapist, a speech therapist, or a vocational counselor may be needed. Some doctors in private practice make evaluations without the assistance of other

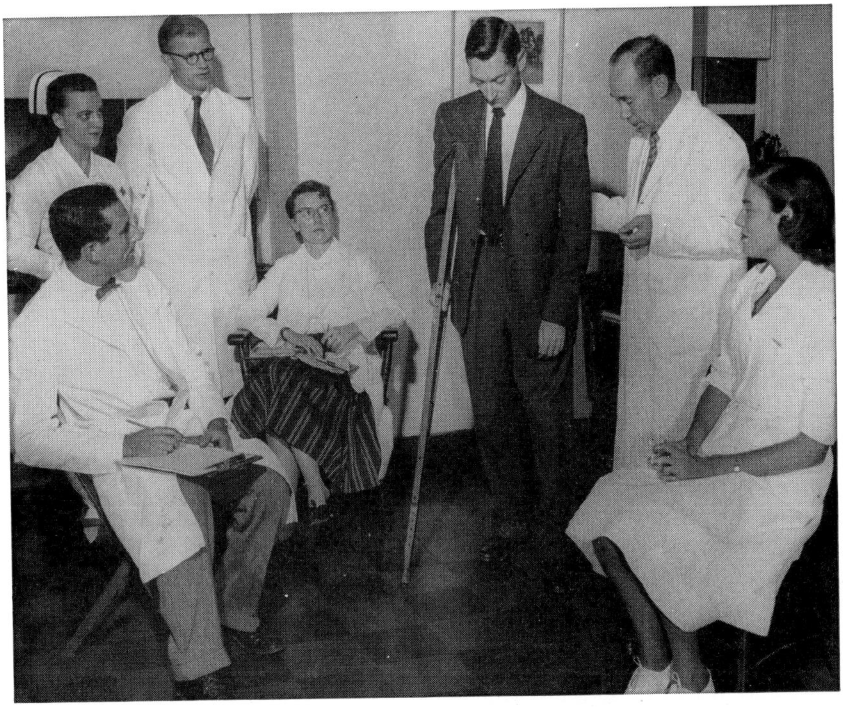

Figure 4

The team approach to rehabilitation is essential. Here the patient, the doctor, the nurse, the social worker, and the occupational therapist review a particular problem.

professional personnel either because such personnel are unavailable or because the doctor may not realize the possible contributions they may be able to make. Teamwork requires that each member of the group be able to use his special knowledge and skill and understand the value of his contribution to the body of information about a patient. To do this effectively each team member needs some understanding of each of the other member's functions.

As a team member, the nurse can make a valuable contribution to total evaluation of the patient because she has the advantage of being with the patient for longer periods of time than any other health worker. Daily she coordinates the many activities needed to help the patient in his rehabilitation. The day-to-day observations made and care given by the nurse can be tremendously helpful if she makes these observations and results available to others. When all the information on the patient, his life situation, and his goals has been carefully interpreted and evaluated by the group, a plan of rehabilitation can be made.

PATIENT MOTIVATION

The most important contribution to his evaluation and rehabilitation must be made by the patient himself. The patient, the doctor, the nurse, the social worker, and sometimes others planning together can arrive at the best goal for his future, but the patient's attitudes, acceptance, and direction of motivation are the most important considerations. If he cannot accept his disability, whatever it may be and however extensive it may be, attempts at rehabilitation usually are hindered. The patient is the person who really makes the decisions, and he changes within himself at his own pace and state of readiness. If he is agreeable to suggestions but makes little or no effort to try them, one should question if he really has accepted the suggestions.

The patient's behavior from day to day in small ways can be the first indications to direction of motivation. For example, if he makes every effort to resume normal daily activities such as feeding himself, bathing, and dressing, one can be quite certain that he is a person with a sincere desire to be independent. As he becomes ready for more advanced activities such as ambulation and work in the occupational therapy shop, he needs continuing genuine interest and support from the nurse and others. As obstacles present themselves, he may be able to accept them and eventually overcome them. However, there are some patients who, faced with an added burden, cannot accept it and give up trying. Those who are truly motivated toward helping themselves seem never to give up and find ways of accomplishing activities which professional personnel might believe impossible.

THE NURSE'S ROLE IN REHABILITATION

The nurse's role in rehabilitation begins with her point of view and her understanding of herself and others. Her point of view can be the stimulus which helps her to be alert to the needs of patients and to make thorough evaluations. If she has a comprehensive approach to each patient, she will be able to work with him much more constructively than if she approaches him with only an isolated part of care in mind. If she gets to know the "person" in the bed, in the clinic, or in the home, she will begin to realize the significance of social and emotional factors and will experience the difference between giving only required care and truly working with and for patients to help them meet their needs.

Planning care. Planning is an essential part of the nurse's comprehensive approach to patient care. Consideration of the patient as a person, what he wants, and what he wishes to do is of the utmost importance in planning. Plans for patient care need to be kept flexible and within practical limits for the patient and his family. With encouragement the patient and his family often will go ahead with future planning but need help and support when any new activity is begun. In the hospital, patient-care plans keep the nurses informed as to what the patient is capable of doing and what he is working toward. Keeping careful, up-to-date plans reduces the number of times the patient has to inform the staff about his capabilities and helps produce a more consistent, united approach toward the patient's goal.

The nurse's evaluation. Since any patient may need rehabilitation, the nurse must learn to evaluate each new patient with whom she has contact. For example, if the patient has been started on a program of self-care in which nurse, occupational therapist, and physical therapist participate, the nurse will need to know the plans of each therapist and must help the patient follow these plans in his usual self-care activity on the ward. A special technique may be required so that the patient can feed himself. The physical therapist will give exercises to strengthen the necessary muscles. The occupational therapist may supply the necessary equipment such as arm slings and built-up utensil handles and may help the patient in using these. The nurse will need to help the patient use these methods at mealtime while he is on the ward.

In making observations of the patient's physical, emotional, and social states, the nurse gradually learns which patients need more thorough evaluation than others. The nurse almost automatically seems to make observations of the patient's physical state such as temperature, pulse, respiration, color, blood pressure, height, and weight. These are usual admission requirements, and some are daily requirements. Patients require bathing, feeding, some facility for elimination, and changes of bed linen. Various medications and treatments are given as needed and as prescribed by the doctor. Most of these procedures involve some physical contact and observation.

Observations of social and emotional factors vary, depending on the patient and the nurse. Nurses need to place more emphasis on these areas and use their opportunities to observe them to a high degree. In a busy situation the physical requirements are always accomplished, but attention to the patient's emotional and social needs may vary. Yet it is in these areas that many patients have the maximum needs.

The following guide can be used by the nurse in evaluating a patient. Her evaluation should not be limited to just the general points listed but should be broken down into specific details. For example, under I, B, 5, (e), "physical setup of the home," one might specifically find out if the patient lives in a house or an apartment, if he has to use stairs (and if so, how many), the number of rooms, exactly where the patient will be sleeping, access to bathroom and kitchen, type of doors and doorways, whether there are doorsills, placement of articles the patient will need to use every day or possibly at night, ventilation, and placement of furniture. Each evaluation requires use of imagination, foresight, and ingenuity.

PATIENT EVALUATION GUIDE FOR THE NURSE

I Physical, emotional, and social observations
- A Physical
  - 1 General appearance
    - (a) Body build, weight, height, posture, gait
    - (b) General day-to-day appearance
    - (c) Changes in appearance
    - (d) Appearance before illness
  - 2 Symptoms and signs
    - (a) Temperature
    - (b) Pulse
    - (c) Respiration
    - (d) Blood pressure
    - (e) Color
    - (f) Specific complaints such as pain, nausea, fatigue, dyspnea
    - (g) Usual pattern of specific complaints; e.g., in cardiac patient, time and nature of chest pain over a period of days, in relation to activity
    - (h) Intake and output
    - (i) Other physical symptoms and signs which occur in relation to self-care (see II, Self-care activities)
  - 3 Previous state of health
    - (a) Number of admissions—present hospital and others
    - (b) Contact with other health agencies—public health nursing, family service
- B Emotional and social
  - 1 Behavior
    - (a) Adjustment—to illness, roommates, staff, therapy
    - (b) Previous behavior—collection of observations made by patient and by family and/or friends
    - (c) Usual day-to-day behavior—interest, occupation, general frame of mind or spirits
    - (d) Changes in behavior—circumstances at time of change and before and after change
    - (e) Family relationships—at home, reaction to visitors if in hospital, reaction to lack of visitors, family interest, family members who seem to help
  - 2 Social activities
    - (a) Usual way patient likes to spend time
    - (b) Amount of free time available and how used
    - (c) Friends or lack of friends
    - (d) Activities at home or outside home or both
  - 3 Family
    - (a) Nationality
    - (b) Birthplace
    - (c) Religion
    - (d) Place in family—mother, father
    - (e) Siblings
    - (f) Children
    - (g) Language spoken in home
  - 4 Mental ability and education
    - (a) Vocabulary
    - (b) Ability to understand explanations
    - (c) Ability to carry out functions in relation to care needed
    - (d) Ability to repeat actions, such as giving self-medication after a demonstration
    - (e) Ability to retain knowledge to be used another time

(f) Ability to make suggestions regarding own care
(g) Amount of schooling
(h) Kind of schooling
(i) I.Q.—if psychologic testing has been done

5 Household
(a) Importance to patient
(b) Importance to family
(c) Patient satisfied or dissatisfied
(d) Location of home
(e) Physical setup of home

6 Finances
(a) Kind of work patient has done
(b) Kind of work patient is doing
(c) Income of patient and family
(d) Attitude toward job—satisfaction, dissatisfaction
(e) Use of income—values of individual in relation to finances
(f) Use of public assistance or private funds—acceptance of, reaction to
(g) Effect of finances on health habits, purchase of prescribed medications, follow-through on prescribed diagnostic tests

II Self-care activities

(Include factors such as patient's interest in doing, specifically how the activity is done, progression in doing activities)

A Personal hygiene

1 Bathing
(a) By patient, nurse, member of family, or combination
(b) Usual method—bed, tub, shower
(c) Frequency

2 Nails
Care of, by patient, nurse, member of family, or combination

3 Hair
(a) Shampoo by patient, nurse, member of family, or combination
(b) Where shampooed and type of equipment used or needed
(c) Usual method

4 Shaving
(a) By patient, nurse, member of family, barber, or combination
(b) Usual method and equipment used
(c) Frequency

B Grooming and appearance

1 General appearance
(a) Neat
(b) Untidy
(c) Interest in

2 Use of cosmetics
(a) Used by self or with help
(b) Interest in

3 Combing hair
(a) By self, nurse, member of family, or combination
(b) Special device necessary

4 Dressing
(a) By self, nurse, member of family, or combination
(b) Special devices used
(c) Difficulties involved, need for practice

C Feeding

1 Type of food
(a) Regular
(b) Special diet

2 Appetite
3 Likes and dislikes
4 Accomplished by self, nurse, member of family, or combination
5 Special devices or setup necessary

D Elimination

1 Continent
2 Incontinent
3 Constipation
4 Amount of urinary output
5 Habit
6 Need for special training schedule and management—bladder and bowel
7 Facility used
(a) Bedpan
(b) Commode
(c) Toilet
(d) Special equipment

E Activity

1 Bed activities
Ability to turn, lift, pull, balance, attain sitting position

2 Special devices for bed activity
(a) Bars
(b) Trapeze
(c) Others

3 Ability to go from bed to chair, from bed to wheel chair, from wheel chair to chair
4 Ability to return to bed
5 Ability to stand
6 Walking and stair climbing
7 Use of any devices in standing and walking
8 Tolerance for activity
9 Amount of activity advised in comparison to that carried out
10 Activity on ward and activity off ward
11 Ability to move about in house and how

12 Ability to go outside house and how
13 Ability in managing transportation

F Rest
  1 Usual habit
  2 Ward habit
  3 Habit since illness
  4 Prescribed amount in comparison to amount taken
  5 Problems of maintaining or securing rest—when and how helped

III Special teachings for future

(Need for special teaching may be in relation to any of above activities)

A Special diet—selection, purchase, and preparation of food

B Administering medication
  1 Purchasing and obtaining medication and necessary equipment
  2 Method

C Household activities
  1 Easier ways of managing
  2 Relocation of articles in home
  3 Scheduling activities

D Care of other members of family by patient

E Care of patient by other members of family

F Provision for follow-up of patient and reevaluation

PREVENTION AS PART OF REHABILITATION

Rehabilitation begins at the time of diagnosis. Part of the aim of patient care should be to preserve the functions and abilities the patient has and to prevent the occurrence of unnecessary limitations such as contractures. If contractures are allowed to develop, months may be added to the patient's course of treatment to correct them and the cost of care is substantially increased. Helping the patient keep as active as possible within his limitations and helping him to keep good body alignment despite disability may enable him to resume usual activities sooner. The nurse should be particularly attentive to these factors in the care of patients who are confined to bed or who have severely restricted activity.

Preserving motion. The nurse can help the patient prevent contracture by teaching him what good body alignment is and how to maintain it in lying, sitting, and standing positions or in motion. Patients confined to bed rest or who are allowed limited activity will have problems of body mechanics. The nurse should have a thorough understanding of joint motion and should either help the patient go through the full range of motion twice daily or should move each joint through its range of motion. The daily bath provides an excellent opportunity for doing this. The nurse should know the motions in a systematic fashion and should familiarize herself with their terminology (see Figures 5 to 7).

If a patient has lost an extremity (amputation) or has loss of function (hemiplegia) careful attention given to bed posture, changes in position, and follow-through on exercise programs will help prevent development of additional disability. Many patients who require extended periods of bed rest but who have less obvious disability (such as patients with cardiac disease or tuberculosis) can be helped to maintain muscle tone by use of a footboard, foot exercises, quadriceps setting, correct position, and adequate turning unless contraindicated. Specific methods of prevention can be checked with the doctor if there is doubt.

Most patients are placed on progressive activity programs as their condition permits. As new activities are to be done, the nurse should give a clear explanation of what the activity consists of, what she will do to help, and what is necessary for the patient to do. Preparation of the patient prior to changes in activity will help to pave the way for better acceptance of the change and will help allay the patient's apprehension. For example, the patient who has pain on moving in bed and has been on bed rest for weeks may become apprehensive and fearful when approached with the idea of being moved out of bed. The nurse can do much to allay fears and apprehension by knowing exactly how the patient can be moved, and moved with the least effort on his part. The nurse with a confident but un-

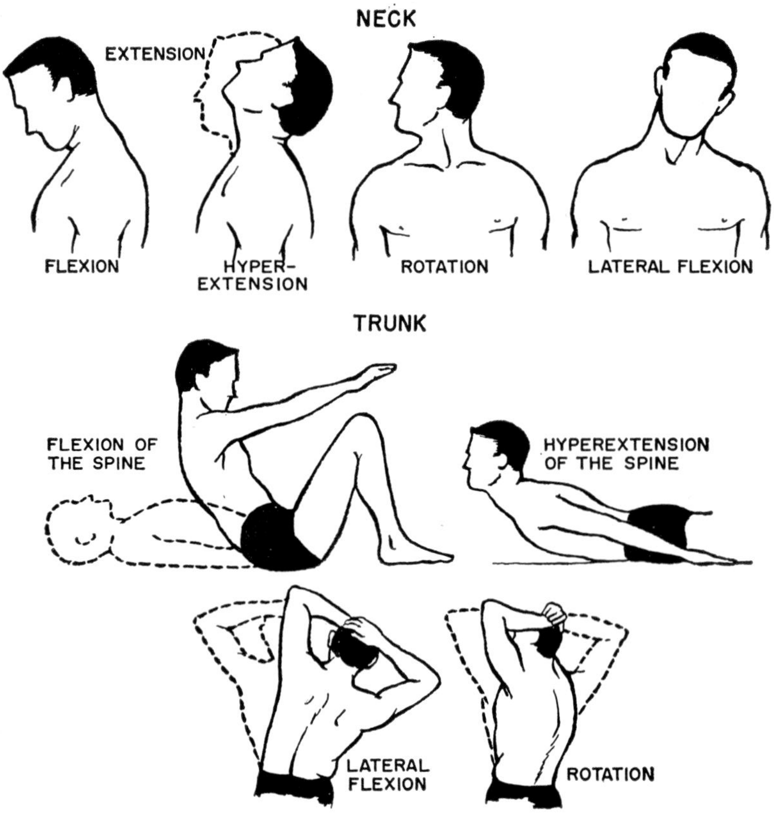

Figure 5

Illustrating range of joint motion for the neck and trunk.

derstanding manner can make a new procedure much less traumatic for the patient than can the competent technically skilled nurse who lacks understanding.

The nurse can be a source of encouragement to the patient in finding new ways to manage necessary self-care. Nurses can learn much about techniques from their patients. Many activities have been developed by the disabled for the disabled. Faced with a problem and knowing that the problem is one to be lived with for the rest of his life has spurred many a patient, as well as doctors, nurses, and therapists, to develop easier ways of managing daily needs as well as meeting occupational needs. Extension handles for combs, toothbrushes, and eating utensils are simple to construct and make it possible for many patients to be self-sufficient. If given a picture or simple drawing with explanations of what is needed, members of the family can often help in making self-help devices. In this day of small gadgets, one can find numerous useful articles already on the market. However, patient and family may need help in recognizing the need for such aids, in learning where to find them, and in learning how to use them effectively.

The nurse can and should contribute suggestions for working out activity problems with her patients. One way of finding a method for a particular body motion is for the nurse actually to assume that she has the same disability as the patient and proceed from there. For example, if the patient has weak upper and lower extremities, it may be difficult for

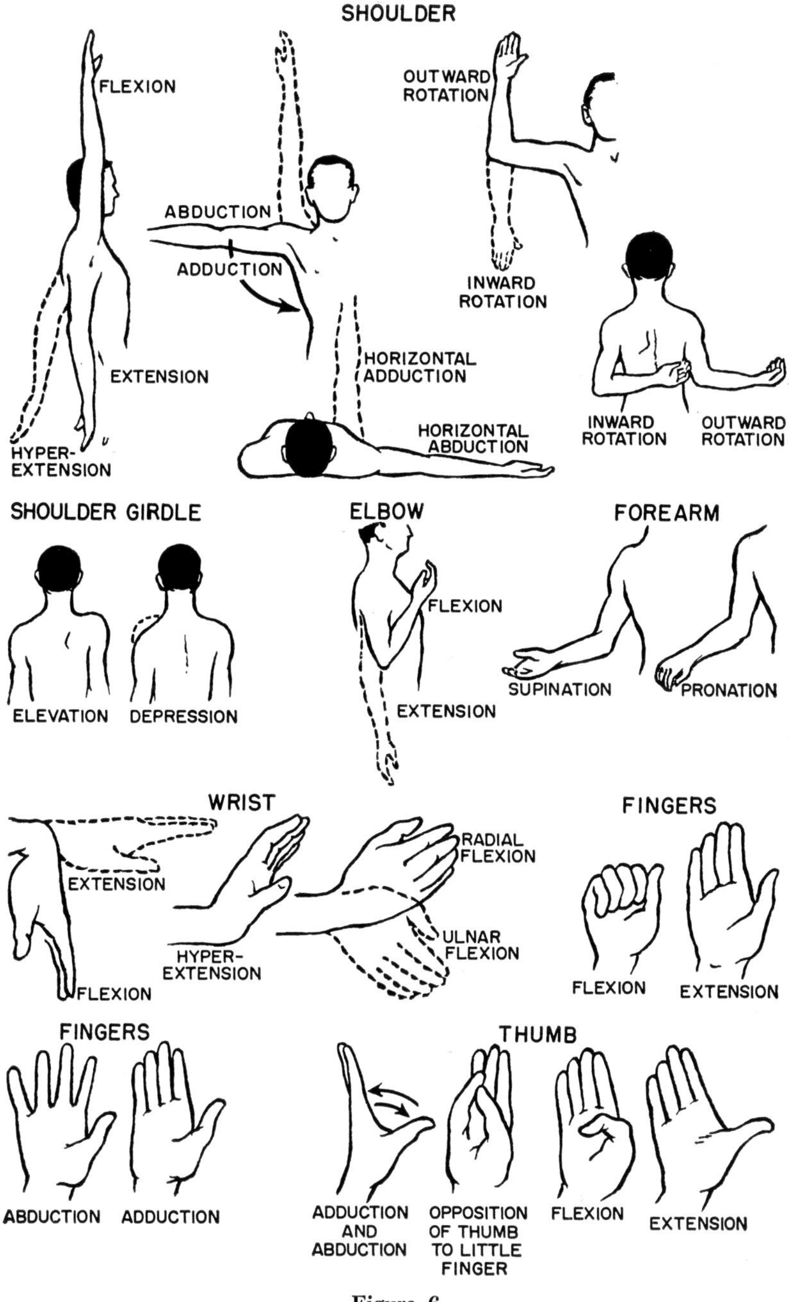

Figure 6

Illustrating range of joint motion for the shoulder and shoulder girdle, elbow, wrist, forearm, and hand.

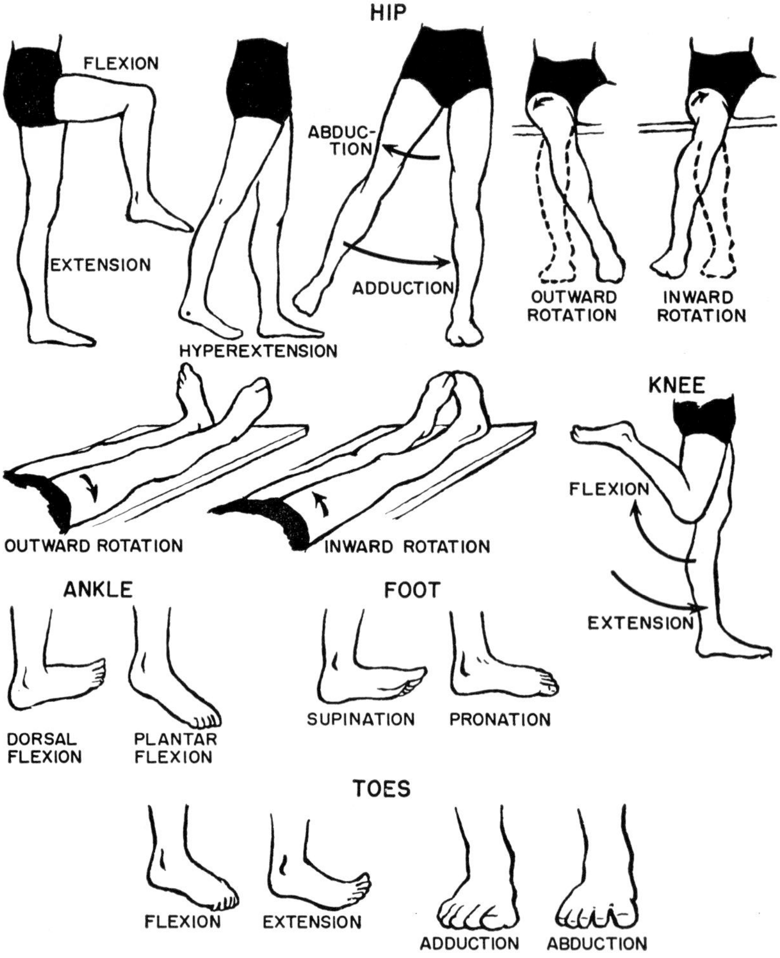

Figure 7

Illustrating range of joint motion for the hip, knee, ankle, foot, and toes.

him to assume a sitting position in bed. Experimenting for herself, the nurse will find that, starting from a back-lying position, she must first place the palms of her hands close to her hips. Then, by pushing on her elbows, she can raise her head and shoulders from the bed. By sliding one elbow back and then the other until both elbows are under the shoulders, she will be in a position in which she is supported but in which the hands are not free. By pushing on the right hand and extending the right elbow, then pushing on the left hand and extending the left elbow, she will find herself approaching a sitting position but not yet in a balanced position. By moving first one hand forward then the other, she can gradually assume a balanced sitting position. While this may be an easy procedure for the nurse who is strong and not hindered by weakness, it may be painstaking and slow for the patient who has weak extremities. However, through a step-by-step demonstration the nurse can teach the patient exactly how he can achieve a sitting position in bed. Since almost all rehabilitation is a slow process, it is important not only to have an ultimate goal, but also to set intermediate goals that may be obtained in a shorter time. Unless patients experience some success, discouragement develops.

Many more considerations of patient care are included in the rehabilitative process than are given in this chapter. However, since rehabilitation is an integral part of all comprehensive patient care, further specific measures have been incorporated in the chapters which follow. The points of emphasis which have been given for the patient and the nurse in the preceding pages apply generally to all patient care. Some references at the end of this chapter give much more specific detail on particular techniques with which the nurse should become familiar.[10,16]

SPECIAL SERVICES FOR REHABILITATION

Many patients require treatment in addition to that provided in the general hospital and that available in the home. Intensive physical therapy and a more extensive program may be necessary for some. Rehabilitation centers and services have developed quite rapidly since World War II. There are various types of centers: teaching and research centers (centers located in and operated by hospitals and medical schools), community centers with facilities for inpatients, community outpatient centers, insurance centers, and vocational rehabilitation centers. Most centers offer a wide range of services, which usually fall into three areas:

MEDICAL AREA

Physical and medical evaluation
Physical therapy
Occupational therapy
Speech therapy
Medical supervision of appropriate activities

PSYCHOSOCIAL AREA

Evaluation
Personal counseling
Social service
Psychometrics
Psychiatric service

VOCATIONAL AREA

Work evaluation
Vocational counseling
Prevocational experience
Industrial fitness of programs
Trial employment in sheltered workshops
Vocational training
Terminal employment in sheltered workshops
Placement

Advantages of organized programs. Patients participating in organized programs of therapy have an opportunity to see and be with others who have similar or more extensive disabilities. Often they progress more rapidly when they realize that others have similar difficulties and are overcoming them. Group therapy often arouses a competitive spirit and a formerly reluctant person may become most willing and diligent. On the other hand, the nurse, doctor, and therapists need to be alert to those patients who have the opposite reaction. A patient who sees others advance in activity while he either does not improve or progresses very slowly may become so discouraged that he gives up trying.

Activities are scaled so that the individual can see his own progress in comparison with his beginning abilities. Patients take an active interest in keeping their "own scores." After a program of therapy has been planned and is scheduled as to time of day, the patient can help to keep himself on schedule by having a copy at the bedside. The nurse can help him gradually to assume more and more responsibility for getting himself ready for scheduled activities. A master plan of activities for all patients on the ward can be a useful device for nurses, doctors, and therapists. The plan can be kept in a central place on the ward and should list name, activity, and time of activity for each patient.

REFERENCES AND SELECTED READINGS*

1 Buchwald, Edith, and others: Physical Rehabilitation for Daily Living, New York, 1952, McGraw-Hill Book Co., Inc.

---

*References preceded by an asterisk indicate material particularly well suited for student reading.

2 Cockerill, Eleanor, and Margolis, H. M.: The Concept of Disability, J. Chron. Dis. **3**:167-169, Feb. 1956.
3 Eisenhower, Dwight D.: Message to Congress, January 18, 1954, Washington, D. C., 1954, U. S. Government Printing Office.
4 Kessler, Henry H.: Rehabilitation of the Physically Handicapped, revised edition, New York, 1953, Columbia University Press.
5 *Kurtagh, Cathryn H.: Which Bed to Buy, Am. J. Nursing **58**:208-210, 1958.
6 Larson, Carroll B., and Gould, Marjorie: Calderwood's Orthopedic Nursing, ed. 4, St. Louis, 1957, The C. V. Mosby Co.
7 Mead, Sedgwick: Rehabilitation of the Geriatric Patient. In Cowdry, E. V. (editor): The Care of the Geriatric Patient, St. Louis, 1958, The C. V. Mosby Co.
8 *Morrissey, Alice B., and Zimmerman, Muriel E.: Helps for the Handicapped, Am. J. Nursing **53**:316-318, March 1953; **53**:454-456, April 1953.
9 *Morrissey, Alice B., and others: The Nurse and Rehabilitation, Am. J. Nursing **54**:1354-1359, Nov. 1954.
10 Morrissey, Alice B.: Rehabilitation Nursing, New York, 1951, G. P. Putnam's Sons.
11 National Health Forum, Changing Factors in Staffing America's Health Services, New York, 1954, National Health Council.
12 *Newton, Kathleen: Geriatric Nursing, ed. 3, St. Louis, 1960, The C. V. Mosby Co.
13 Public Health Service: Restorative Services for Older People, Pub. Health Rep. **71**:1194, Dec. 1956.
14 Redkey, Henry: Rehabilitation Centers in the United States, Chicago, 1953, The National Society for Crippled Children and Adults.
15 *Rose, Donald L., Shipes, Edward B., and Alyea, William S.: Physical Measures in the Aged, J.A.M.A. **162**:1524-1526, Dec. 22, 1956.
16 Terry, Florence J., Benz, Gladys S., Mereness, Dorothy, and Kleffner, Frank R., (Jensen, Deborah MacLurg, editor): Principles and Technics of Rehabilitation Nursing, St. Louis, 1957, The C. V. Mosby Co.
17 U. S. Department of Health, Education, and Welfare, Office of Vocational Rehabilitation: Vocational Rehabilitation for Civilians, Washington, D. C., U. S. Government Printing Office.
18 U. S. Department of Health, Education, and Welfare, Office of Vocational Rehabilitation: New Hope for the Disabled, Washington, D. C., 1956, U. S. Government Printing Office.

Section II

Nursing related to specific medical and surgical care

Nutrition

Chapter 5

Study questions for review

1 Review the average caloric needs for persons of different weights and who participate in different amounts of activity.
2 Study the appetites of two patients on your ward for a forty-eight hour period. List some of the reasons for your findings.
3 What important details have you learned about feeding the critically ill patient or one who cannot feed himself?

The progress of most patients with a medical or surgical condition is profoundly affected by their individual response to the diet prescribed by the doctor. Vital structures, such as the brain and the liver, which have suffered severe damage as a result of prolonged malnutrition and chronic disease may not survive without daily essential fuel. When new disease places an added burden upon such structures, the final outcome of the patient may be determined largely by his ability to take and retain enough food. The nurse cannot separate the rest of nursing care from attention to adequate nutrition. An inherent part of all good nursing is to see that the patient takes and, in so far as possible, enjoys the diet ordered. The nurse's interest in her patient and in his response to food, as well as her whole attitude toward nutrition, greatly affects the patient's acceptance or rejection of his diet.

Dietary prescriptions during illness may require changes from normal eating habits. It may be that the patient is served a regular well-balanced diet when he does not have a normal appetite and when he has not been accustomed to eating such a diet. The ingestion of new and unfamiliar foods and food mixtures in varying amounts may be necessary. Elimination from the diet of certain foods and food seasonings may be quite disturbing to some patients. The nurse does not, at least in the larger hospitals, have an active part in the preparation of special diets. If, however, diets are ordered for her patients, she should know the purpose of these diets and the major adjustments in eating patterns they represent for individual patients. In the patient's home she may be called upon for more specific assistance to the patient and his family in helping the patient to follow a therapeutic diet.

SPECIFIC NURSING RESPONSIBILITIES IN NUTRITION

The nurse has several specific responsibilities in relation to diet. She must see that the right diet is ordered and served to the patient. She should discuss food likes and dislikes with the patient and relay these to the dietition. She must explain to the patient why his desires for specially prepared foods may not always be realized in a large hospital. She must know the essentials of good nutrition and should check the daily food intake of all patients carefully enough to note consistent deficiencies.

Participation in making food attractive and in creating a suitable environment for good appetite is a nursing function. No disturbing articles such as emesis basins should be about when trays are served. Odors should be eliminated by thorough ventilation of rooms before meals, and no disturbing or painful dressings or other treatments should be done either immediately before or after meals. A mouthwash shortly before meals makes food more palatable for some patients. Offering water so that patients confined to bed may wash their hands before eating is a desirable procedure. Most people have been trained over many years to wash their hands after going to the bathroom and before sitting down to the table, yet in many hospitals neither water nor even a damp washcloth is offered after a bedpan has been used. Treatments and other ward activities should be planned so that food can be eaten as soon as served to prevent chilling of hot foods. If the patient can be up, serving meals away from bed and in an area such as the sunporch in the company of other patients often improves appetite. Depending upon the patient's reaction, visitors should be encouraged or restricted during meal hours.

The nurse should appreciate the emotional implications of food for all people and how these may affect the patient who has food denied him. Hunger is perhaps the most fundamental of all human drives and is the basic response to the instinct for personal survival. Prisoners, starving in camps during World War II, report that they had no thoughts whatsoever of sex or of any other satisfactions often considered essential in our lives. Thoughts of food occupied their every waking moment, and during sleep they dreamed almost constantly of food. Food represents association with other gratifying sensations; it is closely related to comfort and companionship and belonging. The infant learns to associate warmth, cuddling, safety, and belonging with food and thus with life. At no time in civilization and in no primitive or civilized society is a gathering of human beings held for pleasant or convivial purposes without food being served. Withholding food, therefore, has meaning for the patient far beyond the actual denial of calories. It is probable that the denial of food, no matter how fully its purpose is explained to the patient and no matter how temporary he may know it to be, affects him much more profoundly than has been generally recognized. Deep-seated uneasiness may not be quickly put to rest by merely telling the patient that soon he may be able to have food.

Different foods mean different things to different people. Cultural groups have developed feelings about and values for particular foods. A good example of this is the Thanksgiving turkey in our modern American culture. Some foods come to be associated with status, with whether or not an individual is a normal and accepted member of his cultural group. Then, also, some foods have negative cultural values for various groups; in one society of the past, green vegetables were considered "vulgar" and suitable for the common people but not for the nobility. Because of the importance of food in all societies, the list of foods that have significance in cultural groups is endless. The patient who is denied certain foods that have social, cultural, and emotional significance for him may suffer keenly. Irritability and apparent lack of cooperation are natural responses to food deprivations and should be understood and accepted by the nurse. She should relay facts learned about the patient's eating habits to the dietitian and the doctor; adjustments can perhaps be made in the diet so that the patient will be happier. Members of the family can often prepare acceptable substitutes for desired foods or even prepare therapeutic diets in the home and bring them to the patient. This practice should be permitted, provided that it is desired by the patient and his family and provided that therapeutic diet orders are followed.

TEACHING NUTRITION

The nurse should be a teacher and should set an example of good nutrition for patients in the hospital, the clinic, the home, and the community. Many people in our country suffer from malnutrition despite the fact that this nation has the potentiality for the best nutrition in the world. It is a commentary on the eating practices of the people of the United States that the best-fed groups, with the exception of the Armed Forces, are those in our federal prisons.[1] It is true that more leafy vegetables and more fruits are consumed than forty years ago. Yet wide consumption of food highly advertised but lacking in basic food value has proved that natural selection cannot be relied upon to ensure that each person will meet his nutritional needs in the best fashion.

Eating patterns are exceedingly difficult to change. The influence of habit and custom and likes and dislikes has not been given enough consideration in the past. It is questionable whether public health educators have been as successful as they would like to believe in changing the eating habits of some groups in our population. Particularly is this true of the older people and the foreign born whose cultural eating patterns have not been too carefully considered. Many people, however, will and do make an earnest attempt to change food patterns, provided they learn what changes to make and provided these changes are not too much out of keeping with their economic circumstances and their cultural and social values. Young mothers are often quite receptive to guidance on how to feed their families properly.

In teaching nutrition, as in any other teaching, the patient must first be motivated to want to learn. The nurse should help the patient recognize and identify the nutrition problem. She, then, should begin to work with the problem as the patient sees it and only gradually hope to help the patient see other perhaps more important implications of the problem. The nurse who is not convinced herself of the need for good nutrition probably will in some way communicate this to the patient and thus be much less effectual in her teaching.

To teach nutrition, the nurse must know the basic essentials of good nutrition: (1) vegetables and fruits—four or more servings a day including a citrus fruit and a green leafy or a yellow vegetable; (2) meat, eggs, fish, poultry, or cheese—two servings or more daily and the use of fats and oils limited to about three teaspoonfuls a day; (3) milk—one pint of whole, skim, or buttermilk daily; (4) breads, cereals or potato—one serving at each meal. These are the basic or so-called protective foods. Additional foods supply caloric needs which vary with size, age, and activity of each individual. The leaflet *Food for Fitness, Daily Food Guide** is helpful in determining caloric needs. The diet for elderly people differs only in that more calcium and fewer calories are needed. Foods high in protein and vitamin contents are often neglected by the aged because of cost and the trouble of preparation.

Posters and pamphlets help a great deal in teaching patients about nutrition, and excellent ones are available. Miniature copies of the poster *Basic 4 Food Groups*† can be given to patients for reference. Pictorial guides, such as *Guide to Good Eating*,‡ and *Essentials of an Adequate Diet*§ are also available. Local health departments and voluntary community agencies are good sources of posters, pamphlets, and other visual aid material in this field.

The nurse should begin teaching nutrition by getting to know the patient and what he likes to eat; the patient should

---

*Issued by Home Economics Research, Agricultural Research Service, Washington, 1957, U. S. Department of Agriculture.

†Issued by the Bureau of Human Nutrition and Home Economics, Washington, 1957, U. S. Department of Agriculture.

‡Prepared by the National Dairy Council, Chicago, 1956.

§Leaflet 425, Agricultural Research, Washington, 1958, U. S. Department of Agriculture.

do most of the talking at first. Learning what he buys each week will give the nurse good basic information. She then needs knowledge and imagination to help the patient fit basic requirements into the foods he likes and to suggest ways by which essential foods may be incorporated into mixed dishes if they are not otherwise acceptable. Above all, she must make her teaching practical. It is useless to recommend certain foods to patients when it is obvious that money is not available for their purchase. It is also fruitless to suggest special methods of preparation when the patient lives in a boardinghouse and cannot prepare his own meals or when he has a job that requires travel and must eat in restaurants or on trains. The nurse should make some effort to know prices of foods in her own locality, and she should be able to give practical suggestions to patients such as buying foods in season, buying canned goods at special sales, buying suitable amounts of perishable foods, and taking advantage of special sales of surplus foods.

Although the nurse often is not responsible for determining special therapeutic diets or for teaching the patient about these, she should understand the basic elements of diet in disease so that she can motivate the patient to be receptive to teaching, reinforce teaching done by the dietitian, and be able to intelligently check whether a patient is following dietary instructions. The nurse should anticipate the need for dietary instruction so that referrals for teaching are made as soon as possible. She also should determine whether members of the family should learn about the patient's diet. The nurse should be familiar with current lay and professional literature concerning diet so that she can answer the patient's questions intelligently.

Some patients are not on special prescribed diets, yet because of their physical condition should be cautious about certain foods or should include certain foods in their menus. For example, a person who has had his gallbladder removed need not necessarily be on a low fat diet; however, a high fat meal may cause him to be uncomfortable since there is no reserve bile to be poured out to assist in digestion of the extra fat. A person who is on a constipating medication such as Amphojel needs to include more fruit and roughage in his diet. This kind of general health teaching is the nurse's responsiblity.

The nurse should recognize the need for a change in diet and should suggest this to the doctor. For example, a person who is on a bland diet for a long period of time may complain of distention and flatulence since the emollient effect of this diet tends to decrease gastric secretion including hydrochloric acid and since its low roughage tends to decrease peristalsis.

A person who returns to work on a special diet may need revision of the caloric content of such a diet. Those with diabetes, for example, often find that although their diabetes was under control previously, they had difficulty upon returning to work.

OBESITY

Obesity is a major health problem in our country. The emotional suffering caused by this condition is very great. In addition, statistics compiled by the Metropolitan Life Insurance Company show that excessive weight after the age of 45 years runs parallel with shortening of the life span. They also show that our life expectancy after 45 years of age is not so good as that in other countries. Our higher death rate is due to the degenerative diseases, and there is evidence that, with our high standard of living, many of us are literally eating ourselves to death. Cardiac disease is known to occur one and one-half times as often in those who are overweight. The overweight person is a greater surgical risk than the lean one, and often weight reduction is necessary before needed surgery can be done.

In most instances obesity is the result of the ingestion of more calories than are necessary to meet daily energy requirements. There are slight variations in the body's ability to extract minimum benefit from food consumed; the short stocky person has a proportionately longer intestinal tract and possibly more efficient absorption of food than does the tall thin one. There are rare instances in which hormone balance interferes with normal metabolism and contributes to weight gain. Generally, it can be assumed that when people are overweight they are eating too much. The cause can usually be traced to three sources: heredity, injury, and unfavorable external factors relating to nutrition or exercise.[7] Obese persons still may be malnourished; many people who are greatly overweight may not be eating enough of the essential foods such as those containing proteins, minerals, and vitamins.

Studies made by the United States Department of Agriculture show an increased consumption of fat in American diets over recent years. In 1910 the average daily American diet (approximated in grams) was composed of carbohydrates, 540; protein, 93; fat, 113—total of 3,189 calories. In 1948 it had changed to carbohydrates, 375; protein, 90; fat, 130—total of 3,030 calories. The disadvantages of a high fat diet are not definitely established, but there is a high incidence of coronary artery disease among sedentary professional men who are overweight and whose fat consumption is high.

Obesity may result from habits of eating that are continued without modification as the person goes from young active years to a more sedentary middle age. Women face the same problem as men. As their children grow up, women often spend more time in activities such as playing bridge and visiting friends, where high caloric snacks are often consumed. Many people, therefore, gain during middle age simply because their energy output is lessened. They may not have given serious thought to the situation, or else they are not sufficiently motivated or well enough informed to make the small modifications that would keep them from gaining weight.

A very large number of obese persons have serious psychologic problems. They may insist that they do not eat much and they really believe that this is so. However, in reality, they often eat large servings of the most fattening foods, and many of them snack almost constantly. Through food they seek to satisfy some very strong, compelling emotional needs that are not otherwise fulfilled. It is useless to advise such persons repeatedly about their eating habits and the consequences of these habits. Sometimes intensive psychotherapy is beneficial if it is accepted by the obese person, but the results of even this treatment may be disappointing. Many people regain weight at the conclusion of long periods of psychotherapy and weight reduction.

Many studies are now being conducted on the effect of various types of diets, and before any stringent dieting of any kind is begun, the person should be urged to seek medical advice. In treatment of obesity by diet, a rate of loss of not more than two pounds a week (roughly a deficit of 1,000 calories a day below what the patient has been eating) is recommended. This allows for three good meals a day and can be used as a basis for the dietary education of the patient. People who lose weight rapidly usually regain it easily and quickly, and there are indications that repeated weight gains and losses may cause greater stress to the body than static obesity.[7]

REFERENCES AND SELECTED READINGS*

1 Bortz, Edward L.: Nutritional Deficiences and Premature Aging, Second International Gerontological Congress, St. Louis, Sept. 11, 1951.

2 Committee on Fats in Human Nutrition, Food and Nutrition Board: The Role of Dietary Fat in Human Health, National Research Council Publication 575, Washington, D.C., 1958.

3 Cooper, Lenna F., Barber, Edith M., Mitchell, Helen S., and Rynbergen, Henderika, J.: Nutrition in Health and Disease, ed. 3, Philadelphia, 1958, J. B. Lippincott Co.

*References preceded by an asterisk indicate material particularly well suited for student reading.

4 Fryer, J. H.: Obesity: Some Theoretical and Practical Considerations, Health News (New York State Department of Health) **35**:10-11, June 1958.

5 *Kelly, Cordelia W.: Nurses, Nutrition, and the General Public, Am. J. Nursing, **58**:217-218, Feb. 1958.

6 MacBryde, Cyril Mitchell: Signs and Symptoms, ed. 3, Philadelphia, 1955, J. B. Lippincott Co.

7 *Mayer, Jean: Obesity, Am. J. Nursing **59**:1732-1736, Dec. 1959.

8 *Morris, Ena: How Does a Nurse Teach Nutrition to Patients? Am. J. Nursing **60**:67-69, Jan. 1960.

9 *National Research Council: Recommended Dietary Allowances, National Research Council Publication 589, Washington, D.C., 1958.

Study questions for review

1 Review the process of diffusion. What is oncotic pressure? Hydrostatic pressure? What happens to the extra salt and water you consume when ham is served for dinner?
2 Review from your physiology notes the normal pH of the blood. What are the body's "buffer systems," and how do they help maintain acid-base balance?
3 Review these procedures: hypodermoclysis, venoclysis, and blood transfusion. What are the special details for the nurse to remember when these procedures are ordered?
4 If you (or a close friend or member of your family) have recently had severe diarrhea, vomiting, or elevation of temperature, what symptoms did you observe that might indicate change in fluid or electrolyte balance?

Fluid and electrolyte balance

Chapter 6

We live in two environments—an external one of heat and cold, noise, dirt, and physical force and a much more constant internal one of fluid, electrolyte, and temperature balance. The human machinery, carefully steered by the hormones and the central nervous system, is constantly adapting to changes in body requirements and to variations in the availability of essential elements. Upon this adaptive quality rests our ability to survive. The nurse must know how normal fluid and electrolyte balance is maintained if she is to carry out her responsibilities in this increasingly important part of medical management.

NORMAL FLUID BALANCE

Body fluid component

In the normal adult, with average fat, approximately two thirds of the body weight is fluid.[3] Since fat is essentially free of water, the body type of the person must be considered in estimating his body fluid component.[4] Thus, 100 pounds (50 liters) of a lean adult weighing 150 pounds is fluid.

Body fluid is contained within three compartments which are separated by semipermeable membranes. Roughly two thirds of the fluid is within the cells (intracellular) while the remainder is divided between the interstitial fluid which surrounds all living cells (three twelfths of the total) and the fluid within the blood vessels (intravascular) (one twelfth of the total). The interstitial fluid acts as the intermediary between the blood and the cells, allowing for diffusion of nutrients, electrolytes, water, hormones, oxygen, and waste products.

Normal exchange of body fluids

Body fluid is constantly being lost and, for normal processes to continue, must be replaced. With an average daily intake of food and liquids, the healthy body easily maintains compartmental balance.

Loss. Fluid normally leaves the body through the kidneys, lungs, and skin with a very small amount being lost through the gastrointestinal tract and negligible amounts being lost in saliva and tears. Two vital processes demand continual expenditure of water—the removal of body

Table 1 Normal fluid intake and loss in an adult eating 2,500 calories per day (approximate figures)

Intake		*Output*	
Route	*Amount of gain (ml.)*	*Route*	*Amount of loss (ml.)*
Water in food	1,100	Skin and lungs	1,000
Water from oxidation	300	Bowel	100
Water as liquid	1,200	Kidneys	1,500
Total	2,600	Total	2,600

*Adapted from Fluids and Electrolytes, North Chicago, Ill., 1957, Abbott Laboratories.

Note that the intake of water in solid food is almost equal to that taken as liquid. Two-thirds as much water is lost from the skin and lungs as from the kidneys. This is significant in the care of patients with severe burns, who have loss of ability to perspire and who have poor pulmonary function.

heat by vaporization of water and the excretion of urea and other metabolic wastes. The volume of water used in these processes varies greatly with external influences. It has been estimated, however, that even with no food or fluid intake an adult of average build loses at least 800 ml. of water daily through the skin and lungs and he excretes about 900 ml. of water daily through the kidneys. This is known as *compulsory fluid loss* which is essential for maintaining normal body processes. The average adult, taking a normal amount of food and fluids, actually loses larger amounts. (See Table 1.) Fluid ingested in excess of need is eliminated through the kidneys which also can conserve fluid if it is needed. Approximately 120 ml. of fluid in the form of blood plasma is filtered through the glomeruli every minute. Normally, however, only 1 ml. per minute is excreted in urine; the remainder returns to the blood stream.

Replacement. The body receives water from ingested food and fluids and through metabolism of both foodstuffs and body tissues. Solid foods such as meat and vegetables contain 60 to 90 per cent water. Metabolic processes release about 12 ml. of water for each 100 calories of fat, carbohydrate, or protein oxidized.[4] Table 1 shows the approximate daily intake for an average adult. Note that the normal daily replacement of water equals the normal daily loss. Easily measurable intake (liquid) and easily measurable output (urine) are also approximately equal. These figures, therefore, serve as guides for determining normal fluid balance and emphasize the great need for recording intake and output accurately.

NORMAL ELECTROLYTE BALANCE

Body electrolyte component

All body fluids contain chemical compounds. Chemical compounds in solution behave in two ways: either they remain molecularly intact such as urea, dextrose, and creatinine, or they break up into separate electrically charged particles known as *ions*. The ions are either positively charged *(cations)* or negatively charged *(anions)*. Chemical compounds which break up into ions are called *electrolytes;* they help to maintain the acid-base balance of the body, and they help to control body water volume. The three fluid compartments contain similar electrolytes, but the concentration of the various electrolytes in each compartment varies markedly. (See Table 2).

In health the ratio of cations to anions in each of the body fluid compartments and the concentration of the various ions in these compartments is relatively constant.

Normal exchange of electrolytes

Electrolytes move more readily between interstitial and intravascular fluids than between intracellular and interstitial fluids. Therefore, normally most of the electrolyte exchange occurs between interstitial and intravascular fluids.

Loss. Electrolyte loss is mainly through the kidneys with normally only minimal losses through the bowel, skin, and lungs. The kidneys selectively excrete electrolytes, retaining those needed for normal body fluid composition. Hormonal influences affect the kidney's selective function. For example, the pituitary antidiuretic hormone tends to promote sodium excretion and to favor water reabsorption. The adrenal cortical hormones favor sodium reabsorption and the excretion of potassium.

Carbon dioxide, bicarbonate, and hydrogen ions are removed from the body through the lungs and kidneys as part of the process of maintaining a normal acid-base balance of body fluids.

The acidity or alkalinity of body fluids depends upon the concentration of the hydrogen ions (H^+) in relation to the concentration of the hydroxyl ions (OH^-) and is expressed as pH. A pH of 7 is a neutral solution. The normal body fluid is slightly alkaline (pH 7.35 to pH 7.45) and is maintained relatively stable by the "buffer systems" in the body. A buffer is a substance which can act as a chemical sponge either soaking up or releasing hydrogen ions so that the normal ratio of acids to bases is maintained. There are several "buffer systems" in the body, but the carbonic acid–bicarbonate system is one of the most important clinically. Two types of carbonate are present in body fluids—carbonic acid (H_2CO_3) and bicarbonate (HCO_3^-). The ability of the body to keep the pH of body fluids within normal limits relies essentially upon maintenance of the normal ratio of one part of carbonic acid to 20 parts of bicarbonate. Since carbonic acid ionizes into a hydrogen ion (H^+) and a bicarbonate ion (HCO_3^-) and bicarbonate ions plus water yield carbonic acid (H_2CO_3) and the hydroxyl ion (OH^-), the normal balance is maintained by removing from the body whichever ion, (H^+) or (OH^-), is in excess.

Replacement. Since most loss of electrolytes occurs from extracellular (intravascular and interstitial) fluids, there is

Table 2 Normal electrolyte content of body fluids and normal daily loss of ions in urine*

Electrolytes (anions and cations)	*Maintenance levels of fluid compartments*			*Daily loss in urine (mEq./L.)*
	Intravascular (mEq./L.)	*Interstitial (mEq./L.)*	*Intracellular (mEq./L.)*	
Sodium (Na^+)	142	145	15	200
Potassium (K^+)	5	4	157	90
Calcium (Ca^{++})	5	3	5	90
Magnesium (Mg^{++})	3	2	27	20
Chloride (Cl^-)	104	116	4	200
Bicarbonate (HCO_3^-)	27	27	10	17
Protein ($Prot^-$)	16	1	72	0
Phosphate ($HPO_4^=$)	2	3	100	26
Sulfate ($SO_4^=$)	1	2	18	22
Organic acids	5	5	0	50

*Adapted from Fluid and Electrolytes, North Chicago, Ill., 1957, Abbott Laboratories.

Note that the electrolyte level of the intravascular and interstitial fluids are approximately the same and that sodium and chloride contents are markedly higher in these fluids; whereas potassium, phosphate, and protein contents are markedly higher in intracellular fluid. Normally most loss of electrolytes occurs through the kidneys, but with high fever or excessive perspiration 25 to 50 additional mEq./L. of both sodium and chloride may be lost through the skin and lungs.

needed a higher daily replacement of those substances found in greater concentration in the extracellular fluid. A healthy person eating a well-balanced diet will easily ingest all the substances needed to maintain electrolyte balance. If more electrolytes than needed are ingested, they normally will be neutralized and excreted.

FLUID AND ELECTROLYTE IMBALANCE

Almost all medical and surgical conditions threaten the fluid and electrolyte balance. The patient who sustains extensive blood loss during surgery may fail in his adaptation to fluid loss and may go into serious and even fatal shock. The patient with colitis loses electrolytes abnormally through the intestines. When the respiratory system does not provide adequate oxygen and carbon dioxide exchange, serious electrolyte imbalance may ensue. Fluid and electrolyte losses as a result of relatively minor illness may themselves give rise to symptoms of more serious disease. Farr[3] cites case histories of seriously ill patients whose conditions were erroneously diagnosed as cerebrovascular accident or coronary artery disease when they were in fact suffering entirely from fluid and electrolyte losses. Any person under stress (emotional or physical) loses excessive amounts of potassium through the kidneys because production of adrenocortical hormones increases. Potassium depletion is, therefore, common in all disease, injury, and surgery.

Fluids and electrolytes may exist in the body in too large amounts causing, for example, edema, acidosis, and alkalosis.

Abnormal fluid and electrolyte loss

Excessive amounts of body fluid and the electrolytes contained therein may be lost through the skin due to profuse perspiration or to oozing from severe wounds or burns. They are lost from the gastrointestinal tract when excessive salivation, vomiting, or diarrhea occur and when the gastrointestinal system is drained by intubation or purged with cathartics or enemas. With hemorrhage body fluids and electrolytes are always lost. Fluids with their electrolyte constituents may be trapped in the body by conditions such as wound swelling, edema, ascites, and intestinal obstruction and therefore may not be available for normal processes. Knowing the common electrolytes found in various body fluids is helpful for nurses in planning to prevent depletion of necessary substances and in noting early symptoms of imbalance. (See Tables 2 and 3.) For clarity of discussion, imbalance of each ion and of body fluid will be considered separately. Actually several imbalances occur simultaneously because of the interrelationship of body fluids and their electrolytes.

Excessive fluid loss. When the body is not supplied with enough fluid to carry on vital processes, a serious chain of events occurs. Abnormal loss of body fluid decreases blood volume, the maintenance of which is essential for life processes. Usually however, except in hemorrhage, the plasma protein is not lost so that the proteins remaining in the blood are concentrated and have a greater protein osmotic or oncotic (pull) pressure than the fluid in the interstitial tissues and in the cells. This causes extravascular fluid to diffuse into the blood stream, first from the interstitial tissue and then from the cells, producing symptoms of *dehydration* such as flushed, dry skin, poor skin turgor, dry lips, a dry coated tongue, excessive thirst, sunken and soft eyeballs, and atonic muscles. If intravenous fluids are given at this stage, they should be given slowly enough to allow diffusion into the extravascular fluid compartments. Running an infusion too rapidly increases the blood volume and, consequently, the hydrostatic pressure, and much of the fluid will be excreted through the kidneys before it can diffuse into the dehydrated tissues. If possible, it is better to give fluids by mouth.

If the cause of dehydration continues unchecked and treatment is not given, anorexia, dyspepsia, and constipation develop as a result of inadequate fluids for proper gastrointestinal functioning. Normally about 8 liters of fluid are used daily

Table 3 Fluid and electrolyte composition of digestive juices*

	Approximate ml. of fluid (daily)	*Chief ions*
Saliva	1,500	Na^+, K^+, Ca^{++}, Cl^-, PO_4^-, $SO_4^=$
Gastric juice	2,500	Na^+, H^+, Cl^-
Intestinal juice	3,000	HCO_3^-, Cl^-, Ca^{++}, $HPO_4^=$
Pancreatic juice	700	K^+, Ca^{++}, Cl^-, HCO_3^-
Bile	500	Na^+

*Adapted from Gamble, J. L.: Extra Cellular Fluids, Cambridge, Mass., 1954, Harvard University Press.

This table shows the electrolyte losses to expect upon losing these juices. Also note that approximately 8 liters of fluid are used daily for digestive purposes; normally most of this fluid is reabsorbed. Some of each of the ions is present in each of the fluids listed although only the predominating ones have been enumerated.

for gastrointestinal fluids (see Table 3) most of which is reabsorbed. As both intracellular and interstitial fluids decrease, cell function is impaired since food, oxygen, and waste products are diffused inadequately. The cells then release potassium and replace it with sodium, causing electrolyte imbalance with all its symptoms. Fluids given at this stage of fluid depletion should contain electrolytes (especially sodium and potassium chlorides) provided that kidney function is normal. Glucose and water are often given first to assure adequate blood volume and to reestablish urinary output since the kidneys play the major role in selection of ions needed for normal electrolyte balance. Intravenous fluids containing electrolytes need to be run slowly to allow the body to regulate their use, and the patient should be carefully watched for signs of intoxication (excess of fluids or electrolytes). If the patient can retain fluid given by mouth, fluids high in potassium content such as orange or pear juice and tea and fluids high in salt content are often ordered.

If, due to lack of treatment or other causes, the blood volume again decreases after having mobilized the reserve of extravascular fluids, the blood pressure falls, kidney function and vaporization then decrease causing body wastes to be retained in the blood stream which disturbs the acid-base balance still further. The heat regulating mechanism also is upset. Unless extensive fluid and electrolyte treatment is given at once the patient may die.

If plasma proteins are lost from the body, as occurs in hemorrhage, or if they are shifted from the blood to the interstitial fluid, as occurs in severe burns, fractures, and crushing injuries, the blood volume drops rapidly and shock follows. Whole blood, plasma, or plasma expanders must usually be given to these patients to replace the protein loss before extensive fluid therapy is effective. If fluid treatment is continued the patient must be carefully watched for early signs of overhydration, since after a few days the plasma tends to suddenly shift back to the blood stream from the interstitial tissues and the patient may develop pulmonary edema from too much circulating blood.

Fluid retention. Retention of abnormal amounts of fluid in the body usually is due to too much sodium chloride being retained in extravascular fluid compartments. The salt holds water causing tissue edema; therefore, reducing salt intake may decrease the edema.

Since adrenal cortical hormones tend to favor sodium reabsorption in the renal tubules, tissue edema can be expected in diseases in which abnormal amounts of these hormones are excreted. Edema in patients being treated with ACTH and cortisone also is due to the hormonal action on the renal tubules.

Inadequate venous return of blood causes fluid with its sodium chloride to be pushed out into dependent tissues because of the increased blood volume (hydrostatic pressure) in these areas. The kidney then retains fluid to bring the total blood volume back to normal. Promotion of venous return by such means as elevating dependent parts and applying supportive stockings not only is preventive of discomfort and of venous disease, but also helps to prevent fluid and electrolyte imbalance.

Some diuretic drugs act by temporarily blocking the reabsorption power of the renal tubules so that large amounts of fluid are lost from the vascular system, increasing its oncotic pressure and causing it to pull fluid back into the blood stream from the tissues. Other diuretic drugs mobilize sodium so that it returns to the blood stream, and fluid, therefore, is no longer held in the tissues. (See discussion of diuretic drugs in Chapter 18, page 234.) Since many electrolytes also are lost when the diuretic blocks tubule reabsorption, the nurse should observe carefully for signs of electrolyte imbalance. Preventive measures such as giving food and fluids high in potassium (orange juice, tea, and pears) may be necessary.

Fluid retention may be caused by overloading the vascular system with fluid. This overloading may be due to increasing the oncotic (pull) pressure of the intravascular system by giving proteins so rapidly that the body cannot eliminate those in excess of its need. This causes fluids to be pulled into the blood stream from other body fluid compartments; the blood volume increases rapidly, neutralizing the oncotic pressure, but increasing the hydrostatic (push) pressure of the vascular system and the (pull) pressure of the interstitial fluid compartments. This may lead to general tissue edema, but, more important, it rapidly leads to death from drowning in one's own fluids as large amounts of fluid are pushed out into the lungs (pulmonary edema). This is a danger in giving fluids such as plasma, plasma expanders, albumin, and blood. Even though only 250 to 500 ml. are given, these fluids must be given slowly unless the patient has lost a large amount of blood. If these intravenous fluids are being given rapidly, the patient should be watched closely for signs of bounding pulse, engorged peripheral veins, hoarseness, dyspnea, cough, or pulmonary râles, and at the first signs of any of these indications of increased blood volume and increased interstitial fluid the rate of flow of the infusion should be greatly reduced and the doctor notified.

Giving large amounts of fluid either by mouth or parenterally to a person with poor kidney function or allowing intravenous fluids to run faster than normal kidneys can filter them (120 ml. per minute) is equally dangerous and can produce pulmonary edema. The nurse should consider this in giving fluids to the elderly patient with circulatory impairment, the patient whose heart is decompensated, the patient with kidney disease, and the severely burned patient. It also should cause her to question the advisability of excessively speeding up the rate of flow when a patient is receiving large amounts of fluid by infusion daily.

The size of the patient is considered in giving fluids. The smaller person normally has less fluid in each of the body compartments, especially in the intravascular system (see Table 4), and therefore may develop pulmonary edema easily. Because he becomes seriously dehydrated more quickly than a larger person, he needs fluid losses replaced promptly. In hemorrhage for example, a person who normally has only 3 liters of blood plasma and has bled extensively needs replacement of blood sooner than one who normally has 5 liters and has lost the same amount. However, age must also be considered since the inelastic vessels of an older person prevent the body from keeping the remaining blood in vital areas.

Since maintenance of normal blood volume is essential to electrolyte balance and the prevention of shock, *blood volume determinations* may be ordered for patients about to undergo surgery. They also may be done to check on the effectiveness of fluid or blood therapy.

One of several substances such as a harmless blue dye, albumin tagged with radioactive iodine, or red blood cells tagged with a radioactive substance such as radioactive phosphorus may be used in making blood volume determinations. A known quantity of one of these substances is injected intravenously, and blood samples are taken from the opposite arm at a specified time and are examined to determine how much the injected substances have been diluted; from this the volume of intravascular fluid is determined. If blue dye is used, the patient should know that his skin may have a slight blue tinge for several days before the dye is completely excreted.

The *hematocrit* is helpful too, since it gives an index of the ratio of plasma to cells and thus indicates need for whole blood or for fluid replacement only.

Sodium deficit. When a patient has lost excessive amounts of both water and sodium chloride, such as may occur with profuse perspiration, drinking too much water may cause *water intoxication*. Also this may occur if excessive amounts of water are drunk when no salt or water has been lost; the blood volume is increased because of inability of the kidneys to excrete the excess fluid as fast as it is taken and the normal salt content of the body becomes diluted. The patient with water intoxication or sodium deficit may have headache, muscle weakness, nausea, vomiting and abdominal cramps, and diarrhea. If salt is not replaced, convulsions may occur, reflexes may disappear, and the patient may go into shock and die since lack of sodium alters conduction of nerve impulses including those to the heart muscle. When fluids are being forced, care should be taken that patients do not drink too much; there is no standard amount since it depends on the size of the patient, the amount of fluid loss, and the circulatory and kidney functions.

A person who is perspiring profusely because of climate, exercise, or fever should take extra salt as well as extra fluids. A person on a restricted-salt diet is especially likely to have difficulty. Under these circumstances most doctors feel that salt intake should be increased slightly. Patients who are having intensive hot-pack treatment may lose too much sodium; if they are able to take fluids by mouth, consommé and hot salty broths should replace some of the fruit juices so often served.

Sodium depletion occurs most often from loss of lower intestinal fluids such as with severe diarrhea. Losing large amounts of bile also depletes sodium stores; symptoms of sodium depletion may appear rapidly in patients with profuse ileostomy drainage. When sodium in the extracellular fluid becomes depleted, potassium moves out of the intracellular fluid to replace it. Therefore, the patient with sodium imbalance is likely also to have potassium imbalance.

Sodium excess. If fluids are markedly limited or if extra salt is retained due to

Table 4 Approximate division of total body fluid into compartments

Body fluid compartments	*Liters of fluid*	
	Lean adult weighing 100 pounds	*Lean adult weighing 150 pounds*
Intravascular (plasma)	2.8	4.2
Interstitial	8.4	12.5
Intracellular	22.3	33.3
Total	33.5	50.0

Note that the smaller the individual, the less fluid he has in each compartment and that plasma is reduced most markedly with decrease in size. The *normal* size and body type of the individual is considered when fluid replacement is ordered.

poor kidney function or hormonal influences, sodium may become concentrated in the body fluids. Excess intravascular sodium causes fluid to be withdrawn from the tissues resulting in dehydration; if fluids are not given to dilute the sodium and if excretion of sodium is not enhanced, manic excitement, tachycardia, and eventual death follow. Pituitary antidiuretic hormones may be used to encourage tubular excretion of sodium. Urine output which greatly exceeds the fluid intake should be reported to the doctor since this may be an early symptom of hormonal imbalance which will lead to sodium excess. Oliguria and minimal fluid intake also should be reported.

Potassium depletion. When cell metabolism is upset or when cells are damaged, potassium tends to move from the intracellular fluid to the intravascular fluid. If the kidneys are functioning normally it is excreted, depleting the body potassium. Withholding a balanced diet for several days, dehydrating a patient or diluting extracellular tissues with potassium-free fluid causes potassium depletion. This accounts for many problems of electrolyte imbalance in the postoperative patient. Patients undergoing elective surgery should be urged to eat well-balanced meals preoperatively. Patients who must remain on nutritionally inadequate diets or nothing by mouth for extended periods of time usually are given intravenous fluids containing proteins and electrolytes as well as glucose; intravenous fat (Lipomul) also may be given.

The nurse should encourage the patient who is taking diuretics to eat foods that are high in potassium. The patient is usually on limited fluids so that he should take his fluid as tea, coffee, orange juice or pear juice; Coca-Cola is high in potassium and low in sodium whereas Pepsi-Cola is low in potassium and high in sodium. Bananas, most fresh fruits, and meats are high in potassium. Since the patient who is being given diuretics is usually on a low sodium diet, foods high in both potassium and sodium cannot be used.

The practice of giving multiple enemas is becoming less common because it is now known that some of the enema fluid is absorbed and dilutes the potassium in the interstitial fluid compartment upsetting the balance between compartments. Solutions for hypertonic enemas may damage cells and cause potassium loss. Potassium also may be lost from the gastrointestinal tract when there is excessive loss of gastrointestinal fluids. Large quantities of potassium-free fluid given intravenously dilutes the intravascular potassium thus changing its concentration and upsetting electrolyte balance.

Since the adrenal cortical hormones favor potassium excretion, prolonged or repeated use of ACTH or cortisone may cause potassium depletion. Extra potassium in tablet form is often given to patients receiving these drugs.

The patient with potassium deficit usually has generalized weakness and apprehension. Since there is a reduction in nerve impulses to the muscles, paralytic ileus may develop; the circulation may slow down and finally, without treatment, shock and death will ensue.

Potassium excess. Whenever there is severe tissue damage, potassium is released from the cells into the extracellular fluids. Since shock usually accompanies this damage, kidney function is reduced and a high plasma potassium level results. This clearly indicates the need to treat shock promptly. The patient with potassium intoxication complains of nausea, colic, diarrhea, and muscular weakness. If the condition is not controlled, the heartbeat eventually becomes irregular and stops. (See Chapter 21 for a complete discussion of the treatment of potassium intoxication.)

There is great danger in giving extra potassium to any patient with poor kidney function. If the patient is dehydrated or has lost vascular fluid, glucose and water or plasma expanders usually are given until kidney function returns. When potassium therapy is contemplated, the nurse should observe the urinary output carefully and report any reduction in it to the doctor. If she is planning the se-

NORMALS:

	AMALYASE	40-120 u
	BUN	9-20 mg %
	CALCIUM	9-11 mg %
	CHOLESTEROL	150-250 mg %
	CO_2	24-32 mcg/L
	CHLORIDE	99-108 mcg/L
	SODIUM	137-147 mcg/L
	POTASSIUM	4-5.6 mcg/L
FASTING	– FBS	70-110 mg %
	LDH	150-450 u
FASTING	– PHOSPHORUS	3-4 mg
	SGOT	8-40 u
	SGPT	5-35 u
	TOTAL PROTEIN	6-8 Gm
	ALBUMIN	3.5-5.6
	GLOBULIN	1.3-3.2
		M! 2.5-7 mg %

quence of intravenous fluids, she should be careful to give hydrating fluids such as physiologic solution of sodium chloride and glucose solution first. Untreated adrenal insufficiency also is a contraindication for giving potassium.

Intravenous fluids containing potassium should be run at a moderate rate to allow the kidneys time to excrete that in excess of body needs. If they are run too fast, pain tends to occur at the site of injection.

Care must be taken in giving whole blood transfusions to a patient with potassium intoxication since the cells in blood which has been kept for several days tend to release potassium and the plasma potassium level will be further increased. The cells in fresh whole blood do not do this, and it should be used. Leaving blood improperly refrigerated speeds the release of potassium from the cells, and the nurse should follow carefully the instructions supplied by the blood bank as to storing blood. The practice of keeping it in refrigerators on the nursing units should be discouraged since the temperature usually is not low enough.

Calcium deficit. Patients who have abnormal openings into the intestines or pancreas lose large amounts of calcium. When renal tubule absorption is impaired, calcium may be lost and the body is unable to utilize calcium when the parathyroid glands are removed. A deficiency of vitamin D in the diet also leads to calcium deficiency.

Early signs of calcium deficiency are numbness and tingling of the nose, ears, finger tips, or toes. Muscular twitching, irritability, tetany, and convulsions may follow (see Chapter 21, page 328, for Trousseau's and Chvostek's signs). The nurse's observations may help the doctor determine the appropriate treatment for convulsions and, if she recognizes early signs, treatment often may be given before severe symptoms develop. Calcium gluconate or calcium chloride is given intravenously or by mouth. Patients who have draining intestinal fistulas with subsequent calcium loss should be encouraged to eat foods that are high in calcium such as milk and foods high in vitamin D such as butter.

Calcium excess. Calcium excess causes few clinical problems related to electrolyte balance.

Bicarbonate deficit. In some conditions, such as uncontrolled diabetes mellitus and starvation, glucose either cannot be utilized or is not available for oxidation. The body compensates for this by using body fat for energy, producing excessive amounts of ketone bodies. In an effort to neutralize the ketones (fatty acids) and maintain the acid-base balance of the body, plasma bicarbonate is exhausted. The resultant acid-base imbalance is known as *metabolic acidosis.* The patient becomes dyspneic and has deep periodic breathing as the lungs fail in their efforts to blow off carbon dioxide, and a *secondary respiratory acidosis* develops with an increasing level of plasma carbonic acid. If the condition is untreated, disorientation, stupor, coma, and death will occur. This type of acidosis is controlled by giving intravenous solutions of sodium bicarbonate or sodium or molar lactate. Soda bicarbonate sometimes is given by mouth if it can be retained. Treatment of the condition precipitating the acidosis is then instituted.

Bicarbonate excess. When excessive amounts of hydrochloric acid and sodium chloride are lost through vomiting or drainage of the stomach or when fluids high in potassium chloride are lost abnormally through biliary drainage, intestinal fistulas or diarrhea, electrolyte imbalance results with an excess of base elements.[1] Rapid ingestion of large amounts of sodium bicarbonate or carbonated drinks or the ingestion of these substances when there is impaired kidney or lung function also causes this acid-base imbalance. This condition is known as *metabolic alkalosis.* Breathing becomes depressed in an effort to conserve carbon dioxide for combination with hydrogen ions in the blood to raise the blood level of carbonic acid. Chloride ions combine with the base ions leaving inadequate chloride to neutralize calcium and it is excreted, reducing the calcium level of the blood and causing tetany and convulsions. Sodium chloride or ammonium chloride intravenously or by mouth helps to relieve metabolic alkalosis. Potassium losses must also be restored. The treatment of this very important condition is discussed more fully in medical textbooks.[1]

Carbonic acid deficit. When for any reason there is inadequate oxygenation of the blood although the gas exchange in the lungs is normal, the lungs blow off excessive amounts of carbon dioxide and thus lower the blood carbonic acid level. This is known as *respiratory alkalosis.* Breathing is deep and rapid and calcium, lacking anions for chemical combination, is excreted. This may cause tetany and convulsions. The treatment is oxygen administration. However, if the oxygen deficiency is caused by anemia, whole blood is given; when extra plasma is undesirable, packed cells are used.

Carbonic acid excess. Primary carbonic acid excess may occur in any medical condition which interferes with gas exchange in the lungs. This is known as *respiratory acidosis* or *carbon dioxide narcosis.* The symptoms are the same as those of respiratory acidosis secondary to metabolic acidosis, but the treatment is to increase respiratory excursion (see Chapter 23).

GENERAL NURSING CARE RELATED TO FLUID AND ELECTROLYTE BALANCE

Determination of loss. An important nursing function is careful observation and recording of fluid and electrolyte losses. Every acutely ill medical patient and every patient undergoing major surgery should have a fluid chart that is thoroughly understood by nurses and all others who may give care to the patient. Space should be provided on this chart for recording urine output and identifying fluid losses from the less common routes such as through wound drainage. Often a daily weight record is requested since it is a good indication of the onset of dehydration or of the accumulation of fluid either as generalized edema or as "hidden" fluid in body cavities. Each day weight must be taken carefully on the same scales, at the same hour, and with the same amount of clothing. Sometimes all clothing and even wound dressings are removed from the patient for this procedure.

Urine output should be carefully recorded as to time and amount. This helps to evaluate the kidney function more accurately. If kidney function is of major concern, for instance if the patient is severely burned, an indwelling catheter is used so that the amount of urinary drainage can be recorded every hour and fluid intake regulated accordingly.

It has been said that nothing is more difficult to obtain in the modern hospital than an accurate record of urine output, and unfortunately this is often true. Conspicuous signs posted on the patient's chart and in the utility room will help to prevent the discarding of urine before it has been measured.

Vomitus should be measured. It is surprising how inaccurate guessing can be in estimating the amount of such fluids. Electrolytes are lost in large amounts with excessive vomiting or when the stomach is aspirated, a procedure which removes gastric secretions that contain electrolytes normally reabsorbed through the intestinal wall. The patient with an indwelling tube in the stomach often complains of thirst, and it might appear a harmless practice to give fluids by mouth since they will immediately be removed through the aspiration equipment. However, this must never be done because it will wash out electrolytes, thus leading to greater electrolyte deprivation. Physiologic solution of sodium chloride is usually used instead of plain water when repeated lavages are necessary. An ileostomy presents a serious problem in loss of fluid and electrolytes because, if the opening is high in the ileum, fluid is lost before complete reabsorption through the wall of the small intestine can occur. Stools should be described as to consistency, and, if diarrhea is present, it is important that the number of stools and the approximate amount be recorded.

Fluid aspirated from any body cavity such as the abdomen or pleural spaces must be measured. This fluid contains protein as well as electrolytes and water. Blood loss should be carefully estimated and measured if possible. Wound drainage such as that from the common bile duct following gallbladder surgery must be measured. If there are draining wounds which require frequent change of dressings, it may be necessary to weigh the dressings and any wet linen at each change. This may be done accurately by weighing the linen and dressing on a small dram scale prior to use. This is recorded as dry weight. Upon the removal of dressings, they are again weighed and the dry weight is subtracted to give an accurate record of the fluid lost. If the drainage is from a fistula, catheters or collection bags may be used so that more accurate recording of fluid loss is possible (see Chapter 8).

Diaphoresis is difficult to measure accurately, but it should be recorded when careful check of fluid intake and output is considered necessary by the doctor. Since elevation of temperature speeds up metabolism and increases loss of fluid through the lungs and the skin, careful checking and recording of temperature help the doctor determine how much fluid the patient needs.

Provision for replacement. The best way to restore water, electrolytes, and food nutrients to the body is by mouth. The nurse needs to know foods which contain large and small amounts of various essential substances. A useful reference book is *Bridge's Food and Beverage Analysis*.[12] The dietitian and nutritionist should be consulted as necessary. When fluids can be tolerated by the stomach but cannot be swallowed, a tube may be passed through the nose into the stomach and fluids containing all the essentials of a balanced diet may be given through the tube.

Normal saline solution or plain water may be given by slow drip into the stomach or in small amounts by rectum and will be absorbed quickly in most instances. Occasionally, fluid is given intraperitoneally; this method is usually reserved for infants and small children. Physiologic solution of sodium chloride or solutions containing other electrolytes may be given into subcutaneous tissues (hypodermoclysis); this method is used most often for those patients who are so restless that keeping a needle in the vein is difficult.

By far the most common method of giving fluids when it is not possible for the patient to take them orally is by intravenous infusion (venoclysis). Occasionally an incision is made and a polyethylene catheter is threaded into the vein, where it remains for several days. This is often called a "cut-down"; it may result in thrombosis of the vein.

The nurse needs to know the common solutions used for infusions. Glucose, 5 per cent, in distilled water is often used to maintain fluid intake. Ascorbic acid and vitamin B (Solu-B) are frequently added. Small quantities (1,000 ml. or less a day) of 5 per cent glucose in saline may be used to maintain the sodium chloride level in the body and potassium chloride may be added to maintain normal intake needs of potassium and to replace losses. A physiologic solution of sodium chloride usually is given only when sodium chloride has been lost in large amounts. One-sixth molar lactate solution may be ordered when sodium but not chloride needs replacement, and ammonium chloride solution may be used to replace chlorides without adding sodium. Balanced solutions containing several electrolytes may be used. Ringer's solution, Hartmann's solution (lactated Ringer's solution), Darrow's solution, and Tyrode's solution are examples.

Body needs for carbohydrates may be partially met by giving fructose or 10 or 20 per cent glucose in distilled water. Since these are slightly hypertonic solutions, there is some danger of their causing blood cell destruction.

Efforts are being made to find a really

satisfactory substitute for protein taken by mouth. The serious problem of transmission of infectious hepatitis in blood and blood plasma, as well as the cost of these fluids, limits their usefulness. Amino acid preparations (Aminosol) are available and are being used rather widely. They have to be given slowly to prevent nausea, and in many patients they cause unpleasant side effects such as peculiar sensations of taste and smell. Plasma volume expanders can be given to substitute for blood protein loss and thereby help to maintain normal blood volume and prevent shock. Dextran, a polysaccharide derived from cane sugar by bacterial fermentation, is the most generally accepted of these substances and has been stock-piled for emergency use in the event of major disaster such as an atomic attack.

There is no satisfactory way of supplying fat when it cannot be taken by mouth. Some intravenous fat substances such as Lipomul are being tried, but side effects are still rather severe. The patient may complain of dyspnea, chest pain, urticaria, chills, fever, nausea, vomiting and abdominal discomfort, dizziness, flushing, or headache. Overloading the blood stream with fat given intravenously may cause clotting defects with resultant bleeding and enlargement of the liver and spleen. If such an infusion is given it should be started very slowly (10 drops per minute) and gradually increased over a period of an hour to 100 drops per minute. No more than two units of 500 ml. are ever given in a day. If any untoward symptoms develop, the infusion should be stopped and the doctor notified.

Whole blood and packed red cells are given to replace erythrocytes and to raise the hemoglobin. Whole blood, plasma, plasma expanders, 5 per cent glucose in distilled water or in saline or a physiologic solution of sodium chloride may be given to re-establish blood volume.

For details of equipment and nursing techniques needed in fluid administration, the student is referred to basic textbooks on fundamentals of nursing. It is imperative that the nurse check fluid bottles carefully for correctness of contents and that she record accurately the fluids given. Too much fluid and too much of any one of the electrolyte substances can be disastrous for the patient. The rate of administration of fluids is usually ordered by the doctor and will depend upon the patient's illness, the kind of fluid given, and the patient's age. Specific principles to follow have already been discussed. The nurse should realize that the various equipment for fluid administration may have varying numbers of milliliters per drop. This is important to know since it is not the drops per minute but the milliliters per minute that are important.

Patients who are receiving fluids intravenously should be observed frequently to check the rate of flow, to note symptoms indicating the need to slow down, speed up, or stop the infusion, and to watch the site of the insertion of the needle for infiltration. Some solutions such as those containing potassium are very irritating to the tissues. Tampering with infusions that are not running properly is an unsafe practice for nurses; fatal emboli have resulted from accidental entrance of air through intravenous tubing.

The greatest care should be taken to see that any needle that enters a vein has been sterilized by autoclaving. Care must also be taken to see that needles which have been removed are cared for so that staff members are not accidentally exposed to infectious hepatitis. (See Chapter 27.)

RELIEF OF THIRST

Thirst is the first and most insistent sign of dehydration, sometimes causing the patient more misery than an operation or the symptoms of a disease. Excessive thirst should be reported to the doctor. If fluids cannot be taken by mouth, thirst can usually be alleviated by increasing the fluid intake by other routes such as intravenous infusion. If the patient is receiving an infusion, it is often helpful to explain to him that he will soon have some relief from his thirst.

Mouth care allays some of the discomfort of thirst. This should include cleansing the tongue and the use of cold mouthwashes; it may be necessary to repeat these procedures every hour. If the patient can be trusted not to swallow, he may be given water or ice chips to be held in the mouth and then expelled. Hard lemon candies (sour balls) are often comforting even though they must be expelled. Chewing gum may be helpful. It is essential that the temptation of a water pitcher at the bedside be removed when fluids by mouth are not permitted.

Discomfort of thirst can be made more bearable by explaining to the patient why fluids are withheld, as, for example, when tests are to be done. Thirst can be such a compelling and disturbing sensation that patients who have had extensive operations may get out of bed and go to the bathroom for water even when their condition may be most adversely affected by so doing. If the patient cannot be relied upon, special precautions are sometimes necessary.

Excessive or prolonged thirst is not normal. In the patient recently returned from surgery, this kind of thirst should make the nurse suspect internal hemorrhage, elevation of temperature, or some other untoward development. In the chronic medical patient it may indicate the onset of disease such as diabetes mellitus in which extra water is used by the kidneys to eliminate glucose in the urine.

NAUSEA AND VOMITING

Nausea and vomiting are often part of the body's response to a large variety of insults to its integrity. Their precise cause is unknown, but there are many secondary causes. Nausea and vomiting usually occur together, but occasionally, as in the case of patients with increased intracranial pressure, vomiting may be sudden and not preceded by nausea or any other warning sensation. Infection, incipient uremia, toxicity from almost any disease, inhalation of foreign gases, systemic absorption of drugs, and irritation from poisons can cause nausea and vomiting. Vomiting during pregnancy may be caused by a toxic factor. Mechanical obstruction anywhere in the gastrointestinal tract, irritation of the posterior pharynx such as occurs in severe coughing, and presence of air in the stomach may lead to nausea and vomiting. Increased intracranial pressure can touch off the mechanism in the medulla which initiates vomiting, and it is well known that emotional states and psychic trauma can often do the same. Vomiting can follow severe pain as a sympathetic reaction. Nausea and vomiting can also occur in well persons under unusual circumstances involving motion (for example, seasickness).

The mechanism of vomiting is not too well understood. It is known that there is reversal of peristalsis in the upper part of the small intestine, although this probably has little to do with the actual act of vomiting. There is relaxation of the gastric cardia and spasmodic contraction of abdominal muscles and of the diaphragm which cause increased intra-abdominal pressure. The breath is held, the glottis is closed, and expulsion of stomach contents takes place.

Treatment of nausea and vomiting depends upon their cause. Drugs or toxic substances known to cause the trouble are usually stopped or eliminated. Most patients will have less vomiting if the emotional components of its cause are removed. For instance, the nausea immediately following an injection of morphine in some patients may sometimes be controlled by deliberately talking with the patient for several minutes. This takes his mind off the injection. Nausea is sometimes relieved if the patient takes deep breaths through the mouth.

Nausea and vomiting are profoundly affected by sights, sounds, and smells. Emesis basins must be removed immediately after use. Empty emesis basins are themselves suggestive of vomiting and should usually be kept out of the patient's sight. At other times, such as postoperatively, it may be a comfort to the patient to have an emesis basin conveniently placed. The patient may become nauseated from seeing equipment being used for another patient or from seeing dressings being changed on himself or on someone else. Food odors, drug odors, and other odors which are part of a hospital setting may contribute to nausea in the person who is ill. Even perfumes and strongly scented soaps may cause nausea. Rooms should be carefully ventilated during both the day and night. Relatives learning to care for a patient at home need help in improvising equipment that will be psychologically acceptable to the patient. For example, an empty coffee can lined with paper may be used instead of a baby's "potty" as a mouthwash basin.

Postoperative nausea and vomiting may be caused by toxic reaction to general inhalation anesthesia, irritation to the stomach from gases swallowed, and psychologic factors, including the smell of the anesthetic. Letting the patient take water and then vomit, thus washing out the stomach, sometimes helps to stop the vomiting. Ginger ale and other effervescent drinks seem to have a remarkable effect in controlling postoperative vomiting and can often be taken and retained long before other fluids are tolerated. Effervescent fluids have been found effective in controlling the nausea and vomiting of motion sickness in some people.

Dimenhydrinate (Dramamine) is the drug widely used in the control of motion sickness. It is also ordered with varying success in the nausea and vomiting associated with illness. The dosage is usually 50 mg. (¾ grain) every four hours orally when it can be tolerated by mouth, or the same amount in a small amount of normal saline (25 ml.) rectally if it cannot be retained in the stomach. Dramamine may cause drowsiness and dizziness, and these reactions must be pointed out to those who are taking it when traveling. Accidents have been known to happen to those who drive cars after taking Dramamine and other antihistaminic drugs. When the drug is being used in the hospital, the patient must be watched carefully to prevent such accidents as falling out of bed.

REFERENCES AND SELECTED READINGS*

1 Cecil, Russell H., and Loeb, Robert F. (editors): A Textbook of Medicine, ed. 10, Philadelphia, 1959, W. B. Saunders Co.

2 *Dunning, Marcelle F., and Plum, Fred: Potassium Depletion by Enemas, Am. J. Med. **20**:789-792, May 1956.

3 *Farr, Hollon W.: Fluid and Electrolyte Balance—With Special Reference to the Gastrointestinal Tract, Am. J. Nursing **54**:826-831, July 1954.

4 Fluid and Electrolytes, North Chicago, Ill., 1957, Abbott Laboratories.

5 Fox, Charles L., Jr., and others: Electrolyte Solution Approximating Plasma Concentrations, J.A.M.A. **148**:827-833, March 1952.

6 Gamble, J. L.: Extra Cellular Fluids, Cambridge, Mass., 1954, Harvard University Press.

7 Gold, Harry (editor): Cornell Conferences on Therapy, vol. VI, New York, 1953, The Macmillan Co.

8 Gropper, Arthur L., and others: Plasma Expanders, Surg. Gynec. & Obst. **95**:521-542, Dec. 1952.

9 Jorgensen, H. E.: Studies in Metabolism of Trauma—Postoperative Sodium Retention, Surg. Gynec. & Obst. **108**:339-342, March 1959.

10 *Lowe, Charles U.: Principles of Parenteral Fluid Therapy, Am. J. Nursing **53**:963-965, Aug. 1953.

11 MacBryde, Cyril Mitchell (editor): Signs and Symptoms, ed. 3, Philadelphia, 1955, J. B. Lippincott Co.

12 Mattice, Marjorie R.: Bridge's Food and Beverage Analysis, ed 3, Philadephia, 1950, Lea & Febiger.

13 Mayer, Carl A.: Fluid Balance, A Clinical Manual, Chicago, 1952, Year Book Publishers, Inc.

14 Preston, F. W., and Henegar, G. C.: Use of Intravenous Fat Emulsions in Surgical Patients, Surg. Clin. North America **39**:145-155, Feb. 1959.

15 *Snively, William D., and Brown, Barbara J.: In the Balance, Am. J. Nursing **58**:55-57, Jan. 1958.

16 Statland, Harry: Fluid and Electrolytes in Practice, Philadelphia, 1954, J. B. Lippincott Co.

17 *Wolf, Edith S.: The Nurse and Fluid Therapy, Am. J. Nursing **54**:831-833, July 1954.

*References preceded by an asterisk indicate material particularly well suited for student reading.

Study questions for review

1 Consult your notes on fundamentals of nursing, and review the descriptive terms commonly used to describe various kinds of pain.
2 Review the analgesic drugs. What are the main classifications? Review the therapeutic benefit and potential hazard of each.
3 Study a patient in pain on your ward. Describe in detail all the physical and emotional manifestations of pain. What are the physical causes of the patient's pain? Do any other factors seem to be involved?

The patient with pain

Chapter 7

Pain accompanies almost all illnesses, and perhaps no sensation is more dreaded by patients undergoing medical treatment or surgery. Pain is a two-edged sword. It warns us to move away from heat, cold, and sharp objects before injury occurs, and sometimes it warns us to seek medical attention. On the other hand, the fear of pain may cause us to delay medical treatment that is really needed.

Care of patients suffering pain demands skill in both the science and the art of nursing. The nurse's responsibility is to make the patient as comfortable as possible physically and emotionally and to observe and report her findings so that they may help the doctor to make a correct diagnosis and to prescribe appropriate treatment. Two important elements must be considered in caring for the patient in pain. The pain perception, or actual feeling of pain, must be recognized and evaluated, and the reaction of the individual patient to pain must be carefully considered and appraised.

Pain has never been satisfactorily defined nor clearly understood. It is known that the sensation of pain often appears only a short time before actual tissue damage occurs. In fact, extensive tissue damage may occur without any pain being experienced. Studies have shown that perception, or feeling of pain, is quite uniform. In other words, the same amount of pain stimulus (heat, for example) will cause the sensation of pain at the same time in the majority of normal persons regardless of age or emotional make-up. Tolerance for pain, however, varies a great deal and is based largely upon subjective reaction to pain. It is this aspect of pain that is usually referred to when the term "pain threshold" is used.

PHYSICAL ASPECTS OF PAIN

When pain fibers are stimulated certain physiologic responses occur. The simplest of these is the *withdrawal reflex* in which impulses are conducted over the shortest nerve pathways from the place of injury to the spinal cord and back to local muscles. This reflex occurs when one accidentally touches a finger to a hot object and immediately withdraws the hand. At the same time, *visceral responses,* involving the vital organs and the glands of internal secretion, prepare one for "fight or flight." These responses account for the increased pulse and respiratory rate, dilated pupils, and muscle tension that often occur in sudden severe pain. The body is prepared for the possible need to flee from the cause of pain. Because blood supply is suddenly withdrawn from the viscera, nausea may also occur.

When pain fibers are stimulated, some of the impulses pass to the thalamus, which in turn conducts them to the cerebral cortex, where the perception of pain takes place. The pain is felt, and, based upon reason, knowledge, and previous experience, the source can be located and action taken. This is known as *voluntary response* because the person experiencing the pain decides what action to take.

There are two types of pain fibers: large myelinated fibers, which carry "fast pain" described as sharp or pricking, and much smaller nonmyelinated fibers, which carry "slow pain" described as lingering or burning pain. This accounts for the sudden sharp or localized pain experienced at once when one hits his thumb with a hammer and the somewhat slower throbbing pain in the entire extremity.

The perception of a pain stimulus may be altered at many points by both normal and abnormal conditions. At the original site it may be altered by such things as tissue damage or inflammatory conditions which increase or decrease the original impulse. For example, slapping a person who has a sunburn may set off a far greater impulse than if the person were not sunburned. On the other hand, if the local nerve endings have been damaged by a severe burn, the patient may not respond at all to what would ordinarily be painful stimuli.

Abnormal conditions within the spinal cord, such as inflammatory diseases, tumors, or injuries, may prevent transmission of nerve impulses. This may occur at either the spinal or the thalamic relay stations. The impulse may also be altered at either of these two relay stations by other activity going on simultaneously within the spinal cord. This probably accounts for the fact that sometimes bruises and cuts sustained during absorbing activity go unnoticed until the activity is over.

Perception, which takes place in the cortex, is also influenced by circumstances. Here, too, abnormal conditions such as inflammatory processes, degenerative changes, and depression of brain function may alter the original signal pattern. An elderly person may have less pain than a younger one because his sense organs have become less acute. Anesthesia and analgesia also cause depression of sensory perceptions.

REACTION TO PAIN

What is perceived as pain will be influenced by the entire life situation of the patient. Previous experiences, childhood training, cultural values, and physical and mental health all act as conditioning influences in the total concept of the pain a person will feel. A pleasant environment, an enjoyable book, stimulating conversation, or other distracting activity of a pleasing nature may serve to lessen the sensation of pain.

People may learn by experience to avoid and, perhaps, to fear pain. This may alter their reaction to it. Persons from cultures in which health teaching and disease prevention are emphasized tend to accept pain as a warning to seek help and expect the cause of pain will be found and cured. They believe that the cause of pain can be found and corrected. Morbid fear of a disease may intensify pain caused by it, or it may lead the individual to deny pain in his eagerness to believe that nothing is wrong. Anticipation of pain based on past experience may intensify pain. For example, the child who enters the hospital for the last of several operations may react more vigorously to postoperative pain than he did on his first encounter with the sensation.

Parents' attitudes toward pain may determine their children's lifelong reaction to pain. Some people, by training and example, are taught to endure severe pain without reacting outwardly. American Indian men have rites in which they show their strength by the amount of pain they can endure. Such individuals would probably tolerate pain from disease or injury better than those from a culture in which free expression of feelings is encouraged. Tolerance for pain seems to be increased by faith, and it is sometimes difficult to judge how much pain persons with deep faith are experiencing. The social setting in which injury occurs may influence the external response to pain. Boys may feel that pain suffered from injury during a football game should be borne quietly, while pain resulting from an automobile accident may be expressed freely.

The personality make-up of a person also influences reaction to pain. An unstable person who reacts hysterically to trying situations may find even a small amount of pain intolerable. People may sometimes use moderate pain as an escape from unacceptable life situations, or they may try to use it to control situations around them. This latter reaction is often demonstrated both in the hospital and in the home.

The pain threshold is lowered by persistent pain such as that sometimes experienced by patients with far-advanced carcinoma. A weak, debilitated patient usually tolerates less pain than a stronger one, although increasing debility will eventually cause mental dulling with a resultant decrease in pain perception. Fatigue, anger, boredom, and apprehension decrease one's ability to tolerate pain.

Pain is less tolerable in the night and early morning hours when there is little distracting activity and the patient's thoughts may easily turn to concern for himself and his loved ones. Persons with strong drives and definite goals tend to tolerate pain well and do not let moderate pain distract them too much.

Age affects tolerance for pain. The young fear it because it may represent an unfamiliar experience and frequently respond to it by crying. The older person may know what to expect and may be withdrawn and quiet while experiencing pain.

TYPES OF PAIN

Cutaneous or surface injuries are usually more painful than injuries of deeper tissues, since the skin is richly supplied with sensory nerve endings. In surface injuries the intensity of the pain is usually proportional to the extent of injured tissue, but this is not always so, as is exemplified by the severe pain caused by neuralgia (herpes zoster).

The visceral organs have no sensory nerve endings, and therefore pain does not exist in normal viscera. It is believed that in diseased visceral organs pain results from traction, pressure, and tension on parietal peritoneum or on mesenteric attachments. These structures refer the visceral pain sensations to the spinal cord through various routes. Visceral pain may be referred to surface areas which have pain fibers or to spinal nerves supplying whole areas; pain thus transmitted is usually not well localized because sensations originate from a wide area. Because of this, extensive tissue damage may occur before pain is felt from visceral disease. Other symptoms often precede pain and the appearance of pain may indicate far-advanced disease.

Visceral pain produces no body defense reaction (visceral response). Severe visceral pain, therefore, can cause shock. The patient becomes weak and prostrate; blood pressure may drop, the skin may become cold and clammy, and nausea and vomiting may occur. Cardiac and kidney damage can follow, and, if the vital organs are already impaired by disease, even death may result.

Pain has already been described as sharp or pricking and lingering or burning. The pain caused by a tension or pressure on the viscera may be described as aching, dragging, or boring. Muscle contractions may cause sensations described as cramping or spasm. Muscles which have peristaltic action frequently cause the pain to be stabbing. A sudden sharp, popping sensation is characteristic of rupture of a visceral organ.

NURSING CARE OF THE PATIENT IN PAIN

Evaluation of pain. In observing a patient in pain the nurse should avoid generalizations and should evaluate the pain and the patient suffering from pain carefully. A specific description of the pain will be most helpful to the doctor in determining the probable cause. The nurse should note its exact location, its type, when it began, how long it has lasted, whether this is its first occurrence, and what activity immediately preceded it. She must determine whether it is constant or intermittent and whether it is relieved or made worse by medication, food, or rest. She must know whether it is affected by change of position or any other activity known to the patient. As the nurse gathers this information, she may make observations on the patient's emotional response to pain. She must not minimize the pain of those who report it with much vehemence, and even noise, or the pain of those who do not reveal it readily. Either reaction may be acceptable in the patient's social and cultural setting. Knowing how the patient feels about pain helps the nurse plan measures to make him more comfortable.

Close observation of the patient often gives clues to his pain. Facial expression is often revealing. Pinched facies, drawn and wrinkled brows, clenched teeth, and tightened fists may indicate severe pain. Profuse diaphoresis and a rapid pulse also are valuable clues. The patient who is curled up in bed or who tosses about frequently is often in pain or at least is uncomfortable.

General care. Patience, tolerance, gentleness, technical skill, and keen powers of observation are needed in giving care to the patient in pain. The nurse and the doctor are the two professional team members to whom the patient turns when pain is one of his major problems. Pain is affected by physical, emotional, and social factors, and in turn its presence disrupts the patient's entire life. The person in pain does not respond in the usual manner to those about him nor relate appropriately emotionally and socially with people; he is not able to because his psychic energy is absorbed by the pain. The nurse must often interpret his reactions and conduct to his family and others. At no time can she let the patient feel that she is lacking in sympathy and understanding of his problem, or that the time and effort spent in attempting to alleviate his pain are not worth while. Although she makes objective observations of the patient's physical and mental reactions and reports these observations, the nurse should not decide that the pain of which the patient complains is not real. The objective observation is, of course, of great importance in the diagnosis and treatment of the patient. There may even be situations in which the patient whose pain is largely based on emotional reactions is more in need of her interest and support than the one whose pain is largely caused by a physical ailment. It is important for the nurse to remember that the patient *feels* the pain regardless of its cause. This recognized fact should guide her in care of the patient.

The patient in pain is often afraid. Fear may be allayed in part by the nurse's calm, quiet manner and particularly by her demonstration of competence. Confidence in those who care for him is a tremendous help to the patient. It is a great comfort to the patient to know, for example, that the nurse will not be so careless that she shakes the bed and thus increases his pain when giving care or so hurried that she forgets his medication as prescribed.

Overtalkativeness and overoptimism are often annoying to the patient who has pain. This is particularly true when the patient knows or suspects that his prognosis is poor. Florence Nightingale gave the following advice on this:

But the long chronic case, who knows too well himself, and who has been told by his physician that he will never enter active life again, who feels that every month he has to give up something he could do the month before—oh! spare such sufferers your chattering hopes. You do not know how you worry and weary them. Such real sufferers cannot bear to talk of themselves, still less to hope for what they cannot at all expect.

If no estimate can be made as to the duration of pain, the patient should be given encouragement that the problem will not become too great for him to accept with the assistance that is available.

Most patients who have prolonged pain with no hope of relief can and do derive benefit from faith. This may help them to consider pain in a more positive way and thus make it more endurable for them. The nurse should be alert for signs that the patient feels a need for strengthening his faith and should help to make desired assistance available to him.

Noise is troublesome to the patient in pain, and there is evidence that unpleasant sounds are more upsetting than unpleasant sights and odors. Sudden unexpected sounds are disturbing to the patient who has, after continued effort, been able to fall asleep. The irritation of being awakened and the fact that he has not slept long enough to relax often make it difficult for him to fall asleep again.

Fear and irritability can sometimes be allayed in part by explaining to the patient why he has pain, thus causing him to relax somewhat and thereby lessen his discomfort. If he can be honestly told that the pain is probably of short duration, this should be done. Sometimes preparation for pain helps to increase acceptance and relaxation which will decrease pain. An example of this is the benefit derived from special preparation for childbirth.

Care and treatments should be planned so that the patient in pain is moved about as little as possible and rest periods between necessary activity are not interrupted. With careful planning it is usually possible to give an analgesic medication and allow time for it to take effect before procedures are performed and to have sufficient help available so that such procedures as the removal of wound packing, an enema, a bed bath, and a change of bed linen can be done in definite sequence. It is distressing to the patient in pain to be moved, bathed, and have his bed linen changed only to find that an enema must be given or that he must be moved for a roentgenogram to be taken. The nurse cannot control all activity around her patient, but she can help a great deal by thoughtful planning for him.

Sometimes if the patient helps to make some decisions regarding his care he tolerates pain better. The nurse must use good judgment, however, in deciding when she should encourage the patient to make decisions and when she must make them for him. Such matters as whether the bed should be changed before or after the nap or whether friends should be encouraged to visit are examples. The patient may feel less helpless by making some decisions, or he may be too uncomfortable to want to be bothered. Pain may alter rational judgment so that the patient may not be able to make sensible decisions.

The patient should be given explanations of why things that must be done are necessary, as, for example, moving postoperatively to prevent complications. The assurance that he will be prepared for procedures that are painful helps to keep the patient from being "on edge" and encourages relaxation and rest. Plans should be made for a minimum number of persons to enter the room of the patient in severe pain. The patient cannot possibly learn to know and trust all the individuals who pop in and out of the average hospital room in the average hospital day. Unless some effort is made to control traffic in and out of his room, the patient may be afraid to relax and rest. The same principle applies to care of the patient in his own home where the problem of neighbors is frequently a real one. The nurse, of all members of the health team, is in the best position to give attention to this real need of the patient. Some patients in pain welcome interruptions and distractions, while others prefer privacy and seclusion. The nurse should see that the patient's wishes are respected.

Every member of the nursing team who gives any kind of care to the patient in severe pain should have access to specific guides to his care. She should know why the patient is in pain, if the cause is known, what aggravates it, how he responds to it, and the special nursing techniques and nursing measures that have been found effective in helping him. The Kardex or other forms of written nursing care plans should contain this information and should be kept up to date and available. Such individual and extremely important matters as how the patient responds to certain visitors, to his spiritual adviser, to food, to other patients, and to ways of moving him should be recorded.

Pain is usually aggravated by activity, and the patient may try to delay necessary moving and treatments. The nurse must decide just how long moving should be delayed in the interest of comfort, rest, and benefit to the patient and how much damage will be done to the skin, the circulation, and other vital functions by not moving the patient or not having him move enough. With skill and adequate help, the patient can usually be moved without causing too much pain. Support to painful parts of the body is essential. Binders, surgical belts, and girdles give support to the abdomen. Body casts, corsets, and braces are used to immobilize the vertebral column and thus decrease pain. A firm bed gives support and thereby lessens pain both when at rest and when moving. Traction, splints, casts, and braces are used to immobilize a painful part of the body such as an ankle. Special beds such as the Stryker frame, the Foster bed, and the Bradford frame allow movement with minimal handling of the body and thereby help lessen pain.

Technique of handling the patient with generalized pain or a painful limb or part of the body is important. Supporting the trunk and limbs in good body alignment will prevent increasing pain by unnatural pulling on muscles, joints, and ligaments. A "turning sheet" is often useful in preventing uneven lifting or pull on patients with severe neck, back, or general trunk pain. Painful joints may be moved with less discomfort if they are placed on a pillow, or otherwise supported, when being moved rather than directly lifted. If there is tenderness or pain in the shaft of the bone, in muscles, or in large skin areas, the limb should be supported at the joints to prevent additional pain when the patient moves.

Appetite is affected by pain. Very gratifying improvement in appetite has followed when surgical procedures or other means have been used to control pain in those with fatal illnesses. When one is in continuous pain, nothing seems quite right, and this applies to meals. Care should be taken that foods the patient likes are prepared in a way which he likes. His appetite may be improved by small attractive servings and by a sincere interest in his response to food. Foods that the patient does not like or that he believes disagree with him should not be offered to him.

When caring for the patient who is experiencing severe, continuous, or intractable pain, the nurse must keep in mind the possibility of suicide. Pain is wearing and demoralizing. This is especially true when it is difficult to control with drugs and when the patient knows or suspects that no permament relief is forthcoming. The patient may dread the danger of a growing dependence upon drugs, he may fear that drugs will no longer help, and he may be depressed by thoughts of being a burden and an expense to his family. He may appear to tolerate pain quite well but at the same time may be planning his own destruction. Plans for protection must be individually made for each patient and will depend on such things as whether or not he is confined to bed. For further discussion on patients who may contemplate suicide, see Chapter 10.

Medications and treatment for pain. The nurse needs to know the precise effect on the body of drugs used in the treatment of pain. She must be aware of the time curve of their beginning effect, the height of their effectiveness, and their declining effect.

The opiates are drugs most widely recognized and used for the control of pain; morphine and codeine are usually ordered. Synthetic narcotic drugs such as meperidine hydrochloride (Demerol) and methadone hydrochloride are also widely used. When given in therapeutic doses, narcotics act by depressing brain cells involved in pain perception without seriously impairing other sensory perceptions. They also affect to some extent the patient's feeling about pain and thus affect both physical pain and the reaction to it. In addition, the synthetic narcotic drugs have some antispasmodic action and thereby encourage relaxation.

Narcotics cause lowering of the blood pressure and general depression of vital functions. This can be an advantage in treating a condition such as hemorrhage in which some lowering of blood pressure may be desirable. It may be a disadvantage in the debiliated patient who may go into shock from too much drug. The narcotic drugs are less likely to cause shock if the patient is up and moving about and taking food and fluids since these activites tend to maintain the blood pressure at a safe level.

Ataractic drugs, or so-called tranquilizers, which affect the mood of the patient have been found helpful in the treatment of pain, particularly when given in combination with narcotics. Thorazine is an example. These drugs tend to dull the sensorium and give the patient a sense of well-being. If they cause lethargy and failure of normal response, this should be reported to the doctor at once.

One of the most useful of all analgesic drugs is acetylsalicylic acid (aspirin). This is the safest of the coal-tar products, and its continuous use over long periods of time has not been found injurious in any way unless excessive doses are taken. The specific action of acetylsalicylic acid on pain is not known. It does not cause clouding of the sensorium. Aspirin is often surprisingly effective when given with codeine, the combined effect being much superior to the use of either drug alone. Other coal-tar analgesics such as phenacitin and acetanilid can be harmful, and their use should be under the direction of a physician despite the fact that they can be purchased without medical prescription.

Before giving medication for pain, the nurse must determine whether the patient's pain is the same as that for which an analgesic drug was ordered. If it should be a "new" pain, analgesics may mask symptoms of disease that are undiagnosed. She must find out whether the patient is really in pain and in need of medication, or if he is in need of company, information, counsel, or acceptance. Knowing the patient as an individual, as well as understanding what disease condition he has and what treatment he has received, will help the nurse to give the most appropriate of the prescribed medications or to seek new orders if she feels that they are needed. So much emphasis has been placed upon the danger of drug addiction (and to be sure, the danger is very real) that nurses sometimes withhold narcotic drugs and allow patients to suffer more than is advisable. When prescribed by the doctor, narcotics should usually be given for pain as often as every four hours for forty-eight hours after the patient has had an operation, provided that his blood pressure, pulse, respiration, and other vital signs do not indicate depression. The patient in really severe pain will not become addicted to narcotic drugs if they are given at frequent intervals for several days.

Sometimes the patient needs a sedative drug instead of additional analgesics. This may permit him to become drowsy and relaxed enough for the analgesic to be effective. Phenobarbital, for example, often enables the patient to be comfortable with less narcotic drug than might otherwise be necessary. The patient with a severe emotional reaction to his illness will often get relief when analgesic drugs are interspersed with sedative drugs. This arrangement has been found useful when the narcotic or other analgesic drug does not seem to quite "hold" the patient for the desired interval.

Pain may be treated by drugs that help to relieve the cause of pain. For example, the belladonna group of drugs (atropine), which cause relaxation of smooth muscle, may diminish the pain caused by spasm of the smooth muscles. If pain is due to impairment of circulation, drugs that dilate the blood vessels, such as papaverine, nitroglycerine, and Priscoline, may do more good than analgesic drugs. Ointments, emollients, and liniments such as ethyl aminobenzoate and methyl salicylate (oil of wintergreen) may be applied locally to alleviate pain. Oil of clove, used for toothaches, is another example.

Measures to diminish pain or remove its cause should be considered before analgesic medications are given. The nurse would, of course, need an order for these. Local applications of heat and cold often bring relief of pain. Hot sitz baths or a heating pad applied to the abdomen may relieve pain such as that caused by menstrual cramps. Hot gargles relieve the pain of a sore throat, and an icecap may be more effective than medication in relief of a headache. If pain in the abdomen is due to gaseous distention, removal of flatus by means of gastric and intestinal drainage may relieve it. Miller-Abbott tubes passed through the nose, carminative enemas, or a rectal tube often gives more relief than the administration of analgesic drugs. Pain may be caused by distention such as that of an overdistended bladder. Sometimes the patient is even aware of the presence of pain but has a sensation of pressure and restlessness. Treatment for this kind of pain is obviously to relieve the pressure.

Placebos are sometimes given patients who appear to use pain as an attention-getting device and for those who are being weaned from narcotics. They should never be used without a physician's order. The patient should be carefully observed to determine the placebo's effectiveness in controlling pain. This will help the doctor determine the best treatment for the patient. The patient should not know whether a placebo has been found effective. Favorable response to a placebo should not lead the nurse to ignore complaints of pain, because the patient who responds to placebos is in great need of her interest and attention. The patient may also have a genuine new physical pain which needs attention.

REFERENCES AND SELECTED READINGS*

1 *Ashbrook, James B.: Not by Bread Alone, Am. J. Nursing **55**:164-168, Feb. 1955.

2 Elman, Robert: Surgical Care, New York, 1951, Appleton-Century-Crofts, Inc.

3 Koch, Dorothy M.: A Personal Experience With Pain, Am. J. Nursing **59**:1434-1435, Oct. 1959.

4 Livingston, W. K.: What Is Pain, Scient. Am. **188**:59-66, March 1953.

5 *MacBryde, Cyril Mitchell (editor): Signs and Symptoms, ed. 3, Philadelphia, 1955, J. B. Lippincott Co.

6 *Mullen, John F., and Von Schoick, Mildred R.: Intractable Pain, Am. J. Nursing **58**:228-230, Feb. 1958.

7 *Nightingale, Florence: Notes on Nursing: What It Is, and What It Is Not, London, 1859, Harrison; reprinted by J. B. Lippincott Co., Philadelphia.

8 Sandove, Max, and others: Chlorpromazine and Narcotics in the Management of Pain of Malignant Lesions, J.A.M.A. **165**:626-628, June 12, 1954.

9 Wolff, H., Hardy J., and Goodell, H.: Pain Sensations and Reactions, Baltimore, 1952, Williams & Wilkins Co.

---

*References preceded by an asterisk indicate material particularly well suited for student reading.

The patient with incontinence

Chapter 8

Study questions for review

1 Review the anatomy of the bladder, urethra, and lower bowel.
2 What is constipation? How may it be prevented and/or treated by diet? Review the mild cathartics and laxatives. Study the indications and contraindications for each. What is the therapeutic effect of glycerine suppositories? How should they be stored? How are they administered?
3 What is a fecal impaction? How may it be prevented and treated?
4 What foods are omitted in a low-residue diet?
5 What are the common drugs ordered for diarrhea? What is the therapeutic action of each?
6 How can decubiti be prevented? If they occur, what are accepted methods of treating them?

Patients with urinary and fecal incontinence may be found in hospitals, homes for the aged, terminal care institutions, and private homes, because this condition occurs in many kinds of illnesses. These patients present baffling problems. The conscious patient suffers from embarrassment and discomfort. Much time and energy must be expended by those who care for incontinent patients, and the task is an unpleasant one. Difficulties in providing an adequate supply of clean linen may even become overwhelming. Unless patients are given meticulous care, skin irritations and decubitus ulcers become additional problems.

Practicability of home care and the possibilities of the family being able to give care to a family member in his own home will be determined many times by whether the patient is continent or whether methods that are reasonably acceptable can be established for care of incontinence. Handling of body excreta can be very unpleasant, particularly to those unaccustomed to management of other than their own normal functions. Incontinence can be so objectionable to family members that they may refuse to care for the patient at home for this reason. They may need a great deal of help in learning ways to control their own reactions as well as in understanding the patient's feelings. The nurse's attitude in teaching families how to keep the patient clean and dry can have a positive effect. Her skill in arranging materials for cleansing the patient and for disposal of excreta very often will set an example of how to handle a situation which would be difficult for the family member to establish himself.

CAUSES OF INCONTINENCE

To solve the problems of incontinent patients, the nurse needs to know the physiologic causes of the incontinence. This will help her determine whether functional rehabilitation of the bladder and bowel is possible or if she should try to make the patient as comfortable and safe as possible, calling upon ingenuity in improvising equipment and using the commercial appliances at her disposal. If the problem is long-standing, the patient or his family may have worked out a satisfactory solution. The nurse should find out if this is so. She may then continue the plan, with modifications if necessary. This will make transition from home to hospital or vice versa easier for the patient, his family, and the nurses who care for him.

Incontinence, which may be urinary, fecal, or both, has many causes. It may result from surgery performed to deflect the urinary or fecal drainage temporarily or permanently through an opening which cannot always be controlled. Examples are nephrostomy, ureterostomy, cystostomy, ileostomy, cecostomy, and colostomy. These procedures will be discussed in the chapter dealing with the diseases for which they are performed. Other causes of incontinence may be disorders involving the central nerve pathways, resulting in loss of conscious control of the bladder and bowel functions; spinal cord damage, resulting in loss of bladder and bowel reflex mechanisms; and actual tissue damage of the bowel or bladder sphincters or of surrounding supportive tissue.

In many instances the very elderly patient is incontinent of both urine and feces because of a lack of awareness of the need to empty the bladder or bowel. This is caused by cerebral clouding which often is not associated with any definite pathology such as a cerebrovascular lesion. These patients often respond remarkably well to simple measures such as getting them up and into a sitting position several times each day which improves general circulation and increases awareness. Occasionally, ephedrine is given in doses of 25 to 50 mg. (3/8 to 3/4 grain) three times a day to improve tonus and increase alertness.[4]

URINARY INCONTINENCE

A person must have bladder sphincter control in order to have urinary continence. Such control requires normal voluntary and involuntary muscle action coordinated by a normal urethro-bladder reflex. During the interval between voidings, the bladder outlet is elevated by the contraction of the levator ani muscle in the perineum, and the muscular walls of the bladder are relaxed. As the bladder fills with urine, involuntary nerve endings at the trigone are stimulated by the weight of the urine and the increased muscle tone of the bladder. (See Figure 8.) This causes the internal sphincter to relax, releasing urine into the posterior urethra. Stimulated by this, the bladder muscles then contract preparatory to emptying the bladder. As these involuntary stimuli occur, some of the charges overflow to the pudendal nerve, which is a voluntary nerve from the sacrospinal cord. This allows the central nervous system to send appropriate stimuli to the levator ani muscle, causing this muscle either to quickly and forcefully pull the outlet higher to prevent voiding or to lower the outlet to permit voiding. If any part of this complex function is upset, the patient is likely to have some incontinence.[12]

Causes of urinary incontinence

The four main causes of urinary incontinence are cerebral clouding, infections in the urinary tract, disturbance of central nervous system pathways caused by a lesion along their course, and local anatomic or tissue changes.

Cerebral clouding. Cerebral clouding is most common in the aged and has already been described. It also occurs in the acutely ill patient who may be so ill and so toxic that cerebration is dulled. He sometimes "doesn't think" or "doesn't care," or he may not have the energy to exercise voluntary control. This condition usually disappears at once with general improvement in the patient's condition. A patient who is comatose is incontinent because he has lost the ability to control voluntarily the opening of the external sphincter. As soon as urine is released into the posterior urethra, the bladder contracts and empties. This is the reason why patients sometimes void under anesthesia.

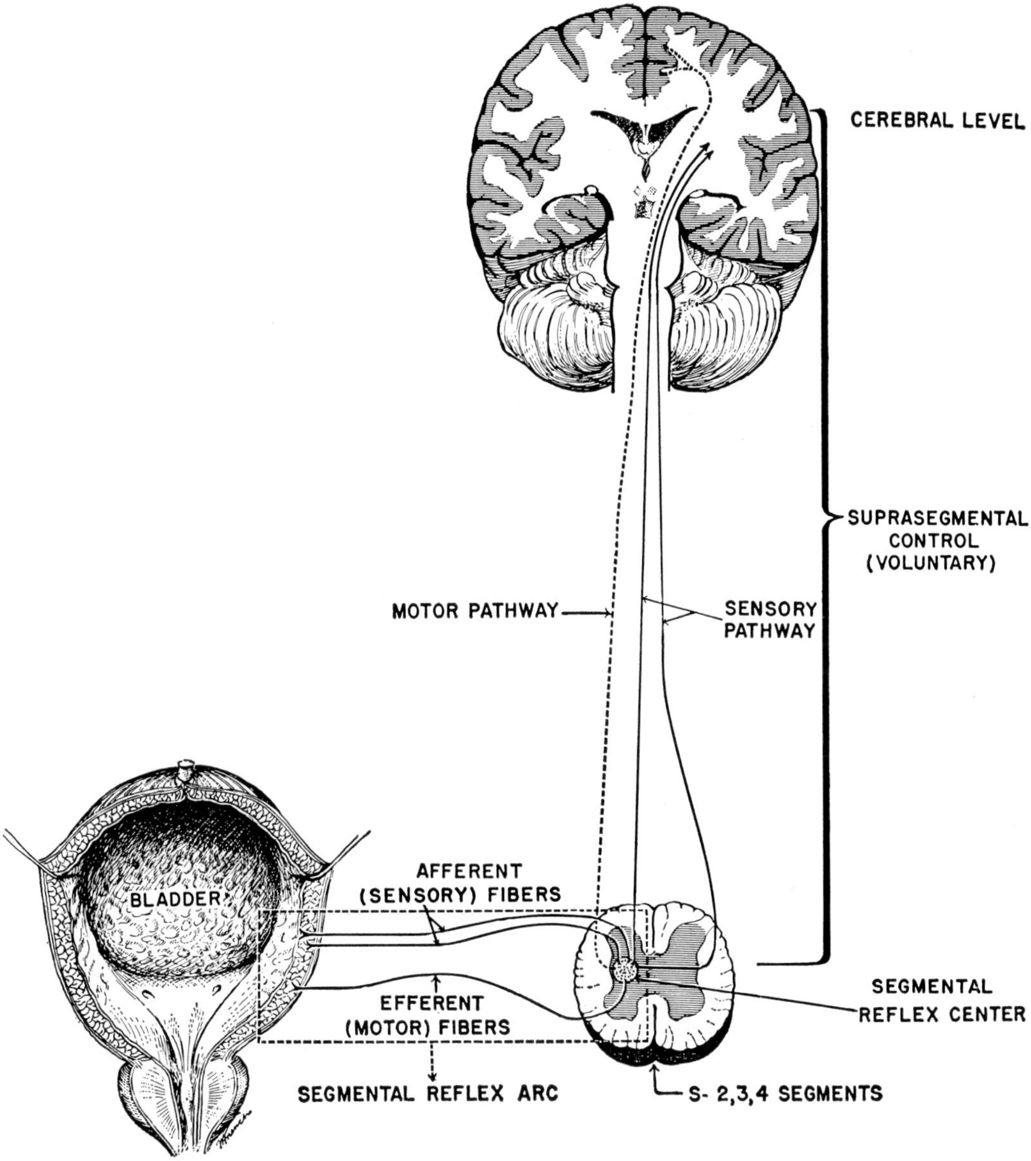

Figure 8

Normal nerve pathways involved in bladder function. (From Cordonnier, Justin J.: Clinical Urology for General Practice, St. Louis, 1956, The C. V. Mosby Co.)

Infection. Infection anywhere in the urinary tract may lead to incontinence since bacteria in the urine cause irritation and stimulate the urethro-bladder reflex abnormally. This condition is quite common in elderly women who have relaxed perineal structures and subsequently poor emptying of the bladder. The physician who is treating urinary incontinence always determines whether or not there is infection before seeking other causes. Infection may be treated systemically with antibiotics and locally by instilling medication such as silver nitrate solution into the bladder at intervals. Specific causes of infection such as obstruction must be found and corrected (see Chapter 21). Many elderly patients who are incontinent respond well to mobilization simply because getting them out of bed and having them move about in an upright position, sit in a chair, and use a commode results in better emptying of the bladder and improvement in the infection. Prevention of urinary incontinence due to infection can sometimes be achieved in elderly patients by getting them out of bed regularly. This is primarily a nursing responsibility.

Disturbance of the central nervous system pathways. Incontinence due to loss of voluntary control may be managed in several ways. An *indwelling urethral catheter* may be inserted into the bladder. However, there are many disadvantages to the use of a urethral catheter, especially if it remains for a long time. As a foreign body, it causes irritation of the urethral and bladder mucosa which, in turn, predisposes to urethritis and cystitis. Indwelling catheters not attached to a closed drainage system have proved to be a source of staphylococcal infection in the urinary tract.[1] When a urethral catheter is used, men are likely to develop epididymitis because the ejaculatory ducts open into the prostatic urethra and organisms easily enter at this point and proceed along the vas deferens to the epididymis. Since epididymitis is a painful and serious infection and frequently is complicated by vasoepididymal strictures, causing sterility (see Chapter 22), it is always best, if possible, to find means other than a urethral catheter to drain the bladder of a male patient. Prolonged use of a catheter also leads to the formation of bladder stones. This is because the urine, instead of maintaining its usual acidity, becomes alkaline as a result of urinary tract infection. This encourages inorganic materials found in the urine, especially calcium and urate crystals, to settle out. A bladder which is continuously drained will eventually lose its muscle tone and its normal capacity. For this reason, when a catheter is being used for a period of weeks in an incontinent patient who is expected to regain normal bladder function, it should be clamped and opened for drainage at regular intervals. Two to four hours is the usual interval. Sometimes a *tidal drainage apparatus* such as the McKenna irrigator is used to provide automatic filling and emptying.[8] A disadvantage of this type of apparatus is that it requires the patient to be on bed rest.

If an indwelling catheter is being used, 3,000 ml. of fluid should be taken daily. This provides for internal bladder irrigation and assures that waste products are well diluted for excretion, thus providing less chance for stone formation. A retention catheter should be changed about every ten days, since mineral deposits collect both within its lumen and at the point where it comes in contact with the bladder and urethra.

It is important that the catheter not be permitted to slip out accidentally. The more often a person must have a catheter inserted, the more likely he is to develop a urinary tract infection. In catheterizing a patient, some organisms from the urethra are always introduced into the bladder where the mucosa, if it is already irritated, is a fertile field for bacterial growth. Therefore, prophylactic doses of sulfisoxazole (Gantrisin) are usually ordered for most patients who have indwelling catheters. To prevent catheters from becoming displaced, they should be anchored securely, and the drainage tubing should be attached to the bed in such a way that the excess tubing is coiled on the mattress and does not pull on the catheter. If the patient is up and about, the use of an "up bottle" prevents undue tugging on the catheter (see Figure 9). If the patient is disoriented, he should be closely observed since he may seriously injure the bladder sphincters and the urethra by pulling on the catheter. It may be necessary to order mittens which make it difficult for the patient to grasp the catheter firmly.

Care must be taken that drainage is not interrupted. Whenever a straight

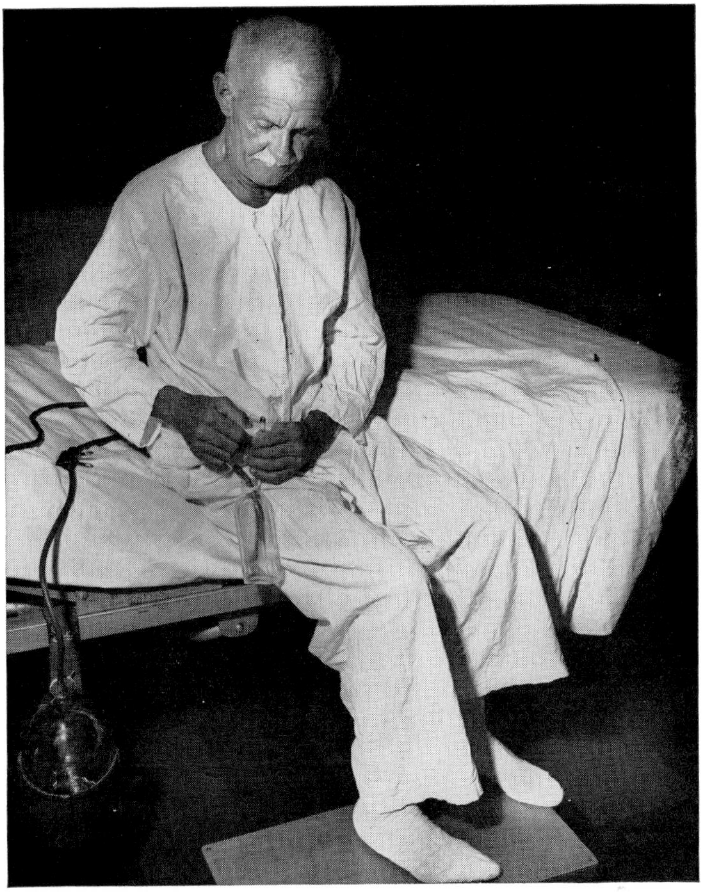

Figure 9

The patient can be taught to detach the catheter from the large drainage bottle and attach it to an "up bottle." This enables him to be more independent.

drainage system is being used, one should remember it functions on the principle of gravity so that the drainage collection receptacle must be placed at a level lower than the cavity being drained. Tubing should run straight from the mattress to the drainage bottle with no loops in the tubing. Leg urinals and "up bottles" do not provide adequate drainage for a patient who is in a reclining position. They either cause the tube to act as a cork, with resultant retention of urine and infection, or cause leakage of urine around the tube or other apparatus.

Because of the contraindications to the use of indwelling catheters, the resourceful nurse will usually try to control incontinence by other means. In *toilet training* children, one takes them to the toilet at regular intervals to void. This same plan can be employed with an incontinent adult. People ordinarily void upon awakening, before retiring, and before or after meals. If a diuretic such as coffee has been taken, it is usually necessary to void in about half an hour. Using this knowledge, the nurse can begin to set up a schedule for placing the patient on a bedpan or taking him to the toilet. Then, if a record is kept for a few days of the times that the patient voids involuntarily, it is usually possible to determine the individual's normal voiding pattern. If the nurse carefully follows this schedule, the problem of incontinence should become minimal. It is important to know the amount the patient voids and to see that the bladder is not distended after voiding. Voiding in frequent small amounts may indicate that the bladder is overflowing as it becomes overdistended; the muscles are not contracting strongly enough to empty it completely. Gentle manual pressure applied downward and backward above the bladder will sometimes give the added impetus needed to stimulate the involuntary nerve pathways. Frequent voiding in small amounts is sometimes due to the pressure of a bowel distended with flatus or feces and can be relieved by the insertion of a rectal tube to release the flatus or by enemas.

Sometimes it is impossible to keep the patient on a voiding schedule. If this is so, an indwelling catheter may be used for women patients since, having a shorter urethra, they are less susceptible to infections from a urethral catheter than are men. If a male patient must have a catheter for several weeks, a cystostomy is frequently done. A cystostomy is a small suprapubic incision into the bladder through which a catheter is inserted. Because the peritoneum is not entered, the operation is a relatively simple one.

A form of *external drainage* can also be used for a male patient because a water-tight apparatus can easily be applied. A satisfactory method is as follows: Tie the closed end of a thin plastic or rubber penile sheath securely over one end of a large glass connecting tube; making a hole in the sheath so that the urine can drain into the connecting tube; carefully cleanse, shave, and dry the penis; pull the foreskin over the glans; invert the sheath and roll it onto the penis, leaving only about one-half inch between the meatus and the connecting tube. Secure the top of the sheath to the shaft of the penis with adhesive tape after tincture of benzoin has been applied to the skin. The adhesive should serve as a seal, yet not be tight enough to cause constriction in case of penile erection. The penis should be checked frequently for signs of skin irritation. The sheath should be changed and the skin thoroughly cleansed once every twenty-four hours.[2] (See Figure 10.) External drainage apparatus, similar to that described, is now available commercially. Rubber incontinence urinals are available, but in using these there is great danger of skin irritation. Unless they are kept meticulously clean and aired daily, there is the additional problem of odor. External drainage may be used with an "up bottle" or leg urinal when the patient is ambulatory. Since it may be embarrassing and upsetting to a man to have a young nurse apply this type of drainage apparatus, someone else may need to do this. If there is no male member of the nursing team, an older, more mature nurse may be called upon, or a member of the patient's family such as a wife, brother, or son may be taught to care for this personal need. At other times the doctor may be willing to do this, or the patient may be able to do it himself.

Diseases such as cerebral embolus, cerebral hemorrhage, brain tumor, meningitis, or traumatic injury of the brain may permanently damage the original pathways which enable the patient to control voiding consciously. New pathways can usually be established if a persistent *retraining program* is carried out. As with the acutely ill or comatose patient, a voiding schedule is set up and strictly adhered to until gradually the patient again learns to recognize and react appropriately to the feeling of having to void. A successful program of this type, leading to complete rehabilitation, requires a mentally competent patient. Otherwise someone else must always remind the patient to follow the schedule.

Disturbance of the urethro-bladder reflex. Any obstruction to the spinal nerve tracts above the level of the sacrospinal cord where the pudendal nerves synapse

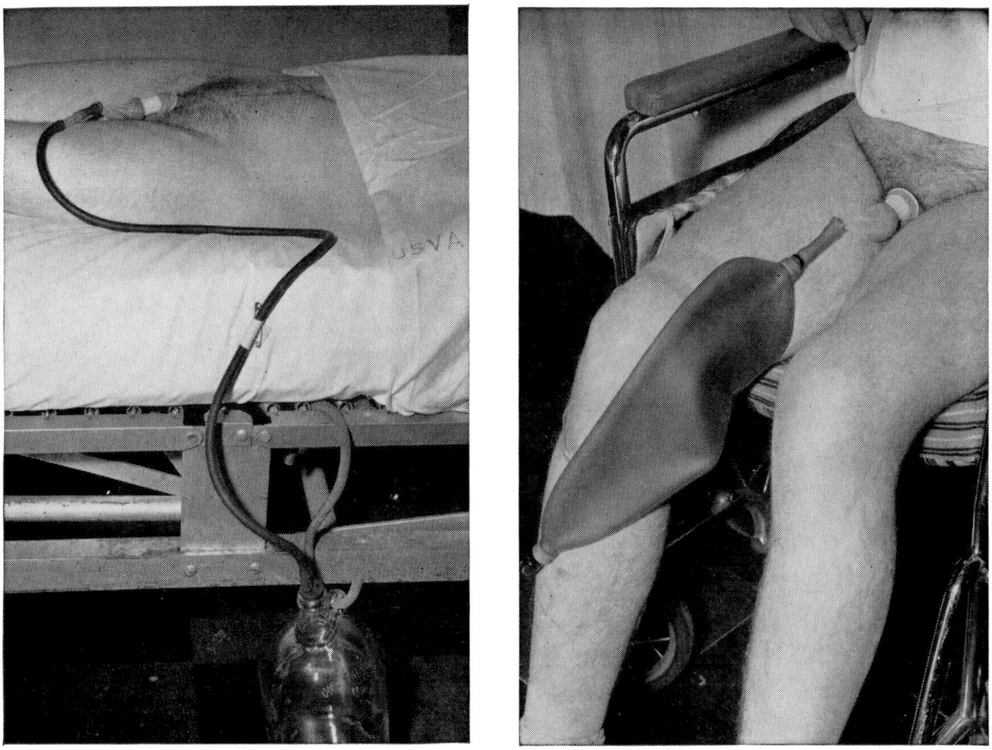

A *B*

Figure 10

Urinary incontinence in a man can be controlled by the use of an external drainage apparatus. *A* shows the arrangement of this apparatus for the bed patient; *B* shows the use of external drainage for the ambulatory patient. (Courtesy Medical Illustration Service, Veterans Administration Hospital, Hines, Ill.)

will cause incontinence. This is because the transmission of the impulse to void does not reach the central nervous system, and thus no conscious control is exercised. This form of incontinence may be seen in patients with cord injuries, cord tumors, tabes dorsalis, and compression of the cord from fractures of the vertebras, herniated disc, metastatic tumor in a vertebra, or postoperative edema. This type of difficulty can result in two types of responses known as "neurogenic bladder." The bladder may be spastic, causing inability to retain any urine, or flaccid, causing the bladder to overflow periodically. Patients with neurogenic bladders have no way of knowing when they are going to void and are frequently embarrassed by this.

Incontinence due to neurogenic bladder can best be controlled by attempting to develop an *automatic bladder*—one which is trained to empty at regular intervals. A regular schedule of both intake and output is worked out with the patient by trial and error. Fluids are spaced in such a way that the bladder is filled and ready to empty at designated times. This can be planned for the convenience of the patient and adapted to his living pattern. For instance, if he wishes to go out, the patient will limit fluids for several hours. Most patients limit fluids in the evening so that the bladder will be less likely to empty during the night. They should plan to force fluids to 3,000 ml. within the twenty-four hour period.

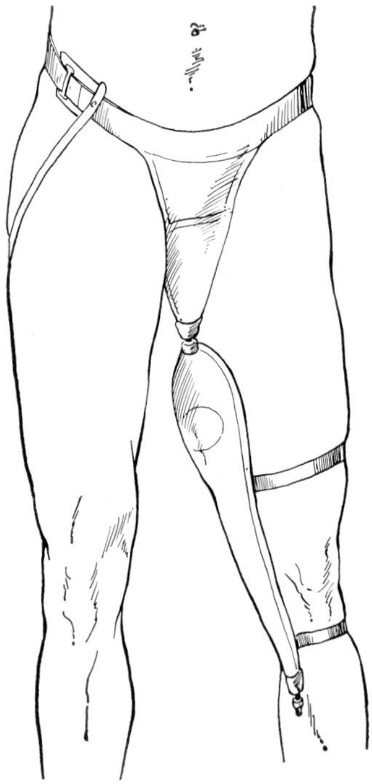

Figure 11

Diagram of a rubber incontinence urinal. Note that it is supported by a strap about the waist and under the buttock and is connected to a drainage bag strapped to the leg. The stopper at the end of the drainage bag can be removed for emptying.

This is necessary because their bladders seldom empty completely, and infection and stone formation may therefore occur. Since alcohol, caffeine, and the theobromine in tea tend to stimulate the kidney and upset the voiding pattern, it is wise to avoid them. Patients may learn to recognize a full bladder by such systemic reactions as restlessness, sweaty or chilly sensations, or high abdominal discomfort. (Restlessness may also serve as a guide to the nurse in knowing when an unconscious patient should be placed on the bedpan.) If the patient has trouble starting to void, brushing motions over trigger areas such as the inner aspects of the thighs or over the bladder may stimulate micturition. Sometimes special positions such as leaning forward will help, or it may be necessary to use the *Credé* method which consists of exerting manual pressure over the bladder. This method may also be used to ensure better emptying of the bladder. It is important for both the patient and the nurse to know that this type of rehabilitation may take weeks and even months to accomplish. The patient often becomes discouraged by recurring accidental voiding and needs a great deal of encouragement. It is helpful if the patient is taught the physiology of voiding so he can better understand and help in his rehabilitation.

Usually the patient will feel more secure if he wears some type of rubber drainage apparatus in case of accidental dribbling. Men may wear a *rubber urinal* (Figure 11) or a *penile clamp* (Figure 12) which mechanically compresses the urethral wall. Penile clamps are usually uncomfortable and must be released and repositioned every two hours to prevent circulatory obstruction. This needs to be especially stressed to the paraplegic patient since he does not have sensation in the penis. Most patients who use clamps alternate them with a rubber urinal and use the clamp primarily when they are going out.

To improvise protection for the incontinent male patient, a shower cap can be used. Cut a hole near the elasticized edge big enough to fit around the penis. Bind the opening with adhesive tape to prevent tearing of the cap and skin irritation. Fill the inside of the cap with absorbent material placed in doughnut fashion. Then, slipping the penis inside, pin the edges of the cap together. If more support is needed, the cap may be pinned to a belt. This improvization may be used if skin irritation has resulted from the use of mechanical devices. It may also be used following a perineal prostatectomy when every effort is being made to have the patient void normally.[5] Other methods which give more protection may decrease his efforts to achieve continence.

Women with incontinence present an extremely difficult problem. At present the most satisfactory method is the use

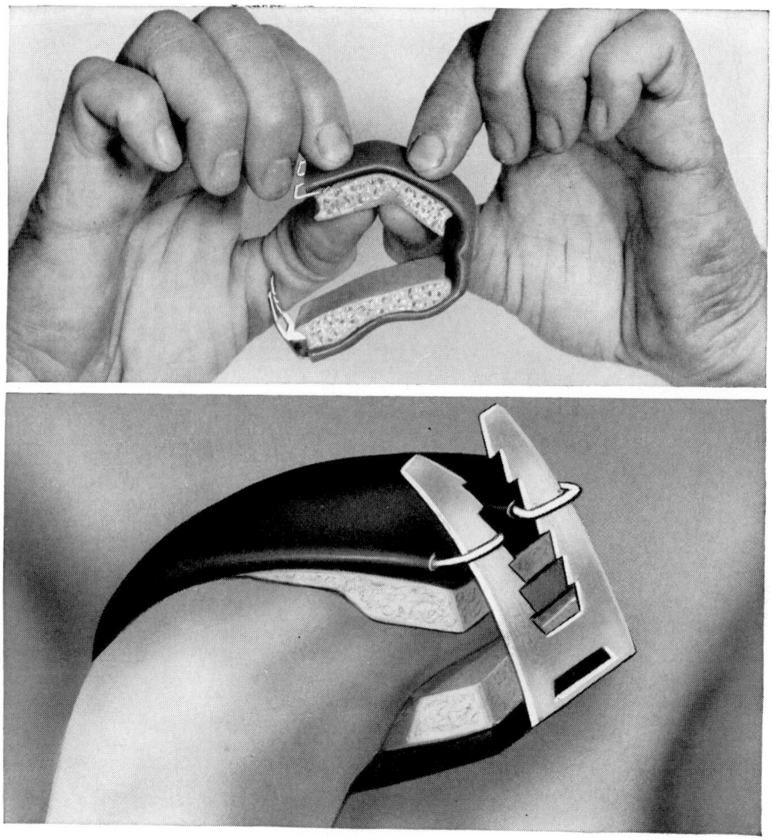

Figure 12

The penile incontinence clamp. Note its flexibility. It should be applied at the base of the penis. (Courtesy C. R. Bard, Inc., Summit, N. J.)

of perineal pads and plastic-lined pants (see Figure 13).

Care of the skin is very important in incontinent patients. The perineal and genital areas should be thoroughly washed several times a day. Tub baths are preferable. Washing the skin with soap and water will help prevent irritation and odor. Exposure to the air is beneficial. Since the acid or alkali in the urine will penetrate any ointment, ointments are useless in protecting the skin. If the skin becomes irritated, a heat lamp should be applied for fifteen minutes after each bath. A zinc oxide powder, such as one used for babies, can be applied and may be helpful in reducing irritation.

Tissue damage. Damage to the sphincters of the bladder from instrumentation, surgery, or accidents, scarring following urethral infections, lesions involving the sphincters, or relaxation of the perineal structures may cause urinary incontinence. The latter cause of incontinence is occasionally seen following childbirth. The problem is local in nature and does not involve the nervous system.

It is practically impossible to repair a sphincter which has been cut. If only the external sphincter has been damaged, the patient will be incontinent on urgency. A voiding schedule may be set up for such a patient so that he will always void before the bladder is full enough to

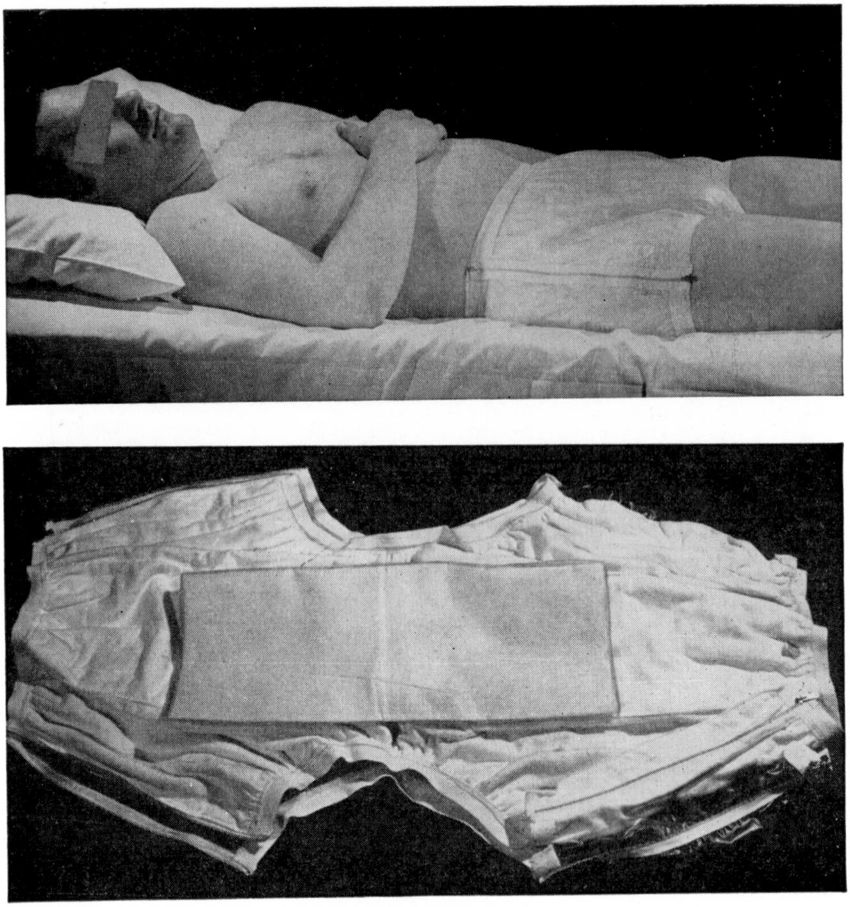

Figure 13

Protective pants for the incontinent patient. The protective pads may be disposable or washable. A cotton jersey liner must be worn under the plastic pants to prevent excoriation of the skin which must have special care. (Courtesy Ferguson Manufacturing Co., Grand Rapids, Mich.)

exert sufficient pressure to open the internal sphincter involuntarily. If only the internal sphincter is damaged, the patient may have no acute feeling of the need to void. Here, there is no problem of incontinence, but one of retention. To assure the regular emptying of the bladder, he, too, should use a voiding schedule. If both sphincters are damaged, the patient will be totally incontinent and will require permanent catheter drainage or the use of external protection.

Some conditions respond to treatment. For example, a levator ani muscle that is shortened by scar tissue, thus holding the bladder outlet at a downward angle and allowing a continuous dribbling or causing frequency of urination, may be treated surgically. Sometimes lesions may be surgically removed or improvements effected by plastic procedures.

Incontinence due to relaxation of the sphincters and the perineum presents serious problems. In men this may follow prostatic surgery or prolonged use of an indwelling catheter. In women, it usually follows childbirth, although some women who have had no children have relaxation of the perineum. Of all adult women 5.5 per cent are reported to have poor control of the bladder outlet.[7] In both sexes old age may cause relaxation of the muscles and consequent incontinence. The patient is taught *perineal exercises* which consist of contracting the abdominal, gluteal, and perineal muscles while breathing normally. This exercise can be explained by asking the patient to hold himself as he would if he needed to void very badly and there were no available facilities. Some times gluteal muscle tone can be increased by having the patient hold a pencil in the fold between the buttock and the thigh. Stopping and starting the urinary stream during voiding will give additional exercise. Women are often instructed to do this while standing in the bathtub or shower with their legs spread apart. The patient should strive eventually to maintain a constant muscle tone. Although operations designed to tighten the muscles are sometimes attempted, the results are not always predictable.

Another serious problem of incontinence occurs in women who have vesicovaginal fistulas. These may result from childbirth injuries or surgical injuries of the vagina or uterus. They also may occur after x-ray therapy for carcinoma of the cervix. The treatment is surgical repair. Frequently this cannot be undertaken for several months because of tissue induration, and it may require several stages. Therefore these women must usually endure long periods of complete incontinence through the vagina. The doctor may recommend that internal douches and sexual intercourse be avoided. These patients need a great deal of encouragement and should be urged to continue their usual activities in so far as possible. If they plan to be away from home for a period of time, it is wise to limit fluids for about four hours before leaving. The use of scented soaps and baths may help their morale. Sometimes the fistula is located so that voiding at regular intervals prevents the bladder from filling to the point at which leakage occurs. Rectovesical fistulas present fewer problems in incontinence since the anal sphincter will usually hold urine. (See Chapter 22.)

FECAL INCONTINENCE

In fecal incontinence the anal sphincter may be relaxed, the voluntary control of defecation may be interrupted in the central nervous system, or messages may not be transmitted to the brain because of a lesion within the cord or external pressure on the cord above the sacrospinal area. The disorders causing breakdown of conscious control are identical with those affecting the bladder. Perineal relaxation and actual damage of the anal sphincter are often caused by injury during childbirth or during perineal operations. Relaxation usually increases with the general loss of muscle tone in aging. Perineal exercises may help some patients.

If fecal incontinence is to be prevented, bowel training or a regular routine of stimulation of peristalsis and of going to the toilet should be carried out. Ordinarily the bowel is trained to empty at regular intervals; once a day or every other day after breakfast is common. Food and fluids increase peristalsis and this may stimulate defecation. The taking of certain food or fluids may be associated with the accustomed time for defecation. For example, coffee or orange juice may provide the stimulus for some people. Most patients will be more relaxed and thus more likely to have a bowel movement if placed in as near the normal position as possible and if they have privacy. Glycerine suppositories (usually two are needed) help stimulate evacuation of the bowel; they should be inserted about two hours before the usual time of defecation. They should be lubricated with petrolatum and pushed well into the rectum with a gloved finger. If the patient is unconscious or has disease of the spinal cord, it may be necessary to use an enema. Usually about two quarts of fluid are needed at one time to stimulate reflex peristalsis. Fluid is more easily retained if the patient is on his side. It may be necessary to pinch the buttocks together securely around the rectal tube in order to retain the fluid in the bowel, or to use a Foley catheter, inflating the balloon to help retain the fluid in the bowel. If a Foley catheter is used, insert it four inches into the rectum and then inflate the balloon with 30 or 40 ml. of fluid. After giving the enema, wait five minutes and then, with the patient on the bedpan or toilet, deflate the balloon. Patients may not get full results for one to two hours or longer following enemas, so they should be provided with protective padding.

Sometimes it is possible for patients with cord lesions to develop *automatic* defecation. They may need to use a cathartic nightly such as milk of magnesia and to dilate the anal sphincter digitally, using a gloved finger. Manual pressure on the abdomen, rubbing toward the sigmoid and rectal areas, stimulates peristalsis. A diet which will form a soft stool should be given. The general welfare of the patient is benefited so much by automatic defecation that the time and energy expended to accomplish this are well spent.

Incontinent patients may have *diarrhea.* This may be a symptom of *fecal impaction.* The doctor should make a rectal examination, breaking up the impaction if necessary, and then an oil enema followed by a cleansing enema should be given. If this does not control the leakage and it is liquid in consistency, a rectal tube (28 or 30 Fr.) may be left in place anchored in the fold under the buttock with adhesive tape and attached to straight drainage. (See Chapter 21 for method of anchoring tubes.) If the diarrhea is not due to an impaction, one should look for other causes. A patient may find that certain foods cause him to have diarrhea. The nurse can help him analyze his diet and avoid foods that cause trouble. Emotional stress may also cause diarrhea, so it is important that this be reduced in any way possible. Diarrhea is a rather common reaction to medications, especially the antibiotics. Camphorated tincture of opium, bismuth subcarbonate, or kaolin may be given in an attempt to control the diarrhea. The camphorated tincture of opium acts as an intestinal "splint" by slowing down peristalsis, and the other two drugs have a soothing effect on the intestinal mucosa because of their coating property. These drugs are usually given after meals and after each loose bowel movement.

UNCONTROLLED URINARY AND FECAL INCONTINENCE

Some patients will have urinary and fecal incontinence despite all efforts. The nurse must see that they are kept clean, odorless, and free from decubiti. Linen must be changed as soon as it is soiled. Newspaper pads covered with a piece of cloth or "chuck" can be used to protect bedding and furniture. Oilcloth and the newer plastic materials can also be used. Linen may be saved and the patient made more comfortable if pants made of some absorbent material backed with plastic are used (see Figure 13). A resourceful person may be able to improvise equipment that will be more comfortable and less costly than commercially manufactured pants. Zippers, snap-tape and ties, elastic, and a variety of fabrics and waterproof materials may be used. Cellucotton for padding is less expensive if purchased in large rather than small rolls. Any padding used must be changed often and the skin thoroughly washed and dried at each changing. If possible, the patient should be bathed in a tub of warm water at least once a day. Zinc oxide powders are also beneficial for these patients.

Commercial preparations, such as Diaparene chloride, which control odor of urine and to some extent lessen its irritating properties are available. For the patient's comfort, however, it is necessary to change protective pads frequently.

Sawdust has been shown to be unusually effective in preventing pressure sores in incontinent patients who are bedridden.[13] It must be changed frequently and is difficult to handle. Probably for these reasons it is not generally used.

Deodorant sprays are available for use on dressings and linen. Deodorants for deodorizing room air may also need to be placed about the room. An electric deodorizer works well.

If the patient can be up, his favorite chair can be equipped with a commode seat. Special commode wheel chairs are also available, making it possible for the patient to be more comfortable and enabling him to mingle socially with others. Thus, he will probably be a happier individual and one with whom it is more pleasant to live.

REFERENCES AND SELECTED READINGS*

1 Adams, Ralph: Prevention of Infections in Hospitals, Am. J. Nursing **58**:344-348, March 1958.

2 Barber, Knowlton E., Adams, John F., and Sosinski, Leonard D.: Control of Incontinent Urine by Use of External Drainage, Am. J. Nursing **49**:526-527, Aug. 1949.

3 *Buchwald, Edith, McCormack, Margaret, and Raby, Emilie: A Bladder and Bowel Training Program for Patients With Spinal Cord Disease, Rehabilitation Monograph III, New York, 1952, The Institute for Physical Medicine and Rehabilitation, New York University-Bellevue Medical Center.

*References preceded by an asterisk indicate material particularly well suited for student reading.

4 Eckstrom, Sten: Urinary Incontinence in Old Persons, Geriatrics **10**:83-85, Feb. 1955.

5 *Hargett, G., and others: Tidal Drainage of the Urinary Bladder, Am. J. Nursing **46**:26-27, Jan. 1946.

6 Hurwitz, Sidney P., Jacobson, Edward B., and Kolman, Isadore L.: Preparation of an Incontinence Bag, J. Urol. **73**:1103-1104, June 1955.

7 Kegal, A.: Physiological Therapy for Urinary Stress Incontinence, J.A.M.A. **146**:915-917, July 7, 1951.

8 *McKenna, William F.: A Simple, Efficient, Automatic Tidal Drainage Apparatus, Urol. & Cutan. Rev. **52**:18-21, Jan. 1948.

9 *Morrissey, Alice B.: The Procedures of Urinary and Bowel Rehabilitation, Am. J. Nursing **51**:194-197, March 1951.

10 Muellner, S. Richard: Special Problems of Urinary Control in Patients With Multiple Sclerosis, J. Urol. **73**:254-259, Feb. 1955.

11 *Robertson, Carolyn: Manual Expression of Urine, Am. J. Nursing **59**:840-841, June 1959.

12 Rose, D. K.: Analysis of Bladder and Related Renal Symptoms in Urinary Obstruction and Incontinence, West. J. Surg. **63**:196-200, April 1955.

13 *Sawdust Bed Therapy, Am. J. Nursing **49**:654, Oct. 1949.

14 *Trainham, Genevieve, and Montgomery, John C.: Developmental Factors in Learning Bowel and Bladder Control, Am. J. Nursing **46**:841-844, Dec. 1946.

The unconscious patient

Chapter 9

Study questions for review

1 As a result of your experience on the wards, list the equipment that you would need in preparing a room for the admittance of an unconscious patient.
2 Review your basic physical needs in a twenty-four hour period. Do these differ from the needs of one who is unconscious? If so, how?
3 Review the following basic nursing procedures: mouth care, gavage, throat suction, enemas, and skin care.

Unconsciousness is an abnormal state resulting from disturbance of sensory perception to the extent that the patient is not aware of what is happening around him. Periods of unconsciousness may be momentary (the common faint or syncope) or may last for months (for example, following a serious motor vehicle accident in which extensive brain damage has been sustained).

The term unconsciousness is relative since there are many degrees or levels of unconsciousness: excitatory, somnolent, stuporous, and comatose. In *excitatory unconsciousness* the patient does not respond coherently but is easily disturbed by sensory stimuli such as bright lights, noise, or sudden movement. He may become excited and agitated at the slightest disturbance. This is the stage of unconsciousness commonly seen in patients who are going under anesthesia or who are partially reacted from anesthesia. In caring for such patients the room should be kept dimly lighted, the environment should be quiet, talking should be avoided, and any necessary moving of the patient or activity about him should be slow and gentle.

The *somnolent* patient is extremely drowsy and will respond only if spoken to directly and perhaps touched. This response is rarely more than a mumble or a jerky body movement in response to a stimulus.

The *stuporous* patient responds only to painful stimuli such as pricking or pinching of the skin. In deep stupor he may respond only to supra-orbital or substernal pressure; this may be a reflex withdrawal from the painful stimulus.

The patient in *deep coma* does not respond to any type of stimulus and his reflexes are gone. He has no gag or corneal reflexes, and he may have an irregular response or complete loss of pupillary reflexes. The thermal, respiratory, or other vital regulatory mechanisms in the brain may be disturbed; in the presence of such a disturbance, the prognosis is poor.

Unconsciousness may be caused by systemic disease or toxemia affecting the brain. In vascular diseases such as cerebral hemorrhage or cerebral emboli there may be enough damage to brain tissue from anoxia to cause unconsciousness. The pressure of expanding lesions such as subdural hematomas and intracranial tumors also may cause unconsciousness. Other causes are head injuries with primary damage to the brain or pressure on the brain from swelling, drugs such as the barbiturates, alcohol, and anesthetizing agents. Unconsciousness is also seen in some functional diseases of the nervous system and in diseases such as epilepsy in which there is a disturbance of brain physiology.

NURSING CARE OF THE UNCONSCIOUS PATIENT

Although special care for the unconscious patient is directly related to the cause of the condition, general care does not vary with the cause. In this chapter, only the general nursing care will be discussed. Nursing problems related to unconsciousness in specific diseases are discussed in the appropriate chapters.

In caring for the unconscious patient, the nurse must make provisions for meeting his physical and spiritual needs and his family's emotional and spiritual needs. The objectives of patient care are to maintain normal body function and to prevent complications which will hamper the patient when consciousness is restored. The nurse must remember that the patient cannot do anything for himself or even ask for help. He cannot, for example, change his position if he is uncomfortable, strained, or cramped. Nurses caring for unconscious patients should keep in mind the bodily needs they meet for themselves each day and should also recall the requests that conscious patients make for little extra comforts.

The environment and the family

The appearance of the unconscious patient and his surroundings is very important to his family. Not being able to communicate with a loved one is very difficult for them. Seeing the patient looking comfortable in a room that is neat and pleasant helps members of his family to remain relatively composed. The room should be well ventilated, and the temperature should be kept at about 21° C. (70° F.) If a member of the family is remaining with the patient, a comfortable chair should be provided. He should be told where the rest room is, where he may eat, and where the public telephone is located. If the patient remains unconscious for an extended period of time, members of the family should be urged to share the "vigil." Sometimes they can be encouraged to come only for short periods of time each day; they should be assured that they will be notified at once if there is any change in the patient's condition. The nurse should help them conserve their physical resources, for the patient who recovers after a period of unconsciousness needs much care and attention during convalescence.

Members of the patient's family frequently have many questions. If the nurse cannot answer them, she should refer the family to others who can. Explanations of treatments, such as would be given to the patient if he were conscious, should be given to members of the family. This helps to allay some of their fears and helps them to understand and to feel they have a part in the patient's care. If the family wishes, the spiritual adviser should be called. He may help the patient and give the family comfort and emotional help. If religious medals are significant to the patient and his family, they may be attached to the head of the bed or secured in such a way that they are not lost. Often the patient wears a medal on a chain around his neck, and many hospitals do not require that it be removed unless necessary for a treatment or examination such as when a roentgenogram is to be made.

Hearing is probably the last of the critical faculties to be lost in unconsciousness. Upon regaining consciousness, many patients have reported conversations that were held near their beds, and many vividly recall conversations they heard when other faculties were obliterated by anesthesia. Conversation of those close to the patient should be no different than if the patient were conscious. Members of the family and other visitors may need to be reminded of this. Because the patient may be able to hear, the nurse should tell him what she is going to do; for example, she should tell him if he is going to be moved onto his other side or given mouth care.

Physical care of the patient

Maintenance of an adequate airway. It is unsafe to leave an unconscious patient unattended if he is lying on his back because the tongue may fall back and occlude the air passages. When the patient is placed on his side or abdomen, a small firm pillow rather than a soft one should be used under the head so that there is no danger of his becoming accidentally smothered as a result of his face being buried in the pillow. Since the patient is unable to blow or otherwise clear his nose, the nasal passages may become occluded with mucus. Cleansing or suctioning of the nasal passages of patients who have had brain surgery or who have suffered a head injury should not be done without a doctor's specific order, but in other instances the nose should be gently swabbed first with a moistened applicator and then with one lightly lubricated with mineral oil. If the mucous membranes of the nose and mouth become unusually dry, a steam vaporizer is useful.

Excess mucus may need to be suctioned from the nasopharynx; a No. 18 or 20 Fr. whistle-tip catheter may be used for this. The mouth should be held open with a gag, and the suction should be shut off until the tube is inserted into the back of the throat. If the tube is to be inserted through the nose, it should be lubricated with water only.

Maintenance of circulation. Circulation of blood is enhanced by muscle movement. The patient must not be left in a position that hampers circulation to any part of the body; for example, lying for any length of time with an acute angle bend at the knee joint will produce enough pressure on the popliteal artery and veins to hamper circulation to the lower leg. Reddened areas should be gently massaged, and they should be noted in the nursing care plan and in the nursing notes of the patient's chart so that they will receive special care. A definite routine for turning and for exercise not only improves the circulation and helps to maintain muscle tone but also helps to prevent hypostatic pneumonia or atelectasis; in addition, it maintains a normal range of joint motion and helps to prevent formation of vascular thrombi. Scheduled turning of the unconscious patient at specific intervals by an assigned team of nurse and/or auxilliary personnel assures maintenance of these physiologic functions. A check list with the patient's name and the position changes needed at specific intervals is also useful.

Moving and position. A "turning sheet" should be used in moving an unconscious patient. It not only helps to maintain the patient's body alignment, by allowing the entire trunk to be moved at the same time, but also lessens the strain on the nurse or attendant's back. A turning sheet is a large sheet folded lengthwise and then in half; it should be placed under the patient so that it reaches from above the shoulders to below the buttocks. In preparing to turn the patient, remove the top bedclothes so that they will not be in the way and so that the alignment of the patient's body can be easily seen. Two nurses are needed to execute the turn—one on each side of the bed. Roll the sheet edges up close to the patient's body and grasp them firmly. Gently roll the patient onto his back, then lift or pull him on the sheet toward the side of the bed opposite to that which he is to be turned. Bend the knee that will be uppermost after the patient is turned. The nurse who will be facing the patient after he is turned should then grasp the far side of the turning sheet and roll the patient toward her onto his side, pulling the hip and shoulder well under him. Check to see that the spine is straight, the neck is not bent, and the lower leg is straight. Place firm rubber covered pillows under the uppermost arm and leg. These should support the entire extremity and be of such a height as to prevent the abduction or adduction of the arm or leg. The uppermost leg should be flexed with the knee at right angles to the hip. To prevent foot drop, the foot of the straightened leg should be firmly dorsiflexed against a foot block at scheduled intervals. The lowermost arm should be flexed at the elbow and placed palm up flat on the bed. The fingers of the hand which rests on the pillows should be allowed to curve gently over the edge of the pillow. The wrist, however, must be supported on the pillow to prevent wrist drop. The fingers should never be continuously hyperextended or tightly clenched, and sometimes it is advisable to prevent this by placing a roll of 3 inch bandage in the palm and curling the fingers around it. If the thumb tends to fall forward, it may be supported in a position of common use by attaching a tab of cloth to the hand roll and using this as a supportive bandage. If the unconscious patient is placed correctly in a side-lying position, a pillow to support his back is unnecessary. (See Figure 14.)

If the patient does not move, all the extremities should be put through the complete range of joint motion at least twice each day. When he is turned each hour, the extremities on one side may be passively exercised. Provided that this nursing procedure is properly carried out, such a routine assures passive exercise to all extremities. In turning the patient, extreme care should be taken to prevent strain on joints.

The patient may be turned directly onto his abdomen for short periods. When this is done, the feet should extend over the edge of the mattress to prevent pressure on the toes, and the head should be turned well to the side. Usually no pillow is necessary under the head, but a small one may be slipped under the abdomen to prevent excessive pressure on the chest; this is sometimes needed to relieve pressure on the breasts of women.

Skin care. The unconscious patient should be thoroughly bathed with warm water each day. The skin should be briskly washed and dried to stimulate circulation. In some hospitals patients who have been unconscious for some time are lifted into a bathtub several times a week since this seems to control the development of decubiti remarkedly well. Three people trained in doing a three-man lift are needed for this. Care must be taken not to injure the patient in moving him to the tub or to place undue strain upon the nurses. Shallow tubs at bed height with access on three sides are preferable but not essential.

If the skin is dry, it should be lubricated daily with lanolin or cold cream; superfatted soaps may be used, or detergents may replace soaps. The feet should be lubricated each day since poor circulation from lack of activity causes the skin to become dry and the nails to harden and become horny. Alcohol is drying to the skin and should not be used. The fingernails and toenails should be short and clean. As the depth of unconsciousness becomes more shallow, many patients scratch themselves.

The hair should be neatly combed. If it is long, a woman's hair is usually more manageable and attractive in braids. If unconsciousness persists, the doctor may permit a shampoo provided the movement involved is not harmful to the patient. Shampoos should be given at least every two weeks to patients who are unconscious for long periods of time.

Mouth care. Since the unconscious patient tends to be a "mouth breather," the mouth often becomes dry. Therefore, mouth care should be given every two to four hours. All dentures should be removed and safely stored until the patient is fully conscious. The patient's own teeth should be brushed at least twice a day; a child's toothbrush is more easily used than an adult's. The inside of the mouth, the gum line, and the tongue should be inspected daily, using a flashlight and a tongue depressor, and the mouth should be cleaned thoroughly every two to four hours with glycerin and lemon juice or an aromatic alkaline mouthwash solution. (See Figure 14.) The mouth will have to be held open with a gag, and it may be cleansed with a piece of gauze wrapped around a toothbrush or a tongue depressor. The nurse should never put her fingers in a patient's mouth because the gag or hold on the jaw may loosen and allow the jaws to close down on the fingers; a human bite may cause severe infection. The lips should be coated with a lubricant such as cold cream to prevent cracking.

Eye care. The patient's eyes should be carefully inspected several times a day. If they appear irritated, if the corneal reflex is absent, or if the lids are incompletely closed, they should be covered with an eyeshield. This may be a plastic

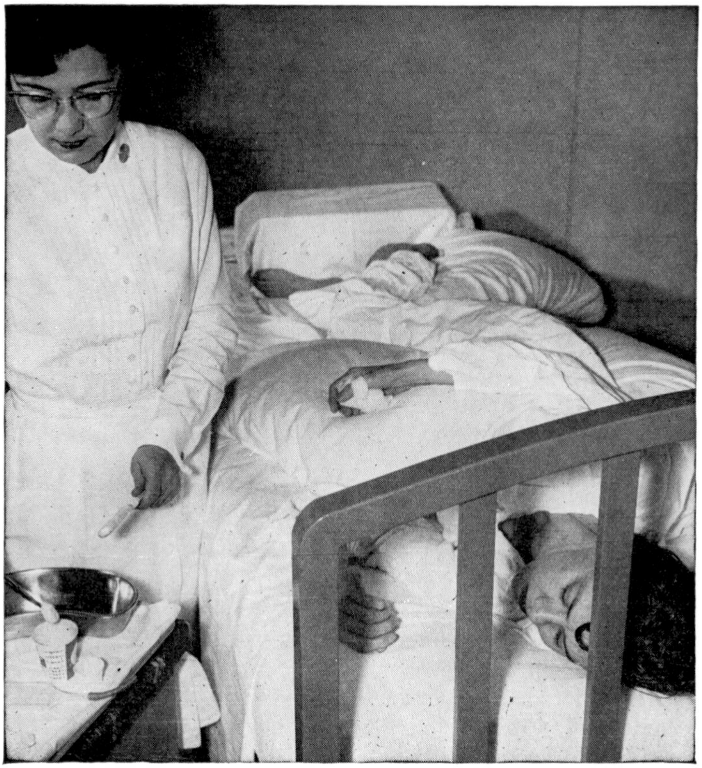

Figure 14

The nurse is preparing to give mouth care to an unconscious patient. Note that she has a padded gag to hold the mouth open. Note also that the patient is supported by pillows at her side and that her hand is curled about a hand roll with the thumb held in pronation.

watch glass, or a circle of transparent x-ray film, 9 cm. in diameter, may be used by slitting it to the middle and overlapping the edges of the slit to make a cone-shaped shield. All the edges of the x-ray film shield should be bound with cellophane tape to prevent irritation of the skin, and the shields may be held in place with cellophane tape. The doctor may order an eye irrigation; physiologic solution of sodium chloride is often used. The eye should always be irrigated away from the inner canthus so that the return flow is away from the other eye. If the patient tends to open his eyes at intervals there also may be an order for instillation of a drop or two of mineral oil in each eye daily to protect the cornea from lint and dirt. Neglect of this may lead to drying of the cornea and eventual blindness.

Food and fluids. The comatose patient cannot be given fluids or food by mouth since he does not swallow normally and would surely aspirate fluid into the lungs. He may be fed by intravenous infusion or hypodermoclysis. While protein and carbohydrates can be administered parenterally, fats are not yet being routinely used intravenously and it is therefore difficult to meet all his nutritional needs in this way. In most instances it is preferable to use a gastric tube and to give small amounts of liquid containing all essential foods. Only about 100 to 200 ml. should be given at each feeding, and feedings should be spaced every two to three hours. If the stomach is overfilled, the patient may vomit and aspirate with serious consequences. All feedings should be followed with about 50 ml. of water to clear the tube. The tube should be removed at least every five days and reinserted into the other nostril. Usually the doctor inserts the tube. If he does not, the nurse must be certain that she can perform the procedure without damage to the patient. After the tube is inserted, it is customary to test its placement in the following ways: by placing it under water and checking for the presence of air bubbles, which would indicate that it is in the lungs instead of the stomach; by aspirating a little fluid to prove that it is in the stomach; by having a second nurse check the tube to be certain it is in the stomach before feedings are given; by inserting a small amount of clear water first since this would cause the least harm if an error had occurred. For details of care of the equipment and of technique of this procedure, see textbooks on fundamentals of nursing. The patient who has a gastric tube passed into the stomach needs special care of the nose to prevent crusting and ulceration. (See Common diagnostic tests and procedures in Chapter 26.)

If the patient responds to verbal stimuli and has a gag reflex, fluids may be put into the back of the mouth through an Asepto syringe to which is attached about two inches of rubber tubing to obviate the danger of the patient's biting down on the glass tip of the syringe. He may have to be reminded to swallow each mouthful. Suction should be readily available in case he shows signs of choking; if signs of choking do occur the nurse may have to apply pressure on the jaws to insert the suction tube.

Hyperthermia. When the heat-regulatory center in the hypothalamus is disturbed, the patient's temperature will rise suddenly. This is known as hyperthermia. It may occur after trauma to vital centers, and it often occurs in the last stages of chronic medical illness (such as uremia) when the body relinquishes vital controls prior to death. The temperature of any unconscious patient should be taken rectally every four hours, and, if it is elevated, it should be taken every two hours. Elevation of temperature may also be a sign of complications such as pneumonia, wound infection, dehydration, or urinary tract infection. The nurse should carefully observe the patient for any signs that might indicate the onset of complications.

When elevation of temperature is caused by the improper functioning of the heat-regulatory center, the nurse must help in efforts to compensate for this natural control. If the temperature is over 38° C. (101° F.), some bedclothes should be removed and sometimes the patient should be covered only by a sheet. Occasionally the patient's gown and sheet are removed and only a loin cloth and breast covering used. Aspirin may be dissolved and passed though a gastric tube into the stomach, or it may be introduced into the rectum as a suppository or dissolved in a small amount of water as a retention enema. The dosage for drugs given by rectum is usually double that given orally. Fluids may not be forced if the doctor feels that increasing fluid intake may increase intracranial pressure. If the temperature continues to rise despite conservative treatment, icecaps may be applied to the groins and axillas. Alcohol sponge baths are often ordered, and fans placed slightly to the side of the patient may be used to increase evaporation. If the fever still persists following this treatment, ice-water enemas may be given, and the patient may be packed in ice or placed in a tub of cool or cold water. In very hot weather he may be placed in an oxygen tent for its air-conditioning effect. The room should be kept cool so that body heat will be used for evaporation of perspiration. If the patient's temperature goes over 40° C. (104° F.), it should be taken every hour until it returns to and remains at a lower level. Sometimes, if the elevation is due to increased intracranial pressure, a lumbar puncture is done. Unabated high

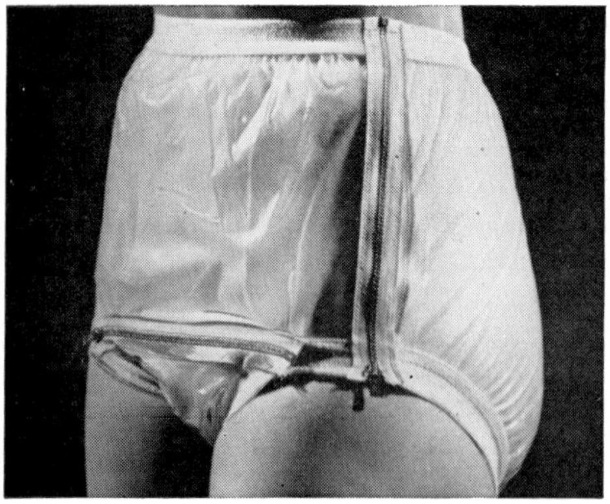

Figure 15

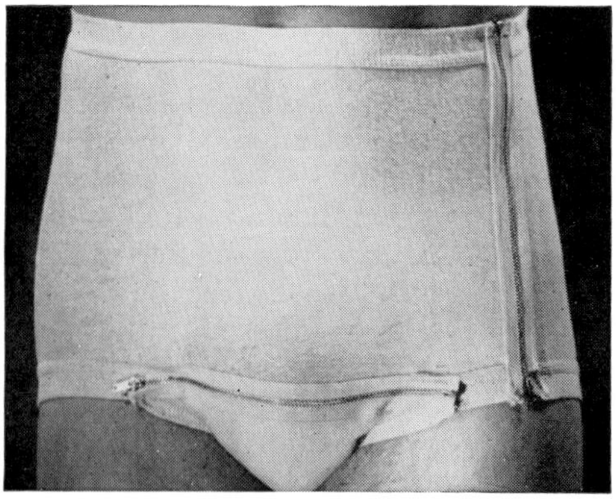

Figure 16

Outside plastic pants for a woman, and the cotton jersey liner for a man. Note that both the liner and the plastic outer pants open at the crotch so that the protective pads can be easily changed. (Courtesy Ferguson Manufacturing Co., Grand Rapids, Mich.)

temperature eventually will cause death because of damage to the respiratory center in the brain.

The family often becomes concerned lest the patient treated for hyperthermia develop "pneumonia." It must be explained that the fever is associated with the unconsciousness and is not related to infection, that the treatment the patient is receiving is the usual one for this complication, that there is little danger of pneumonia from chilling because the high temperature is keeping the patient warm, and that excessive bed covering will increase the temperature of even the normal person.

Hypothermia. The unconscious patient may have a temperature which is too low; this may happen when vital centers are depressed but control has not yet been lost. The unconscious patient who does not move produces less normal body heat and is likely to have a low temperature and to need extra covering. The nurse should feel the patient's feet to determine circulation in the extremities and to judge whether or not adequate external warmth is being supplied.

Problems of elimination. The unconscious patient often has both urinary and fecal incontinence. A Foley catheter or external drainage apparatus may be used to control urinary incontinence. If these are contraindicated, the nurse should try to determine the patient's normal voiding schedule and place him on a bedpan or put a urinal in place according to this schedule. The skin should be kept dry and clean to prevent decubiti and add to comfort. (See Figures 13, 15, and 16.) The urinary output should be measured. If this is impossible because of incontinence, it should be estimated by recording each time the patient is incontinent and whether or not a large amount of urine was voided. (See Chapter 8.)

The unconscious patient usually is given an enema every two or three days to help prevent fecal incontinence and formation of impactions. The patient who is fed through a gastric tube may be given juices, such as prune juice, which have a laxative effect. Sometimes a mild cathartic such as milk of magnesia or citrate of magnesia is given through the tube the night before the enema is scheduled. In giving the enema, the buttocks may need to be held together to prevent premature expulsion of the fluid. The patient should never be placed on the bedpan before the enema is given, for if the enema is expelled immediately it merely serves as an irrigation; and the procedure, which is tiring to the patient, must then be repeated.

When it is desirable for the enema to be expelled, the patient should be turned onto a bedpan, with special care taken to support the back and to prevent pressure damage to the skin from weight against the pan. A firm pillow protected with water-resistant material is best for this. The lower abdomen should then be massaged gently from right to left. Sometimes it is necessary to siphon fluid from the lower bowel, in which case the enema may have to be repeated.

If the patient has a vaginal discharge, it should be reported to the doctor. Sometimes cleansing douches are ordered. The patient who is menstruating will need perineal care every few hours.

Prevention of accidents. Precautions should be taken to prevent accidents to unconscious patients. No external heat such as hot-water bottles or heating pads should be used. Padded side rails should be kept on the bed, since the patient might have a convulsion or suddenly move when not expected to do so. If a convulsion is anticipated a mouth gag should be kept at the bedside; if a convulsion occurs, the gag should be inserted at the side of the mouth between the molar teeth, since the front teeth are easily loosened or broken. Manual pressure at the angle of the jaw sometimes makes it easier to open the mouth. The unconscious patient should be observed at least every half hour; if his condition is critical, he may need to be observed every fifteen minutes or to be attended constantly.

If the patient is semiconscious, he may be placed in a chair twice a day; this improves circulation and prevents pulmonary and circulatory complications. To prevent him from falling, the nurse should apply a chest harness type of Posey belt or tie a drawsheet about his waist and to the back of the chair. She must make certain that he is placed in as near a proper sitting position as possible. The spine should be straight, he should be sitting on his buttocks, and his feet should be flat on the floor. The head and arms will need to be supported. The reason for getting the patient out of bed should be carefully explained to the family since they may feel that this is "cruel."

Observations

The nurse should make and record detailed observations of an unconscious patient. The diagnosis may be obscure, and the nurse who notes such things as stiffness of the neck and flaccid limbs or who carefully reports the course of a convulsion may provide the doctor with essential information. Observations over and above those made while giving patient care may be ordered. The doctor may wish the vital signs, the pupillary response, and the level of consciousness determined at periodic intervals. A rising blood pressure correlated with a slowing of the pulse rate is indicative of increasing intracranial pressure and should be reported at once. Any marked change in the character of the pulse or respirations or any decrease or increase in the level of consciousness should be reported.

The pupillary response is checked by opening the upper eyelid and flashing a light into the eye from the outer aspect inward toward the nose. Each eye should be tested separately. Irregular reaction of either eye or "fixed" pupils should be reported, since these responses suggest intracranial hemorrhage.

The corneal response is tested by the doctor. He will need a wisp of sterile absorbent cotton for this. The patient who has lost the corneal reflex will not blink when the cornea is touched.

Convalescence

A patient may recover completely after being unconscious for several weeks. If he has been well cared for during this time, he will not have as extensive a hospitalization period as if decubiti, contractures, or blindness are allowed to develop. The patient will gradually return through the stages of unconsciousness, and he often first responds verbally to a familiar face or voice. Efforts should not be made to arouse him until the level of unconsciousness has lightened. He may be unable to speak, be partially paralyzed, or have other losses, and the rehabilitation program will be planned accordingly. During convalescence, definite rest periods should be planned each day. If the patient becomes overtired, he will tend to regress. He will need the encouragement and security of knowing that family and friends are concerned and interested in his getting well. He also will need to be reoriented since his memory will be "blank" for the time immediately before and during unconsciousness.

Death of the patient

Many patients die without regaining consciousness. When this happens, members of the family often need emotional support, since they are not only upset emotionally but also may be worn out physically. If the patient has been unconscious for some time, the sudden release of the tension of "not knowing" may cause some people to respond inappropriately. If this happens, they should be assured privacy and be protected from the embarrassment of having others aware of this reaction.

REFERENCES AND SELECTED READINGS*

1 Best, Charles H., and Taylor, Norman B.: The Physiological Basis of Medical Practice, ed. 5, Baltimore, 1950, Williams & Wilkins Co.

2 *de Gutiérrez-Mahoney, C. G., and Carini, Esta: Neurological and Neurosurgical Nursing, ed. 3, St. Louis, 1960, The C. V. Mosby Co.

3 *Fuerst, Elinor V., and Wolff, LuVerne: Fundamentals of Nursing, ed. 2, Philadelphia, 1959, J. B. Lippincott Co.

4 MacBryde, Cyril Mitchell: Signs and Symptoms, ed. 2, Philadelphia, 1952, J. B. Lippincott Co.

5 Meyers, Emma Mary: Nursing the Comatose Patient, Am. J. Nursing **54**:716-718, June 1954.

6 *Richardson, Henry: Patients Have Families, New York, 1945, Commonwealth Fund, Harvard University Press.

7 *Trowbridge, L., and Trowbridge, W.: Measures Used in Controlling Central Hyperthermia, Am. J. Nursing **53**:1092-1094, Sept. 1953.

---

*References preceded by an asterisk indicate material particularly well suited for student reading.

The patient with personality disorder

Chapter 10

Study questions for review

1 Study the behavior of several selected patients on your ward. What impression can you get about their mental health from observing their posture and facial appearance, their grooming, their bedside unit, and their relationships with other patients?
2 What provisions does your ward have for the safety of a patient who develops symptoms of mental illness? What is the policy of your hospital regarding care of such patients?

Patients with personality disorders are often encountered in the medical and surgical units of general hospitals. Many patients who are physically ill suffer from psychoneuroses; others may develop acute organic or toxic psychoses while undergoing medical or surgical treatment. Because their mental illness is either of short duration or does not require the facilities of a special hospital, the trend is toward housing these patients in the general hospital. Sometimes, patients who are mentally ill develop a medical or surgical condition that requires temporary care in a general hospital. For example, a mentally ill patient who fractures a bone in attempted suicide may need care on the surgical or orthopedic service of the general hospital. Many general hospitals have set aside a few rooms with special safety provisions to meet the particular needs of mentally disturbed patients.

Basic courses in personality development now offered in many schools help the nurse to understand the normal behavior of all her patients. However, she needs specialized help in caring for those with mental illness. If the hospital has a psychiatric division, it may be possible for the psychiatric nurses to consult with the medical and surgical nurses regarding the care of patients who are mentally ill. Since many hospitals do not have such experts available, however, nurses must depend largely upon their own knowledge and resources. When the nurse is assigned to care for patients with acute psychoses, she should refer to the many good textbooks on psychiatric nursing. The following pages contain only a brief discussion of a few important principles or guides to follow in caring for patients with mental illness.

THE PATIENT'S BEHAVIOR

The nurse who encounters a mentally ill patient for the first time may be truly unprepared for the behavior demonstrated. She has been accustomed, in her daily living and in her dealings with patients, to meeting persons who are able to face challenges to their security with a normal amount of assurance, thus keeping themsleves in harmonious association with others. In the hospital the patient is expected to repress his fears, irritations, and aggressive impulses and to be a "good patient." Because the "normal" patient has a reasonably well-integrated personality and because he anticipates a short stay in the hospital, he usually is able to live up to these expectations.

The patient with mental illness has a serious defect in his personality and usually is no longer able to live in relatively normal harmony with his human environment. Personality means more than that one has a "pleasing personality" or a "difficult personality"; it means more completely what a person does, feels, and is, either consciously or subconsciously, in all emotional interactions with others. When mental illness occurs, there is a breakdown in this mechanism of normal interaction to a point where the patient may be conspicuous among others. His behavior, therefore, is sometimes, although not always, very different from that of the nonpsychotic patient.

Man's entire life, from birth to death, consists of a continuous series of adjustments. The adjustment must be made in the face of definite biologic and emotional needs that cannot always be met, since man is a social being and depends upon acceptance by his social group for the feelings of security so essential to his personality integration. The person who has a mental illness has failed in his adjustment and has given up trying. He may have passively retreated into a dream world where the realities of living need not be faced, or he may be trying to protect himself from others by combative or other behavior.

Regardless of how they may appear to others, almost all mentally ill patients are lonely and afraid. They have strong feelings of inferiority and have lost the assurance and self-esteem derived from measuring oneself against the yardstick of one's associates and receiving a favorable report. A patient's efforts to augment his self-esteem may take the form of hostility toward authority and of general behavior that would be considered preposterous were it not viewed with the knowledge that it has some meaning for the patient. It is imperative for the nurse to realize that the patient's behavior, regardless of how bizarre it may appear, has meaning to him. Relatively minor deviations from "normal" behavior may be viewed with annoyance by nurses who do not realize this. Thus, the patient who worries about tests, talks endlessly about his operation with doctors, nurses, or anyone who will listen, and hesitates to sign his operative permit may be regarded as a "problem." Those giving him care may not realize, until the operation is over and the patient goes into an acute psychotic episode, that his behavior demonstrated a terrible fear that he could not verbalize as such and that was not recognized.

PERSONALITY DISORDERS

Organic and toxic psychoses. Organic psychoses are due to disease processes which have produced physical changes. Among the common causes of organic psychoses are neurologic syphilis, arteriosclerosis, and epilepsy with deterioration. Brain tumors, brain trauma, Huntington's chorea, and encephalitis are other examples of organic origins of mental illness.

Toxic reactions or *toxic delirium* may occur when high temperature is present or when toxins have accumulated in the body from disease (for example, nephritis). When such factors are the cause, the toxic reaction is called an endogenous one. When psychosis results from a reaction to drugs such as bromides, anesthetics, and alcohol, the cause is termed an exogenous one.

Toxic reactions are the most common of the psychoses seen in general hospitals. They usually come on suddenly and may disappear as quickly, particularly if the cause can be found and eliminated. Patients with toxic reactions almost always suffer from confusion, hallucinations, and delusions that usually cause fear. The environment is often misinterpreted, and the patient may try to escape from what he imagines is acute danger around him. This may lead to physical injury such as may be sustained from falling out of bed, removing drainage tubes, or falling from an open window. The patient may not be intent upon suicide but may destroy himself as he attempts to flee from imagined danger unless special precautions for his safety are taken. The patient with a toxic psychosis may attack hospital personnel in the belief that they are endangering his life. He acts quickly and impulsively and therefore should be watched most carefully. A good rule to follow is never to turn one's back on any mentally ill patient.

Alcoholism is fairly common in our society. Sometimes the patient does not give his doctor a true report of his habits in the use of alcohol, and he may develop delirium tremens while hospitalized for a medical or surgical condition. The patient who has taken large amounts of alcohol over a long period of time usually requires large doses of sedative drugs, and his tolerance to anesthetics is often extremely high. The patient who does not respond to preoperative medication or to anesthetics in the usual manner should be observed very carefully as he reacts from anesthesia. Signs of an acute alcoholic psychosis include tremor and hallucinations; the patient often imagines that he sees insects on the wall and that rats or mice are on his bed and perhaps biting him. Alcohol may be prescribed for these patients during their hospitalization. Close observation is necessary because the patient may be extremely resourceful in obtaining additional alcohol.

Functional psychoses. Functional psychoses have no demonstrable organic cause, though it is suspected that eventually one may be found. Classification of these diseases as distinct entities is no longer the practice in many psychiatric clinics since many patients have a mixture of reactions. The most common functional disturbance is *dementia praecox*, or *schizophrenia,* which accounts for almost a third of all admissions to mental hospitals.[14] Schizophrenia is a very serious mental illness requiring skilled and intensive psychotherapy. The patient with a medical or surgical condition who develops the acute symptoms of this psychosis is usually transferred to special psychiatric facilities as soon as his physical condition permits.

Manic-depressive psychoses are characterized by marked swings from a state of euphoria (feeling of well-being) and elation to one of depression. These swings are much beyond those experienced in varying degrees by normal people. Some patients have only the elation; others, only the depression. During periods of elation the patient is manic in his activity and his reactions; he flits quickly from one thing to another, and it may be impossible to capture his attention for more than a moment. During the stage of depression he feels tired and is dejected in his posture, his facial expression, his gait, and his verbal reactions. He loses interest in his physical surroundings and his personal appearance; his appetite is poor and constipation may develop. During this stage the patient may mention and often contemplates suicide. Patients with manic-depressive psychoses have a fairly good prognosis for recovery from an attack, but attacks tend to recur. If the nurse knows that the patient has a history of the disease, she should be alert for early signs of either phase, since mental health is taxed by physical illness.

Psychoneuroses. The psychoneuroses differ from the psychoses in that the patient suffering from a psychoneurosis conforms to social standards and is able to appreciate the rights of others. He is oriented as to time and place. Psychoneurosis is the most common of all mental illnesses and affects a very large number of persons who seek medical care. In psychoneurosis the emotional problem is predominant and is the one that is really important to the patient, even though he may have physical disease which may or may not be related to his basic emotional disturbance. The patient has failed to make a satisfactory emotional adjustment in bringing his desires into a satisfactory compromise with social demands. He seeks to escape from his problem in the development of psychoneurotic behavior which may seem implausible to others but which offers a satisfactory escape for him, or the best escape he is able to achieve without treatment. He is less upset by his symptoms than would be expected. Even when extensive diagnostic procedures and surgery are performed, he is usually surprisingly philosophic about the whole experience.

There are many types of psychoneuroses. *Anxiety states* are common. The patient may have an abnormal fear of impending disaster, and this fear may be expressed in bodily signs such as flushing, tachycardia, and excessive perspiration. A word or two picked out of a statement made by his physician may serve as a basis for worries and fears which are only temporarily relieved by rational explanation. *Hysteria* is another form of psychoneurosis and has been recognized for centuries. The patient may not be able to move a particular limb, may have areas of numbness, may have convulsions (however, he never injures himself as may be true of the patient with epilepsy or other organic disease who has a convulsion), or may have a large variety of other complaints.

Hypochondrial reactions constitute another type of neurosis. In this form there is an abnormal concern and preoccupation with body function. *Obsessive* and *compulsive neuroses* are those in which the patient is compelled to follow certain rituals or behavior patterns which are far beyond the normal but which in some way serve to relieve inner tensions. For example, it is normal for many persons to count fence posts as they walk down the road; however, it becomes a compulsion neurosis when a person cannot ever walk down a road without counting and touching each post. Ritualistic compulsions in such matters as bathing, handwashing, and dressing in certain sequence are common and, even when carried to great extremes, may sometimes be successfully concealed from the outside world.

Patients with psychoneuroses are seen most often in general hospitals. This is because their behavior, although exasperating to the physician and to all who must help them solve their health problems, is seldom such that care in a mental hospital is necessary. It is probable, however, that the economic cost to society of this group of patients is greater than the cost for all the psychoses combined.[14] Psychoneurotic patients are large consumers of medical care and all related services. Just because the patient is suffering from a psychoneurosis does not mean that he may not also have a physical ailment, and it is the possibility of both conditions being present that makes management very difficult.

The nurse or anyone else caring for psychoneurotic patients should not assume that these patients are willfully sick. Unfortunately they are too often considered problems by members of the staff who lack the insight to recognize their need to be ill. The patient does feel real pain and discomfort even though no physical cause may be found.

The patient with a psychoneurosis requires infinite patience and understandstanding. He also needs careful, firm, and studied management. Usually he has told his physical symptoms endless times to numerous people and has worn out his welcome with all. The nurse should listen attentively for a reasonable time and should then try to direct the patient's conversation away from discussion of himself. She must not be trapped into implying that she thinks there is nothing wrong with the patient, and it is well to avoid discussion of any medical subject. Occupational therapy which can be undertaken at the bedside is often very beneficial in slanting conversation away from the patient and may also result in creative activity that earns recognition for him.

The nurse should watch for any attempts the patient may make to aggravate his physical ailment or to produce symptoms. So great may be his need to maintain an acceptable outlet for his problems through illness that he may go to surprising length to delay a cure. Patients have been known to drink hot water before an oral temperature is taken, tamper with their wounds in order to produce infection, deliberately take toxic drugs, and even to subject themselves to needless operations. The nurse, however, must never under any circumstances assume that the patient is attempting to prolong illness; such an assumption will be harmful to the patient. If suspicions that the patient is making deliberate attempts to delay his recovery are confirmed, it is important that the patient not be told of this directly. To tell him would only embarrass him, increase his insecurity, perhaps cause him to find a new and less satisfactory outlet for his tensions, and delay any progress he may have made toward overcoming his psychoneurosis. Help of a psychiatrist is advisable.

GENERAL PRINCIPLES OF NURSING CARE

Care of the mentally ill patient on medical and surgical units places special responsibilities upon the nurse. She is largely responsible for the patient's safety and physical care, she must observe his behavior closely and record her observations carefully, and she must modify nursing procedures to fit the individual patient.

Physical care. When a patient in a general hospital becomes mentally ill, there is a tendency to become overconcerned with his behavior and to neglect his physical needs. It must be remembered that the patient needs good general nursing care, including mouth care, attention to *cleanliness,* and *good grooming.* Dressings must be changed and medications given. For some time before hospitalization the depressed patient may have eaten too little or improperly. He may refuse to eat, or he may hide his food to give the impression that he has eaten. The hyperactive patient may be too busy, frightened, or preoccupied to eat, yet he may require more than the usual amount of food. A careful record of *food* and *fluid intake* should be kept on all patients with mental illness. A record of *urinary* and *bowel elimination* is also necessary; the patient who is depressed often suffers from constipation, and the hyperactive patient may delay going to the bathroom because of his many preoccupations.

Medications are often refused by the mentally ill patient, who may be exceedingly clever at concealing the drugs not swallowed. Pills should be crushed and dissolved unless their bitter taste precludes this, because otherwise they can easily be held in the back of the mouth for some time and then expelled. Such a patient finds it much more difficult to retain fluids in his mouth if the nurse remains to see that he takes several swallows of water after the medication. Serious problems in giving medications by mouth must be reported to the physician so that he may order a more effective route.

Sleep is necessary for the mentally ill patient but is sometimes hard to achieve. Plenty of sleep and good general physical health make it easier for him to face his problems and attempt to solve them. Patients with acute mental illness may require large doses of sedatives or tranquilizers and even these do not always succeed in producing sleep. Exercise outdoors, a quiet environment, a backrub or warm bath, and warm drinks are often surprisingly helpful.

Prevention of suicide or other injury requires alert attention on the part of the nurse. Pocketknives, objects such as nail files, razor blades, and all other pieces of equipment that might be used either impulsively or with premeditation must be removed. If the patient is known to be suffering from mental illness, such belongings should be removed on admission, as is done in mental hospitals; otherwise, this must be done as inconspicuously as possible. If windows can be raised enough so that the patient could crawl through them, they must be equipped with "stop" devices to prevent complete opening, and occasionally protection over the glass is necessary. Doors must be fitted with locks that cannot be turned from the inside. Electric fixtures must be out of reach of the patient who might attempt to electrocute himself by tampering with the socket or who might injure himself with glass from bulbs or shades.

The physician is responsible for ordering constant observation if this is necessary because of the danger of suicide or of injury to others. The order, if issued, must be carried out to the letter. The newspapers bear testimony to many instances of patients leaping from windows or otherwise destroying themselves in the few brief moments when the nurse's back was turned. A decrease in the patient's tension should not cause relaxed vigilance since decision on a plan of action may be its cause. The patient may resent constant observation; he may believe that he is being spied upon or that he is in danger from the observer. The least conspicuous way to observe a patient is by observing him in a group, but this may not be feasible on the medical and surgical unit because of the patient's other illness. The nurse may appear to busy herself with a patient in an adjoining room while watching the mentally ill patient; sometimes locating the observer outside the patient's room may cause the least annoyance.

It is not true that persons who talk about suicide rarely attempt it. Studies have shown that at least a third of those committing suicide talked about it. Mention of suicide intent by the patient should be taken calmly by the nurse but should be reported to the physician at once and recorded in the nurse's notes. It is exceedingly important that the nurse not answer the patient in a way that appears to dare him to carry out his threat. Such a comment as "I know you don't mean that" leaves the patient with little choice but to carry out his threat to prove the seriousness of his statement.

Patients with personality disorders may have decreased sensation or may be so occupied with their activities and their thoughts that they are oblivious to pain. They may, for example, lean against a hot radiator and sustain a severe burn or step into a tubful of very hot water without flinching. They must be protected from injuries that would normally be avoided by the well person.

Observations and recording. The nurse's notes are very important in the care of the mentally ill patient. She is around the patient longer than any other professional person, and she may be the only one who observes him during evening and night hours. Her recorded observations can be of great help to the psychiatrist in his management of the patient. These notes should be remarkable for their quality rather than their length, but it is best to err on the side of length rather than of brevity. They should contain actual expressions of the patient, using quotation marks and taking care that the words recorded are exactly those of the patient. Notes should be recorded immediately after significant conversation or behavior has been noted, so that details will be fresh in mind. The specialty of psychiatry has a complete vocabulary of its own. For example, hallucinations refer to false sensory perceptions; delusions, to fixed false beliefs. Rather than to label the symptoms of the patient, it is better to write factual statements, such as "States over and over, 'I see men at the window, they are wearing red, they have come to kill me.' " The nurse's notes should also contain detailed accounts of what the patient does, such as "Sat at the window grimacing and smiling for two and one-half hours this P.M.," "Keeps saying as he smiles, 'I'll be dead tomorrow'."

Management of behavior. The patient with mental illness benefits from calmness, consistency, and uniformity in his environment. Procedures should be explained to him calmly, and sometimes repeatedly, even though he may not appear attentive or concerned. Even the smallest details of necessary medical or surgical treatment should be explained before they are undertaken. The equipment used for procedures should be reduced to a minimum, but basic principles, such as aseptic technique used in changing dressings, should not differ from those used in good nursing anywhere. The patient must also be prepared for routine nursing measures; e.g., when lights are to be turned out, a meal is to be presented, or a visit to the bathroom is to be made, the patient should be told what is going to occur.

Anything that increases the patient's anxiety may be harmful to him. Use of of technical language and discussion of disease and technical procedures should be avoided. Subjects that appear to increase the patient's anxiety should be carefully noted, and mention of these should be made in the nurse's notes. Religion is commonly associated with anxiety or feeling of guilt. Sexual maladjustment is common in those who are mentally ill. Mention of close members of the family may produce anxiety; often the final failure in interpersonal relationships occurs in the family setting, among those whose acceptance was most valued by the patient. It is safest to let the patient volunteer the information he wishes. If he divulges personal information, the nurse must let him know that his confidences will be kept and that his disclosures, regardless of their nature, do not lessen her opinion of him. It is impossible to tell anyone how to respond to a mentally ill patient; indeed, no written words could ever transmit this skill which can be mastered only through practice. Certainly calmness and matter-of-factness combined with a genuine interest in the patient and in trying to help him are positive qualities for the nurse to develop.

At all times, the nurse must avoid the temptation to develop a personal relationship with the patient. Her position is that of a nurse, or a friend in the professional sense, of one who is interested and willing to listen and to help. She cannot take the place of the patient's family and she should realize this. The patient may hope that she can replace his emotional attachments to his family as he gropes for relationships that are satisfying and yet not too demanding. The inexperienced nurse may encounter serious difficulties and do real harm to the patient if she does not seek help from those with more experience when patients become too dependent upon her.

It is useless to argue with the mentally ill person or to attempt to talk him out of his delusions by reasoning with him. He has lost the ability to understand the psychotic nature of his ideas or to see the fallacies in them. No attempt should be made to explain the patient's behavior to him. This belongs in the realm of psychotherapy. Very often the patient's behavior reflects his reactions to a life situation which has become unbearable, and by drawing his attention to this the nurse may lose her effectiveness in helping to bring about his improvement. She must never let the patient know that she knows anything about any past mental illness or his present problems; if she does let him know, the usefulness of her relationship with the patient will be destroyed.

Reassurance, in the general sense, should be avoided. Simply telling the patient that he is not going to die or that he is worthy of his family may do more harm than good, since it may destroy a picture of himself that it is necessary for him to have at the moment. Reassurance, however, used in the sense of producing a calm, quiet, accepting environment is always of value. The patient should feel that he can behave largely as he wishes without fear of censure or rejection. He should be given security by assurance of consistency of routine, of the conduct of others toward him, and of the limitations that are placed upon him. He may gain reassurance from consistency in the way in which he is encouraged to express negative feelings. He may show such feelings by disliking the nurse, for example. He may dislike the nurse without the fear of retaliation that would be present if he disliked his wife or any other close member of the family. Thus, hostility toward personnel may be a healthy sign and should be accepted as such by the nurse. Effort should be made to have the patient feel that his behavior is understood, even though it may not be approved. The right of the patient to want to behave as he does is acknowledged. For example, the patient may have the right to want to hurl his water pitcher, but he should know that the staff will continue to prevent him from harming himself or others.

Restraints should be avoided if possible since anxiety is almost always increased by any kind of physical restraint, and real panic may be caused their use. For this reason, psychiatrists usually try to control agitated patients by such means as warm baths, isolation in a quiet room, and drugs and resort to physical restraints only if the patient's life or the lives of those around him are in danger. If restraints have been ordered and are to be used, it is imperative that enough help be available to carry the procedure through quickly once it has been started. In the general hospital a quick effective restraint can be made by two persons holding a drawsheet at opposite corners and twirling it to form a soft rope. This procedure should never be performed in the presence of the patient.

REFERENCES AND SELECTED READINGS*

1 *Cohen, Sidney, and Klein, Hazel: The Delirious Patient, Am. J. Nursing **58**:685-687, May 1958.
2 Faddis, Margene O., and Hayman, J. M.: Care of the Medical Patient, New York, 1952, McGraw-Hill Book Co., Inc.
3 *Fernandez, Theresa: How to Deal With Overt Aggression, Am. J. Nursing **59**:658-660, May 1959.
4 *Godek, Isabelle: 3 Keys to Significant Behavior, Am. J. Nursing **59**:1564-1565, Nov. 1959.
5 Golin, Milton: Robber of Five Million Brains, J.A.M.A. **167**:1496-1503, July 19, 1958.
6 Karnosh, Louis J., and Mereness, Dorothy: Psychiatry for Nurses, ed. 5, St. Louis, 1958, The C. V. Mosby Co.
7 *Lemkau, Paul V.: Followup Services for Psychiatric Patients, Nursing Outlook **6**:149-150, March 1958.
8 Mann, Marty: New Primer on Alcoholism, New York, 1958, National Council on Alcoholism, Inc.
9 *Matheney, Ruth V., and Topalis, Mary: Psychiatric Nursing, ed. 2, St. Louis, 1957, The C. V. Mosby Co.
10 *McCarthy, Raymond: Alcoholism, Am. J. Nursing **59**:203-205, Feb. 1959.
11 Peplau, Hildegard E.: Interpersonal Relations in Nursing, New York, 1952, G. P. Putnam's Sons.
12 *Quiros, Alyce: Adjusting Nursing Techniques to the Treatment of Alcoholic Patients, Nursing Outlook **5**:276-279, May 1957.
13 Steele, Katherine McLean, and Manfreda, Marguerite Lucy: Psychiatric Nursing, ed. 5, Philadelphia, 1955, F. A. Davis Co.
14 Strecker, Edward A.: Basic Psychiatry, New York, 1952, Random House, Inc.
15 Ulett, George A., and Goodrich, D. Wells: A Synopsis of Contemporary Psychiatry, St. Louis, 1956, The C. V. Mosby Co.

*References preceded by an asterisk indicate material particularly well suited for student reading.

Study questions for review

1. What is a normal white blood count? Distinguish between the various types of white blood cells. What is the normal proportion of each? What are the main functions of the polymorphonuclear leukocytes?
2. In disease what is the significance of a leukocytosis? Of a leukopenia? Study the laboratory findings of a patient on your ward who is (or has been) acutely ill; compare repeated white blood count reports. What circumstances or treatments appear to have contributed to these changes?
3. Review the physical care necessary for the acutely ill patient who has a high temperature.
4. Consult your notes on fundamentals of nursing, and review the principles that apply when changing sterile dressings.

The body's reaction to injury and disease

Chapter 11

Injury and disease of the body may be caused by external or internal factors. The external causes may be physical, resulting from mechanical trauma such as surgery or accident, exposure to extreme heat or cold, or radiation, or they may be chemical such as those caused by the ingestion of poisons or by excesses or deficiencies in the diet. Living organisms (bacteria, viruses, or parasites) or foreign inanimate material (such as foreign proteins, which cause allergies) may enter the body.

Internal causes may be classified as those due to the normal aging process of the body cells, constitutional anomalies (patent ductus arteriosus, coarctation of the aorta), glandular deficiencies (diabetes mellitus and hypothyroidism), psychosomatic factors (such as may cause the development of a peptic ulcer), and changes of tissue structure or function resulting from a previous disease. The latter may prepare the way for the development of another disease; for instance, the scar following the healing of a duodenal ulcer may cause pyloric obstruction.

When the causes are known, disease and injury can often be prevented. It is easier to prevent a disease than to cure it, and the additional factors of loss of time from work or school, emotional and psychological trauma, financial problems, and residual disabilities are major socioeconomic considerations. The nurse should take an active role in teaching accident and disease prevention in school, industry, home, clinic, and hospital.

EXTERNAL DEFENSES

Skin. The skin is the first line of defense against injury and disease. It is not only very effective in preventing bacteria from entering the body, but it also protects the body from some external forces such as heat or cold. The normal acid secretion of the skin (pH 5.5) tends to inhibit the growth of disease-producing microorganisms, and bacteria which are normally present on the skin (resident bacteria) are usually nonpathogenic. Staphylococci are the exception. Of the transient organisms, only the bacilli causing anthrax and tularemia are able to live or multiply in the acid flora of the skin. If the skin is not broken, and if the glands secrete normally, pathogenic bacteria cannot enter the body through the skin to produce disease. Resident bacteria, however, are present on the skin in great numbers and penetrate the hair follicles and the glands. Because perspiration continuously brings bacteria out onto the skin, scrubbing with soap and water removes surface bacteria but cannot remove all bacteria. The skin, therefore, can never be considered sterile (free from all organisms). For this reason, even though the hands are thoroughly scrubbed, the surgeon wears gloves to prevent contamination of the wound when performing an operation. Preoperatively, the patient's skin is scrubbed in an attempt to mechanically remove most of the bacteria, and the hair to which bacteria may cling is shaved. The use of a skin disinfectant, hexachlorophene in soap (pHisoderm or pHisoHex), is now advocated for scrubbing the skin because of its long-lasting bacteriostatic effect. The additional precautions of cleansing the skin with ether, painting it with a disinfectant such as benzalkonium chloride, and of using sterile instruments minimize the possibility of introducing bacteria into the body when the incision is made.

Mucous membrane. The eyes, including the conjunctivas, are protected from the entrance of bacteria and particles of dirt by the lavage action of the tears. Tears also have the ability to destroy some microorganisms.

The vaginal secretions contain lactic acid which usually destroys all pathogenic bacteria that enter the vagina. Frequent vaginal irrigations should not be given because they wash away these protective secretions. Bacteria are also carried away by the menstrual flow. Since these secretions are not present in children, vaginitis from various organisms is a fairly common disease among very young girls.

The mucous membranes of the nose and mouth normally contain many pathogenic bacteria such as streptococci and pneumococci. These organisms normally are not harmful. They cannot be removed by mouth rinses, gargles, or irrigations. Bacteria that enter through the mouth usually are washed back into the throat by saliva and are swallowed into the stomach where they are destroyed by the gastric juices. When giving mouth care to a delirious or unconscious patient, care should be taken that the patient does not bite the nurse's hand, since pathogenic bacteria from the mouth, when introduced into the soft tissues, may cause an extremely virulent infection. Human bites should be treated immediately with thorough cleansing and antibiotics.

Respiratory system. Bacteria that are inhaled into the nose are usually blocked by the cilia in the anterior nasal passages. If they succeed in passing through this barrier, the mucous secretions of the nose move the bacteria back into the nasal pharynx, where they are swallowed and destroyed by gastric juices. If these bacteria are aspirated into the lungs instead, the movement of the cilia and mucous secretions normally propel them forward into the pharynx where they are expectorated or swallowed into the stomach. To prevent the spread of bacteria from the nose and throat, people are taught to cover the nose and mouth when sneezing or coughing and to blow the nose and expectorate into disposable handkerchiefs. A dry, double-thickness mask worn over the nose and mouth helps to decrease the spread of bacteria to others. Therefore, when there is known respiratory disease, a dry mask worn by the patient may prevent contamination of others. Masks are worn in the operating room to decrease the possibility of introducing pathogenic organisms from the nose and throat into wounds.

Gastrointestinal tract. Most of the organisms entering the bowel are destroyed by the proteolytic enzymes. *Escherichia coli,* although normally present in the bowel, frequently cause infections of the urethra and bladder, especially in women. Therefore, after a bowel movement, the anus should be cleansed away from the vagina and urethra. Under normal conditions there are also organisms in the anterior urethra, but unless they are very virulent, massive in numbers, or enter a bladder containing residual urine, they will be washed out with the urine on voiding.

If the hands are not washed after using the toilet, bacteria that exist in or pass through the bowel or urethra may be transmitted to eating utensils or food. Pathogenic organisms sometimes found in the rectum are the typhoid and paratyphoid bacilli, the virus causing infectious hepatitis, *Bacillus welchii* which causes gas gangrene, and *Entamoeba histolytica,* which causes amebic dysentery. All employees of food establishments are required to have physical examinations, including stool specimens, before employment to determine whether they have an infectious disease or are carrying infectious organisms. The employer is responsible for instructing them in proper hygienic measures and for providing approved toilet and hand-washing facilities. Eating utensils must be thoroughly washed after use in restaurants. All restaurant kitchens and meat-handling establishments are inspected regularly by community health officers in an attempt to decrease the spread of infectious diseases.

Natural defenses in prevention of external causes of disease. The best prevention against the invasion of disease-producing bacteria is the maintenance of health and nutrition, the practice of good hygienic measures, and the avoidance of exposure to people with known infections. Although people are continuously exposed to an environment in which there are many organisms, most of these are nonpathogenic, and the bacteria that are normally harbored in the body do no harm. When the skin is broken, the glands stop secreting, there is exposure to an excessive number of virulent organisms, or the resistance is low owing to debilitation, malnourishment, or being overtired, disease generally occurs.

INTERNAL DEFENSES

When body tissue is injured by trauma or invaded by bacteria, a local reaction called *inflammation* occurs. This inflammatory reaction is caused by the body's attempt to localize the effects of the injury or the invading bacteria. There is first an accelerated blood flow to the site of injury or bacterial invasion and dilatation of the surrounding capillaries. The vasodilation is thought to be caused by a histamine-like substance which is liberated by the tissue as it is destroyed. As blood cells and serum escape into the tissues because of the increased permeability of the capillaries, the part becomes red, hot, and swollen. It is also painful because of the pressure of the increased intercellular fluid on nerve endings. Because of the swelling, loss of function in the part may develop. Redness, heat, swelling, and pain are called the cardinal signs of inflammation.

The increased blood flow brings with it polymorphonuclear leukocytes (neutrophils) which also are mobilized by the histaminic toxins of tissue destruction. These leukocytes ingest the bacteria (phagocytosis) at the site of the tissue damage. Having engulfed the dead bacteria and the dead tissue cells, they then carry them away through the blood and lymph streams. The inflammatory process subsides as the leukocytes remove the debris and as the blood, serum, and lymph are reabsorbed into the blood vessels and lymphatics.

If the bacteria are picked up by the lymph stream, which drains all the tissues and organs of the body, they will be carried to the nearest lymph node. These nodes are located along the course of all lymph channels, and here, too, bacteria can be ingested and destroyed. If the bacteria are strong enough to resist the action in the lymph nodes, leukocytes are brought in by the blood stream to attack and engulf the bacteria in the node. The node then becomes swollen and tender because of the accumulation of phagocytes, bacteria, and destroyed lymphoid tissue. This is known as *lymphadenitis.*

If the bacteria are picked up by or introduced into the blood stream, there are large phagocytic cells called *tissue macrophages* located along the course of the blood stream, in the spleen, liver, lungs, bone marrow, and adrenal glands which function similarly to lymph nodes and which will engulf and digest these blood-borne organisms as well as any dead cells or other foreign particles that may pass through the blood stream.

INFECTION

The external defenses are usually effective in preventing pathogenic bacteria from entering the body, and if they do gain admittance, the internal defenses usually prevent them from causing disease. However, the bacteria or their toxins may be strong (virulent) enough to destroy many leukocytes and tissue cells before they themselves are ingested and destroyed. On coming in contact with the leukocytes, certain pathogenic bacteria are able to destroy them by ingestion, to discourage their approach by the production of chemical substances which repel them, or to kill them with their toxins or poisons. These bacteria are then able to produce disease by destroying the tissues in which they are located or by causing a toxic reaction in the body. The toxins are soluble proteins which are rapidly carried by the blood and the lymph to organs and tissues which are especially susceptible to their action. For instance, the toxins from bacteria causing diphtheria choose tissues of the heart. Bacteria, themselves, also choose specific tissues to attack. Typhoid bacilli elect lymphoid tissue, the tubercle bacilli usually attack the tissues of the respiratory tract, and dysentery bacilli choose the gastrointestinal tract. This process by which bacteria enter the body and cause disease is called *infection.* The length of time it takes for the symptoms of the disease to appear after the bacteria have entered the body is called the *incubation period.* Infection is more likely to occur if the person is debilitated, tired, or malnourished so that organisms easily gain a foothold.

A local accumulation of dead phagocytes, dead bacteria and their chemicals, and dead tissue may occur and is called *pus.* The bacteria most commonly causing this reaction are the staphylococci found on the skin and the streptococci normally found in the mouth and nose. Pus that is localized by a zone of inflamed tissue is called an *abscess.* Pus that spreads in sheets into the surrounding tissue is called *cellulitis,* while that collecting in a pre-existing cavity such as the pleura, gallbladder, or appendix is called *empyema.* An infection that spreads along the tissues and ruptures onto the surface is called a *sinus.* If the infection opens onto two different surfaces and there is a communication between the two openings, it is called a *fistula.*

The systemic reaction to generalized infection and severe organic disturbances is a toxic condition which results from the absorption into the blood stream of products of tissue destruction and toxins from bacteria and viruses. The patient has a fever, a hot, dry skin, coated tongue, rapid pulse, general malaise, anorexia, and chills. Sweating and delirium may also occur. There is an increase in the white blood cell count and in the sedimentation rate of the red blood cells. The high temperature is thought to be an attempt by the body to destroy the circulating bacteria by stimulating an increase in white blood cells to engulf and digest the invading organisms. High temperatures or prolonged elevations may be lowered to safe levels by the administration of acetylsalicylic acid and by alcohol sponge baths; ice bags may be applied to the groins and axillas. Antibiotics are given to help the body fight the infection. When a severe infection is present and the body does not respond with fever, the prognosis may not be good since the natural body defenses are not being mobilized.

Most doctors advise that the patient with a temperature over 38° C. (100.4° F.) be kept in bed since the respiratory and pulse rates are increased. He is often, however, allowed bathroom privileges. Since there is a tendency to headache and irritability, the room should be kept quiet; the patient may wish his eyes shielded from bright light. He should be encouraged to sleep. A warm sponge bath, a back rub, and a smooth bed may relax him so that he will sleep. Frequent baths may be needed to keep the skin clean since many body wastes may be excreted through excessive perspiration. The mucous membranes of the nose and mouth may become dry, and crusts may form. To prevent this, the anterior nasal passages should be lightly lubricated with a vegetable oil, the teeth should be thoroughly cleansed three or four times a day, the lips should be lubricated with cold cream, and fluids should be given freely. Since the toxins are often excreted through the kidneys, the patient should be urged to take 3,000 ml. of fluid a day. The urinary output should be measured, for there always is danger of kidney damage. If fluids are being forced and the urine becomes concentrated or if there is less than 1,000 ml. voided daily, the doctor should be notified. The patient is usually kept in bed until the temperature has been normal for twenty-four hours. After fever he often feels weak, perspires on physical exertion, and easily becomes tired. For several days he should have extra rest and should eat foods high in caloric value. As the fever subsides, the patient will appreciate visitors, radio, television, reading, or other activities which help to pass the time.

The systemic reaction due to the absorption of toxins in the blood stream is called *toxemia.* If both bacteria and toxins are absorbed into the blood stream, the infection is called a *septicemia.* Pus in the blood stream is known as *pyemia.* Bacteria circulating in the blood stream may lodge at points distant to the original source of infection and cause a *secondary infection.* This is the process by which infections of the heart and kidneys usually occur.

TISSUE HEALING

Injury to tissue cells and inflammatory changes stimulate the regeneration of cells. This process begins after tissue debris has been removed. The new cells fill in the space left by the injury. They may be the normal structural cells, or they may be fibrotic tissue cells. Some body cells readily regenerate; for instance, after the bowel has healed, it is almost impossible to find the injured area. The respiratory tract also regenerates its tissues readily. Liver tissue and some nerves, however, are always replaced with fibrous tissue. If the inflammatory or infectious process is severe and if a large amount of tissue is destroyed, structural cells may not be replaced regardless of the type of tissue. Instead, fibrous tissue known as *scar tissue* fills in the gap. Some people, especially Negroes, are prone to excessive scar tissue formation. Such a tissue formation is known as a *keloid.* It may cause disfigurement and need to be surgically excised.

Instead of healing, there may be necrosis or death of the tissue, and if putrefaction occurs in the necrosed areas, the process is called *gangrene.* Serous membranes sometimes become adherent during inflammatory and healing processes. As the inflammation subsides, fibrous tissue forms; this is called an *adhesion* and commonly occurs in or about the intestinal tract, causing it to become obstructed.

When the wound edges are pulled together and the space caused by the tissue destruction is obliterated, *healing by first intention* occurs. This is the type of healing that usually occurs in a clean, incised wound that is sutured. The skin edges are glued together by shreads of fibrin, a thin layer of blood clot, and a crust of dry, protective plasma. Within three days fibroblasts multiply and grow across the gap while leukocytes, blood, and lymph continue to remove the debris. Collagen fibrils are then formed to replace the fibrin, and the injured area is quickly filled with granulation tissue composed of new capillaries, fibroblasts, and collagen fibers. Meanwhile, epithelial cells bridge the gap from each side of the wound. As the fibrous connective tissue increases in amount, shrinkage of the tissue occurs and the scar increases in strength. The rapidity with which this occurs is influenced by the maintenance of a good blood supply, adequate lymph drainage, a high protein diet, and a continuous supply of vitamin C. The care of clean wounds is discussed in more detail in Chapter 14.

When the wound is infected or when there is excessive loss of tissue and the skin edges cannot be brought together, healing by granulation tissue must occur—*healing by second intention.* This healing process is similar to that in healing by first intention, but takes longer since a larger area must be filled with granulation tissue. When there is infection, pus and dead tissue must first be removed before healing will occur. The area then fills in with soft, red, insensitive, granulation tissue which bleeds easily. It is composed of minute, thin-walled capillaries which are surrounded by cells that later form the fibrous connective tissue. The scar from healing by second intention is usually large and unattractive and, since it contains no nerve endings, it is numb. As the healing progresses, the scar tissue shrinks, and, if the injured area is large enough (such as following burns), contraction of surrounding tissue may occur and lead to malfunction and deformity of that part of the body.

Wound irrigation and packing. The nurse is often asked to irrigate or pack infected or gaping wounds. It is important that these wounds heal from the bottom since, if the skin and superficial layers of tissue heal first, a collection of pus may form in the unhealed space. When irrigating deep wounds or sinus tracts, a catheter is usually first placed as deep into the wound as possible; then, with an Asepto syringe, the irrigating fluid is instilled until the returns are clear. The doctor should be consulted as to the direction and depth the catheter should be inserted. This information should be recorded on the nursing care plan. In irrigating fistulas the fluid instilled in one opening should return from the other. The patient should be turned so that all the irrigating solution drains back, or the solution should be aspirated from the wound with an Asepto syringe, since fluid that is left in a deep wound becomes a culture medium for bacterial growth.

If the wound is to be packed, the packing also should be placed into the bottom of the wound cavity to prevent surface healing. Packs should be kept moist; if they become dry, they should be moistened with normal saline solution before being removed to prevent damage to the newly formed granulation tissue. Such tissue will ooze readily, and it should be handled gently. The doctor often trims this tissue with scissors to stimulate further healing; the patient feels no pain from this since there are no nerve endings.

Sodium hypochlorite solution, 0.45 per cent (modified Dakin's solution), often is used to irrigate or pack infected wounds. It is a powerful germicide and dissolves necrotic tissue, preparing the area for granulation. It is usually not used if sutures are still in place, since it may dissolve them. The skin around the wound should be protected with zinc oxide paste. Since Dakin's solution decomposes rapidly, it should be freshly made every forty-eight hours. Hydrogen peroxide solution may be ordered for the irrigation of infected wounds; it acts as a cleansing agent, removing organic debris. Its bactericidal action is limited in the presence of blood or pus. Antibiotic solutions and solutions containing proteolytic enzymes, such as *streptokinase* and *trypsin* which digest the necrotic tissue, may be instilled into the wound. Open wounds that are exposed frequently to the air may become infected with the air-borne bacteria *Bacillus pyocyaneus.* Their presence may be detected by the characteristic blue-green watery drainage. Such infected wounds are treated with irrigations and packs of acetic acid, 0.25 per cent.

IMMUNITY

When a patient has an acute infectious disease, he is usually very ill, and he may develop complications such as pneumonia, nephritis, pericarditis, and other secondary infections. These complications increase the length of convalescence and may leave the patient with residual disabilities. When bacteria are virulent enough or the patient's resistance is low, he may die as a result of the disease. However, in most instances he does recover, and after some infections such as typhoid fever, diphtheria, scarlet fever, smallpox, measles, whooping cough, mumps, and chickenpox, he may develop an immunity which will prevent his ever getting that particular disease again. This immunity occurs when, as a result of being exposed to the bacteria or its toxins, the reticuloendothelial system produces a chemical protein substance called an *antibody*. This substance is circulated in the blood plasma, and it becomes part of the globulin fraction of the plasma. This is called an *active immunity*. If the bacteria or their toxins ever again enter the body, the antibodies that were produced against these bacteria will make them clump together so that they cannot multiply or live, and they will render the toxin impotent. The phagocytic leukocytes will then be able to engulf the bacteria and carry them away. This action takes place in the tissues at the point of bacterial invasion and prevents the bacteria from entering the blood stream.

A *permanent* immunity against a particular kind of bacteria or a virus exists as long as the body continues to circulate antibodies against it in the blood stream. A permanent immunity may last a number of years or for the patient's lifetime. To prevent a person from getting an infectious disease such as typhoid fever or smallpox, the body can be artificially stimulated to produce antibodies against the causative organisms. This is done by injecting into the person a dose of dead bacteria suspended in saline solution. Typhoid bacilli, paratyphoid bacilli, and the bacteria causing whooping cough are injected after being killed by heat. The virus causing poliomyelitis is killed by exposure to a chemical, formalin, before being injected if the Salk vacine is used. The body can also be stimulated to produce certain antibodies by the injection of bacteria whose virulence has been decreased by heat, cold, or chemicals. This *attenuation* of the bacteria prohibits them from producing disease in the body but permits the body to manufacture antibodies against them. This is done in rabies immunization (the Pasteur treatment). The body will also manufacture antibodies against some more virulent bacteria and viruses if it is exposed to a less virulent form with similar characteristics. For instance, an injection of cowpox virus will produce an active immunity against the smallpox virus.

The procedure of injecting an infectious agent in one form or another into the body so that disease is not produced but so that antibodies can be built up is called *vaccination*. The fluid containing the organism is called a *vaccine*. It is used in the prevention of disease, not for treatment.

When the toxin secreted by the bacteria is dangerous, the body must be stimulated to produce *antitoxins* against it. This is done by injecting modified toxins from the organism. For example, diphtheria toxoid usually is routinely given to babies to protect them against contracting diphtheria. Tetanus toxoid, staphylococcus toxoid, and scarlet fever (streptococcus) toxoid also are on the market. If a year has elapsed since the vaccination and the patient is exposed to the causative organisms, a booster dose of toxoid usually is given to ensure adequate protection. To maintain immunity, a booster dose is required at least every five years.

Although antibody stimulation against many bacteria or their toxins can be produced by immunization, this is a slow process and may take several months to become fully effective. Therefore, if the person has been exposed to an infectious disease or has the disease, he may be given an injection of an immune serum which will provide a *passive immunity;* this serum contains antibodies produced against the specific organism in the serum of other human beings, in horse serum, or sometimes in rabbit or bovine serum.

This immune serum is known as *antitoxin* and gives *temporary immunity* which lasts only one or two weeks; it does not stimulate antibody formation by the patient. Immune serums are available against the toxins of diphtheria and tetanus bacilli and the venom of snakes. Immune serum is also available for pneumococci, staphylococci, dysentery bacilli, and the influenza bacilli. For effectiveness, the patient must receive the serum early in the course of the disease before the bacteria or their toxins damage the body tissues. Antibiotic therapy is now being used instead of immune serum for pneumococcal and staphylococcal infections. Diphtheria antitoxin or tetanus antitoxin is administered to patients with diphtheria or tetanus to neutralize the toxins and to modify the course of the disease. The whole blood or serum of a patient who has recently recovered from either of these diseases also may be used to modify the course of these diseases. Immune serum is especially effective with measles, whooping cough, or scarlet fever. Immune serum globulin *(gamma globulin)* often is given to a child who has been exposed to measles, scarlet fever, or poliomyelitis since it tends to make the disease less severe. It may also be given to women who have been exposed to German measles in the first trimester of pregnancy since this disease often causes the baby to have congenital anomalies and to women who have been exposed to viral hepatitis in the third trimester of pregnancy since they are particularly susceptible to the disease at this time. In addition, it is given to men exposed to mumps in an effort to prevent the complication *orchitis* (inflammation of the testicle). Gamma globulin is the fraction of the plasma which is thought to contain the antibodies. It is obtained by pooling the plasma of a large number of normal people and injecting a small portion into the patient. The rationale is that someone among the donors will have had these diseases and will have developed antibodies against them. A temporary immunity is produced in the patient. A passive immunity against measles, smallpox, and diphtheria also is passed on to the newborn child by his mother through the placenta.

While a temporary passive immunity can be obtained by the use of immune serum, every person should be taught the advantages of acquiring an active immunity against the common and more virulent infections. Prevention by vaccination is easier and less costly than an attack of these diseases. The patient may have a slight febrile reaction, some backache, and general malaise for a day or two following a vaccination, but these effects quickly subside. Occasionally a patient will develop a severe local reaction, with redness, swelling, and tenderness about the site of the injection. This is treated with hot wet dressings. The United States Public Health Service recommends that all children be immunized against diphtheria, whooping cough, tetanus, smallpox, and poliomyelitis. Mothers should be encouraged to have their babies immunized since infectious diseases are particularly serious in the young child. The injections are started when the baby is 3 months old and are given monthly for three months. A vaccination against smallpox is then given and repeated before the child enters school. The cooperation of mothers in having their children immunized has practically eliminated diphtheria and smallpox from the American scene and has greatly reduced infant and child mortality.

HYPERSENSITIVITY

Some persons are sensitive to certain foreign proteins such as pollens, animal danders, and animal serums. Some are sensitive to substances such as house dust, cosmetics and an endless variety of commercial products. Some may also be sensitive to certain foods or to drugs. Such sensitivity is called an *allergy,* and the substances causing the allergic state are called *allergens.* Although allergies to specific substances are not inherited, the tendency toward hypersensitivity seems to run in families. When a person who

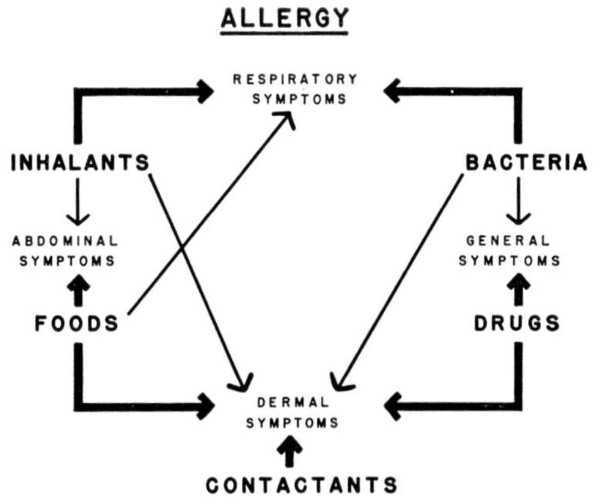

Figure 17

This diagram illustrates the causes of allergic responses and their relative severity. (Courtesy Dr. Paul F. deGara, New York, N. Y.)

has a tendency to become allergic first comes into contact with the specific allergen to which he is sensitive, antibodies are formed. When this allergen is again introduced into the body, the antibodies will combine with it, liberating histamine, and reactions such as sneezing, tearing of the eyes, watery discharge from the nose, wheezy breathing (asthma), skin eruptions, and urticaria may occur. (See Figure 17.) Nausea, vomiting, and diarrhea may also be allergic reactions. Antihistaminic drugs such as epinephrine, Pyribenzamine, Benadryl, and Chlor-Trimeton may provide temporary symptomatic relief. Since these drugs have a tendency to produce drowsiness, persons who must drive motor vehicles or work around machinery should be instructed when to take these drugs and, with the doctor who prescribes the drug, should work out a suitable dosage if drowsiness occurs. The patient usually can be desensitized by the administration of the allergen in graduated doses, beginning with minute amounts diluted with saline solution and gradually increasing the dosage and decreasing the time interval between doses.

The patient may be so sensitive to an allergen that its subcutaneous injection will cause a severe allergic reaction known as *anaphylactic shock.* The initial symptoms of anaphylactic shock are edema and itching about the site of the injection, apprehension, and sneezing. These mild reactions are followed rapidly by edema of the face, hands, and other parts of the body, asthma, cyanosis, and dyspnea, dilation of the pupils, rapid and weak pulse, and falling blood pressure, and death may follow in a few minutes. Epinephrine hydrochloride (Adrenalin) 1:1000, an antihistaminic drug, will counteract the effects if given immediately. The patient may need to be placed in the Trendelenburg position, and a general systemic stimulant such as caffeine sodium benzoate, or Coramine may be given in an attempt to elevate the blood pressure. He should be protected from biting his tongue by the insertion of a mouth gag between his back teeth. No patient who has received horse serum or an antigen of any type should leave the clinic or the doctor's office for at least twenty minutes, since an untoward reaction is most likely to occur during this interval. If any untoward symptoms occur, the patient should be seen by the doctor immediately.

In an effort to prevent anaphylactic shock, all patients should be questioned about sensitivity to drugs and to foreign proteins such as horse serum. People have been known to develop anaphylactic reaction to acetylsalicylic acid as it is absorbed into the blood stream. Therefore, this drug may not be as innocuous as many people think it is. Patients with a history of allergies are more likely to develop anaphylactic reactions than are those without such a history. Before any serum, such as horse, bovine or rabbit, is injected into the body, these patients should be tested for sensitivity. One skin test for sensitivity to serum consists of the injection of a small amount of serum (0.1 to 0.2 ml.) into the skin of the forearm (intradermal). A similar amount of saline solution is injected into the skin of the other forearm to serve as a control. A reaction to the serum is indicated by the appearance of a reddened, itching wheal or hive about the site of the serum injection within five to fifteen minutes. Another test for sensitivity to serum consists of the instillation of one drop of the diluted serum into the conjunctival sac. If the patient is sensitive to the serum, redness of the conjunctiva and a watery discharge will appear within ten to twenty minutes. Sensitivity to other antigens may be tested in a similar manner. These sensitivity tests are used on people who have allergic reactions such as urticaria, hay fever, and asthma to determine the substances to which they are sensitive.

SHOCK

Shock is a failure of the peripheral circulation, regardless of the causes or of the multiplicity of causes.[5] It may be caused by a variety of unrelated conditions such as severe infections, toxemia, anaphylaxis, severe dehydration, hyperinsulinism, severe physical or psychic trauma, massive hemorrhage, or loss of blood plasma such as occurs in burns. Severe cardiac disease may also produce symptoms of shock because of the inability of the heart to pump sufficient blood to the body.

Shock is sometimes classified as primary and secondary. Primary shock is a fleeting type caused by spinal anesthesia, operations on the sympathetic nervous system, and psychic trauma such as worry, fear, and emotional tension. Fainting is the commonest form. The symptoms are caused by sudden vasodilation of the blood vessels, especially the peripheral vessels, into which much of the circulating blood rushes; there is no actual loss of blood. The symptoms of primary shock are similar to those of shock due to any cause, but they appear suddenly and will readily disappear when the patient is placed in a recumbent position.

Secondary shock may be caused by a decrease in the total blood volume resulting from the loss of large quantities of whole blood or plasma from a traumatized area or from the loss of large quantities of plasma from the blood vessels into other body tissues owing to the immobilization or actual loss of electrolytes and extracellular fluid.[11] Some authorities believe that shock may be due to an increased permeability of the capillaries through which large quantities of plasma escape. This is thought to be caused by the liberation of a histamine-like toxin at the site of the injury and the circulation of this toxin through the blood stream.[13] Shock also may be caused by vasodilating drugs such as histamine and alcohol or by foreign proteins such as those causing anaphylactic shock.[11] Vasodilation caused by psychic trauma (primary shock is considered an important contributory factor of secondary shock.[13]

The treatment of shock is based on its cause. When there has been loss of fluid from the circulating blood, the venous return to the heart is slowed and the cardiac output is therefore decreased. A compensatory vasoconstriction due to the excretion of epinephrine by the adrenal glands maintains the blood pressure at a normal level for a short time; however, as fluid losses increase the vasoconstriction becomes ineffectual and the blood pressure drops markedly, decreasing the blood supply to vital body tissues. This leads to tissue anoxia, and, if it is allowed to persist, the shock becomes irreversible. The liver, kidneys, and nervous tissues tolerate a lack of oxygen for only a very short time before permanent tissue damage occurs. If the systolic pressure remains below 50 mm. Hg for long, the patient usually dies.[11] Therefore, one of the main aims in treating shock caused by fluid loss is to replace the fluid. If the loss is due to internal or external loss of blood or plasma, whole blood is the fluid of choice. Plasma or plasma substitutes such as albumin, dextran, or normal saline solution are sometimes used to maintain the blood volume until whole blood can be obtained. The blood is given in sufficient quantities and as fast as is safe to restore the systolic pressure to at least 80 mm. Hg.[11] Oxygen may be given by mask to increase the oxygen saturation of the blood and tissues. If the shock is due to electrolyte imbalance, appropriate fluids and electrolytes are given either intravenously or orally to restore the normal balance. When shock is caused by vasodilation, vasoconstricting drugs such as Neo-Synephrine or levarterenol bitartrate (Levophed) may be given, but they must not be used until blood volume has been restored. When shock is due to cardiac insufficiency, digitalis usually is administered.

Very young patients, elderly patients, and patients with cardiovascular diseases and metabolic disorders such as diabetes are more likely to develop shock following trauma, disease, or surgery than is a young, healthy adult.[11] A patient who has recently been on cortisone therapy may have a rapid onset of primary shock because the adrenals may have atrophied. These patients may be given cortisone intravenously. To prevent the occurrence of secondary shock following elective surgery the patient is prepared so that he is in the best physical and emotional state possible.

Typing and crossmatching of blood are done before surgery so that if blood is needed to combat shock, it will be available. An infusion is usually started in the operating room to keep the veins patent so that if blood is necessary, it can be easily administered.

Symptoms of secondary shock usually do not appear until it is well established. Restlessness, apprehension, coldness, and pallor may be the first noticeable symptoms. The blood pressure and pulse usually are within relatively normal limits for a short period as a result of the compensatory vasoconstrictive action. It is only by careful observation of the vital signs and the general physical appearance of the patient that early shock may be recognized and treatment started. In shock, regardless of the cause, the blood pressure drops below 100 mm. Hg, the pulse increases in rate and becomes weak and thready, the patient becomes extremely weak, and the skin is pale, cold, and covered with perspiration. As shock progresses, the respirations become rapid and shallow and the temperature becomes subnormal. The patient may be apprehensive and restless or he may become apathetic, indifferent, and finally unconscious.

The patient in shock should be kept quiet and warm, but he should have only enough covering to maintain his body heat. If he perspires, he is too warmly covered and the peripheral blood vessels have become dilated, dissipating the available blood to the surface vessels. Any movement of the patient in shock is contraindicated. All physical care, except for essentials such as using the bedpan and comfort measures such as washing the face and hands, should be omitted until the blood pressure stabilizes. The patient often is placed in the Trendelenburg position (a head-low position), since this increases the flow of blood to the vital organs. This position should be used only on a doctor's order, however, since elevation of the foot of the bed may increase bleeding in some instances, and it may cause the visceral organs to press against the diaphragm, thus inhibiting respirations. The patient should be kept flat until medical orders are received. Barbiturates may be needed to quiet the patient. His questions should be answered and all procedures explained in an attempt to decrease his anxiety. Since the relief of pain also decreases shock, morphine sulfate is often ordered; usually it is given by the doctor intravenously since subcutaneous injections may be ineffective because of the decreased circulation to the tissues. Repeated injections of any drug given subcutaneously during shock may cause symptoms of overdosage on the return of normal circulation. If the patient is receiving such drugs as levarterenol bitartrate (Levophed) by infusion, the nurse must take his blood pressure every 5 to 10 minutes so that rate of flow of the drug can be adjusted according to rise and fall of blood pressure. The site of injection should be watched for signs of infiltration because the drug can cause tissue necrosis.

HEMORRHAGE

Hemorrhage is a loss of blood from the body due to rupture or injury of a blood vessel, slipping of a ligature from a blood vessel postoperatively, erosion of a vessel by a drainage tube or tumor, or from some interference with the clotting mechanism of the blood such as occurs in hemophilia (a disease of males inherited through the mother). The patient may lose small amounts of blood over a long period of time, or he may lose a large amount of blood in a short period of time. The bleeding may be arterial (bright red and spurting), venous (continuous flow of dark red blood), or capillary (oozing). The blood may be expelled from any body orifice, from an incision, or from the site of an injury, or it may collect under the subcutaneous tissue as a tumor mass (hematoma) or in a body cavity such as the peritoneum.

Symptoms of massive hemorrhage, both internal and external, are apprehension, restlessness, thirst, paleness, cold moist skin, drop in blood pressure, increased pulse rate, subnormal temperature, and rapid respirations. As hemorrhage continues, the lips and conjunctivas become pale and the patient complains of spots before the eyes, ringing in the ears, and extreme weakness. If the hemorrhage is not controlled, death will occur.

The treatment of hemorrhage is to stop the flow of blood if possible and to replace the lost blood. When bleeding occurs, the vessel walls contract, narrowing the lumina of the vessels, and a clot forms over the end of the bleeding vessel. In arterial bleeding this clotting phenomenon is not possible until there has been enough blood loss to decrease the pressure of the blood circulating through the bleeding vessel. Pressure against the artery proximal to the bleeding point decreases the flow of blood through it and permits clotting to take place. Direct pressure at the site of the bleeding also decreases the blood flow and encourages clotting. This method is frequently used in superficial wounds, and a gelatin sponge (Gelfoam) also may be applied to help form the clot. The principle of direct pressure may also be used to control hemorrhage from esophageal varices and from the prostate. In the former, an esophageal balloon is inserted and then inflated until it compresses the bleeding vessels. In prostatic bleeding, a Foley catheter is inserted and the balloon inflated to compress bleeding vessels. Elevation of the part may decrease arterial bleeding. Cold applications are often used to control bleeding into tissues or internal bleeding, since the cold causes the small vessels to contract. In uterine hemorrhage, an ice bag may be applied to the abdomen over the uterus; in gastric hemorrhage, it may be placed over the epigastric region; and in hemorrhage from the lung, it is usually applied over the sternum. Very hot applications also control bleeding temporarily. This method is often used during an operation in which there is considerable vascular oozing. To control the bleeding permanently, large vessels usually have to be ligated, and smaller ones may be electrically cauterized. A ruptured organ such as the spleen may have to be removed to control bleeding. Removal of the spleen may also be necessary to control bleeding due to a blood dyscrasia such as idiopathic thrombocytopenic purpura. When the bleeding is caused by a prothrombin deficiency such as occurs in liver diseases in which hepatic ducts are obstructed or in biliary duct obstruction, vitamin K is given parenterally. Vitamin K cannot be manufactured in the intestinal tract to be absorbed into the blood without the presence of bile. Vitamin K may also be helpful in controlling hemorrhage following overdoses of Dicumarol.

Blood replacement usually is started before complete hemostasis has been accomplished, since the restoration of blood volume is imperative in preventing the occurrence of irreversible shock. The blood loss should be measured and immediately replaced. Dressings saturated with blood can be weighed, and blood in vomitus, both that which is bright red and that which is coffee-ground color, should be measured and the amount of loss reported to the doctor. If possible, tarry stools and bright blood discharged from the rectum should be measured; if this is not possible, the blood loss should be estimated. The doctor often will want to see such evidence of bleeding as bloody stools, vaginal clots, and bloody vomitus. Whole blood is given until the systolic pressure is between 85 and 100 mm. Hg, and it may be necessary to administer from 2,500 to 3,500 ml. of whole blood before this is accomplished. Blood plasma may be given until whole blood is available. The speed at which blood is given during this time depends upon the patient's condition. If the blood pressure is very low, the blood may be given very rapidly and may even be pumped in under pressure by the doctor.

The patient is usually very apprehensive during the course of the hemorrhage and because of the emergency measures that follow it. Every attempt should be made to keep him quiet, reassured, and comfortable. Barbiturates and morphine sulfate are often ordered as sedatives. Evidences of bleeding should be removed from the bedside, and stained linen and clothing should be replaced. Noise and excitement should be kept to a minimum, and all treatments and procedures such as frequent blood pressure readings, transfusion, restriction of food or fluids if this is necessary, and use of Trendelenburg position should be explained to the patient. The patient with a serious hemorrhage usually is given nothing to eat or drink until the hemorrhage is controlled since he may have to be taken to the operating room.

Transfusions. Before blood is given to the patient, a sample of his blood is drawn for typing and crossmatching. This blood is matched with blood of possible donors to see if they are compatible. If the bloods are compatible, the red blood cells do not clump together or agglutinate when the serum of the donor and the red cells of the recipient are mixed and vice versa. The blood also is tested for the Rh factor. Approximately 85 per cent of the population is Rh positive, which means that their blood contains agglutinins that will sensitize and later cause agglutination of the red cells of those persons (15 per cent of the population) who are Rh negative (who do not have these agglutinins).[2] The donor's blood also is tested for syphilis.

The administration of the blood transfusion is the responsibility of the physician, but the nurse gathers the equipment and prepares the patient. When the blood is ready, the label should be checked against the accompanying card by both the nurse and the doctor for name, type, and Rh factor. When the doctor is assured that the blood is intended for the patient, he will give it intravenously. This is an indirect blood transfusion. The patient's arm should be secured to an arm board, and it can be propped on a pillow if necessary to prevent muscle strain. The patient should be advised to rest quietly and not to move his arm. The nurse should check the flow of the blood frequently and should observe the patient for signs of possible reaction to the blood.

Transfusion reactions. Mild transfusion reactions (pyrogenic reactions) can occur as a result of improperly prepared anticoagulant (sodium citrate) or improperly cleaned tubing or needles. After the transfusion is received, the patient has a rise in temperature, headache, nausea and vomiting, weakness, and lumbar pain. These symptoms do not last, and the patient is treated symptomatically.

Allergic reactions to blood transfusions may occur and are due to a reaction of the patient to specific allergens contained in the donor's blood. Urticaria is the first symptom that usually appears. This may be followed by dyspnea and cyanosis. The transfusion should be discontinued at once if any of these symptoms occur. Epinephrine hydrochloride, 1:1000, will cause prompt disappearance of the symptoms. Benadryl or Pyribenzamine also may be ordered to relieve an allergic reaction.

The most serious reaction to blood transfusion is caused by giving the patient incompatible blood. When this is done, the donor's blood is agglutinated and dissolved (lysis) by the recipient's serum, and the product of this hemolysis is circulated throughout the blood stream. After he receives about 50 ml. of incompatible blood, the patient complains of fullness in the head, severe pain in the back, and a sensation of constriction in the chest. Nausea and vomiting may occur, the pulse becomes rapid, and the blood pressure drops. If the transfusion is discontinued at this point, the generalized symptoms will disappear, but a few hours later the urine will become red (port-wine urine) and will contain red blood cells and albumin; the urinary output will diminish. This kidney reaction is thought to be due to the release of a toxic substance from the hemolyzed blood. This causes a temporary vascular spasm in the kidneys, resulting in kidney damage and in blockage of the renal tubules by hemoglobin precipitating out in an acid urine.[13] If the patient is allowed to receive more than 100 ml. of the incompatible blood, irreversible shock with complete kidney failure will usually occur and death will follow.

If the patient has a transfusion reaction, the blood should be discontinued immediately. If the symptoms indicate that incompatible blood was given, epinephrine hydrochloride, 1:1000, is given at once and the urine rapidly alkalinized by an intravenous injection of sterile one-sixth molar sodium r-lactate solution. This minimizes the precipitation of hemoglobin in the kidneys. The patient may be treated with an artificial kidney for a few days to help the kidneys to recover. (See Chapter 21.)

SPECIFIC INJURIES AND INFECTIONS

Common wounds

An incision is the type of wound which the nurse in the hospital sees most often. However, when she is working in the emergency room, the outpatient department, the industrial health clinic, the school, or in the community, she may be called upon to care for patients with wounds that are sustained through injury. She needs to recognize the seriousness of various types of wounds, to know what emergency care to give, and to know when to advise the patient to seek medical attention.

An *incised wound* is one caused by a sharp, cutting object such as a knife, glass, or razor blade. Several layers of tissue are cut and the wound gapes apart. A *laceration* is similar to an incised wound except that it has jagged, rough edges. It may be caused by animal bites, wire, or machinery. Both of these wounds usually bleed profusely, and bleeding may have to be controlled by pressure over the wound or at pressure points. (See Chapter 15.)

A *puncture wound* is one caused by a sharp, pointed, narrow object such as a nail, pin, bullet, or splinter of wood. As the tissues are penetrated by the object, pathogenic organisms may be introduced. Since the skin quickly seals over and the wound rarely bleeds extensively, enough to wash these organisms out, a good medium for the growth of those bacteria that thrive without air (such as the bacilli causing tetanus) is created. This type of wound, therefore, should be made to bleed for several minutes by "milking" the vessels away from the heart. If the object was dirty or rusty, tetanus toxoid or antitoxin usually is given by the doctor. Any puncture wound should be watched for subsequent swelling, redness, or pain; if any of these symptoms occur, medical attention should be sought at once.

A *stab wound* is one caused by a sharp, cutting, pointed instrument such as a knife.[11] Deep tissues are usually penetrated, and the instrument may be plunged into a body cavity or into an organ. When a stab wound is of the chest, the instrument should never be removed unless a "sealing" dressing such as petroleum jelly gauze is available for immediate application; otherwise air may be drawn into the pleural cavity, causing a *pneumothorax* (collapse of the lung). (See Chapters 15 and 23 for further discussion.) All stab wounds require medical attention since they are deep and should be well débrided. If the injury has been on the trunk, the patient should be carefully examined and observed to determine whether an organ has been perforated.

A wound caused by a blunt force which breaks the skin and bruises the surrounding tissues is known as a *contusion.* There is hemorrhage into the tissue with a resultant *hematoma* (swelling caused by leakage of blood into the tissues). The immediate application of ice to the area and elevation of the injured part may reduce swelling due to superficial tissue bleeding.

Since all accidental wounds may be infected, they should be washed well with running water, soap and water, or an antiseptic such as hydrogen peroxide which bubbles up and helps to débride the wound. Excessive bleeding should be controlled. If wounds do not bleed, bleeding should be encouraged to help wash away bacteria. Patients with large or deep wounds should seek medical attention because sutures may be needed to prevent unsightly scarring. If a finger tip has been amputated, the amputated part should be brought to the doctor with the patient, since he may be able to suture it in place, and union may occur. For even minor wounds that have been caused by bites or by dirty or rusty material, the patient should seek medical attention. The wound may need to be surgically incised and drained. If there is any danger of its being infected with *Clostridium tetani,* tetanus toxoid or antitoxin is given. *Clostridium tetani* is especially likely to be present in areas where there are horses since they permanently carry the organism in their intestinal tracts. It may also be present in any soil since this organism can survive for years in soil or dirt. If the tissue around wounds becomes reddened, swollen, or painful, medical attention should be sought since these are symptoms of infection.

Wound complications

Staphylococcic infections. Wounds are most often infected by staphylococci. Both the pathogenic strain *(Staphylococcus aureus A)* and the nonpathogenic strain *(Staphylococcus aureus B)* normally live in the mucous membranes of the nose, throat, hair follicles, and sweat glands of man. While most people have a high tolerance for these microorganisms, the very old, the very young, and those with metabolic disease, acute infections, wounds, or abrasions are very susceptible to staphylococcal infections. Although staphylococci are responsible for most suppurative infections of the skin, streptococci and enteric organisms also may infect wounds.

The incidence of serious staphylococcic infections in hospitals is increasing and poses one of the most difficult aspects of care of hospitalized patients today. In recent years, staphylococcic organisms have become increasingly resistant to antibiotic drugs; pathogenic strains appear to have become more virulent as many other organisms have been destroyed by modern antibiotic therapy. Personal contact with infected persons *within the hospital* is the most common means of spread. Staphylococci can be isolated from other patients and from staff members as well as from dust, hospital equipment such as blankets, pillows and mattresses, and the air. Many authorities feel that the best hope of controlling staphylococcal infection lies in strictest attention to good aseptic techniques and in a return to full use of all the precautions that were more carefully followed before so much reliance was placed upon antibiotic drugs. Stress is being placed on cleanliness. Hospital housekeeping is being examined for adequacy and for spread of dust. The nurse is primarily responsible for teaching other staff members and supervising good aseptic technique in matters such as handwashing, care and handling of linen and of all other hospital equipment that may be active in transfer of infection. Patients with active infection are isolated, with the strictest medical asepsis being observed, and hospital personnel are now having nose and/or throat cultures; those who are carriers of staphyloccocci should not be in contact with patients.

When the staphylococci are implanted in susceptible tissues, the body defenses attempt to ward them off or eradicate them. Unless body defense mechanisms overcome the infection quickly, the staphylococci produce coagulase and certain toxins which destroy tissue cells and phagocytes and which cause a dense, hard fibrinous wall to surround the infected area. This wall protects the staphylococci from body defenses, allowing the infection to spread to adjacent tissues, and necrosis of tissue develops. The degeneration and liquefaction of the cells in the zone of inflammation results in abscess formation.

Local infections caused by pathogenic staphylococci are usually treated by hot soaks, incision and drainage of the abscess, and the administration of antibiotics. Surgical incision of the abscess is necessary since antistaphylococcal drugs are less effective in the presence of pus. If the infection is allowed to progress without adequate treatment, necrosis of soft tissues may occur, underlying bone may become infected, the lymph nodes may become involved, and generalized bacteremia may occur and cause death. (Treatment of infected wounds by packing and by irrigation has been discussed under tissue healing.)

Tetanus. Tetanus, or lockjaw, is an infectious disease caused by the gram-positive, anaerobic, spore-forming bacteria, *Clostridium tetani.* These bacteria are normal inhabitants of the intestinal tracts of men and animals, and they can survive for years in soil and dirt. They are introduced into the blood stream of human beings through wounds. They produce a powerful toxin which, by its action on neuromuscular end organs, causes maintained muscular contractions. This toxin also travels through the blood and lymph streams to the central nervous system.[4]

The symptoms of tetanus appear from four days to four weeks after the introduction of the bacteria into a wound. The patient first notices stiffness of the jaws, and then he develops difficulty in opening his mouth. He complains of rigidity of the facial and sternocleidomastoid muscles which become hypertonic and cause stiffness of the neck and spasm of the facial muscles which produces the characteristic sardonic smile *(risus sardonicus).* The abdominal and lumbar muscles also become rigid, and opisthotonos (arching of the back) occurs. Painful muscle spasms may occur upon the slightest stimulation (a draft, jarring the bed, or touching the bedclothes). Death may occur as a result of spasm of the respiratory muscles, or the cause of death may not be apparent.[4]

Even with rigorous treatment, about 50 per cent of patients with tetanus die. Prophylaxis is the only sure treatment. Everyone who is likely to sustain injuries that are contaminated with soil should receive tetanus immunization. Children, farmers, artisans, and military personnel should all be immunized.[4] It is recommended that children and adults be immunized against tetanus by three subcutaneous injections of 0.5 ml. of fluid toxoid at three to four week intervals or two injections of 0.5 ml. of alum precipitate toxoid four to six weeks apart. Another injection of 0.5 ml. of either toxoid should be given six months to one year later and every four years thereafter. If the patient follows this plan and sustains an injury he would only require a booster injection to protect him against tetanus infection. If he has not received a booster dose within five years, he may be given both 1,500 units of tetanus antitoxin and 0.5 ml. of fluid toxoid.[4] Before tetanus antitoxin is given, the patient must have a skin test for sensitivity to horse serum. If he is sensitive, the tetanus antitoxin is given in divided doses over a longer period of time, or he may be given a bovine serum.

Once tetanus has developed, treatment is directed toward neutralizing the toxin with large intravenous doses of tetanus antitoxin. The area around the wound is infiltrated with tetanus antitoxin, and then it is widely excised and débrided, flooded with zinc peroxide, and left open. Prevention of muscle spasms limits the spread of the toxin; therefore, the patient should be kept in a warm, quiet, darkened room removed from external stimuli. If bedclothes or pajamas cause spasm, they should not be used, and the patient should not be disturbed during the acute stage of tetanus for such routine nursing measures as bathing and bedmaking. He should be protected from injuring himself during muscle spasms by padded side rails on the bed and a padded headboard. If possible, a mouth gag should be inserted between the back teeth to prevent biting of the tongue; no attempt should be made to pry the jaws apart, however. The muscle spasms also may be controlled by the administration of sedatives which may be given by infusions containing barbiturates or by giving Avertin, curare, chloral hydrate, or paraldehyde by rectum. A temporary tracheotomy may be necessary to prevent respiratory difficulty due to laryngeal spasm. The fluid and caloric intake must be maintained to prevent electrolyte imbalance. It may be necessary to give intravenous feedings because of the dysphagia. A high caloric, fluid diet sometimes is tolerated without ill effects; a nasal catheter may be used for feeding if it does not cause spasm of the throat muscles. Penicillin is given in massive doses to combat concomitant infection. The nurse must observe the patient at least every half hour, and it may be necessary for him to be attended at all times. He should be observed for signs of respiratory distress, and the type and length of all the muscle spasms should be recorded. Any change in his condition should be reported to the physician.

Gas gangrene. Gas gangrene is a much feared wound infection that usually occurs following traumatic wounds in which there is damage to the muscle tissue. It is caused by *Clostridium welchii*, which is found in the intestinal tract of human beings and domestic animals. These bacteria are able to survive for indefinite periods of time in dust, dirt, and clothing made of sheep's wool.

Gas gangrene is characterized by a rapid onset of pain and swelling in the infected area. These symptoms occur within seventy-two hours after the introduction of the Welch's bacilli into the wound. The patient becomes prostrated with extreme weakness, exhaustion, and pallor, the pulse and respirations become rapid, and the blood pressure falls. The temperature may be only slightly elevated. The infected area is extremely tender, and there may be gas bubbles within the wound and under the skin. A thin, brownish, odorous, watery discharge comes from the wound; this drainage contains large numbers of the bacteria. The involved muscle tissue is swollen, brick red, and necrotic, and the surrounding area at first is blanched and then may become a mottled purple. Because not all wounds containing gas bubbles are infected with gas gangrene, the diagnosis can be made only by culture of wound discharge or of the muscle tissue.

The treatment of gas gangrene consists of radical excision of the wound to remove necrosed tissue, dirt, and debris, packing of the wound with zinc peroxide dressings, and administration of large doses of antibiotics. Gas gangrene antiserum also is available. Since precautions must be taken to prevent the spread of the infection to the wounds of other patients, the patient should be isolated, his soiled dressings burned, and any instruments used for wound care washed and sterilized immediately after use. Sterilization should be with steam under pressure for twenty minutes. If this is impossible, fractional sterilization should be used.[11] Soiled linen also should be autoclaved or fractionally sterilized before it is sent to the laundry. The policy of the hospital may demand that the nurse wear protective gowns and gloves while caring for the patient to prevent contamination of the clothing and hands since the organisms may easily be carried to other wounds. If gown and gloves are not used, the nurse should be careful that she does not contaminate her uniform with drainage from the wound, and all dressings should be handled with instruments. Whether or not gloves are used, the hands should be well scrubbed with soap and water after caring for the patient or his belongings. Anyone with hangnails or open wounds on the hands should not care for a patient with gas gangrene.

The patient is usually very ill but very alert and aware of the seriousness of his condition.[4] He requires constant supportive nursing care to keep him comfortable and as free from pain and apprehension as possible. Care also must be taken to prevent complications due to prolonged bed rest. (See Chapter 14.) Gas gangrene, fortunately, is less prevalent and less serious since the advent of antibiotic therapy.

Infections of the hand. Infections of the hand occur frequently because the hands are functionally involved in most activities and thus are likely to be injured or infected. Since these injuries and infections are usually painful, they incapacitate the patient so that he is unable to work, and thus cause loss of time and money. Most patients with infections of the hand are treated in an industrial health clinic, in the outpatient department of a hospital, or in the doctor's office. The nurse should become familiar with some of the more common types of infections of the hand so that she may teach patients how to prevent them and how to give prescribed treatment at home.

A *paronychia* is an infection involving the soft tissues around and underneath the nail. It usually results from the infection of a hangnail. The involved finger is very painful, and the patient complains of a continuous throbbing sensation in it. The pain is immediately relieved by lifting the soft tissues away from the nail with a scalpel and draining the pus from under the tissues. The patient then usually is given an antibiotic, instructed to soak his finger in warm sterile saline solution for fifteen to twenty minutes several times a day, and told not to use his hand.

A *felon* is an infection that involves the soft tissue of the finger tip. It often is caused by staphylococci which are introduced into the finger usually by a pinprick. Pins from babies' diapers are commonly contaminated with pathogenic organisms. The finger tip becomes swollen and painful, and a throbbing sensation may prevent sleep. In the early stages the infection responds to antibiotics and warm soaks. If it is allowed to progress untreated, however, the swelling may cause obstruction of the arterial blood supply to the soft tissues of the finger, and necrosis of the tissue and underlying bone may occur. The infected area will then have to be surgically incised and drained and the necrotic tissue excised. Felons sometimes can be prevented by making pinpricks bleed. A pricked finger should be carefully watched; if swelling or pain develop, the patient should seek immediate medical treatment.

Infection of the tendon sheath on the palmar surface of the hand usually follows puncture wounds of the fingers or hand. Streptococci are the organisms that most often cause the infection. The hand becomes red and swollen along the tendon, and movement is very painful. This kind of infection usually responds to early treatment with antibiotics and hot soaks, but surgical incision and drainage may be necessary. Untreated infections of the tendon sheath lead to destruction of the tendon, with resulting finger and hand deformities. If the tendon has been damaged, a tendon graft to correct deformities may be necessary after healing has occurred.

Lymphangitis and lymphadenitis. Lymphangitis is an inflammation of the lymphatic vessels. It is usually of streptococcal origin and is a sequela of other infections of the legs, feet, hands, or palms. The first symptom is a red, tender streak under the skin of the leg or forearm. This is an important symptom, since it warns that the local infection is spreading; unless it is controlled, septicemia may presently occur. The lymph nodes above the infection (in the knee, groin, elbow, or axilla) rapidly become swollen and tender as the infectious organisms invade them. This condition is known as lymphadenitis. If the infection continues uncontrolled, chills, fever, malaise, and increase in the pulse rate occur. Infections of the lymph channels are treated by drainage of the original infection, antibiotics, hot wet dressings, and rest.

Furuncles and carbuncles. A furuncle, or a boil, is a circumscribed, suppurative, inflammatory lesion of the skin and its immediate subcutaneous tissue.[4] A carbuncle is a furuncle with multiple foci infection. It occurs in thick inelastic skin, such as that on the neck, and spreads into the deeper layers of fibrous tissue.[4] Both furuncles and carbuncles are caused by *Staphylococcus aureus.* Furuncles are likely to occur on the face, neck, forearms, groins, and legs, while carbuncles are usually limited to the nape of the neck and the back. The infection usually begins as a small pustule at the base of a hair follicle or, in the case of carbuncles, at the base of several hair follicles. Local swelling and redness soon occur, and there is some pain in the area. Within three to five days the boil becomes elevated or "points up," the surrounding skin becoming shiny, and the center or "core" turns yellow. A carbuncle has several "cores." The boil will usually rupture spontaneously and, as drainage occurs, the pain is immediately relieved. The drainage soon changes from a yellow, purulent material to a serosanguineous discharge. All drainage usually subsides within a few hours to a few days,[4] and the redness and swelling gradually subside.

As the boil drains, care must be taken to keep the infected drainage off the surrounding skin, or *furunculosis* (multiple boils) may occur because of secondary infection. Although hot wet dressings are used to help bring the boil "to a head," the patient should be warned to discontinue them as soon as drainage starts since they tend to macerate the skin, making it easily infected. The patient should also be cautioned to keep his hands away from the draining area to prevent spread of the infection.

To prevent infections such as boils from developing, patients should be advised not to traumatize the skin by manipulating pimples with their hands and advised to keep the skin free of oil and dirt by thorough washing with mild soap and water. Local irritations and pimples should be treated with hot wet dressings—not by squeezing or picking. It is especially dangerous to manipulate infected areas about the nose and lips, since the blood supply from these parts drains directly into the venous sinuses in the head. The infection may spread to these sinuses, causing meningitis.

Ulcerations. An ulcer is a superficial loss of skin due to death of cells. It may be caused by infection, second-degree burns, or an inadequate blood supply to the part. If the ulcer does not become secondarily infected, it will heal by granulation tissue. Because of their location, however, skin ulcers usually become infected with staphyloccocci or streptococci and require extensive treatment with both systemic and local antibiotics. Saline dressings, bed rest, and elevation of the part usually are prescribed. If the ulcer does not heal, as often occurs in arteriosclerotic diseases or varicose veins, a skin graft may be necessary to close the area. The treatment of arteriosclerotic and varicose ulcers is discussed more fully in Chapter 19.

Home care of common infections

Since patients often ask the nurse for advice on minor infections involving the superficial tissues, she must be able to recognize the more common infections and to know when medical attention is indicated. She will also often be asked to give patients instructions on applying hot dressings, soaking the hands and feet, providing rest for the part by splinting or elevating with a sling or pillows. Sterile normal saline solution is most often used for hot dressings and soaks to open wounds. The patient can make this in the home by adding 8 ml. (2 teaspoons) of table salt to each quart of water and boiling the solution for ten minutes. It must be allowed to cool until it can be used without danger of causing a burn.

If hot wet dressings are to be applied, the area covered by the dressing should be lubricated with petroleum jelly to prevent burns. Sterile dressings are placed in the solution and wrung out with forceps, eyebrow tweezers, or two sticks. These should be boiled before the initial use and the instruments should be stored in a jar containing 70 per cent alcohol or benzalkonium chloride. If sterile dressings are not available, the dressing material can be boiled with the solution. Unsterile hot dressings can be prepared by immersing a bath towel in hot water and wringing it out. Heat will be maintained for longer periods if the wet dressing is covered with a piece of plastic and flannel. A hot-water bottle may also be placed over the dressing to maintain the heat. The length of time hot dressings are to be kept in place will be determined by the doctor, but twenty minutes to half an hour, four times a day, is the usual time.

If hot soaks are being used, a basin large enough to immerse the part completely should be obtained. If the soak is to an open wound, the basin and solution should be sterile. Soaking is usually ordered for fifteen to twenty minutes, three or four times a day. Soaks are often done with the dressing left in place. However, outside layers of the dressing should be removed. The wound usually is redressed after the soak.

Rest for a finger is often accomplished by wrapping it in a bulky dressing. This prevents bending of the joints. A *splint* may sometimes be made by placing a tongue blade under the finger before applying the dressing. If the wound is on the finger tip, a splint of this type is helpful in preventing accidental trauma. *Slings* are frequently used to provide elevation and rest for an infected finger or hand. A large handkerchief or a triangle of muslin will serve as a sling. The sling should be applied so that the hand is supported with only the tip of the little finger showing, and it should be tied so that the hand is elevated above the elbow. In order to prevent pressure sores, care must be taken to avoid knotting the sling over the spinous processes. Elevation of arms or legs on pillows should be done according to the principles of good body mechanics, making sure that the part is in proper body alignment and is supported along the entire length of the limb. Care should be taken that drainage of the vessels is not impeded rather than enhanced by the position.

If the infection involves the leg or foot, the patient may not be able to be up and about to care for himself and a family member may need to be taught to prepare the dressings or soaks. However, if no such assistance is available, the patient may be admitted to the hospital. The nurse should discuss plans for home care with the patient and consult the doctor if home care seems inadvisable.

REFERENCES AND SELECTED READINGS*

1 *Adams, Ralph: Prevention of Infections in Hospitals, Am. J. Nursing **58**:344-348, March 1958.

2 Carter, Charles F., and Smith, Alice L.: Microbiology and Pathology, St. Louis, 1953, The C. V. Mosby Co.

3 *Caswell, H. Taylor: Staphylococcal Infection Among Hospital Personnel, Am. J. Nursing **58**:822-823, June 1958.

4 Cecil, Russell L., and Loeb, Robert F. (editors): A Textbook of Medicine, ed. 10, Philadelphia, 1959, W. B. Saunders Co.

5 Davis, Loyal (editor): Christopher's Textbook of Surgery, ed. 6, Philadelphia, 1956, W. B. Saunders Co.

6 Eliason, Eldridge L., Ferguson, L. Kraeer, and Sholtis, Lillian A.: Surgical Nursing, Philadelphia, 1950, J. B. Lippincott Co.

7 Elman, Robert: Surgical Care, A Practical Physiologic Guide, New York, 1951, Appleton-Century-Crofts, Inc.

8 Emerson, Charles Phillips, and Bragdon, Jane Sherburn: Essentials of Medicine, ed. 18, Philadelphia, 1959, J. B. Lippincott Co.

9 Fuerst, Elinor V., and Wolff, LuVerne: Fun-

*References preceded by an asterisk indicate material particularly well suited for student reading.

damentals of Nursing, ed. 2, Philadelphia, 1959, J. B. Lippincott Co.

10 Haggerty, Robert J.: Levarterenol for Shock, Am. J. Nursing **58**:1243-1244, Sept. 1958.

11 Harmer, Bertha, and Henderson, Virginia: Textbook of the Principles and Practice of Nursing, New York, 1955, The Macmillan Co.

12 Hicks, Mary L., and Cannell, Ina June: Decubitus Ulcers, Am. J. Nursing **58**:1243, July, 1958.

13 Ilgenfritz, Hugh C.: Preoperative and Postoperative Care of Surgical Patients, St. Louis, 1948, The C. V. Mosby Co.

14 Lam, Conrad R.: What is "Shock"? Am. J. Nursing **51**:116-117, Feb. 1951.

15 *Landrum, Faye L.: Nursing in an Allergist's Office, Am. J. Nursing **58**:677-678, May 1958.

16 Moseley, H. F.: Textbook of Surgery, St. Louis, 1956, The C. V. Mosby Co.

17 Miller, Joseph M.: The Proteolytic Enzymes, Am. J. Nursing **58**:1410-1412, Oct. 1958.

18 *Prout, Harry C.: Modern Concept of Surgical Shock, Am. J. Nursing **58**:78-79, Jan. 1958.

19 *Sister Mary: Open Injuries of the Hand—Nursing Care, Am. J. Nursing **52**:1106-1107, Sept. 1952.

20 *Thompson, LaVerne: Staphylococcus Aureus, Am. J. Nursing **58**:1098-1100, Aug. 1958.

21 Thompson, LaVerne: Viruses—Old and New, Am. J. Nursing **59**:345-351, March 1959.

22 U. S. Department of Health, Education, and Welfare: Staphylococcal Disease—Selected Materials on Nursing Aspects, Atlanta, 1960, Communicable Disease Center, U. S. Public Health Service.

23 *Wilson, Judson D.: Open Injuries of the Hand, Am. J. Nursing **52**:1104-1106, Sept. 1952.

Preoperative care

Chapter 12

Study questions for review

1 What general reactions do you believe you would have if told that you must have an immediate operation? Have you observed these reactions in any close member of your family? If so, describe them.
2 What general physical deficiencies can you identify that might necessitate delay of an operation?
3 What are safe and effective ways to cleanse the skin? Can the skin be made sterile?

The purpose of care during the preoperative period is to prepare the patient, both physically and psychologically, to withstand the effects of anesthesia and surgery. The time allowed for this preparation depends upon the condition of the patient and the type of operation to be performed. It may be very short, or it may extend into weeks. The physician is primarily responsible for this preparation, but he relies upon the nurse for much assistance and delegates certain responsibilities to her. She can contribute substantially to the patient's physical and emotional welfare and can influence the progress and outcome of the preoperative period. She should study the doctor's orders for preparation for surgery and be certain she has the necessary knowledge before she carries them out. She must use sound judgment and carry out these orders in such a way as to provide the greatest possible comfort and safety to the patient.

SOCIOPSYCHOLOGIC PREPARATION FOR SURGERY

Preparation for hospital admission

Preparation for surgery should begin as soon as the doctor has decided that an operation is necessary. The doctor tells the patient and his family that the operation is necessary and explains why it must be performed, what will be done, and what the probable outcome will be. He discusses cost, duration of hospitalization, length of absence from work, and disabilities or residual effects that may be expected. An appointment for admission to the hospital is then made. The date for admission is influenced by the acuteness of the patient's illness and by the amount of time the patient requires to make necessary arrangements regarding his family, financial matters, and work.

The nurse must know what information has been given to the patient so that she can answer his questions intelligently and can begin the preoperative instructions. Many patients hesitate to ask the physician to repeat information and are often too upset to understand all they have been told or to ask questions. Thus they frequently turn to the nurse for clarification and reinforcement of such information. The nurse may also be questioned about the surgeon's competence, the number of people she has seen recover from a similar operation, and about the hospital. She can answer these questions in such a way that the patient acquires confidence in the surgeon, the nursing staff, the hospital, and the outcome of the operation.

The patient needs to know when to arrive at the hospital, where to go, and what information to give. The admitting clerk will ask about his employment, insurance, and hospital plans. He should know that the business office can help him make arrangements for paying his bill and that he can consult social service about family, financial, and convalescent problems.

He should be told what toilet articles and clothing to bring with him. He will be interested in knowing the visiting hours and how his family may contact him. He should be encouraged to think through any problems that may arise and to plan for them.

Preoperative instruction

The patient and his family should also be informed about the preparation he will undergo in the hospital before surgery is performed. The responsibility for giving preoperative instructions to the patient is primarily that of the nurse who cares for him in the hospital. However, the nurses in the outpatient department, doctor's office, and public health agency also share this responsibility and should tell the patient as much as they can about the preoperative period. The patient and his family should be told how extensive the preoperative preparation will be and approximately how long it will take. The purpose of the physical examination, roentgenography, and other tests should be explained to them. The patient should be told about the preoperative enema, medications, and shave and why foods and fluids will be withheld. He should know if he will wake up in a recovery room, if an oxygen tent is to be used, and if intravenous fluids will be given. He should be instructed in any special exercises that he must do postoperatively, such as coughing, contracting and relaxing the leg muscles, deep breathing, and turning. He should know the reasons for the frequent blood pressure readings and other special observations and treatments. Patients and their families are more frightened by what they do not know or by the unexpected than by what is planned with them.

Sometimes when the patient is scheduled to remain in the hospital for only a few hours postoperatively, he and his family should be given instructions for postoperative care at home preoperatively while the patient is alert. These instructions often must be reviewed postoperatively.

Fear of surgery

Although patients may or may not express it, almost all of them have some fear of surgery. It can be a fear of the unknown, or it can be a fear based on something they have heard friends or relatives say about their operative experiences. They may have had personal contact with someone who died as a result of an operation. They may be afraid of the diagnosis. They may have fears about anesthesia, pain, disfigurement, or disability. The older patient often worries about becoming a burden to his family.

The nurse may be able to help the patient talk about his fears. She should be with him as much as possible and give him every opportunity to ask questions. If staffing conditions permit, the same nurse should be assigned to care for the patient in order to develop a good patient-nurse relationship. The nurse can keep the patient and his family well informed and explain each procedure and examination. She can inspire confidence in the nursing staff by a competent manner. If it is desirable, she can make arrangements for the patient to talk with other patients who have successfully recovered from similar operations. She can explain to the family the need for them to visit the patient frequently to show him that he is wanted and loved. Very often the patient has great confidence in his spiritual adviser and gains much comfort from speaking with him. If the patient wishes, the nurse can make arrangements for a visit from the hospital chaplain. If the patient shows signs of apprehension or depression by crying, withdrawing from his visitors and other patients, refusing to eat, or not sleeping, the nurse should consult with the physician and with his help try to ascertain the cause of the patient's behavior.

OPERATIVE PERMIT

The patient will be asked to sign an operative permit before undergoing surgery. "The main purpose of this permit is to protect the physician and the hospital against claims of unauthorized operations and to guard the patient against unsanctioned surgery."[5] The patient should be made fully aware of the type of surgery to be performed. Permission should be obtained for each operation and for every procedure which involves entering a body cavity, such as a thoracentesis or a cystoscopy. Written permission is safest and should be witnessed by the nurse, physician, or other authorized personnel. In an emergency, the surgeon may operate without written permission of the patient or his family, although every effort is made to contact some family member. Consent in the form of a telegram or letter or by telephone is permissible. If the patient is a minor, permission must be obtained from either parent or from his legal guardian. The signature of the husband or wife of a married minor is acceptable. An emancipated minor, that is, one who is mature, married, reliable, and earning his own living, can sign his own operative permit.

The nurse is usually responsible for seeing that the operative permit is signed and attached to the patient's chart when he goes to the operating room. The signature should be obtained without pressure and before the patient is sedated. The patient may refuse to undergo an operation and it is his priviledge to do so.

PHYSICAL EXAMINATION AND PREPARATION FOR SURGERY

Both surgery and anesthetics produce changes in the body, and the patient must be in the best possible physical condition to withstand these changes. The heart and the circulatory, respiratory, and urinary systems are depressed by anesthetics and therefore are carefully evaluated before surgery is attempted. A history of the patient's past and present illnesses is obtained, and a complete physical examination, including laboratory tests, is made to ascertain the patient's physical status and to discover coexisting diseases. Routine roentgenograms of the chest are taken to be sure that the patient does not have tuberculosis or pneumonia, since these diseases are aggravated by anesthetics. The urine is examined to eliminate the possibility of urinary tract infections and diabetes mellitus, since these conditions may become increasingly troublesome in the postoperative period. Blood tests, such as a complete blood count and hemoglobin and bleeding and clotting time determinations, will help establish the presence of anemias or other blood dyscrasias which may interfere with wound healing and thus prolong convalescence. A blood sugar test is made to determine the presence of diabetes mellitus which, if present and untreated, may lead to such postoperative complications as delayed wound healing and infections. Electrocardiograms are taken on older patients since they are more likely to have cardiac diseases. When the preliminary examinations establish that there is a coexisting disease, a more intensive study is done. While it is not always possible to cure existing diseases before surgery, knowledge of their presence will influence the care given to the patient in the preoperative period, during the operation, and postoperatively. For instance, efforts are made to bring cardiac diseases and diabetes mellitus under control prior to surgery or general anesthesia. Patients with bronchiectasis or emphysema are frequently treated with aerosol inhalations and postural drainage of the lungs for several days preoperatively. The nurse must see that all treatments are carried out and that the patient is prepared for all tests. She should assist with the tests when necessary and see that they are completed and that the results are reported before the operation is scheduled.

Nutrition

The patient should be in the best possible nutritional state before undergoing surgery, for when he is malnourished and dehydrated, he is more prone to postoperative complications. Wounds heal more slowly, bedsores are more likely to occur, and there is less resistance to infection when there is protein deficiency. Hemorrhage may be caused by a deficiency of vitamin K, which is necessary in the production of prothrombin for blood clotting. A lack of vitamin C will retard wound healing. Excessive vomiting or diarrhea preoperatively will dehydrate the patient and cause electrolyte imbalance.

Every effort is made to correct nutritional deficiencies before surgery. A well-balanced diet will be ordered for the patient, and he may receive supplementary proteins and vitamins. When he cannot tolerate food by mouth, he will be given intravenous fluids containing glucose, proteins, vitamins, and salts. The nurse should make the patient aware of the importance of maintaining good nutrition and should encourage him to eat the proper foods. When he expresses likes and dislikes or does not eat well, the nurse can have the dietitian consult with him so that satisfactory adjustments can be made. The doctor may give the patient's family permission to bring in special foods that the patient particularly enjoys. The nurse should always know how well her patient is eating and should report to the physician any problems that may arise.

CARE OF THE PATIENT THE DAY BEFORE OPERATION

Preoperative orders

When the patient is ready for surgery, the physician will write orders for the immediate preoperative preparation. In many hospitals the writing of these orders cancels all previous orders. The nurse should consult with the physician at this time to see that the orders meet all the patient's needs. Care must be taken that orders for important treatments such as postural drainage or medications such as digitoxin and insulin are not inadvertently cancelled. After the physician tells the patient and his family that the operation is scheduled for the next day and gives them any other information that they may wish to have, the nurse may begin preparing the patient. She explains the procedures and treatments that will be done and supplements the information given to the patient by the doctor.

Diet

Unless the patient is on a special diet, he may have a regular meal the evening before the operation. If the operation is scheduled late the next day or is going to be done under local or spinal anesthesia, the patient may have a light breakfast and fluids up to six hours before the operation. If the operation is to be under general anesthesia on the following morning, fluids are permitted until midnight, and the patient is told that he must not take anything by mouth after this time since there is danger that he may vomit while under anesthesia and aspirate stomach contents into his lungs. If the patient's mouth becomes very dry while waiting for surgery, the nurse should give him mouth care. The patient is often given intravenous fluids during this period to maintain his fluid intake and to supply caloric needs. If the nurse discovers that the patient has taken food or fluids immediately before the operation, she should inform the surgeon. He will either pass a stomach tube to empty the stomach or will postpone the operation.

Preparation of the skin

Thorough cleansing of the skin surrounding the operative area helps to reduce the incidence of wound infection. Although the skin can never be made completely free of bacteria, it can be cleansed so that when the incision is made, there are few bacteria present. The skin is usually scrubbed with soap and water and then shaved. The cleansing agent most commonly used is green soap, but a detergent agent, hexachlorophene (G-11), has been found to be very effective and is thought to be superior to green soap. It has antibacterial properties which have a cumulative effect, and with a short scrub the skin can be made relatively germ free. PHisoderm, which is a mixture of hexachlorophene in a synthetic detergent, and Septisol, which is a mixture of hexachlorophene in soap, are often used. Neither rinsing with water nor drying will remove hexachlorophene from the skin; alcohol or ether (organic solvents) will remove it, however, and should not be used as a rinse.

Shaving the skin also reduces the incidence of wound infections because it removes the hair to which bacteria may cling. Extreme care must be taken that the skin is not cut during shaving, because cuts are open wounds which can become infected. An autoclaved razor and a new blade should be used on each patient since it is believed that viral hepatitis may be transmitted through razor cuts. The skin should be lubricated with soap, and the hair should be shaved in the direction that it grows. The nurse should teach all personnel who shave patients the correct technique and the importance of not cutting the skin. Occasionally doctors permit patients to shave themselves. The nurse should check to see that the preparation is adequate. Many surgeons prefer to have the skin preparation done in the operating room immediately after the patient has been anesthetized. The patient is thus spared this sometimes embarrassing procedure, and there is less risk of infection.

The surgeon will usually leave instructions on how large a skin area he wishes prepared. The area to be prepared will be more extensive than actually required for the incision. In other instances, the nurse prepares an area specified by hospital procedure for a particular operation. The following guide may be used in preparing the skin for specific operations.

Abdominal operations. If the patient is a woman, shave the skin from below the breasts to and including the pubic area; if the patient is a man, shave from the nipple line to and including the pubic area. Cleanse the umbilicus with soap and water and remove any material collected there.

Chest operations. Shave the skin on the affected side from the spine to beyond the midline of the anterior chest and from the clavicle to the umbilicus.

Radical mastectomy. Shave the skin from the spine on the affected side to beyond the midline anteriorly and from the clavicle to the umbilicus. The axilla and the arm on the affected side down to the elbow should also be shaved.

Rectal operations. Shave the skin within a 6 to 8 inch radius around the rectum.

Gynecologic operations. Shave the skin from the umbilicus to and including the pubic area and the perineum.

Kidney operations. Shave the skin on the affected side from the spine to beyond the midline anteriorly and from the nipple line to the pubic area.

Neck operations. Shave the skin from the chin to the nipple line and to the hairline of the face on both sides.

Head operations. The head is usually shaved in the operating room by the surgeon. Long hair should be saved and given to the patient or his family.

Other operations. Areas to be prepared for other operations will be specifically ordered by the surgeon. Operations for amputations and spinal surgery require preparation dependent upon the extent of the patient's disease and the preference of the surgeon.

Preparation of the bowel

An enema is given preoperatively so that the lower bowel will be free of feces. This prevents the possibility of fecal incontinence during the operation as a result of muscle relaxation following anesthesia. The preoperative enema also eliminates the need for the patient to have a bowel movement for several days after surgery. The enema should be effectual; if it is not, the doctor should be consulted and another enema may be ordered. If the enema is to be given until the returns are clear, the nurse should ask the doctor how many enemas he wishes the patient to have. Excessive enemas tire the patient and irritate the rectal and bowel mucosa. Rest periods between enemas are beneficial to the patient, and enemas given slowly may produce better results and thus reduce the number necessary.

Sedation

It is important that the patient rest the night before the operation. Barbiturates such as Seconal, Nembutal, Amytal, and phenobarbital are ordered for this purpose and are usually effective. They are given after all preoperative treatments have been completed. Barbiturates sometimes cause the patient to become confused, and it is advisable to put side rails on the bed, especially if the patient is elderly. Chloral hydrate is somtimes given to older patients to avoid the confusion caused by barbiturates. The nurse should instruct the patient to call her during the night instead of getting out of bed if he wishes something. She should observe the patient frequently during the night, and if he cannot sleep she should try to make him comfortable and spend as much time with him as possible. If a second barbiturate or any medication for pain is needed, it must be given at least four hours before the preoperative medication is due. This will avoid any respiratory depression caused by the cumulative effect of these drugs. If it is too late to give the patient medication safely and he is apprehensive or has pain, the doctor should be consulted. Unless the patient is scheduled for an operation early in the morning, he should be permitted to sleep and should not be disturbed by routine procedures.

CARE OF THE PATIENT ON THE OPERATIVE DAY

The activities of the nurse on the day of the operation center about the patient and his immediate needs. The nurse is chiefly concerned with observing the emotional state of the patient, checking his physical condition, safeguarding his belongings, and physically preparing him to receive anesthetics. She should visit him early and ascertain his emotional and physical status. Although the average patient may not express his fear, it probably exists. This fear may be allayed by explaining all procedures to the patient, and if the operation is to be delayed even for as short a time as one-half hour, the patient and his family should be so informed. The members of the family should be permitted to see the patient before the operation and stay with him if they wish. If the patient is very concerned about the operation and expresses fear about its outcome, the nurse should notify the physician. Patients who are extremely apprehensive tolerate surgery poorly, and the operation may have to be delayed or canceled.

The patient's temperature is taken and the nurse checks to see that it is within normal limits. If it is elevated, she should report this to the surgeon. She observes the patient's respirations, inspects his color and skin, and questions him about his health. Signs and symptoms of upper respiratory infections and expressions of new or different pain should be referred to the physician. Anesthetics and surgery aggravate such conditions and cause postoperative complications.

The patient should be given sufficient time to bathe, brush his teeth, and change to a hospital gown before he is called to the operating room. The woman patient is advised to braid her hair if it is long, and it can be secured with a bandana or towel to protect it from the anesthetic agents and from vomitus. Hair pins are removed because they may become dislodged and injure the patient's scalp and because they may cause sparks during administration of anesthetics. Since the nail beds are very sensitive to a lack of oxygen and some anesthetists check them for the presence of anoxia, the patient may be asked to remove nail polish. Religious medals or rosary beads taken to the operating room should be taped to the patient's wrist or secured to the bedpost. All jewelry and money should be taken from the bedside and locked up. The patient is permitted to wear a wedding ring, but it should be taped or tied securely to the hand.

Most anesthetists prefer that dentures and removable bridges be removed before the patient goes to the operating room, since, as the muscles relax under anesthesia, these prostheses may fall away from the gums and drop back into the pharynx, causing respiratory obstruction. The removal of dentures also prevents them from accidentally being broken when intubation is done. Dentures taken from the patient should immediately be put into a container in a safe place. If the patient is permitted to retain his dentures for the sake of appearance until he is in the operating room, the nurse who accompanies him there must see that they are removed. The nurse is responsible both to the patient and to the anesthetist for seeing that the dentures are removed and that they are protected against loss or breakage. Other prostheses, such as false limbs or eyes, should also be removed and placed in safekeeping.

The patient should void shortly before going to the operating room to prevent urinary incontinence due to muscle relaxation during the operation. An empty bladder permits the surgeon a better view of the abdominal cavity and decreases the chances of inadvertent injury to the bladder. Since restriction of fluids causes dehydration, the patient may not need to void immediately before surgery. Voiding during the preoperative night should be recorded, for this may help the nurse determine whether or not the patient who is unable to void immediately prior to surgery needs to be catheterized. Catheterization may be necessary if the patient has not voided. If the bladder must be kept collapsed throughout the operation, an indwelling catheter is inserted and attached by tubing to a collection bottle.

Preoperative medication

A preoperative medication is given to the patient to reduce reflex irritabilities caused by pain, fear, and increased metabolic rate. These reflex irritabilities make the induction of general anesthesia more difficult and decrease the effectiveness of the anesthetic agent. The preoperative medication also lessens the undesirable systemic action of the local anesthetic drugs. Examples of the medications given for these purposes are morphine sulfate, meperidine hydrochloride (Demerol), codeine sulfate, and the barbiturates such as soluble phenobarbital, and sodium Amytal.

Atropine sulfate and scopolamine are also given preoperatively. These drugs decrease the formation of mucous secretions and are used when ether and other mucus-producing anesthetic agents are to be administered. Atropine sulfate and scopolamine also depress the vagus nerve and thereby decrease circulatory and respiratory depression caused by surgical trauma.

The nurse must give the preoperative medications at the scheduled time, since the full effect of these respiratory depressant drugs must be obtained before anesthetics may safely be given. The opiates have their maximum effect one to one and one-half hours after administration. In the event that the nurse cannot or does not give the medication when ordered, she should notify the surgeon and/or the anesthetist. They may decide to omit the medication or to give it intravenously. The maximum effects of the drug given by this route are reached in three to five minutes. After the medication is given, the patient should be carefully observed for signs of respiratory or circulatory depression caused by a sensitivity to the drug or by an overdosage. Because opiates make the patient feel drowsy, lightheaded, and unsteady on his feet, he should stay in bed after they are administered. If atropine is given, the patient should be told to expect that his mouth will feel dry. The nurse should have completed all preoperative procedures before the medication is given. Rush, noise, and confusion should be avoided and the patient's environment should be kept quiet until he is taken to the operating room.

Charting

The preoperative charting should be accurate and complete. It is essential that the nurse chart the time the medication was given, the temperature, pulse, and respirations, the time the patient last voided, whether the dentures were removed, and any treatments that were done. The operative permit should be attached to the patient's chart. All laboratory tests should be reported and roentgenograms and charts of previous admissions should be available.

Transportation to the operating room

The patient is transported to the operating room in his bed or on a stretcher. He should be made comfortable and be protected from drafts. Cotton blankets should be used; woolen blankets must be removed because they are a source of static electricity. The bed or stretcher should be inspected ahead of time to see that it is freely movable. The stretcher must have straps to protect the patient from falling. If the bed is used, a name tag must be used so that the patient will be returned to his own bed postoperatively.

The patient should be accompanied to the operating room by a nurse with whom he is familiar. There should be a minimum of delay, noise, and physical disturbance. The nurse should remain with the patient until she is relieved by a member of the operating room staff, since the patient should not be left alone in this strange and sometimes frightening environment.

The patient's family

If members of the patient's family so desire, and if there are accommodations, they may wait in the hospital for the patient's return from the operating room. If they are going outside the hospital, it is wise for them to leave a telephone number where they can be reached, since the doctor usually wishes to speak to a member of the family following surgery. If the patient is to go to a recovery room, the family should be told; in any event they should be given some idea of when they might expect information about the patient or be allowed to visit him. They are usually less disturbed on seeing the patient postoperatively if they are told that he may be very groggy, and if they are warned that such things as an oxygen tent, a stomach tube, or an intravenous infusion may be used. The nurse should urge that only one member of the family visit the patient on the operative day.

REFERENCES AND SELECTED READINGS*

1 *Bird, Brian: Psychological Aspects of Preoperative and Postoperative Care, Am. J. Nursing **55**:685-687, June 1955.

2 *Cantor, Alfred J., and Foxe, Arthur N.: Psychosomatic Aspects of Surgery, New York, 1956, Grune & Stratton, Inc.

3 Elman, Robert: Surgical Care, A Practical Psychological Guide, New York, 1951, Appleton-Century-Crofts, Inc.

4 Harmer, Bertha, and Henderson, Virginia: Textbook of the Principles and Practice of Nursing, ed. 5, New York, 1955, The Macmillan Co.

5 Hayt, Emanuel, Hayt, Lillian R., and Groeschel, August H.: Law of Hospital, Physician, and Patient, New York, 1952, Hospital Textbook Co.

6 Ilgenfritz, Hugh C.: Preoperative and Postoperative Care of Surgical Patients, St. Louis, 1948, The C. V. Mosby Co.

7 Litin, Edward M.: Mental Reactions to Trauma and Hospitalization of the Aged, J.A.M.A. **162**:1522-1524, Dec. 22, 1956.

8 Van Schoick, Mildred R.: Emotional Factors in Surgical Nursing, Am. J. Nursing **46**:451-453, July 1946.

9 Wagner, D. H.: The Preparation and Care of Diabetic Patients Requiring Surgery, Surg. Clin. North America **39**:161-168, Feb. 1959.

*References preceded by an asterisk indicate material particularly well suited for student reading.

The patient receiving anesthetics

Chapter 13

Study questions for review

1 Review the charts of several patients on your ward who have received anesthetics. What kinds of anesthetics were used? How were they administered?
2 Talk to two patients on your ward who have recently received anesthetics. Did they express fear? What vivid recollections do they have?
3 What is the significance to the circulatory system of a sudden drop in blood pressure?

USE OF ANESTHETICS

The nurse should be able to answer a patient's questions about the anesthetic he is to receive; she should understand the preparation of the patient for anesthesia during the preoperative period; and she should know the effects of anesthetics so that she can help the patient recover from them quickly, safely, and with a minimum of complications. She must also be able to assist the physician intelligently when he is administering regional anesthetics.

An anesthetic produces a loss of sensation in a part of or in all of the body. If it also produces unconsciousness, it is called a *general anesthetic.* If it produces a loss of sensation in only a part of the body while the patient remains conscious, it is called a *regional anesthetic.*

General anesthesia is produced by inhalation of gases or vapors of highly volatile liquids or by injection into the blood stream or introduction into the rectum of anesthetic drugs in solution. Certain drugs that produce general anesthesia, such as Pentothal sodium, do not always produce the complete muscle relaxation that is a requirement of surgical anesthesia. Other general anesthetics such as ether, do produce surgical anesthesia but are very irritating to mucous membranes of the respiratory tract. Such irritation prolongs the introductory stages of anesthesia. Therefore, the patient may receive two general anesthetic agents during the course of the operation: one that quickly produces anesthesia and one that produces surgical anesthesia. General anesthesia affects all the physiologic systems of the body to some degree. However, it chiefly affects the central nervous, respiratory, and circulatory systems. The anesthetist judges the depth of anesthesia by the changes produced in these systems. These changes are used in describing the stages of anesthesia. Stage I extends from the beginning of the administration of an anesthetic to the beginning of the loss of consciousness. Stage II, often called the stage of excitement or delirium, extends from the loss of consciousness to the loss of lid reflex. If the patient is very apprehensive or was not given premedication correctly or on time, this stage, usually of short duration may last a long time. The patient may become markedly excited and struggle, shout, talk, laugh, or cry. Stage III, the stage of surgical anesthesia, extends from the loss of the lid reflex to cessation of respiratory effort. The patient is unconscious, his muscles are relaxed, and most of his reflexes have been abolished. Stage IV is the stage of overdosage or the stage of danger. It is complicated by respiratory and circulatory failure. Death will follow unless the anesthetic is immediately discontinued and artificial respiration given. The nurse may find that some patients recovering from the effects of general inhalation anesthesia pass through Stage II before becoming fully conscious and will be very noisy and restless. It is important to remember that hearing is the last sense to disappear before consciousness is lost and the first to return.

Regional anesthesia is produced by the injection or application of a drug along the course of a nerve, thus abolishing the conduction of all impulses to and from the area supplied by that nerve. The patient experiences no pain in the operative area and remains awake during the entire procedure because the effect of the anesthetic is regional only and does not affect essential sensory function.

The choice of anesthetic is based upon many factors: the physical condition and the age of the patient; the presence of coexisting diseases; the type, site, and duration of the operation; the personal preference of the surgeon, the anesthetist, or the patient; the skill of the anesthetist; and the effects of various agents and methods upon the patient. For example, Avertin is not given to a patient with advanced liver disease because this drug is detoxified in the liver. An apprehensive patient may not respond well to a regional anesthetic. The older patient tolerates depressant drugs poorly. Cyclopropane interferes with cardiac conduction mechanisms and is not given when cardiac diseases are present. The anesthetist evaluates each patient carefully and chooses the anesthetic that is best for him.

ANESTHESIA AND THE PATIENT

Patients have many anxieties and fears about anesthesia. They may be afraid of going to sleep and not waking up. They fear the unknown. They frequently express a dislike of ether because of previous experience with it, and they remember its pungent odor. They may worry that the anesthetic will not be effective and that they will feel pain during the operation. Many patients are concerned about the nausea and vomiting that may occur postoperatively as a result of the anesthetic. Some fear that they may talk while under the effects of an anesthetic and reveal facts that they do not want known. Others are frightened by the anticipation of having a mask placed over their face. Many do not want a spinal anesthetic because they do not wish to be awake during the operation.

Many fears can be dispelled if the patient and his family are given information about the anesthetic he is to receive. If the patient expresses concern about the anesthetic he should be told that the anesthetist carefully studies each patient's physical condition and administers the anesthetic that is best for him. The patient does not always see the anesthetist, however, because he may determine which agent is best by talking to the patient's surgeon and studying the patient's medical record. The nurse can assure the patient and his family that accidents resulting from the administration of anesthetics are rare and that his chances of recovering from its effects are excellent. The patient and his family should be told that he will be carefully watched while he is under anesthesia and that he will not be left alone until he is fully recovered from its effects. The nurse can further explain that most anesthetizing agents are now administered in such a way that little vomiting occurs postoperatively. Very few patients talk while under anesthesia and what is said is usually unintelligible, so that this need not be of great concern to any patient. The nurse should relay any persistent anxiety of the patient concerning anesthesia to the physician or to the anesthetist.

The preoperative nursing measures that increase the effectiveness of the anesthetic drug and make anesthesia possible have been discussed in detail in Chapter 12. Specifically they are as follows: instructing the patient about the preoperative and postoperative period, accurately weighing the patient, administering the preoperative enema, withholding food and fluids as ordered, reporting any changes in the patient's physical condition, giving the preoperative medication on time, and removing all prostheses before taking the patient to the operating room.

PREVENTION OF FIRE AND EXPLOSION

Certain anesthetizing agents such as ether, ethylene, and cyclopropane are inflammable and explosive. Therefore, extreme precautions must be taken at all times so that electric charges are not produced to ignite or explode these agents. When the nurse enters the operating room for any reason, she should be aware of these dangers. She should dress according to operating room regulations and should wear conductor bands on her shoes to ground possible electric charges and use any other protection that is required. She should never approach the anesthetist or the head of the table, and she should never touch any of the anesthetist's equipment unless specifically instructed to do so.

GENERAL ANESTHESIA

Inhalation anesthesia

Inhalation anesthesia is produced by having the patient inhale the vapors of certain liquids or gases. Oxygen is usually given with these anesthetics. The gas mixture may be administered by mask or be delivered into the lungs by a catheter or a tube that is inserted into the trachea or into the bronchi. The use of the catheter or tube is called *intubation.* The intubation method provides for an airway that can be easily suctioned and that can be used to aerate the lungs when the chest wall is opened.

Ether. Ether is a volatile, inflammable liquid. It has a very pungent odor which is disagreeable to many patients. It is very irritating to the mucous membranes of the pulmonary tract; this irritating quality prolongs the first and second stages of anesthesia. For this reason, a rapid-acting, nonirritating drug such as Pentothal sodium often is used to produce sleep before ether is administered. Ether is a relatively inexpensive drug. It is used for many operations because it provides excellent muscle relaxation and has a great margin of safety. Ether is generally not used for patients who have acute or chronic disease of the respiratory system, the liver, or the kidneys.

When caring for patients who have had ether, the nurse will discover that recovery from anesthesia may be prolonged, especially if a large amount of the drug was used. The patient will require constant supervision until completely awake. Because of ether's irritating qualities, large amounts of mucus may be present, in which case the patient must be suctioned frequently. Since vomiting often occurs after the administration of ether, the patient should be placed on his side to prevent aspiration of any vomitus. If the foot of the bed is elevated, gravity will aid the flow of mucus and vomitus from the throat and mouth. Mineral oil or a similar lubricant is dropped into the patient's eyes before anesthesia is begun to prevent possible irritation of the eyes by ether. If an irritation does occur, a lubricant may be used postoperatively. Redness or blistering of the skin which sometimes occurs around the site of the mask is caused by the combination of ether, moisture, and pressure. This can be unsightly and uncomfortable for the patient. Petroleum jelly or other ointments may be applied as ordered to relieve discomfort. When the patient has recovered from the anesthetic, he should be encouraged to breathe deeply and to cough productively to clear secretions from the bronchi. Since the odor of ether may be disturbing to others, patients recovering from anesthesia should be segregated.

Nitrous oxide. Nitrous oxide is a nonirritating, sweet-smelling, noninflammable gas. It is used for operations that do not require deep anesthesia. Nitrous oxide is always given with proportionate amounts of oxygen. The patient becomes anesthetized quickly and recovers rapidly. This gas is used largely for dental surgery and as a preliminary anesthetic when ether is to be administered. It is relatively inexpensive to use. Patients who have hypertension and associated cardiovascular diseases or those with diseases of the respiratory tract tolerate nitrous oxide poorly. If an excessive amount of this gas is given, there is always the possibility of anoxia, and patients with cardiovascular and respiratory diseases tolerate a reduction in oxygen poorly.

Ethylene. Ethylene is a nonirritating, inflammable gas used for procedures not requiring deep anesthesia. Its odor is rather similar to that of ether and this may disturb some patients. Ethylene produces unconsciousness quickly, and recovery takes only two or three minutes. It is often used to produce sleep before ether is administered. Since ethylene must be given in high concentrations, oxygen must be concurrently given to prevent anoxia. Patients who have mild anoxia from pulmonary diseases or who have liver and renal diseases do not tolerate this anesthetic. Vomiting may occur after this drug, but little mucus is produced.

Cyclopropane. Cyclopropane is a nonvolatile, inflammable, pleasant-smelling gas which quickly produces unconsciousness. The patient recovers rapidly from its effects because most of the gas is eliminated from the body about ten minutes after the anesthetic is stopped. It is not so potent as ether but does produce adequate relaxation for most abdominal surgery. Since it increases cardiac irritabilities and causes arrhythmias, it is contraindicated in all patients with cardiac diseases. The nurse should frequently check the pulse rate and rhythm for any irregularities that might occur as a result of having received this gas. Vomiting may occur postoperatively. Cyclopropane is highly inflammable and explosive. When it is being administered, great care must be taken to prevent the production of any electric charge which might ignite it.

Vinyl ether. Vinyl ether is a highly volatile, inflammable liquid. Its vapor quickly produces unconsciousness, and recovery is rapid. It is usually used to produce sleep before ether is administered. It may also be used for minor surgical procedures in which deep anesthesia is not required. (for example, dental extraction or incision and drainage). This drug is expensive to use. It is irritating to the respiratory mucosa and causes a large amount of mucus to form, thus making frequent suctioning necessary. Its use is contraindicated in patients who have pulmonary diseases.

Chloroform. Chloroform is rarely used because of its toxicity and narrow margin of safety. A very small amount can cause death. It may cause liver function derangement, cardiac depression, and serious biochemical disturbances. It produces anesthesia quickly and does offer excellent muscle relaxation, but it must be administered with great caution and skill.

Intravenous anesthesia

Thiopentothal sodium (Pentothal) is the drug used most frequently for intravenous anesthesia. It produces unconsciousness quickly, recovery is rapid, and the patient has amnesia for the preanesthesia period. Pentothal sodium is used for brief, minor procedures in which pain is not anticipated, such as dilatation and curettage of the uterus. It frequently is used to produce sleep before an inhalation anesthetic is administered. If a patient is very apprehensive about the operation, Pentothal sodium is sometimes given in his room before he goes to the operating room. It may also be given to relieve severe prolonged convulsive states. Patients who have received this drug should be watched carefully for laryngeal spasms. Signs of laryngeal spasm are restlessness, apprehension, stridor, retraction of the soft tissue about the neck, and cyanosis. The nurse should notify the physician when these signs begin to develop, for the patient may require an emergency tracheostomy. If large amounts of Pentothal sodium have been used, the patient may sleep for a long time and should be observed for signs of respiratory depression, such as shallow, slow respirations. The blood pressure should be checked frequently because it may fall suddenly. Patients who receive this drug often have generalized muscle twitching. The cause of this is not known, but if it continues for any length of time, it should be reported.

Pentothal sodium is detoxified in the liver and excreted by the kidneys. Therefore, patients with diseases of the liver or kidneys may not tolerate this drug.

Rectal anesthesia

Some drugs can be given rectally to produce anesthesia, analgesia, or amnesia. *Tribromoethanol (Avertin)* is the drug usually given for these purposes. This clear, colorless, nonirritating liquid is instilled into the rectum, where it is absorbed. Since dosage is based on body weight, the nurse must weigh the patient carefully and record his weight accurately. Tribromoethanol induces sleep but, if major surgery is planned, must be followed by a drug that produces a deep anesthesia. It is used to "steal" patients for surgery who are extremely apprehensive preoperatively. The patient is put to sleep in his room so that he does not know when he is taken to the operating room. Although he knows he is to be operated upon, he does not know the exact time. If such is the case, the following procedure is carried out. For several days preceding the day of operation the patient is given a small saline solution or tap water retention enema every day at the same time. Then, on the day of the operation, the anesthetist prepares a solution of Avertin to be substituted for the daily retention enema and instructs the nurse in its administration. After the solution has been instilled, the tube is clamped and left so that none of the fluid can escape. Deep sleep is produced in minutes. The nurse remains with the patient until he is asleep, checking carefully to see that he has a clear airway at all times. The anesthetist then assumes responsibility for the patient.

The patient who has received Avertin may remain unconscious for some time after its administration, since the rate of its elimination from the body varies with each patient. Depression of respirations is common, and the patient should be placed in a position that enables him to breathe freely. When the patient does awaken, he is very drowsy and should be protected from injury by the use of side rails on the bed. Since hypotension may also occur, the blood pressure should be taken frequently. Avertin is detoxified by the liver and eliminated by the kidneys and, therefore, is contraindicated in patients with liver or kidney disease. It also is not given to patients who have pulmonary tract infections or diseases of the heart and other circulatory disturbances. Elderly and cachectic patients tolerate Avertin poorly.

REGIONAL ANESTHESIA

Regional anesthesia is used for treatments, diagnostic measures, examinations, and surgery. The nurse usually assembles the equipment necessary for the administration of the drugs used to produce regional anesthesia. She assists the physician during the procedure and observes the patient for reactions to the anesthetic or to the procedure.

The drugs used to produce regional anesthesia are usually called *local anesthetics.* Examples are procaine, cocaine, Pontocaine, Nupercaine, Butyn, and Metycaine. When these drugs are absorbed into the blood stream, they cause stimulation of the central nervous system and depression of the heart. Care, therefore, is taken that they are given in a localized area and in the smallest dose necessary to produce anesthesia. A barbiturate is usually given before the drugs are administered to reduce their action on the central nervous system. Epinephrine may be added to the solution of local anesthetic drugs to produce vasoconstriction in the area of the injection. Vasoconstriction tends to reduce the rate of absorption and to extend the length of anesthesia.

The nurse must carefully observe the patient for signs of excitability, twitching, pulse or blood pressure changes, pallor of the skin, and respiratory difficulties. When the first signs of these toxic reactions occur, an intravenous injection of a short-acting barbiturate such as Pentothal should be ready for the physician to administer. Oxygen may also be necessary, and it is important that an airway be maintained. If the reaction is due to an idiosyncrasy to the drug given, circulatory failure may occur and emergency measures such as artificial respiration must be started. Patients should be questioned regarding any previous sensitivity to these drugs, and skin tests are usually advocated before their administration.

Topical anesthesia

Topical anesthesia is accomplished by spreading or spraying a local anesthetic drug directly on the part to be anesthetized. It is used for diagnostic procedures or treatments of the nose and throat, and it may be used for minor skin operations.

Infiltration anesthesia

Infiltration anesthesia is accomplished by the injection of the anesthetic drug directly into the area to be incised or manipulated. This method is used for minor procedures (incision and drainage, thoracentesis). Another method of infiltration anesthesia is the *nerve block*, in which the drug is injected into the nerve a short distance from the site of the operation. This method is employed in tonsilectomies or plastic or dental surgery.

Spinal anesthesia

Spinal anesthesia is accomplished by the injection of a solution of a local anesthetic drug into the subarachnoid space, where it acts upon the nerves as they emerge from the spinal cord. Depending upon the type of anesthesia desired, the injection is made through the second, third, or fourth interspace of the lumbar vertebras. Anesthesia is quickly produced and provides good relaxation of muscles. Spinal anesthesia is used for abdominal surgery and as an aid in the diagnosis of disease of the autonomic nervous system. For example, following spinal anesthesia some patients with poor circulation of the lower extremities due to spasms of the arteries show signs of increased blood flow; such patients benefit from a sympathectomy, an operation that severs the nerves which keep these blood vessels contracted. Spinal anesthesia cannot be used for operations on the upper part of the body because it can cause paralysis of the diaphragm. One of the limitations of this type of anesthesia is that the patient is awake throughout the operation, although the preoperative medication does make him less aware of his surroundings and a towel is placed over his eyes. In addition, the conversation and activities of the members of the operating room staff are restricted. The patient may be conscious of pulling sensations throughout the operation although he experiences no pain.

Following spinal anesthesia, the patient should be kept flat in bed with a pillow under his head. Since sensation may not return to the anesthetized area for an hour or two, the nurse must see that the patient sustains no injuries such as burns from hot-water bottles during this time. He will need to be turned, and he should not be placed in a strained or unnatural position which might cause him later discomfort. The nurse must always be alert for signs of respiratory or circulatory depression. Although the patient is conscious, the blood pressure, pulse, and respiration should be checked frequently. Hypotension does occur as a result of relaxation of the vascular bed, but, because of the danger of the anesthetic traveling up the spinal canal and paralyzing the diaphragm, the patient should not be placed in the Trendelenburg position until this is ordered by a physician.

Some physicians request that the patient remain flat in bed for from six to twelve hours following spinal anesthesia to reduce the possibility of a "spinal" headache. This headache is thought to be due to leakage of spinal fluid from the puncture in the dura or to sterile chemical meningitis. It usually occurs twenty-four hours after the puncture and is more common in women than in men. It may last several days, and occasionally it persists for weeks or months. The nurse should not suggest the possibility of this complication to the patient. If it does occur, the patient complains of a throbbing, pulsating headache which is aggravated by a change in position. He should remain flat in bed and move about as little as possible. An ice bag may bring relief. To lessen discomfort, analgesics and sedatives should be given as ordered. Other measures that are sometimes used are the forcing of fluids and the use of drugs such as vasodilators to stimulate the production of spinal fluid.

When the effects of the anesthetic wear off, the patient occasionally complains of a backache. This may be due to the position he was in on the operating table or to the insertion of the needle at the time of the puncture. This complaint is treated symptomatically, and heat applied locally often brings relief.

Refrigeration anesthesia

Insensibility to pain may be produced by the application of ice or iced water. This may be the anesthesia used for the amputation of a limb and is called refrigeration anesthesia. Advantages are that physical shock to the patient is minimal, no inhalation anesthesia is required, and the lowered temperature reduces cell metabolism.

Patients requiring refrigeration anesthesia are generally quite ill and in pain. Since the procedure is cumbersome and the weight of the ice makes the patient uncomfortable until anesthesia is obtained, a sedative such as phenobarbital is usually given to lessen the patient's reactions to the procedure. Occasionally a few whiffs of a short-acting anesthetic such as trichloroethylene are given to lessen initial discomfort.

Before anesthesia is begun extra rubber or plastic sheets are placed under the patient to protect the bed. One half hour before the ice is applied, ice bags are placed around the limb at the sites where tourniquets will be applied. Tourniquets are used to prevent chilling of the rest of the body by curtailing blood flow out of the affected limb. After the tourniquets are applied by the doctor and secured with clamps to prevent their slipping, a layer of crushed ice is placed in a metal trough and the extremity is placed upon it. If a suitable trough is not available, one can be made from a rubber sheet covered with a bath blanket by rolling it from either side toward the patient's leg. The rubber sheeting should extend 8 to 10 inches over the edge of the bed into a bucket to permit drainage of water. The leg is then covered with ice from the area above the tourniquets to below the extremity. The bath blanket and rubber sheet are wrapped around the ice-covered limb and secured with bandages to keep the ice in place and to prevent it from melting too fast. Elevation of the head of the bed on blocks will facilitate drainage of melted ice. Anesthesia is obtained in about one and a half hours if only the lower leg is involved and two and one-half hours if the entire limb is to be anesthetized. The refrigeration equipment is removed in the operating room.

The nurse should supplement the doctor's and/or the anesthetist's explanation of the procedure to the patient and to his family. She should move the affected limb as carefully and gently as possible, work quickly in applying the ice, and arrange for someone to stay with the patient until he goes to the operating room. Emotional reaction to necessity for an amputation may be further aggravated by general illness and pain which increase the patient's uneasiness if he is left alone.

HYPOTHERMIA DURING ANESTHESIA

Hypothermia during anesthesia is the lowering of body temperature after the patient is anesthetized for an operation on the heart or the major blood vessels. Because lowering the temperature reduces total oxygen consumption, this procedure permits interruption of circulation for as long as thirty minutes without causing irreversible damage to tissues.[4]

The patient is given premedication about an hour before anesthesia is started, usually with a narcotic and an anticholinergic drug, for example, atropine sulfate. After the patient is anesthetized, an intratracheal catheter is inserted into the trachea. A thermometer is inserted into the patient's rectum to record his temperature, electrocardiographic leads are applied to the patient's legs and arms since ventricular fibrillation during hypothermia does occur, and the patient is placed on a cooling blanket. This blanket contains multiple coils through which ice water circulates. Usually the patient is cooled to 26° C. (78.8° F.); this requires approximately an hour. When the desired temperature is reached the operation is performed. Hypothermia may also be induced by placing ice packs about the patient or by placing him in a quick-freezing unit or immersing him in a tub of ice water.

When the operation has been completed, the patient is rewarmed by running warm water through the blanket, by immersing him in warm water, or by use of diathermy coils. Care is taken to prevent burning the patient while his body is rapidly warmed until his temperature reaches 32° C. (89° F.) at which time consciousness usually returns. The patient is then removed from the warming agent and his temperature permitted gradually to rise to normal.

The rectal thermometer is left in place for several hours after the operation. The patient's temperature is checked frequently, and if it rises above normal the doctor may order ice bags or cool sponges to lower the temperature. The patient's pulse and respiratory rate are also checked frequently since cardiac irregularities may occur. Electrocardiographic tests are also frequently done to check heart action further.

CURARE

Curare is a drug which has a powerful relaxing action on skeletal muscles. It is given when anesthetics that are to be used do not provide for sufficient relaxation of the abdominal muscles. It can cause respiratory depression or paralysis, and the patient must be watched very carefully for signs of respiratory difficulty during and after its administration.

GENERAL POSTANESTHESIA NURSING CARE

The immediate postanesthesia period is a critical one for the patient. He must be watched carefully until the effects of the anesthetic have worn off, his reflexes have returned, and his vital signs are stable. The nurse is largely responsible for the care of the patient during this period, and she must be prepared to meet his specific needs as they arise. It is the practice in many hospitals to have all postanesthesia patients taken to a recovery room where they can be given undivided attention. All the equipment that may be necessary is available in a recovery room: oxygen, suction machines, sphygmomanometers, infusion fluids, shock blocks, airways, emergency medications, respirators, side rails, and cardiac massage trays. Ideally, recovery rooms are located on the same floor as the operating room or in its immediate vicinity. If there is no recovery room, the nurse prepares the patient's unit with as much equipment as may be needed. In either instance, the bed is made according to hospital routine. Details may vary, but it is usually prepared so that the patient can be easily returned to it and so that it is protected from any drainage or emesis that may occur. The patient is placed directly into his bed from the operating table or is transferred very gently onto a stretcher. The move should be done with a lift sheet or by the three-man lift so that all parts of the patient's body are supported. The patient should be accompanied to the recovery room or to his room by the anesthetist and another member of the operating room professional staff because of the danger of respiratory embarrassment or the aspiration of vomitus enroute.

The nurse assumes the responsibility for the care of the patient after she receives a report on the patient's condition from members of the operating room staff. Her first responsibilities are to make certain that the patient has a clear airway until his pharyngeal reflexes have returned, to prevent and to be alert for any circulatory depression, to remain with

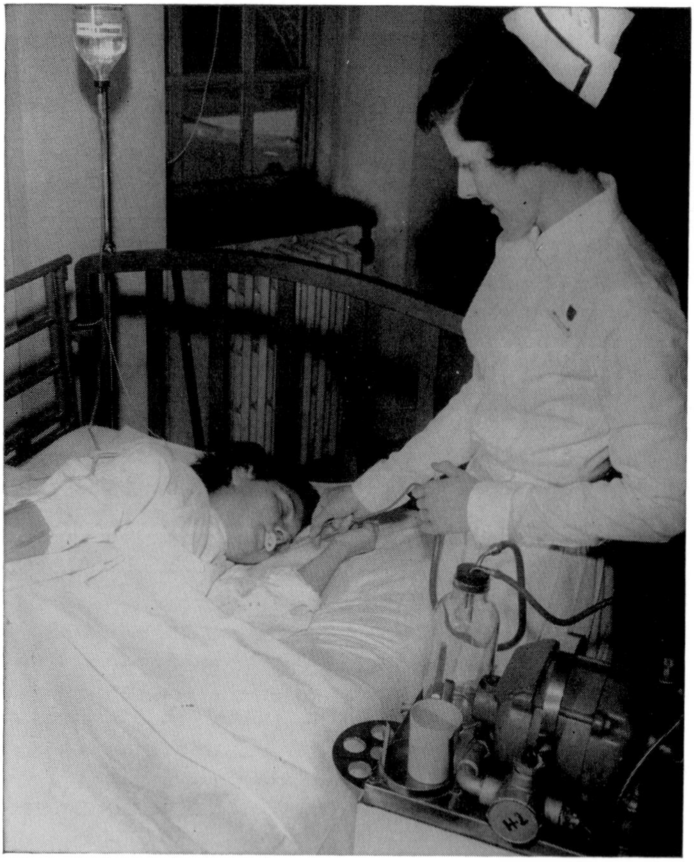

Figure 18

Suctioning the unconscious postoperative patient. Note the position of the nurse's thumb over the free end of the Y glass connecting tube. In practice, to prevent trauma to mucous membranes by the suction, this opening is not covered until the catheter is inserted.

the patient until he is rational and oriented, and to protect the patient from any physical injury.

Maintenance of an airway. In order to maintain a clear airway, the nurse should place the patient in a position so that he can breathe normally and so that emesis, blood, and mucus can drain and will not be aspirated. This can best be accomplished by turning the patient to one side or by placing him in a semiprone position. Compression of the chest of the patient in a semiprone position can be avoided by flexing the patient's uppermost arm and leg or by placing rolled sheets or blankets under his abdomen. If the patient cannot be turned onto his side or if he does not move, he may be placed on his back with the chin up and the jaw forward or with the head turned slightly to one side.

Excessive secretions in the nasopharynx, trachea, and bronchial tree may also obstruct the airway and interfere with respirations. These secretions are usually caused by the anesthetic, by other drugs that have been administered, or by irritation to the mucosa of the throat due to intubation or suctioning. They are removed from the posterior pharynx with a lubricated rubber nasal catheter (see Figure 18). If suction is on, the catheter should be pinched off as it is inserted so that the nasal mucosa is not irritated or traumatized. If the secretions are in the tracheobronchial area and cannot be reached by the catheter, intratracheal suctioning must be done.

When the tongue is relaxed from anesthesia, it may fall back and prevent free passage of air. This condition can be prevented by holding the patient's jaw up and forward or by placing him on his side. If it should occur, however, the nurse must turn the patient over onto his side or onto his abdomen with his head hanging down over the side of the bed. This position will bring the tongue forward. If it is not possible to turn the patient, the nurse can open the mouth by pushing at the angle of the jaw with her thumbs and have someone insert a padded tongue depressor between the back teeth. The tongue can then be brought forward by grasping it with a compress or with a clamp. A metal, rubber, or plastic airway is often left in place following the administration of an anesthetic to keep the passage open and to keep the tongue forward until the pharyngeal reflexes have returned. This tube should be removed as soon as the patient begins to wake up since its presence is irritating and leads to vomiting.

Maintenance of circulation. As soon as the nurse is certain that the patient's airway is clear, she should check the blood pressure and pulse reading. Moving the patient from the operating room table to his bed, reaction to drugs and anesthesia, loss of blood during the operation, and postoperative bleeding all will cause circulatory changes. The blood pressure should be taken frequently until it reaches a satisfactory level and remains there. The pulse is also checked for rate, volume, and rhythm. When the blood pressure drops, the pulse rate usually increases, pulse volume becomes thin and thready and the skin becomes cold, wet, and pale. The physician should be notified as soon as there is a change in blood pressure. He will examine the patient and probably order intravenous fluids, blood, or plasma to increase the blood volume. Oxygen may be given to increase its concentration in the available circulating blood. The Trendelenburg position may be used to help increase the blood flow to the vital organs unless its use is contraindicated because the patient has had spinal anesthesia. Shock resulting from lowered blood volume must be prevented because the liver, kidney, and brain tissues do not tolerate long periods of anoxia.

Protection from injury. Following anesthesia, side rails are usually placed on the bed and are left until the patient is fully awake. Although the patient is constantly watched, it is possible for him suddenly to turn and throw himself from the bed. Hot-water bottles, heating pads, or heat lamps must be used with care while the patient is unconscious, so that burns do not occur. If infusions are being given, the patient's arm should be secured so that the needle does not become dislodged and cause injury. Physical restraints are seldom used if the patient is restless, and the nurse must guide the patient's movements so that he does not hurt himself. His position in bed should be watched so that there is no possibility of nerve damage resulting from pressure or from his being in an unnatural position for a long time. The patient under anesthesia has complete muscle relaxation with loss of sensation and is unable to indicate discomfort. The nurse must be constantly aware of this when moving or turning him.

Additional considerations following surgery. The nurse must check the patient's dressing for any drainage or bleeding. If drainage is noted, she must check the dressing frequently, and, if it increases in amount, she must report to the doctor. Although drainage is expected when a drain has been inserted, a closed wound should not stain the dressing very much, and the nurse must be alert for hemorrhage. She can outline the first evidences of bleeding on the dressing with a pencil and then watch carefully to see if it spreads beyond this marking. The bed and the patient's gown should be inspected frequently, and the patient should be turned at intervals to check for seepage of blood under his body or down the side of the dressing. If he cannot be turned, the nurse must then put her hands under him to check for bleeding.

The nurse should also check for tubes of any kind and connect them as indicated: gastric tubes to suction and Foley catheters or other tubes to straight drainage. She should also inspect any infusions that are being given and add to them as ordered. The doctor's order sheet must be checked for other treatments and medications that must be given.

It is important that the nurse caring for the patient during the postanesthesia period accurately chart and report all medications, fluids, and treatments that the patient receives during this time so that there will be no duplication that might prove harmful to him.

The nurse can ascertain the return of reflexes and the rationality of the patient by asking him his name and other questions that would indicate he is oriented to time and place. The patient may be returned to his room and left alone as soon as his blood pressure is stable and he is breathing freely, is not vomiting, and is fully awake. Although he does not need constant supervision at this stage, he should be observed frequently by the nurse. His vital signs should be checked until they become stable. The dressing should be checked for signs of bleeding and the tubes for drainage. He should be given the necessary physical care such as a partial bath, mouth care, and a change of linens. Nursing measures for the prevention of complications should be begun at this time. These will be discussed in Chapter 14.

REFERENCES AND SELECTED READINGS*

1 Adriani, John: Techniques and Procedures of Anesthesia, Springfield, Ill., 1956, Charles C Thomas, Publisher.
2 Beal, John M. (editor): Manual of Recovery Room Care, New York, 1956, The Macmillan Co.
3 *Cantor, Alfred J., and Foxe, Arthur N.: Psychosomatic Aspects of Surgery, New York, 1956, Grune & Stratton, Inc.
4 Cullen, Stuart C.: Anesthesia; A Manual for Students and Physicians, Chicago, 1957, Year Book Publishers, Inc.
5 Elman, Robert: Surgical Care, A Practical Physiologic Guide, New York, 1951, Appleton-Century-Crofts, Inc.
6 *Greisheimer, Esther M.: The Physiological Effects of Anesthesia, Am. J. Nursing **49**:337-343, June, 1949.
7 Lennon, Benjamin B.: Before and After Anesthesia, Am. J. Nursing **41**:534-537, May 1941.
8 McMahon, Janet, and Fife, Gertrude L.: Nursing Problems in Recovery From Anesthesia, Am. J. Nursing **45**:616-622, Aug. 1945.
9 *Nugent, G. Robert, and Graves, Nancy: Prolonged Hypothermia and Nursing During Prolonged Hypothermia, Am. J. Nursing **60**:967-970, July, 1960.
10 Sheldon, Thomas H., Lundy, John S., and Adams, R. Charles: Nursing Care as Related to Anesthesia, Am. J. Nursing **44**:747-750, Aug. 1944.

*References preceded by an asterisk indicate material particularly well suited for student reading.

Postoperative care

Chapter 14

Study questions for review

1. Review the circulation of the blood and the physiology of respiration.
2. Consult your notes on fundamentals of nursing and review the dangers of prolonged bed rest. What techniques have you learned for helping patients to get in and out of bed? What safety measures should be taken in helping patients to get in and out of bed?
3. What disturbances of physiology can occur when the patient cannot take solids or liquids by mouth?
4. List the nursing measures you have learned that may assist a patient to void.

The aim of postoperative care is to restore the patient to normal function without the development of complications. The nurse who knows the physiologic and emotional responses to anesthesia and surgery and who understands the program prescribed by the doctor can plan and carry out nursing care which will support, protect, and comfort the patient until normal functions are restored and which will prevent complications from developing. The average patient's response to such care is a rapid return to the activities of daily living. Much of the nursing care in the postoperative period is concentrated upon the prevention of complications, and this care should be started as soon as the patient returns from the operating room. The nurse should know what complications can develop, how she can help prevent them, and their early signs and symptoms. Prevention and recognition of complications will be discussed in this chapter. Treatment of the various complications is discussed in more detail in chapters dealing with the specific disorders.

IMMEDIATE POSTOPERATIVE NEEDS

The nurse must know what operation was performed and what pathology was present so that she can plan the nursing care accordingly. She also needs to know what information was given to the patient and his family so that she will be able to answer their questions intelligently. The patient and his family frequently are too upset to hear or to understand all that the surgeon tells them, and they often ask the nurse for repeated explanation. Most surgeons discuss the results of the operation with the family immediately after surgery. They also visit the patient, telling him briefly what was found and reassuring him about his condition. Although the surgeon often tells the family when a malignancy is found at operation, he usually withholds this information from the patient in the immediate postoperative period. However, he may tell the patient that a tumor or infection was found and removed.

When the postoperative patient returns to the unit, the nurse should immediately check his blood pressure, pulse, and respirations, the dressing and drainage tubes, and his orientation. If the vital signs are relatively stable and there are no indications of hemorrhage or abnormal drainage, she should then make him as comfortable as possible. The patient usually is concerned about the outcome of the operation, the whereabouts of his family, and his general discomfort. By washing his face and hands, giving him mouth care, rubbing his back, changing his gown and bed linen as necessary, and changing his position to provide support for all dependent parts, the nurse can help to relieve his general discomfort. A pillow usually is placed under his head and the head gatch on the bed is raised to a low Fowler's position. If necessary, medication for pain should be given. Since the patient often is rather "groggy," side rails should be placed on the bed. At this time nursing measures designed to prevent complications are begun, and other treatments are given as ordered.

As soon as the patient's condition is satisfactory, some member of the family should be permitted to see him and talk with him briefly. Such a visit will usually reassure the family and will make the patient feel secure and loved.

PREVENTION OF RESPIRATORY COMPLICATIONS

The most common respiratory complications are bronchitis, atelectasis, and pneumonia. Bronchitis is an inflammation of the bronchi. Atelectasis is the blockage of air to a portion of the lung, causing this portion to fail to expand. Pneumonia, a bacterial infection, often follows atelectasis. Signs and symptoms of these complications usually develop within twenty-four to forty-eight hours after surgery. There is usually a rise in the patient's temperature and in his pulse and respiratory rates. He may or may not complain of chest pain, cough, or difficulty in breathing. Cyanosis may be present, and the patient may be restless and apprehensive. These complaints should be brought immediately to the doctor's attention.

While most patients experience some respiratory irritation following intubation and inhalation anesthesia, respiratory complications most frequently occur in patients who smoke heavily, who suffer from chronic respiratory diseases such as bronchitis or bronchiectasis, or who are elderly, debilitated, or obese. They are most likely to occur after high abdominal operations or prolonged inhalation anesthesia.

If all postoperative patients are suctioned when necessary, turned frequently, and encouraged to breathe deeply and to cough productively, most respiratory complications can be prevented. Following inhalation anesthesia, bronchial secretions usually are increased. Unless the mucus is removed, the bronchioles will become obstructed and *atelectasis* will occur. Preoperative and postoperative medication, anesthesia, and shock tend to depress respirations and thus encourage the development of atelectasis because the ability to expel bronchial exudates is decreased. As the air is absorbed from the lung tissue behind the occluded bronchioles, exudation and consolidation of this lung substance usually occurs. This is known as *pneumonitis,* or inflammation of the lung. The patient may aspirate nasopharyngeal secretions containing pathogenic bacteria, and, since his resistance to disease tends to be lowered by anesthesia and operative trauma, these organisms may invade the lung tissue, causing *bronchitis* or *pneumonia.* The lungs may be inadequately aerated because of incomplete excursion of the chest muscles. Tight abdominal dressings or binders tend to immobilize the abdominal muscles and the diaphragm, causing the lung bases to remain uninflated. In the elderly patient, firming of the rib cage and loss of elasticity of chest structures increases this problem. Surgical trauma, especially after high abdominal operations, may lead to injury of fibers of the phrenic nerve, causing the diaphragm to become flaccid and relaxed. Pain in the incision or fear of pain may prevent the patient from fully expanding his chest cavity on inspiration. Such a patient tends to breathe rapidly, and the respirations become shallow to compensate for the restricted intake of air; bronchial secretions collect in the lung bases and, because they are expelled with difficulty, lead to atelectasis and pneumonia.

Position also influences the development of respiratory complications. If the patient is permitted to lie in one position with continuous pressure against his chest, proper ventilation of the dependent lung tissue and drainage of secretions are not possible, and atelectasis ensues. There is danger that an unconscious or very drowsy patient may aspirate vomitus into his lungs. Gastric fluid is very irritating to the lungs and may cause respiratory distress. Pneumonia may develop, or the lung tissue may become necrotic and gangrenous *(lung abscess).*

Turning. To prevent atelactasis from occurring, the patient's position should be changed frequently while he is on bed rest. Turning and changing of position provide for better ventilation of the lungs by encouraging deep respiration and drainage of secretions. The patient should be turned at least every two or three hours. His position may usually be rotated in the following manner: side, back, side, abdomen. When turning is restricted by the nature of the operation, he should be moved within the specified limitations. Although turning increases pain in the incision, the nurse can use techniques that will cause as little discomfort as possible, such as turning the patient in one smooth movement. This can be accomplished by three nurses working in unison or by the use of a lifting sheet. When the patient is able to cooperate in the turning, the nurse can help him by first moving the head and trunk to the side of the bed and then by moving the buttocks and the lower extremities. The patient then is in a position to roll onto his side or abdomen. Good body mechanics should be used to protect both the patient and the nurse from injury, and the nurse should not attempt to move a helpless or very heavy patient without assistance. Once the desired position is attained, the patient should be placed in good body alignment with all dependent parts supported to prevent pull on the incision and unnatural strain on muscles. Pillows placed against the back and abdomen and between the legs may make the patient more comfortable in a side-lying position. If not contraindicated by the type of anesthesia or surgery, the head of the bed should be slightly elevated. The schedule for turning the patient should be interrupted only when he is out of bed for several hours at a time and should be discontinued only when ausculation and roentgenograms indicate that his lungs are clear and fully expanded.

Deep breathing and coughing. When the patient coughs productively, he expels any mucous secretions blocking the bronchi. Deep breathing often causes the patient to cough, and it assures complete ventilation of the lungs. All postoperative patients, therefore, are asked to breathe deeply and to cough at least every two hours. Unless specifically contraindicated, this should be done routinely by all patients. Coughing may be contraindicated following brain, spinal, or eye surgery, but deep-breathing exercises should be done.

The patient can be taught to breathe deeply by pulling in his abdominal muscles as he breathes. The nurse can determine whether or not he is doing this correctly by placing her hand on his abdomen as he breathes. This type of breathing permits the diaphragm to descend fully and the entire lung to expand. If there are secretions in the bronchi, deep breathing will stimulate coughing and expectoration of the mucus. The patient should be asked to do the breathing exercises at frequent intervals himself.

Since most patients find coughing painful after surgery, they will need supervision and assistance. Some surgeons advocate the administration of narcotics before coughing is begun. Narcotics decrease the cough reflex, however, and heavily sedated patients should be encouraged to cough more frequently. The nurse can best assist the patient to cough by placing her hands firmly on either side of the incision and exerting pressure. She can also splint the operative area with a drawsheet or towel. Such splinting prevents excessive muscular strain around the incision. If the patient must remain flat in bed while he coughs, restraining bedclothes and pillows should be removed from around the chest. If he is permitted to sit up in bed, a pull rope attached to the foot of the bed will help him get up into and maintain a sitting position while coughing. The patient should be encouraged to cough deeply and productively. If the first attempt is not successful, he should rest and then try again. If he is unable to cough productively and if his attempts only lead to fatigue, the physician may use intratracheal suction to stimulate the cough reflex, or a bronchoscope may have to be passed to remove pulmonary secretions. Routine coughing should be continued until the lungs are clear of all secretions. The doctor determines this by auscultation, percussion, and roentgenographic examination.

PREVENTION OF CIRCULATORY COMPLICATIONS

The formation of clots in the veins of the lower extremities is a common postoperative complication. It is thought to be due to retardation of the venous flow, increased tendency of the blood to coagulate, and inflammatory changes in the walls of the veins. Venous stasis occurs in the lower extremities as a result of muscular inactivity, postoperative respiratory and circulatory depression, and increased pressure on blood vessels due to tight dressings, intestinal distention, and prolonged maintenance of a sitting position. Other contributing factors are old age, obesity, cardiovascular diseases, debility, malnutrition, foci of infection, and varicose veins. *Femoral thrombophlebitis* and *phlebothrombosis* are the most prevalent circulatory complications, and they may be prevented by exercise and ambulation.

In phlebothrombosis the clot usually forms in one of the deep veins of the calf or the foot. The thrombus is soft, is loosely attached, and floats in the blood. The patient may or may not complain of pain and tenderness in the leg. The pain usually is noticeable upon dorsiflexion of the foot. As the thrombus becomes larger, it is easily separated by the circulating blood from its attachment to the vein wall and may be carried to the lungs as a massive embolus *(pulmonary embolism).* When this occurs, the patient usually complains of a sudden, sharp, upper abdominal or thoracic pain and difficulty in breathing. He goes into shock, and death often follows in a few minutes.

In thrombophlebitis the clot becomes firmly attached to the vein wall and grows until it occludes the lumen of the vein. It usually forms in the femoral or iliac veins, and fever, local tenderness, and pain develop. The entire leg becomes swollen, pale, and cold. There is usually exquisite tenderness along the course of the vein. The swelling and coldness are caused by lymphatic obstruction and arterial spasm. If the thrombophlebitis is confined to the saphenous vein, the accompanying edema is not so marked, but pain and tenderness are just as severe, and heat and redness can be noted along the inflamed vein. The development of the thrombi prolongs the patient's convalescence. He is confined to bed, and extensive treatment is begun. (See Chapter 19.) He is extremely uncomfortable and his leg may still be swollen for some time after discharge.

Postoperative exercises and early ambulation. Nursing measures to prevent thrombus formation should be initiated at once after the operation.

Bed exercises and early ambulation are known to minimize the effects of venous stasis caused by bed rest, and they usually are contraindicated only in the presence of thromboembolic diseases or after vascular surgery such as anastomosis of a blood vessel. Specific exercises for the upper extremities are not usually necessary since the patient uses his arms in eating, bathing, combing his hair, and reach-

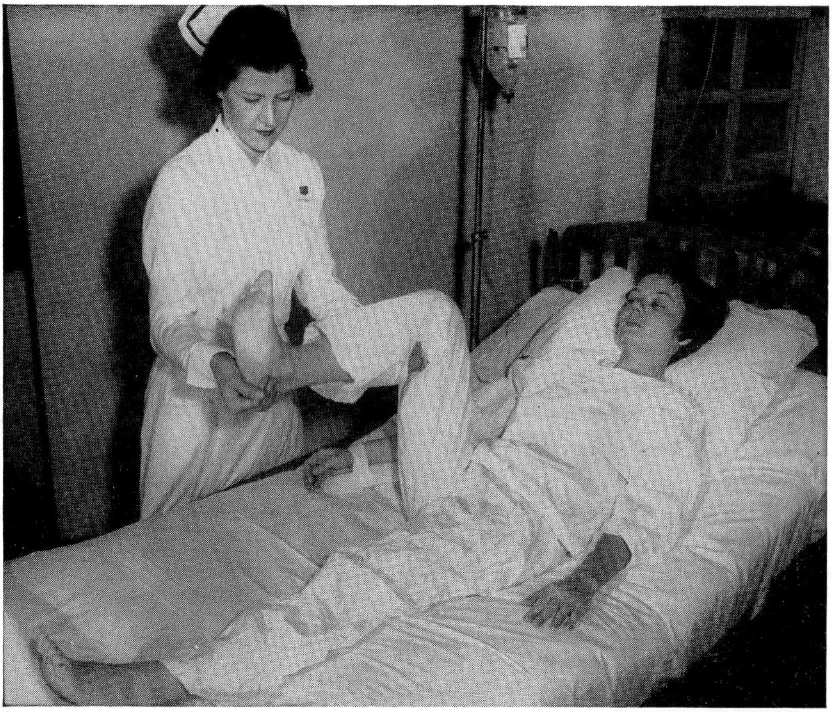

Figure 19

Supervising the postoperative patient in bed exercises. Here the nurse assists the patient as she bends the knee and dorsiflexes the foot.

ing for articles on his bedside stand or overbed table. If exercises are indicated, they should consist of flexion and extension of the fingers, rotation of the hand on the wrist, flexion and extension of the elbow, and thrusting of the arms forward, backward, to the side, upward, and out. Exercises of the lower extremities are particularly important in the prevention of venous stasis and should be performed until the patient is up and walking about several hours a day (see Figure 19). He should be taught to bend his knees, to lower them, and to push the backs of the knees hard against the bed. The nurse can slip her hand under the popliteal area and have the patient push hard against it. The same thing can be accomplished by having the patient alternately contract and relax his calf and thigh muscles. This should be done at least ten times, and a brief period of rest should follow each contraction and relaxation. The cycle is contract, relax, rest. Leg exercises should also include flexion, extension, adduction, and abduction of the leg and extension, flexion, and rotation of the foot. A footboard placed at the bottom of the bed, against which the foot can rest in the normal walking position and against which the patient can push, will help prevent foot drop and provide additional exercise. Whenever possible, the patient should lie on his abdomen for one-half hour two or three times a day to prevent blood from pooling in the pelvic cavity and contracture at the hip joint. Until he is permitted out of bed, he should have supervised exercise at least every four hours, but he should be encouraged to do the exercises more frequently than scheduled and to move his legs about in bed as much as possible. The bed should be made so that the bed linen does not restrict the patient's movements. If the patient is unable to do these exercises ac-

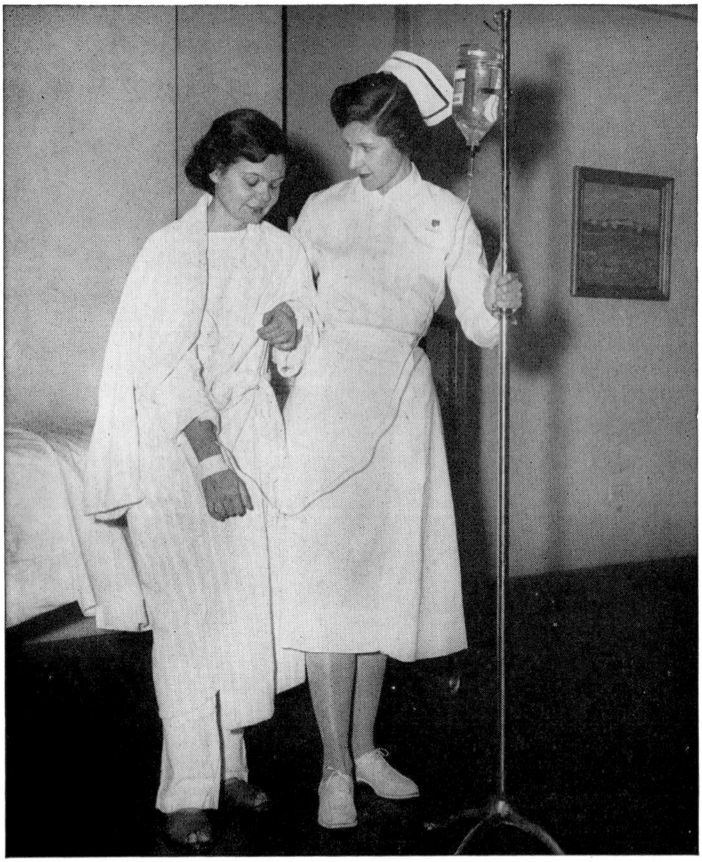

Figure 20

The patient who is receiving an infusion can be assisted to be ambulatory.

tively, they should be done passively by the nurse.

To be effective in preventing venous stasis, ambulation should be initiated within twenty-four hours after surgery. At first the patient should walk a short distance at least twice a day, but he should not be pushed beyond his physical ability. The distance walked should be increased each time, and when the patient becomes tired he should return to bed. The nurse should assist and supervise the patient in getting out of bed and walking until he is able to do this without difficulty or injury to himself. Early ambulation should not include only sitting in a chair at the bedside since this may cause increased stasis of blood in the lower extremities. If the patient is permitted to sit in a chair, he should be advised to get up frequently and walk about. When he is sitting, he should elevate his legs on another chair to prevent pooling of venous blood in the lower extremities. The legs should be supported from the knees to the ankles, but there should be no pressure against the popliteal area.

When the nurse must get the patient up for the first time, she should evaluate his condition carefully to see what problems are involved. The aged patient usually has difficulty getting up because of stiff joints and muscle weakness. Patients who have arthritis or arteriosclerosis or who have been on prolonged bed rest may need to be ambulated gradually.

They should be permitted to sit on the edge of the bed and dangle their feet for short periods before walking is attempted. Their progress may be slow. Treatments need not interfere with getting the patient out of bed. If the patient is receiving an infusion, his arm can be secured to an arm board, and the bottle of infusion fluid can be hung on a movable pole which can be pushed along by the nurse as the patient walks (see Figure 20). Permission is usually given by the physician to clamp off gastric tubes for a short period of time. Urethral catheters and other tubing can be attached to small, portable drainage bottles.

By using good body mechanics, one nurse can get most postoperative patients out of bed for the first time without injury to herself or to the patient. Most patients, however, are more confident if there are two people present when they first get out of bed. The nurse should walk close beside the patient and link her arm with his so that his palm is up and her palm is down. If the patient becomes weak, the nurse can then slide her arm up into the patient's axilla and, by moving her outer leg to the side, provide herself with a wide enough base of support to balance the patient against her hip until help arrives.

PAIN

Pain in the incision is a common postoperative complaint. The patient often becomes aware of this pain as soon as he awakens from anesthesia. It usually lasts twenty-four to forty-eight hours after surgery, but it may continue longer, depending upon the surgery performed, the pain threshold of the patient, and the personality of the patient. Most of this pain arises from trauma to the somatic nerve fibers in the skin. It is sharp and localized. Muscles and fascia are also supplied with somatic nerve fibers, and extensive dissection or prolonged retraction of these tissues will produce deep, long-lasting pain. Pain in the operative area may be aggravated by skin sutures, tight dressings, swelling of the incision during healing, and the presence of infection or hematomas in the wound. Continuous and severe pain can produce anxiety, restlessness, sleeplessness, anorexia, and irritability. Its presence can also prolong convalescence since it may interfere with the performance of certain activities.

It is not always possible to prevent the occurrence of pain, but it can be alleviated so that the patient is relatively comfortable. Patients who have had adequate preoperative instructions and who have confidence in the surgeon, in the nurses, and in the outcome of the surgery usually have less postoperative pain than the apprehensive patient. Pain can be relieved by nursing measures and/or by the administration of narcotics. The patient's position often aggravates wound pain. A change of position, elevation of the head of the bed, loosening of restraining sheets, and support of dependent parts of the body may give relief. Dressings that are binding or casts that are too tight should be reported to the doctor so that they can be loosened or removed.

In addition to making the patient as comfortable as possible, it may be necessary to administer a narcotic. Before it is given, however, the nurse should decide whether the patient's pain is a reasonable result of the operation or whether it is a new development. The latter must be reported to the physician. The nurse should also check the patient's physical condition. Since most narcotics depress the respiratory center, the patient's respirations should be above fourteen before these drugs are administered. Narcotics, especially meperidine hydrochloride (Demerol) cause the blood pressure to drop; therefore, if the blood pressure is low or unstable, they should not be given without consulting the doctor. A very drowsy patient should not receive a narcotic because it will further depress his respirations and activity. Since aged patients usually do not tolerate narcotics well and have a high pain threshold, these drugs should be given to them in small doses and as infrequently as possible.

When the nurse decides that the need

for a narcotic is justified and that the patient's condition is satisfactory, she should give the medication as ordered to keep him comfortable. Narcotics can be given every four hours during the first twelve to thirty-six hours postoperatively without danger of addiction. Narcotics, however, besides causing respiratory and circulatory depression, may cause urticaria, restlessness, nausea, and vomiting. Therefore, the patient should be observed for any untoward reaction. Patients who have received a narcotic shortly before getting out of bed to walk should be closely supervised since the action of the drug may cause them to become dizzy or faint. The need for narcotics should decrease after forty-eight hours, and continuous, severe pain after this time should be reported to the physician.

CARE OF THE WOUND

Most surgical wounds are clean, closed wounds that heal rapidly with a minimum of scarring. After the incision has been sutured, the incised skin surfaces are quickly glued together by strands of fibrin and a thin layer of clotted blood. Plasma seeps onto the surface, forming a dry protective crust. There should be a minimum of serous drainage from such a wound, and after twenty-four hours all seepage onto the dressing should cease. The dressing does not need to be changed until the sutures are removed. The wound is weakest during the third to sixth day after surgery. After this time there is union of the deep tissues as a result of fibroplasia and collagen deposition. Increase in wound strength progresses rapidly from the sixth to the fourteenth day and then continues slowly for some months. Although wound union is only relatively firm until after the sixth postoperative day, the sutures permit the patient to cough, turn, and get out of bed without danger of wound separation. It is important for the patient to know this; otherwise he may be reluctant to participate in such activities for fear of injuring the incision. Skin sutures (black silk thread, fine wire, or metal skin clips) are removed from abdominal wounds on about the seventh postoperative day, from neck and face wounds on about the third to the fifth postoperative day, and from wounds of the extremities on the eighth to tenth postoperative day. Retention sutures made of heavy wire and placed deep into muscle tissue usually are not removed until the fourteenth to the twenty-first postoperative day. Most patients become apprehensive when they know the sutures are to be removed. They may be told that they will have little, if any, pain during the procedure. Unless there is some seepage of fluid after the sutures are removed, a dressing is not necessary, and the area may be washed.

Drains inserted at the time of surgery may exit directly from the incision or through a separate small incision known as a stab wound. These allow fluids such as bile, pus, and serum to drain from the operative site and prevent the development of deep wound infections. Drainage from stab wounds may be profuse. The nurse should check with the doctor or look on the operative sheet to determine the exact location of drains so that she will know the type of drainage to expect. The dressings which cover wounds containing drains usually are changed within twenty-four hours postoperatively. Until this time the dressing may be reinforced only as necessary; after the initial dressing is changed, however, the nurse may be allowed to make further changes as often as necessary to keep the patient dry and comfortable. Care must be taken that a drain is not inadvertently removed when the dressings are changed. The use of Montgomery straps will make the dressing more comfortable for the patient and will eliminate the repeated removal of adhesive tape from the skin. If the drainage is irritating to the skin, the skin should be washed frequently with soap and water and a protective ointment such as zinc oxide applied. (Refer to a textbook on nursing arts for the correct technique in changing dressings.) The character and the amount of drainage should be recorded, and any change in the amount or consistency should be reported to the surgeon. The patient should be told the reason for the drainage so that he does not become alarmed when he sees it on the dressing or his gown. Drains are shortened gradually and are removed when the drainage has diminished. The opening caused by the drain heals in a few days.

Hemorrhage. Hemorrhage from the wound may occur within the first forty-eight hours postoperatively, or it may occur as late as the sixth or seventh postoperative day. It may be caused by the slipping of a ligature due to inadequate tying, by infection, or by the erosion of a vessel by a drainage tube. The nurse should inspect every postoperative dressing frequently; if bright red blood is present, she should outline it with a pencil so that the rate of increase can easily be determined, and she should report it to the doctor. The dressing should be checked at fifteen-minute intervals to determine the rapidity of bleeding, and the patient should be observed for other signs of hemorrhage such as fall in blood pressure, rise in pulse and respiratory rates, restlessness, pallor, weakness, and cold, moist skin. When the bleeding is profuse, the nurse should apply a pressure dressing until the doctor arrives. Her actions should be efficient, and she should remain calm so that the patient is not unduly alarmed. She should take the patient's blood pressure at fifteen-minute intervals since this will help the doctor to determine the extent of the hemorrhage, and she should gather equipment that the doctor may need, such as infusion fluid, material for drawing blood for typing and cross-matching, shock blocks, and dressing equipment. The doctor usually treats a hemorrhage by applying pressure on the wound to occlude the bleeding vessels and administering a blood transfusion to replace blood lost. A hemostatic gelatin sponge, such as Gelfoam, soaked in saline solution is sometimes used to control surface bleeding. This sponge is applied with pressure to the bleeding site for two to four minutes, and then it is left in place. It is absorbed in one to five weeks. When severe wound hemorrhage occurs, the patient is taken immediately to the operating room, where the wound is opened and the bleeding vessel ligated. If a preoperative medication is ordered, the nurse should check to see when the last narcotic was given. Under pressure of the emergency, there is danger that the patient may receive an overdose of narcotic, thus causing respiratory and circulatory depression and prohibiting the administration of an anesthetic. Since the patient often becomes frightened by the hemorrhage and the subsequent emergency procedures, the nurse should make every effort to reassure him and to keep noise, confusion, and technical discussions at the bedside to a minimum.

Infection. Wound infections are a fairly common postoperative complication. The causative organisms often are staphylococci and streptococci and are usually introduced into the wound as the incision is made. (See Chapter 11 for discussion of staphylococcal infections.) Wound infections are more prevalent in debilitated and obese patients since the blood supply to the incisional area tends to be inadequate. From three to six days after surgery the patient begins to have a low-grade fever and the wound becomes painful and swollen. The nurse should report complaints of persistent pain in the incision to the physician, and she should be alert for purulent drainage on the dressing. If spontaneous drainage of the wound does not occur, the surgeon may choose to open a section of the healed incision to facilitate drainage. Wound discomfort usually disappears after this is done, and the patient is much more comfortable. The nurse usually is asked to change the dressings as they become soiled; she should use sterile technique to prevent further contamination. The patient should be cautioned not to touch the wound at any time.

A culture is made of the fluid obtained from the wound, and the administration of appropriate antibiotics is started. If it is a superficial wound infection, sterile, hot wet dressings may be ordered. These must be applied at the correct temperature and only for the prescribed period of time since prolonged soaking causes maceration of the skin. Petrolatum usually is applied to the skin around the infected wound to protect it from burns. The wet dressing should be covered with a Koroseal or plastic sheet to maintain the heat and moisture and to prevent the bed linen from becoming damp.

Dehiscence and evisceration. Wound dehiscence is a partial to complete separation of the wound edges. Wound evisceration is protrusion of loops of the intestine through the incision onto the abdominal wall. These complications often are brought to the nurse's attention by the patient's complaint of a "giving" sensation in the incision or of a sudden, profuse leakage of fluid from the incision. Upon inspection, the dressing will be found to be saturated with clear, pink drainage. The wound edges may be partially or entirely separated, and loops of intestine may be lying on the abdominal wall. These complications may occur at any time through the fourteenth postoperative day, but they usually occur between the sixth and the eighth day. They are thought to be due to cachexia, anemia, advanced age, hypoproteinemia, dehydration, infection, or excessive vomiting, retching, and coughing.

If the nurse discovers either of these complications she should put the patient to bed in a low Fowler's position and caution him not to cough. She should try not to alarm him but he should be told to remain quiet and not to eat or drink anything until the doctor has seen him. While awaiting the doctor's arrival, the nurse may apply warm, sterile dressings over the protruding intestines to keep the serous membrane from becoming dry if this is the policy of the hospital; otherwise, she should apply sterile dressings and secure them loosely with a scultetus binder or adhesive tape. She should then gather the equipment that the doctor will need, such as dressing equipment and infusion fluid. The patient's blood pressure, pulse, and respirations should be taken to determine if he is in shock.

The treatment for wound dehiscence and wound evisceration is immediate closure of the wound under local anesthesia. The patient is taken to the operating room in his bed. Preoperative medication usually is not given since the patient is likely to be in shock. These are serious complications because they involve a second operation, are potential threats to the patient's life, and prolong convalescence.

RETURN OF URINARY FUNCTION

If the patient is well hydrated, urinary function usually returns within six to eight hours after surgery. Although 2,000 ml. of intravenous solution usually is given on the operative day, the first voiding may not be more than 200 ml., and the total urinary output for the operative day may be less than 1,500 ml. This is due to loss of body fluid during surgery and to perspiration, hyperventilation, and vomiting. As body functions stabilize and fluid and electrolyte balance return to normal, however, the ratio of intake to output should also return to normal. This may take about forty-eight hours, and during this time a record is kept of the intake and the time and amount of each voiding. If the urinary output is less than 500 ml. in twenty-four hours, this must be reported to the doctor, since the decreased urinary output may be due to kidney failure caused by shock or a reaction to the anesthetic or other drugs.

Some patients are unable to void after surgery, and this is an annoying and uncomfortable sensation. The difficulty may be due to the recumbent position, nervous tension, the remaining effects of anesthetics such as Avertin or spinal anesthetics which interfere with bladder sensation and the ability to void, the use of narcotics which reduce the sensation of bladder distention, or the pain caused by movement onto the bedpan. Inability to void is a common occurrence following operations on the rectum or colon and following gynecologic procedures since the innervation of the bladder musculature may be temporarily disturbed. The desire and the ability to void may be facilitated by nursing measures such as forcing fluids, placing the patient on the bedpan at regular intervals, running the water in the sink while the patient is on the bedpan, pouring warm water over the pelvic area, and assuring the patient of privacy. Most patients are able to void if they are gotten out of bed. Walking tends to increase the ability to void, and if the patient is allowed to be up, the use of the toilet or a commode may be more conducive to voiding than a bedpan. If these measures are not effective, the doctor may order the patient to be catheterized. Because of the emotional trauma to the young child and the possibility of reproductive tract infections in men, catheterization may be delayed longer than the usual eight hours postoperatively in these patients in the hope that voiding will take place. If the bladder is palpable over the pubic bone and suprapubic pressure causes discomfort, however, the patient must be catheterized to prevent stretching of the vesical wall. Distention of the bladder may cause infection of the urinary system and atony of the bladder muscles, resulting in inability to void later. If the patient must be catheterized more than three times after an operation, a Foley catheter usually is inserted into the bladder and the patient is given sulfisoxazole (Gantrisin) and fluids are forced.

Occasionally, a patient voids frequently but in small amounts. This is known as "retention with overflow." The overdistended bladder expels just enough urine to relieve the pressure within it temporarily. This condition should be reported to the physician, who will probably order the patient catheterized for residual urine. Since a large volume of residual urine is a good medium for bacterial growth, a Foley catheter may be left in place for several days. Otherwise, catheterization usually is done every six to eight hours until the residual urine left in the bladder after voiding is less than 50 ml.

Postoperative urinary tract infection can usually be avoided by the complete emptying of the bladder at each voiding, the prevention of bladder distention, and the use of sterile, nontraumatic technique when catheterizations are necessary. Staphylococcal infection of the urinary tract, a common complication of catheterization, is thought to be most often caused by poor technique in doing the procedure. Patients who must be on prolonged bed rest, who have had urinary tract infections in the past, who are elderly, or who have had operations on the pelvic organs are especially prone to bladder and kidney infections. Special attention should be given to the amount and quality of their urinary output, and they should drink at least 3,000 ml. of fluid a day. Symptoms such as a burning sensation in the bladder and urethra during or after urination, frequency, chills, fever, malaise, and anorexia can be indicative of urinary tract infection and should be reported to the doctor.

RETURN OF GASTROINTESTINAL FUNCTION

Gastrointestinal function usually returns to normal within twenty-four to forty-eight hours after surgery. The slowing down or absence of peristalsis is caused by anesthesia, handling of the bowel, and pressure on abdominal organs. Bed activity and early ambulation are thought to stimulate the return of peristalsis. The return of normal peristalsis is determined by hearing bowel sounds upon auscultation of the abdomen. The passage of flatus by rectum or a spontaneous bowel movement also indicates the return of peristalsis.

Until bowel sounds are heard, the patient is not permitted to have food or fluid by mouth; his fluid intake is maintained by parenteral fluids. The ingestion of food or fluids before peristalsis returns causes vomiting, and the patient is not only uncomfortable but his electrolyte balance is also upset by the loss of gastric juices. If he is well hydrated, his thirst should not be excessive, but he will be made more comfortable if given frequent mouth care and allowed to chew gum and suck on small pieces of ice or hard candy to increase salivation. This also will help to prevent the occurrence of *"surgical parotitis,"* a swelling and inflammation of the parotid glands seen most often in debilitated patients. This may occur because of the invasion of an inactive gland by organisms from the mouth. If the gland is secreting normally, the organisms will be unable to gain entrance or will be washed back into the mouth by the saliva. Parotitis is extremely painful, and it may be unilateral or bilateral. If it occurs, it is treated with antibiotics. Warm gargles and an ice collar usually are ordered as comfort measures.

When peristalsis returns, the patient is permitted to have clear fluids by mouth. It is preferable that iced fluids, milk, and fruit juices be omitted at first, since if the peristalsis is still rather sluggish, these fluids tend to cause gas formation. If the patient tolerates fluids well, he can usually progress rapidly to a regular diet. Some surgeons believe that the patient should eat solid food as soon as gastrointestinal activity returns because solid food stimulates the stomach to empty, whereas fluids tend to cause distention.[10]

Since it is desirable that he regain a good nutritional status as soon as possible so tissue healing will readily occur, the patient should be encouraged to eat a well-balanced diet as soon as he can tolerate one. It is estimated that a caloric intake of 50 per cent more than the basic caloric requirement for the individual is needed to provide for energy expended in early ambulation and for reparative processes.[10] An attractive, well-balanced general diet should be served, and the patient should be allowed to select what appeals to him. Even after a few days of enforced starvation, the patient may be somewhat indifferent to food, mentally depressed, and weak; it may take two or three days on a well-balanced general diet to overcome this condition brought on, in part at least, by lack of food. Special surgical diets usually are ordered only after gastric surgery. Special diets for medical conditions, such as diabetes mellitus or cardiac insufficiency, should be resumed as soon as possible after surgery.

Vomiting. Postoperative vomiting is one of the most distressing problems that the patient encounters. It leaves him weak and uncomfortable, with a bad taste in his mouth, and it usually aggravates incisional pain. Postoperative vomiting is usually of short duration and is due to the effects of anesthetics such as ether and ethylene, from an accumulation of fluid in the stomach, or from eating food or drinking water before peristalsis returns. It is not unusual for the patient who expects to vomit postoperatively to do so.

To prevent danger of aspiration, the patient who is vomiting should lie on his side. He should be advised not to take food or fluid for several hours and to lie quietly in bed. The emesis basin and soiled bed linen should be removed, and mouth care should be given. When vomiting has subsided, sucking on chips of ice or taking sips of gingerale or hot tea may help to relieve the nausea. Sometimes small amounts of solid food such as crackers or cooked cereal may relieve nausea.

Persistent postoperative vomiting is usually a symptom of pyloric obstruction, intestinal obstruction, or peritonitis. This type of vomiting tires the patient, puts a strain on the incision, and causes excessive loss of fluids and electrolytes. Projectile vomiting of gastric contents occurs in the presence of pyloric obstruction. In intestinal obstruction, the vomitus is fecal in nature, and it usually flows continuously and effortlessly from the patient's mouth. If persistent vomiting occurs, a gastric tube is passed into the stomach and the stomach is lavaged. The tube may be left in place and attached to a suction apparatus to keep the stomach empty. The patient is not given anything by mouth, and intravenous fluids containing electrolytes are administered to replace the fluid and electrolyte loss.

Hiccoughs. Hiccoughs are among the most exhausting postoperative complications. They weaken the patient and interfere with eating, talking, and sleeping. The exact cause of postoperative hiccoughs is not known, but it is known that dilatation of the stomach, irritation of the diaphragm, peritonitis, and uremia each causes either reflex or central nervous system stimulation of the phrenic nerve. Fortunately, hiccoughs are not too common a postoperative complaint. They usually disappear within a few hours, and they may respond to such a simple measure as having the patient breathe his own carbon dioxide at five-minute intervals by having him inhale and exhale into a paper bag held tightly over his nose and mouth. Carbon dioxide inhalations, using 5 per cent carbon dioxide and 95 per cent oxygen, may also be given for five minutes every hour. If dizziness occurs, these should be discontinued, since an overdose of carbon dioxide may cause convulsions and coma. Aspiration of the stomach will stop hiccoughs caused by gastric dilatation. Chlorpromazine (Thorazine) has recently been used with good results in mild cases of hiccoughs. If the hiccoughs are persistent and do not respond to these treatments, local infiltration of the phrenic nerve with 1 per cent procaine may be necessary, or in extreme cases surgical crushing of the phrenic nerve may be done.

Abdominal distention. Postoperative distention is a result of an accumulation of nonabsorbable gas in the intestines caused by handling of the bowel during surgery, swallowing of air during recovery from anesthesia and as the patient attempts to overcome nausea, and from the transudation of gases from the blood stream to the atonic portion of the bowel.[11] Distention will persist until the tone of the bowel returns to normal and peristalsis resumes. It is experienced to some degree by most patients after abdominal and kidney surgery.

"Gas pains" are caused by contractions of the unaffected portions of the bowel in an attempt to move the accumulated gas through the intestinal tract. The patient is uncomfortable and, if the distention is high in the abdomen, he may have difficulty in breathing. High distention may be due to stomach dilatation and can be relieved by aspiration of the stomach contents with a gastric tube. Ambulation often stimulates the return of peristalsis and the expulsion of flatus. Gas also may be removed by a lubricated rectal tube inserted into the rectum. This tube should be inserted just past the rectal sphincter and should be removed at the end of twenty minutes. If necessary, it may be used every four hours. Heat applied to the abdomen in the form of a hot-water bottle, heating pad, or flaxseed poultice may be ordered in conjunction with the use of a rectal tube. Small carminative enemas of milk and molasses or glycerine, magnesium sulfate, and water sometimes are ordered to stimulate the expulsion of flatus. If the distention progresses and the flatus is not expelled after forty-eight hours, a *paralytic ileus* is suspected. This is complete absence of bowel tone caused by the anesthetic, by a generalized infection such as peritonitis, or by other causes. The patient is kept on "nothing by mouth," and gastric suctioning is started and continued until peristalsis returns.

Defecation. The first spontaneous bowel movement usually occurs four to five days after surgery and indicates that normal gastrointestinal function has returned. Unless there are symptoms of fecal impaction or intestinal distention, no attempt is made to hasten bowel evacuation. The patient who is eating normally, drinking adequate fluid, walking about, and taken to the bathroom routinely will usually have a bowel movement without an enema. When an enema seems necessary, a small soapsuds enema usually will stimulate defecation. If the patient is constipated, an oil retention enema followed by a soapsuds enema may be necessary. Patients who are prone to constipation should be given prune juice at least once a day.

While caring for the postoperative patient, the nurse should question him about the expulsion of flatus or the occurrence of a bowel movement, since a delay in bowel evacuation beyond four or five days postoperatively may be a symptom of paralytic ileus or intestinal obstruction.

Postoperative diarrhea may occur; since this may be caused by a fecal impaction, it should be reported to the physician. If the patient has severe burns of the buttocks or has undergone extensive rectal surgery, bowel movements may be intentionally delayed for several days by the administration of lead and opium pills, paregoric, or bismuth subcarbonate by mouth.

PREPARATION FOR DISCHARGE FROM THE HOSPITAL

Preparation of the patient for discharge from the hospital is an important part of the nursing care in the postoperative period. Plans for discharge may have been discussed and begun in the preoperative period, but most of the teaching, arrangements, and preparations are done after surgery. The patient, his family, and the members of the health team responsible for the care of the patient during his hospitalization should participate in the long-range planning.

As a result of the early resumption of ambulation and a nutritious diet, most patients regain their strength rapidly, and the average hospital stay following surgery is less than two weeks. During this time the patient and his family should be prepared for any care that must be given at home, and any necessary arrangements for convalescent care should be completed several days prior to discharge. The patient should be helped to become as self-sufficient as possible before being discharged so that he does not have to depend any more than necessary upon the assistance of relatives and friends. Upon returning home he should be able to perform all the activities of daily living and be able to do his own treatments. Early in the postoperative period the nurse should consult with the doctor regarding the anticipated discharge plans for the patient so that she can evaluate his needs, his ability to participate in the care to be given at home, the interest and the desire of the family to help, and the home situation and its facilities. Whenever possible, both the patient and a member of his family should be taught all treatments and exercises that must be done at home. Arrangements should be made for a member of the family to come to the hospital to watch and learn procedures, to talk to the dietitian, to consult with the doctor, to discuss problems with the social service worker, and to plan with the nurse about home care. Ample opportunity should be given the patient and his family to ask questions. The nurse should try to anticipate any problems that might arise and help the patient and his family plan for them. If a colostomy irrigation must be given and there are no bathroom facilities, extra equipment will be necessary so that it can be done in the room available. If the patient is reluctant or unable to give himself an injection, some member of the family must be taught how to give injections or arrangements must be made for a visiting nurse to do this. If the patient does not understand English, an interpreter may be needed to explain diets, medications, or treatments. If he lives alone, has no relatives, or is unable to be cared for by his family, he may have to be sent to a nursing home to receive the required care. Admittance to another hospital or to a nursing home for further treatment or for terminal care takes time, and since there is usually a long waiting list, arrangements should be begun as soon as the decision to do this is reached by the doctor, the patient, and the family.

On discharge the patient is given an appointment for a follow-up examination in the doctor's office or in the outpatient department of the hospital. This appointment is usually for one or two weeks after discharge. The nurse should make sure that the patient understands the importance of returning for the medical examination and that he can make arrangements to come in at this time.

With modern surgical techniques the wound is sutured securely and is usually well healed by the time of discharge from the hospital. Therefore, the convalescent period usually is relatively short, and most patients may return to their usual activity and occupation within two to four weeks postoperatively. During the convalescent period the patient should rest when he becomes tired and increase his activity gradually. Permission to return to work is given after the patient returns to the doctor for his follow-up examination. At this time the doctor checks the healing of the wound and the patient's general physical condition. Depending upon the outcome of this examination and the type of work the patient does, the doctor will decide when it will be desirable for him to resume his occupation.

REFERENCES AND SELECTED READINGS*

1 *Adams, Ralph: Prevention of Infections in Hospitals, Am. J. Nursing **58**:344-348, March 1958.

2 Beal, John M. (editor): Manual of the Recovery Room, New York, 1956, The Macmillan Co.

3 *Calabro, John J.: Hiccups, Am. J. Nursing **55**:1365-1366, Nov. 1955.

4 Cooper, Lenna F., Barber, Edith M., Mitchell, Helen S., and Rynbergen, Henderika J.: Nutrition in Health and Disease, ed. 13, Philadelphia, 1958, J. B. Lippincott Co.

5 *Covalt, Nila K.: Early Exercise for the Convalescent Patient, Am. J. Nursing **47**:544-546, Aug. 1947.

6 *Dripps, Robert D., and Waters, Ralph M.: Nursing Care of Surgical Patients—The "Stir-Up," Am. J. Nursing **41**:530-534, May 1941.

7 Elman, Robert: Surgical Care, A Practical Physiologic Guide, New York, 1951, Appleton-Century-Crofts, Inc.

8 Fuerst, Elinor, and Wolff, LuVerne: Fundamentals of Nursing, ed. 2, Philadelphia, 1959, J. B. Lippincott Co.

9 Hanson, Donald: The Salivary Glands, Am. J. Nursing **58**:240-241, Feb. 1958.

10 Hayes, Mark A.: Postoperative Diet Therapy, J. Am. Dietetic Assn. **35**:17-18, Jan. 1959.

11 Ilgenfritz, Hugh C.: Preoperative and Postoperative Care of Surgical Patients, St. Louis, 1948, The C. V. Mosby Co.

12 *Leithauser, Daniel J.: Early Ambulation, Am. J. Nursing **50**:203-206, April 1950.

13 *Stanton, Joseph R.: Venous Thrombosis and Pulmonary Embolism, Am. J. Nursing **55**:709-711, June 1955.

*References preceded by an asterisk indicate material particularly well suited for student reading.

The nurse's role in

accidents, emergencies, and disaster

Chapter 15

Study questions for review

1 Based on reports in the daily papers, list what you believe to be the most common causes of accidents.
2 What provisions are there in your hospital for the reporting of accidents within the hospital? What action is taken when an accident occurs? By whom is the action taken?
3 What are some precautions taken in your unit to prevent accidents to patients?
4 List potential accident hazards that are found in the average home.
5 What is the Civil Defense program in your hospital, in your community, and in your state?

Accidents

The accident death rate showed a downward trend from 95,300 in 1957 to 91,000 in 1958. The cost to the nation of these accidents, including wage loss, medical care, claims, and property damage, is estimated to be at least 12 billion dollars.[1] This figure does not record in any way the tremendous suffering and loss in social contribution of the injured, many of whom spend months and years seeking total or partial rehabilitation.

Accidents are the leading cause of death for persons 1 to 24 years of age and the second cause for those 25 to 44 years of age. In the more conservative years of life, from 45 to 64, accidents rank in fourth place. After age 65 accidents rank sixth as cause of death, being exceeded by heart disease, vascular lesions of the central nervous system, cancer, arteriosclerosis, and pneumonia. These figures are shocking since accidents are, for the most part, preventable and require only public education and individual caution for their control. This is in sharp contrast to cancer which is among the three top causes of death in all age groups from 5 years of age on, but which is, to a much greater extent, beyond our control.

The accident picture has changed in recent years. There are now proportionately fewer accidents sustained while earning a living. The shorter work day and better industrial safety programs have accounted for this. In 1958 only 13,300 persons were killed at work, in contrast to 1951 when 16,000 were killed.[1] Home accidents in 1958 (27,000) decreased slightly over previous years, reflecting better public education and the fact that accidental deaths in nursing homes are now listed as deaths occurring in public places, whereas previously they had been listed as home accidents.[2] Many accidents now occur during leisure-time activities.

PREVENTION OF ACCIDENTS

Prevention is the keynote to success in dealing with the problem of accidents. Accident control has been acknowledged as a major public health goal, and the American Public Health Association has had an active subcommittee on accident prevention since 1943. In 1955 this subcommittee made a survey and prepared a report entitled "Suggested Home Accident Prevention Activities for Health Departments." Some communities have local citizens' committees that have been helpful in conducting surveys of accident hazards in homes.

Teaching accident prevention and participating in programs for accident prevention are responsibilities of all members of the health team, including doctors, nurses, health educators, and others. The nurse is an essential member of this team. Her influence can be felt in many areas, since she is represented in schools, in industry, in the home, in the hospital, and in the community. Space does not permit a detailed description of the many ways in which a nurse can contribute in this important health field, but a few examples will be given for some areas. Many references are available. The nurse can turn to the National Safety Council which has a monthly publication, *Home Safety Review*, and a yearly bulletin, *Accident Facts*. An excellent way for the nurse to keep informed in this field is to get her name placed on the mailing list to receive the *Statistical Bulletin* of the Metropolitan Life Insurance Company. She can turn to her local health department for health education materials and for information on other sources of materials, such as the many excellent materials on accident prevention prepared by life insurance companies and industrial organizations. Engineers are often invaluable resource people for consultation on structural hazards at home and in the community. The safety committee in the nurse's own hospital or public health agency may be of help. Finally, she must use her own resourcefulness and imagination in preventing accidents.

Home and community

The nurse can help in accident prevention whether she is actively practicing nursing in a hospital or in a community nursing agency or whether she is a full-time mother and homemaker. Lay individuals and lay groups often turn to her for assistance and guidance in learning of community needs and of how they may best contribute in accident prevention. She should be able to point out good sources of general information on the national level, such as the reports of the National Safety Council. The local or county health department, the local police department, the Visiting Nurse Association, the Welfare and Health Council, or similar agencies are all good sources of help. The nurse should assure the layman that his voice will be heard provided it is directed to the right authorities, and she may point out that groups have a stronger voice than individuals. Parent-teachers associations, various religious and social organizations, and many other groups are interested in the problem of accident control. Efforts should be made to use existing agencies and groups and to work with them in order that the sincere efforts of small groups of enthusiastic citizens will not be dissipated. Phases of accident prevention that should be of community interest include the following: how accident prevention can be taught in the public school, how better control and inspection of homes for the aged may be fostered by law, how rigid enforcement of driving regulations can be enforced, how better street lighting and wider use of light signals at busy intersections can be brought about, how regular checking and inspection of all cars can be done, and what laws pertaining to fireproof features in buildings are needed.

Accidents in and about the home cause almost a third of all accidental deaths each year. Falls account for about half the number, and fires, burns, and poisonings account for most of the remainder. Many aged persons who fall do so merely walking from room to room; some fall because of slippery floors, loose rugs, poor lighting, scattered toys, and other circumstances that could have been corrected. A fair number of fatal home accidents occur as a result of the recently intensified "do it yourself" movement. People are falling from roofs, windows, high ladders, and steps and are being fatally burned or otherwise injured while using solvents and cleansing agents without proper knowledge of their hazards. The number of electrical appliances used in the home has increased the danger of electric shock and of fire from overloaded circuits. Each year the consumption of cigarettes increases, and many persons die in fires caused by burning cigarette ashes left on furniture or rugs and by falling asleep while smoking. More rigid control measures are needed to prevent death in the home from escaping gas. More caution should be taught to persons living in rural areas who use gas to heat their homes and who are not prepared to care for equipment that is not functioning properly.

The public health nurse is frequently called upon to evaluate the patient's home for accident hazards prior to his leaving the hospital. Very often such patients are those with physical disabilities. This kind of request provides the nurse with an ideal opportunity to teach not only the patient but also members of his family about general accident prevention as well as specific measures for the safety of the patient.

Hospital

In the hospital the nurse should take an active part in accident prevention. The doctor looks to her to help devise means to protect each individual patient from accidents. The hospital administrator depends upon her for suggestions on how the hospital can be made a safer place for patients. Every nurse should be on the alert for accident hazards and should use her initiative in suggesting ways to prevent them. She should submit her suggestions verbally or in writing to her nursing supervisor so that they may go through appropriate channels to those who can put them into general use.

The danger of accidents to hospital patients has increased in recent years. The turnover of patients is much more rapid and the patient has less time to adjust to his new environment. Early ambulation of patients has added to accident hazards. Most important is the great increase in the proportion of elderly patients; many are in their eighties and even their nineties. An infinite number of improvements could be made in general hospitals which might reduce accidents, and they vary with each situation. For example, hand rails should be installed in the corridors of medical and surgical units where patients now walk about each day. Stools should be placed in showers, beside tubs, and in washrooms; chairs with arms should replace the straight armless ones so often used.

Careful study of nursing practice and of the quality of nursing care may reveal good suggestions for accident prevention. For instance, one large hospital* analyzed a group of accidents in which patients fell out of bed. The two main causes of the falls were attempts to climb over the side rails and attempts to reach for a bedpan or other piece of equipment in the bedside table when the table or the bed had free-rolling casters. Obvious solutions seemed to be the use of high-low beds (this must be done gradually, since few hospitals can afford to replace all beds at once) and the removal of casters on beds and bedside tables.

Study of the patients who attempted to climb over side rails showed that most of them were aged and that many had received barbiturate sedation. Again, measures for prevention of accidents seemed obvious. Aged patients should be placed in high-low beds and in a location where they will have frequent observation. After having slept for forty years in a low bed, they cannot remember that they are in a high hospital bed; like Rip Van Winkle, they awake to find many changes. Fewer sedatives should be given to elderly patients than to younger ones. It is better to rely upon nursing measures such as a warm drink, a backrub, a cheerful word, attention to ventilation, and control of noise to ensure a good night of sleep.

Emergency care

Every nurse should be conversant with the general principles of first aid and if a physician is not present should be prepared to assume leadership when accidents occur. First aid is defined as immediate and temporary care given the

*Unpublished study, The New York Hospital-Cornell Medical Center.

victim of an accident. Some general principles have application to most accident situations; the nurse can teach these to patients and to their relatives. Printed booklets such as *When the Unexpected Happens** should be useful in helping the public to learn the practical steps in first aid.

In the following discussion a distinction will be made between the first aid given by the nurse at the scene of an accident and the nursing care she may give or help to give in the hospital. Usually standing orders guide her actions in schools, industries, and public health agencies. Emergency treatment of medical emergencies, including postoperative shock, pulmonary embolism and edema, heart attack, convulsions, cerebrovascular accident, and severe burns, will be considered in chapters relating to the body systems involved.

EMERGENCY MANAGEMENT IN GENERAL

The first thing to do when an accident occurs is to stop for a moment and remember to keep calm and to think before acting. The nurse may then quietly step forward, observe the patient, and take his pulse. This often establishes the nurse as someone with experience, and it may discourage the eager individual at the scene of an accident who tends to "take over" and create more excitement, sometimes causing additional harm to the patient. Onlookers who wish to help can be asked to call a doctor, the local police department, and an ambulance. They may stop traffic or direct people away from where the patient lies. Whoever calls the doctor must be prepared to give the location of the scene, the nature of the accident, and the first-aid materials available.

The patient must be kept flat. Often the first act of the uninformed is to try to raise the patient to a sitting position and to induce him to respond. What is done first in an emergency depends upon the situation. Signs of hemorrhage or of breathing difficulties are looked for first. A quick survey may be made for signs of poison, for electric wires, and for murder or suicide weapons.

Hemorrhage. Severe hemorrhage must be treated at once, since it is possible to bleed to death from a severed large artery in less than one minute. It is important to look under the patient for signs of bleeding and to remember that bleeding may be internal and not apparent. The bleeding point should be covered with a sterile dressing. If this is not on hand, a freshly opened handkerchief or the cleanest material available must be used. Bleeding may be controlled in various ways, depending upon its location and severity. Pressure on the wound, pressure within

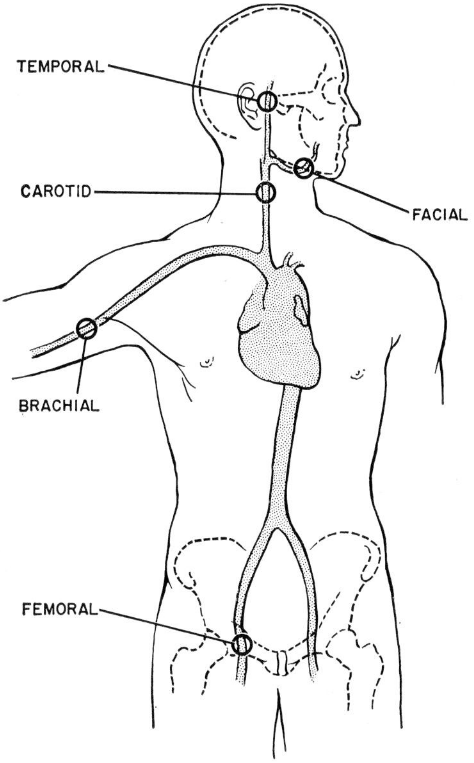

Figure 21

This diagram illustrates the pressure points or locations where large blood vessels may be compressed against bones to help control hemorrhage.

*Prepared by the John Hancock Mutual Life Insurance Co.

the wound, pressure on major blood vessels where they lie over bony prominences (pressure points, Figure 21), elevation of the part, or a tourniquet may be used. Tourniquets have been used too often by the inexperienced and in circumstances in which they were not needed, and serious damage has been done. It is now recommended that they be used at once however when it is apparent that elevation and pressure will not stop the bleeding.[21] Tourniquets should be carefully applied as low on the limb as possible and tightly enough to stop the flow of blood.[1] Ties, belts, and torn pieces of clothing may be used as tourniquets, but wire and rope should not be used because they are too damaging to tissues. Tourniquets, once applied, should not be removed until a doctor is present; provided they have been correctly applied, it is not true that they must be released every fifteen or thirty minutes. The time that the tourniquet is applied and its location must be recorded, and this information must be attached to the patient if he is transported.

Breathing and consciousness. The best way to tell whether or not the patient is breathing is to watch the movement of the chest and the nostrils and to feel for flow of air from the mouth or nose. Any obstruction to breathing must be removed at once, and if the patient is vomiting, his head must be turned to one side. State of consciousness should be determined by questioning the patient. Ask him where he is hurt and where he has the worst pain; if he does not respond, check his ears and nose carefully for signs of bleeding or draining serous fluid both of which indicate the probability of fracture of the base of the skull. Loss of consciousness immediately following an accident by trauma usually indicates a head injury.

Evidence of fracture. Check carefully to see whether the patient moves all parts of his body or whether an extremity is limp or flaccid. If paralysis of a limb is apparent or if any definite evidence of skull or other bone fracture is present, do not, under any circumstances, permit the patient to be moved until skilled help and suitable equipment have been secured.

The injured part must not be moved when fracture of a bone is suspected or known to have occurred. The first inclination of many well-meaning persons at the scene of an accident is to try to put the injured part into normal alignment. This can cause great harm. Nerves, blood vessels, and other tissues may be damaged, and pain and shock will be increased.

Moving the patient. If the patient must be moved before an ambulance with suitable splint materials has arrived, it is imperative that some form of temporary splint be improvised. The purpose of splinting is to preserve position and prevent motion; the materials used will depend upon the part of the body involved. Pillows, pieces of board, the leaves of dining room tables, rifle barrels, golf clubs, and tennis rackets have been used as splints by resourceful persons. A heavy magazine makes an excellent splint for the wrist; lacking even this, many pages of the daily newspaper serve almost as well.

Before the patient is moved, the splints should be prepared and all persons who are to help must know what to do and how to work together. If the fracture is within a joint, the entire limb may be very carefully supported, placed upon a splint such as a pillow, and bandaged securely. If the fracture is in the shaft of the bone, traction and countertraction will usually be needed. One person may support the part above the fracture and one may exert a steady firm pull until the splint has been applied and secured with improvised bandages. In some instances (for example, when strong muscle pull is involved, as in fracture of the femur), a steady pull away from the body must be maintained.

Injury of the spine. The patient with injury to the spine requires the most exact care in handling if he must be moved. Forward bending of the spine must not be allowed to occur, since this may cause pressure on the spinal cord and immediate death. A door makes the best temporary splint. It takes at least six persons working in perfect harmony to move the patient safely. The patient with a fracture of the neck or of the lower spine should not be rolled if he is lying on his back; he should be slid carefully sideways onto the board or splint. One person kneels at the patient's head and, holding the head securely with his hands under the jaws, exerts a firm steady pull. A second person supports the patient's feet, again exerting a firm steady pull. The other members of the team draw the patient's body onto the stretcher or splint. At no time must his head be allowed to bend forward or to the side; his head and body must move as one piece, and there must be very firm support under his shoulders so that sagging, which will cause forward-bending of the neck, cannot occur. If the patient is found lying on his face, he is usually rolled very carefully onto his back and onto the splint. Again, traction is applied to his head so that his spine is kept straight, and forward bending is avoided. A pillow or folded blanket is laid on the splint at the level of the injury before the patient is placed on it so that hyperextension of the spine is maintained when the patient is in a backlying position. For hospital care of patients with fractures see Chapter 36.

Wounds. Wounds should be exposed, and enough clothing must be removed to do this. A gaping or blowing wound in the chest must be covered immediately and manual pressure applied to seal off the opening. Open wounds of any kind must be kept as clean as possible, covered with the cleanest material available, and left untreated until a doctor sees the patient. If the patient is conscious, do not permit him to see his wounds.

Warmth. The victim of an accident, no matter what the cause, should be kept warm. Body warmth should be preserved, but extra heat should not be applied, because it causes vasodilation and further loss of body heat. Coats, blankets, and other coverings can be used, but hot stones, hot-water bottles, and the like should be avoided. It is often difficult to decide whether or not to risk harming the patient by moving him slightly to place protection under him since he cannot be kept warm when lying directly on damp ground. The apparent nature of the injury must determine this decision.

The patient found unconscious. If a person is found unconscious either in his home or on the street, he should be examined for signs of having bitten his tongue, as so often happens in convulsions, and for a fruity odor to the breath, which may indicate diabetic acidosis. Patients subject to convulsions and those with diabetes are usually advised to carry identifying information on their persons. The odor of poisons such as phenol and iodine can be detected on the breath. When an odor of alcohol is detected, it should not be assumed that the cause of unconsciousness has been determined. The environment should be carefully inspected for evidence of the cause of the patient's condition, and the patient should be examined for signs of injury particularly of the head. Do not attempt to give anything by mouth to an unconscious person; notify a doctor and make immediate arrangements to get the patient to a hospital. Unconsciousness with marked decrease in respiration is common in patients with morphine and barbiturate poisoning and in carbon monoxide poisoning. Artificial respiration may be given while awaiting arrival of an ambulance.

BITES

Animal bites

The most common animal bites are those of dogs and cats. Dog bites are particularly dangerous, since dogs are the most common carriers of the deadly disease hydrophobia or rabies. Cat bites are likely to cause infection because the cat's mouth contains many pathogenic bacteria and because the long sharp teeth make a deep wound which may become sealed off. Human bites, although rare, do occur and easily become infected because of the very high bacterial count in the human mouth.

The first-aid treatment for all animal bites is extremely thorough washing with soap and hot water for from ten to fifteen minutes. Running water should be used. If the bite is deep and if the animal is suspected of having rabies, the wound must be made to bleed and may even be probed, depending upon circumstances and how soon medical aid will be available. Strong caustic medications should not be applied; detergent solutions, however, have been found to be very effective in cleaning wounds from animal bites. The wound should be covered with a piece of sterile gauze and the advice of a doctor sought at once. He will decide whether or not treatment for rabies is necessary. The offending animal should always be kept alive until the advice of a doctor has been obtained; if it is a household pet and the circumstances indicate that the bite was accidental, the animal will usually be confined and observed for a week to ten days. If the animal must be killed immediately for the protection of others, the brain should not be damaged and must be sent to a laboratory for examination. If an animal suspected of having rabies is at large, the police department and the health department must be notified at once. For further discussion of prevention and treatment of rabies see Chapter 17.

Insect bites

Insect bites are more serious in children than in adults. It is well to remember that multiple bites have caused serious systemic reaction and even death of children. The bites of wasps and bees are among the most common of insect bites. A poultice of sodium bicarbonate and water often gives relief, since formic acid is present in the material injected by these insects. A weak solution of household ammonia also decreases pain and is safe to use.

A tick is best removed by holding a lighted match to it, thereby causing it to withdraw its mouthpiece; sudden removal of a tick will result in its mouthpiece being left in the skin. A drop of turpentine placed on the insect is also effective and without fire hazard. Ticks are the vectors of Rocky Mountain spotted fever and Colorado tick fever. If the person bitten lives in an area where these diseases are endemic, the advice of a doctor should be sought.

Mosquito bites are important because one species of mosquito (Anopheles) is active in the transmission of malaria and because the bites of mosquitoes and similar insects sometimes cause troublesome infections. The greatest danger of infection is in elderly persons with poor circulation in whom bites on the legs may lead to infected ulcers which heal with extreme difficulty. The best treatment for the nuisance and discomfort of mosquito bites is prevention, largely by avoiding highly infested areas and wearing protective clothing when one must be exposed. A mosquito net worn over a broad-brimmed hat when outdoors and the use of a large net canopy when sleeping provide good protection. Oil of citronella and many trade preparations are useful as repellents, but none are completely effective. Lotions containing calamine and phenol help to allay the itching and discomfort accompanying the bites.

The bites of poisonous spiders and other poisonous insects such as scorpions are treated in a manner similar to treatment of snakebite.

Snakebites

There are four kinds of poisonous snakes in the United States. Three of these, the copperhead, the cottonmouth moccasin, and the rattlesnake, belong to the group known as pit vipers and are distinguished by a pit resembling a second nostril between the eyes and the nostrils and by a broad, flat, triangular head. Everyone should know the kinds of poisonous snakes found in the part of the country in which he lives and how to recognize them. The copperhead is named for its color, is about 3 feet long, and is found in the eastern and southern states. The cottonmouth moccasin is grayish in color and blends with its surroundings; it is found in marshy country in the southeastern states. Rattlesnakes are probably to be found in every state in the United States and are responsible for the largest number of bites and the largest number of deaths. One antivenin is effective for all pit vipers. The fourth poisonous snake, the coral snake, is small and brilliantly colored. It is found in North Carolina and other southern states, particularly around the Gulf of Mexico. The snake is shy and seldom bites, but its venom is deadly and affects the nervous system. No specific antivenin is prepared for the bite of the coral snake, but the cobra antivenin kept in most zoos is effective.

Poisonous snakes in North America will almost always move away when disturbed and will not bite unless suddenly molested without warning. Snakebites can often be prevented by wearing high leather boots and thick trousers when walking through snake-infested areas. Heavy gloves should be worn and the greatest care taken when climbing, because hands may be placed on ledges that cannot be seen and reptiles often sun themselves on rocky ledges.

The bite of a poisonous snake is distinguished by two fang marks above the horseshoe-shaped array of tooth marks. Immediate severe pain and swelling distinguish the bite of a poisonous snake from that of a nonpoisonous one, even when swelling and discoloration are so sudden as to make the fang marks impossible to see. The wider the space between the fang marks, the larger the snake (sometimes unseen) and the more intensive the treatment should be.

The first-aid treatment for snakebite is the immediate application of a tourniquet just above the bite. This tourniquet should not be tight enough to prevent blood circulation in deep vessels but should be tight enough to prevent superficial circulation of blood and lymph, thus stopping absorption of the poison. In severe cases, if swelling appears above the tourniquet, the tourniquet is reapplied above the level of edema, or a second tourniquet may be used. Incision into the bite must be made immediately, with care being taken not to injure nerves and blood vessels by cutting in the direction of the vessels and nerves. A pocket knife or any sharp instrument, sterilized, if possible, by flaming with a match, can be used. If emergency snakebite equipment* is not available, suction must be applied by mouth; this is safe since the venom is not poisonous if swallowed. The patient should lie down and be kept warm. Medical aid should be sought at once; about 15 per cent of those bitten by poisonous snakes die without treatment.[33] If a snakebite kit is available, antivenin should be given at once; if a physician is not available or is delayed, whoever is at the scene should inject at least half of the ampule into the tissues around and above the bite and the rest intramuscularly. Warm fluids can be given; alcohol is contraindicated since it may speed up the absorption of venom. The patient must be kept quiet because moving about may also increase the absorption of venom. Signs of poisoning are palpitation, weakness, shortness of breath, nausea and vomiting, and dimness of vision. Occasionally the venom from the snake is injected directly into a blood vessel and severe fatal reaction may occur within fifteen minutes.

When the patient who has been bitten by a snake arrives at the hospital, the nurse should anticipate that stimulants such as strychnine and caffeine may be ordered. Intravenous infusions of glucose and physiologic solution of sodium chloride may be ordered for those patients who are dehydrated, who have low blood pressure, and in whom liver damage is suspected. Tetanus toxoid is usually administered, and antibiotics are given to combat infection. Since there is horse serum in antivenin, a reaction may be anticipated in some patients who have been treated at the scene of the accident. Usually skin testing for sensitivity to horse serum is done before additional antivenin is used in the hospital. Occasionally massive sloughing of tissue occurs following

*Snakebite kits contain a suction cup, tourniquet, razor blade, iodine, ampule of antivenin powder, vial-syringe of sterile distilled water, and instructions.

snakebite; this heals very slowly and in severe cases may necessitate amputation.

POISONING BY DRUGS AND CHEMICALS

More than four-fifths of all fatal accidents from poisoning occur in the home. Although poisoning is the third ranking cause of home accidents among children under 14 years of age, deaths from poisoning in this age group scarcely exceed those in persons 45 years of age and over.[1] In small children, poisoning usually results from accidental ingestion of poisonous substances; in adults it commonly occurs from not checking medications and from suicide attempts. Most large cities now have poison centers in the emergency departments of hospitals where emergency information and supplies are kept. This program is sponsored by health departments and is under the supervision of specialized pediatricians. These centers act as resources for physicians and provide immediate telephone directions to citizens.

Barbiturates are most often recorded as the cause of accidental death by poisoning. Their consumption has increased so tremendously in the last three decades that serious thought is now being given to much stricter supervision of these products; many states now have laws prohibiting the dispensing of barbiturates without medical prescription. The nurse should discourage the public from injudicious use of barbiturates and should urge safekeeping of these drugs where they will not be accessible to children. Acetylsalicylic acid (aspirin) and petroleum products are sources of poisoning for many children.

Drug cabinets, kitchen cupboards, and laundry closets are the places from which poisons most often are taken. In one large hospital it was strychnine poisoning that brought young children to the hospital most often.[13] The poisoning resulted from swallowing several laxative tablets, each containing a relatively large amount of the drug. Disinfectants such as phenol, iodine, bichloride of mercury, and cresol are easily taken by children if these substances are not locked away. Bromides and sleeping tablets left on bedside tables and in handbags are a potential source of trouble. The "do it yourself" movement has brought more paints, solvents, dyes, stains, turpentine, bleaches, and paint removers into the home. The public constantly needs to be reminded to keep poisons of all kinds conspicuously labeled, stored in cupboards, separate from foods, and placed out of the reach of children. Most manufacturers list the constituents of their products on the outside of the container. Some do not. The public should be encouraged to buy only those products whose contents are noted on the container, since medical treatment in the event of accidental poisoning may be delayed while the doctor attempts to learn what poison must be dealt with.

First-aid treatment in poisoning consists of trying to find out what poison was taken, diluting the poison, removing it from the stomach if possible, and getting in touch with a doctor. Lives have been saved by quick common-sense treatment while awaiting the doctor. For example, if bichloride of mercury, a deadly poison, can be removed from the stomach within fifteen minutes, the patient will usually live. On the other hand, when a strong acid such as phenol or a strong alkali such as lye has been taken, further damage and even rupture of the esophagus may be caused by vomiting; if strychnine has been taken, convulsions may be brought on by vomiting. If in doubt, give something bland by mouth and seek a doctor.

When poisoning is suspected, first examine the mouth of the patient for signs of burns and for any poison that can be removed and saved for study. Note the breath for an odor such as that of kerosene or phenol. The poison can be diluted by giving large amounts of fluid by mouth, provided the patient is conscious and able to swallow. Do not try to remember the specific antidote for each poison, but, if the container is nearby, naturally one would read the label for the antidote recommended. Give milk, egg, soap and water, plain water, soda and water, mustard and water, or other fluid that is on hand. The important thing to do is to give plenty—usually 6 or 7 glasses—and then produce vomiting by tickling the back of the throat. After a few minutes, repeat the process. If it is known that an alkaline substance has been taken, give an acid such as vinegar or lemon juice; if an acid has been taken, give an alkaline substance such as baking soda or starch and water. After the stomach has been washed out thoroughly, give a bland liquid such as milk. Then get in touch with the doctor, who will give directions as to what to do next and may suggest that a saline laxative be given.

In the hospital the nurse need not know the specific antidote for each poison. The emergency wards of most general hospitals have a list and keep the common antidotes, as well as equipment for washing out the stomach, on hand. A few of the more common poisons and their antidotes are given in Table 5.

Good nursing care of the acutely poisoned patient may make the difference between a favorable and a fatal outcome. The patient should be kept warm and watched extremely carefully for changes in physical signs such as rapid thready pulse, respiratory changes, cyanosis, diaphoresis and other signs of collapse, shock, or impending death. Pulse rate, respirations, and blood pressure reading should be recorded every fifteen minutes for several hours. Nausea, vomiting, and abdominal pain should be noted, and all vomitus should be observed for signs of blood and should be saved for study. Stools must be checked for abnormal constituents such as blood. Intravenous infusions which have been ordered must be administered at the prescribed rate.

When poisoning has resulted from an overdose of opiates, barbiturates, bromides, or other sedatives, efforts must be made to keep the patient awake. A cup of strong coffee may be given every hour if it can be swallowed and retained. Strong coffee may also be ordered to be given as a retention enema. It is not good treatment to walk the patient about, since this simply tires him and may cause complete exhaustion. The artificial kidney may be used in an effort to speed up excretion of the drug (see Chapter 21).

If the patient has marked depression of respiration, oxygen may be given, and sometimes a respirator is used. A suction machine should be on hand at all times, for sometimes deep suctioning of the bronchial tree is necessary in an effort to prevent pneumonia. If the patient is unconscious, his position must be changed every hour, and he should be turned completely on alternate sides to provide drainage from each bronchus; occasionally, the head of the bed is lowered to encourage drainage of bronchial secretions. Death from barbiturate poisoning is likely to be a long, drawn-out affair; many patients live two or three days before death occurs. Death from poisoning by gas, however, is much more sudden. The patient who is in the hospital recovering from

Table 5 Common poisons and their antidotes*

Poison	*Antidote*
Mercury and heavy metals	Milk and egg albumin
Barbiturates	Amphetamine sulfate and caffeine
	Picrotoxin
Arsenic	BAL (2,3-dimercaptopropanol)
Lead	Calcium in large doses
	Milk diet
Alkaloids (strychnine, quinine, nicotine)	Potassium permanganate 1:10,000 by mouth
Cyanide	Sodium nitrite and sodium thiosulfate intravenously

* From Gold, Harry, and others: Cornell Conferences on Therapy, vol. IV, New York, 1951, The Macmillan Co.

carbon monoxide poisoning must be observed very carefully for the first twenty-four hours; some patients who appear to have responded favorably to artificial respiration and oxygen die of heart failure several hours after some level of consciousness has been restored.

The person who has been known to take poison in a suicide attempt presents additional nursing problems. Such a patient must not be left alone under any circumstances; he should be in a room whose windows are equipped with bars or stops if this is available. Upon awakening the patient has not only his original problem to face but also the discomfort and the emotional impact of learning that he has failed in his suicide attempt. Patients in these circumstances have been known to get up and jump out a window when it was not thought possible that they had the strength to get out of bed. Others have attempted to electrocute themselves or to carry out their original aim of self-destruction by other means. The routine precautions used for mentally ill patients should be observed (see Chapter 10).

FOOD POISONING

Acute food poisoning. Each year a large number of people many of whom eat away from home suffer acute gastrointestinal upsets due to food poisoning. Acute food poisoning, until recently termed "cholera morbus" and "ptomaine poisoning," is usually caused by a toxin produced by certain strains of staphylococci. This toxin causes immediate irritation to the gastrointestinal tract, hence the name enterotoxin. Illness is not caused by eating foods that are simply "old" and that have been subject to bacterial action. In many parts of the world (for example, in England, where "seasoned" game is popular), "spoiled" foods are ingested without harm. Pathogenic organisms must be present and active to produce disease. Cooking will destroy the organisms and stop the production of enterotoxin but will not destroy the poison that has already been formed.

Acute food poisoning can be prevented by rigorous enforcement of sanitary practices in eating establishments and by teaching the public to take sensible precautions, particularly when eating in restaurants and attending picnics during hot weather. Staphylococci are carried on the hands of workers and inadvertently deposited on food; food handlers should not be allowed to work if they have even minor infections on their hands or if they do not meet hand-washing requirements. Foods that are handled and allowed to remain without refrigeration before being cooked or eaten are the most dangerous. For example, chicken that has been removed from the bone and left for some time before creamed chicken is prepared, potatoes which have been peeled and left standing before potato salad is prepared, and sea food that has been removed from the shell by hand some time before being eaten all provide excellent opportunities for the pathogenic organisms to produce enterotoxin.

Signs of acute food poisoning include salivation, cramping, nausea, vomiting, and diarrhea. Signs and symptoms usually appear from one to six hours after eating the offending food, the length of time depending upon the amount of food eaten and the amount of enterotoxin present. In severe cases there may be lassitude, headache, dehydration, rapid pulse, and prostration. Treatment may be the same as for drug poisoning, although a laxative is seldom given since the contents of the gastrointestinal tract are largely evacuated. Usually fluids such as tea, boiled milk, and broth are tolerated within a short time. If diarrhea is severe, drugs such as bismuth and camphorated tincture of opium are ordered and intravenous fluids may be given.

Mushroom poisoning. Poisonous mushrooms are the most common cause of death from poisoning by food. It is best to teach the public that there is no sure way to tell whether or not a wild mushroom is safe to eat. All mushrooms found in the free state should be looked upon with suspicion, and only those grown under cultivation should be eaten. Deaths occur each year from the consumption of mushrooms by persons who either thought they were experts in determining a safe variety or else listened to other so-called experts.

Signs and symptoms of mushroom poisoning are severe abdominal pain, nausea, vomiting, diarrhea, and prostration occurring usually within one-half hour to twenty-four hours after eating the mushroom. The first-aid treatment should be the same as for drug poisoning: give fluids and induce vomiting, keep the patient warm, and notify a doctor at once. One ounce of magnesium sulfate should be given in water by mouth, and enemas can also be given.

In the hospital, the care is symptomatic. Fluids are given intravenously. The Trendelenburg postion and suctioning may be ordered, and side rails are used if convulsions occur. Moist compresses may be ordered if lacrimation is excessive. The patient should be attended constantly, since he is fearful of death.

Botulism. Botulism is a very serious form of food poisoning caused by a neurotoxin produced by an anaerobic spore-forming organism, the *Clostridium botulinum.* Improper home canning is often the cause of the poisoning, since the spores can resist several hours of ordinary cooking. Even intermittent cooking is not considered safe. People should not can foods at home unless pressure-cooking methods are used. Agricultural colleges in most states distribute booklets on home canning, and the nurse should encourage their use. The neurotoxin, unlike the enterotoxin produced by a strain of staphylococcus, is destroyed by cooking but not by mere heating. Foods should be cooked for ten to fifteen minutes, depending upon the density of the solid food, before they are safe to eat.

There is no emergency first-aid treatment suitable for botulism poisoning except to notify the doctor at once and to make preparations to move the patient to a hospital. If the symptoms are severe, the patient may not tolerate being moved. All persons who are suspected of having eaten the contaminated food should be reached, for it is in early treatment of those least affected that the best results are obtained. Symptoms usually appear within twelve to thirty-six hours after ingestion of the food, and their severity depends upon the amount of infected food eaten. There may be constipation, lassitude, headache, and double vision. Nausea and vomiting are often absent. As further damage to the nervous system occurs, there are difficulty in swallowing, lowered voice, and finally inability to talk or to swallow and muscular incoordination. Treatment consists of supportive care and the administration of large doses of antitoxin. Antitoxin cannot undo damage that has been done, but it helps to prevent further damage. The mortality rate from botulism in the United States is approximately 65 per cent, with patients usually dying within three to sixteen days of the onset of symptoms.[5] Fortunately, this poisoning is now quite rare.

Nursing victims of botulism poisoning includes keeping the patient quiet, usually in a darkened room. Fluids are given intravenously, and sometimes a tube is passed through the nose into the stomach. The patient should be attended constantly since he is fearful of choking to death. Suctioning and postural drainage may be used to remove the accumulated mucus and in an effort to prevent the regurgitation of fluids and aspiration into the lungs. It must be remembered that the patient is fully conscious up to the time of death and hears whatever is said by those near him, although he may not be able to speak.

REACTIONS TO THE SUN'S HEAT

Sunburn. Sunburn can occur even when the sun cannot be seen, since rays are able to filter through clouds. Reflection of rays from water increases the danger of burning. The best prevention for sunburn is careful, gradual exposure to the sun's rays, avoiding the midday hours when the rays are hottest. Some trade preparations are helpful in keeping out harmful rays, and olive oil, cocoa butter, and many creams and ointments are useful. Compresses of magnesium sulfate or sodium bicarbonate may be used to ease discomfort from sunburn. If chills, fever, edema, or blistering occur, the advice of a doctor should be sought.

Heat cramps. Heat cramps are sudden muscle pains caused by excessive loss of sodium chloride in perspiration during strenuous exercise in hot weather. The best treatment is prevention by taking extra salt when severe exertion is anticipated. The immediate treatment consists of salty fluids and foods by mouth, extra water, and rest for a few hours.

Heat exhaustion. Heat exhaustion is vasomotor collapse due to inability of the body adequately to supply the peripheral vessels with sufficient fluids to produce the perspiration needed for cooling and yet meet vital tissue requirements. The condition usually follows an extended period of vigorous exercise in hot weather, particularly when the person concerned has not had a period of acclimatization. The symptoms are faintness, weakness, headache, and sometimes nausea and vomiting; the skin is pale and moist. Heat exhaustion can often be prevented by taking extra salt and extra fluid during hot weather and by tempering physical activity during very hot weather. Emergency treatment consists of lowering the patient's head, preferably by placing him with the head lower than the body. He should be in the coolest spot available. Fluids should be given, and preferably these should contain salt. If the attack has been severe, the patient should rest for several hours before resuming activity.

Heatstroke (sunstroke). Heatstroke is a serious condition requiring immediate emergency treatment. It is due to a failure of the regulating mechanism of the body which controls perspiration. The person undergoing vigorous exercise in intense heat may perspire profusely for some time and then become dehydrated and fail to produce sufficient perspiration to maintain normal body temperature. The skin is dry, hot, and flushed in contrast to the pale moist skin of the person suffering from heat exhaustion. The patient becomes confused, dizzy, and faint, and may quickly lose consciousness.

There is probably no greater medical emergency than heatstroke. Without treatment almost 100 per cent of heatstroke victims will die, but with prompt and vigorous treatment almost as many will recover. The patient must be moved to the shade, preferably to a cool room, and a doctor must be notified at once. Every effort should be made to secure a thermometer. Treatment to reduce the temperature must be started immediately. The best method of doing this is to place the patient in a tub of cold water and to massage the skin vigorously to bring more blood to the surface for cooling. Spraying the body with cold water from a garden hose is often effective. Ice should be placed on the head and cold drinks given by mouth if the patient is conscious and can swallow. Pouring cold water on the patient and fanning him helps in the absence of tubs and sprays. If the elevated temperature is allowed to persist, serious permanent damage is done to the brain and the entire nervous system. A temperature of 40.5° C. (105° F.) or more means that treatment is essential; treatment should be continued until the temperature has been lowered to 39.9° C. (102° F.) and it must then be checked carefully for several hours for sudden rise. The patient should respond when the temperature lowers; failure to do so may indicate that brain damage has occurred. Patients do not recover from heatstroke so quickly as from heat exhaustion. Ofter there is faulty heat regulation for days and a lowered tolerance to heat for years and sometimes for the rest of the patient's life. The person who has had heatstroke should be advised to plan his living so that repeated long exposures to heat are avoided.

FROSTBITE

Frostbite occurs most often on the nose, cheeks, ears, toes, and fingers. Sometimes the patient will not know that he has been frostbitten since he cannot see the part, although it will feel numb and will appear white upon inspection. The frozen parts should not be rubbed with snow or cold water as was formerly thought desirable, because if this is done, the frozen crystals of body fluid will traumatize cell walls and may cause serious damage to them. Good first-aid treatment consists of taking the patient to a warm room, keeping him warm, and giving him warm drinks; alcohol is sometimes recommended. The frozen part should be thawed as quickly as possible by immersing it gently in warm, but not hot, water or by wrapping it in warm blankets. Massage must be avoided, and the use of heat lamps and heated objects and the placing of the part near a warm stove have been found to be harmful since they increase metabolism, thereby taxing blood supply demands which are already seriously reduced. When the part thaws, the patient should be advised to exercise it gently. Blisters that form should not be disturbed. As thawing occurs, pain may be severe; aspirin may be given for this. The patient should be taken to a doctor or a hospital as soon as possible. The care for frostbite is then similar to that needed in vascular disease of the extremities (see Chapter 19). Efforts are made to decrease the oxygen needs of the tissues while heating takes place, to improve blood supply by the use of drugs, and to prevent infection if there are open lesions. Some tissues may eventually die and have to be débrided as healing occurs.

Frostbite can usually be prevented by better attention to the clothing worn out-of-doors in intemperate weather. It is more likely to occur in the aged and debilitated person or the one with poor circulation. In the colder states of the United States it also occurs fairly often among teen-agers who conform to local styles in regard to clothing, such as no hats or covering for the ears.

ASPHYXIATION

The common causes of asphyxiation are inhalation of carbon monoxide gas, inhalation of fumes from burning buildings, drowning, and electric shock. If carbon monoxide or toxic fumes are encountered, it is useless to hold a cloth over the nose, as is so often done by persons who enter burning buildings. While this procedure may screen out some smoke and smoke particles, it does not screen out carbon monoxide or other toxic fumes. The victim of carbon monoxide or other toxic gas poisoning should be moved at once into fresh air and artificial respiration should be started. Emergency aid, including a pulmotor, must be sent for.

The drowning victim should be placed on his back with his chin forward. It is not necessary to elevate his feet in an attempt to drain water out of the respiratory passages. The important thing to do is to begin artificial breathing while other aid is being sought. Nothing takes the place of artificial respiration.

Electric shock accidents become more numerous as man puts up more electric wires to operate equipment in his home and at work. Immediate first aid consists of removing the person from contact with the live wire, with the rescuer being careful to avoid contact with the electric charge. The rescuer must never have direct contact with the body of the victim since the charge may be transmitted. He should use a long dry stick and stand on a dry board; also, asbestos or some other material or heavy dry gloves should be used when moving the victim away from the wire. Artificial respiration should be started at once and a doctor summoned. Artificial respiration should be continued even when there is no evidence of response; some patients have responded after as long as several hours.

The accepted method of artificial respiration at the present time is mouth-to-mouth or mouth-to-nose breathing.[33] First, any foreign matter in the victim's nose and mouth must be removed with a finger or a finger covered with cotton material. The procedure is then as follows: (1) Tilt the victim's head back and pull or push the jaw into a jutting-out position. (2) If the victim is a small child place your mouth over his mouth and nose and blow gently. If the victim is an adult open your mouth wide and place it over vic-

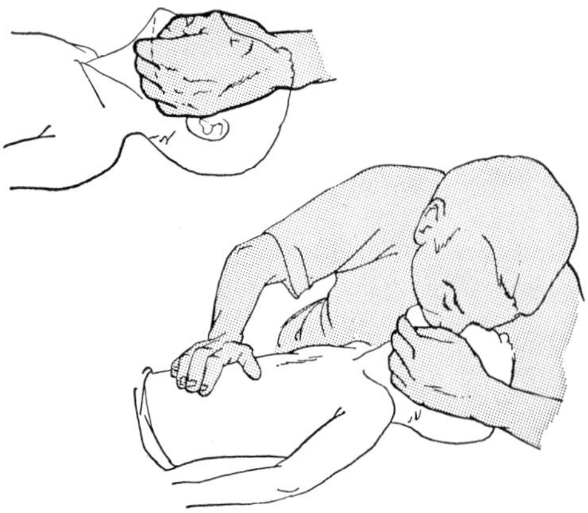

Figure 22

This diagram shows the correct method of mouth-to-mouth breathing. Note that the victim's chin is held forward.

tim's mouth while pinching his nostrils, or close his mouth and place your mouth over the victim's nose; blow vigorously. (3) Remove your mouth, turn your head to the side and listen for return rush of air. (4) If there is no air return check position, turn the victim quickly on his side and slap him between the shoulder blades to loosen foreign matter. Return him to the back-lying position and remove any material from his mouth or nose. (See Figure 22.)

For a child the rate of blowing should be approximately twenty times per minute blowing shallowly. For an adult it should be twelve times per minute blowing vigorously. A piece of gauze or other material such as a handkerchief can be placed between your mouth and the victim's and, with vigorous blowing, diminishes the air blown into the victim's lungs very little.

Artificial respiration should be continued until the patient has started to breathe or has been pronounced dead. It may be continued for four or more hours. Whereas a few gasping breaths on the part of the patient are most heartening to the person giving artificial respiration, they should not be taken as an indication that artificial respiration can be stopped. Patients may take one or two breaths and then stop breathing again. The patient must be watched carefully for at least an hour, and assistance must be given as needed. A cyanotic and then deep red flush will suffuse the entire face when breathing is resumed.

FOREIGN BODIES IN THE EYE

The eye should not be rubbed when a foreign body has entered it. Hands should be thoroughly washed before attempting first-aid measures. The inner surface of the lower lid should be examined first. If the foreign object is not there, then gently bring the upper lid down over the lower lid (many foreign bodies lodge on the undersurface of the upper lid). If this is not effective, lavage the eye, using an eyecup, a medicine dropper, or a drinking glass; this often suffices to wash away the offending material. The patient can usually feel and tell approximately where the irritation is. If it appears to be under the upper lid, the lid should then be inverted. The procedure for this is as follows. Prepare an applicator by anchoring a shred of clean cotton on a toothpick and moistening it with tap water. Then, preferably standing behind the patient, grasp the upper lashes firmly and invert the lid over a matchstick, pencil, or other convenient object. Standing behind the patient is favored because it allows for better control if he should jerk and permits one to use a sidewise approach to the lid with the applicator, again avoiding danger if the patient should move quickly. Many persons experienced in removing foreign bodies from the eye prefer to approach the patient from the back if they are to work on the patient's right eye and from the front if dealing with the left eye, assuming that they are right-handed.

If the foreign body is on the cornea and is not removed by irrigation, or if marked irritation remains but no foreign object is seen and removed, it is best to close the eye, cover it with a piece of cotton, and anchor the cotton with tape such as cellophane tape. The patient should then seek a doctor at once. Foreign bodies embedded in the cornea can lead to serious consequences because of the danger of infection and ulceration. They should never be removed by the uninitiated. Metallic objects are of particular danger because rusting may occur, and this is extremely irritating to eye tissues.

Chemicals accidentally introduced into the eyes should be washed away with copious amounts of plain water. Many persons whose vision could have been saved by this simple remedy are now blind. Use a cup or glass and pour the water from the inner to the outer part of the eye; the eye must be held open since the patient will not be able to do this himself. Sometimes it is best to put the victim's head under a faucet if one is available and to use large amounts of running water. A drinking fountain is ideal for this purpose. Lavage should be continued for several minutes, and after fifteen minutes the procedure should be repeated. The patient should then be taken at once to a doctor.

FOREIGN BODIES IN THE EAR

When a foreign object has entered the ear canal, the first thing to do is to attempt to identify it. In this connection the outer ear is held up and back in an adult and down and out in a child. This straightens the ear canal and makes it possible, with good lighting, to see as far as the eardrum. The patient must be cautioned not to try to dislodge the object since such an attempt may push it further in; children must be constantly observed and may need to be restrained. Occasionally, the foreign object (for example, a wad of material or cotton) may be removed with tweezers if it can be readily seen and has free ends. Some authorities[6] believe that it is permissible in first-aid treatment to attempt to get behind the object with a bent hairpin, but this practice may be dangerous in the hands of the uninitiated. Irrigation of the ear is often a fruitless practice, since it seldom dislodges a foreign body that is firmly anchored. If the object turns out to be a bean, a pea, or any other substance that swells, irrigation may cause further damage. The best thing to do is to take the patient to a doctor.

The best treatment for insects in the ear is to drop a little oil or strong alcohol into the ear canal; water should not be used because it makes the insect more active and this will increase pain. Insects can sometimes be enticed out of the ear canal by a flashlight held to the ear; the light from matches should not be used because of the danger of burns.

FOREIGN BODIES IN THE NOSE, THROAT, AND ESOPHAGUS

Foreign bodies in the nose are usually placed there by children during play. If they are visible, one may attempt to remove them with a fine forceps or a pair of tweezers. Again, some authorities recommend use of a curved hairpin.[6] If a foreign body has passed into the posterior nose or pharynx, it is best to take the patient to a doctor.

Food and other material may become lodged in the throat and interfere with breathing. This requires emergency treatment. The best thing to do is to place the patient on his face, with the head lower than the feet, and to slap him briskly between the shoulders. Children may be treated by picking them up by their heels, which usually suffices to cause them to cough and dislodge the foreign object.

Surprisingly large objects can pass the larynx and go into the trachea and bronchi. Sometimes these cause immediate respiratory difficulties, while at other times the aspirated object (a peanut, for example) may remain in the lungs for some time and lead to a mistaken diagnosis of asthma or cause an abscess before it is discovered. The procedure for removal of these objects is discussed in Chapter 23.

Foreign objects which lodge in the esophagus are usually fish and chicken bones. The symptoms of these are most distressing. First aid consists of keeping the patient as quiet as possible and encouraging him not to swallow or struggle to dislodge the object. A doctor should be notified at once. Foreign objects in the esophagus are relatively easily removed by means of esophagoscopy. The danger of fatal mediastinitis following perforation of the esophagus by a foreign object is not so great as it was before the use of bacteriostatic drugs, but mediastinitis still may be a serious complication.

Disaster nursing

Disaster nursing has become increasingly important because of the occurrence of a relatively greater number of natural disasters such as hurricanes and floods in recent years and because each year finds nations of the world with larger and more powerful means of mass destruction. The main differences between damage caused by atomic attack and that caused by other major disasters, such as severe explosions, are extent of damage and the spread of radioactive substances. In the following discussion consideration will be given particularly to nursing preparation for, and conduct during, disaster resulting from atom bombing. Emphasis will be placed upon the principles of disaster nursing that remain relatively constant from year to year and which apply, in varying degrees, to all major disasters. It is a foregone conclusion that information confined within the covers of a book cannot possibly be completely up to date. However, pamphlets are released at frequent intervals by national, state, and local agencies responsible for keeping professional workers and the public informed about new dangers that may have to be faced and include changes in methods of treatment and management in the event of disaster.

The nurse cannot begin too early in her professional preparation to think seriously of her own particular responsibility in national disaster. In general this consists of knowing what over-all plans are being made on national, state, and local levels, and how she may best fit in with these plans. She should help the public to learn some simple facts that may save lives, and she should understand what will be encountered in the event of bombing and what services she may be required to give. The professional nurse will be looked to by others for leadership and guidance in time of disaster. She is a member of the largest single professional group in the health field and will, therefore, be in contact with many people. Her sphere of activity covers a wider range than that of members of most other professional groups who will be in positions of leadership. In time of disaster her duties will include direct care of the sick and injured, the teaching of lay persons to care for themselves and others, administrative duties, supervision of practical nurses, medical aids, and other workers, and assistance in the field of sanitation and disease prevention. Decentralization of cities and relocation of perhaps millions of people will present challenges to all health workers because there will be interruption of sanitary controls for milk and water and for the disposal of wastes.

OVER-ALL PLANS

Over-all disaster planning for a country as large as the United States is a major undertaking and is dependent upon public and private organizations working in close cooperation with each other. The Federal Civil Defense Administration, with national headquarters in Battle Creek, Michigan, is the official national agency concerned with all aspects of national defense. Within this administration are several divisions, such as the Medical Care Division, which has a nursing branch. Some functions of the Federal Civil Defense Administration are to encourage states to establish civil defense commissions, to furnish part of the funds needed for supplies, and to arrange for civil defense forces from one state to aid those of another state in the event of bombing within its boundaries. This Administration works closely with other groups, including other governmental departments such as the Department of Agriculture, the military services, the United States Public Health Service, the American Medical Association, the National Red Cross, the American Hospital

Association, and the national nursing organizations. It serves regional, state, and local civil defense organizations in a guidance capacity. Specific activities include helping to prepare literature and helping to develop courses for professional groups such as doctors, dentists, and nurses. It also sponsors the assembling of improvised hospitals, each of which will be able to care for over two hundred patients. These will be located close to probable target areas. It is assigned the responsibility for assembling such essential equipment as transfusion sets, dressings, plasma and blood volume expanders, and drugs and equipment to determine radiation contamination (survey meters, dosimeters, dosimeter readers, and dosimeter changers). The state civil defense commissions carry out similar functions on a state level, providing supplies and developing plans for training professional workers as well as for educating the public. Responsibility for civil defense within states is usually delegated to the state health department. Local communities may have their own organization, the Emergency Medical Service.

Certain highly populated cities and industrial areas throughout the country have been designated as target areas because they are most likely to be attacked. Communities near these target areas have been designated as support areas, and in the event of an attack their medical forces will act as automatic aid in that they will go immediately to the assistance of the attacked area without direction from the state. Additional help will be sent as needed by the state and is termed state-directed aid. If further help is needed, the Federal Administration will direct aid from other nearby states.

Every nurse should learn about the Emergency Medical Service in her community. This can usually be done by enrolling in courses in medical and nursing aspects of medical defense offered by the local civil defense organization. Here, her knowledge can be tested to some extent in practical experience. Membership in local units of the National League for Nursing and the American Nurse's Association is important as a means of learning of new developments in disaster nursing; local organizations of the two associations, sometimes assisted by the state, may sponsor and conduct institutes and refresher courses for their members. The professional nurse may contribute to lay education and refresh her own knowledge by teaching courses sponsored by the Federal Civil Defense Administration and the American Red Cross (for example, home nursing and first-aid courses and courses for nurses' aids).

The nurse's attendance at local civil defense meetings is valuable for her and for others. She should not, however, offer her services as a plane spotter or a Geiger count checker for instance. The reason for this is simply that her special training in care of the injured will be so badly needed if disaster occurs that she will not be available for duties which can be handled by laymen. She should know specifically where and how she reports in the event of disaster and should be prepared to go quickly. Most nurses who work in general hospitals should be quite well oriented by their institutions. In March, 1956, the Joint Committee on Accreditation of Hospitals issued a statement that all hospitals wishing to qualify for accreditation must have a written plan for their institutions in the event of disaster. It is probable that in the future there will be more detailed planning within general hospitals and better orientation of the professional members of the staff for their particular assignments.

Nurses who are not attached to a hospital or an emergency medical unit should listen for radio instructions and proceed immediately to the nearest assignment depot in the area in which they happen to be. Nurses who live a good distance from their place of regular work should know the location of the assignment depot and of secondary-aid stations in their living area. Married nurses should make some provisions for care of their children so that they may make themselves available in the shortest possible time.

The nurse who reports in time of disaster and for emergency drills should not wear a uniform. It has been suggested that a canvas apron with six pockets in the front be worn over slacks and blouse or sweater.* The nurse should carry her personal identification as a nurse and wear a Civil Defense armband if she has one. In addition, it is advised that she have with her a flashlight with batteries, bandage scissors, a dozen safety pins, a hypodermic syringe and needle, indelible pencil, matches, a small package of tissues, a small notebook, and lipstick for skin marking.

EDUCATING THE PUBLIC FOR PROTECTION

Everyone should know the basic rules for self-protection in the event of sudden enemy attack, how to prepare for disaster, and how to protect oneself immediately following a bombing. The nurse should include this information in teaching health education to all patients and in all her contacts with laymen.

The American public is strangely apathetic about learning to cope with the hazards which will be present in atomic disaster. Despite the thousands of booklets and pamphlets distributed on the subject and the pages in the daily papers devoted to a description of the proper courses of action, the average citizen does not know the most fundamental steps that may be necessary for his survival. Just as the patient often delays going to the doctor when he fears cancer lest his suspicions be confirmed, so he fails to heed the constant public reminders of what he should know to help assure his survival.

Many pamphlets give simple but complete explanations and rules to go by in preparation for disaster and during disaster. *Survival Under Atomic Attack*, a pamphlet released by the United States Government in 1950, is excellent for the average layman.

*Emergency Treatment and Techniques in Aid Stations, Supplement to the "Guide for Nurses" (V-C-2).

Families living in or near target areas should set aside materials for an emergency. These should include two flashlights, a battery radio, a first-aid kit, canned food to last several days, bottled and canned fluids, a can opener, a bottle opener, and spoons. A large bottle of drinking water should be stored and changed weekly. In addition, a container of water should be available for washing in case any one is exposed to radiation dust, since water may suddenly be cut off or contaminated.

Every citizen should know the radio station numbers (1240 and 640) that will be used in a national emergency. These will use frequency waves that cannot be intercepted by enemy planes. The radio should be tuned to one of these stations and instructions awaited if a bombing is threatened. Windows and doors should be closed and blinds drawn, all electric equipment except the radio should be turned off, and pets should be brought indoors. The family should then proceed to the basement. Many people fear they may be trapped in the cellar, but it has been shown that this danger is much less than that which will be encountered by staying above ground in the event of an atomic bombing. When a bomb is known to have been exploded, the family should remain in the basement until advised by radio that it is safe to go outdoors.

It is important to know what to do when at work or out-of-doors at the time of a bombing. Despite the tremendous fear of radiation in this country, by far the greatest number of deaths and severe injuries in an atomic bombing will come from blast and heat. The following three rules, if followed, will save many lives. (1) Try to put a wall between yourself and the bomb, judging that the bomb will be dropped in the most industrialized area. Even a ditch or a gutter is better than no protection. (2) Fall flat on your face, bury your face in your arm, and if possible pull something over your head and hair. (3) Stay there until things are quiet. Do not rush out to look around. Explosive radiation lasts for about a minute after a bomb has exploded and may easily affect those within a mile of the center of the attack unless they have been quite well protected.

Lingering radiation is due to the presence of many fine particles of "ashes" or left-over fission products which may remain in the vicinity of the bombing for an indefinite time. These particles usually rise high in the air and spread over a wide area and may not be concentrated enough to do harm to those a few miles from the site of the bombing. Lingering radiation dust is extremely difficult to remove from houses, and it is advised that windows broken by the blast be covered with a blanket or cardboard to prevent as much dust as possible from entering the house. If a large amount of radiation dust is present, some will undoubtedly filter into the house. If the explosion has been under water or if water reservoirs have been exposed to large amounts of radiation dust, the water will be seriously contaminated. So far there is no known simple or effective method for decontaminating such water, and if a major bombing occurs this may present an extremely serious problem, although use of shale, coagulant, and settling gives promise of effectiveness. Those persons at home should immediately draw water and put it into covered clean containers, because the water in the immediate mains will not be contaminated by radioactive substances and may suffice for emergency needs. Thereafter it is not advisable to use water from taps until advised by radio of its safety. Even if water is not contaminated by radioactive substances, it may be contaminated by bacteria following damage to sewer systems. Bacterial contamination can be overcome by boiling the water, but boiling will not remove radioactive contamination.

Although radiation is a real danger following a bombing, it should not prevent one from assisting others. Anyone who is out in the open shortly after a bombing should keep his head and other parts of the body covered. Upon coming into the house, he should shed his outer clothing, including his shoes, at the doorway and should scrub thoroughly with soap and water. If it is possible, he should then be checked for the amount of radioactive contamination still present, particularly on exposed parts of the body, and the scrubbing process should be repeated if necessary.

The public is urged not to telephone during a disaster. The radio will give instruction for the precautions and cleanup measures that are necessary for each vicinity. A safe rule to follow if in doubt, however, is to err on the side of caution. Food that has been uncovered during a bombing should be discarded. Food in wrappers is safe, though the outer wrappings should be carefully removed and discarded. The outsides of cans, as well as utensils, furniture, and any equipment that has not been in tightly closed cupboards or drawers, should be washed thoroughly.

The public should know that mass evacuation of cities may seriously affect water and other sanitary facilities. Foods and fluids of all kinds should be cooked if there is any doubt about contamination. Disaster conditions often threaten mass epidemics of diseases such as typhoid. It may be that those living in target areas will soon be urged to receive immunization against typhoid and tetanus so that it will not be necessary in time of a national disaster. Personal identification, which includes blood type, may also be encouraged for those who live in target areas.

IMMEDIATE SERVICES IN EVENT OF BOMBING

Patients whom the nurse will encounter in disaster will not differ too much from those seen in her everyday practice. It will be the numbers of injured and the severity of the injuries that will be different, as well as the conditions under which she will work. It is estimated that one atomic bomb (A bomb) could kill 80,000 persons and wound 80,000 more. Of the injured it is estimated that approximately 12,000 will be in shock, 12,000 will suffer radiation illness, 27,000 will be severely burned, and 13,000 will have fractures, open wounds, and crushing injuries. It is almost impossible to think in these numbers and to plan how work can be carried out with the confusion and tensions that will be present. Major obstacles will be dislocation of transportation, communication, light, and water supply.

It must be understood by all nurses that tremendous adjustments in basic thinking will have to be made if atomic bombing should occur. It will not be possible even to begin to do all that might be desirable for everyone. Whatever is best for the largest number must be done; the dying should be made as comfortable as possible, but the available facilities must be directed to those whose possibility of survival is best. Careful techniques will have to be discarded, and the nurse will have to rely heavily upon her knowledge of basic principles rather than specific procedures. She will have to improvise and use whatever is available. For example, one syringe may have to be used for several patients, with only the needle being changed. She must remember that prompt action will save many lives. Those who are available to help will be less likely to suffer emotional reactions if they are kept busy with definite tasks. In the first few hours of disaster, treatment will have to be routine and simple; much of it will have to be performed by unskilled workers, while nurses will have to do many things usually done by physicians. Perhaps the nurse's ability to keenly appraise the physical condition of people will be her greatest asset in time of disaster. She is the only person with this skill with the exception of the physician. For example, by observing a group of patients, she will be able quickly to determine which one is not responding to fluid therapy, which must be constantly attended lest he attempt to remove an artificial airway, and which is responding well and can tolerate being moved.

All nurses should willingly serve where most needed in time of disaster. There will not be time for consideration of choices and probably not even time to use all skills to the best advantage. It is hoped that physicians will be in charge of all aid stations. It is possible, however, that a nurse may have to take charge until a doctor arrives. Nurses will be assigned from their designated assignment depots to secondary-aid stations, permanent hospitals, improvised emergency hospitals, and holding stations. Secondary-aid stations are established at designated places outside target cities as part of preparation for disaster. First-aid stations will be determined by groups sent out from the secondary-aid station after the bombing. Permanent hospitals will be hospitals in the target city that are suitable for use. Improvised emergency hospitals will be temporary facilities set up in school buildings, garages, or any other place with suitable space at a considerable distance from the bombed area.

Stretcher teams will go from the first-aid station, give first aid, and bring the wounded to the secondary-aid station, where the important function of sorting and identifying casualties is done. This is called *triage.* Injuries may be any of the following: injury caused by blast of the nuclear weapon, traumatic injuries resulting from flying parts of physical structures, burns from the initial bombing or from the heat from explosions, radiation injuries from explosive radiation, or poisoning from nerve gas or other poisons. Emotional reactions will also occur. The doctor should be responsible for triage and should decide which patients should receive immediate treatment, which should be sent to secondary-aid stations, or which should be sent to remote stations. He should also determine which should be transported by litter and which may be treated as "walking wounded." If no doctor is available, a nurse will have to substitute. She should follow the general rules taught in all first aid: treat severe hemorrhage, suffocation, shock, severe wounds, burns, fractures, and dislocations in that order. Judgment in estimating the severity of the injury must be used along with this rule. Treatment will not usually be given at the triage station, but each patient will be tagged and the injuries noted on the tag.

In first-aid stations and secondary-aid stations nurses may be called upon to do things usually done by physicians, such as prescribing medications, starting intravenous infusions, giving anesthetics (if she has had some preparation for this), suturing lacerations, débriding wounds, applying pressure dressings, dressing burns, applying and readjusting splints, and directing the disposition of patients. It is to be hoped that the nurse will not be so occupied with medical procedures that observing patients for changes in vital signs is neglected. She may also be needed to search for and help persons who are injured and in need of care yet who are too frightened to leave their homes or places of hiding.

Morphine has been stockpiled in disposable syrettes, each containing 30 mg. (1/2 grain). Penicillin in oil has also been stockpiled, and Aureomycin, 250 mg. or 0.25 Gm., and Terramycin, 250 mg. or 0.25 Gm., are available. Dried plasma has been stocked in containers ready for the addition of sterile distilled water and normal saline solution. Sodium citrate has been stocked in powdered form, ready for use by addition of unsterile water; this is given by mouth to those who can take fluids orally.

Shock. Shock will be a major problem, particularly in the first few hours following the explosion, and should have second priority in treatment, sometimes even taking precedence over hemorrhage. Shock will probably be due to trauma which may or may not have caused external laceration. Blood loss may be external or internal and may be due to crushing injury or fluid loss from burns. Shock may be partially prevented and controlled by stopping hemorrhage, giving medication for pain if the patient is not already in shock, splinting fractures before moving patients, covering burns, dressing open wounds, preventing loss of body heat, and giving fluids by veins, by hypodermoclysis, or by mouth. The head should be lowered unless a head injury has also been sustained.

Hemorrhage. The care of the patient with hemorrhage will not differ from that given in any emergency situation. Once applied, a tourniquet is not removed until a nurse or doctor checks the patient for cessation of bleeding. This must be done where facilities are available to control the bleeding. Whenever a tourniquet is applied in the field or in a first-aid station, a large "T" is marked on the forehead of the patient with a skin pencil; these patients receive priority in transportation to secondary-aid stations.

Burns. Patients burned in disaster have been classified into three groups: the hopelessly burned, the severely burned, and the moderately burned. Attention in disaster will be given first to the severely burned, since the hopelessly burned will not be expected to survive. Treatment includes prevention of infection by giving antibiotics, alleviation of pain, and replacement of body fluids. A special burn dressing has been stockpiled in large quantities as part of civil defense emergency medical supplies. It consists of a cellulose pad covered with a layer of cotton and faced with extremely fine gauze. The gauze is placed next to the burn, and the dressing is then held in place with a tensile yarn roller bandage, included in the burn package. Burn dressings are provided in two sizes. When applying dressings it is important to bandage the neck loosely, never to leave two skin surfaces in contact, to cover the burned area completely, and to avoid overlapping of the cellulose dressing, since this may cause uneven pressure. The pressure of the outer yarn bandage should be firm, gentle, and even. For further details in care of patients with severe burns see Chapter 30.

Wounds, lacerations, and fractures. Many patients will have open chest wounds, wounds of the face and neck, and penetrating abdominal wounds, as well as fractures of the skull and other bones of the body. Abdominal viscera must be kept moist. If sterile water or normal saline solution is not available, plasma or even unsterile water must be used. No penetrating objects or debris should be removed, the patient should not be given fluids by mouth, and he should be sent at once to a secondary-aid station.

Open chest wounds can sometimes be closed by applying wide adhesive tape (three-inch) in a criss-cross fashion. A small dry dressing should be placed over the opening, and the adhesive tape should extend approximately four to six inches on each side of the wound so that good traction can be obtained and the wound can be kept air tight. If the patient is having difficulty in breathing, he should be placed on his injured side, with the head and shoulders elevated. If he does not have difficulty in breathing, he should be placed in shock position.

Severe wounds of the mouth and jaw often cause obstruction of breathing after an hour or so when swelling occurs. Under no circumstances should tight bandages or slings be applied to severe wounds of the jaws, mouth, or throat since they may cut off passage of air as edema occurs. Patients should be transported in a face-down position. In some instances it is safest to insert an airway before the patient is moved; airways are stocked in the supplies for emergency medical units.

Blood clots and obstructions must be removed before an airway is used. The airway is inserted by directing it along the tongue, with the concave side down, and by moving it carefully back and slightly from side to side until the guard comes in contact with the teeth. It is then tied in place or anchored with adhesive to prevent its slipping out in transit.

Some débridement of large open wounds is necessary to prevent infection. Even with large doses of antibiotics, infection cannot be prevented if much dead tissue is left. The nurse who is not familiar with suturing or who does not have suture equipment may make excellent use of strips of adhesive tape to hold wound edges together. Pieces of adhesive tape are notched and folded over in the center portion and are applied so that the center part passes over the wound. This center portion is flamed before the adhesive tape is applied. Adhesive tape of any width can be used, depending upon the location and size of the wound. The skin must be dry, and usually several strips, or "butterflies," are used (see Figure 23). Wounds on the lips and other parts of the face are often very satisfactorily cared for in this way. Skin clips can be easily used by nurses who are not familiar with the technique of suturing.

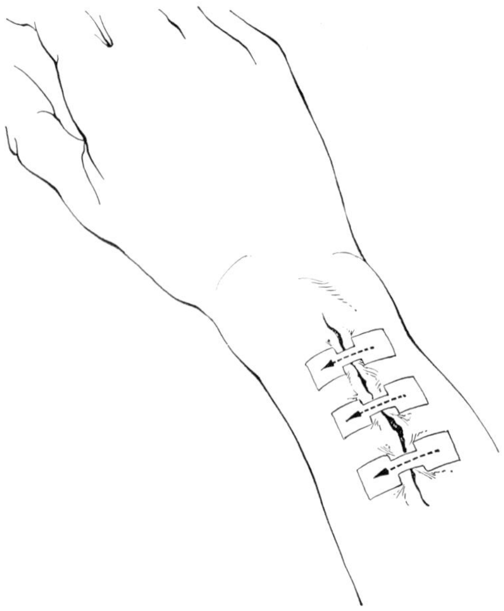

Figure 23

Schematic drawing showing the use of "butterfly" adhesive strips to approximate the skin edges in a laceration of the forearm. Note the irregular wound edges and the placement of the adhesive. Arrows indicate the direction of pull used to partially close the wound.

The care of fractures is similar to that necessary in any accident situation, with the exception that many patients with fractures will also have severe burns and may be suffering from radiation effects or other injuries. The enormous number of persons with fractures will make the need for improvised equipment very great. Pieces of wood from destroyed buildings, doors, canes, umbrellas, ironing boards, and magazines are a few of the materials that may be used.

Obstetric emergencies. A bombing disaster will cause many women to abort and many to deliver their babies prematurely. They will be sent to the secondary-aid stations to be delivered, and the nurse may be the only professional help available. No materials have been stockpiled for this situation, and the nurse or person in attendance will have to improvise to the best of her ability. A shoelace, a piece of string, or a piece of bandage may have to be used to tie the cord. A lay person may be called upon to watch the fundus for an hour or more, and the patient may then be treated as a "walking wounded" and returned to her home or sent to a permanent hospital. It is most important that the mother and baby be identified. Identification bands for both mother and baby can be made of cloth, and information on each should include the name of the father, the address, the sex of the baby, and the time and place of birth. If at all possible, the baby should be kept with the mother. If the delivery has been such that there is danger of infection, penicillin will probably be given.

Radiation sickness. Radiation sickness usually does not make its appearance until several hours or even days after exposure. Persons affected may have nausea, vomiting, and malaise within a few hours of exposure. Since it may be difficult to distinguish the person with early and severe radiation sickness from the one with severe emotional reaction, all those suspected should have immediate bed rest and should be sent as quickly as possible to a hospital where transfusions and fluids can be given if necessary.

Nerve gas damage. Nerve gases are the means of chemical warfare that are most likely to be used. They are colorless to light brown substances that can be released in either liquid or vapor form. They have a slightly fruity odor or else are odorless. If inhaled in large amounts, they may cause death within a few minutes by producing overstimulation of the centers of respiration and circulation. Symptoms include excessive salivation, constriction of the pupils, dimness of vision, pain in the eyeballs, coryza, cyanosis, coughing, circulatory disturbances, and convulsions. Atropine sulfate should be given at once in large doses (1/30 grain or 2 mg.); it has been stockpiled in tablets of this strength. Clothing should be removed and the skin washed with sodium bicarbonate in water. If sodium bicarbonate is not available, plain water should be used. Since clothing is highly contaminated by liquid gas, care should be taken to avoid contamination of others with such clothing. The victim of nerve gas poisoning should be hospitalized as soon as possible.

Emotional reactions. The stresses and strains placed upon all who survive a major disaster are almost beyond our imagination to think through and plan for. They will affect the doctor, the nurse, and all others giving aid, as well as all other survivors. Members of the medical and related staffs will be less likely to show signs of emotional effects than others because they will have more knowledge of what is happening and will be kept busy. The American Psychiatric Association has outlined the major types of reactions that are likely to occur and has suggested methods of management.

1. Normal reaction. There may be a normal reaction of tremor, profuse diaphoresis, pallor, and nausea which soon disappears.

2. Acute panic. This reaction is one of the most serious of the reactions and must be dealt with immediately, since in time of crisis it is acutely "contagious." It has been demonstrated repeatedly that in times of disaster one person in panic can set off a chain reaction and cause untold damage. The person in panic is devoid of judgment and is inordinately but not purposefully active; he cannot be reasoned with and makes wild attempts to flee. Horses in panic have been known to rush back into a burning barn and be killed,

and such behavior is not too different from that of human beings in panic. Panic must not be confused with rapid exit from a point of danger; this is sensible, provided it is orderly and purposeful. The person in true panic must be restrained, usually by force, and should be firmly held by medical aids until he can be removed to a place where his influence upon others will not be dangerous. Those who have experienced disaster should be segregated from those who have not, since they may easily become panicky at threat of further disaster.

3. Depressed reactions. Persons who have depressed reactions will be slowed down or numbed. They will sit and stare into space and will be completely oblivious to what is going on around them. These patients must be protected, since they will not move to help themselves.

4. Overly active response. The patients will be very active, possibly joking inappropriately or laughing hysterically, be unable to concentrate on one job, and be a disturbing influence upon the person in command of the location.

5. Severe bodily reactions. The patient may not be able to use a limb and may have nausea and vomiting as a result of fear of radiation exposure.

In management of patients and others who are suffering from emotional effects, the nurse should apply the basic principles of psychiatric nursing. She must remember that there will be serious limits to what she can do. She should evaluate each patient and decide what can be done in the particular situation and what is best for the patient and the group. It is useless to argue with the patient, to expect him to stand up better under strain than he has done, or to imply that any of his beliefs or physical limitations are not real. Kindness and gentleness are important. Most patients with emotional reactions are afraid, and they respond to a genuine kindly interest in them and an honest attempt to understand how they feel. Patients should be kept busy if this is at all possible. The patients in panic must be restrained, the dazed ones given routine things to do in as quiet an environment as possible, the overly active ones assigned to tasks which require moving about. Those with an imagined major physical defect can often help with a task with which their imagined problem does not interfere, such as writing identification tags if they believe that their lower limbs are affected.

Chlorpromazine has been stockpiled for use by medical workers primarily and may be used to treat those who have severe or prolonged emotional reactions. This drug relieves nausea and vomiting, releases tension, and lessens anxiety.

The most important point in nursing management and in prevention of emotional reactions is the poise and conduct of the nurse herself. Just as one person in panic can upset a crowd, so one calm, collected person can quiet a group.

REFERENCES AND SELECTED READINGS*

1* Accident Facts, Chicago, 1959, The National Safety Council.

2 Accident Hazards in the Home, Statistical Bulletin, Feb. 1956, Metropolitan Life Insurance Co.

3 American Public Health Association: Control of Communicable Disease in Man, ed. 8, New York, 1955, The American Public Health Association.

4 Anderson, Gaylord, W., and Arnstein, Margaret G.: Communicable Disease Control, New York, 1950, The Macmillan Co.

5 Cecil, Russell L., and Loeb, Robert F. (editors): A Textbook of Medicine, ed. 10, Philadelphia, 1959, W. B. Saunders Co.

6 Cole, Warren H., and Puestow, Charles B.: First Aid–Surgical and Medical, ed. 4, New York, 1951, Appleton-Century-Crofts, Inc.

7 Committee on Civil Defense of the American Psychiatric Association: Psychological First Aid in Community Disasters, Washington, 1954, American Psychiatric Association.

8 Conley, Bernard E.: Insecticide Vaporizers and Fumigators Can Be Dangerous, Nursing Outlook 2:266-267, May 1954.

*References preceded by an asterisk indicate material particularly well suited for student reading.

9 Costa, P. James, and Dews, Mary Jane: Mushrom Poisoning and Nursing Care, Am. J. Nursing **56**:998-1000, Aug. 1956.
10 Crawford, Ora E.: Eye Injuries in a Chemical Plant, Nursing Outlook **3**:447-449, Aug. 1955.
11 Eckelberry, Niel E.: Electric Burns, Am. J. Nursing **55**:836-838, July, 1955.
12 *Getting, Valdo A.: Food-Borne Diseases, Nursing Outlook **2**:364-366, July 1954.
13 Gold, Harry, and others: Cornell Conferences on Therapy, vol. IV, New York, 1951, The Macmillan Co.
14 *Goldstein, Joseph D., and Werley, Harriet H.: Care of Casualties Caused by Nuclear Weapons, Am. J. Nursing **56**:1576-1582, Dec. 1956.
15 Harrison, T. R., and others (editors): Principles of Internal Medicine, ed. 2, New York, 1954, The Blakiston Co.
16 Hollister, William Gray: Some Mental Health Aspects of Civil Defense for Public Health Workers, Am. J. Pub. Health **46**:1275-1282, Oct. 1956.
17 Holthaus, Louise Sharko: Cooperation in Prevention of Home Accidents, Am. J. Nursing **56**:1160-1162, Sept. 1956.
18 Home Accident Prevention Activities in State Health Departments, The News, Feb. 1956, American Public Health Association.
19 Hornibrook, John W.: Snake Bites, Am. J. Nursing **56**:754-755, June 1956.
20 Wilson, William J.: Heat Injury, Am. J. Nursing **60**:1124-1125, Aug. 1960.
21 *Lindsey, Douglas: The Case of the Much-Maligned Tourniquet, Am. J. Nursing **57**:444-445, April 1957.
22 *Lindsey, Douglas: Effective Emergency Splinting, Am. J. Nursing **56**:1120-1124, Sept. 1956.
23 *Lueth, Harold G.: Meeting Disaster, Am. J. Nursing **56**:1135-1138, Sept. 1956.
24 *Magnussen, Ann K., and Schafer, Margaret K.: Nursing in Disaster—Red Cross Service and Civil Defense Service, Am. J. Nursing **56**:1290-1292, Oct. 1956.
25 New York State Department of Health: Guide for Nurses, Emergency Medical Services, March, 1954, V-C-1.
26 New York State Department of Health: Supplement to the Guide for Nurses, Emergency Treatment and Techniques in Aid Stations, Feb. 1956, V-C-1.
27 New York State Department of Health: Guide for Venipuncture and Intravenous Therapy in Emergency Medical Services, 1952.
28 News Note: J.A.M.A. **161**:242, May 19, 1956.
29 *Phillips, Elisabeth Cogswell: A Nurse With Many Jobs, Nursing Outlook **6**:580-583, Oct. 1958.
30 Rayner, Jeanette F.: How Do Nurses Behave in Disaster? Nursing Outlook **6**:572-576, Oct. 1958.
31 *Ridgway, James M.: The Nurse in Disaster Medical and Health Program, Nursing Outlook **5**:41-42, Jan. 1957.
32 *Steele, James H., and Carroll, L. Dorothy: Animal Diseases Transmissible to Man, Nursing Outlook **4**:156-161, March 1956.
33 *American Red Cross: First Aid Textbook ed. 4 (and 1957 Supplement on Artificial Respirations), Washington, 1953, The American National Red Cross.
34 Thomas, Harold Allen: The Public Health Implications of Radioactive Fallout in Water Supplies, Am. J. Pub. Health **46**:1266-1274, Oct. 1956.
35 *Sullivan, Catherine, M., Elliman, Virginia B., and National League for Nursing: What Price Survival, The Bridge Between Disaster and Mass Casualty Nursing: Nursing Outlook **8**:128-135, March 1960.
36 *Toyan, Angela: The Nurse's Role in Poison Control, Am. J. Nursing **58**:96-102, Jan. 1958.
37 When the Unexpected Happens, Boston, 1956, Health Education Service of the John Hancock Mutual Life Insurance Co.
38 Whitney, J. M.: National Medical Civil Defense Planning and Requirements, J.A.M.A. **160**:1195-1201, April 7, 1956.
39 Linden, Maurice E.: Rescue Breathing, Am. J. Nursing **60**:971-974, July 1960.

The patient with cancer

Chapter 16

Study questions for review

1 Review the differences between benign and malignant tumors. What are the important characteristics of malignant growths?
2 How are tumors classified, and how are they usually named? What features of a growth help to determine the degree of malignancy? What is meant by metastasis, and how does it occur?
3 Since principles of medical aseptic technique are used in care of some patients receiving radioisotope therapy, review these principles and techniques.
4 What facilities, such as home-care programs and hospitals for chronically ill patients, are available in your community for care of the patient with cancer in the terminal stages.

CANCER AND THE NURSE

The professional nurse can take a very active part in the prevention and control of cancer, as well as in the care of patients who have the disease. She may contribute to the prevention of cancer as she works in industry; she may do case finding in the community and educate the public to report early suspicious signs to competent physicians; she may give care to patients hospitalized for treatment of cancer; she may be a team member in a research center; she may assist the patient's family in giving him terminal care at home or help those who give such care in nursing homes.

The nature of many nursing functions fosters a close personal feeling on the part of patients toward the nurse. As a result, the nurse is often the recipient of confidences when fear or other emotions keep the patients from seeking help from others. Cancer is a disease that is much publicized and greatly feared in our society. The nurse herself shares this fear. Fear of cancer must be faced squarely and dealt with intelligently by using present knowledge of prevention, control, and treatment satisfactorily. The nurse must examine and, perhaps, alter her own feelings about cancer if she is to be alert to signs of the disease and be effective in helping the patient to secure medical attention. To be effective the nurse needs mature attitudes and reactions, knowledge of the disease and of its treatment, and a knowledge of the community resources available to those who have cancer.

Cancer incidence is highest during the middle years of life. It is estimated that one of every eight persons reaching 45 years of age will develop cancer by the age of 65 years. More women than men die of cancer; however, figures for the last decade show less difference than previously, partly because more early cancers of the cervix are being diagnosed and effectively treated and because the incidence of lung cancer is much higher in men than in women. It is probable that the actual incidence of cancer is not increasing, although there is some evidence that it is occurring more often in certain parts of the body in certain peoples, such as cancer of the lung among men in the western hemisphere.

Cancer ranks second only to heart disease as the cause of deaths in the United States; in 1958 there were about 252,000 deaths from cancer in the United States.[22] In the decade from 1945 to 1955, the deaths from cancer among men aged 55 to 64 increased by almost 50 per cent, and this rise is attributed largely to increase in lung cancer.[15] Cancer results from abnormal cell growth and is found in other animals besides man and also in plants. The disease is not new. It was recognized in ancient times by skilled observers who gave it the name cancer (crab) because it stretched out in many directions like the legs of the crab. Cancer is no respector of race or social status. As death from other causes are reduced, cancer is becoming much more prevalent and is a much more common cause of death. For example, since in the United States the death rate from pneumonia has been appreciably lowered mainly due to the antibiotic drugs and since many deaths from communicable disease in childhood have been prevented by immunization, the life span has been considerably lengthened. Therefore, there is a higher prevalence of cancer in the United States because more of our people are living to the age when cancer is most likely to develop.

Cancer occurs relatively frequently in children. It now follows accidents as the leading cause of death in the age group from 4 to 15 years. The leukemias and Hodgkin's disease are now statistically included with other forms of cancer. This gives a more realistic picture of the incidence of malignant disease in children than was possible before these conditions were included.

RESEARCH

Although a tremendous amount of money and research effort goes into attempts to learn the cause and true nature of cancer, the cause of the disease is unknown. However, each year more is learned about cell behavior and cell growth, and it is to be expected that eventually the actual cause of abnormal cell growth will be found.

Cancer research workers are active in a variety of fields, and it may finally be shown that several factors act together in the development of abnormal cell growth. Many years ago it was noted that certain substances caused skin cancer. It was observed that skin cancers developed in men who were employed to sweep the chimneys in English homes in which coal was burned in fireplaces; skin cancer was considered an occupational hazard in chimney sweeping. It was then learned that when the suspected substance (methylcholanthrene) contained in the sweepings was repeatedly painted on the ears of experimental animals, it caused cancer. Then it was noted that this carcinogen was somewhat similar in chemical structure to some of the hormones. This observation led physicians to experiment with removal of the ovaries in women who had cancer of the breast and later to give male hormones. Hormone treatment is used at the present time for many forms of cancer in both sexes, and, although it does not cure the disease, it sometimes retards the activity of abnormal cell growth to a remarkable degree.

There appears to be a genetic factor involved in the predisposition to develop cancer and in determination of the part of the body attacked. This has been conclusively demonstrated by repeated breeding of mice from cancerous and noncancerous strains. A strain of mice has been developed in which almost all the mice develop breast cancer, and this would certainly indicate that heredity may affect the tendency to develop cancer, although many other factors may also be involved. Evidence obtained through animal experimentation does not necessarily prove that the same thing occurs in human beings, but it raises the possibility that this may be so.

The possibility that viruses may contribute to the development of cancer has been raised repeatedly. In the animal laboratory it has been demonstrated that something in the milk of the mouse from a carcinogenic strain can be transmitted and in some way affects the young who ingest this milk. In a high proportion of cases, baby mice from a noncarcinogenic strain put to nurse immediately at the breast of a mouse from a carcinogenic strain will later develop cancer.

It is believed that certain chemical compounds may have cytotoxic effects that contribute to the development of cancer. It is known that certain toxic damage to cells, such as is caused by repeated exposure to substances containing radium, can cause cancer. It is also known that cancer may follow chronic irritation to any part of the body. Examples are cancer of the lip in pipe smokers and cancer of the skin over the bridge of the nose or behind the ears in people who wear glasses. Also, cancer of the bone has been known to occur following bone injuries caused by sudden blows.

PREVENTION AND CONTROL

Prevention and control of cancer depends largely upon use of the knowledge that we now have in avoiding those conditions which we know predispose to the development of the disease, education of the public to encourage prompt treatment when signs of cancer appear, and repeated follow-up examination of those who have had cancer of any kind so that signs of recurrence may be dealt with promptly. The nurse is important in any program for prevention and control of cancer. Charles S. Cameron, the Medical and Scientific Director of the American Society for the Prevention of Cancer, says: "If cancer control is to make the progress so urgently called for, the nurse will have to assume more and more responsibility, as a community-minded citizen, for the development of broad cancer education programs among the general public. The success of control measures depends in large measure on developing a public with higher awareness, better understanding, and a more constructive attitude toward the disease."*

Prevention. Sources of chronic irritation that may lead to cancer should be avoided. Effort is being made in industry to protect workers from coal-tar products known to contain carcinogens. Masks and gloves are recommended in some instances, and workers are urged to wash their hands and arms thoroughly to remove all irritating substances at the end of the day's work. Industrial nurses participate in extensive educational programs to help the workers understand the need for carrying out company rules which may help to prevent cancer.

There are many small things that can be done to prevent irritation that may lead to cancer. It is possible that cleanliness of the skin is helpful particularly for those who live and work in highly industrial environments where the soot content in the air is high. Prolonged exposure to wind, dirt, and sunshine may lead to skin cancer; skin cancer on the face and hands is particularly frequent among those farmers and cattle ranchers who have fair complexions and who do not protect themselves from exposure.

Any kind of chronic irritation to the skin should be avoided, and moles that are in locations where they may be irritated by clothing should be removed. Shoelaces, shoe tops, girdles, brassieres, and shirt collars are examples of clothing that may be a source of chronic irritation. Glasses, earrings, dental plates, and pipes that are in repeated contact with skin and mucous membrane may contribute to cancer. Chewing food thoroughly is recommended to lessen irritation in the throat and stomach. Cancer in the mouth seems to have been sometimes caused in part by rough jagged teeth and by the constant aggravation of tobacco smoke. The habit of drinking scalding hot or freezing cold liquids is thought to be irritating to the esophagus. Indiscriminate use of laxatives, particularly mineral oil, is thought to have possible carcinogenic effects upon the large bowel.

Encouraging women to breast feed their babies, if there are no contraindications, may contribute to the prevention of cancer of the breast. Cancer of the breast is found among women who have had children and those who have never become pregnant, although it is more common in the latter. For some reason cancer of the breast is relatively rare among Japanese women, most of whom marry and have childen whom they breast feed.

---

*From a Cancer Source Book for Nurses, New York, 1950, The American Cancer Society, Inc.

There seems to be little question but that excessive smoking is linked in some way with the increased incidence of lung cancer in recent years. More and more reports appear to incriminate moderate and heavy cigarette smoking as a predisposing factor in the development of lung cancer. It may eventually be shown that the smoky air of our industrial age is also a causative factor, although at the present this is merely speculation.

Control. More widespread knowledge of cancer and a more positive attitude toward the disease are essential for the control of the disease. Despite all the public announcements that have been made in the last few decades, there are still people who think of cancer as a disgraceful disease that must be hidden from others. Cancer is talked about in whispers by many people who look upon it as a punishment for past sins, a shameful disease, or a disgrace to the family. Part of this is because cancer, in its terminal stages, often is a painful and demoralizing disease, accompanied by body odor and other signs of physical decay that are deeply etched upon the consciousness of friends and relatives. Actually there is no characteristic odor of cancer, although diseased tissue that breaks down and becomes infected with odor-producing organisms will be as unpleasant as any other infected wound. The essential point—so often missed by the public—is that this tragic situation is by and large an unusual one.

Some people fear cancer and shun those with the disease because they believe it is contagious. Scientific speculation as to the possibility of a virus being the cause has added to this fear. At this time there is no conclusive evidence that a virus or any other communicable agent contributes in any way to the development of cancer.

The positive aspects of cancer should be emphasized. It is estimated that approximately one third of those in whom a diagnosis of cancer is made are cured by medical treatment and never have recurrences. Another third usually can be cured by medical treatment if diagnosis is made early enough. Another third have cancer occurring in locations in which the disease advances beyond permanent medical aid before sufficient signs appear to warn the patient of trouble.[15] In spite of these facts, however, some patients think it is useless to report symptoms early, since they believe that if they do have cancer they cannot be cured.

Early signs and symptoms. Everyone should know the seven danger signs of cancer and should report them immediately to his physician: (1) Any sore or lesion in the mouth or anywhere else in the body that does not heal within two weeks. (2) A lump or mass in the breast or anywhere else in the body. (3) Any unusual bleeding or discharge from any body orifice. (4) Any change in size, color, or appearance of a wart or a mole. (5) Persistent indigestion or difficulty in swallowing. (6) Persistent hoarseness or cough that does not clear up within two weeks. (7) Any change in normal bowel habits.

A very common misconception which leads the patient to ignore symptoms is a belief that a disease as serious as cancer must be accompanied by weight loss. Weight loss is usually a late symptom of cancer, yet the patient often remarks, "I wasn't losing weight so I thought nothing serious could be wrong." Another reason for early neglect of cancer is that it may not cause pain, and, again, the patient takes this as a sign that his indisposition is minor. It must be repeatedly emphasized to the public that pain is not an early sign of cancer and that cancer may be far advanced before pain occurs. All women should know the most common sites of cancer in women: the breast, the uterus (cervix), the skin, and the gastrointestinal tract. They should be taught to examine their breasts each month immediately after the menstrual period. Such self-examination is a much better method of detecting early cancer than is an annual physical examination. (See Chapter 31 for details of self-examination of the breast.)

Women of all ages should know the importance of reporting any abnormal vaginal bleeding or other discharge occurring between menstrual periods or after the menopause. (See Chapter 22 for details of early symptoms of cancer of the female reproductive system.)

It is recommended that all women over 35 years of age have a pelvic examination annually and that a cervical smear be taken for testing by the Papanicolaou method. The Papanicolaou test represents an enormous step forward in the early diagnosis of cancer of the cervix. It is also useful in diagnosing cancer in other parts of the body, such as the lungs. The value of the test lies in the fact that abnormal malignant cells that are sloughed off in the early stages of a cancer of the endothelium may be identified from secretions about the lesion. This usually occurs before the lesion has invaded the deeper structures, and, if the test is done early, the cancer may be diagnosed and removed before metastasis occurs.

The most common sites of cancer in men are the skin, lungs, gastrointestinal tract, and prostate gland. All men 40 years of age and over should have an annual physical examination that includes search for diseases in these locations. In many cancer-detection clinics, proctoscopic examinations are done on all men 35 years of age or over because of the high incidence of cancer of the lower bowel in men in this age group.

Facilities for education and care. The nurse needs to teach that there is no quick or certain cure for cancer. Despite all the public education and all efforts of the medical profession to control the extravagant claims of a few unethical practitioners, there are still some people who rely on quick "cure" remedies prescribed by quacks. The best hope for cure of cancer lies in immediate medical attention if danger signs appear. If a person who suspects he has cancer has no private doctor or feels that he cannot afford one, he should report to his local health department and seek referral to a suitable hospital or to a local cancer-detection clinic.

In dealing with a patient who has delayed seeking early medical treatment, the nurse must give hope and encouragement to him and his family. Sometimes guilt, a feeling of hopelessness, or a fatalistic attitude will cause further delay in pursuing a suggested course of medical diagnosis.

The nurse must know of sources of information and help for those who have the disease. There is one large national voluntary organization, the American Cancer Society, Inc.,* which has branches in all states and in eleven major cities. It was organized in 1913 as the National Society for the Control of Cancer with the major objective of combating the fear, shame, and ignorance which were outstanding obstacles in the control of the disease. This huge organization, which receives large annual bequests and gifts, has expanded its functions and now has several objectives. It finances research to seek the cause of cancer and to develop better methods of treatment. It publishes booklets and pamphlets for the use of doctors and nurses, and it stimulates better preparation of professional people in the care of patients with cancer by sponsoring institutes and special group programs. Information about booklets and pamphlets may be obtained by writing directly to the main office of the Society or to the state or local offices.

In addition, the American Cancer Society, Inc., has a division known as the Woman's Field Army which strives constantly to educate the public. It works intensively through magazines, women's clubs, insurance companies, state departments of health, and medical and nursing organizatins in an effort to reach all the population with the educational message of how cancer may be prevented and controlled. Through the Woman's Field Army, a large amount of literature for the laity is prepared and distributed annually. Also, many excellent films for use in public education are made available.

---

*Headquarters: 47 Beaver Street, New York, N. Y.

The American Cancer Society, Inc. also performs services for the cancer victim. Branches in most communities provide assistance for cancer patients who cannot afford to pay for adequate care and for those who, although they can presently afford to pay, will eventually leave their families medically indigent. Depending on how much local support is given to the Cancer Society, this may include dressings, transportation to and from clinics and doctors' offices, special drugs such as expensive hormones, blood, and the loan of expensive equipment such as hospital beds. In some communities homemaking, visiting nurse, and rehabilitation services are also provided. Of the money collected, 60 per cent remains with the local chapter for the community's use. Patients and their families should know about these services before their own resources are depleted, and local citizens should be urged to support the Society generously. Many of these agencies do not use the term cancer in their title so that patients who do not know their diagnosis may be safely referred to them.

In addition to the American Cancer Society, Inc., some large cities have other voluntary organizations which serve only cancer patients; e.g., Cancer Care, a large voluntary organization in New York City, confines its activities solely to the tremendous needs of patients with advanced cancer and to the needs of their families. The nurse who works in a small community or a rural area may learn of the resources available to cancer patients through her local or state health department.

Lists of available films for both professional and lay use can be obtained from the American Cancer Society, Inc., and state and local health departments. Some insurance companies, such as the Metropolitan Life Insurance Company and the John Hancock Insurance Company, prepare very useful pamphlets on control of cancer and the care of those with the disease. These are useful to nurses in conducting health education programs and in teaching relatives of a patient with cancer how to care for the patient.

Federal recognition of the need to give intensive assistance to educational programs in cancer was evident in 1926 when Congress proclaimed April of each year as National Cancer Control Month. In 1937 the National Cancer Institute was created within the National Institutes of Health. This Institute, with generous support from the federal government, conducts an extensive program of research in the field of cancer.

GENERAL NURSING CARE

A sound personal philosophy and an objective positive attitude toward the disease based on real knowledge will help the nurse caring for the patient with cancer. She should be able to give encouragement, support, and hope to the patient and to his family. While she may have compassion, she should avoid inspiring false hope. She must try to understand the fears experienced by the patient as he awaits diagnostic procedures or other treatment—fear of hospitals, fear of pain, fear of radical surgery with mutilation, fear of expense that cannot be met, and fear of death, with all that it means to him. In working with the patient, the young and inexperienced nurse should not hesitate to turn to her instructor, head nurse, or supervisor with problems which appear too great for her to handle alone.

A nurse's kindly interest in the patient as an individual often helps him. Many patients must undergo extensive diagnostic examination and surgery in large medical centers a long distance from their homes. Some patients have reported that, although they were confident that they were in "good medical hands," such confidence did not make up for the feeling that they were not always known as individuals. They needed desperately to feel that at least one person knew and understood them as individuals. Some patients experience near panic at the thought of their loved ones coming to visit and being unable to locate them. The nurse who works with the patient in the community, in the small hospital, or in the doctor's office can help the patient by preparing him for what he may experience in the large center. In most instances it is best for the patient to be accompanied by a relative or close friend. It should also be recognized that even a patient in familiar surroundings may feel very much alone when awaiting diagnostic tests or surgical treatment for known or suspected cancer.

The nurse must know whether or not the patient has been told that he has cancer. She should know quite specifically what he knows so that he may not be upset by conflicting impressions. He may receive several different answers to the same questions from doctors, nurses, social workers, physical therapists, and others, or he may receive no answer to his questions. This is one of the most upsetting experiences for patients in today's busy hospitals. It is unfortunate in any situation, but it is doubly so when a threat of cancer hangs over the patient. Some hospitals have almost completely overcome this problem by having regular meetings of all the members of the professional staff at which the information given to each patient is reviewed by the professional team members. The nursing group taking care of patients with cancer should be careful in their communications with each other and plan a consistent approach so that the patient's daily care will proceed as swiftly and with as little stress to him as possible.

The emotional climate produced during the period of diagnostic examination and initial treatment is very important in determining whether or not the patient will continue diagnostic examination, treatment, or repeated follow-up care after discharge. The care he receives in the hospital may shape his attitudes toward his disease and determine whether or not he can care for himself at home or whether his family will be able to give the care that is needed. An important nursing function in care of the patient with cancer is building up his faith in the doctor and in the clinic or the medical center where he receives care. The patient needs to feel certain that everything possible is being done for him and that new measures will be tried if there is any promise of their being helpful.

Members of the medical profession differ in their opinions as to whether or not the patient with cancer should be told the diagnosis. Decision usually depends upon the patient, his family, and the physician. The present trend is toward telling the patient he has cancer; many spiritual advisers recommend this. Some patients obviously do not want to know the diagnosis; they may ask and then answer their own question negatively. Some do not ask for the diagnosis since they do not wish to have confirmed what they already suspect. Some insist on knowing the diagnosis and are preoccupied with every detail of their progress and treatment in a detached but completely abnormal fashion. Finally, there are some who wish to know the facts and who can accept them in a realistic way. Some physicians prepare the patient over a period of time and tell him the complete truth when they feel it is best to do so. Psychologic reactions depend upon the emotional make-up of the individual and are as varied as man's ability to face stresses and threats throughout life. Since disclosure of the diagnosis lies entirely with the discretion of the doctor, the nurse cannot tell the patient or his family. She can, however, refer to the doctor any questions, misinformation, or apprehensions that the patient or his family have expressed to her. This will often help the doctor to decide what course of action seems best. Any sudden severe depression or expressed thoughts of suicide should be reported at once. Often a patient's fears are communicated to a nurse long before he "gets up courage" to question the doctor.

The patient needs something to keep him occupied while he is awaiting completion of diagnostic tests and treatment and between steps of treatment such as surgery or x-ray therapy. Usually he fares best in a room with others, where there is more going on and less time for introspective thought. Conversation, music, newspapers, and light games are about all most patients can concentrate on at this time. Some patients may like to do work with their hands, such as crocheting or working with leather. If there is no occupational therapy department from which supplies may be obtained, the nurse may arrange for members of the patient's family to provide them.

The family also needs to keep busy while awaiting the results of diagnostic tests and the outcome of surgery or of other treatment. One woman, upon learning that her husband had far-advanced carcinoma, went home immediately and made his favorite cake, even though he was in the hospital and unable to enjoy it. Psychologic relief may sometimes come from keeping occupied with usual daily activities. Anxious relatives also get satisfaction from doing things that the patient would do if he could and thus preserving parts of cherished routines. Taking the dog for his daily walk is an example. Members of the family often need direction in their activity when they have just learned that a loved one has cancer. They may need to talk over immediate and long-term plans with someone not close to the family situation. The nurse can sometimes be this listening person; at other times she should refer the family to a social worker who will help them talk through and think through a course of action.

SURGICAL TREATMENT

The best treatment for cancer at the present time is complete surgical removal of all malignant tissues before metastasis occurs. Surgery must often be extensive and may require adjustment for the patient beyond that needed in many other conditions. The patient with cancer does not have the privilege of electing surgery, as he may in some diseases. This fact alone makes him feel trapped and seriously threatened. Immediate extensive surgery is often imperative if there is to be any hope of saving the patient's life; he does not have time to accustom himself gradually to the idea of how the surgery may change him and how it may affect his way of life. What is more, the patient must often face the prospect of mutilating surgery with only the hope and not the certainty that this will cure the cancer and save his life. He may be more concerned about his family than he is about himself. Obviously he needs sympathy and understanding when he and his family are attempting to accept the news and the immediate surgical treatment that the surgeon recommends. The operative procedures and nursing care for cancer involving the particular systems are discussed in the appropriate chapters and will not be included here.

RADIOTHERAPY

Radiotherapy has been used in the treatment of cancer for a little over fifty years, whereas surgery has been used for hundreds of years. The principal agents used are x-ray, radium, and artificially induced radioactive isotopes. Radioactive cobalt is now partially replacing radium because of its lower cost.

Radiotherapy is effective in curing cancer in some instances; in others it controls the cancer cells for a time. Because it may deter the growth of cancer cells, it may relieve pain even when extension of the disease is such that cure is impossible. Radiotherapy is based upon the known fact that malignant cells are more sensitive to radiation than normal cells. Usually the less well differentiated the tumor cell, the more it will respond to treatment, while the more closely it resembles its parent cell, the more resistant it is to treatment. Therapeutic doses of radiotherapy are calculated to destroy or delay the growth of malignant cells without destroying normal tissues.

To many people, radiotherapy and cancer are synonymous. It is natural, then, that the patient may react with panic to news that this treatment is necessary. Sometimes the patient is told that the treatment is necessary "to cure a growth that may become cancerous if not so treated." Often he does not really believe this. The nurse should give the patient a chance to talk. She should find out how he feels about the treatment and ask the doctor to discuss it further if she thinks it is necessary.

X-ray therapy. The patient who is to have x-ray therapy needs explanation so that he will know what to expect before, during, and after the treatment. He may have heard that the treatment causes nausea or skin "burns or irritation." If he asks about these the nurse should explain simply and clearly what they are and why they *sometimes* occur or she should refer the question to the doctor; usually patients are not told of these possible complications unless they occur. The nurse's course of action must depend upon her knowledge, her experience, and her judgment. The patient should know that he will be placed on a table in a room by himself and that the equipment, although somewhat similar to what he has probably seen during a routine x-ray examination, will be larger and more complicated. He should know that the radiologist or the radiotherapist will be stationed outside the room, will observe him throughout the treatment, and will communicate with him if he wishes. He must be told how he can assist by remaining in the exact position in which he is placed so that the rays will be correctly directed. He should be told that the treatment will not be painful.

X-ray dosage may be difficult to estimate accurately if the growth is deep within the body. In giving treatment, rays can be directed at the tumor from several different angles so that, normal tissue has a minimum of exposure. The areas through which rays pass are known as *ports*. Different ports may be used on different days; the position may be changed at intervals during a daily treatment so that only a certain amount is given through each of several ports, or the patient may be placed on a rotating device such as a rotating chair so that, although the tumor mass receives the full dose of radiation, skin areas receive less exposure.

The patient may be curious as to how many treatments he will receive. It is best not to give a definite answer. Sometimes treatment must be discontinued because of local skin reaction or other reasons; thus the patient who has been told the number of treatments planned to assure successful recovery may become depressed when treatment is discontinued. The patient also becomes concerned if he learns he is to receive more treatments than were originally planned. If he shows apprehension, the doctor should be notified so that he may give needed reassurance.

Skin preparation for x-ray therapy includes removal of any ointment and dressings and thorough cleansing of the skin. This usually is followed by an alcohol rub. After this preparation, nothing should be used on the skin. The area to be treated is usually outlined by the radiologist at the time of the first treatment. Occasionally a small tattoo mark is used instead of the conspicuous skin markings when treatment is given to exposed parts of the body. Marks must not be washed off until the treatment is completed since they are important guides to the radiologist (see Figure 24). If the patient is ambulatory, he is instructed not to wash the skin or remove the marks; sponge bathing of other parts of the body must replace showers and tub baths. A vegetable fat such as Crisco should be used to protect the skin.

Medicated solutions or ointments and even powders which may contain heavy metals such as zinc are not permitted on the skin until the series of x-ray treatments is completed because they may increase the dosage. Starch may be used instead of powder.

When treatment is directed toward abdominal organs or any deep tissues, there is almost always some skin reaction. There may be itching, tingling, burning, oozing, or sloughing of the skin. The term "burn" should never be used in referring to this reaction since it implies incorrect dosage, which is not the case. Reddening may occur on or about the tenth day, and the skin may turn a dark plum color after about three weeks. The skin may also be-

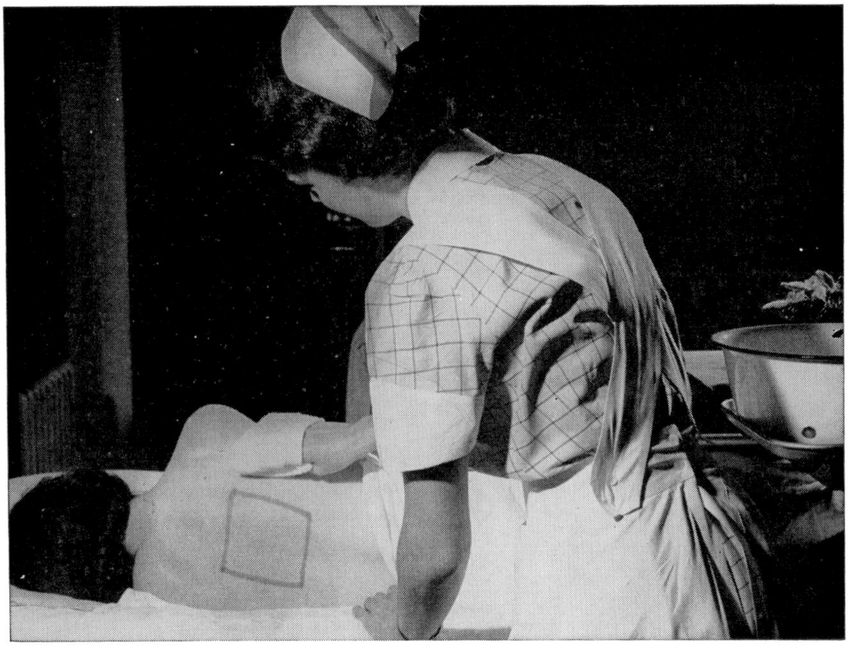

Figure 24

When the bath is given, care must be taken not to remove skin markings used to guide the radiologist in giving x-ray treatment.

come dry and inelastic and may crack easily. The area may be gently cleansed with sterile mineral oil but crusts should not be removed. Lanolin or petroleum jelly may be used to protect the area, and healing ointments containing vitamins A and D and healing oils such as cod-liver oil may be used if breakdown of superficial tissues occurs. Healing usually starts approximately in the fifth week of treatment and should be complete about a month later.

Ointments are best applied by spreading them on a piece of sterile gauze and fastening the gauze to the patient's clothing. If this cannot be done, dressings may be bandaged loosely or anchored to good healthy skin outside and beyond the treatment ports. If tape must be used instead of bandage, cellophane tape should be used instead of adhesive since it is less irritating to skin. In removing dressings the greatest care must be taken to pull toward the middle of the area and thus avoid any pull on affected skin. Dressings should be loose to permit circulation of air and to avoid pressure on the skin.

The skin exposed to treatment should be protected from constricting clothing or friction of any kind. For example, the patient receiving treatment to the trunk should not wear a girdle, garter belt, or a constricting trouser or skirt belt during the period of treatment and for several weeks thereafter. During the period of treatment, the patient should avoid excesses of heat and cold to affected skin surfaces; hot-water bottles and icecaps should not be used, and exposure to the sun should be avoided. Some doctors advise that no water be used on the skin for at least two weeks after the completion of treatment.

If the x-ray dosage has been high and blanching or discoloration of the skin results, the doctor may advise the patient to avoid exposure to temperature changes for several years. The patient may have to take much cooler baths or showers than he is used to, and he may have to avoid sun bathing or any other extreme of temperature. If x-ray treatment has been given to a woman's face, she must be cautioned regarding the use of cosmetics to cover discolored skin. These may contain heavy, irritating oils and should not be used until the doctor believes they are safe.

Gastrointestinal reactions to x-ray therapy are more common when treatment includes some part of the gastrointestinal tract or when the ports lie over this system. The patient may have nausea, vomiting, anorexia, malaise, and diarrhea. This difficulty is not discussed with the patient before treatment is started because it is thought that the power of suggestion may contribute to symptoms. However, almost all patients who receive moderate or large doses of radiation have these symptoms in various degrees. Liver extract, vitamin B, and intravenous solutions of glucose in physiologic solution of sodium chloride are used for nausea, anorexia, and dehydration. Pyriodoxine, folic acid, and dimenhydrinate (Dramamine) give symptomatic relief in some patients. Camphorated tincture of opium (paregoric) may be used to control the diarrhea, but drugs such as bismuth subcarbonate are not given because they contain heavy metal that will increase radiation dosage.

Many patients find that rest just before meals and lying down immediately after eating help to control nausea and vomiting. Frequent small meals instead of regular ones should also be tried. Some patients find that it helps to withhold food for two to three hours before and about two hours after each treatment. Sour beverages and effervescent liquids may also prevent nausea. Usually breakfast is the meal best tolerated. Therefore, it should be substantial and the patient should be encouraged to eat as much as possible.

Problems related to x-ray therapy in specific diseases are discussed in the appropriate sections of this book.

Radium. Radium and its emanations are used in the treatment of established cancer. Radium is extremely costly and, if incorrectly used, is dangerous to both the patient and those who handle it. The nurse must help maintain accurate dosage, see that radium does not become lost or stolen, and carry out certain essential nursing procedures.

Radium is usually kept in a lead-lined container in a locked cupboard or room in the radiology department. It must never be handled with bare hands. When the nurse handles radium products, she should use a pair of forceps at least fourteen inches long and should hold the radium at arm's length. If boiling is the method of sterilization used, great care must be taken to wrap the materials so that they cannot under any circumstances be lost down the drain. To prevent accidental loss, radium that has been removed from a patient is cleansed in a basin of water instead of in an open sink. If a brush must be used for cleansing, it must be grasped with forceps so that close contact with the radium is avoided. Radium should be cleansed and returned to the radiology department as soon as it is removed from the patient so that it may not be accidentally thrown away or unknowingly handled.

The patient who receives radium treatment should be told the importance of lying in the desired position. He should be instructed not to do anything that might shift the position of the radium and thereby alter the dosage to affected tissue or injure normal tissue. For example, when several small radium needles are inserted into the cervix, the patient must be instructed not to permit any traction on the strings protruding from the vagina. She must report at once if one of the needles should become dislodged; the strings may be fastened together to the thigh where they may be quickly counted. Patients who have radium treatment of this kind are not permitted to use the bathroom because of the danger of losing the radium and because movement displaces tissues which alters dosage. The nurse should check the contents of the bedpan after each use. When radium is used, it is part of routine nursing care to check all linen, general equipment, dressings, and drainage from wounds or body orifices before removing them from the room to be certain that no radium is misplaced.

The patient who has had radium or x-ray treatment in the abdominal or pelvic area should be advised to report any difficulty in voiding or any unusual bowel function. Occasionally adhesions form which interfere with normal function of the urinary and intestinal systems. Because of sloughing of neoplastic tissue, a vesicovaginal or rectovaginal fistula can also follow this treatment. This condition presents serious nursing problems, since incontinence, infection with odor, irritation, and discomfort usually follow. Douches followed by warm sitz baths or compresses soaked in a solution of sodium bicarbonate are sometimes helpful. Medicinal zinc peroxide solution may be used to control odor, reduce inflammation, and combat infection; it may be used as a douche, to soak gauze packing to place in the wound, or as compresses to external sloughing wounds.

Radon seeds are tiny sealed tubes (usually gold) which contain the emanations of radium but which have a relatively short life. While radium takes about 1,600 years to lose half of its strength (its half-life), the half-life of radon seeds is about four days, and most of the emanations have disappeared at the end of thirty days. Radon seeds may be inserted to remain indefinitely in tissue such as the tongue when the cancerous lesion cannot be removed surgically. The patient who receives radon treatment must be cautioned about seeds that may slough from the tissue, since even the relatively few remaining emanations may be dangerous. Such seeds should be buried in the ground or returned to the hospital or the doctor's office.

Sloughing of tissue and subsequent hemorrhage are complications that must be considered when radium is used in any form. Hemorrhage is not mentioned to the patient, but, if he is ambulatory, he is told that he should report to the doctor at once should any sloughing of tissue occur.

Radioactive isotopes. Radioactive isotopes or radioisotopes are isotopes of elements which have been rendered radioactive by bombardment with highly energized particles in a cyclotron. Each element has a number of natural isotopes which are variations of the element having different molecular weights. With developments in the field of nuclear energy, it has been possible to produce radioactive isotopes of a number of the elements, although only a few of them have medical application at the present time. The nurse needs to know the behavior of the more commonly used radioactive isotopes and the precautions that must be taken in giving care to patients being treated with these substances. The precautions necessary will depend upon whether only a tracer dose has been given or whether larger doses have been used. There is not complete agreement at the present time regarding how much exposure to radioactive substances is safe. Most hospitals have set up specific procedures and guides for those who care for patients receiving radioactive materials. The nurse should familiarize herself with the procedures used in the hospital in which she is employed.

When radioactive isotopes first became available, it was believed that tremendous strides had been made in the treatment of cancer. Both the public and the medical profession anticipated more progress than has so far been made. For example, it was hoped that radioactive iodine (I^{131}) might be given for cancer of the thyroid in the form of an "atomic cocktail" and that malignant cells would be satisfactorily destroyed. Results of this have been disappointing because malignant thyroid cells do not concentrate iodine as well as normal thyroid cells, and therefore the treatment to the original tumor in the thyroid or to its areas of metastasis is limited. It is most often used in conjunction with surgical removal of the thyroid gland.

Radioactive iodine (I^{131}) is used in the study and diagnosis of disease of the thyroid, and it is used to treat hyperthyroidism. It is being experimented with in other diagnostic tests. Radioactive iodine–tagged albumin has proved useful in locating tumors in the brain, and it is frequently used to determine blood volume. In diagnostic procedures, the radioactive iodine is taken either by mouth or injected intravenously as radioactive iodine–tagged albumin. The Geiger-Müller counter, an instrument which is very sensitive to radioactivity, is then passed over the body to locate areas that have retained the radioactive substance. Sometimes the tests are dependent upon the percentage of the dose picked up (blood volume) or on the rate of excretion (hyperthyroid studies). The use of radioisotopes in specific diseases is discussed more fully in the appropriate chapters.

Other radioactive substances that are being used are radioactive phosphorus (P^{32}) in the treatment of polycythemia vera and leukemia, radioactive gold (Au^{198}) for cancer of the lung with effusion into the pleural cavity and for peritoneal ascites due to generalized carcinoma, and radioactive cobalt (Co^{60}) as a substitute for radium. Radioactive phosphorus is given orally as a liquid; radioactive gold is injected into body cavities as a liquid; and radioactive cobalt is given as a ray using equipment somewhat similar to that used for x-ray therapy. None of these cure cancer, but they sometimes control the disease to some extent and lessen pain. It is now believed that they should be used in selected cases of cancer along with other forms of treatment such as surgery and x-ray therapy. Early surgical treatment is a better form of treatment than any treatment with radioactive substances.

Nursing care. It is believed that care of patients receiving radioactive substances presents no particular hazards to personnel provided certain measures similar to those employed in isolation technique are used. The nurse caring for patients receiving radioactive isotopes should be given instructions in how to care for herself and how to use the special equipment provided. She should know the nature of the radioactive isotope with which she is working. For example, if the patient has received radioactive iodine, the nurse needs to know that this substance has a half-life of eight days and is eliminated largely in the urine.

Most radioactive isotopes emit either beta or gamma rays or a combination of the two. Beta rays usually confine their effects to areas close to the site where the isotope has been placed, whereas gamma rays penetrate further to other parts of the body. If the patient has received a radioactive isotope that emits both beta and gamma rays (I^{131} is an example), the isotope is eliminated mainly through the urine, but small amounts will be present in sputum, vomitus, and perspiration. Special precautions must be taken if more than a tracer-diagnostic dose has been given, and these precautions should be explained to the patient. The patient is placed in a single room with a sign on the door identifying him as having had radiation treatment and stating that no visitors are permitted. The nurse and all who come in direct contact with the patient for any length of time must wear isolation gowns and rubber gloves and film badges under the isolation gowns to determine the amount of exposure received.

It is important to explain the routine to the patient. He must remain in his own room for the period of isolation so that danger of contamination to others is minimized and so that his reaction to the radioactive substance can be better studied and controlled. He should know that visitors will not be permitted in his room for forty-eight to seventy-two hours, so that he may notify relatives and friends and thus be spared the embarrassment of their coming to the hospital and being confronted with the sign on his door. A radio should be provided so the patient may keep in contact with others. He should know how the radioactive substance he takes is eliminated; otherwise he may fear that he will be dangerous to others indefinitely and may become panicky about social isolation or about the possibility of harming his loved ones when he returns home. The nurse explains to him that she will be available for anything he needs but that she will work quickly while in the room and will remain only long enough to carry out essential nursing activities. Many patients anticipate cure from radioactive isotopes. The nurse can learn what the patient understands about the treatment as she gives essential care and should report this to the doctor.

Since most radioactive iodine is eliminated through the kidneys, the care of urine is important. A lead-encased container is usually used. An indwelling catheter may be inserted before the substance is given, and this may be released at intervals to drain directly into the jug which is transported daily on a cart to the radioisotope laboratory, where it is stored until it can be disposed of safely. Male patients may be instructed to empty their urinals directly into the container if the insertion of a catheter is not considered advisable. It is important that all urine be carefully collected since it is the quantitative determination of the amount of radioactive substance excreted that determines when the patient may be removed from isolation. The amount of contamination of equipment in the room is determined by monitoring with a Geiger counter. If the isolation gown and linen show contamination, they are placed in a special container labeled "radioactive" and stored in lead containers in the isotope laboratory, or they are burned. Since dishes are usually kept in the room, the patient must be placed in a room that has running water. Dishes are thoroughly washed and then monitored. In some institutions they are sent to the kitchen if the monitor reading is less than 6 milliroentgens per hour. If the nurse's skin should become contaminated, it is thoroughly washed with soap and water and then monitored. If contamination remains, the skin is washed again until monitoring shows that additional cleansing is of no use.

When the patient is removed from isolation, all equipment is monitored and carefully scrubbed by attendants who have been instructed in safe methods to use by those who are in charge of the administration of the radioactive substance. It is then remonitored. The room is aired for at least twenty-four hours and sometimes longer until monitoring shows that radioactivity is negligible and that the room is safe to use for any other patient.

Strict isolation procedures are not always carried out when radioactive gold is used, although a film badge is worn by all who attend the patient and rubber gloves are worn when applying dressings over the site of injection. The Au^{198} is injected into the pleural space, and contamination is possible only at the point of injection. When a purple stain appears, it indicates that some of the material is escaping. The patient is turned every fifteen minutes for two hours so that the radioactive gold will be spread evenly within the pleural cavity. If Au^{198} is escaping, linen that has been in contact with the chest wall should be placed in a special container clearly marked for care in the isotope laboratory or other facilities provided by the hospital. Dressings and cleansing tissues should be burned immediately. The patient who receives radioactive gold is usually terminally ill. If he dies soon after receiving Au^{198}, a notation that the patient was receiving radioactive gold immediately before death should be made on a tag, and the tag should be conspicuously placed on the body. This is for the protection of the coroner and the mortician. If the nurse has any questions about precautions that should be taken, the doctor in charge of radioisotopes in the institution should be consulted.

CARE OF THE PATIENT WITH UNCONTROLLABLE CANCER

When all possible surgery and maximum radiation therapy have failed to control cancer, the patient and his family have many special problems. They need encouragement and help in living as normally as possible, in planning for the late stages of the patient's illness, and in adjusting to death and its implications for the family.

The patient who knows he has cancer with uncontrollable metastasis often asks about the length of time he may expect to live. Since life is precious to every normal person, it is safe to assume that this question is on every patient's mind even though he may not ask it directly. Although no absolute answer can be given, the doctor can give the best estimate of life expectancy, and questions about this should be referred to him. The nurse must know what the doctor tells the patient since the patient may also ask her or mention what the doctor has said, and she must be prepared to clarify misunderstandings. Very occasionally there is a mistake in diagnosis, or the disease is in some way arrested for a long time. If the patient assumes that this may happen in his case, the nurse should not try to help him face probable reality. She must, however, avoid encouraging false hopes. Many patients accept their prognosis philosophically with the hope that a cure for cancer will be found before their disease is far advanced. Some patients are better able to accept the situation if their religious faith can be strengthened. The nurse must encourage the patient and his family to live each day as fully as possible without looking too far ahead. Sometimes patients with cancer have few symptoms and are able to carry on quite well until shortly before death. It is useless for them to concern themselves with problems that may not arise.

Patients with uncontrollable cancer should resume their regular work if they can possibly do so for this makes them feel still an active part of their group and worthy of the approval of others. It was said many centuries ago that employment is man's best physician, and this applies particularly to those whose existence is seriously threatened by cancer. Social activities and all experiences associated with normal family life should be continued whenever possible.

The patient with uncontrollable cancer worries about whether or not he will have severe pain and whether or not such pain can be alleviated. He should know that medical science now has several ways of controlling pain. Hormones, radiation therapy, and a number of analgesic drugs are available and helpful in most instances. Synthetic substitutes for the opiate drugs make it possible to alternate drugs so that the benefit of each is not lessened by individual tolerance and so that toxic reactions can be avoided. Members of the patient's family are sometimes told of operations that can be done if pain becomes too severe to control by other means. (For details of care of the patient with pain, see Chapters 7 and 34.)

The patient may be haunted by fear of brain involvement, loss of mental faculties, and the possibility that he may become completely helpless and dependent upon others. By these fears he expresses one of man's basic wishes—the wish to leave the world with as much dignity as possible. The nurse should urge the patient and his family to discuss such fears with the doctor. The patient may feel that the doctor is too busy and that his questions are too trivial to justify the use of the doctor's time. Such questions, however, are not trivial at all, and a satisfactory answer to them adds tremendously to the patient's peace of mind. Metastasis to the brain in those who have other metastases is somewhat rare, and some patients suffer more from fear of this than is justified. The patient should know that good general hygiene, good nutrition, being up and about for part of each day, and doing deep-breathing exercises with attention to posture all help to prevent helplessness. A positive approach to all problems certainly shortens the time of helplessness and makes the patient more content.

At least half of all deaths from cancer occur in the patient's home. Planning for home care of the patient without completely disrupting the rest of the family takes the concerted efforts of many people. The patient must always be consulted, and his wishes should be respected in the early stages of the disease; in the final stages, he is too ill to be bothered or concerned with making decisions. In the hospital, the doctor, the social worker, and the nurse must work together with the local community nursing agencies, such as the American Cancer Society, Inc., to ensure continuity of care from the hospital to the home. The principles governing suitability for home care are similar to those for any patient receiving home care, although the patient with cancer may not live so long as many others with chronic long-term illnesses. The patient must be under medical supervision and it must be possible to give the care he needs in his home, he must want to be at home, his family must want him home and be able to assist with care, and the home facilities must be suitable. (For further details on home care, see Chapter 3.)

REFERENCES AND SELECTED READINGS*

1 *Alston, Frances, and others: Perfusion, Am. J. Nursing **60**:1603-1607, Nov. 1960.

2 *American Cancer Society, Inc.: A Cancer Source Book for Nurses, New York, 1950, American Cancer Society, Inc.

3 *Barckley, Virginia: What Can I Say to the Cancer Patient? Nursing Outlook **6**:316-318, June 1958.

4 *Best, Nelliana: Radiotherapy and the Nurse, Am. J. Nursing **50**:140-143, March 1950.

5 *Bouser, Mary M.: When Cancer Can Be Cured, Nursing Outlook **5**:138-140, March 1957.

6 *Burns, Patricia, and Parker, Helen: When Radioactive Iodine or Gold Is Used, Am. J. Nursing **56**:1404-1406, Nov. 1956.

7 Cameron, Charles S.: Progress in Cancer Research, Am. J. Nursing **50**:209-211, April 1950.

8 Crile, George, Jr.: Radioactive Iodine in Treating Thyroid Disease, Am. J. Nursing **54**:825, July, 1954.

9 Duffy, Benedict J., Jr.: Atomic Energy in the Diagnosis and Treatment of Malignant Diseases, Am. J. Nursing **55**:434-437, April 1955.

10 *Golbey, Robert B.: Chemotherapy of Cancer, Am. J. Nursing **60**:521-525, April 1960.

11 Harmer, Bertha, and Henderson, Virginia: Textbook of the Principles and Practice of Nursing, ed. 5, New York, 1955, The Macmillan Co.

12 *Karnofsky, David A.: Cancer Quackery: Its Causes, Recognition and Prevention, Am. J. Nursing **59**:496-500, April 1959.

13 *Knapp, Margaret F.: How Do You Feel About Cancer? Nursing Outlook **2**:350-352, July 1952.

14 *Lee, Marjorie Mackay: The Nurse in Cancer Epidemiology, Nursing Outlook **6**:160-162, March 1958.

15 Metropolitan Life Insurance Company: Statistical Bulletin, June 1956.

16 National Cancer Institute, Federal Security Agency and New York Department of Health: Cancer Nursing, 1955, New York Department of Health.

17 *Peterson, Rosalie I.: Knowledge of Cancer—Equipment for Nursing, Am. J. Nursing **54**:463-466, April 1954.

18 Reagan, James W.: Cytological Studies, Am. J. Nursing **58**:1693-1695, Dec. 1958.

19 *Rhoades, Cornelius P.: Cancer Control—Present and Future, Am. J. Nursing **58**:516-519, April 1958.

20 *Scott, Wendell G.: The Clinical Radiologist and the Problems of Radiation Hazards, J.A.M.A. **170**:421-428, May 23, 1959.

21 Shields, Warren: Ionizing Radiation and Medicine, Scientific American **201**:154-176, Sept. 1959. (Entire issue devoted to radiation, including articles on what it is, its circulation in the body, and how it affects the cell, evolution, and the whole animal.)

22 Cancer Facts and Figures, New York, 1960, New York City Cancer Committee of the American Cancer Society.

*References preceded by an asterisk indicate material particularly well suited for student reading.

The patient with communicable disease

Chapter 17

Study questions for review

1 What are the most common means by which diseases are transferred from one person to another? How are they transferred from animals to man?
2 What are some of the provisions of the sanitary code in your community and of the laws in your state that protect against communicable disease?

The development of immunizing agents and the introduction of antibiotics have changed nursing in the communicable diseases. Duties of the nurse are to participate in prevention and control of these diseases and to give, or assist in giving, the best possible care to those who are ill. Her responsibility for control of the communicable diseases includes leadership in education of the public and of individual patients and their families. This may be done at the bedside of the hospitalized patient, in the clinic, in the school, in the patient's home, or in some other community setting. She helps to interpret to the public the necessary control measures and thereby helps to ensure their support of recommended measures. She may also direct investigation of persons suspected of having contracted communicable diseases, and of their relatives, friends, or other contacts. The nurse's role in the control of communicable diseases has become relatively more important as demands for bedside nursing of the patient with a communicable disease have decreased. (See Chapter 11.) The nurse must help to ensure that gains of the past fifty years are maintained. This can be accomplished by teaching sanitary practices in the home, interpreting community efforts in sanitation, and encouraging immunization against diseases for which this protection is available. She must know more than she did previously about epidemiology and about general facts concerning the spread of communicable diseases. Particularly, she must know about those diseases that have, so far, eluded scientific efforts in their control by immunization or by specific means of treatment.

This chapter deals with a few of the communicable diseases that affect large numbers of our population and that are controlled by methods promoted largely through health education. They are, therefore, of particular importance to nurses. These diseases may be encountered in the general hospital, in the clinic, in industry, in the doctor's office, or in the patient's home. The acute contagious diseases, so well described in nursing texts on the subject, are not included. The student is referred to texts on fundamentals of nursing for the basic principles and procedures in isolation technique which are necessary for the care of patients with communicable diseases. Tuberculosis, pneumonia, poliomyelitis, encephalitis, viral hepatitis, tetanus, gas bacillus infection, and various venereal diseases are discussed in the chapters dealing with the body systems most often affected by these diseases.

SYPHILIS

Development and diagnosis of the disease

Syphilis is caused by the spirochete, *Treponema pallidum,* a delicate spiral-shaped organism that is between a protozoan and a bacterium in form. The spirochete is destroyed by soap and water and by drying and can live only a few hours outside a warm environment such as that provided by the human body. It is transmitted from person to person largely through direct contact and less often by transfer from the mother's blood to that of the unborn child. Live spirochetes can also be transmitted through blood transfusions, although they die after refrigeration for more than three hours.

Syphilis is diagnosed by the observation of live treponemes in the material obtained from an early syphilitic lesion and by tests on blood and spinal fluid when the disease is well established. Blood and spinal fluid tests are of two kinds but the underlying principle of both is the fact that an antibody-like substance, *reagin,* is present in the blood of the infected person. This reagin reacts with certain prepared cells of animal tissue which are termed *antigens.* If a precipitate is obtained, the test is termed a *flocculation test,* an example of which is the *Mazzini test;* if all complement in the serum is bound by the test so that none is left to combine with other antibody substances, it is known as a *complement-fixation test,* an example of which is the *Wassermann test.* These tests have a variety of names, having been named after the men who modified and improved them. False positive reactions in the serologic tests occur fairly often, particularly after recent infections or immunization, or in the presence of early collagen disease. A new test, the *treponema-fixation test,* or *Nelson test,* is proving valuable in ruling out false positives in the serologic test for syphilis (often abbreviated S.T.S.).

Syphilis differs from most infectious diseases in its slow progress, its tendency toward chronicity, and its invasion of a large number of organs and body systems. Eventually about one fourth of those persons infected are crippled or die if the disease remains untreated.[5] In 1958 syphilis was the fifteenth cause of death in the United States, with a mortality of 3,896.[12] The disease is described in stages. *Early syphilis* includes the time during which the initial lesions or *chancre* develops at the site of exposure and the time of early spread of the disease throughout the body, when a rash and other secondary lesions may appear and may persist for as long as two years. *Early latent syphilis* refers to the interval from two through four years when body defenses have not yet been fully mobilized and infectious exacerbations may occur. *Late latent syphilis* designates the disease after four years of infection when reappearance of infectious lesions is unlikely.

Persons who are untreated usually transmit the disease to others through sexual contact during the first three years of infection, although in rare instances it appears that lesions in latent syphilis may also be infectious. It is uncertain how long spirochetes can be carried in the seminal fluid, but there seems to be evidence that untreated persons have transmitted the disease during sexual intercourse as long as ten years after infection.[2] There is no evidence that an infection in the father can in any way affect an unborn child when the mother is not infected. Spirochetes may pass through the placental barrier to the fetal blood stream at or after the fourth month of fetal life. This transfer occurs in approximately one half of the instances in which treatment is not given to the expectant mother with active syphilis. Active syphilitic infection in the fetus leads to its death in many instances and to malformations of various kinds in many of the infants born alive.

Syphilis is almost always acquired through sexual contact. The spirochetes pass through minute breaks in the mucous membrane and skin, where they begin to multiply within an hour. Within three days the organisms have entered the blood stream and, at the end of the incubation period of about three weeks (ten days to ten weeks), the initial lesion or chancre appears. This lesion, a painless indurated ulcer, is usually found on the genital area but may appear on the lip, in the mouth, or on the nipple. It may develop on the wall of the vagina, on the cervix, or within the male urethra where it will be unobserved by the patient. Adjacent lymph nodes are almost always somewhat tender and enlarged, but these symptoms, together with malaise and headache, may not be recognized as more than a minor indisposition if the chancre is not evident.

While the chancre is present, the serologic blood test is negative because insufficient reagin has been produced to render it positive. The chancre is, however, teaming with live spirochetes, and fluid obtained from the lesion will reveal them easily under a dark-field microscope. It is unfortunate if the patient is given penicillin before this test is done, because this antibiotic causes disappearance of the spirochetes within twenty-four hours, and the opportunity to make a definite diagnosis by observation of the living organisms is thus lost. Diagnosis must then be made by means of the serologic test which must be delayed for a few weeks and is subject to the hazards of false negative reactions which will cloud the laboratory picture. The patient may then remain inadequately treated and develop complications of latent syphilis.

If not treated, the chancre heals within three to eight weeks. The *secondary* manifestations usually occur immediately after the healing of the chancre or about six weeks after the initial infection, although they may be delayed for months and may never appear as a distinct stage. A *rash* resembling that of almost any dermatitis may appear. *Mucous patches* (condyloma lata) may be present in the mouth and on the mucous membrane of the genital area and the perianal skin. These signs may be accompanied by headache, malaise, and sore throat. *Acute iritis* and *retinitis* sometimes occur as secondary metastatic manifestations of the disease, and occasionally there is patchy *loss of hair* (alopecia). The disease is highly infectious during the time when secondary manifestations are present. Lesions on the skin and mucous membrane contain large numbers of spirochetes which are readily transmitted to others, organisms are in the seminal fluid, and organisms are in the milk of lactating mothers. The serologic test will be positive. The secondary manifestations of early syphilis usually disappear after a few weeks even without treatment, although they have a tendency to recur at intervals.

The late stage of syphilis may be characterized by the development of *gummas* or cellular deposits in various parts of the body such as the bones, mucous membranes, skin, and organs. Gummas seldom contain live spirochetes but are disturbing because they tend to break down and form ulcers or abscesses which eventually heal spontaneously even when no treatment is given. In the late stage the disease is seldom infectious since the spirochetes have retreated to inaccessible places in the body as body defenses have been further mobilized. The serologic test is positive in untreated late syphilis.

During the chronic stage of syphilis, the heart and blood vessels are often affected. Lesions may develop in the heart muscle or valves, and aneurysms may occur in the large blood vessels, particularly in the aorta. Damage may occur to the central nervous system, causing optic atrophy, tabes dorsalis, and general paresis. There may be some racial differences in either vascular or central nervous system diseases, although both complications may occur in either the white or Negro race. The chronic manifestations may occur as early as a year or two after the initial infection, they may be delayed until as many as twenty years have elapsed, or they may never occur at all.

Treatment

Hospitalization is seldom necessary for those who have contracted syphilis. The disease is usually treated in the doctor's office, in the hospital clinic, or in community clinics or in homes of patients by doctors and public health nurses. The year 1943 was a revolutionary one in the treatment of syphilis. Before that time the treatment had been tedious and had required weekly injections of arsenicals and other "heavy metal" drugs for twelve to eighteen months and sometimes longer. In 1943 it was shown that penicillin was remarkably effective in treating early infectious and early latent syphilis. The ideal dosage and distribution of dosage has not been conclusively established, but 2,400,000 to 6,000,000 units of sodium penicillin are given in a period of one to three weeks, depending upon the stage of the disease. This effects a cure in 80 per cent of all patients with early syphilis.

Patients in whom diagnosis is made and treatment started in the early chancre stage never experience the signs and symptoms described for untreated syphilis. It is established almost beyond doubt that biologic cure can be effected by adequate treatment in the early stages of the disease. This means that all living spirochetes within the body are destroyed. Results of treatment have been difficult to analyze because reinfection is possible and is rather frequent in those treated for early infectious syphilis. Whether or not reinfection is possible in late latent syphilis and whether or not the disease is completely eradicated in this stage have not been determined. The blood and spinal fluid may remain negative for a long time and then become positive even when reinfection has not occurred, although this is exceedingly rare. Possibly the organisms are harbored somewhere in the body and released at intervals under certain conditions not yet understood.

Incidence, prevalence, social significance, and control

Syphilis is probably as old as civilization, although the country of its origin is debatable and uncertain. Hand in hand with civilization, it has gone to new lands and taken a heavy toll on peoples whose natural defenses were low. There is evidence that some host resistance is transmitted through generations, since the disease is not so virulent in western countries as it was centuries ago. Of course the decreased virulence of the organism may account for part of this. There is, however, no natural immunity, and no way to produce an artificial immunity has been found.

The incidence and prevalence of syphilis are high in the United States. Despite intense public interest after World War I, tremendous effort by the United States Public Health Service under Surgeon General Parran in 1936, and renewed interest with support from the federal government in 1947, our control of this disease is still woefully behind that of other enlightened nations. Public education, legislation, and easily available treatment without cost have made the control quite effective in some countries. In the United States, 4.89 per cent of the second million persons registered under the Selective Service Law in 1941 were infected with the disease.[15] This prevalence is probably higher than that for the population as a whole, since the incidence of syphilis is highest between the ages of 15 and 35.[5] It is believed that there are at least 500,000 infections coming to medical attention each year[5] and probably a large number of new infections occur that are not reported and are, therefore, not treated. The cost of syphilis is high despite the newer methods of treatment. It is estimated that the disease among veterans of World War II will cost 328 million dollars in the next twenty years.[15] Probably no disease costs more in peace of mind and in the effects of disruption of family life.

Syphilis has no respect for class or person. The prevalence is higher in the Negro than in the white population, but this is thought to be due to social rather than biologic causes. The disease is more common in men than in women, probably because of greater exposure. The incidence and prevalence of syphilis are increased by war and by frontier migration, both of which take young people away from their homes and lead to increased promiscuity. Since the disease is so often spread by casual sexual encounters, it increases in any situation in which promiscuity is common as, for example, in social and cultural groups in which mores do not require rigid adherence to monogamy and in adolescent groups in unfavorable home and community environments.

Syphilis is not simply an infectious disease caused by spirochetes that responds quickly to the administration of penicillin. It is caused by a social and emotional unhealthiness as well as by spirochetes. Therefore, it has not responded well to methods of mass control which have been effective in other aspects of public health such as typhoid control. The disease thrives among emotionally immature persons in poor environments. Incidence is high among young people from broken homes who seek affection, acceptance, love, and security in unsound sexual relationships. These young people attempt to justify or "prove" themselves or try to achieve acceptance by promiscuous sexual behavior. Its incidence is high among sexual deviates who are often lonely and out of the common stream of human contacts.

The public's attitude toward syphilis is a major obstacle in its control. Often the immediate assumption is that anyone who has the disease has been guilty of moral wrongdoing. The average person thinks of the method of exposure and not of the complex social and emotional climate that made the disease possible. Actually, syphilis may be contracted congenitally or by an innocent married partner. Fear of detection leads many persons to fail to report symptoms. Lack of education is another obstacle to control; many young people do not know the symptoms and do not know the dangers of failure to receive treatment. Complete ignorance of the fact that a person under treatment is not infectious leads employers to dismiss workers without reason. This seriously militates against efforts to have patients remain under treatment, since many of them are reluctant to ask for time off for treatment lest the nature of their medical problem be discovered.

Several practices in this country help in the detection and control of syphilis. Thirty-eight states now require that a serologic test for syphilis be made before a marriage license is issued (one state, Louisiana, requires only that men have this examination).[24] In some states the law requires that physicians order serologic tests for syphilis for all pregnant women under their care; all approved hospitals and almost all recognized physicians order a serologic test for all antenatal patients and for all persons who give blood for transfusion. Most hospitals require a serologic test for syphilis for all patients admitted for care, and these tests reveal a significant number of persons with the disease. Industrial health services usually incorporate multiphasic screening tests which almost always include the serologic test for syphilis.

The nurse's role

The nurse's responsibilities include assisting in programs for the prevention of the disease, case finding, assisting with education and treatment of those infected, interviewing patients for contacts, helping to secure medical care for contacts if this is necessary, and giving nursing care to patients who have not had adequate treatment and are in advanced stages of the disease.

Before the nurse can be effective in working with patients with syphilis, she must face her own emotional reactions squarely. The patient is often young, fearful of pain, and unaccustomed to his surroundings in the clinic or the doctor's office. Above all, he fears that his family and friends will learn of his predicament and that they will think less of him because of it. He must be certain that information he divulges will be kept in strict confidence, and he should be treated as a patient who has a medical problem and not as one who has sinned. In all contacts with patients who have syphilis, regardless of the circumstances that may unfold, the nurse must refrain from passing moral judgment. The nurse who is successful in working with these patients is the one who can create an atmosphere in which the patient feels free to discuss all aspects of the problem. This need not mean that the nurse accept the patient's standard of conduct for herself but that she show sincere professional concern. She is interested in whether or not the patient is under treatment and in teaching him why he should remain under medical care. Other concerns are who the contacts are, how they may be brought under treatment if necessary, and how the situation may be improved so that events such as those encountered are less likely to recur.

The patient should know that syphilis is a reportable disease and that he, as well as those whom he names as contacts (if they are shown to have the disease), must be reported to the department of health. He should know that numbers instead of names are used in public places such as clinic waiting rooms so there is little danger of others learning the nature of his disease unless he chooses to tell them. He should recognize the importance of reporting at intervals for checkups as recommended by his doctor because a few persons either are resistant to the drugs or have but slight resistance to the disease. Serologic tests, made at intervals as specified by the doctor, reveal whether or not a relapse of active infection has occurred.

The nurse should not only re-examine her own attitude toward the disease, but also make use of every opportunity to change the attitude of the public. Group meetings of citizens or patients, association with her less informed colleagues, and face-to-face relationships with patients all afford opportunities for this. All young people should know about the disease. In educational programs conducted in venereal disease clinics, patients themselves have stated that they wished they had known more about syphilis at an earlier age.[2] Since good family relationships are so important in preventing syphilis, the nurse should help parents to solve their own problems and to prepare their children to be good members of the family and of the community. Premarital counseling, including sex education, is important in the prevention of syphilis. The *Social Hygiene News,** a monthly publication, is helpful in keeping the nurse informed in the field of venereal disease. The dangers of reinfection by spirochetes should be stressed in all health teaching. The effectiveness of penicillin in treatment of syphilis has produced mixed results. It has been a boon in making treatment easier, cheaper, safer, and more convenient and in rendering the patient noninfectious much more quickly than with any other treatment. On the other hand, according to some authorities, treatment has become so simple that patients tend to take the disease too lightly, to believe that they are immune to reinfection, or to believe that they need not worry about reinfection since they can again be easily cured. The incidence of reinfection in patients treated early is quite high, again demonstrating that not only must the spirochete be killed but also that the causes of promiscuity must be controlled if the disease is to disappear. The nurse should participate in community activities which are designed to improve environment for young people. For example, better recreational opportunities for teen-agers tend to lessen sexual promiscuity and thus aid in the prevention of syphilis.

Contact investigation. The nurse often interviews the patient and reviews with him his understanding of the disease. Her success in obtaining the names of contacts and in securing the patient's confidence and cooperation in treatment depends largely on her objectivity, her sincerity, and her discretion. (See Figure 25.) With the appropriate outlook and attitude she is often surprisingly successful in getting information that is difficult for the patient to impart to anyone. If the nurse is to win the patient's confidence, she must make him feel that she is concerned about the disease and what it is doing to him as a person and to his associates. The patient should be given the opportunity to inform his contacts of the

*Published by the American Social Hygiene Association.

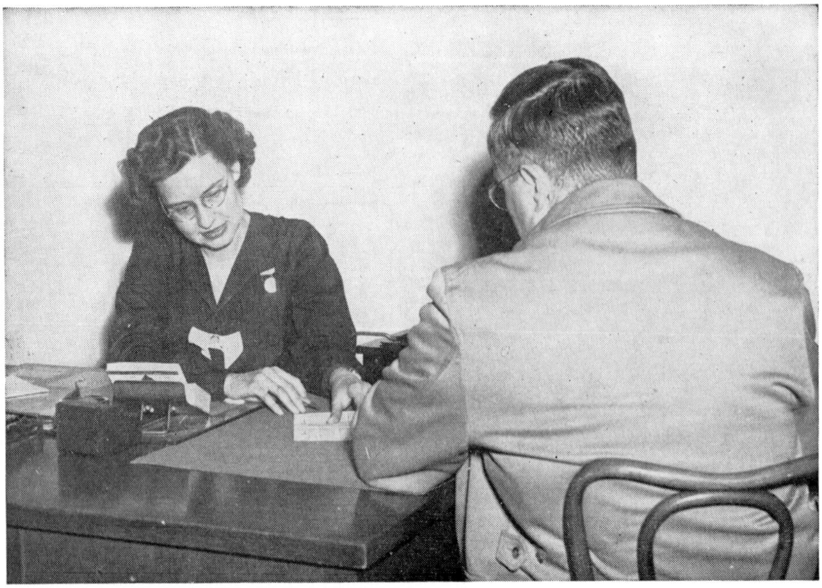

Figure 25

The nurse with a mature, sincere, and objective outlook is often surprisingly effective in obtaining needed information from the patient. (Courtesy Visiting Nurse Association of Plainfield and North Plainfield).

urgency to seek medical care voluntarily. Many situations in contact investigation become exceedingly complex and difficult (in the case, for instance, of a married patient who has contracted the disease extramaritally). Although the real burden of contact investigation in many clinics rests with the nurse, she may occasionally refer a patient to the social worker, to a community agency, back to his doctor, or to his spiritual adviser, depending upon the particular circumstances.

In contact investigation it is necessary to identify and bring under medical supervision all sexual contacts of the past three months if the patient has a primary lesion, all contacts for the past six months if secondary manifestations are evident, and all contacts for the past year if the patient is in the stage of latent syphilis.[7] In late latent syphilis effort is made to determine the contacts at the time the disease was probably acquired, since such persons may also be suffering from latent syphilis which should be treated in the hope of preventing cardiovascular, neurologic, and other late complications. In latent and congenital syphilis all members of the immediate family should be considered. It is not always necessary to examine the children of the patient, since the likelihood of congenital syphilis may already have been ruled out by routine blood tests done premaritally, upon induction to the armed services, or at the time of a hospital admission. Because the problem of syphilis is such a personal one, most clinics designate one nurse to handle phone calls and appointments for further information requested by the patient's contacts; this nurse's extension number is also given to the patient for distribution to his contacts in the event he notifies them first. Form letters and individual letters are sent out to those who fail to report to the clinic as arranged. Telegrams have been effectively used by some clinics and health departments. In the event that contacts fail to report or patients with infectious disease fail to report for follow-up, law requires that the names be submitted to the local health department which assumes the legal responsibility for the control of communicable disease.

Chronic disease. The nursing care of patients with chronic organic pathology from syphilis is similar to nursing in other conditions except that it is given within the framework of the patient's and his family's guilt about the original cause of his trouble. *Gastric* crisis is one late manifestation that is most distressing to the patient. He has severe abdominal pain and nausea and vomiting; the pathology is in the nervous system, not in the stomach. *Optic atrophy* is sometimes treated by fever therapy, usually induced by giving a foreign protein such as milk intramuscularly or by placing the patient in a fever cabinet. *General paresis* occurs when there has been extensive and permanent damage to the brain. Patients with this condition occupy a large number of beds in mental hospitals throughout the country; in 1944 there were 25,450 man years of hospitalization in mental institutions from this cause.[12] Fever therapy and the new drugs such as chlorpromazine are of some benefit in controlling violent behavior, but far more important than any kind of treatment is prevention of the original infection and early and complete treatment when it occurs.

GONORRHEA

Gonorrhea is a venereal disease that has been prevalent since ancient times. In the United States it is estimated that 1 million new reportable cases occur each year.[1] Many persons are infected several times during their lives since one attack does not confer immunity.

The initial symptom of gonorrhea is burning on urination, usually forty-eight hours after exposure. This is followed by a thick yellowish-green discharge from the urethra in men and women and from the vagina in women. Women may also complain of redness and tenderness of the labia and of the vaginal and urethral orifices. Pain on walking and on sitting is common. Diagnosis is made from the history of exposure by sexual contact and by identification of the gonococcus organism in the discharge.

The treatment of gonorrhea consists of the administration of 300,000 units of penicillin daily for three or four days as soon as diagnosis has been made. Usually cultures are taken from the urethra or the vagina daily, and the antibiotic is given until three negative cultures have been obtained. Since organisms can be harbored and cause reinfection, cultures are often taken weekly for three months; if the cultures are negative over this period of time, the patient is considered cured. If treatment with penicillin is begun within a day or two of the onset of symptoms, patients rarely develop the complications such as epididymitis and salpingitis which were common before the antibiotics were discovered.

In women the organism may lodge in Skene's glands on either side of the urethral meatus or in Bartholin's glands in the vulvovaginal region. It may then be necessary to dilate the urethra with sounds to facilitate drainage from areas where the organisms have become lodged. The formation of a *Bartholin's gland abscess* which must be incised and drained is not unusual in patients who have delayed seeking medical attention. It is important that the disease be successfully treated before the onset of the woman patient's next menstrual period because at this time the infection may ascend through the uterus to the fallopian tubes. This may lead to pelvic inflammatory disease, and salpingitis with subsequent sterility.

In men the gonococci may be harbored in the glans penis, causing a *balanitis* which may require surgical drainage and circumcision when the inflammation has subsided. Circumcision of male babies definitely decreases the possibility of local infection of the penis. Infection may travel up the reproductive and urinary tracts, causing urethral strictures, prostatitis, seminal vesiculitis, and epididymitis. The long tortuous path of the epididymus becomes bound down with adhesions, and the lumen of the duct becomes closed by strictures, resulting in sterility. If urethral strictures occur, the patient has difficulty in voiding and may require periodic dilation of the urethra with sounds; occasionally an external or internal urethrotomy or a plastic repair of the urethra is necessary (see Chapter 22).

The doctor emphasizes to the patient that sexual contact must be strictly avoided. Sexual stimulation should also be avoided, since it may produce congestion of blood in the area and increase the discomfort.

Patients with acute gonorrhea are rarely hospitalized. The nurse, however, is responsible for teaching the patient in the hospital clinic, in the doctor's office, and in the home. The patient must be taught to care for himself and to protect himself and others. Anything that comes in contact with discharge, such as bedclothes, washcloths, towels, and underclothing, must be used only by the patient, must be separated from other linen, and must be washed well with soap and hot water. The gonococcus, although it thrives in dark, moist, protected parts of the body, does not long survive sunshine, exposure, drying, and soap and water. The patient should wash his hands thoroughly each time he goes to the bathroom or otherwise contaminates his hands. Women patients usually wear a protective pad; they should not use tampons which may obstruct free flow of drainage. Men patients occasionally wear an athletic support to protect their clothing.

The greatest care must be taken to protect the eyes from infection. The mucous membrane of the eyes is particularly susceptible, and before the use of penicillin and the sulfonamide drugs, gonorrheal ophthalmia was the cause of much blindness. The patient must be cautioned to wash his hands thoroughly before washing his face and to wash his face under running water.

Very young girls are extremely susceptible to gonorrheal infection of the vagina; they should never be permitted to share the same bed with persons who have the disease and must be carefully protected from exposure when members of their family have gonorrhea.

The patient with gonorrhea should take large amounts of fluid by mouth. This helps to "wash out" the organisms and decreases irritation of concentrated urine on the inflamed tissues of the meatus and surrounding area. Hot douches may be ordered for their cleansing effect and to stimulate circulation and therefore stimulate healing. In giving a douche, the nurse usually wears gloves but the patient, giving her own, should be instructed to rely on careful handling of equipment and thorough washing of her hands. Sitz baths or warm tub baths twice a day or more often may also be ordered for their stimulating effect. The tub should be thoroughly cleansed with hot water and soap, and, if at all possible, should not be used by the rest of the family.

The patient must understand the importance of keeping his appointments for medical care. Unfortunately, gonorrhea occurs more commonly in those who are not always too responsible in their conduct. One of the difficulties in the management of this disease is due to its common occurrence among certain groups of people who almost take it for granted; getting the disease may even be considered a sign of manhood. The serious results of failure to secure treatment are not too well understood and the startling success in treatment of gonorrhea by chemotherapeutic and bacteriostatic agents has resulted in overconfidence of patients. Some of them have become careless about reporting a fresh exposure since they are so certain of cure when symptoms become troublesome for them. Complications sometimes develop while they are delaying treatment or are ignoring instructions to return to the doctor.

BRUCELLOSIS

Brucellosis is a disease caused by a gram-negative, rod-shaped bacillus which is widespread among animals. There are three strains which cause different diseases in animals, but the same disease in man: *Brucella melitensis*, which occurs primarily in goats; *Brucella abortus*, which causes contagious abortion in cattle (Bang's disease); and *Brucella suis*, which causes abortion in swine and cattle. The *Brucella suis* strain gives rise to the most virulent symptoms in man.[2] Other names for brucellosis are undulant fever and Malta fever.

In the late 1940's many cases of brucellosis were reported annually in the United States, and it is suspected that many remain undetected.[8] In the early 1950's the incidence of the disease dropped markedly as a result of an accelerated program to eradicate the disease in cattle. The organisms are carried in the tissues, blood, milk, urine, feces, and vaginal discharges of infected animals. Animals may appear well, yet continue to be carriers transmitting the disease for years to other animals or to human beings. Brucellosis is transmitted mainly through drinking unpasteurized milk containing the bacilli, handling infected meat and other animal products, and coming into contact with the organisms in the discharges of infected animals. The disease is found among food handlers, farmers, and veterinarians; farmers and veterinarians who assist at calving may easily become infected. In farming areas brucellosis occurs more often in men than in women, since it is usually the men who help with animal deliveries and who dispose of animal excreta. One report showed that 55 per cent of 1,086 slaughter house employees showed positive skin tests as evidence of past infection.[2] The causative organisms are resistant to prolonged exposure outside the body and have been shown to survive several months in animal feces and at least a month in cheese and other dairy products.[5] They are, however, sensitive to heat and are destroyed by pasteurization.

Brucellosis can be controlled and finally eradicated by careful pasteurization of milk and milk products, examination of all cows, swine, and goats and destruction of infected animals, immunization of calves between 6 and 12 months of age, examination of all animals sold by animal dealers, and education of those who handle meat products and who tend animals. In urban areas pasteurization has decreased the prevalence of the disease, but the disease is still widespread among rural and animal-handling populations and in places where unpasteurized milk is consumed.

The nurse working in a rural area has excellent opportunities to teach people the importance of pasteurizing milk products and otherwise protecting themselves from infection. In schools, children can learn of the danger of infection in handling farm animals, and this knowledge will often be communicated to their parents. Sometimes nurses may work through the local farm bureau or the grange to stimulate an educational program that will help to control the disease.

The organisms causing brucellosis gain entrance to the body through the skin and the alimentary tract, and sometimes are inhaled with dust. The incubation period varies from five to twenty-one days but is usually about ten days. Frequently the symptoms are not severe enough to lead to laboratory study and diagnosis; many people simply feel under par and may even be thought to be suffering entirely from emotional troubles or to be malingering.

The symptoms of brucellosis are malaise, headache, muscle aches, joint pains, backache, and fever which is usually higher in the afternoon. The patient may feel fairly well in the morning and then develop fever, muscle and joint pain, and profuse diaphoresis. Chills, cough, and marked depression and apathy can also be part of the clinical findings, although by far the most pronounced symptom is severe and unexplained fatigue upon the slightest exertion. In very severe infections there may be inflammation throughout the body, and a rash may occur. There is usually some enlargement of the liver and spleen, and in about 50 per cent of all patients the cervical lymph nodes become enlarged. Rare complications are encephalitis, meningitis, peripheral neuritis, and destructive suppurative arthritis.

Diagnosis of brucellosis is made by finding the organisms in the excreta of those suspected of having the disease and by an agglutination test of the blood. Usually blood cultures are also made. If untreated, the disease usually lasts from two to eight weeks, although it may persist for months or years. Eighty-five per cent of all patients recover within three months, and less than 20 per cent have the disease for over a year.[5] Treatment of brucellosis has been aided to some extent by the administration of antibiotics. Dihydrostreptomycin, 0.5 Gm. (7½ grains), may be given intramuscularly every twelve hours, accompanied by chlortetracycline (Aureomycin), 0.5 Gm., or oxytetracycline (Terramycin), 0.5 Gm., given orally every six hours.

Nursing care of the patient with acute brucellosis depends upon the severity of the infection and the symptoms present. There is no agreement as to whether disinfection of excreta is necessary. Precautions should be taken in the handling of all body discharges even though there is no evidence that the disease has ever been spread from a patient to a person giving him nursing care. The patient should be urged to take fluids. If diaphoresis is marked, frequent sponge baths are refreshing and add to the patient's comfort. An icecap is often greatly appreciated by the patient who has severe headache. Acetylsalicylic acid is often prescribed for the joint pains, and warmth provided by extra covering or a heating pad is helpful. If pain in the joints is severe, care should be taken to avoid jarring the bed and to avoid jerky movements in handling affected parts. The patient's mouth may need special care if the temperature is high and appetite is poor. The mouth should be rinsed after meals with a mild alkaline solution. If bleeding of the gums occurs, the doctor should be notified; hot saline solution rinses are often ordered.

Since brucellosis is a prolonged disease and often occurs in rural areas, it is likely that the patient will spend most of the time during his illness at home. The nurse may teach the family how to care for the patient while he is in the hospital for diagnosis or for treatment during the acute stage of illness, or she may be called upon to teach the family in the home. They should be taught to give the symptomatic care already described. It is important that they realize that depression and discouragement are due to the disease and are likely to occur when convalescence is prolonged. All practical measures that can be devised to keep the patient happily occupied are beneficial and should be used. Television and radio are helpful diversions, but it must be remembered that people need to do things with their hands as well as to watch others perform.

TRICHINOSIS

Trichinosis is one of the greatest uncontrolled public health problems of the present time since autopsy reports show that at least 16 per cent of the population of the United States is affected. No immunization is possible and no specific treatment is available, yet the disease could be eradicated with the knowledge that we now possess.[5] The disease is caused by the larvae of a species of roundworm, *Trichinella spiralis,* which become encysted in the striated muscles of man and hogs and other animals, particularly those (such as rodents) that consume infected pork in garbage. Trichinosis is transmitted through inadequately cooked food; pork is the most common source of infection. When infected food is eaten, live encysted larvae develop within the intestine of the host, mate, and produce eggs which hatch in the uterus of the female worm. The larvae are discharged in huge numbers (approximately 1,500 per worm) into the lymphatics and lacteals of the host's small intestine at the rate of about two an hour for about six weeks. They pass to the muscles of the host, where they become encysted by the reaction of the host's body and may remain for ten years or longer.

Signs and symptoms of trichinosis are varied. If a very large number of larvae have been ingested, nausea, vomiting, and diarrhea due to intestinal irritation usually occur about four days after the infected food has been eaten. On about the seventh day, when the larvae migrate throughout the body to the muscles, there are usually muscle stiffness, weakness, and remittent fever; the extent of these symptoms depends upon the number of larvae present and the resistance of the host. There may be pain in the back, the muscles of the eyeballs, the muscles of chewing, and elsewhere in the body; muscles of the diaphragm are often affected, causing pain on breathing. Although the reason is unknown, edema appears as puffiness about the eyes, particularly involving the upper lids. An increase in the eosinophil count is a characteristic finding in trichinosis and persists for several weeks after the onset of acute symptoms. In some small epidemics the mortality has varied from 5 to 30 per cent;[5] death usually occurs from pneumonia or cachexia from four to six weeks following the onset of symptoms.

The incidence and prevalence of trichinosis are higher in the United States than in any other country in the world. Swine are the commonest source of the infection. Trichinosis is common on the east coast of the United States, where hogs are fed uncooked garbage. In the middle west, where hogs are fed mostly on grain, the infection is much less common. Only about 70 per cent of the pork in this country is processed in plants that are under close supervision, and it is known that at least 10 per cent of the sausage sold in large city markets is infected.[5] The larvae do not form cysts in pork and therefore are not visible to the naked eye and are not noticed by food inspectors.

Basic scientific facts necessary for the complete prevention of the disease in human beings have been known for years. Trichinae can be killed by cooking and freezing; they are not killed by smoking, pickling, or other methods of processing. Sausage and other infected pork products carelessly prepared in eating places are a common source of infection in man. The nurse has an important responsibility to teach the need for thorough cooking of all pork products consumed at home regardless of how sanitary the local meat market may appear to be. A safe rule to follow is never, under any circumstances, to eat pork products in a restaurant—only at home, where adequate cooking can be assured.

RABIES

Rabies is a fatal acute infectious disease caused by a filtrable virus which travels along nerve pathways to the brain. The disease has been known for centuries. In the twentieth century B.C. the Eshnunna code of ancient Mesopotamia set forth strict regulations about the obligations of dog owners who let mad dogs bite others, thereby causing death.[14] Rabies is most commonly acquired from dogs, but it can be carried by any animal that nurses its young; in the United States it is fairly common in dogs, cats, rats, cows, skunks, foxes, and even bats. The economic loss from rabies among cows is significant, even though the cow is not a common source of the disease in man.

Infection always occurs through an open break in the skin and usually through the bite of an animal. Clothing gives some protection, since the animal's teeth are wiped by the garments. For details of the first-aid treatment see Chapter 15. The saliva is infectious for several days before the onset of symptoms in the affected animal, so it is exceedingly important that all suspected animals be caught and kept under inspection for ten days. If the animal must be killed for the protection of others, the brain should not be damaged and must be sent to a laboratory for examination. The presence of Negri bodies in the brain of an animal is conclusive evidence of rabies.

Acute rabies can be prevented in man by the *Pasteur treatment.* Some persons who are exposed will not contract the disease; however, since if it develops the disease is always fatal, the treatment is always given if the offending animal is known or suspected to have rabies. If bites have been sustained about the head, the injections will most likely be started at once, since the incubation period seems to be shorter than when the bite is on other parts of the body. Antirabies treatment is usually given if the animal has escaped and is suspected of having rabies.

The Pasteur treatment, which is painful and expensive, consists of fourteen to twenty-one injections of antirabies vaccine given daily. These injections may cause severe local reaction, and sometimes evoke serious and even fatal complications. This happens often enough to make rigid control of wandering animals imperative. Furthermore, since a series of injections of antirabies vaccine gives protection for a maximum of only six months, a child might have to have more than one series in a year. It is recommended that two additional injections be given if a questionable bite is received later than three months after a series of injections has been given. If six months has elapsed since the Pasteur treatment was given, the complete series must be repeated.[22] Passive immunization is now attempted by giving hyperimmune antiserum. To be effective, this must be given within seventy-two hours of exposure to the disease and is usually given in combination with the vaccine.

The control of rabies is a public health problem. The police and health departments must be notified at once if a rabid animal is thought to be at large. In England and the Scandinavian countries the disease has been almost entirely eliminated by rigid enforcement of laws controlling dogs running about unleashed. Rabies could be controlled by compulsory vaccination of all dogs and cats kept as household pets, capture and confinement of stray animals, and destruction of wild animal reservoirs under the supervision of wildlife experts. Annual vaccination of all dogs is required in some states and counties; recent improvements in the vaccine have resulted in the decision in one state (New York) to permit dogs to run loose twenty-one days after inoculation, whereas prior to this, thirty days was required. How long the immunity lasts following vaccination is not known for certain; immunization in man is thought to last about a year and in animals up to thirty-nine months.

The public should know that not all rabies-infected animals are "mad." There are two types of rabies. In one type the animal may be restless, barking, and biting. In the other so-called "dumb" rabies, the animal may be quiet and stay close to its master. In the latter type, paralysis which begins in the throat and lower jaw may lead the animal's owner to suspect that something harmful has been swallowed. In his efforts to investigate the trouble, he may get the highly infectious saliva into an abrasion on his hand.

Another name for rabies is *hydrophobia*. The incubation period of the disease in man is from ten days to more than a year.[4] The involvement, as in animals, is in the central nervous system. The disease is ushered in with a few days of melancholia, depression, pain at the site of the animal bite, and a feeling of impending danger. Acute symptoms—difficulty in swallowing, excessive salivation, muscle spasm, often maniacal fear, difficulty in breathing, and convulsions—then appear. A terrific, painful spasm of the muscles of deglutition occurs when there is an attempt to swallow water, hence the name hydrophobia; even the mention of water is often enough to bring on an attack. Aerophobia is also present, and convulsions can be produced by a draft of air on the skin. Occasionally acute bulbar poliomyelitis is confused with rabies.

The nursing care of the patient with acute rabies is difficult but of short duration. Most patients die from heart failure or respiratory difficulty within three or four days of the acute onset of symptoms. The patient is restless, irritable, and fearful, with episodes of uncontrolled fear and mania alternating with periods of calm. Every effort is made to keep the patient quiet; the room is darkened, and noises in the halls outside the room should be eliminated. Side rails are placed on the bed, and sometimes these are padded to help prevent injury during episodes of uncontrolled thrashing about. Sedatives, including chloral hydrate, morphine, and the barbiturates, are given. Magnesium sulfate may be given intramuscularly to help produce relaxation, and anesthetics may be given intravenously. Fluids may be given intravenously, and it is important to bandage the arm securely on a board to prevent injury in the event of a convulsion or an attack of mania while a needle is in the vein. The head of the bed is sometimes lowered in an attempt to facilitate drainage of saliva, and often suctioning must be used. The nurse should wear gloves when giving immediate care, and some authorities believe that doctors and nurses caring for a patient with rabies should receive antirabies serum. Relatives of the patient must be prepared for the fact that the patient cannot talk. Sometimes the visits of relatives bring on severe painful muscle spasm in the throat of the patient who is usually conscious up to the time of death, even though he is unable to speak.

INFECTIOUS MONONUCLEOSIS

Infectious mononucleosis is a disease probably caused by a virus, although this has not been conclusively proved. It is more common in younger persons, the largest number of cases occurring in those between 20 and 30 years of age. It is sometimes more or less epidemic among closely associated groups and also may be sporadic in its appearance; hospital personnel seem to be the most often affected by the disease. The infection is thought to be transmitted from one person to another by means of the secretions of the nose and throat, although repeated efforts to transmit it to man in this fashion have failed; symptoms presumably appear five to fifteen days following exposure.

Signs and symptoms of infectious mononucleosis are many and varied. By and large, it is a benign disease with a good prognosis. Malaise is the most frequent complaint and is often accompanied by elevation of temperature, headache, sore throat, increased nasal secretions, aches and pains resembling those of influenza, and moderate enlargement of the liver and spleen. On some occasions jaundice, rupture of the spleen, encephalitis, and even death have occurred. Diagnosis can be conclusively established by means of a test of the blood—the heterophil agglutination test. This test, developed in 1932, makes use of the fact that a certain substance is present in the patient's blood which causes clumping or agglutination of the washed erythrocytes (antigen) of another animal (in this case, sheep cells are used). The test is almost always positive at the end of a week of illness. Another conclusive laboratory finding is a marked increase in mononuclear leukocytes, which leads to the name of the disease. At the height of the disease, the white blood count usually ranges between 10,000 and 20,000 cells per cubic milliliter of blood. So far, no modern antibiotic is effective in treating infectious mononucleosis, and no immunization is available.

Nursing care of the patient with infectious mononucleosis is purely symptomatic. If sore throat is severe, hot gargles may be ordered and glucose solutions often give greater relief than saline solution. Liquid and soft foods may have to constitute the patient's entire menu. An icecap may be helpful if headache is severe. Acetylsalicylic acid is usually given for headache and generalized discomfort, and the patient is encouraged to remain in bed; if he is allowed to be up, he is advised to stay indoors and engage in little activity. The disease usually disappears within two weeks, but it may continue in a chronic form for several weeks and even months. Relapses do occur, and this explains the need for rest at the time of acute illness even though the patient does not feel ill and resents the time spent away from his work or regular activities.

REFERENCES AND SELECTED READINGS*

1 *Albert Neisser and the Gonococcus, Am. J. Pub. Health **45**:95-97, Jan. 1955.
2 Anderson, Gaylord W., and Arnstein, Margaret G.: Communicable Disease Control, ed. 2, New York, 1950, The Macmillan Co.
3 *Busse, Geraldine: Promiscuity and Venereal Disease, Nursing Outlook **4**:223-225, April 1956.
4 *Carroll, Dorothy L.: Problems in Acute Communicable Disease Control, Nursing Outlook **2**:593-595, Nov. 1954.
5 Cecil, Russell L., and Loeb, Robert F. (editors): A Textbook of Medicine, ed. 10, Philadelphia, 1959, W. B. Saunders Co.
6 *Chatman, Frances Patterson: Serving Patients With Veneral Disease, Pub. Health Nursing **44**:92-95, Feb. 1952.
7 Control of Communicable Disease in Man, ed. 8, New York, 1955, The American Public Health Association.
8 *Cromwell, Gertrude E.: The Teenager and Venereal Disease, Am. J. Nursing **59**:1738-1739, Dec. 1959.
9 Donohue, James F., and others.: Venereal Disease Among Teenagers, Pub. Health Rep. **70**:453-461, May 1955.
10 DuBos, René J.: Bacterial and Mycotic Infections of Man, ed. 3, Philadelphia, 1958, J. B. Lippincott Co.
11 Evans, A. C.: Brucellosis in the United States, Am. J. Pub. Health **37**:139-151, Feb. 1947.
12 Facts About Syphilis, 1952, Federal Security Agency, The United States Public Health Service.

*References preceded by an asterisk indicate material particularly well suited for student reading.

13 *Getting, Vlado A.: Food-Borne Diseases, Nursing Outlook **2**:354-366, July 1954.
14 Harrison, T. R., and others (editors): Principles of Internal Medicine, ed. 2, New York, 1954, The Blakiston Co.
15 Lynch, Theresa I.: Communicable Disease Nursing, ed. 2, St. Louis, 1949, The C. V. Mosby Co.
16 Modell, Walter, and Schwartz, Doris R.: Handbook of Cardiology for Nurses, ed. 2, New York, 1954, Springer Publishing Co., Inc.
17 Parrino, Paul S., O'Shaughnessy, Edward J., and White, John D.: Standardization of Diagnostic Methods for Gonococcal Infections, Am. J. Pub. Health **45**:457-463, April 1955.
18 Rivers, Thomas M., and Horsfall, Frank L.: Viral and Rickettsial Infections of Man, ed. 3, Philadelphia, 1959, J. B. Lippincott Co.
19 *Roueché, Berton: Eleven Blue Men, New York, 1953, Berkley Publishing Corp.
20 *Smith, Carl H.: Infectious Mononucleosis, Am. J. Nursing **56**:776-777, June 1956.
21 Social Hygiene Committee, New York Tuberculosis and Health Association: The Epidemiology of Syphilis, Am. J. Med. **5**:655-669, Nov. 1948.
22 *Steele, James H., and Carroll, Dorothy L.: Animal Diseases Transmissible to Man, Nursing Outlook **4**:156-161, March 1956.
23 *Steele, James H., and Lester, Mary R.: Rabies and Rabies Control, Am. J. Nursing **58**:531-536, April 1958.
24 World Almanac and Book of Facts for 1960, New York, 1960, New York World-Telegram and the Sun.

Study questions for review

1 Diagram the main chambers of the heart and the adjacent blood vessels. Trace the flow of blood through these structures, and review the normal physiology of the cardiovascular system.
2 What drugs improve, regulate, or stimulate heart action? How are these administered?
3 What is the normal daily intake of sodium chloride? What common foods are high in salt content?
4 Review the nursing care needed by a patient receiving oxygen.

The patient with cardiac disease

Chapter 18

Diseases of the heart have become the leading cause of death in the United States.[32] It is estimated that heart disease was responsible for 38.4 per cent of all deaths in the United States in 1957.[23] More than 10 million persons in this country are known to have some form of cardiovascular-renal disease, and undoubtedly there are many more with undiagnosed cardiovascular disease.[37] Although there are over twenty different kinds of diseases of the heart and circulatory system, the most common are hypertensive, coronary, and rheumatic heart disease. Hypertensive and coronary heart disease usually occur in persons over 40 years of age, while rheumatic heart disease occurs in children and in young adults. The increase in cardiac disease is attributed in part to a reduction in premature deaths from diseases such as tuberculosis and the communicable diseases of childhood. Control of communicable disease has caused an increase in the population and an increase in the number of elderly people. Of the 578,270 who died from heart disease in 1955, one third were men and women over 75 years of age.[32]

PREVENTION

Although at this time a "cure" is not usually possible for patients with heart disease, heart disease can be prevented from developing in many persons, and many of those who have heart disease can be helped to live happy, useful, and long lives. Immunization against many of the acute infectious diseases, such as diphtheria and scarlet fever, and successful treatment of other infections with antibiotics have lowered the incidence of infectious complications such as pericarditis, endocarditis, and myocarditis. Early case finding and treatment of syphilis have helped to decrease the incidence of syphilitic aortitis. State health departments now provide physicians with gamma globulin for women who are exposed to German measles in the first trimester of pregnancy in an effort to prevent congenital heart disease or other malformation of their babies. The incidence of rheumatic heart disease is being markedly decreased by concentrated educational and prophylactic programs. Through the joint efforts of local heart associations and local health departments, penicillin for prophylactic use has been made available at a cost within the means of families who have children with rheumatic heart disease. Prevention of streptococcal infections seems to decrease the recurrences of rheumatic infections. By working closely with the parents of children with rheumatic disease, public health nurses help them to care for the children and encourage them to cooperate with medical follow-up and with long-term programs for prevention of recurrences. Since streptococcal infections are frequently complicated by rheumatic fever and inflammatory heart conditions, educational programs stressing the importance of early and adequate treatment of these infections have been aimed at the medical professions and the general public. Since dental extractions and surgery may activate a bacterial infection in the heart, efforts have been made by dentists and surgeons to prevent bacterial endocarditis in persons with known valvular and congenital heart disease. Antibiotics are usually given prophylactically both before and following surgery.

The informed nurse can play an important role in public education concerning heart disease, in the prevention of heart diseases, and in case finding. She is often in a position to give advice that may prevent cardiac complications. For instance, she should impress upon parents the importance of seeking medical care for children with diseased tonsils and carious teeth; she can advise parents to have children immunized against infectious diseases; she can encourage people with infectious disease to stay in bed and to have medical care. She, herself, should set an example of good hygienic practices by avoiding overwork, undue mental strain, obesity, and lowered resistance due to poor dietary habits, lack of rest, and irregular patterns of living.

A fatalistic attitude about heart disease and a conviction that nothing can be done about heart attacks, which "just happen," prevent many persons from reporting early signs of heart disease to their physicians. Since early medical treatment could often prevent or delay progress of the condition, this is doubly unfortunate. Nurses can help to prevent the development of serious heart disease by teaching the public the early signs of possible heart disease and by urging prompt referral to physicians when these occur. For example, attacks of shortness of breath or unexpected dyspnea on exertion, feeling of pressure in the chest, awakening in the night with consciousness of heart action or discomfort, and discomfort resembling indigestion that is relieved by sitting up are reasons to see a doctor even though the cause may be found to be trivial. Most persons have read magazine articles about anginal attacks with pain. They should be taught that pain is *not* a common sign of coronary artery disease; dyspnea and signs of cardiac decompensation are much more often found.[31] Many elderly persons hesitate to report symptoms because they believe that nothing can be done for them because of their age. Again this is very seldom true. A friendly interest on the part of the nurse and her assurance that medical care can be helpful will often lead them to seek medical treatment.

Research in prevention

Although the causes of many types of heart disease are not yet known, extensive epidemiologic studies and research are being carried on currently in an attempt to determine preventive measures. Organizations such as the American Heart Association are financing research to uncover further information on the causes of heart diseases and to develop new methods for its treatment. As part of the National Institutes of Health, supported by the federal government and under the United States Public Health Service, the National Heart Institute is conducting an intensive study on the cause, control, and treatment of heart disease. Vital statistics are being carefully studied in an attempt to discover whether such factors as sex, occupation, constitutional make-up, ethnologic background, or dietary patterns are associated with certain types of heart disease. Grants have been made to study the effects of new drugs on the heart, to perfect techniques which will make cardiac surgery possible for more patients, and to study the mechanisms by which heart diseases affect the tissues.

Overcoming fear

Fear is one of the biggest problems to be met in educating the public on heart diseases. Although 40 per cent of those who have heart attacks recover almost completely, and another 25 per cent are able to live relatively normal lives;[35] fear of another attack prevents many persons from ever again becoming useful members of society. Others cannot find work because employers are afraid to hire them. Heart associations, health departments, and insurance companies spend large sums of money each year for educational publications on heart disease in an attempt to overcome this problem.

The nurse needs to overcome any fear of heart disease that she may have before she can be effective in caring for patients during acute heart attacks, in assisting with the rehabilitation of cardiac patients, in helping families to care for elderly patients with chronic heart disease, and in assisting with the prevention and control of heart diseases. She should know the signs and symptoms of heart diseases and the kind of emergency care to give. In working with patients and their families, she should not only gain their cooperation in following medical advice, but she should also help both the patient and his family develop a "matter-of-fact" attitude toward his condition so that they can lead a relatively normal life.

DIAGNOSTIC PROCEDURES

Routine procedures

Heart diseases are diagnosed by the clinical signs and symptoms. Although the patient may undergo various procedures (laboratory tests and x-ray examination), these are mainly helpful in confirming the diagnosis, determining the course of the disease, indicating complications, showing residual effects, and predicting the results of treatment. The nurse can help in the diagnosis by carefully observing and recording signs and symptoms as she works with the patient. The character, as well as the rate, of the *pulse* is important. The pulse may be markedly irregular, or there may be a regular irregularity that recurs in the same patterns. The pulse may be abnormally rapid or unusually slow. The heartbeat and the radial pulse may not be the same, since sometimes the heart beats ineffectually and little blood is pushed out into the arteries. The *respirations* may be labored, and this difficulty may be increased by certain positions or activities. The patient may have *pain* in his arms, chest, neck, shoulders, or epigastrium. It is important for the doctor to know the location and type of pain, as well as the activity which caused it. The patient's *color* and its relationship to activity, position, dyspnea, and pain should be observed. The presence of *edema* of the tissues and increase or decrease of edema related to activity, position, or fluid and salt intake should be recorded. Many of these signs and symptoms are subtle and will be missed if one is not looking especially for them.

In addition, the nurse helps to prepare the patient for special examinations and laboratory tests by explaining what will be done and why it must be done. This helps to decrease the anxiety and fear which can impede the recovery of a patient with heart disease. The nurse also may assist with some of the procedures.

Blood count. A complete blood count is made on all patients with heart disease. In bacterial endocarditis an anemia persists as long as inflammation is active; the blood count, therefore, guides the doctor in determining when the patient's physical activity can be increased. The red blood cell count and the hemoglobin level are carefully observed in patients with heart disease that involves intracardiac shunts, for such observations enable the doctor to determine how well the blood is being oxygenated. Adequate oxygenation of the blood is a major problem in cardiac disease. If there has been a myocardial infarction, which causes death of a portion of the heart muscle, the white blood cell count is usually elevated since necrotic tissue anywhere in the body will cause leukocytosis.

Blood sedimentation rate. A determination of the blood sedimentation rate is ordered for many patients with heart disease. It is used to follow the course of acute rheumatic heart disease, infectious disease of the heart, and acute myocardial infarction. Since the sedimentation rate is elevated during the acute phase of an inflammatory process and gradually falls to normal as the infection abates, it is useful to the doctor in determining when physical activity can be increased following acute infections.

Prothrombin time determination. A prothrombin time determination is a blood test which indicates the ability of the blood to form intravascular clots. This test may be done routinely on all patients with heart disease, especially if there is reason to believe that blood clots may form within the blood vessels or the chambers of the heart. Patients who are being given Dicumarol to prevent intravascular blood clotting must have daily prothrombin time determinations to determine how much of the drug should be given each day. It is the nurse's responsibility to see that the blood is drawn and sent to the laboratory. Patients who are on maintenance doses of Dicumarol may have prothrombin time determinations made at longer intervals.

Blood urea nitrogen test. A blood urea nitrogen test, used to determine kidney function, is usually made to determine whether kidney function is disturbed as a result of impaired cardiac output or is due to other causes.

Urinalysis. A urinalysis is made to learn if there is albuminuria. Albuminuria may occur in patients with heart failure and in those whose heart disease is complicated by kidney damage. It often is present in patients with hypertension and shows that stress is being placed upon the kidneys.

Transaminase test. A transaminase (serum glutamic oxaloacetic transaminase) test is helpful in diagnosing acute myocardial infarctions, especially when the results of other tests such as the electrocardiogram are inconclusive. The transaminase level of the blood serum rises within twenty-four hours after an acute myocardial infarction and falls to normal by the sixth day. The number of transaminase enzymes in the blood serum is also increased in diseases of the liver and skeletal muscles.

Electrocardiogram. An electrocardiogram (ECG or EKG) is a record of the electric activity of the heart muscle. On the electrocardiogram, certain drugs such as digitalis and quinidine produce changes similar to those seen in disease; therefore, if the patient is receiving such a drug, the electrocardiologist should be informed of this.

Three or more electrodes or leads are placed against the patient's skin on the extremities and the thorax and then connected by wires to a recording galvanometer. They are usually placed on both forearms and on one or both lower legs and over the precordial area, but many variations may be ordered. A special electrode jelly is rubbed onto the skin over which the lead, a small strip of metal, is strapped. The patient lies down or sits reclining while the electrocardiogram is made, and he should be relaxed. If it is his first EKG, an explanation of the procedure should be given. If the patient is hospitalized, a technician usually comes to the bedside to do this procedure. The recording machine may be brought to the bedside, but in some institutions the wires are plugged into special wall outlets, and the recording is taken by remote control. The patient may be assured that he will feel no sensation during this examination and that he is in no danger of receiving an electric shock. Many patients fear electric shock when they see the equipment to be used.

The electrocardiogram is used to identify types of myocardial damage and to determine the mechanism of rhythmic disturbances of the heart. Since the rhythm may be normal even in the presence of serious heart disease, a single electrocardiogram often is not significant, and repeated tracings may be necessary before evidence of disease can be detected. Electrocardiograms may also be done at intervals to follow the course of disease. These repeated examinations may be upsetting to the patient who does not understand why so many must be made.

Roentgenogram of the chest. A roentgenogram of the chest may be taken to determine the size and shape of the heart and the aorta. Calcifications in the pericardium, heart muscle, valves, or large blood vessels also can be visualized in such an x-ray film, which is sometimes called a *cardiovascular film.*

Special tests

Special procedures and tests may be ordered to gain additional information concerning certain heart diseases. If known infection is present or if the patient has a transient fever of unknown origin, a *blood culture* is usually made to determine the causative organism and the antibiotic that will be most effective in treating it. The doctor frequently orders multiple blood cultures for patients who have suspected endocarditis. The most scrupulous attention to aseptic technique must be observed in any procedure in which a blood vessel is entered. The nurse has a major responsibility for this as she prepares equipment and assists during the procedure. Some procedures may be done, for example, in the x-ray department, where the nurse and the doctor are the team members most aware of the aseptic precautions that are necessary.

Venous pressure. Venous pressure is the pressure exerted by the circulating blood against the venous walls. It is elevated in congestive heart failure, in acute or chronic constrictive pericarditis, and in venous obstruction caused by a clot in a vein or external pressure against a vein such as occurs when the juglar vein is manually compressed. The normal venous pressure ranges from 6 to 12 cm. of water. To test it, the following equipment is necessary: a 10 ml. syringe, a No. 19 needle, a manometer, a three-way stopcock, sterile normal saline solution, a tourniquet, a solution such as benzalkonium chloride, and sponges to cleanse the skin. The patient lies or sits so that his arm is supported at a level with his heart. He may be flat in bed with the arm outstretched on the bed, or, if he must remain in a sitting position, the arm can be supported slightly below shoulder level with pillows. A stopcock is attached to the hub of the syringe and, with the needle attached to one side of the stopcock, 5 ml. of sterile normal saline solution are drawn into the syringe. The doctor then does a venipuncture drawing 2 or 3 ml. of blood into the syringe. The manometer is attached to the other side of the stopcock, the tourniquet is released from the arm, the blood and saline mixture is run into the manometer, and then the stopcock to the vein is opened. The pressure is recorded when the level of the fluid stabilizes in the manometer. The nurse assists by encouraging the patient, placing and holding the manometer, and recording the readings. It is important that the patient be relaxed.

Circulation time determination. Circulation time is a test used to determine the amount of time it takes a patient to taste a substance, such as Decholin, injected intravenously. The normal arm-to-tongue time is 15 seconds or less. Circulation time is prolonged in congestive heart failure. To do this test, the following equipment is necessary: a stop watch, a sterile 5 ml. syringe, a No. 19 needle, a tourniquet, an ampule of Decholin, sucrose or calcium chloride, a solution such as benzalkonium chloride, and sponges to cleanse the skin. The nurse should carefully explain to the patient his part in this test, and she may be asked to record the time interval between the injection of the drug and the time that the patient tastes it. Special variations on this test are used occasionally.

Angiocardiogram. An angiocardiogram is a roentgenogram of the heart and its vessels made after the intravenous injection of a radiopaque medium such as Urokon. It outlines the chambers of the heart and the large blood vessels. The meal preceding the x-ray procedure is omitted, and the patient is given a sedative such as phenobarbital sodium about one-half hour before going to the x-ray department. The sedative helps to alleviate apprehension. After injecting a local anesthetic, the doctor makes a skin incision over the antecubital vein and then inserts a No. 19 needle, attached to a syringe, into the vein. The dye is forced rapidly into the vein, and a series of roentgenograms are taken as the solution flows through the heart, pulmonary vessels, and aorta.

Some patients are sensitive to drugs containing iodine, such as Urokon and Diodrast. Nausea is a frequent untoward reaction, and urticaria, dyspnea, or severe anaphylactic reaction may occur. If the patient has a history of asthma or other allergic reactions, this test is seldom done. Any systemic reaction to the drug usually occurs immediately, and antihistaminic drugs such as Pyribenzamine, Adrenalin, and oxygen should be readily available.

Leakage of the dye outside the vein may cause irritation and sloughing of tissue. Thrombosis of the vein at the site of the injection may occasionally occur. When the patient returns from the x-ray department, the incision should be checked for bleeding and irritation. The vein will be tender, and the patient may have difficulty bending his arm; he should be reassured that this is temporary and will probably disappear within twenty-four hours. If irritation or thrombosis of the vein occurs, warm sterile compresses are usually ordered.

Cardiac catheterization. Cardiac catheterization is done especially when congenital heart disease is suspected. Blood samples and blood pressure readings are taken, electrocardiographic studies are done, and roentgenograms of the right heart chambers and the pulmonary arterial circulation are made. The doctor who obtains the patient's written permission should explain the procedure to him. The nurse should reinforce this explanation as necessary, and she must know what the doctor tells the patient since often the latter is not told exactly what will be done lest he become unduly anxious. Even with careful explanation most patients are apprehensive. The meal prior to the procedure is withheld, and about one-half hour before the patient is scheduled for the procedure he is given a sedative such as phenobarbital sodium. It is preferable that he not be given drugs such as morphine sulfate that will slow down heart action. Young children usually are given a general anesthetic for this examination. Local anesthetic is injected over the vein to be used, and a cut-down similar to that for an angiocardiogram is done, usually using the antecubital vein. A sterile x-ray-opaque catheter similar to a ureteral catheter, but 100 to 125 cm. in length, is passed into the incision in the vein and through the vein into the superior vena cava, through the right auricle and the right ventricle, and into the pulmonary artery. The course of the catheter is followed by fluoroscopy, and roentgenograms may be taken at any point. A continuous electrocardiogram is made. As the catheter is passed through the various vessels and cardiac chambers, samples of blood are taken to study the oxygen content, and blood pressures are recorded. When there is an interauricular septal defect, the oxygen content is higher in the blood of the right atrium than in the superior or inferior vena cava. In certain heart conditions, such as pulmonary or mitral stenosis, the pressure readings within the heart may be elevated three to four times above normal.

The patient has no pain during a cardiac catheterization, but he usually is extremely alert and anxious. He may feel the passage of the catheter, and he may complain of a feeling of warmth and of a fluttering sensation around the heart. He also may have a tendency to cough as the catheter is passed up the pulmonary artery. When he returns from the special x-ray room, he is usually quite exhausted and needs rest since the procedure takes from one to three hours. He may resume his regular activity as soon as he desires, but his pulse is usually taken every fifteen minutes for one hour and then every half hour for three hours. Tachycardia or arrhythmia should be reported to the doctor. The temperature may be slightly elevated for four to six hours after the procedure, and the patient may complain of some discomfort at the site of the cutdown. It should be checked at hourly intervals for several hours to note any bleeding or inflammation. If a local thrombophlebitis occurs, it is treated with warm moist compresses. Fluids should be given freely, and the doctor usually orders an antibiotic before and for several days after cardiac catheterization to prevent the complication of infection.

Although the risk during cardiac catheterization is slight, patients often speak apprehensively of it even after it is done. Memory of the experience often is vivid, and they can describe in detail what was done. This may be due to the amount and size of the equipment that is used, the number of personnel needed to do the procedure, fear of the catheter and its placement in the blood vessels and heart, the anticipation of something going wrong, and thoughtless discussion by those performing the procedure. The patient should be allowed to talk about his reactions since this may help to relieve his preoccupation with them.

Ballistocardiogram. When a ballistocardiogram is ordered, the patient is placed on a special table which is so delicately balanced that any vibration of the body, caused by the systolic ejection of blood from the heart into the aorta and pulmonary arteries, can be recorded by a machine attached to the table. There is no special preparation for this test. The patient simply lies quietly on the table. He may be aware of the vibrations and may be startled by them. This is a relatively new examination which is thought to be more sensitive in some instances than an electrocardiogram but which gives a very different kind of information.

CLASSIFICATION OF HEART DISEASES

Heart diseases are often classified as those caused by etiologic factors, such as rheumatic fever, bacterial endocarditis, pericarditis, myocarditis, and hypertension; those caused by anatomic change, such as valvular scarring and congenital anomalies of the heart; and those caused by physiologic change, such as heart failure and the arrhythmias. Heart failure and some types of arrhythmias occur as complications of many kinds of heart disease which damage tissue and thus prevent normal function of the heart. Systemic infection either is or has been present in patients with inflammation (pericarditis, myocarditis, or endocarditis) of any of the heart structures. This inflammation may lead to scarring of the heart structures and may cause serious residual problems, such as scarring of the heart valves following endocarditis, with resultant cardiac insufficiency. Whenever the valves are unable to open or close completely, the heart, which is the pump for the body's cardiovascular system, cannot work efficiently. A decrease or absence of the blood supply to the heart muscle, such as occurs in a myocardial infarction and in coronary artery disease, also decreases the efficiency of the "pump." In congenital anomalies, blood may be unable to circulate normally through the heart and the pulmonary vessels so that the heart is overworked in an attempt to supply the body with adequate oxygen and nutrients. Spasm or thickening of the smallest arterioles causes elevation of the blood pressure within the arterial system. This, in turn, causes the heart to overwork in pumping the blood against increased resistance. The heart hypertrophies and eventually enlarges, losing its efficiency as a "pump." When for any reason the heart is unable to pump an adequate supply of blood to the rest of the body, congestive heart failure occurs. Congestive heart failure is also known as *cardiac decompensation, cardiac insufficiency, heart failure,* and *cardiac incompetency.* Since cardiac insufficiency and cardiac arrhythmias are the cause of many of the symptoms commonly associated with various cardiac diseases, these conditions will be discussed before the specific diseases.

CONGESTIVE HEART FAILURE

Physiology

In congestive heart failure the heart is unable to receive its normal flow of blood from the venous system and to pump out the required amount through the arterial circulation. The left ventricle does not empty completely into the aorta, and the blood that would normally enter the right auricle from the superior and inferior vena cavae cannot do so. Pressure rises in the venous circulation, and the organs and tissues which are normally drained by the veins become congested with the blood which is flowing slowly against increased pressure. The left ventricle, meanwhile, tries to do extra work to pump this blood, and it becomes enlarged. This is usually a gradual process, occurring over a period of months or years.

Congestive heart failure is often classified as right-sided or left-sided according to the side of the heart at fault. Most often it begins in the left ventricle and later becomes a combination of left-sided and right-sided failure. Heart failure may temporarily disappear as soon as the mechanisms causing it are rectified; it may be present for the rest of the patient's life and require continuous care and medication; or, despite treatment, it may quickly become worse and cause death.

Symptoms

The symptoms of heart failure are caused by the congestion of fluid throughout the body. *Edema,* which is an excessive amount of fluid in the extracellular tissues and body cavities, is a common symptom of congestive failure. It may occur in the legs, the liver, the abdominal cavity, the lungs, the pleural spaces, or other parts of the body. When the heart becomes an inefficient pump, venous stasis occurs and venous pressure increases. Because of this fluid remains in the venous system rather than circulating normally to the kidneys where the excess sodium would be excreted. If the patient consumes more salt in his diet than can be excreted, the excess is stored in the body. Sodium is a water-fixing ion; i.e., it holds water to prevent body fluids from becoming too salty. Therefore, the more salt in the body, the more water will be retained. Some of this fluid passes into the interstitial spaces and causes generalized edema.

In *right-sided heart failure* the right auricle cannot accommodate blood returning to it through the inferior and superior vena cavae, thus causing the blood to dam back into the veins of the systemic circulation and causing edema to appear in the legs. This edema is of the pitting type (can be depressed by touching) and is nontender. It is known as dependent edema and almost always disappears at night when the legs are not lower than the rest of the body. As the edema becomes more pronounced, it progresses up the legs into the thighs, scrotum, abdomen, and sacrum. If the tissues become too engorged, the skin may crack and fluid may "weep" from the tissues. The liver may also become engorged with blood, causing it to enlarge and producing tenderness in the right upper quadrant of the abdomen. As the venous stasis increases, increased pressure within the portal system often forces serum through the blood vessels into the abdominal cavity; this is known as *ascites.* As much as 8,000 or 10,000 ml. (8 to 10 quarts) or more of serous fluid may accumulate in the abdominal cavity, and, unless removed by a paracentesis, it may cause severe respiratory distress as a result of pressure on the diaphragm.

In *left-sided failure* the weakened left ventricle of the heart cannot accept the complete return of blood from the pulmonary veins, and serum passes out through the pulmonary vessels, thus causing *pulmonary edema* and *pleural effusion.* The fluid may be present in the lower interstitial tissues of the lungs, in the alveoli of the lungs, in the bronchioles, or in the lower pleural cavity.

Dyspnea or shortness of breath is an early symptom of left-sided congestive heart failure. This is caused by a decreased vital capacity owing to the fluid level in the lungs. Dyspnea may occur or may become worse only on physical exertion, such as climbing stairs, walking up an incline, or walking against a wind, since these activities require increased amounts of oxygen. Sometimes dyspnea occurs upon lying down. This type is called *orthopnea.* When the patient is lying flat on his back, there is decreased vital capacity and the blood volume to the pulmonary vessels is increased; patients with orthopnea often must sleep propped upright in bed or in a chair. Although orthopnea may occur immediately upon lying down, it often does not occur until several hours later, when it causes the patient to wake up with severe dyspnea and coughing. This is known as paroxysmal nocturnal dyspnea and is probably triggered by such things as a nightmare, a noise, or a full bladder, which causes the output of the right ventricle to be increased for a short time and increases the need for oxygen.[7]

In cardiac failure the patient may have periods of apnea and *hyperpnea* (Cheyne-Stokes respirations). Often an insufficient amount of oxygen is carried by the blood to the brain. This apparently makes the respiratory center in the brain insensitive to the normal amounts of carbon dioxide in the arterial blood, and respiration ceases until the carbon dioxide content in the arterial blood increases enough to stimulate the respiratory center. The carbon dioxide content of the arterial blood is also decreased by the periods of overbreathing. Periodic breathing often begins as the patient goes to sleep and decreases as sleep deepens and ventilation decreases.[7] Morphine sulfate may relieve Cheyne-Stokes respirations because it slows the respiratory rate.

Pulmonary edema caused by left-sided heart failure may be very severe, and râles (moist breath sounds) sometimes may be heard across the room. This condition is known as *acute pulmonary edema.* The patient is extremely dyspneic, is apprehensive and struggles for breath, has a persistent cough and may expectorate frothy or even blood-tinged sputum, is usually cyanotic, and his heart pounds rapidly. Acute pulmonary edema is a medical emergency, since, if it is not immediately treated, the patient may "drown" in his own secretions. Treatment will be discussed more fully later in this chapter.

A persistent hacking cough and expectoration of mucoid material are frequent symptoms of left-sided heart congestion. These are usually caused by the congestion of the lungs and bronchi. Cardiac pain is not common in congestive heart failure, although some patients develop discomfort in the chest on lying down. This is often described as a "heavy feeling" or a "feeling of pressure" and is caused by the blood being less completely oxygenated when the patient is lying flat than when he is sitting, standing, or even walking. This discomfort arises in patients with a diseased heart which is sensitive to a deficiency in the oxygen content in the coronary circulation.

Fatigue is a common sign of congestive failure and is one of the earliest to develop. The patient notices that he becomes tired after doing things that ordinarily would not tire him. This fatigue results from the impaired circulation of blood to the tissues and thus the cells do not receive sufficient oxygen or nutrients for their needs. In addition, the slow-moving blood does not carry off wastes with sufficient speed to permit the muscles to regain their power.

Because of the edema, weight loss may not be noticed in patients with congestive heart failure. Often 5 to 10 kg. of fluid may be retained. The patient, however, may have lost much muscle tissue because of inadequate nutrition; on reduction of the edema, he may appear as emaciated as a patient with an advanced malignancy.[7]

Medical treatment and nursing care

Cecil and Loeb[7] state that the principles of treatment for congestive heart failure are to bring back into balance the demand for blood and the supply of blood and to remove and to prevent the reaccumulation of excess fluid and excess blood volume when the output of the heart cannot be made to meet near normal requirements of the body. This is accomplished by reducing the requirements of the body for oxygen, by increasing the cardiac output, and by eliminating the edema.

Rest. The body's oxygen requirements can best be reduced by providing the patient with both physical and mental rest. The patient with congestive heart failure is usually kept in bed until he is free from the signs and symptoms of the disease; that is, until the heart rate has been slowed, venous engorgement has disappeared, dyspnea and orthopnea have lessened, pleural effusion, ascites, and generalized tissue edema have decreased, and the liver has become smaller and is no longer tender. This may take days, weeks, or months. If the attack is mild, with only edema of the legs or minimal signs of pulmonary edema, the patient may be treated on an ambulatory basis with only a regimen of less activity and more rest than usual. If the attack is severe, however, a program of strict bed rest may be maintained for some time.

Rest may be difficult to provide, and sometimes it takes the ingenuity of all concerned to obtain this for the patient. Providing rest is one of the major responsibilities of the nurse in caring for the patient who is acutely ill with congestive heart failure. A restless, anxious, disturbed patient is not at rest, and the nurse must employ measures that will help such a patient to relax. His environment is important. He should be alone in a room; however, if this is impossible, he should be with convalescing patients rather than with those who are acutely ill. The room should be away from the elevator and busy traffic areas. If the patient is more relaxed with his wife or some other relative nearby, such a person should be permitted to stay with him. Other visitors should be prohibited. If the presence of the family disturbs the patient, members of the medical and nursing staff should explain this to the family and gain their cooperation. The family should be kept well informed of the patient's condition, since the need for such a restriction is usually upsetting to them. The patient's mail should be screened by a close member of the family so that disturbing communications will not reach him.

Almost every cardiac patient is extremely apprehensive and anxious, both about his own physical condition and about the welfare of his family. Many times the doctor feels that it is best to tell the patient what he wishes to know since this will often quiet him. The family should be urged to visit the patient regularly or to keep in touch with him. While they should be encouraged not to worry him, mention of daily problems should not be avoided since he may suspect that information is being withheld. No news often is worse than bad news, and the patient may imagine that things are much worse than they are.

The nurse should listen carefully to the patient to find out what concerns him and makes it difficult for him to rest. During evening and night hours, she should visit the acutely ill cardiac patient often to see whether he is awake and to give him a chance to mention worries that are interfering with sleep and rest. It may help if he can be in daily contact with a social worker to whom he can talk about his family, his job, and his plans for the future. Although the social worker will not make extensive plans with him at this time, she often can take care of immediate problems, and this helps to relieve his mind. Visits from a spiritual adviser may be quieting to some patients. Visits from other patients who are progressing satisfactorily from the same condition sometimes give reassurance. Reading, watching television, and listening to radio for short periods of time may be relaxing for some patients. Others find this most distracting, so that provisions for patients should be made on an individual basis. Occupational therapy that does not require extensive arm movements and which is not so intricate as to tire the patient may be a valuable pastime as the patient improves.

Sedatives. The patient should have adequate sleep, and it is better for him to sleep at night and to be awake during the day. Cardiac patients are likely to be apprehensive during the night. Pentobarbital sodium, 0.1 Gm. (1½ grains), at bedtime and repeated if necessary, or phenobarbital, 30 to 60 mg. (½ to 1 grain), may be ordered by the doctor. Whiskey, 30 to 60 ml. (1 to 2 ounces), at bedtime may be ordered to increase the effectiveness of the barbiturates. For older patients and patients with liver damage, paraldehyde by mouth, by rectum, or by intramuscular injection may be necessary. Chloral hydrate or sodium bromide may also be used. If the patient is unable to sleep, time should be taken to talk with him, and nursing measures such as rubbing his back and straightening the bedclothes may help him to relax. It is usually impossible to give warm milk because of fluid and salt restrictions, but, if this seems desirable, it may be possible to plan for it with the dietitian. Sometimes other warm fluids may be given when milk is not permitted.

If dyspnea under sedation is marked, if the patient complains of pain, or if he is very restless and anxious, the doctor may order morphine sulfate, 10 mg. (1/6 grain). If necessary, the drug may be given as often as every four hours for two or three days. The nurse should give it before the patient becomes agitated, since worry and excitement normally cause constriction of the blood vessels, and this increases the heart rate. Although a normal heart can accommodate to this, the diseased heart may be overburdened by the increase in pressure and activity. Some patients are allergic to morphine sulfate and develop nausea and vomiting. The doctor may also order meperidine hydrochloride (Demerol) or Pantopon.

Position in bed. A comfortable position in bed can best be determined by the patient. Since no two patients are alike, the nurse must be guided by the patient's habit patterns and his symptoms in finding a position that is most conducive to rest. Most patients with congestive heart failure are more comfortable and can breathe more easily with the head of the bed elevated in a high Fowler's position. A pillow may be placed lengthwise behind the shoulders and back in such a manner that full expansion of the rib cage is possible. The patient who is in proper position for comfortable breathing will also be in correct body alignment. A foot block is needed to prevent the patient from slipping toward the foot of the bed. Patients who must be in a high Fowler's position are usually more comfortable and have less pull on their shoulder muscles if pillows are used to support the lower arms. A small pillow slipped under the "small" of the back also may make the patient more comfortable. If the patient must remain upright all the time, his position may be changed occasionally by allowing him to rest his head and arms on pillows placed on an overbed table pulled up close to him (see Figure 26). Both the pillows and the table should be tied to prevent them from slipping. Side rails should be kept on the bed to give the patient something firm on which to hold during brief changes of position and to prevent accidents.

Oxygen. The patient with congestive heart failure may be more comfortable and more relaxed in an oxygen tent, since oxygen helps to relieve the dyspnea and cyanosis by providing a higher concentration of oxygen in the blood stream. In cardiac failure the oxygen content of the blood stream may be markedly reduced because of the less effective oxygenation of the blood as it passes through the congested lungs.

If pulmonary edema is severe, a high concentration of oxygen under pressure may be given by means of a positive-pressure mask. This helps to prevent further transudation of serum from the pulmonary capillaries by exerting pressure on the pulmonary epithelium during expira-

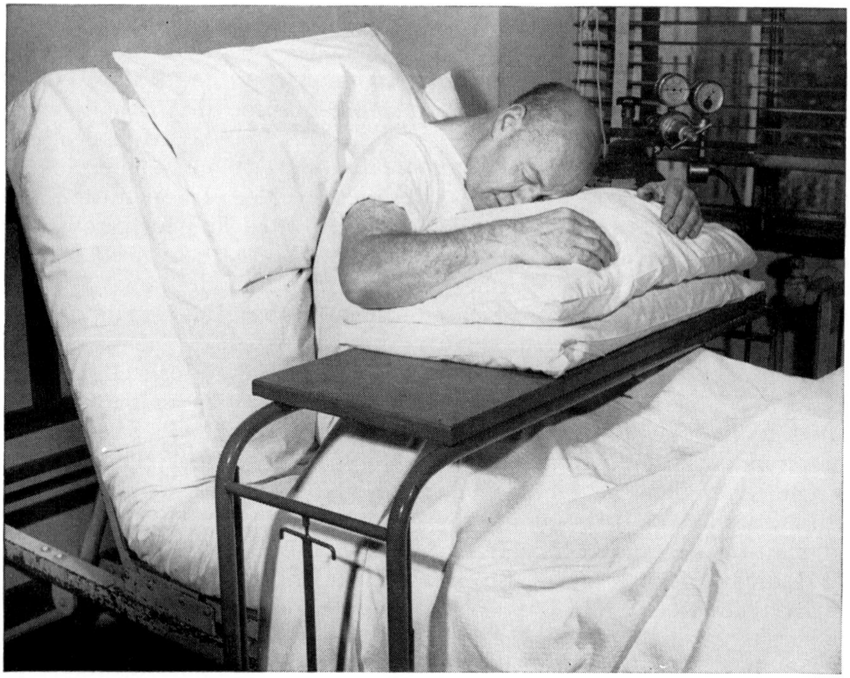

Figure 26

Pillows placed on the overbed table provide a comfortable support for the patient who must sleep in a sitting position.

tion. The doctor must determine the concentration of oxygen, the desired pressure, and the frequency of use. Fifty to 100 per cent concentrations of oxygen are usually given at a pressure of 3 to 4 ml. of water, and later, although the oxygen is continued, the positive pressure may be used only every one to four hours for short periods of time. The patient receiving this treatment needs attention to the skin where pressure from the mask may cause irritation. The skin should be massaged, sponged, and powdered between treatments if they continue for some time. The nurse must protect the patient with pulmonary edema from *any* exertion since any activity increases the body's need for oxygen.

Activity. Restricted physical activity is necessary for the patient with congestive heart failure, and the nurse should find out from the doctor how much activity the patient may be allowed. Some patients are not even permitted to turn or to feed themselves. Because dependence on nursing personnel for even these simple tasks is disturbing to some patients, they should be carried out without apparent rush, and the patient's needs should be anticipated so that he will not have to ask for things.

Most patients with heart failure are not allowed to bathe themselves, and, while they are acutely ill, they should not be disturbed more than is necessary for their safety and comfort. If special attention is given to the back and to bony prominences, a partial bath may suffice for several days. The patient's head often cannot be lowered to change bedclothes; thus, when the lower sheets need changing or tighening, he may need to be supported in an upright position while the head of the bed is lowered and made. The sheets are more easily changed from the top to the bottom than from side to side. If the patient is permitted to use a commode once a day, the bed can be changed at this time. Occasionally it seems best to have several people lift the patient to a stretcher and support him in a sitting position while the bed is completely changed.

If the patient must remain on complete bed rest, he should move his legs about occasionally and tighten and relax his leg muscles, to prevent phlebitis and extensive muscle wasting. While the patient is being bathed, the joints should be put through complete range of motion. When the patient is acutely ill, this should be done passively by the nurse; later, when he is convalescing, he is taught to do this for himself. The patient is also encouraged to breathe deeply five to ten times every one to two hours to expand the lungs and help to prevent hypostatic pneumonia.

Skin care. Since there may be generalized edema, special skin care should be given to the patient with congestive heart failure. The patient may be thin, malnourished, or elderly. Bony prominences should be carefully inspected for any signs of irritation and should be massaged frequently. The elbows should be carefully observed and a lubricant applied to the skin, since irritation often occurs especially if the patient must be kept in high Fowler's position. Patients also easily develop decubiti in the sacral region because of continual pressure and the edema caused by the upright position; heavy rubber drawsheets that wrinkle and retain moisture should not be used; light plastic materials are available. Soft tissue areas are not massaged without an order from the doctor. It is best to use an alternating air pressure mattress or a sponge rubber mattress, but, if these are not available, pieces of sponge rubber are very helpful when placed under areas receiving pressure.

Feeding the patient. The nurse should try to make mealtime as pleasant an occasion as possible; few people like to be fed and the appetite of a patient with heart failure may be poor. During the acute stage of congestive failure the diet should be soft or liquid and the foods served should be easily digested. The work of the heart is increased during digestion, since blood is needed by the digestive tract for its functions. Several small meals a day may be better tolerated than three large meals. When the patient is allowed to feed himself, his appetite may improve as morale improves with his feeling that he is making progress toward recovery.

Defecation. It is advisable for the patient with cardiac disease to avoid straining at defecation since this places an extra burden upon the heart. The feces are kept soft by giving a mild cathartic daily; milk of magnesia, 30 ml. (1 ounce), is usually effective. If the feces tend to become hard, mineral oil may be ordered in small doses to be given with the milk of magnesia. If an oil enema is necessary, it should be given with a small rectal tube inserted only three to four inches. Most patients dislike using the bedpan, and the effort required to get onto the pan and to maintain a satisfactory position on it often puts a real strain on the heart. Therefore, some doctors prefer that the patient slide off the bed onto the commode to have a bowel evacuation. Commodes raised to bed height are now available so that little moving is necessary to get the patient onto them. The patient with cardiac disease should not be left alone when on the commode or on a bedpan, although the nurse or attendant may leave the room or step outside the curtain for a few minutes. Since it is extremely upsetting to the patient to know that someone is waiting while he uses the commode or pan, it often helps to let him know that there is no need for hurry.

Ambulation. Ambulation for the patient with cardiac disease is started slowly to avoid overburdening the heart and to determine how much activity the heart can tolerate without again showing signs of failure. The regimen differs according to each patient and according to the doctor's orders. Even though they are acutely ill, older patients may be put on a modified schedule of bed rest after several days to prevent them from developing hypostatic pneumonia or thrombophlebitis; the doctor may allow them to be out of bed in a chair for several hours a day.

The usual procedure for ambulation of a cardiac patient is to allow him to dangle his legs from the side of the bed fifteen minutes twice a day and then to progress to sitting in a chair at the side of the bed twice a day for gradually increasing periods of time. The patient who is dangling his legs should have support at his back and a chair to place his feet on if he so desires. If being up in a chair is tolerated well by the patient, walking is then allowed. This should also be increased very gradually and should be closely supervised. The patient may only tolerate a few steps around his room the first few times he walks. The activity permitted is slowly increased, and most patients are fairly self-sufficient before discharge from the hospital, having climbed stairs, taken a bath or shower, and performed all the activities of daily living.

The patient should be observed closely during each step of the ambulation program. The nurse should be alert for signs of fatigue, increased pulse rate, and dyspnea. If at any point the patient shows that he cannot tolerate the activity or shows signs of distress, he should return to bed. If he is at all dyspneic, the head of the bed should be elevated. The doctor should be consulted before further ambulation is attempted. The plan for ambulation should be explained to both the patient and his family. They should understand that if activity tires the patient excessively, it may be curtailed. Overactivity can produce physical and mental setbacks that delay ultimate recovery. In the early stages of ambulation it is important to begin stressing to the patient the importance of rate of activity; that is, the decrease in demand on the heart when a normal activity is performed more slowly than before.

Digitalization. When digitalis, one of its derivatives, or drugs with similar action on the heart muscles are given to patients with heart failure, the cardiac rate decreases and the contraction of the heart muscles becomes stronger. This increases the cardiac output and also helps to increase the output of excess fluid from the body. Over a twenty-four to forty-eight hour period, the doctor may order that the patient with congestive heart failure be given an amount of digitalis that will slow the ventricular rate to between 70 and 75 beats per minute. This is called a digitalizing dose or the optimum therapeutic dose. In some instances this amount of digitalis may approach the toxic level so that the nurse should carefully watch the patient for symptoms of toxicity. She should be especially alert for this when the heart and circulation return to normal under treatment because the full effects of these drugs will then be realized. Since digitalis preparations have a cumulative effect and are slowly eliminated, early recognition of toxic symptoms and discontinuance of the drug will decrease their severity and duration. After the optimum therapeutic dose has been determined, the patient is placed on a daily maintenance dose of digitalis. The selection of the drug is determined by the rapidity of action desired, the route by which it is to be given, and the response of the patient.

Before digitalis preparations are given, the pulse rate should be taken. If the radial rate is below 60, an apical rate should be taken. If this also is below 60, the drug should be withheld until the doctor has been consulted. The pulse rate of patients with cardiac disease should always be taken for a full minute since the pulse may be irregular. The patient who is being digitalized is placed on recorded fluid intake and output, and, if possible, he is weighed before treatment is started and daily thereafter. A record of daily weight is a helpful guide to the doctor in determining if edema is being decreased. The weight should be taken at the same time each day, preferably early in the morning, since it is more accurate when the patient has not eaten or had a bowel movement. The patient's color, the amount of edema, and the amount of dyspnea should also be observed and recorded. When the color is otherwise normal, cyanosis may be noticeable in the nail beds, the ear lobes, and lips.

Powdered digitalis, or the whole leaf digitalis, is a potent oral preparation to which many patients develop toxic reactions. Usually 1.5 Gm. (22 grains) of the drug are given in divided doses over a twenty-four to forty-eight hour period in order to achieve initial digitalization. The usual maintenance dose is 0.1 Gm. per day. Toxic symptoms of any preparation of digitalis are loss of appetite, nausea and vomiting, diarrhea and abdominal pain, a drop in the pulse rate below 60, development of an irregular cardiac rhythm, headache, malaise, drowsiness, blurred or colored vision, and hallucinations. If toxic symptoms appear, the drug is stopped, morphine sulfate and atropine sulfate are given to relieve the vomiting and abdominal pain, and the patient is kept quiet with sedatives. Often potassium chloride is ordered to be given orally or intravenously. When the drug has been eliminated from the body, treatment may be resumed.

Several types of purified glycosides of digitalis have been developed for use when the patient cannot tolerate powdered digitalis. The effects are the same, but the speed of action and the rate of elimination is different. Although the toxic symptoms are the same, severe toxicity is less likely to occur.

Digitoxin is a glycoside of digitalis. It may be ordered under the following names: Purodigin, Digitaline Nativelle, Crystodigin, and Unidigin. Digitoxin is excreted slowly. The usual digitalizing dose is 1.5 mg. (1/40 grain) given over a period of twenty-four to forty-eight hours. The maintenance dose is 0.1 or 0.2 mg. (1/600 to 1/300 grain) a day. This drug may be given either orally or intravenously.

Lanatoside C (Cedilanid) is also a purified glycoside of digitalis. It comes as an oral preparation only, and the usual maintenance dose is 0.5 mg. (1/120 grain) a day.

Deslanoside (Desacetyl-lanatoside C; Cedilanid-D) is a glycoside of digitalis for intravenous use. An initial dose of 1.2 to 1.6 mg. (1/50 to 1/40 grain) is usually given, followed by a maintenance dose of 0.2 to 0.6 mg. (1/300 to 1/100 grain) each day.

Digoxin is a purified glycoside of digitalis that produces effects more rapidly than does digitoxin. It is also eliminated more rapidly. It may be given either orally or intravenously. The average digitalizing dose is 4 mg. (1/16 grain) orally or 0.5 to 1.5 mg. (1/120 to 1/40 grain) intravenously. The maintenance dose both orally and intravenously is 0.25 to 0.75 mg. (1/250 to 1/90 grain) daily. If any of the drug infiltrates into the tissues during intravenous injection, sloughing may occur since digoxin is a tissue irritant. Heat should be applied to the infiltrated area immediately to encourage absorption of the drug into the blood stream.

Digalen is very similar to digitalis. It can be given both orally and intravenously. The usual maintenance dose is 0.5 to 1 U.S.P. unit three times a day.

Digilanid is a drug which has an action similar to digitalis. It can be given orally, rectally, intramuscularly, and intravenously. Two to four tablets (0.67 to 1.33 mg.) are given daily until the patient is fully digitalized, and then one or two tablets are given daily as a maintenance dose.

Digifolin is also a form of digitalis leaf. It can be given orally and intravenously. Until the desired effects are obtained 0.8 U.S.P. unit is given daily.

Gitalin (amorphous) is excreted more slowly than digoxin but more rapidly than digitoxin. It is given by mouth, and two or three tablets are given daily for three or four days or until 4 to 6.5 mg. (1/16 to 1/10 grain) have been given. The daily maintenance dose is then usually 0.25 to 0.75 mg. (1/250 to 3/250 grain).

Strophanthin is a drug with an action identical to that of powdered digitalis, but it acts more rapidly. It can only be given intravenously or intramuscularly since it is not absorbed from the gastrointestinal tract.

Ouabain (G-Strophanthin) is the drug often used for emergency treatment of patients with congestive heart failure. It acts very rapidly when injected intravenously or intramuscularly, but it is quickly excreted. Therefore, it is not suitable for a maintenance drug and usually is used in conjunction with some other digitalis preparation. Usually no more than 0.5 mg. (1/120 grain) of this drug is given daily because of its potency.

Scillaren is another drug with an action similar to digitalis. Until the heart becomes compensated 1.6 mg. of the drug are given three times a day, and then a smaller maintenance dose is ordered. *Scillaren B* is available for intravenous use.

The nurse should be familiar with the usual dosage of the digitalis preparation being given. Since these are very potent drugs and thus are given in small units, an overdose is extremely serious. Many of the preparations have similar names, and some come in milligram doses while others come in gram doses. An error between 0.1 Gm. and 0.1 mg. might mean that the patient would be given 1,000 times the dose ordered.

Treatment with diet. Edema is most effectively controlled in patients with heart failure by restriction of salt intake. The degree of restriction depends on the severity of the failure.[7] In mild failure the doctor may order that salt be restricted only to 3 Gm. per day. If this does not control the edema, however, salt may be restricted to as little as 150 mg. of sodium chloride a day. It is difficult to maintain an adequate protein intake on a salt-free diet so that Lanalac, a salt-free milk, may need to be used to supplement the diet. Since the vitamin B intake may also be inadequate because of low protein in a salt-free diet, vitamin supplements are usually ordered. A salt-free diet is unpalatable, and special efforts should be made to use other seasonings. If the patient does not have kidney involvement, the doctor may permit the use of salt substitutes such as potassium chloride. See the second part of Chapter 21 for suggestions for making salt-free diets more palatable. If the patient is on diuretic drugs, salt may not be limited below 3 to 5 Gm. because of the danger of sodium chloride depletion in the blood. (See Chapter 6.)

Fluids are often limited to 1,800 ml. a day for patients with congestive heart failure. This means that the patient may have only about six glasses of fluid a day in addition to fluids contained in food. Soups are usually not served because they tend to make the patient thirsty. Watery foods also must be restricted as they may appreciably increase the fluid intake. If the patient finds this amount of fluid restriction intolerable, the nurse should be sure that foods which might make him more thirsty are not being served, that fluids are spaced throughout the day, and that he is given frequent mouth care, using an iced mouthwash.

Some physicians feel that fluids need not be restricted as long as the patient is on a low-salt diet and is receiving diuretics and digitalis. They feel that in this instance fluids actually act as a diuretic and are beneficial in helping to remove fluids from the tissues. The nursing care would then be based on this theory, and fluids would be forced.

The reason for diet and fluid restrictions should be explained to both the patient and his family so that the patient does not become unduly upset and so that the family does not bring him food or fluids that are unacceptable. The patient often must continue the diet and fluid restrictions after discharge from the hospital; therefore, when he feels better, mealtime may be used to teach him about the type of foods he may include in his diet at home. If he does not eat well, efforts should be made to find food preparations that he will eat to maintain normal nutrition.

Diuretic drugs. If restrictions of salt and fluids and the administration of digitalis do not appreciably relieve the tissue edema and the pulmonary edema, the doctor may order diuretic drugs. A diuretic also may be used to give prompt relief to the patient who is in acute distress because of "waterlogging" of the tissues. The mercurial diuretics are the most effective. They are available for both intramuscular and intravenous use, but most doctors prefer to give them intramuscularly since rare deaths due to ventricular fibrillation following intravenous injections of these drugs have been reported.[7] The patient may complain of discomfort and tenderness about the site of the intramuscular injection. These complaints are usually only temporary, however, and are relieved by a hot application to the area which hastens the absorption of the drug. In giving mercurial diuretics, care must be taken that none of the drug is injected into the intradermal tissues since this will cause sloughing of the skin. Mercurial diuretics usually are given only every second or third day, but the patient who is receiving them should be weighed daily at the same hour and under the same circumstances. By closely following the patient's weight, the doctor can determine the amount of drug to give and the frequency with which it is needed. Bed scales are available for weighing patients who cannot be moved from their beds. If the patient is at home, arrangements will need to be made to provide scales, and the patient or his family must be taught to record the weight daily. When a patient is given a mercurial diuretic, the urinary output may be 2,000 to 4,000 ml. a day, with a corresponding weight loss.[7] Mercurial injections, therefore, should be given in the morning so that the greatest diuresis will take place during the day and not interfere with sleep.

Some patients have toxic reactions to mercurial preparations. These are caused by salt, calcium, or potassium depletion, since salt, calcium, or potassium may also be lost in large amounts through the kidney while its reabsorptive powers are depressed by the mercurials. Nausea, vomiting, fever, and cramps in the calves of the legs and the stomach are due to salt depletion. Potassium depletion causes extreme weakness and symptoms of paralytic ileus; calcium depletion may cause the patient to develop tetany, with muscle spasm. Skin rashes may also occur. The patient who is receiving both diuretic drugs and digitalis needs to be watched closely for toxic reactions to digitalis since toxicity occurs much sooner if the serum potassium is low. If a reaction to a mercurial preparation occurs, the doctor will institute measures to replace the depleted electrolytes. Reactions often can be prevented by giving the patient a little more salt in his food (if medically approved) and by encouraging him to take food and fluids high in potassium and calcium. (See Chapter 6.) Another form of the drug often can be substituted later without untoward reactions. Mercurial diuretics are usually considered contraindicated if the patient has acute kidney disease.

Mersalyl (Salyrgan) is a potent mercurial diuretic for parenteral use. Before a full dose of this drug is given to a patient, a small test dose usually is given to determine sensitivity to it. The usual dosage is 0.1 Gm. (1½ grains) not more than two or three times a week. *Mersalyl and theophylline tablets* (Salyrgan-theophylline) is an enteric-coated mercurial for oral use. *Sterile mercaptomerin sodium* (Thiomerin sodium) is an injectible form of mercurial, and it is less toxic than Salyrgan. *Mercurophylline injection* (Mercuzanthin) and *meralluride sodium solution* (Mercuhydrin) are mercurial preparations commonly used for intramuscular injection. Usually 1 to 2 ml. of the drug are given one to three times a week.

The patient who is receiving any mercurial over a long period should be watched for signs of stomatitis, gingivitis, increased salivation, diarrhea, albuminuria, hematuria, and skin eruption. He may also complain of flushing and have febrile reactions to the drug. Toxic signs must be reported to the doctor at once.

Acetazolamide (Diamox) is a relatively new preparation which depresses the tubule of the kidney, promoting excretion of the bicarbonate ion rather than the chloride ion. It is given orally once a day in 250 to 500 mg. doses and remains active for six to eight hours. It often is given every other day, being alternated with a mercurial preparation. This drug may make the patient drowsy, and he may complain of numbness and tingling in the face and extremities.

Chlorothiazide (Diuril) is a new and effective oral diuretic. It inhibits the reabsorption of sodium from the glomerular filtrate by the kidney tubules and thereby causes less reabsorption of water and other electrolytes. It is often given in two doses of 0.5 to 1.0 Gm. (7½ to 15 grains) daily although only one daily dose may be given; the drug is effective for about twelve hours. Chlorothiazide is well absorbed orally and has shown no appreciable toxicity to date. When the patient has cardiac failure, usually it is given in conjunction with one of the mercurial diuretics.[25]

If good diuresis is not obtained from the mercurials, the doctor may order *ammonium chloride* in enteric-coated tablets to be given on the two or three days prior to and on the day of the administration of the mercurial preparation. For the best results it should then be omitted for a day or two. The ammonium chloride has an acidifying effect which enhances the potency of the mercurial drugs because, in an effort to prevent acidosis, the sodium from the tissues unites with the chloride to neutralize it. This mobilizes both the salt and the water for excretion by the kidney.[7] The usual dosage is 6 to 10 Gm. a day given in four doses.[7] Ammonium chloride should be taken after meals or with food since it may cause gastric irritation.

Occasionally xanthine derivatives are used as diuretics. They act by increasing the rate of salt elimination from the kidneys. *Theobromine calcium salicylate* and *theophylline ethylenediamine* (aminophylline) are the drugs most often used. Theobromine usually is given in 0.5 Gm. (7½ grains) doses, and 0.25 Gm. (4 grains) of aminophylline may be given. Aminophylline may be given orally, rectally, or intravenously. Xanthine derivatives given orally cause gastric irritation and, therefore, should be given with food. These drugs may be used if smooth muscle relaxation is also desired; for example, they are often prescribed for patients who have angina pectoris to help relax the smooth muscles of the coronary vessels.

To relieve an abdominal ascites or a pleural effusion, sometimes it is necessary for the doctor to aspirate fluid. This is done through an abdominal paracentesis and a thoracentesis, respectively. (For the nursing care of patients undergoing these procedures, see texts on fundamentals of nursing and Chapters 23 and 27.)

ACUTE PULMONARY EDEMA

Acute pulmonary edema is a medical emergency in patients with heart disease. It is caused by additional or prolonged strain on an already damaged heart, with resultant failure. Fluid rapidly pours from the circulating blood into the alveoli, bronchioles, and bronchi, and the patient begins to be drowned in his own secretions. Acute pulmonary edema also may follow such conditions as inhalation of irritating gases, cerebral vascular accident, fractures of the skull, too rapid absorption of plasma, serum albumin, administration of whole blood or intravenous fluids, and barbiturate poisoning. Severe dyspnea, cyanosis, and restlessness are usual symptoms.

The patient with suspected acute pulmonary edema should be placed in bed in a high Fowler's position, and the doctor should be summoned immediately. He usually orders morphine sulfate, 15 mg. (¼ grain), to be given at once to quiet breathing and to allay apprehension. This may be given intravenously since circulatory collapse may hinder its absorption from the tissues. Aminophylline usually is given because it helps to increase the cardiac output and to lower the venous pressure by relaxing the smooth muscles of the blood vessels and it relieves bronchial spasm. Digitalization usually is started immediately, either ouabain or lanatoside

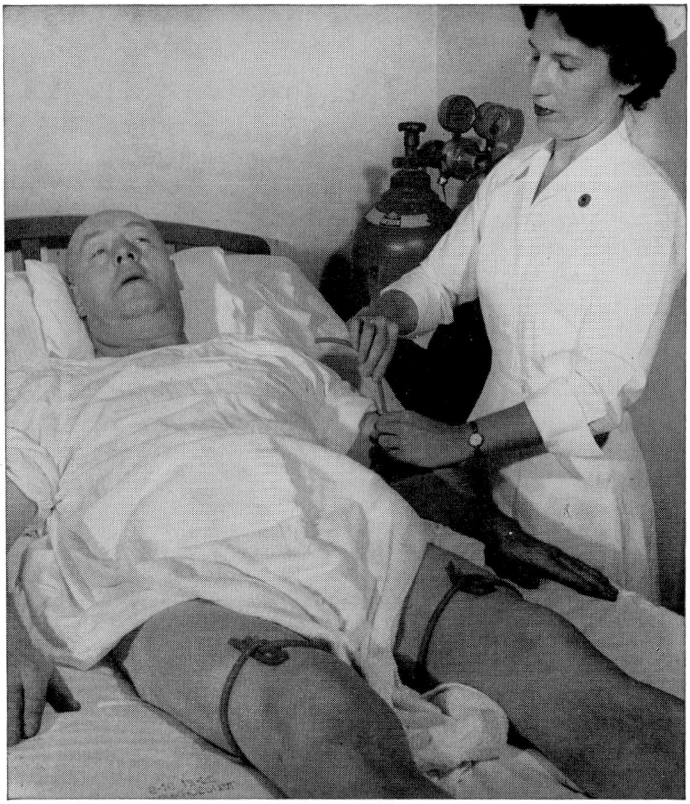

Figure 27

Here the tourniquets are being applied in a clockwise order. The nurse has removed the tourniquet from the right arm and is applying it to the left arm.

is used because of the quick action of these drugs. Since it is dangerous to give either of these if the patient is routinely taking digitalis, the nurse should try to ascertain from the patient or his family whether he takes any heart medicines, and she should inform the doctor of her findings. Oxygen under pressure is usually ordered to prevent further escape of fluid from the blood stream into the lungs. A mercurial diuretic also may be given.

The doctor may order rotating tourniquets to relieve acute pulmonary edema. The tourniquets are placed on three of the extremities at a time, thus reducing the amount of blood that must be circulated by the overtaxed heart. (See Figure 27.) Every fifteen minutes, in clockwise or counter clockwise order, one tourniquet is removed and placed on the extremity that has had no tourniquet on it. In this way the vessels of each extremity are occluded for forty-five minutes at a time, and then the tourniquet is released from the extremity for fifteen minutes. Care must be taken that no tourniquet is left on longer than forty-five minutes lest the tissues be permanently damaged, and the tourniquet should not obliterate arterial pulses in the extremity. The use of a prepared diagram and time schedule kept at the patient's bedside helps ensure the proper changing of the tourniquets. This procedure may be done by either the doctor or the nurse, and it is continued until the acute pulmonary edema subsides. If the patient is alert, the procedure should be explained to him. He may need a narcotic to make him less conscious of the pressure of the tourniquets and of the uncomfortable sensation in the extremities caused by venous engorgement. If the procedure must be continued over a long period, the skin should be carefully watched for beginning signs of irritation from pressure. The tourniquet may be placed over the patient's gown or a towel to prevent damage to the skin. If the extremity does not readily return to normal color on release of the tourniquet, this should be reported to the doctor. When treatment is to be discontinued, one tourniquet is removed at a time, according to time intervals, until all tourniquets have been removed. Sometimes, if the patient is not in shock, the doctor will remove 500 to 800 ml. of blood by a *phlebotomy*. The decrease in the amount of circulating blood decreases pulmonary engorgement. This procedure is similar to that for taking blood from a blood donor.

Home care

If possible, patients with acute pulmonary edema are hospitalized; however, if it is impossible to move them from their homes, improvisations can be made to care for them adequately. Oxygen can be obtained from fire stations or ambulances for emergency use, and hospitals or medical supply houses will provide equipment for continued use. Other sickroom equipment usually can be borrowed from the local public health nursing agency. The local health department office often knows where equipment is available. The patient can be put in a high Fowler's position in the home by use of an inverted straight chair placed on the bed and padded with blankets and pillows. Six-inch blocks placed under the legs of the bed to raise the height makes it easier to care for the patient, although side rails should then be used. The patient with acute pulmonary edema needs continuous nursing care. As he improves, his care will be that of any patient with heart failure.

CARDIAC ARRHYTHMIAS

Cardiac rhythm, the sequence of heartbeats, is normally controlled by the sinoauricular node, sometimes called the "pacemaker." The stimulus initiating the beat arises in the sinus node located in the right auricle, spreads over the auricles, inducing their contraction, and then spreads over the auriculoventricular bundle to stimulate simultaneous contraction of both ventricles.[7] Both the rate and the rhythm of the heartbeat are usually regular but under certain circumstances may vary. These variations may be a normal physiologic response, may have no clinical importance, or may be a symptom or a complication of organic heart disease. Although some arrhythmias do not cause any symptoms, they are noticeable to the patient and cause apprehension. He may describe the sensations as a "flutter," a "turning over" of the heart, "pounding" or "palpitation" of the heart, or "skipping" of the heart. He often feels weak or faint. If he feels his pulse, he may be aware that it is very rapid and irregular or perhaps very slow. Patients with extremely slow pulse rates, however, are less likely to have symptoms.

Patients with cardiac irregularities should be urged to seek medical attention. If, after a thorough examination, the doctor finds nothing organically wrong, the patient should be urged to live normally.

Cardiac irregularities in patients with organic heart disease should be reported to the doctor immediately, since they may become incompatible with life. The pulse rate of a patient with cardiac disease should be taken by a professional nurse for a full minute several times a day to note any marked increase or decrease in the rate, the presence of alternating strong and weak beats (pulsus alternans), coupling of beats (two together followed by a pause), or other irregularities in the rhythm. Abnormal rates and rhythm in a patient with heart disease often mean that the ventricle is not pumping adequate blood into the systemic circulation to take care of body needs. Congestive heart failure may then occur.

Sinus tachycardia

The most common rhythm disturbance of the heart is sinus tachycardia. This is characterized by a heartbeat of more than 100 contractions per minute. This is a normal physiologic reaction to exercise, fever, fear, and excitement, or any other condition in which the basal metabolism is increased, thus necessitating a greater supply of blood. For example, tachycardia is common in patients with fever, anemia, pulmonary tuberculosis, rheumatic fever, hyperthyroidism, myocardial infarctions, congestive heart failure, and hemorrhage. The patient may be unaware of the speeded up heart rate, or he may complain of palpitations. The doctor may order sedatives to relieve annoying symptoms. When the underlying cause is eradicated, the heart rate returns to normal.

Sinus bradycardia

In sinus bradycardia the heart rate falls to 60 beats per minute or slower. A heart rate as slow as this is common in young adult men and in athletes. Bradycardia also normally occurs during sleep. It may occur in patients with brain lesions. It may also occur in patients receiving digitalis because of its action in slowing the heartbeat. On withdrawal of the drug, the heart rate will return to normal. There is no treatment for bradycardia other than removal of the cause.

Heart block

In heart block the pulse rate drops markedly, often to as low as 30 to 40 or fewer beats a minute. In this condition normal stimuli arise in the sinoauricular nodes, but they are blocked or delayed on their way down the auriculoventricular bundle. The passage of a stimulus from its point of initiation in the auricle to the ventricle normally takes less than 0.2 second.[7] If there is any interference in its passage, the ventricles do not contract as expected, and this is known as heart block. It may only be partial or it may be complete. The patient with complete heart block may have no symptoms once the block is established because, although no impulses from the auricles reach the ventricles, the ventricles have adjusted to this by setting up their own rate. This rate is usually very slow (30 to 40 beats per minute). During the period before complete block occurs, however, the patient may have symptoms known as the *Adams-Stokes syndrome.* He may faint and have convulsive seizures, and on exertion he may feel dizzy and weak. This syndrome may be treated by giving Adrenalin 1:1000 (0.5 to 1 ml.), during acute seizures and then ephedrine sulfate, 20 to 30 mg. three times a day. A new preparation frequently used is Isuprel, administered sublingually. Doctors usually advise patients with heart block to avoid strenuous exercise but otherwise to lead normal lives. Heart block in a patient with arteriosclerosis or a myocardial infarction is indicative of progressive heart damage.[7]

Electric pacemaker. The electric pacemaker is an electrically operated mechanical device which stimulates ventricular heart action. It can be adjusted to stimulate the ventricular contractions constantly at a normal rate or else to do this only when normal impulses are not forthcoming or fall below a rate set by the doctor. The machine can also be set just to monitor the heartbeat. If the heart stops beating, in this instance, an alarm will sound and the pacemaker will send two charges of electricity through the heart at 8 second intervals. The medical staff, responding to the alarm, will then decide whether further stimulation is necessary. The electric pacemaker may be used as an emergency measure in event of sudden heart block, as a safety measure following cardiac surgery or in medical illness when it is suspected that heart block may occur.

An electrode paste is applied to the skin and three electrodes from the machine are placed across the anterior chest and secured with adhesive tape. The patient on whom this device is used usually is critically ill and needs constant nursing attention. He needs repeated reassurance when he becomes aware of his condition and of the significance of the machine. The skin beneath the electrodes should be kept clean and dry and the paste is renewed every two or three hours. This is to prevent burning of the skin since the paste dries in that time. The position of the electrodes is changed daily by the doctor. The greatest care must be taken in turning the patient lest the electrodes become loosened.

The maintenance and operation of the electric pacemaker is the responsibility of the physician, but the nurse must understand its use and be able to care for the patient when it is used. A continuous high-pitched beep is heard as the electrical activity of the heart is picked up and amplified, and this serves to inform those in attendance that the equipment is working properly.

The patient is usually quite apprehensive when being weaned from the machine and again needs almost constant nursing attention and repeated reassurance for a time.

Portable pacemakers are now available for use by patients who need this apparatus for long periods but who otherwise need not remain at bed rest in the hospital.

Sinoauricular block

In sinoauricular block the sinus node pauses momentarily, causing an interruption in the discharge of impulses over the auricles and into the ventricles. This is caused by increased activity of the vagus nerve and may be precipitated by quinidine, potassium salts, or digitalis.[8] It may also follow stimulation of an oversensitive carotid sinus by sudden turning of the head, pressure of a tight collar, or bending forward. The heartbeat will be irregular, and if no stimuli are discharged for several seconds, the patient may faint. This condition may be treated with such drugs as atropine sulfate, tincture of belladonna, ephedrine, and phenobarbital. Sometimes the carotid sinus must be denervated to relieve the symptoms.

Ventricular and auricular premature contractions

The irregularity in rhythm of both the auricles and the ventricles gives similar symptoms, but auricular arrhythmia occurs more often in young persons, whereas ventricular arrhythmia occurs more often in older persons. In both conditions there is a premature contraction of the chamber due to abnormal stimuli. The beat is coupled and the patient is often aware of the irregularity, complaining of palpitation and "flutter." He may have a "catch" in his throat and a cough. This premature beat may occur only occasionally, it may occur in a regular pattern, or there may be several beats in sequence. Auricular and ventricular arrhythmias may be of no significance, or they may be associated with organic heart diseases such as mitral stenosis and coronary artery disease.[8] Triple bromides, 1 Gm. (15 grains), may be given three times a day to relieve intolerable symptoms. The patient taking this drug should be warned that he will be drowsy and therefore should neither drive on long trips nor work with or near machinery or in any situation where his safety depends upon alertness. A rash may occur and, if so, the drug is discontinued. If sedation fails to relieve the symptoms in a patient with auricular arrhythmia, digitalis may be given. The patient with ventricular arrhythmia, however, is often not digitalized since this might increase the irritability of the ventricle, thereby causing greater irregularity in the heartbeat. Quinidine is sometimes given to patients with this condition.

Paroxysmal tachycardia

Paroxysmal tachycardia may be either auricular or ventricular in origin. Auricular paroxysmal tachycardia is seen more frequently in young people, and ventricular paroxysmal tachycardia in older patients. An attack is often precipitated by the consumption of excess amounts of alcohol, by excessive smoking, by a gastrointestinal upset, or by an acute infection.[7] Both forms are characterized by a sudden onset and offset of rapid, regular heartbeats. The rate frequently increases to over 150 beats a minute. The patient complains of palpitation and flutter of the heart, feels weak and faint, and is short of breath and apprehensive. Patients often arrest attacks of auricular paroxysmal tachycardia by holding the breath, inducing vomiting, bending forward, or pressing on the carotid sinuses. The latter is dangerous and should only be done by a doctor. He may suggest that the patient try other measures himself. If the attack persists over an extended period of time, the patient is put to bed, and the doctor may order digitalization and sedation. The treatment for ventricular paroxysmal tachycardia is bed rest and quinidine sulfate. The doctor may also order *procaine amide hydrochloride* (Pronestyl hydrochloride). This decreases the irritability of the ventricular muscle and when given orally acts in thirty to sixty minutes. If given intravenously, it must be given very slowly and the blood pressure taken as it is administered. If hypotension occurs, the rate of administration must be slowed down. The usual oral dose is 1 Gm. (15 grains), followed by 0.5 Gm. (7½ grains) every four to six hours.

Fibrillation

Auricular fibrillation is a common irregularity of cardiac rhythm. It usually is associated with organic heart diseases such as rheumatic heart disease, mitral stenosis, and myocardial infarction, but it may follow the excessive use of alcohol, excessive smoking, large meals, and anesthesia.[7] In this disorder the sinus node no longer controls the rhythm of the heart, the auricles no longer contract in coordination, and there is a complete irregularity of the ventricular beats. The auricles may receive as many as 400 to 600 stimuli a minute, but the ventricles rarely contract more than 130 to 150 times a minute, since not all the stimuli are carried over the auriculoventricular bundle and the ventricles do not respond to all the impulses that are sent through. When the ventricle beats this fast, there is little blood in the ventricle when systole occurs, and not enough blood is pumped into the aorta with each beat to produce radial pulsation. This accounts for the pulse deficit (the difference between the apical pulse and the radial pulse). The pulse deficit represents wasted cardiac energy. The nurse often is asked to record the apical-radial pulse rate several times a day since this gives an indication as to how well the patient is responding to treatment. In taking an apical-radial pulse rate, one nurse counts the apical beat, using a stethoscope, while a second nurse simultaneously counts the radial rate. One must be responsible for indicating the beginning and ending count so that results will be accurate. As the patient improves, the apical beat should gradually decrease until it is the same rate as the radial beat.

The patient who is fibrillating usually is put to bed and given either digitalis or quinidine sulfate. Digitalis acts by blocking the impulses that pass from the auricles to the ventricles, increasing the interval between the heartbeats so that the ventricles will contain more blood before they contract. *Quinidine sulfate* restores the normal rhythm by increasing the rest period of the auricular muscles. The doctor may order the pulse rate to be taken before quinidine sulfate is given; if there has been a marked slowing of the rate, it should be withheld. The usual dose of quinidine is 0.2 to 0.4 Gm. (3 to 6 grains) by mouth. It may be repeated every four hours for two to three days. When quinidine is first given, the patient should be watched carefully for toxic signs since many persons are allergic to it. If he becomes flushed, complains of ringing in the ears, or becomes nauseated or faint or if the pulse rate increases, the drug should be withheld until the doctor is consulted. In the patient with a diseased heart there is also the danger that the sudden return to a regular auricular heartbeat may cause emboli to break away from the auricular walls; thrombi are likely to have formed there while the blood has been pumped inadequately.

In *ventricular fibrillation* the coordinated contraction of the ventricles is replaced by rapid irregular twitching of the ventricular muscles.[7] Continued ventricular fibrillation is incompatible with life, since these twitchings do not force enough blood into the systemic circulation to meet body needs. Ventricular fibbrillation is often the cause of sudden deaths in patients with coronary artery disease and during or after the administration of some anesthetic agents. This condition is known as *cardiac arrest* and requires immediate and drastic emergency measures. The doctor may give procaine amide hydrochloride intravenously, or he may give it directly into the heart muscle. Cardiac massage may be done; the chest cavity is surgically incised directly over the heart, the ribs spread apart, and the heart massaged with the hands or stimulated with an electric current. A 100-volt alternating current with an amperage of 1.5 is used. Occasionally a patient is saved by these measures, but they must be employed within several minutes after the cessation of cardiac function.

REHABILITATION OF THE PATIENT WITH CARDIAC DISEASE

To help patients with diseases of the heart and circulatory system learn to live within the limits of their cardiac capacity, the nurse needs to know as much about the patient's condition as possible. She will need to know what the doctor has told the patient and his family and what limitations he has set for the patient. This information should be shared with others, such as the family, the social worker, the occupational therapist, the physiotherapist, the public health nurse, the industrial nurse, the employer, or the school teacher, who may assist in the rehabilitation program.

It is helpful to prepare a list of the activities that the patient usually engages in at home and at work so that the doctor can check those that he considers appropriate to resume. As the patient improves, more of the activities may be added to the approved list. Such a list serves as a guide for the patient and his family, and it may help him strike a balance between too many and too few restrictions. The patient, however, must use judgment and discretion in carrying out these activities, especially the pace at which they are performed. If they cause him to be tired or out of breath, they are too strenuous. Moderation should be the guiding principle. All activities should be carried out at a slower pace, and extra rest periods should be taken. The cardiac patient should not jump out of bed, should not run or walk fast, and should avoid climbing. Walking against a high wind and exercising at a higher altitude than usual also cause additional strain on the heart.

Patients with cardiac disease should strive for equanimity. All removable burdens such as those imposed by fatigue, obesity, infections, and emotional upsets should be removed. It is often difficult for a patient to achieve this without the help of his family. Cardiac disease usually affects the lives of others besides the patient. The entire family's mode of living may have to be changed, responsibilities may need to be reapportioned, and another member of the family may even have to become the wage earner. The life of a child should be planned so that he is not continually frustrated by restrictions. Major adjustments cannot help but disturb the patient, especially if the patient is a mother or a father. The nurse should find opportunities to talk to the family while the patient is still in the hospital since it is better if the family can begin to make adjustments at this time so that life will be smoother for the patient on his return home. They may be unaware of the changes that may be required in their lives or, if they are aware of the changes, they may need help in planning for them. They should realize that adjustments are not just temporary but must be permanent. Their successful adjustment to a new way of life may have a direct effect on how long and how happily the cardiac patient will live.

The doctor will prescribe the patient's diet. On discharge from the hospital some patients will be allowed to eat a regular diet but are told to eat in moderation since large meals increase the work of the heart during digestion. If the patient is overweight, a low-calorie diet will probably be ordered. A diet low in fat may be ordered for patients with a high blood cholesterol level since there is a possibility that this may be a factor in the development of coronary artery disease. The most common diet restriction, however, is a low-salt or a salt-free diet. Both the nurse and the dietitian should work closely with the patient and the family to be sure that they understand the dietary restrictions, why they are essential, and how to prepare acceptable meals. Plans should be worked out with the homemaker so that special food will not need to be prepared for the patient. If salt is restricted, for instance, the simplest method is to cook the food for the entire family without salt, set aside the patient's portion, and season the remainder. If the patient is on restricted salt intake, he should be advised not to take medications or other substances containing salt or sodium, such as saline cathartics, sodium bicarbonate, or soft drinks containing soda water. The teaching program should be started well in advance of the patient's discharge from the hospital; usually a public health nursing referral should be made, listing the specific problems to be checked.

Many patients with heart disease and their families can profit from regular health supervision visits by a public health nurse. If arrangements need to be made because the patient cannot climb stairs, for example, it may be helpful for the public health nurse to visit the patient's home before he is discharged. After seeing the situation, she may be able to make suggestions that will make him more comfortable and will make his care easier. If the patient happens to be the mother and housewife, minor changes especially in the work area of the kitchen may be possible so that she can sit down and carry out many of her housekeeping duties (see Figure 28). After the patient has arrived home, problems and questions often arise with which the nurse can help. This additional help may reduce the patient's fear and the uncertainty of his family so that he will accept his restrictions more readily. If the patient cannot return to full activity, the family may need help in providing nursing care in the home. For instance, sometimes one knows that elderly patients will be semi-invalids. If one or more members of the family take a course in home nursing offered by the American Red Cross, it is easier for the family to give essential care. Sometimes it is possible to do this while the patient is still hospitalized.

Provision for follow-up care should be made, and the patient should understand how important this is. The patient with heart disease should remain under medical supervision for the remainder of his life. In this way he may be kept in the best possible physical condition, one which will cause the least burden on his heart. He should also avoid the danger of additional damage and burden on the heart imposed by infections. If possible, he should avoid colds and other upper respiratory infections. If he does develop an infection, he should go to bed and call a doctor. The patient with cardiac disease will have a longer convalescence from any illness than the normal person and should return to full activity gradually.

When the cardiac patient is ready to return to school or work, the health service, if one is provided, should know exactly what the patient can and cannot do. Most patients will be allowed to return to normal activity unless it is too strenuous or they have a marked incapacity. If the nurse in the health service becomes aware that normal activity tires the patient, she should report this to her medical adviser so that further medical follow-up can be given and necessary job adjustments made. While many patients may return

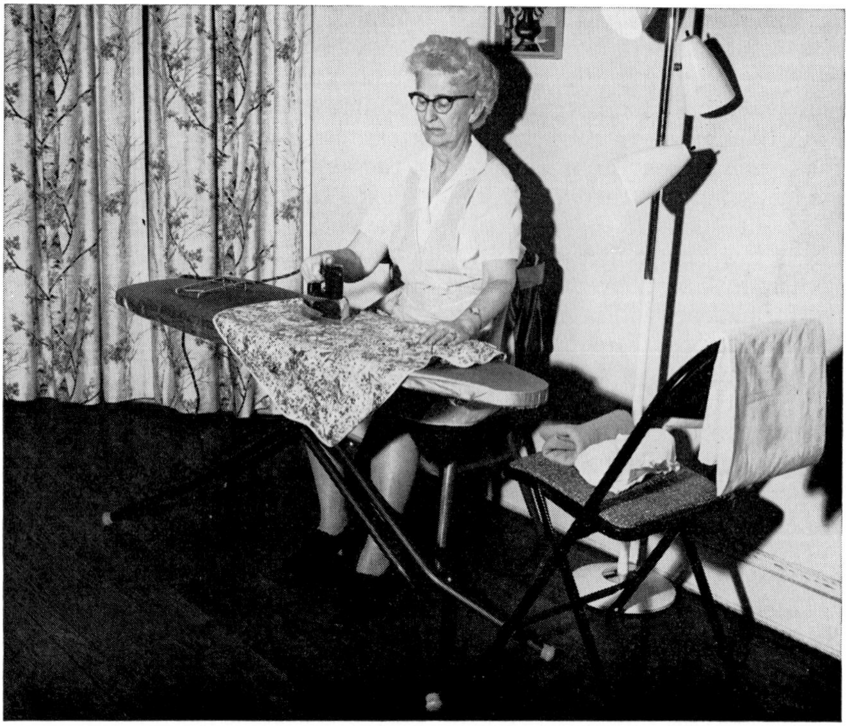

Figure 28

The patient with cardiac disease can be helped to make household activities easier. Note the comfortable position and the placement within easy reach of articles to be ironed.

to their former work, some must change their type of work.

Because heart diseases do cause loss of time at work and because the financial strain placed on the family is great, every effort should be made to evaluate each patient's condition and to place him in a position where he will be gainfully employed within his physical limitations. Help in locating a suitable position for the cardiac patient may be obtained from the local branch of the American Heart Association, from the division of vocationally handicapped in state employment services, and occasionally from adult cardiac clinics in hospitals. Using the functional and therapeutic classifications set up by the Criteria Committee of the American Heart Association, the doctor places the patient in the appropriate categories. There are four functional classifications and five therapeutic classifications.

Functional classification

Class I—No limitation of physical activity
Class II—Slight limitation of physical activity
Class III—Marked limitation of physical activity
Class IV—Unable to carry on any physical activity without discomfort

Therapeutic classification

Class A—Physical activity not restricted
Class B—Ordinary physical activity need not be restricted but patient should be advised against unusually severe or competitive efforts
Class C—Ordinary physical activity should be moderately restricted and more strenuous habitual efforts should be discontinued
Class D—Ordinary physical activity should be markedly restricted
Class E—Complete rest, confined to bed or chair

In some communities special workshops (such as the Altro Workshops in New York City) have a demonstration and research program for cardiac patients requiring rehabilitation.

The housewife with cardiac disease should also be considered, and some rehabilitation centers and hospitals have developed programs to help her adjust to her limitations and still be able to function in her role of wife and mother. Kitchen facilities similar to those found in most homes have been provided so that she may practice work-simplification measures and plan possible adjustments in the physical setup of her own kitchen. In a booklet entitled *Heart of the Home,* prepared by the American Heart Association, work simplification is discussed and changes that can be made in the physical facilities are outlined so that the housewife with cardiac disease can manage with a minimum of effort.

Most communities do not have extensive rehabilitative help available in any organized fashion, but no patient with heart disease should be without this type of assistance. Nurses and doctors can do much to help each patient, and this kind of assistance may be more important than medication.

SPECIFIC DISEASES OF THE HEART

Hypertensive heart disease

Hypertension is one of the most common causes of heart diseases, and it affects all age groups. The patient is said to be hypertensive when the resting systolic blood pressure reading is consistently over 140 mm. Hg, the diastolic pressure is over 90 mm. Hg, and any of the symptoms of hypertensive disease are present.[8] The elevation of the diastolic pressure is of greater significance than that of the systolic pressure. The diastolic pressure more closely indicates the pressure exerted on the arterial walls by the circulating blood exclusive of the additional pressure caused by the contraction of the left ventricle, the pulse pressure. In hypertension there is increased peripheral arteriolar resistance. The systolic pressure is the combination of diastolic pressure and pulse pressure.

Hypertension may be caused by chronic kidney infections such as glomerulonephritis and pyelonephritis, by polycystic disease of the kidneys, by coarctation of the aorta, and by certain adrenal and pituitary lesions. However, there is no known cause in 75 per cent of the patients,[7] and their condition is called *essential hypertension. Malignant hypertension* is no different from other types of hypertension except that it occurs most often in people in their twenties or thirties, and it characteristically progresses rapidly, with symptoms appearing within a few months.

Hypertension may be present for years before the patient has any symptoms. Since no prevention or specific treatment is known, doctors feel that it is best only to tell patients that they have a tendency toward high blood pressure and to reassure them that it may not cause any difficulties for ten or more years. Until symptoms appear, follow-up examinations may be suggested for only every six months to a year. No restrictions are placed on activity, except that young people are encouraged to participate in individual sports instead of group sports lest they feel impelled to overexert themselves so as not to let down their teammates. Moderation in all activities should be the rule, as it should be for all people. Excess in food, alcohol, tobacco, tea, and coffee should be avoided, and adequate rest should be obtained. If the patient has a tendency to become tense, he should be encouraged to talk to someone who will listen to his problems—a medical doctor, a member of his family, a friend, a minister, a nurse, a social worker, or a psychiatrist. The doctor may discuss the problem with members of the family to get their cooperation in freeing the home environment from tension-creating situations since emotional upsets increase the constriction of the already narrowed arterioles.

One of the first symptoms of hypertension may be headache. There may be fatigue, dyspnea upon exertion, failing vision, or symptoms of uremia. When tissues beyond the constricted arterioles receive too little blood or when a constricted arteriolar wall ruptures, symptoms appear. The heart, the brain, the kidneys, and the eyes most often give rise to symptoms. The patient may become blind, have a cerebral vascular accident, develop kidney failure, or develop heart failure.

Hypertensive heart disease occurs because the left ventricle gradually has to work harder and harder to push the blood against the increased arteriolar resistance. Sometimes the walls of the arteries all over the body become thicker and their lumens narrow; this is a form of arteriosclerosis. Arteriosclerosis is not necessarily present, however, and the arterioles may be normal except that they are constantly constricted. As the narrowing of the arteries increases, the left ventricle enlarges, and eventually it may no longer be able to adequately pump the blood out of the heart, causing congestive heart failure to develop. Inadequate blood supply through the coronary arteries may cause symptoms of angina pectoris, or an acute myocardial infarction may occur.

A variety of laboratory tests may be made on patients with hypertension in an attempt to determine the cause; complete kidney and endocrine studies often are done. If the cause cannot be found, the status of the heart, eyes, kidneys, and nervous system are determined and recorded on the patient's record as a guide in evaluating the course of the disease.

If the cause of the hypertension can be determined and if it is amenable to treatment, curative treatment is started. The treatment of essential hypertension and of hypertension caused by irreversible causes is usually palliative, and it may be divided into medical therapy and surgical therapy. The purpose of both types of treatment is to decrease the blood pressure, thus delaying the onset of serious complications. Sometimes the patient may be hospitalized, but often he is treated on an ambulatory basis.

Medical treatment. Bed rest may lower the blood pressure slightly, and it is usually part of the initial treatment of a patient with severe symptoms of hypertension. Sedatives such as phenobarbital are often given to relieve tension and to foster rest. In the past few years several new drugs have been used to lower the blood pressure. They all are potent and may cause undesirable side effects, which lessen their usefulness.

Rauwolfia serpentina (Raudixin) or partially purified fractions from it such as alseroxylon may be used in treating mild or moderate forms of hypertension. *Alseroxylon,* 4 mg. orally, is usually given at bedtime each day. It takes several weeks to obtain a maximum effect from this drug, and severe hypotension is not likely to occur. Both the systolic and the diastolic blood pressures are lowered. The drug is thought to act by depressing the hypothalamus and central sympathetic centers and by stimulating parts of the parasympathetic nervous system. Dizziness and headache are relieved, but the patient often complains of nasal congestion in the morning. This is relieved by antihistaminic drugs. Since alseroxylon may make the patient drowsy, he should be cautious while driving or working around machinery. The appetite is stimulated, and the patient may gain weight. Since the stimulation of the parasympathetic nerves causes increased bowel motility, nausea, vomiting, and diarrhea may occur. The side effects of the drug subside readily on reduction of dosage or withdrawal, but the hypotensive action continues for several weeks. Marked mental depression may necessitate stopping the drug. *Reserpine* is a purified alkaloid of *Rauwolfia serpentina.* Trade names for this drug are Serpasil, Rau-Sed, and Reserpoid.

Hydralazine hydrochloride (Apresoline hydrochloride) is used for patients with moderate or early malignant hypertension. It is thought to reduce the blood pressure by acting on the midbrain and by inactivating some of the pressor substances found in the blood. It increases the blood flow through the kidney, but this action is often transient. The drug is given orally in gradually increasing doses. The patient is usually started on 40 to 50 mg. of the drug a day, given in divided doses; the dosage may be increased to as much as 800 mg. a day. While the patient is receiving this drug, his blood pressure should be checked frequently. Nausea, vomiting, headache, tachycardia, tingling of the extremities, malaise, nervous tension, depression, and hypotension on standing may be toxic reactions. Any of these symptoms should be reported to the doctor. While the depression is often very distressing for the patient, the doctor may decide not to discontinue the drug, since with continued treatment the depression seems to improve.

Hexamethonium bromide (Bistrium bromide) is given for severe essential hypertension. It inhibits the transmission of nerve impulses through both the sympathetic and parasympathetic ganglia. The inhibition of impulses through the sympathetic ganglia prevents vasoconstriction and thereby causes an increased blood flow and a drop in the blood pressure. This drug is most effective when given subcutaneously. The dosage may vary from 15 to 200 mg., and the effects last from four to six hours. Patients may be taught to administer this drug to themselves. Some doctors have the patient or a member of his family learn to take the blood pressure so that the dose of the drug to be taken can be determined by checking the patient's blood pressure against a chart prepared for him by the doctor. Other doctors instruct the patient to stand still for one minute before taking the drug; if he becomes dizzy, he takes only half a dose of the drug. When the blood vessels cannot constrict normally, blood pools in the legs as the patient stands still, causing him to feel dizzy or to faint.

The patient must be taught sterile techniques, how to measure the dosage, and how to administer a subcutaneous injection. See the section on caring for the patient with diabetes for the principles of teaching patients to administer subcutaneous medications (Chapter 28). The patient who is taking Bistrium may have difficulty with constipation, and difficulty in voiding because of blockage of the nerves to the bowel and bladder by the drug. He may need to take a mild cathartic such as milk of magnesia every night. Manual pressure over the bladder may stimulate voiding. Bethanechol chloride (Urecholine chloride), orally or subcutaneously, relieves urinary retention and paralytic ileus; if the problem is not controlled by the more conservative measures, the doctor may order this. Bistrium also may cause dilated pupils, blurred vision, dry mouth, and transient nausea. Severe hypotension is the most dangerous complication.

Pentolinium tartrate (Ansolysen), mecamylamine hydrochloride (Inversine) and chlorisondamine chloride (Ecolid chloride) are more potent hypotensive drugs in the group producing ganglionic blockade, with action similar to that of hexamethonium, but they are more suitable for oral use.

Alkavervir (Veriloid) is a potent antihypertensive agent that causes a dilatation of the arterioles and constriction of the venous vascular beds. It causes a prompt lowering of the blood pressure, and it slows the heart. It should be given only under the direct supervision of a physician, since bradycardia, severe hypotension, respiratory depression, and collapse may result.[20] The blood pressure and pulse rate should be taken frequently; if the blood pressure falls too rapidly, if the pulse becomes irregular, or if vomiting occurs, the drug should be stopped. The patient may complain of epigastric burning and an increased flow of saliva. Usually 9 to 15 mg. of alkavervir is given daily in divided doses. Administration of this drug is usually given in a series with a short interval of time between doses.

Protoveratrine A and B (Veralba) is a drug used to lower the blood pressure of patients with tachycardia, renal failure, or convulsive episodes. The patient should be hospitalized during treatment with this drug. Usually 0.5 mg. is given by mouth after meals and at bedtime. It may also be given intravenously or intramuscularly. The patient may complain of flushing and excessive salivation, and he should be checked carefully for cardiac arrhythmia and hypotension. Complaints of substernal pain and chest tightness should be reported to the doctor, and the drug should be withheld until he has examined the patient.

Salt-restricted diets are sometimes ordered for patients with hypertension. Patients with associated renal disease and heart failure are often placed on this regimen. Two types of diet are commonly used: the 2 or 3 Gm. salt diet and the rice diet (Kempner diet). The rice diet contains less than 0.5 Gm. of salt, only 20 Gm. of protein, and little fat. For six weeks the patient may have only rice, fruit, and sugar. Other foods are then gradually introduced. Unless it relieves their symptoms, few patients will eat this type of diet. Since there is no evidence that this regimen slows down the progress of hypertension, doctors rarely order it until symptoms appear. In the summertime patients on these diets may need to take extra salt to prevent sodium depletion. If they develop abdominal or leg cramps, weakness, nausea, and vomiting, one should suspect that more salt is needed for normal body processes. A low-calorie diet may be ordered for obese patients, and if patients with symptoms of hypertension use alcohol, tobacco, tea, or coffee they are usually advised to use them in moderation.

Surgical treatment. Bilateral resection of some of the sympathetic fibers (sympathectomy) may be done to block stimuli to the blood vessels which they innervate. This, in turn, causes the vessels to dilate, increasing the flow of blood through the body and lowering the blood pressure. However, a sympathectomy does not always give the desired result in the patient with hypertension. Now that drugs are available to lower blood pressure, the operation is seldom done for hypertension. The nursing care of patients undergoing sympathectomy for hypertension is described in other nursing publications.[12]

Coronary artery disease

Coronary artery disease is caused by a narrowing or obstruction of the coronary arteries, resulting in a reduction of the blood supply to the myocardium. This may cause a temporary anoxia of the myocardium such as occurs in angina pectoris, or it may cause a complete obstruction of the blood supply to a portion of the myocardium such as occurs in myocardial infarction. The resultant damage to the heart muscle may cause severe cardiac complications such as congestive heart failure and arrhythmias, or it may cause cardiac standstill and immediate death. hi cholesterol a factor

In most instances atherosclerosis is the cause of coronary artery disease. Yellowish, fatty material composed largely of cholesterol is gradually deposited along the walls of the arteries, causing them to become fibrotic, thick, calcified, and narrow. The resultant reduction in blood supply to the body tissues first affects the myocardium.

If the atherosclerosis develops gradually, with progressive narrowing of the coronary arteries but no thrombus formation, a collateral circulation may develop to minimize the amount of anoxia to the myocardium although the blood supply through the coronary arteries decreases. The collateral circulation is seldom able to circulate enough blood, however, to maintain an adequate supply of oxygen to the heart muscle during excessive exertion. When an *acute coronary occlusion* occurs, it is thought that some of the cholesterol may break away from the wall of one of the coronary arteries, causing the wall to become ulcerated and a thrombus to form. As this thrombus increases in size, it completely closes off the circulation to a portion of the heart muscle *(myocardial infarction)*.

Atherosclerotic changes may occur at any age, but they are more common in people over 40 years of age. Symptoms of coronary heart disease usually do not appear until 50 or 60 years of age. Men are six times more prone to it at an early age than are women, but with increase in age both men and women are affected about equally.[8] Men who are muscular seem to be prone to the disease at an early age. Coronary disease seems to be most prevalent among sensitive, mentally overworked, stout men engaged in professional work and in business. It also is more prevalent in people who have a family history of coronary diseases.

At the present time the only possible prevention of symptoms of coronary artery disease is to "slow down" as one reaches early middle age. Activities which cause one to become excessively tired should be omitted, and vigorous activity after a heavy meal should be avoided. Recurrent pain above the waistline associated with activity or recurrent indigestion after meals suggests the advisability of a medical examination, since these symptoms may be caused by inadequate blood supply to the myocardium during periods when the heart is called upon to pump larger quantities of blood. Much research and speculation about prevention of atherosclerosis are being done, but effective measures are not yet established.

Angina pectoris. Angina pectoris is a serious cardiac disorder. Although it is usually caused by atherosclerosis of the coronary vessels, the incidence of angina pectoris is high in patients with hypertension, diabetes mellitus, thromboangiitis obliterans, polycythemia vera, periarteritis nodosa, and aortic regurgitation due to syphilis or rheumatic heart disease. It is characterized by paroxysmal retrosternal or substernal pain, often radiating down the inner aspect of the arm. This pain is usually associated with exertion and is relieved through vasodilation of the coronary arteries by means of rest or medication. It is believed to be caused by the blood supply being temporarily inadequate to meet the needs of the heart muscle. Variations of the location and severity of the pain frequently occur, but the same pattern recurs repeatedly in a given individual. The frequency and severity of the attacks usually increase over a period of years, and less and less exertion may cause an attack. No matter how mild the attacks, they may be complicated at any time by acute myocardial infarction, cardiac standstill, or death. The diagnosis of angina pectoris is made by history, but it may be confirmed by an electrocardiogram at rest, after exercise, or preferably during an attack.

Treatment. Treatment of the patient with angina pectoris is based on the symptoms and the predisposing factors. The success of the treatment in achieving a comfortable and worth-while existence for the patient depends upon educating him to live within his limitations, being guided by the pain. The nurse, as well as the doctor, should participate in the teaching program. Since the patient often is not hospitalized, the nurse in the doctor's office or in the clinic carries the major nursing responsibility for helping the patient with angina pectoris. He is taught to cease effort immediately upon experiencing pain, and to rest for several minutes after the pain has subsided. *Nitroglycerin tablets* placed under the tongue and allowed to dissolve in the saliva before swallowing often relieve the pain by causing vasodilation of the coronary arteries. Usually tablets containing 0.4 mg. (1/150 grain) of the drug are prescribed. Effects should be noticed in two or three minutes, but if pain persists the dose may be repeated two or three times at five minute intervals. Other nitrate preparations are available, but most patients prefer nitroglycerin since it is less expensive and causes fewer side effects. Perles of *amyl nitrite* come in 3 ml. doses and are preferred by some patients because the action is immediate. The perle is crushed into a handkerchief, and it should be inhaled no more than three times. Nitrite preparations cause flushing of the skin because of capillary dilation. The pulse and respirations increase, and the blood pressure may fall slightly. Many patients develop severe headaches from the use of nitrites; this can usually be overcome by decreasing the dosage. Some patients use nitroglycerin prophylactically when they have no choice but to undertake some activity which causes pain; the action lasts for about one-half hour. The patient with angina pectoris should always carry a nitrite preparation with him. He may use it freely since the effects do not decrease with usage, and it is not habit-forming. Many patients are reluctant to use the medication for various reasons and must be encouraged to do so by careful discussion of their objections.

Xanthine preparations such as theophylline ethylenediamine *(aminophylline)* or theobromine calcium salicylate may be given three or four times a day to produce a prolonged vasodilation. Since these preparations frequently cause nausea and vomiting, they should be given after meals or with food.

Diet. If the attacks or anginal pain are precipitated by eating, six small meals at evenly spaced intervals rather than three average meals may give relief. If the patient is overweight, a low-calorie diet may be prescribed. The doctor may suggest that the patient drink 15 to 30 ml. (½ to 1 ounce) of brandy or whiskey several times a day since this tends to dilate the blood vessels. Doctors usually advise the patient to smoke very little if at all.

Activity. Most patients with angina pectoris can tolerate mild exercise such as walking or golfing, but exertion such as running, climbing hills or stairs rapidly, and lifting heavy objects causes pain. The pain is likely to be more easily invoked in cold weather since the vessels normally constrict to conserve body heat. When the patient with angina pectoris must be exposed to the cold, he should err on the side of being too warmly clad. It is unwise for him to sleep in a cold room, and walking against the wind and uphill should be avoided since these require additional energy and cause pain.

Since excessive emotional strain also causes vasoconstriction by releasing epinephrine into the circulation, emotional outbursts, worry, and tension should be avoided. The patient may need continuing help in accepting situations as he finds them. The family, spiritual adviser, business associates, and friends can sometimes give help in this. An optimistic outlook helps to relieve the work of the heart. Many patients who learn to live within their limitations live out their expected life span in spite of the disease. Helping a patient to adjust to living with this disease can be most rewarding for the family, the patient, the doctor, and the nurse. Fear of impending catastrophe is almost a characteristic of anginal pain, and many patients believe each episode of pain is a "heart attack"; therefore, reassurance and education are extremely important.

Acute myocardial infarction. Acute myocardial infarction is caused by sudden blockage of one of the branches of a coronary artery. This may be extensive enough to interfere with cardiac function and cause immediate death, or it may cause necrosis of a portion of the myocardium, with subsequent healing by scar formation or fibrosis. The blood supply may be interrupted by the formation of a thrombus in the coronary artery; this is called *coronary thrombosis.* Coronary occlusion is a more general term including other causes of blockage of a coronary artery. Blockage may be caused by sudden progression of atherosclerotic changes or extended constriction of the arteries. Myocardial infarction usually follows an acute occlusion of a coronary artery.

Acute myocardial infarction is the most common cardiac emergency.[7] The patient typically complains of a sudden, severe, crushing or viselike pain in the substernal region. This pain may radiate into the left, and sometimes the right, arm and up the sides of the neck. At other times it may simulate indigestion or a gallbladder attack, with abdominal pain. The patient often becomes restless, gets up and paces about the room, throws open the windows, or has a sudden urge to have a bowel movement. He often feels that he is dying, and his skin becomes ashen and clammy. He may become dyspneic and cyanotic and show signs of severe shock. The pulse is usually rapid, and it may be barely perceptible; the blood pressure usually falls, and the patient may collapse.

Treatment. The patient who has had an

acute myocardial infarction is put on absolute bed rest immediately, and the doctor usually orders morphine sulfate or meperidine hydrochloride (Demerol) to be given at frequent intervals until the pain is relieved. If the patient is at all dyspneic or cyanotic or has severe pain, he is usually placed in an oxygen tent. If pain continues, the doctor may order theophylline ethylenediamine (aminophylline) or papaverine hydrochloride. Since both of these drugs relax smooth muscle, they help to dilate the coronary vessels.

Within the first twenty-four hours the temperature may become slightly elevated, and leukocytosis occurs. It is unusual for the temperature to be over 38.5° C. (101° F.), and any elevation over this should be reported to the doctor since it may be caused by a complication such as a pulmonary infarction. The fever and leukocytosis are normal reactions to tissue necrosis.

To confirm the diagnosis, blood sedimentation rate is determined, and an electrocardiogram is made. The electrocardiogram may show no changes for several days, but then usually shows changes indicative of a myocardial infarction. The blood sedimentation rate is elevated, and the blood cholesterol is often elevated.

The major objective in caring for the patient who has had an acute myocardial infarction is to provide him with physical and mental rest. The damaged heart may be able to maintain basal activity, but additional strain may cause it to fail. The patient is usually kept in bed for three or four weeks, and then, if the sedimentation rate has returned to normal and if he has no complications, he may gradually return to normal activity. During this period a collateral circulation has had a chance to develop, and the necrotic tissue in the myocardium has healed, forming a fibrotic scar. The convalescent period for most patients following a coronary occlusion is two or three months.

To decrease the possibility of further extension of the thrombus or embolic complications, the patient who has had a myocardial infarction is usually given an anticoagulant, such as Dicumarol, for three or four weeks. While he is receiving this drug, the doctor will order a daily prothrombin time determination; the dosage of the anticoagulant is based on this. The prothrombin time is maintained at approximately thirty seconds or 10 per cent of normal.[7] If the prothrombin time should drop below 10 per cent, there is danger that the patient will bleed profusely from minor cuts such as shaving nicks or from gum injuries suffered while brushing his teeth. Hematuria may also occur. The nurse should be alert for any signs of excessive or unusual bleeding and report them to the doctor. If bleeding should occur, the patient may be given vitamin K or a small blood transfusion.

The prognosis of a patient who has had an acute myocardial infarction is always guarded until about four weeks after the attack; 25 to 35 per cent of the patients die from the acute attack.[7] There is danger of such complications as pulmonary or systemic embolism, cardiac rupture, cardiac standstill, ventricular fibrillation, irreversible shock, and acute pulmonary edema. The first two weeks are considered the most dangerous, and patients who survive the third week usually recover from the attack.[7] The degree of residual disability cannot be predicted, however, and some patients are permanently incapacitated with severe angina pectoris or congestive heart failure. Many patients may return to normal or near-normal activity, and perhaps 60 to 80 per cent of patients who have recovered can return to some employment.

Nursing care. The patient who has had a coronary occlusion needs the best possible nursing care. The nurse must anticipate his needs so that he can rest; she must keep the environment conducive to rest and help the patient to obtain peace of mind. All the aspects of nursing care discussed under congestive heart failure and suggestions for the rehabilitation of cardiac patients in general and for the patient with angina pectoris in particular should be considered in caring for the patient who has had a myocardial infarction. Too often the patient is allowed to do too much for himself and to return to activity too quickly since, unless he has complications, he may appear quite well. His appearance may also make it more difficult for the family to comprehend fully the seriousness of the situation and the very real possibility of repeated attacks or death for the patient who does not respect his condition and live in moderation both physically and emotionally. During the first several days following an attack, however, the family usually is most concerned. The patient is likely to be quite apprehensive, perhaps for the rest of his life, and he may have many vague complaints. The nurse should listen carefully to his complaints and try to evaluate the situation. The symptoms may be caused by anxiety, or they may herald complications. Changes in the cardiac rate or rhythm, changes in blood pressure, and symptoms suggestive of congestive failure or embolic activity should be reported to the doctor at once.

Since the patient who has a myocardial infarction is quite likely to be in the prime of life and to have become suddenly ill, the nurse should anticipate that he may have many worries and concerns related to his business and to his family. It is often better for the patient if he is allowed to make some arrangements or at least told what arrangements are being made. The family, a business partner, or the social service worker may be able to give the help needed so that the patient can be more relaxed. The decision in this regard, however, is the doctor's. He often orders rather heavy sedation for the patient who seems exceedingly upset over business or family matters.

Before the patient is discharged, he and his family should have been instructed as to appropriate activities, how to follow a pattern of living in moderation, and how to recognize when activity or emotional strain is too great. The patient should know that, if he should have any further symptoms, rest is of prime importance and that the doctor should be contacted at once. He should remain under close medical supervision, and he should follow the doctor's suggestions and instructions. His chance of living for many years following an attack of coronary occlusion is good, provided he gives his heart special consideration. However, this does not mean constant concern over it, and, since this is a common problem, it is recommended that these patients read *Don't Worry About Your Heart.**

Rheumatic heart disease

Some inflammation of the heart almost always occurs during an attack of rheumatic fever. Since symptoms of heart involvement may not be evident, or they may not be present until late in the course of the disease, the patient with rheumatic fever must be kept on bed rest until all evidence of active disease has disappeared. Return of the blood sedimentation rate to normal is the guide most often used to ascertain when he may get up.

Rheumatic fever may occur in persons of any age between 4 and 50 years, but it seems to be most prevalent in children about 11 years old. It is slightly more common in girls than in boys. The disease in adults results in more cardiac complications and fewer joint symptoms than in children. Attacks of rheumatic fever in adults probably are recurrences. With each recurence further cardiac damage is likely to occur. (Care of the patient with rheumatic fever is discussed in Chapter 35.)

Cardiac involvement, such as myocarditis, endocarditis, pericarditis, or a combination of all of these, may be present. *Myocarditis* may be manifested by tachycardia, by changes in the character of the heart sounds, by enlargement of the heart, or by the onset of congestive heart failure. Irregularities of rhythm may occur, and the patient may complain of precordial pain.

Endocarditis is usually detected by the appearance of heart murmurs. As the in-

---

*Weiss, Edward: Don't Worry About Your Heart, New York, 1959 Random House, Inc.

flammation of the lining of the heart heals, scar tissue may form along the cardiac valves, preventing their complete closure or causing stenosis (narrowing) of the valve. These defects may be compensated for by the heart until its work is increased to such an extent that it cannot maintain an adequate output of blood. Congestive heart failure then occurs. This complication of endocarditis (congestive heart failure) often does not become evident, however, until the patient reaches young adulthood.

Pericarditis is associated with precordial pain, dyspnea, increased heart rate, and pericardial friction rub that may be heard on auscultation. It may eventually result in constriction of the heart motion because of scar tissue formation (adhesions). This may cause serious symptoms of heart failure. Pericardial adhesions may sometimes be excised surgically to release the constriction (see pericardectomy, page 256).

Prevention of complications and recurrences. Because recurrence of rheumatic activity may be precipitated by further streptococcal infections, the patient who has had rheumatic fever should avoid people with colds and sore throats, and he should keep his resistance high by eating a well-balanced diet, getting adequate sleep and rest, and protecting himself against exposure to dampness and cold. Oral penicillin may be prescribed in prophylactic doses for five years or longer after an attack of rheumatic fever, and all streptococcal infections are vigorously treated with penicillin and bed rest. Since tooth extractions, dental surgery, and gynecologic and rectal operations may activate rheumatic activity or initiate bacterial endocarditis, patients are often given antibiotics preoperatively, and they may be kept in bed for several days postoperatively.

Since rheumatic heart disease is the leading cause of death from disease among teen-agers in the United States, and since it is one of the most common types of heart disease, great efforts have been made to control it. Extensive studies have been carried out by the Division for Study and Control of Heart Disease of the United States Public Health Service and by the American Heart Association, so that much more is now known about how to prevent heart damage from occurring during an attack of rheumatice fever and how to prevent recurrent bouts of the disease. With the help of the Crippled Children's Division of the Federal Children's Bureau, twenty-five states have established approved rheumatic fever programs. Programs of instruction for parents in the home care of children with rheumatic fever have been organized, and in many large communities special hospitals or sections of hospitals have been set aside to care for children with rheumatic fever. Visiting teachers are available so that the child with rheumatic heart disease may continue his studies, and some communities have arranged for occupational and recreational therapists and volunteer workers to teach handicraft in the home and to provide recreation in other ways. The program for rheumatic children usually is coordinated by the public health agency, and the public health nurse is active in this.

Treatment. To keep a young child or an adolescent confined to bed for months and perhaps a year or more can be a traumatic experience both for the child and for his parents. The child who is accustomed to being active may be deprived of association with his playmates and schoolmates for most of the time. Unless the situation is handled carefully, the child may become resentful and may begin to feel that he is abnormal. Every effort must be made to keep his life as normal as possible and at the same time to give him rest. Very young children are not able to understand the situation and the teen-ager may become very resentful or he may become overconcerned with his health. The child should be kept busy and interested. Books, a phonograph, goldfish, parakeets, television, games, toys, and art work and handicraft may help to stimulate his interests and to keep him occupied. He should be comfortably propped up in bed and should have an overbed table at a height that maintains good body posture while he works or plays. If possible, he should continue his school studies, not only to give him something worth while to do but also to allow him to maintain his school status. Controlled visits with his friends will keep him from losing contact with their activities and help him to continue more normal social development.

When increased activity is allowed, the child may need to be closely supervised to prevent him from overdoing. Few activites are entirely prohibited, but the day's program needs to be planned to include frequent periods of less strenuous activity and periods of actual rest. If his heart has been seriously damaged, some activities such as sports and stair-climbing may be prohibited. The doctor, nurse, parents, and teacher should all work closely to help the child become a stable individual, working and playing within the limits of his physical capacity. When the child is older, the disease and the program should be more fully explained to him. This usually makes him more willing to accept limitations, and it guides him in setting up realistic goals for himself. This may prevent unnecessary frustrations from inability to carry through plans and activities. Since overprotection of the child and alarm over his condition is readily transmitted to him, most parents need help from both the doctor and the nurse in understanding their role in caring for the child with rheumatic fever.

The adult with acute rheumatic heart disease must learn to do everything slowly. He should not walk up stairs when elevators are available; if he must walk up stairs, he should do so slowly, resting frequently. He should avoid situations that do not allow him to rest when he needs rest. His job should not strain his physical capacity. He should avoid infections, and he should maintain good health practices, avoiding excesses in everything. He should remain under medical care and conscientiously carry out the doctor's suggestions. His health program should be one that will prevent the development of cardiac complications such as heart failure, yet one that will allow him to lead as happy and as full a life as possible. The patient who has only a murmur should be allowed to lead a normal life, but he should be given instruction related to prophylaxis.

Complications. The complications of rheumatic heart disease are serious, and they often incapacitate or cause the death of the patient. The most common complications are auricular fibrillation, the formation of thrombi in the chambers of the heart which may break off and be circulated in the blood stream as emboli, subacute bacterial endocarditis, and congestive heart failure caused by the narrowing and stenosis of the heart valves, especially the mitral valve. Auricular fibrillation usually is treated with digitalis or quinidine sulfate. The patient may be kept on anticoagulant therapy (Dicumarol) to prevent the formation of thrombi, and the patient who develops subacute bacterial endocarditis usually is vigorously treated with penicillin. Bacterial endocarditis is more fully discussed later in this chapter. If, because of mitral stenosis, symptoms of congestive heart failure become severe, mitral commissurotomy (surgery to enlarge the mitral valve) may be considered.

Mitral commissurotomy. Mitral commissurotomy is the fracturing (breaking apart) of the stenosed leaves (commissures) of the mitral valve, which is located between the left auricle and the left ventricle. In this operation, the thorax is entered through a left anterior lateral incision. The fourth rib is partially resected to give a better exposure, and then the heart is entered through the left auricular appendage. The surgeon inserts his finger through the incision into the auricle and through the mitral valve (see Figure 29). He then makes several attempts to release the leaves of the mitral valve either with his finger or with a special knife known as a valvulotome. At this point he will know whether or not the operation can be expected to relieve the

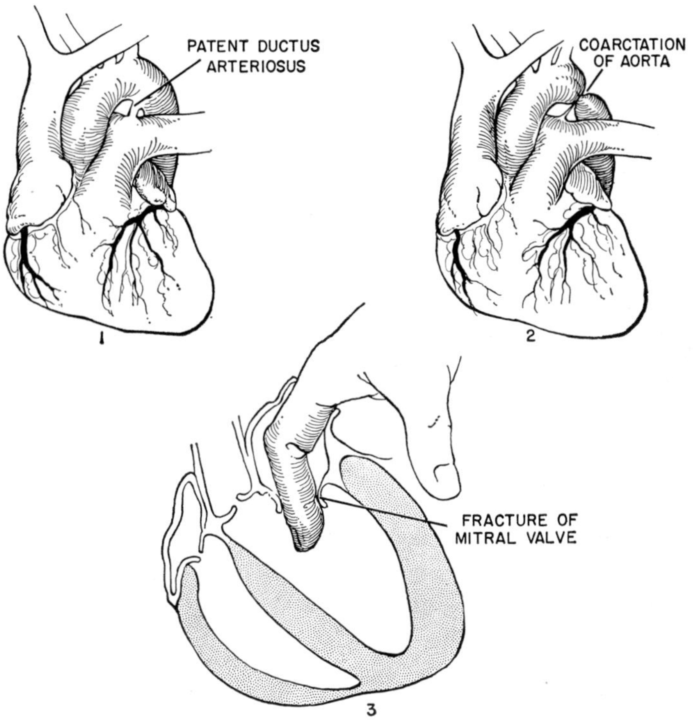

Figure 29

1, Illustrates the communication between the aorta and the pulmonary artery found in patients with ductus arteriosus. *2,* Illustrates the abnormality found in coarctation of the aorta. Note the engorgement above the constriction. *3,* Illustrates the technique used in a mitral commissurotomy.

patient's symptoms. Sometimes it is impossible to release the stenosed valve because of excessive calcium deposits around it or because of other pathology. If any clots are found, they are flushed out to prevent their escape into the general circulation.

The operation on the mitral valve is one of the most successful of all operations on the heart, and there is a low mortality rate associated with it. If the operation has been successful, there will be a decline in the pulmonary pressure, reduction of the heart size, and a gradual diminishing of the symptoms previously experienced. Many patients who have been semi-invalids are able to return to a relatively normal life. In some patients, however, the stenosis may recur after varying periods of time, and the symptoms may become worse than preoperatively.

The nursing care of the patient undergoing mitral commissurotomy is similar to that of other patients having other cardiac surgery. It is discussed in detail later in this chapter.

Chronic constrictive pericarditis

In chronic constrictive pericarditis, dense scar tissue, often impregnated with calcium deposits, forms over the heart, compresses the organ, and interferes with its function. The cause of this disease is unknown although it is suspected that the disease is infectious in origin and that perhaps a virus may be the cause.[7] The average age of patients with chronic constrictive pericarditis is 35 years, and 75 per cent of all patients are men.[7] Signs and symptoms may include an enlarged liver, venous distention, ascites, dyspnea, generalized edema, pleural effusion, cough, and cyanosis. The circulation time usually is prolonged, the venous pressure elevated, and the vital capacity moderately reduced. Physical activity usually is restricted by the symptoms. Chronic constrictive pericarditis may be cured or markedly improved by *pericardial resection.*

Pericardectomy (pericardial resection, decortication of the heart). A pericardectomy is the removal of the scar tissue that forms over the heart in the pericardium. The operation is performed through either a long, left, anteriolateral incision in the fourth intercostal space or through a sternum-splitting incision. The pericardium is carefully separated from the myocardium and removed. As the restricting tissue is removed, the constricted heart bulges through the opening and is able to contract more effectively. Almost at once many of the patient's symptoms are relieved. A chest catheter is usually inserted for drainage postoperatively. The nursing care of patients undergoing a pericardectomy is similar to that of those having other cardiac surgery. It is discussed in detail later in this chapter.

Congenital heart disease

Congenital heart disease no longer always has an unfavorable prognosis. More accurate diagnosis and evaluation of cardiac defects is now possible by means of angiocardiograms and cardiac catheterization. In the last decade advances in anesthesiology and surgical techniques have made correction of some congenital anomalies possible, and subacute bacterial endocarditis, one of the most frequent complications, can now be arrested with penicillin. The prognosis in congenital heart disease, however, is entirely on an individual basis. Patients who are treated before development of serious cardiac complications have a better prognosis. The nurse should urge parents of children with suspected anomalies of the heart to seek early medical care.

Only a few of the more common cardiac anomalies will be discussed here. For further information, see medical textbooks. Only variations from general principles of preoperative and postoperative care of patients undergoing cardiac surgery are given under each condition.

Patent ductus arteriosus. The ductus arteriosus is a blood vessel connecting the pulmonary artery and the aorta. In fetal life it is used to bypass the pulmonary circulation which is not yet being used. Normally this vessel closes soon after birth and becomes a fibrous band. When it does not completely close, it is said to be patent; that is, blood can flow through it. The lumen may vary in width from a few millimeters to the size of a large aneurysm.

Patent ductus arteriosus is more common in girls than in boys, and children with this defect are usually smaller in build than others of the same age. There are usually no other noticeable symptoms, and the lesion is often detected incidentally during a general physical examination. A typical murmur described as a "machinery murmur" or an "in-the-tunnel-murmur" can be heard on auscultation. The left ventricle is usually slightly enlarged, and the pulmonary vessels may be prominent on x-ray examination. On cardiac catheterization increased blood pressure and oxygen content are demonstrated in the pulmonary artery. This is due to the communication with the aorta which normally has a high pressure.

Without treatment, the life expectancy of a patient with patent ductus arteriosus is about twenty-five years.[10] Many patients contract subacute bacterial endocarditis, but most of them die from heart failure. The left ventricle eventually fails to compensate for the increased blood flow that it must provide, and left-sided heart failure ensues. Because of the serious complications of patent ductus arteriosus, surgery usually is advised for any patient between 5 and 35 years of age. It is difficult to make the diagnosis in children under 5 years of age, and after 35 years it is felt that the operation should not be attempted because of arteriosclerotic changes in the vessels which cause increased intravascular pressure and make ligation of the vessel difficult.

In performing the operation, the surgeon enters the left pleural cavity anteriorly between the second and third rib. The patent ductus is exposed and temporarily compressed to observe the effect of this on the blood pressure and the heart rate (see Figure 29). The procedure of choice in occluding the ductus usually is division of the ductus and suture of the ends.

Postoperatively the patients are given penicillin prophylactically. They are usually allowed to be up and walking by the fourth or fifth postoperative day, and they are discharged from the hospital about two weeks after the operation.

Coarctation of the aorta. Coarctation of the aorta is a narrowing of the aorta; it usually occurs in the distal portion of the aorta or just below the arch (see Figure 29). Because of this defect there is an elevation of the blood pressure in the upper extremities, and the pressure is lower than normal in the vessels below the constriction. The pulses in the lower extremities may not be palpable. To provide an adequate blood supply to the lower extremities, the intercostal vessels become dilated so that a collateral circulation is set up. On x-ray examination, the lower margin of the ribs may appear eroded; this is because of the marked dilatation and pulsation of the intercostal arteries. The patient may have no symptoms, or he may complain of throbbing in the head, frequent nosebleeds, and leg weakness. Because of the hypertension in the vessels above the constriction, complications usually begin to develop by the time the patient is 20 years of age. Death is usually caused by a cerebral vascular accident or a rupture of the aorta above the constriction.

Operations for the repair of this defect are most effective if done during childhood since the hypertension is relieved sooner, preventing irreversible changes in the vessels of the heart. The operation, however, can be performed safely up to the age of 20; after this age arteriosclerotic changes in the vessels may make the operation very difficult. The purpose of the operation is to resect the constricted portion of the aorta and to anastomose the vessel. Fortunately, because of the large collateral circulation, clamping of the aorta is possible while surgery is being done. When it is impossible to anastomose the vessel, an arterial graft of a human blood vessel or of plastic material may be inserted to replace the excised aorta.

Postoperatively, the patient who has undergone surgery for coarctation of the aorta usually is given penicillin, and he is kept flat in bed for ten days to two weeks to ensure a firm aortic scar before blood pressure in the aorta is increased by activity. The nurse may be asked to take the blood pressure in both the upper and the lower extremities. There should be a gradual fall in the pressure in the arms and a corresponding increase in the legs. Hemorrhage and thrombus formation are the most serious postoperative complications. Emboli may break away from the thrombus and cause infarction of the kidney or other organs and tissues. Arterial emboli to the vessels of the leg are not uncommon. Any sudden sharp pain, coolness or pallor of the extremities, dyspnea, changes in mentation, weakness of an extremity or the facial muscles, or a decrease in urinary output should be reported to the doctor at once. The symptoms of hemorrhage are the same as those of any internal bleeding. A doctor should be summoned immediately, since if the bleeding is extensive the patient will become exsanguinated shortly.

Patients for whom operation is not feasible are warned to avoid physical exertion such as straining and lifting heavy objects and to avoid excitement since these place extra strain on the heart and the vessel walls. They should avoid infections, and doctors will usually give them penicillin prophylactically before and after tooth extractions and operations of any kind since they are prone to develop subacute bacterial endocarditis.

Tetralogy of Fallot. Tetralogy of Fallot is a congenital anomaly of the heart in which there usually are four structural defects: stenosis near the pulmonary valve, an abnormal opening between the right and left ventricles, malposition of the aortic opening so that part of its blood is from the left ventricle and part from the right ventricle, and hypertrophy of the right side of the heart. Babies with this condition are often called "blue babies" since the outstanding symptom is cyanosis. This is primarily a pediatric condition and will not be considered further here.

NURSING THE PATIENT UNDERGOING CARDIAC SURGERY

Preoperative period

Before a heart operation is attempted, the patient's general health, and particularly the condition of the heart, is carefully evaluated and he is built up to the best physical condition possible for him. He must undergo many tests, and although these patients usually have had previous experience in hospitals because of their heart condition, they should be given an adequate explanation of all procedures. When it has been decided that benefit can be derived from an operation, the doctor discusses the procedure with the patient and his family. He usually tells them why the operation must be done, what he hopes it will accomplish, and what will be done.

In some instances patients have read or heard about heart operations and have come to the surgeon asking to have the procedure done. Some men and women, faced with increasing invalidism, decide that they would like to risk an operation in the hope of being able to live more normally.

Preoperative teaching. Although the doctor has thoroughly prepared the patient for the operation and the patient has prepared himself emotionally, he is still anxious and apprehensive. Surgery on the heart carries a risk; the patient realizes that there is no substitute for the heart and that life without it is impossible. Provision should be made for him to visit with his spiritual adviser and with his family during the preoperative period and on the morning of surgery. Many patients will wish to prepare a will. The anesthetist's visit to the patient preoperatively, usually gives him some reassurance.

All preoperative procedures should be explained to the patient. For example, blood pressure, apical-radial pulse, and temperature may be taken at very frequent intervals for a day or two preoperatively as a basis for comparison postoperatively. Explanation of all that will happen to him postoperatively has been found to make the patient less frightened and to help him to be more cooperative in carrying out the postoperative treatments. He is told that he may wake up in an oxygen tent since this is routine for many patients who have had cardiac surgery. A tent is used to give additional oxygen concentration so that the heart does not have to work so hard postoperatively, and the air-conditioning action makes the patient more comfortable. The patient is told that he will be asked to cough postoperatively to bring up mucus. He is shown how to do this and is asked to practice it under supervision. He should tighten his abdominal muscles, lower the diaphragm, and force himself to cough. Taking a breath that is deep enough to elevate the abdomen will lower the diaphragm and stimulate coughing. Coughing is essential to dislodge any plugs of mucus in the bronchi and, therefore, to allow full expansion of the lungs. The patient needs to know that he will have a heavy, tight feeling in his chest postoperatively. This is a normal reaction after cardiac surgery, but the patient often feels as though he is suffocating. If the patient asks about pain, he should be told that he will feel pain but that he will receive medication to alleviate it. He should be told that postoperatively the nurses will be taking his blood pressure and pulse frequently since this serves as a guide to his condition. If the doctor wishes, the patient may be told that he will have a tube in his chest wound for several days postoperatively to drain any fluid that may collect in the chest. Preoperatively the nurse should evaluate how much activity the patient is able to engage in without becoming tired, for this will serve as a guide in determining his postoperative condition.

Immediate preoperative care. The doctor orders a sedative so that the patient will sleep on the preoperative night. If necessary, this usually can be repeated. In the morning before the patient leaves for the operating room the doctor usually will start an infusion. A *venesection* (cut-down) is usually done; the vein is exposed through a small incision and a polyethylene tube is inserted into the vein. This obviates infiltration of the fluid and assures a patent vein in the event of circulatory collapse. A vein in the ankle is usually used because of the proximity of the arm to the operative area. A narcotic usually is not ordered as a preoperative medication for the patient undergoing cardiac surgery since it depresses respirations. Often phenobarbital sodium, 130 mg. (2 grains), is ordered, and only 0.2 mg. (1/300 grain) of atropine sulfate is given to decrease secretions since a larger dose might block the vagus nerve, increasing the stimuli to the sinoauricular node and causing fibrillation.

Postoperative period

Postoperative unit. While the patient is in the operating room, the nurse should prepare the unit for his return. It is preferable that he be in a room by himself since he will need constant observation for several days. An oxygen tent may be set up. If Alevaire is routinely used to loosen secretions, a setup for this is attached to the tent. Chest suction apparatus should be ready to attach, and a thoracentesis set and a cardiac arrest tray (scalpel, hemostats, and rib spreaders) should be readily available in the event that air or fluid must be withdrawn from the chest cavity or cardiac massage done as emergency measures. Infusion poles, a sphygmomanometer, and a stethoscope should also be at the bedside. Nasal suction apparatus should be available since the patient may need to be suctioned to remove mucus. Some cardiac surgery is done while the temperature of the body is lowered (hypothermia). If this is so, equipment to apply external heat will be needed. (See Chapter 13 for a discussion of hypothermia.)

Postoperative care. After cardiac surgery, the patient is kept flat in bed until he has reacted from the anesthesia, and then he usually may be put in a semihigh or high Fowler's position. The doctor usually will allow him to lie on either his back or the side operated on and will order that he be turned at least every two hours. Following cardiac surgery it is generally advisable to keep the unoperative side uppermost so that the lung on this side will be able to maintain its full expansion. The chest catheter is attached to closed drainage or to chest suction apparatus (Chapter 23, page 474). The patient is placed in the oxygen tent, and the doctor may want the blood pressure reading and pulse rate taken every fifteen minutes for twenty-four hours; the frequency is gradually decreased until they are only taken twice a day. The patient should be observed for any signs of shock, hemorrhage, spontaneous pneumothorax, mediastinal shift, cardiac arrhythmias, or congestive heart failure. Following heart surgery, the patient may need constant attendance for twenty-four to seventy-two hours; if left alone he may become extremely apprehensive and mental stress increases the work of the heart.

Although the patient is usually allowed clear fluids as soon as nausea subsides, supplementary intravenous fluids are given for two or three days or until he takes adequate fluids by mouth. Depending upon the postoperative cardiac condition, the doctor usually places some restriction upon the amount of fluids the patient may take. He usually is permitted to have about 1,500 to 1,800 ml. a day. The nurse, members of the auxiliary staff, and the patient should be aware of this and keep accurate measurement of the fluid intake. Intravenous fluids should be administered slowly to prevent overloading the circulatory system and placing additional strain on the heart. The patient usually resumes a diet containing 2 or 3 grams of salt and remains on this until all signs of congestive heart failure have disappeared, which may not be until some time after his discharge from the hospital.

A narcotic such as meperidine hydrochloride (Demerol) may be ordered to relieve the pain; some surgeons order small doses given frequently (Demerol, 25 or 50 mg. every two hours) since the pain is very severe and since larger doses may inhibit respirations. Pain usually persists for three or four days and is caused by severance of the intercostal nerves. The chest catheter may also irritate the pleura and cause pain. If pain in the incision persists over a long period of time, the doctor may infiltrate the area above and below the incision with procaine. Since the pain is often made more severe by coughing, the patient may refuse to cough or take deep breaths. The pain experienced during an attempt to cough may frighten the patient so that he is afraid to try again. Because of this, coughing should be encouraged about half an hour after the narcotic is given, and whenever coughing is encouraged, the incision should be splinted manually or with a towel or drawsheet (see Figure 68). If the patient does not cough productively and if his breathing sounds moist or "rattley," the doctor should be notified, for he may wish to use endotracheal suction. After the chest catheter has been removed, coughing and turning usually are easier. There is no definite day on which the chest catheter is removed, for this depends on the amount of drainage and air present in the pleural cavity and on the re-expansion of the lungs. Usually however, it can be removed two or three days postoperatively. Antibiotics are given routinely to prevent infection.

Postoperatively the pulse should be checked carefully for rhythm, strength, and rapidity of beat. The doctor may order the apical-radial pulse rate taken since auricular fibrillation often develops about the third day in patients who have had heart surgery. The patient may be aware of palpitation; since this may frighten him, the doctor may tell him it can be expected. When auricular fibrillation occurs, it is controlled by medication. Depending upon the doctor's findings, digitalis or quinidine sulfate is used. If the patient has been on digitalis and/or mercurial diuretics preoperatively, these medications are usually resumed.

While the patient is bedfast, the nurse should encourage him to do arm and leg exercises. These may be done passively by the nurse at first; however, as the patient becomes stronger, the doctor usually wants him to be encouraged to tighten his leg muscles, move his feet up and down, and move his arms through the full range of motion. The patient usually will not use his left arm without being urged, since motion causes pain in the operative area. To prevent a stiff, unusable shoulder, however, exercises should be gradually instituted. The nurse should supervise the exercising of the left arm and shoulder until the patient has regained full range of motion.

Many patients have profuse diaphoresis after cardiac surgery. This may be more pronounced at night. The exact reason for this is not known. The patient should be kept dry and comfortable, and be reassured that this is a fairly common occurrence and that it will gradually subside. The temperature may rise markedly and remain elevated for several days. It is believed that this may be due to the presence of blood within the pericardium.

Some patients experience a period of depression or even disorientation after cardiac surgery, although this does not generally last very long. The patient may become very excited and fearful or he may have hallucinations. Other patients complain of varying degrees of depression. This reaction often occurs in the early postoperative period, and the nurse should be aware of this possibility. The cause is unknown, but it is thought that it may be caused by medication, fear, or some cerebral disturbance. The family also should be prepared for this possibility. During this period, the patient needs a calm environment and much reassurance and understanding. He should be protected from anything or anyone that seems to upset him further.

Ambulation. Mobilization of the patient depends upon the operation and the status of the heart. In general, patients who have had surgery for a coarctation of the aorta or any other surgery on the aorta are kept flat in bed for about ten days to prevent unnecessary strain on the vessel since the blood pressure is lower when the patient is flat. Some doctors do not permit the patient to be turned for several days. Before getting out of bed, the patient must gradually become accustomed to having the head of the bed elevated. When this is first attempted, he may complain of dizziness and faintness. If so, he is returned to a flat position, and elevation is attempted again later. Patients who have had surgery for patent ductus arteriosus and mitral stenosis are kept in Fowler's position postoperatively and are encouraged to move their arms and legs. Unless the cardiopulmonary status is very poor, they are allowed to begin ambulation by the fifth or seventh postoperative day.

The time of ambulation for each patient depends upon his progress and condition, but it usually proceeds as follows: The first day he dangles his feet over the side of the bed for fifteen minutes in the morning and afternoon. The second day he is allowed to sit in a chair at the side of the bed for fifteen minutes in the morning and afternoon. The third day he walks around the room while he is up. The fourth day he is allowed to walk around the room and to sit in the chair for gradually increasing periods of time. By the fifth day he may walk increasing distances. He should be closely supervised during ambulation, and no activity that causes fatigue, dyspnea, or an increased pulse or respiratory rate should be continued. If any of these symptoms appear, he should return to bed and the doctor should be consulted before further activity is attempted. Definite instructions are left by the doctor regarding when the patient may attempt to climb stairs. This should be done slowly under the supervision of a nurse. Only two or three steps should be attempted the first time, gradually increasing this until a flight or more, if ordered, are accomplished. The patient should rest two or three times while climbing one flight of stairs.

Long-term postoperative care. The patient and his family need to be told that no marked improvement will be noticed immediately after the operation—that it will be at least three to six months before the full result of the surgery can be ascertained. It is essential that all patients be given this information so that they will not be depressed by dyspnea or pain that is still present postoperatively. Sometimes even when the patient has not benefited from surgery, he may think he feels better, and this is to be encouraged.

In preparation for discharge from the hospital, the patient is asked to make a list of activities usually carried out at home. This is discussed with the doctor to ascertain the activities he feels are appropriate. The woman usually will want to know if she can dust, make beds, wash dishes, and do other household chores. The man may wish to know exactly what he may do—how much he can walk, what he can do about the house and the yard, and when he can report to work. Patients are usually advised to start slowly and progress gradually to more complicated tasks. The doctor will want them to return for frequent medical follow-up examinations, at which time he will advise them regarding additional activities. The patient should not think of himself as an invalid and should be allowed to do anything that does not tire him. On the other hand, he must be restrained from attempting too much.

The family of the patient who has undergone cardiac surgery should be aware of his condition and how much he can do. Since the patient has often been an invalid preoperatively, the family may be as fearful as he about his activity. They should understand how important it is for him to continue to see his doctor regularly and why he must continue to take his medication and remain on his diet. A public health nurse is often asked to supervise the home program.

OPEN HEART SURGERY

Open heart surgery is now being done on patients who have had unsuccessful results from closed operations on the heart, and on certain selected patients with pulmonic stenosis, aortic stenosis, atrial septal defects and ventricular septal defects. The open heart approach can be used only if the patient is under hypothermia and/or if an extra corporeal circulation is maintained by means of the heart-lung (pump-oxygenator) apparatus. The risks involved with open heart surgery is higher than with closed heart surgery.

Extracorporeal circulation (heart-lung machine, pump-oxygenator apparatus)

The use of the pump-oxygenator as a temporary substitute for the heart and lungs permits the surgeon to see the defect with which he is working, gives him a relatively bloodless field in which to work, and provides him with more time in which to correct the defect (sixty to eighty-five minutes). There are a variety of extracorporeal oxygenator systems in general use for open heart surgery. The most widely used are the bubble method and the screen or rotating disc types. The purpose of the method is diversion of the blood which normally goes to the heart into the machine where carbon dioxide is removed and the blood is oxygenated and then pumped back into the general circulation.

Immediately before the operation the pump-oxygenator is prepared for use by filling it with approximately 2,500 ml. of blood which has been freshly drawn from donors on the morning of the operation. Heparin is added to the blood to prevent it from clotting. The patient is then anesthetized with a general anesthetic, an intratracheal catheter is inserted, a bilateral thoracotomy incision is made, the sternum is transected, and the pericardium entered. The patient is then given heparin intravenously and catheters are inserted into the superior and inferior vena cavae. The catheters are attached by a Y connecting tube to rubber tubing which enters the pump. These catheters deliver the venous blood to the pump-oxygenator. A catheter is inserted into the common femoral artery and connected to tubing attached to the pump. This catheter will return the blood that has been oxygenated by the machine to the systemic circulation. When all catheters are inserted and attached, the machine is set into operation, the vena cavae are occluded, and correction of the cardiac defect is undertaken. Blood is returned to the patient's body at the rate of 50 to 60 ml. per kilogram of body weight per minute to maintain the peripheral pulse at 80 to 90. The blood is kept at body temperature by means of a heating unit in the machine. The blood is oxygenated by means of an oxygen inlet within the machine, and a chemical bath, through which the tubing runs, removes the carbon dioxide.

After the defect has been corrected, the vena cavae are unclamped, the pump is stopped, and the venous catheters are removed. Protamine sulfate is given to counteract the heparin and restore the coagulation time of the blood to normal.

Nursing care

The patient who has undergone open heart surgery requires constant nursing care. The nurse must be alert for signs of hemorrhage, hypotension, fibrillation, arrhythmias, sudden chest pain, and pulmonary edema. Mortality is highest within the first forty-eight hours.

Upon return from the recovery room, the patient is placed in an oxygen tent in low Fowler's position. The two chest catheters from the right and left pleural spaces are attached to a closed drainage system and the color and amount of drainage is checked routinely. There will be some bleeding during the first forty-eight hours, but any increased amount must be reported to the surgeon immediately. The dressings should be inspected frequently for blood. Because of the large amounts of heparin used, hemorrhage is rather common. Drugs such as vitamin K, protamine sulfate, Premarin, or Adrenosem are given to counteract the bleeding tendency caused by the heparin.

The blood pressure, apical-radical pulse, and respiratory rate are taken every fifteen minutes to detect signs of hypotension, fibrillation, and arrhythmia. The nurse should be alert for sudden hypotension with sharp pain which would indicate a coronary occlusion. Blood tinged or frothy sputum usually indicates pulmonary edema. A mucolytic agent such as Alevaire is usually administered by means of the Bennett breathing apparatus, and the patient should be encouraged to breathe deeply and to cough productively every two hours. Roentgenograms of the chest taken with a portable machine and electrocardiograph readings of the heart will be taken daily to evaluate lung expansion and determine heart function.

A self-retaining (Foley) catheter is inserted into the bladder, urine is collected every hour and checked for specific gravity, color, and amount. The patient should excrete 15 to 30 ml. of urine every hour. This frequent observation of his urine helps detect signs of kidney shut-down or failure and bleeding.

The patient usually is permitted clear, low-salt fluids by mouth as soon as desired, but his total fluid intake is restricted to between 2,000 and 2,200 ml. of fluid daily for a few days postoperatively to prevent overloading the circulation. He may be turned from side to side every hour to a 60 degree angle. Care must be taken that the catheters are not compressed by the body or by pillows.

The patient who has undergone open heart surgery is given antibiotics almost routinely, and these are often given intravenously. Meperidine hydrochloride (Demerol) is the drug most often used for pain.

If the patient progresses satisfactorily, after the first few days, he is placed on the postoperative cardiac regimen described earlier in this chapter.

SUBACUTE BACTERIAL ENDOCARDITIS

Subacute bacterial endocarditis is a serious complication of heart diseases. Organisms in the blood stream invade the heart. The valves are most often involved, being covered with vegetations or products of bacterial degeneration. The most common organism affecting the heart is the streptococcus, and its invasion is usually preceded by rheumatic involvement of the cardiac valves or a congenital heart anomaly. Diseased teeth and gums also seem to predispose to subacute bacterial endocarditis.

The patient usually complains of recurring bouts of fever, often dating from an attack of "grippe." He may have petechiae (small capillary hemorrhages) in the conjunctiva, in the mouth, and on the legs, and his fingers are often clubbed if the infection occurs in the presence of congenital heart anomaly. If the disease is untreated, it progresses rapidly, and death may follow within one or two months of onset as a result of emboli to the lungs, kidneys, brain, or spleen or as a result of heart failure. Ninety per cent of patients with subacute bacterial endocarditis can now be cured by the administration of massive doses of penicillin or other antibiotics. It is important to obtain the organism by blood culture prior to treatment to aid in selection of proper antibiotics. Treatment is usually continued for from two to six weeks, and the patient is kept on bed rest during this time and for some time afterward. Prevention of bacterial endocarditis by early and adequate treatment of infections, especially streptococcal infections, and by the administration of prophylactic doses of antibiotics to patients with known heart disease before and after tooth extraction or operation is more important than treatment of the disease. During healing after active infection, the cardiac valves may become scarred, resulting in functional difficulty and eventual heart failure, although the infection itself is cured.

CARDIOVASCULAR SYPHILIS

Cardiovascular syphilis usually occurs from fifteen to twenty years after the primary syphilitic infection. Since the highest incidence of primary syphilis is in the 20-year-old age group, patients with symptoms of cardiovascular syphilis are usually over 35 years of age. If the primary infection is not treated, 5 per cent of the patients will develop aortitis; 2 or 3 per cent, aortic insufficiency; and 1 or 2 per cent, aortic aneurysms.[33]

It is the aim of health organizations and medical personnel to treat all persons with syphilis before they develop cardiovascular disease or any of the other complications of late syphilis. Primary syphilis can be arrested; however, once syphilis has affected the aorta and the valves of the heart, little can be done except to treat the patient symptomatically. The treatment of primary syphilis is discussed in Chapter 17.

In cardiovascular syphilis the spirochetes attack the aorta, the aortic valve, and the heart muscle. The portion of the aorta nearest the heart usually is affected, and the elastic wall of the aorta becomes weakened and bulges. This bulge is known as an aneurysm. As the aneurysm grows, it may press on neighboring structures, such as the intercostal nerves, and cause pain. Aneurysms may also be present without symptoms; evidence may be discovered on x-ray examination. There is possibility of the aneurysm rupturing as it increases in size, and little can be done for the patient except encourage him to avoid excessive and strenuous activities which might cause a sudden increase in the pressure exerted against the bulging vessel.

Syphilis may also attack the aorta more diffusely, causing aortitis. The aorta becomes dilated, and small plaques containing calcium are laid down. Patients may complain of substernal pain associated with exertion due to constriction at the orifices of the coronary arteries. Thrombi may develop along the aorta, causing death. An embolus or myocardial infarction may develop.

The spirochete may also attack the aortic valve, causing it to become scarred. This causes aortic insufficiency, and the patient may have a bounding pulse and a high systolic blood pressure because of the extra effort expended by the ventricles to pump blood into the systemic circulation. Heart failure eventually occurs.

The use of penicillin in the treatment of the patient with cardiovascular disease is thought possibly to prolong life, since penicillin destroys any active organisms and permits healing to occur. Treatment at this stage, however, will not restore damaged aortic tissue or damaged aortic valves, and extensive scarring may occur. The patient with cardiovascular syphilis should be given guidance in planning his activities of daily living and in selecting work that places the least possible burden on the damaged heart and aorta. In certain cases of aneurysm or aortic insufficiency, surgery is possible. A more complete discussion can be found in recent publications.

REFERENCES AND SELECTED READINGS*

1 *Beveridge, Robert J.: Cardiac Catheterization, Am. J. Nursing 49:214-216, April 1949.
2 *Blakeslee, Alton: How to Live With Heart Trouble, New York, 1950, American Heart Association.
3 *Blakeslee, Howard: Know Your Heart, New York, 1948, American Heart Association.
4 Brown, Amy Frances: Medical Nursing, ed. 3, Philadelphia, 1957, W. B. Saunders Co.

*References preceded by an asterisk indicate material particularly well suited for student reading.

5 Bullen, Stanley A.: The Important Uses of Electrocardiography, Am. J. Nursing **55**:1378-1380, Nov. 1955.

6 Cardiovascular Surgery, A Symposium, Bull. New York Acad. Med. **29**:665-708, Sept. 1953.

7 Cecil, Russell L., and Loeb, Robert F. (editors): A Textbook of Medicine, ed. 10, Philadelphia, 1959, W. B. Saunders Co.

8 Cooper, Lenna F., Barber, Edith M., Mitchell, Helen S., and Rynbergen, Henderika: Nutrition in Health and Disease, ed. 13, Philadelphia, 1958, J. B. Lippincott Co.

9 *Creighton, Helen, and Hufragel, Charles A.: Aortic Insufficiency and Its Surgical Treatment, Am. J. Nursing **58**:547-550, April 1958.

10 *Crystal, Dean K.: The Operable Cardiac Anomalies, Am. J. Nursing **49**:587-589, Sept. 1949.

11 *Davidson, Sidney: Diet and Cardiovascular Disease, Am. J. Nursing **57**:194-196, Feb. 1957.

12 *Fedder, Helma: Nursing the Patient With Sympathectomy for Hypertension, Am. J. Nursing **48**:643-646, Oct. 1948.

13 *Fletcher, Anthony P., and Sherry, Sol: Fibrinolytic Therapy for Coronary Heart Disease, Circulation **22**:619-626, Oct. 1960.

14 *Frohman, I. Phillips: Digitalis and Its Derivatives, Am. J. Nursing **57**:172-175, Feb. 1957.

15 *Gaughan, Laurette: Cardiac Workers in Industry, Am. J. Nursing **57**:210-212, Feb. 1957.

16 Glenn, Frank, and O'Sullivan, Ward D.: Coarctation of the Aorta, Ann. Surg. **136**:770-776, Nov. 1952.

17 *Hansen, A. E.: Rheumatic Fever, Am. J. Nursing **53**:168-171, Feb. 1953.

18 *Henderson, Lilian: Nursing Care of the Patient With a Valvulotomy, Am. J. Nursing **54**:424-428, April 1954.

19 Keown, Kenneth K., and others: Open Heart Surgery—Anesthesia and Surgical Experiences J.A.M.A. **165**:781-787, Oct. 19, 1957.

20 Krug, Elsie E.: Pharmacology in Nursing, ed. 8, St. Louis, 1960, The C. V. Mosby Co.

21 *Liberson, A. Theodore: The New "Tranquilizing Drugs," Am. J. Nursing **55**:1465-1466, Dec. 1955.

22 Modell, Walter, and Schwartz, Doris R.: Handbook of Cardiology for Nurses, New York, 1954, Springer Publishing Co., Inc.

23 Monthly Vital Statistics Report, Aug. 22, 1958, U. S. Department of Health, Education, and Welfare.

24 *Moyer, John H.: Diuretics, Am. J. Nursing **59**:1119-1124, Aug. 1959.

25 Musser, Ruth A., and Bird, Joseph G.: Modern Pharmacology and Therapeutics, New York, 1958, The Macmillan Co.

26 Nurse, Amy G.: But Why Can't I Get Up? Am. J. Nursing **53**:172-174, Feb. 1953.

27 *Overholser, M. T.: Congenital Cardiac Program and the Nurse, Am. J. Nursing **53**:1470-1480, Dec. 1953.

28 Price, Constance: Mitral Stenosis, Am. J. Nursing **51**:72-74, Jan. 1951.

29 *Sachs, Bernard A.: Arteriosclerotic Heart Disease, Am. J. Nursing **55**:838-841, July, 1955.

30 *Silber, Earl N.: Medical Management of Angina Pectoris, Am. J. Nursing **55**:168-169, Feb. 1955.

31 Sprague, Howard B.: The Normal Senile Heart. In Stieglitz, Edward J. (editor): Geriatric Medicine, ed. 3, Philadelphia, 1954, J. B. Lippincott Co.

32 Statistical Abstract of the United States, 1956, U. S. Department of Commerce, U. S. Bureau of Census.

33 Stewart, Harold J.: Cardiac Therapy, New York, 1952, Paul B. Hoeber, Inc.

34 Todd, James C., and Sanford, A. H.: Clinical Diagnosis by Laboratory Methods, ed. 12, Philadelphia, 1953, W. B. Saunders Co.

35 White, Paul Dudley: Heart Disease, ed. 4, New York, 1951, The Macmillan Co.

36 *Wood, Edwin C.: Understanding the Patient With Heart Disease, Nursing Outlook **7**:90-92, Feb. 1959.

37 Wright, Irving Sherwood: Vascular Diseases in Clinical Practice, ed 2, Chicago, 1951, Year Book Publishers, Inc.

38 *Zoll, Paul M., and others: Use of External Electric Pacemaker in Cardiac Arrest, J.A.M.A. **159**:1428-1431, Dec. 10, 1955.

The patient with peripheral vascular disease

Chapter 19

Study questions for review

1 Review the anatomic structure of the arteries and veins. What are the major differences? What forces work to assist the return of blood from the veins to the heart?
2 What is meant by collateral circulation? Is it uniform throughout the body?
3 Consult your notes on pathology, and review the major differences between arteriosclerosis and atherosclerosis. What vessels are primarily affected by these two conditions?
4 Review the basic procedures for warm and hot soaks and for continuous warm packs. What are the general precautions to be taken in care of patients having these treatments?

Peripheral vascular diseases are usually only part of a complex disease syndrome that affects the entire body. Cardiovascular-renal disease is one of the most widespread conditions of our times and, indeed, it is rare for anyone to live to old age without undergoing some pathologic change in the cardiovascular system. It has been estimated that at least 60 per cent of all persons in the United States who are 50 years of age or over will die of cardiovascular-renal disease. Because peripheral vascular disease of the extremities is so often associated with other cardiovascular diseases, it is difficult to determine statistically how many persons die primarily of the former condition. It is obvious, however, that this is one of the most important disease groups with which the nurse will work and one in which her greatest effort toward early control is well justified.

Peripheral vascular disease is actually a general term which refers to all disease of blood vessels outside the heart. This chapter, however, will be concerned largely with peripheral vascular disease of the lower extremities. There are certain aspects of nursing care common to most patients with peripheral vascular disease. To avoid repetition, general nursing care that applies to patients with the more common peripheral vascular diseases will be considered before individual disease conditions and related nursing responsibilities are discussed. Lower limb amputations are considered in this chapter because, unfortunately, they are necessary for some patients who have peripheral vascular disease. Techniques of treatment and nursing care are similar to those used for the patient who has had an amputation following trauma, although rehabilitation of the latter is usually less difficult because he usually does not have a chronic medical disease.

GENERAL NURSING CARE

At present there is no specific way to prevent peripheral vascular disease. However, many general measures may be helpful, and much can be done to control the disease and thus enable the patient, in many instances, to live out his life in reasonable health and comfort. Much of the general nursing care of those with peripheral vascular disease is concerned with limiting progress of the disease and with the prevention of complications if mild symptoms appear. The nurse must teach health conservation measures to those who have early signs of vascular disease. In industry the nurse who helps the employees find chairs of a suitable height so as to prevent sharp knee flexion is contributing to prevention of disease. Long hours of sitting with the knees bent causes pressure on the arteries and veins of the legs, resulting in slight swelling and discomfort. The nurse may plan with supervisors in industry to provide short rest periods at frequent intervals for those who must stand still or sit with knees bent while they work. Since walking and moving about improve circulation, such activities should be encouraged during these periods. The nurse caring for a patient hospitalized for acute peripheral vascular disease should use this opportunity to teach the patient general preventive measures. The nurse making an antenatal home visit is contributing to prevention of vascular disease when she questions the patient about her posture and the kind of girdle and the shoes she wears and when she reminds the patient of the need for periodic rest periods with legs elevated above the heart level.

Psychologic and emotional problems

Peripheral vascular diseases are demoralizing for a variety of reasons. The nurse should understand these reasons because they vitally affect the patient's response to preventive teaching and his adjustment to hospital care and necessary treatment.

Age. The patient with peripheral vascular disease is often in the older age group. Although some relatively infrequent conditions, including Raynaud's disease and thromboangiitis obliterans (Buerger's disease), usually occur in younger persons and varicose veins are fairly common among those who are young, the vast majority of patients who develop peripheral vascular disease are over 50 years of age. The person at this age faces many serious emotional problems in addition to illness. He may be adjusting to the idea that his children have grown up and established homes and families of their own and no longer are dependent upon him. For the first time, he may be meeting younger workers whose decisions and judgments are taking precedence over his, or he may fear approaching retirement. He is at the age when friends are beginning to die, and this leads to loneliness and introspection. At this time of life other diseases often appear, so that the patient may have not just one but a number of physical ailments, thus leading to further discouragement. It is to be expected that the patient will have many psychosocial and emotional problems that will color his response to the new illness and make his adjustment to its restrictions difficult.

Chronicity of illness. Peripheral vascular diseases are chronic or lead to chronic illness. They are usually slow in onset, and much permanent vascular damage may be done before symptoms are severe enough to bring the patient to a doctor. Treatment is often long and tedious. The period of hospitalization is usually longer than for many other conditions. The patient with varicose ulcers, for example, may also have arterial insufficiency which makes healing slow and uncertain despite the best of care. Months of hospital or convalescent care may be necessary for this seemingly trivial but extremely discouraging condition. During this time the patient worries about finances, curtailment of normal social outlets, and innumerable other problems. Even if he is being treated on an ambulatory basis, he still faces a long period of medical treatment, probable loss of income from absence from work, and the possibility of becoming even more incapacitated and becoming a burden to his family or to others as he grows older.

Discouraged by the chronic nature of his ailment and its attendant problems, the patient may seek a quick cure by following the advice of nonprofessional persons or by using patent remedies. Some of these only waste the patient's money and others are actually harmful. Mechanical devices are sometimes advertised as being successful in restoring normal circulation; massage and other physical modalities may be recommended by those who have no real evidence of their effectiveness. Thus, the nurse should encourage the patient to remain under the supervision of one physician in whom both he and his family have confidence and should encourage him to take newspaper clippings describing miracle treatment to his physician for explanation. Well-meaning friends and relatives may do the patient harm by describing more rapid progress of someone with the same condition. The nurse can help by explaining that each patient is different and that the blood vessels of one person cannot be accurately compared with those of another. Again, she should refer the patient to his own physician for reassurance.

The patient's main worry may be the expense of hospitalization. The nurse should learn to know the patient and should know the nursing resources of her community. The patient with a varicose ulcer may be able to leave the hospital and return to his home if a responsible relative can come either to the hospital ward or to the clinic and learn to give the necessary care safely. The doctor may feel that the patient can be discharged if he is assured, for example, that a relative can be relied upon to do necessary errands and see that the patient remains off his feet as required for improvement. Even the person living in a rural area and the one living alone may be able to leave the hospital if community nursing service is available to give or to supervise care and to report changes to the doctor.

Pain. Most peripheral vascular diseases cause pain, but the pain may vary as to kind. For example, it may be sudden and excruciating, as in embolic thrombosis; constant and gnawing, as in arteriosclerosis; "heavy" and burning, as in varicose veins; or steady and throbbing, as when gangrene threatens. The characteristic symptom of pain is doubly significant because of the chronicity of most vascular diseases. Having lived with pain for a long time, the patient has suffered from its demoralizing effects. His outlook on his surroundings, his attitudes regarding medical treatment, and his response to improvement and rehabilitation may be affected by constant pain. The patient is greatly in need of people who show a real interest in him as a person and who have a positive approach to his physical ailment. The nurse cannot expect a mental outlook developed over weeks or months to change in a day or two. Some patients feel more protected and "privileged" in a single room and benefit from this deference; others do better in open wards with patients whose varied problems may give them a new perspective on their own.

The patient who has a long history of continuous pain or who is in intense pain may be irritated easily. A tardy medication, sugar missing from the breakfast tray, or a neglected errand are incidents that may upset him unduly and increase his discouragement. Knowledge of the disease, of how it has affected the individual patient, and of the particular problems of the patient will help the nurse understand the patient's behavior.

Physical care

Warmth. Warmth is advised for most patients with peripheral vascular disease because it causes vasodilation and thereby improves circulation to the affected part. Extra warmth in the form of direct heat is seldom, if ever, applied locally because it so easily speeds up metabolism in the extremity already suffering from depleted circulation. Another reason for not applying local heat is that many patients with peripheral vascular disease also have peripheral nerve degeneration which lessens the sensitivity of the skin to heat, thus predisposing to burns. A safe rule to follow is: never, under any circumstances, apply hot-water bottles, heating pads, or other forms of local heat to the legs or feet without a doctor's specific order. Soaking the feet in hot or even very warm water is seldom advised. The patient must be cautioned not to attempt to warm his feet by placing them on a warm radiator or in the open oven.

General body warmth is usually recommended. It must be remembered that exposure of a part of the body to cold can cause chilling of the entire body. This in turn causes vasoconstriction and lessens circulation in a diseased extremity. In cold weather the patient with peripheral vascular disease should wear warm clothing such as long underwear, fleece-lined shoes, ear muffs, scarf, and extra heavy coats, suits, or dresses. If chilling has been experienced, the patient should drink something hot and get to a warm room as soon as possible. Warmth to the extremities can also be increased by placing a hot-water bottle or heating pad on the abdomen or by immersing the entire body in a warm bath at 37° C (98.6° F.). Loose woolen bedsocks can be worn at night.

The patient should be in a warm environment whenever possible. The temperature of the room should be at least 21° C. (70° F.), and hospitalized patients may need even more warmth than this for maximum comfort. The patient must then be in a single room, and sometimes electric heating units, deflected away from the patient, are used to raise the room temperature. The patient should be able to sense that he is rather warm but should not be warm enough to perspire more than usual.

Cleanliness and avoidance of infection. Because resistance to infection is low when circulation is poor, all patients with vascular disease need instruction in the care of their feet and in prevention of infection. The ambulant patient should be advised to check the bath water carefully with his elbow before stepping into the tub; this simple practice would prevent many patients from being burned. A daily bath is recommended unless the patient is quite elderly, in which case two or three baths a week are sufficient. A small amount of a mild soap, a detergent, or a superfatted soap should be used. The skin should be dried by gentle rubbing; vigorous rubbing should be avoided. While bathing, the patient should look for any skin changes on his legs and feet. A dry scaling over the tibia may be the beginning of "bath itch" which is common in older people who have dry skin and who bathe too often with harsh soaps. Blueness or swelling around varicosities, and hard, reddened, or painful areas which may indicate phlebitis should be reported to a physician at once. Trophic changes such as a dry, cracking hardness, thickening, and brownish discolorations of the toenails indicate impairment of blood supply.

If the patient does not bathe each day, he should wash his feet in tepid water, dry them thoroughly, being particularly careful to dry between the toes, and inspect them for calluses, blisters, or any other abnormalities. If he is old and has failing vision, a member of the family should inspect his feet periodically and cut the toenails for him. The skin should be patted dry. Since alcohol is drying to the skin it is not recommended in vascular disease. The skin should be gently massaged with lubricants such as lanolin or other mild creams. In the daily routine care of his feet, the patient should include gentle massage of each toe from the distal end proximally, since this stimulates circulation. Powder should be used between the toes, with care being taken that it does not cake and that it is thoroughly removed at the next washing. Authorities maintain that epidermophytosis (athlete's foot), which is often a precursor of gangrene in the feet of those with arterial insufficiency, will seldom develop if the toes and feet are kept dry at all times. The patient who perspires profusely should powder between his toes more than once a day and should change his socks at least daily. Any kind of powder is satisfactory, although preparations containing undecylemic acid are now widely used. Small pieces of lamb's wool or cotton can be placed between the toes to absorb the perspiration. If the skin is dry, lanolin cream or other softening lotions or creams should be rubbed gently into the skin and the base of the nails. Oil such as "baby oil" or perfumed preparations put into the bath water leave a protective film on the skin.

The best treatment for ingrown toenails is prevention. The feet should be soaked in tepid water before the nails are cut. The nails should be cut straight across and slightly rounded at the sides. They must never be cut down to the level of the tissue. Pocket knives, razor blades, or scissors should never be used. The patient should equip himself with a pair of toenail clippers. Files are usually considered safe; however, tissues can be traumatized by emery boards and files, particularly when the patient lacks normal sensation in the toes. Elderly persons with poor vision should not cut their own toenails; a member of the family should do this for them.

With daily care a toenail that has a tendency to "curl under" at the side of the toe can be trained to grow more normally. With the rounded end of an ordinary toothpick, a small wisp of cotton should be gently inserted under the edge of the nail. No efforts should be made to "straighten" the nail by vigorous treatment; it may be weeks before any improvement is seen. The cotton must be changed daily. With patience and persistence most nails that tend to grow under can be made to grow more normally provided that the condition is not aggravated by such conditions as pressure from shoes.

Medical care should be sought for blisters and for corns, calluses, and thickened skin areas that cannot be rubbed away with a washcloth and an emery board after having been soaked. The patient with circulatory disease of any kind should be advised to seek medical advice before going to a chiropodist. Soap poultices, made of any soft soap such as shaving cream, may be used to soften corns and calluses before rubbing is attempted.

The patient should be warned about injury and infection following trauma. He should not walk barefoot for fear of splinters causing injury. When circulation is impaired, it is dangerous to scratch bites or other minor skin lesions. Many stubborn ulcers of the leg have followed the vigorous scratching of mosquito or other insect bites. The warning not to scratch the skin is hard to heed at times. Venous stasis may cause itching that can be most annoying. This itching usually follows long periods of standing and will subside if the patient rests with the feet elevated for a few minutes every hour or two. Calamine lotion is sometimes prescribed by the doctor when pruritus is troublesome. Any minor infection of the legs or the feet should be viewed as a major one by a patient with peripheral vascular disease; he should never attempt self-treatment when any signs of infection develop.

Socks or stockings should be washed daily. If they are wool or have a tendency to shrink, they should be stretched over a dryer. Frames can be purchased at most notion counters, or a simple inexpensive dryer can be made from a metal coat hanger. The patient should have at least two pairs of shoes and should wear them on alternate days, thus giving each pair a chance to air. If shoes become wet, they should be dried slowly on shoe trees to help preserve their shape. New shoes should be broken in gradually. Leather shoes are best because they give good support to the feet. Canvas, linen, or perforated nylon shoes provide ventilation, are comfortable in warm weather, and are safe if they have leather soles. Rubber-soled shoes are not advised for those who have any kind of vascular disease since they retard evaporation and thus may contribute to the development of fungus infection. Shoes should be carefully fitted by experienced persons; they should extend about one-half inch beyond the longest toe and should be wide enough to avoid pressure anywhere on the foot and to allow fairly free movement of the toes within the shoe. The inner last of the shoe should be straight, and the longitudinal arch of the shoe should support that of the foot. Playshoes and "ballet slippers" which afford little or no support are not recommended for persons with peripheral vascular disease, although there is no objection to women wearing pumps with moderately high heels. In fact, pumps are good inasmuch as the feet can be slipped out of the shoes and the toes wiggled at intervals.

However, they should be roomy enough so that the shoes can be put on again easily. The patient should be advised to shun economy when buying shoes. Ill-fitting bargain shoes may cause blisters and lead to serious and costly illness.

Rest, exercise, and posture. A careful balance of rest and exercise is necessary for the patient with peripheral vascular disease. Some exercise is essential in all peripheral vascular diseases because it improves venous and arterial circulation; exercise is most important for satisfactory return of venous blood from the extremities to the heart. Too much exercise, however, increases metabolism, thereby increasing the demands placed upon the circulation to take nutrients to the tissues and to remove the products of metabolism. Complete rest may be necessary in the presence of associated medical illness such as heart disease or gangrene.

In regard to posture, the following is a safe guide for all patients with peripheral vascular disease (or indeed, for anyone): Do not stay in *any* position too long. This is particularly important for the elderly patient who often has both arterial and venous disease. Much emphasis has been placed upon elevation of the feet, and many patients believe that this will benefit them. However, damage may be done by this when the patient has arterial insufficiency. The nurse must *clearly understand* the patient's condition and the doctor's orders before she attempts to give instructions in this regard. Whereas the patient with good arterial circulation but with venous disease such as lymphedema may safely rest for an hour or more with the feet above the level of the heart, the patient with arterial disease and venous disease should remain in this position for only a few minutes to permit venous blood to drain yet not hinder arterial flow.

It is safe to assume that the flat position is best over an extended time unless the doctor has ordered otherwise. Long periods of standing still should be avoided by those with either venous or arterial disease, and short periods should be alternated with exercise such as rapid walking. Those who have venous disease should alternate standing and walking with elevation of the affected limbs.

The importance of posture must be stressed in the care and teaching of patients with peripheral vascular disease. The patient should sleep on a firm mattress. A soft mattress may allow enough flexion of the trunk at the hips to impede circulation to the lower extremities. It may also permit the lower limbs to be higher than the heart, which is undesirable in arterial disease. The height of a chair should be such that the knees are not bent at more than a right angle, and the depth of the seat should permit two fingers between the chair seat and the popliteal spaces. Both of these provisions will help to prevent pressure on the popliteal vessels which would both prevent good arterial flow to the limbs and interfere with venous return. Furthermore, the patient should never cross his legs at the knee, since this also causes pressure on the popliteal vessels. He should develop the habit of rotating his foot at the ankle, bending the foot up and down, and straightening the knee at intervals. Attendance at movies, for example, can sometimes be made safe and comfortable for patients with impaired circulation by the use of these simple measures to improve circulation.

Exercises (Buerger-Allen). Specific exercises to empty blood vessels and to stimulate collateral circulation are sometimes prescribed for those with arterial disease such as arteriosclerosis obliterans and thromboangiitis obliterans (Buerger's disease). These are often called Buerger-Allen exercises (after the physicians who first used them). They consist of elevating the feet until they blanch, lowering them until redness appears, and then remaining flat for a few minutes, repeating the procedure a prescribed number of times. The length of time the exercises are to be performed varies with each patient and the changes in foot color, but up two to three minutes, down five to ten minutes, and flat five to ten minutes is often ordered. If the nurse is asked to supervise these exercises, she should know their purpose and should not permit the feet to remain elevated longer than necessary to produce whiteness. If she is teaching the patient to do these exercises at home or is instructing his family, she must emphasize that they must watch the color of the feet while they are elevated and lower them as soon as the normal color leaves. In the hospital the overbed table covered with a pillow may be used to support the elevated limbs. At home the patient may lie on the sofa and support the elevated feet against the wall or on the arm of the sofa. A chair inverted on the bed and covered with a blanket provides a comfortable support for elevation of the feet. A 45- to 90-degree angle may be used. If the legs are elevated at 90 degrees, the period of elevation may be shortened; for example, one to two minutes may cause blanching. Exercises are usually prescribed to be repeated five to ten times at least three times a day.

Avoidance of constriction of circulation. The patient with peripheral vascular disease must not wear anything that constricts circulation. Rolled garters, knitted hose designed to stay up without garters, and girdles that cause constriction around the thighs and groin should not be worn. Some doctors also believe that tight waistbands should not be worn. Men may be advised to wear suspenders instead of belts, and women should select garter belts that do not constrict. Socks that do not require garters should be worn by men. Shoelaces should be tied loosely. If edema of the feet occurs at the end of the day, the shoelaces should be loosened and relaced several times each day. Elastic shoelaces are preferred by some patients who have a moderate amount of edema of the feet or ankles at the end of the day or when standing at work.

Diet. The patient with peripheral vascular disease should avoid becoming overweight. Excess fat places an added burden on diseased arteries which already have difficulty in keeping up with tissue demands. Obesity in the patient with venous disease increases congestion and probably lessens the effectiveness of muscles in assisting with the return flow of blood. If the patient has limited cardiac capacity in addition to vascular disease, the heart and the entire vascular system are taxed to such an extent that distribution of blood to the extremities is curtailed. Reducing diets, however, must always be under the direction of the physician. Harm can be done, particularly to the elderly patient, by too rapid loss of weight, which may alter pressure within sclerosed arteries and make it possible for a clot to form, and cause further depletion of the nutrient supply to tissues supplied by them.

When the doctor has prescribed a reduction diet, the nurse can be of real assistance in helping to plan meals that are satisfying to the patient and yet within his caloric restrictions and financial means. The patient with peripheral vascular disease is usually advised to have a diet high in protein because this should help to prevent breakdown of tissues; for example, if he has an ulcer, such a diet should help promote healing. Vitamin B is important in maintaining normal health of blood vessels, and vitamin C is essential in healing and in the prevention of both internal and external hemorrhage.

The nurse should learn about the patient's circumstances of living and their effect on his diet. For example, she should find out whether he has to climb several flights of stairs with groceries. If he is elderly and lives alone, she should find out whether there is someone in his building or neighborhood who can shop for him; she should try to learn what he eats in a usual day. She may find that the young mother with a stubborn ulcer, that complicated phlebitis before delivery, is so harassed with feeding the baby and getting other children off to school or otherwise attended to that she neglects her own breakfast and lunch. She may discover that the elderly man with arteriosclerosis develops intermittent claudication when he walks from his rooming house to the nearest restaurant, so skips one or two meals each day. The nurse in the clinic may find that an individual record for each patient helps her to continue a teaching plan for the patient on successive visits. She often encounters problems that suggest the need for referral to a medical social worker or that should be brought to the attention of the doctor.

It is generally recommended that patients with peripheral vascular disease take larger amounts of fluids than the normal person. As many as fifteen to twenty glasses of water or equivalent fluids are often recommended. This may improve the quality of the limited blood supply to the limbs by improving elimination of waste products. It is also believed that it may lessen the viscosity of the blood and thus help to prevent the formation of thrombi.

Drugs. In addition to medications for pain, the two important types of drugs given to patients with peripheral vascular disease are vasodilators which dilate blood vessels and anticoagulants which lessen the tendency of the blood to clot. Newer drugs, which dissolve thrombi that are already formed, are now being used. These drugs show promise of extreme value although their use at the present time is still experimental. Vasodilators may be given when toxic drugs such as ergot have caused vasospasm, when arteriosclerosis has caused narrowing of the lumen of the vessel, or when a thrombus has formed in an artery and caused partial or total obstruction. If a clot is adherent to a blood vessel, an anticoagulant drug may be given with the vasodilator to prevent further clot formation. While several drugs are useful for vasodilation, the excellent effects of warm baths, heat to the abdomen, and hot fluids by mouth should not be overlooked.

Papaverine, an alkaloid of opium, has long been known to have a relaxing effect on the smooth muscle of the blood vessels. It is not habit forming. The usual dose is 0.03 to 0.06 Gm. (½ to 1 grain) orally or intravenously three to four times a day. In acute arterial occlusion it is injected into the artery above the occlusion; for example, in occlusion of the popliteal artery, it may be injected into the femoral artery; 1 Gm. of the drug is given in 5 ml. of distilled water by the doctor.[27]

Priscoline hydrochloride, 25 to 50 mg. (5/12 to 5/6 grain), given orally three to five times a day, acts by negating the action of epinephrine and therefore aids in vasodilation. It may also be given intravenously. Dibenamine hydrochloride and *beta-pyridyl-carbinol* (Roniacol) are adrenolytic and also block the sympatholytic pathways. Toxic reactions to these drugs include palpitation, nausea and vomiting, pruritus and abnormal skin sensations, and drop in blood pressure. The patient who cannot tolerate one of these drugs may be able to take another without untoward reactions. Toxic signs should be carefully watched for in any patient receiving these drugs and must be reported to the doctor at once.

Alcohol is a very useful drug in dilating the blood vessels. The usual dosage is 30 to 60 ml. three to four times a day. Whiskey and soda is often the alcohol preparation ordered, but any of the common beverages containing alcohol can be used. Some doctors order a double dose at bedtime to produce maximum effect during the hours when muscle action is not assisting with the flow of blood to the legs.

Caffeine (contained in tea and coffee) and *theobromine* (found in chocolate) are peripheral vasodilators.[17] Although these drugs are seldom given for their vasodilating effect, there is no need to eliminate tea, coffee, and chocolate from the diet of the patient with peripheral vascular disease if he enjoys them and if there are no contraindications to their use.

Methacholine chloride (Mecholyl chloride) is a choline derivative which intensifies the action of the parasympathetic system and thus produces vasodilation. The usual dosage is 50 to 100 mg. given orally. This drug can also be given hypodermically, but it is not given intravenously because of the danger of severe toxic reaction. The signs of toxic reaction include nausea and vomiting, fainting, and dyspnea. Atropine is the best antidote available.

Anticoagulants are extremely valuable drugs in the treatment of vascular disease. They act therapeutically by prolonging the clotting time of the blood. They are widely used in the treatment of both venous and arterial thrombosis and are used prophylactically in those with a threatened thrombosis or threatened recurrence of a condition such as thrombophlebitis. *Heparin* and *bishydroxycoumarin* (Dicumarol) are two of the preparations used. Heparin is an expensive drug, costing about $10 a day, whereas Dicumarol costs only a few cents.

Anticoagulant drugs require very careful regulation as to amount and continuity of dosage, and the nurse has a responsibility in this. If too much is given, the patient may have a hemorrhage in a vital area such as the brain. If too little is given, he may have no relief from symptoms of thrombosis and may have additional thrombus formation with perhaps fatal consequences.

Heparin is obtained from the lungs and livers of animals. Its advantage is that its effect is almost immediate. Disadvantages are that it can only be given parenterally, since it is destroyed by the gastric secretions of the stomach, and that its action ceases after three to four hours. Heparin dosage is expressed in units or milligrams and is calculated individually for each patient; 50 mg. or 5,000 units may be given at three- to four-hour intervals, or a continuous drip of 100 to 200 mg. in 1,000 ml. of physiologic solution of sodium chloride may be administered. The average rate of flow should be about 20 to 25 drops per minute. When a patient is getting this drug by infusion, the nurse must watch the rate of flow very carefully and report to the doctor if the solution stops dripping or if its rate cannot be regulated satisfactorily.

Dicumarol was first isolated from spoiled sweet clover after it was observed that cattle eating this food had abortions and hemorrhage. It acts by suppressing the formation of prothrombin.[17] The usual maintenance dosage is 50 to 150 mg. per day administered by mouth. Frequent determinations of the prothrombin level must be obtained and most physicians believe that the prothrombin level should be kept between 10 and 30 per cent of normal. Dicumarol is widely used in the treatment of thrombophlebitis. It takes twelve to twenty-four hours to take effect, and its action persists for twenty-four to seventy-two hours after the drug is discontinued. Cumarin is a newer anticoagulant drug now widely used. Ethyl biscoumacetate (Tromexan) is another synthetic drug which has action similar to Dicumarol except that it acts more quickly and lasts for a shorter time. Determinations of prothrombin levels must be taken carefully since the responses of individual patients to anticoagulants differ widely.

Anticoagulant therapy undoubtedly has prolonged the lives of many persons and enabled them to live quite satisfactorily and productively. The patient who must remain on this drug indefinitely, however, needs encouragement and sympathetic medical and nursing care. Unfortunately the vein must be punctured to obtain blood for a prothrombin determination, and this must be done at least two to three times a week and sometimes daily, depending upon the success achieved in stabilizing the prothrombin level. This is an unpleasant experience for the patient, and its continuance over weeks and months may place a real restraint on the activities of the ambulatory patient. He may begin to feel trapped and hampered beyond endurance. Vacations, for example, present real problems, and even short trips must be carefully planned. Also, since it is so important that the patient keep his appointments for prothrombin determinations, it is difficult for the physician to emphasize this sufficiently without the patient realizing or suspecting that his life may be in real danger. This, of course, causes further depression.

The patient must be taught to recognize the signs of hemorrhage and to report them immediately. He should carry an identification card stating that he takes anticoagulant drugs so that, in the event of accident, those who give him medical care will know this. The identification card should also contain the name and telephone number of the physician prescribing the drug.

Streptokinase, an enzyme, and *SK activated human plasmin* preparations (Thrombolysin) are substances which are fibrinolytic in that they can dissolve fibrin which is an essential constituent of a thrombus. It is believed that plasmin exists in the blood as a precursor in the form of plasminogen or profibrinolysin. Either activated enzyme (streptokinase) or plasminogen activators can be used. Urokinase which occurs naturally in urine is a possible source of the activator needed to convert plasminogen to plasmin (fibrinolysin). Fibrinolytic drugs are either given intravenously or injected above the thrombosed vessel. Comprehensive reports on the trial use of these new drugs are now available.[6,10]

Smoking. Smoking is contraindicated in all vascular diseases, since the nicotine causes spasm of the peripheral arteries. The relationship between arteriospasm and smoking is so definite that many doctors feel it is useless to try to treat the patient unless he gives up smoking. Smoking should be immediately discontinued in any kind of arterial vascular disease and is also contraindicated in venous disease because the arteries surrounding a thrombosed vein often develop spasms, and gangrene has even been known to develop from this.[27]

Smoking has become a major problem with the staggering increase in cigarette consumption in recent years. There is no evidence that chewing tobacco or using snuff contributes to vasospasm.

Ridiculous as it may seem to the nonsmoker, giving up cigarettes is almost impossible for many people. The urge to smoke is almost as compelling as the urge to obtain narcotics. It is just as difficult for women as for men to stop smoking once they have become confirmed smokers. Many patients continue to smoke even after they have lost a toe or even a foot as a result of vascular disease and know that the disease can be definitely arrested if they will only stop smoking.

Unfortunately there seem to be few substitutes for smoking. Candy, nuts, or raisins can be tried (if the patient is not on a reducing diet) and sometimes gum or coffee helps. Occupational therapy may help to divert the patient. Sometimes constant reminders and strict discipline do more harm than good. The need to smoke seems to be related to such deep-seated needs for gratification by this means that the nurse should be guided by the doctor in her individual approach to each patient. He should decide whether she should ignore the patient when he is smoking or whether she should reprimand him, report to his family, or take other action. Members of his family seldom seem able to help in getting the patient to stop smoking; often the patient will promise his family (or his doctor) that he will not smoke and then will do so surreptitiously. Reiteration of the doctor's and the nurse's faith in the patient's ability to stop smoking may yield better results than showing disapproval of his lapses.

The oscillating bed. The oscillating bed (Sanders) is used to stimulate circulation particularly in those with leg or foot ulcers or other conditions that make walking impossible. In the home the bed can also be used with benefit by those who have arterial disease which interferes with sleep. The electrically operated bed seesaws in a cycle which usually takes one to two and one-half minutes but can be regulated according to need or preference. The foot of the bed rises six inches above the horizontal and descends twelve to fifteen inches with a smooth transition from one motion to another. (See Figure 30.) The patient should be given adequate explanation of why the bed is rec-

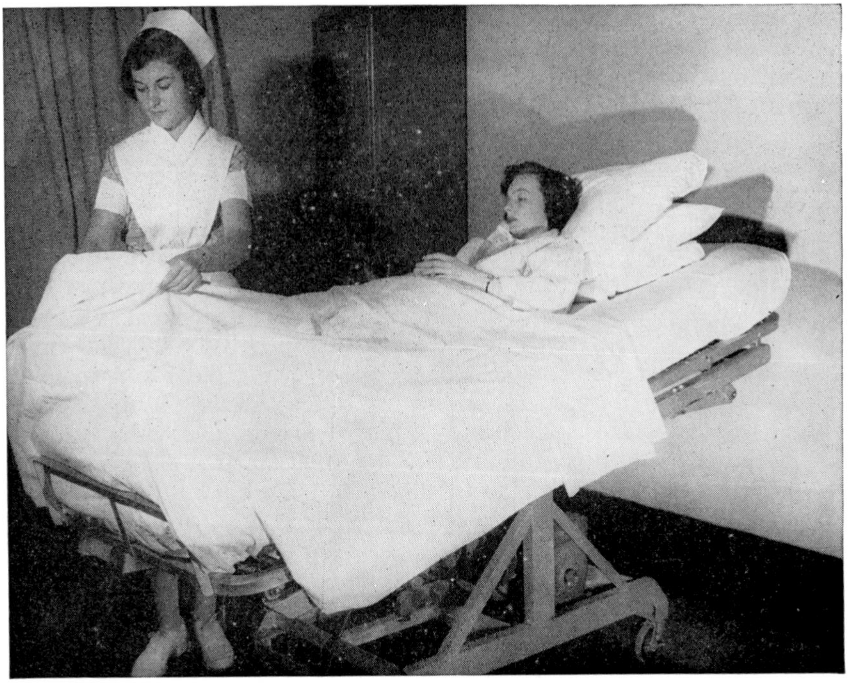

Figure 30

The oscillating bed is used to improve circulation. Here the student nurse checks the temperature and color of the affected limb. Note that a cradle is being used to protect the feet from weight of the covers.

ommended and may need time to become adjusted to the motion. Dizziness, nausea, and headache are probably of psychic origin, but the patient is encouraged to stop the bed for a few minutes should these symptoms occur. He is given the switch and is instructed how to use it. The bed is usually stopped for meals and other necessary care, but otherwise the patient is encouraged to keep it operating both day and night. Since some patients tend to slide downward as the foot of the bed lowers, and pressure of the feet against the footboard causes pain, a padded footboard should be placed on the bed. The bed should be checked weekly by an electrician; it should work smoothly without disturbing sounds or vibration.

Care of ulcers. Ulcers occurring in any patient with vascular disease require meticulous care to prevent infection or to prevent further infection with new organisms. Since local tissue resistance to infection is lessened and the rate of healing is slowed, a long period of repair must be anticipated. Wet dressings are seldom used because they cool quickly, and this cooling may cause arteriospasm, which is harmful. If they are ordered, it is usually for short periods of time, and the nurse must be in constant attendance to change them frequently. They may be used to loosen crusts and facilitate drainage. Foot soaks are used, although this procedure cannot be sterile because it is impossible to cleanse the entire foot sufficiently.

The patient with a foot ulcer is usually required to remain off his feet, although there is not complete agreement on the value of this. It may be reasoned that, provided there is no direct weight-bearing on the wound, the arterial circulation and healing are improved by a moderate amount of moving about and by keeping the limb in a dependent position for a part of the day at least.

Light cradles are used with extreme caution when ulcers are present. In instances in which the physician believes that dry warmth will improve healing, the wound is left exposed with a cradle and light. The bulb should never be larger than 25 watts, and there should be a definite order from the doctor as to how long it should be left on and how far from the limb it should be placed. Too much heat will increase the arterial needs of the tissues and thus will be injurious. Cradles are seldom used for the patient with vascular disease who has painful feet because of the danger of his accidentally hitting a foot when the bed is made and because the patient finds them irritating and restraining when he attempts to move about in bed. Footboards and pillows are usually better to keep the weight of blankets off the feet. If a cradle is used, extra bath blankets should be used to cover the cradle and should be tucked securely under the mattress to prevent drafts on the feet.

A wide variety of drugs are used in the local treatment of ulcers in an effort to stimulate healing and prevent further infection. Castor oil and zinc oxide, nitrofurazone (Furacin), and scarlet red ointment, as well as a wide variety of bacteriostatic preparations, are often used. Special treatment of ulcers occurring in conjunction with varicose veins will be described in the section dealing specifically with that condition.

Since many patients who have chronic ulcers of the legs and feet are not hospitalized, they must be taught how to bathe and otherwise care for themselves without contaminating the ulcer. Many elderly patients have lived with a chronic ulcer for so long that they become careless about their technique in changing soiled or loosened dressings. The patient will often benefit from a periodic visit from a public health nurse who can reemphasize essentials of care both to the patient and to members of his family.

Tests and examinations

Several specific procedures help the physician to diagnose vascular disease and to determine the progress in treatment. Most tests are relatively simple and require no particular preparation. The patient, however, usually is in pain and fears any procedure that he believes may even temporarily increase his pain. The nurse should explain to him what is to be done if the doctor has not already done this. Since spasm of the vessels will diminish pulsations and alter circulation, the nurse should see that the patient is in a warm room and that he has sufficient clothing if he is going to a special room for a test. It should be explained that the tests are painless; nervousness sometimes causes spasm of blood vessels and sensations of chilliness which would interfere with the accuracy of the test.

Test for intermittent claudication. Intermittent claudication is pain in the muscles of the lower limb (primarily in the calf and the thigh) caused by inadequate circulation to the muscle. It may be severe enough to make the patient stop walking and disappears with rest. Knowing the amount of walking that can be done before claudication occurs helps the doctor determine the severity of the condition and the improvement made. Unfortunately this is not easy to measure in the hospital or the clinic. One method is to have an attendant walk with the patient and time with a stop watch the number of steps taken before pain occurs. Sometimes mechanical devices are used; the patient stands with his foot on a pedal which he presses down, thereby lifting a weight of 6.3 kg. (13.6 pounds). This is done at the rate of 120 times per minute until the onset of pain. A normal person may continue this for from five to ten minutes before he has severe fatigue, whereas one with vascular disease may be able to continue only for a few seconds. While these methods of testing are not too accurate, they are still more reliable than the patient's statement of the number of city blocks he can walk before the onset of

Table 6 Generally accepted normal oscillometric readings

Extremity	*Oscillometric reading*
Lower extremity	
Mid thigh	4 to 16
Upper third of leg	3 to 12
Above ankle	1 to 8
Foot	0.2 to 1
Upper extremity	
Upper arm	4 to 16
Elbow	3 to 12
Wrist	1 to 10
Hand	0.2 to 2

pain, since city blocks vary so much in length.

Oscillometric studies. Oscillometric readings help to determine the effectiveness of the larger arteries by measuring their pulsations; collateral vessels cannot be measured by these means. A cuff is wrapped about the limb at the desired level and is connected to a delicate diaphragm, which transmits pressure to a needle moving across a dial that measures in units what is called the oscillometric index. The generally acepted normal oscillometric readings are given in Table 6.

Skin temperature studies. Attempts are made to record the skin temperature as a gauge to the effectiveness of the circulation to an extremity. These tests are not done too often since they must be done in a carefully prepared room with controlled temperature and humidity. A potentiometer which measures the temperature immediately after a thermocouple has been applied to the skin and various kinds of thermometers with wide mercury bulbs have been devised. The physician usually considers the skin temperature readings as only suggestive, because many factors (for example, a rise in metabolic rate) increases the temperature of the skin surface. The patient who is excited or upset by the anticipated test may have increased skin temperature. Normal persons have a wide range of temperature difference in various parts of the body. For example, the forehead and the thorax are usually five to eight degrees warmer than the toes. The test is usually done several hours after a meal since eating alters the skin temperature. Smoking also affects the accuracy of the readings. With a humidity of 40 per cent the surface temperature of the skin usually varies from 24° to 35° C. (73° to 93° F.).

A test of circulation in the extremities consists of immersing one of the limbs in water heated to 42° to 44° C. (107.6° to 112° F.). In the normal person with no vascular disease, temperature of the unimmersed limb will rise to a minimum of 34° C. (93° F.) within thirty-five minutes. The nurse may be asked to assist with this test. An accurate bath thermometer is needed to measure the water temperature, and sufficient blankets should be used to protect the patient from chilling during and after the test.

A simpler way to test circulation in a limb is to place a hot-water bottle or heating pad on the abdomen and then manually test both extremities for change of skin temperature. Many doctors rely on this test since it is simpler, and the hands of the experienced person are quite skillful at judging skin temperature of each limb.

Angiography. Roentgenograms may be taken to show calcification and other anomalies of the arteries. They may show the location of calcified atherosclerotic plaques at the site of an occlusion. By these means calcification can sometimes be traced throughout the entire length of the artery and can even be seen as far distally as the great toe. The information revealed by such an examination is not, of itself, evidence of arterial insufficiency, for some patients who have extensive calcification of the small arteries evidently have sufficient collateral circulation to permit good blood supply and have no symptoms of arterial insufficiency.

Radiopaque substances such as Urokon may be injected into an artery and roentgenograms taken during the last few seconds of the injection and immediately thereafter. For example, the radiopaque substance may be injected into the femoral artery to visualize abnormalities in the femoral and popliteal arteries. Usually this test is done in the x-ray department. The substances used contain iodide, and the patient may have a severe reaction to the dye with dyspnea, nausea, vomiting, numbness of the extremities, diaphoresis, and tachycardia. Any signs of a reaction should be reported at once; occasionally a delayed reaction occurs after the patient returns to his room. Antihistaminic drugs, Adrenalin, and oxygen are used. The site of injection of the dye must be observed for signs of irritation or local thrombosis which may occur if any of the irritating dye gets into the surrounding tissue.

Veins can also be studied by injecting radiopaque substances and taking roentgenograms. The substance is injected into an artery and the roentgenogram is taken (carefully timed) as the material flows back through the veins; if the substance becomes too diluted, the x-ray examination may reveal little. The radiopaque substance may be injected directly into the vein distal to the part of the vessel that is to be visualized. The same materials are used as for arterial studies.

Capillary fragility. The most common way to test capillary fragility is to apply a sphygmomanometer and to increase the pressure within vessels distal to the cuff. This is often called the Rumpel-Leede method and the appearance of petechiae is sometimes called the *Rumpel-Leede phenomenon.* The cuff is inflated to approximately halfway between the systolic and diastolic readings and maintained for fifteen minutes. Five minutes later the number of petechiae in a marked circle on the limb distal to the cuff are counted. Abnormal conditions within the blood, such as decreased number of platelets and lack of vitamin C, will affect the readings from this test. There is no special nursing care during this test; if the nurse applies the cuff and checks the readings, she must be extremely careful to keep the pressure in the cuff at the desired level, time the test accurately, and count the petechiae carefully. If many petechiae appear, the patient may need reassurance from his physician.

Sympathetic block. The most frequently used procedure is the injection of procaine into the area surrounding the sympathetic nerve ganglia supplying the extremity in question. This test is usually done by the anesthetist and is almost always done as a test procedure when a surgical sympathectomy is being considered. The patient should be told that there will be little pain associated with the test beyond the first needle prick and that there may be a sensation of tingling and warmth for several hours following the test. Skin temperature studies are usually made to test the effectiveness of the block of sympathetic nerves in causing vasodilation.

DISEASE CONDITIONS

Only disease conditions that occur quite often are discussed here. For discussion of other important, though less frequently occurring, diseases, the student is referred to specialized texts. Reactions to drugs, for example, can only be mentioned. Ergot is one drug that can cause symptoms of severe vascular embarrassment. This reaction is widespread among certain European peoples who consume rye on which the ergot grows. It is occasionally seen in patients who attempt abortion by taking large doses of ergot and in those particularly sensitive to the vascular effects of ergot who take headache remedies containing the drug. Nursing care of the patient suffering frostbite is included in Chapter 15.

Arteriosclerosis obliterans

Some arterial changes occur in almost all persons over 50 years of age. Those who have diabetes mellitus usually develop vascular impairment more rapidly than others. Men are more often affected by arteriosclerosis obliterans than are women. Symptoms appear when the blood vessels can no longer provide enough blood to supply oxygen and nutrients to the limbs and to remove the waste products of their metabolism.

Changes in the arteries include arteriosclerosis and atherosclerosis. Arteriosclerosis is a hardening primarily of the middle layer of the vessel with the deposition of calcium, causing an inflexibility of the vessel and permanent narrowing of its lumen. The amount of narrowing does not always determine whether or not symptoms will occur; this depends upon blood pressure within the vessel and the effectiveness of the collateral circulation. Arteriosclerosis affects the peripheral arteries more than the large vessels of the trunk.

Atherosclerosis affects the large vessels of the trunk more than the peripheral ones, although atheromatous changes in arteries of the thighs and legs often occur and predispose to thrombosis and obstruction of the vessel lumen. Atheromatous plaques containing cholesterol, fatty acids, and other substances form in the intima or inner wall of the artery. Occasionally calcium is deposited. These plaques cause distortion of the vessel and sometimes project far enough into the lumen to cause a thrombus to form which cuts off the blood flow.

Race is not thought to affect the incidence of arteriosclerosis and atherosclerosis, although it has been reported that some oriental groups have a lower incidence of the disease than some occidental peoples. Nutrition has been thought to have a great influence on the development of atherosclerosis, and this subject is presently undergoing close scientific study. Although there seems to be some evidence that the total fat in the diet and the kinds of fat eaten may have a relationship to the amount of cholesterol in the blood and, in turn, to the development of atheromatous plaques, the relationship is not clear at present. It is known that the body can and does manufacture cholesterol quite independently of that consumed as food. Until the relationship is more definitely established, the patient should be advised to consult his physician concerning the restriction of fat in his diet. A diet fairly high in protein and high in vitamins with only a moderate amount of fat is probably best for everyone.

Signs and symptoms. Signs and symptoms of arteriosclerosis obliterans include pain, skin temperature changes, differences in color and in size of the lower limbs, and trophic changes. The patient may have intermittent claudication and pain on rest. Pain on rest often occurs at night, and the patient may report that it subsides with movement and particularly with walking. Very elderly patients may be awakened by excruciating cramplike pains in the muscles of the calf and the thighs which are believed to be due to lack of oxygen to the tissue (ischemia). Tingling and numbness of the toes may be mentioned by the patient, and a very common complaint is difficulty in keeping the feet and hands warm enough for comfort. Occasionally the first sign of limited circulation is necrosis following mild trauma, such as cutting the skin when trimming the nails. The disease is usually present to some extent in both limbs, although symptoms may be grossly apparent in only one; they may follow an occlusion of a fairly large artery by a thrombus. This will cause numbness, marked coldness, and a chalky-white appearance to the part of the limb supplied by the obstructed vessel.

Medical treatment and nursing care. Medical treatment for arteriosclerosis obliterans includes warmth, use of drugs to produce vasodilatation, specific exercises to stimulate collateral circulation, carefully prescribed general exercise to maintain circulation yet not tax the arterial system, encouragement, and general instruction to avoid injury, prevent infection, and maintain nutrition. Pain on rest may be treated by having the patient sleep with the head of the bed elevated on blocks six to ten inches in height since this aids gravity in carrying arterial blood to the legs and feet. The patient is advised not to walk about during the night unless he is warmly clothed and to avoid sitting with his legs over the side of the bed since this may cause chilling and since right-angle knee flexion further hampers circulation. He should not rub the extremity because of the danger of trauma or of releasing an embolus into the circulation. Vigorous massage is always contraindicated in any patient with vascular disease, although gentle stroking may be permitted. All nursing measures discussed earlier in this chapter under general nursing care may be necessary in caring for the patient with arteriosclerosis obliterans. Arteriosclerosis obliterans is a chronic progressive disease for which there is no cure. Nursing care must be directed toward helping the patient to live within his limitations and encouraging him and his family to carry out medical instructions so that the disease may be held in check for an indefinite time. If the condition cannot be checked, gangrene of the extremity may eventually occur.

Thromboangiitis obliterans (Buerger's disease)

Thromboangiitis obliterans (Buerger's disease) causes an inflammation, thrombus formation, and subsequently destruction of both arteries and veins. It affects men more often than women and is largely a disease of younger people, patients often being between 20 and 35 years of age when symptoms appear. The cause of inflammation is not known, but smoking definitely aggravates the condition and may even be the only cause in those patients sensitive to inhaled smoke. Although the feet usually are first affected, vascular changes may occur in the hands and eventually throughout the entire body. As the inflammation subsides in an area, there is partial or complete replacement of blood vessels with scar tissue. The outcome of acute exacerbations, therefore, depends upon the size of the area deprived of normal blood supply and the amount of collateral circulation that can be established. Collateral vessels attempt to keep pace with the destruction, but over a period of years this is usually not possible without treatment, and gangrene develops.

Signs and symptoms. The disease causes numbness, tingling, and vague abnormal sensations in the extremities involved. It is aggravated by general chilling and by exposure of the hands and feet to cold. There may be hardened, red, and painful areas along the affected vessels and the patient often reports that there is a burning or boring pain which is aggravated by chilling, smoking, and nervous tension. There is often edema about the areas of inflammation, and the entire limb may be cooler to touch and whiter than normal except where there is acute inflammation. Cyanosis may occur when the feet are lowered.

Medical treatment and nursing care. It is often possible to arrest the disease completely and indefinitely by merely having the patient stop smoking. This is considered the one, single, most important aspect of treatment. Tobacco must be given up immediately, completely, and forever. Other measures are prescribed to foster circulation and to help make use of limited resources. These may include warmth, use of vasodilating drugs such as alcohol and Priscoline, moderate exercise, the oscillating bed, and instructions to prevent infection and to avoid trauma. Some doctors believe that a lumbar sympathectomy is helpful when the lower extremities are involved; other doctors report little confidence in this treatment. In some instances the administration of typhoid vaccine to produce hyperpyrexia seems to have a beneficial effect in causing relaxation of blood vessels and improvement of circulation; typhoid vaccine is most often used and is given intravenously (see Chapter 34 for details of nursing care of patients receiving fever therapy and the latter part of this chapter for care following sympathectomy).

Severe pain may require narcotics, but effort is made to limit their use since there is real danger of drug addiction in young patients with a chronic disease such as thromboangiitis obliterans. The nurse can often help by emphasizing to the patient the precautions he should take to prevent the onset of acute symptoms, including pain. Sensitivity to cold should be anticipated, and the patient must be advised to equip himself with warm footwear and warm gloves in the fall. Those who drive cars should wear warm, comfortable driving gloves, and those engaged in outdoor work should take extra precautions to avoid general chilling as well as exposure of their hands and feet.

Raynaud's disease

Raynaud's disease affects young women who are usually of fairly high-strung temperament. Its cause is unknown. There is spasm of the arteries in the extremities which lessens the blood supply. Often the hands and arms are affected before the feet. The condition may lead to coldness, numbness, cyanosis, pain, dryness and atrophy of the nails, and eventually gangrene of the ends of the fingers. The symptoms are intensified by exposure to cold and by emotional excitement. Patients often respond well to a sympathectomy in which the nerve control of blood vessels to the hands is removed. Those in whom the condition is mild may be treated with drugs which inhibit sympathetic nervous system activity, such as Dibenamine hydrochloride. The patient is advised to avoid smoking and to keep the hands and the rest of the body warm.

Raynaud's disease is sometimes associated with scleroderma, a condition in which there is disturbance in the collagen content of the body and in which the skin becomes tightly stretched, firm, partially atrophied, and fibrosed (see Chapter 29).

Thrombophlebitis

Thrombophlebitis is the occlusion of a vein with a thrombus and subsequent inflammation. Many relatively simple circumstances contribute to the development of thrombophlebitis in those who are perhaps particularly susceptible to congestion in the venous system. For example, thrombophlebitis of superficial leg veins may follow a trip during which long hours were spent sitting in a plane or car with the knees sharply bent. Flying at high altitudes in nonpressurized cabins seems to predispose to recurrence of thrombophlebitis in those who have a tendency toward this condition. Pregnancy is often complicated by thrombophelebitis due to interference with venous return in the lower abdomen. Thrombophlebitis may occur from inactivity following surgery, and before the days of early ambulation and emphasis on bed exercises it was a dreaded complication of surgery. Despite early ambulation, some patients still develop thrombophlebitis postoperatively, and occasional deaths from this cause are reported. For prevention of postoperative thrombophlebitis see Chapter 14. Thrombophlebitis is also caused by trauma to venous walls, with subsequent inflammation and congestion, and the irritating effects of certain drugs. Changes in blood pressure, blood volume, and abnormal substances in the blood, such as bacteria, may also contribute to development of the condition.

Signs and symptoms. Thrombophlebitis of superficial veins is easily apparent. Upon palpation, the veins appear hard and thready and are sensitive to pressure. There may be edema, and the area may be reddened and feel warm to the touch. Deep veins in the legs may be affected, and the pain they cause when the patient dorsiflexes his foot in bed or walks is known as *Homans' sign.* Thrombophlebitis may be accompanied by reflected pain in the entire limb, and systemic reaction to the infection, which sets in rapidly in any blood vessel when free flow of blood is interrupted, may cause symptoms such as headache, malaise, and elevation of temperature. Sometimes a thrombosis in a vessel may be "silent," giving no signs or symptoms until an *embolus* is released, floats in the blood stream, and lodges in a vital structure such as the lungs, the heart, or brain. This may cause death within a few seconds or an overwhelming shock reaction that is followed by death or by slow recovery (see Chapter 23).

Medical treatment and nursing care. Superficial thrombophlebitis is usually treated by rest. Occasionally the doctor does a ligation of the vein above the involvement (usually at the femoral juncture). Continuous warm moist heat may be used for both deep and superficial thrombophlebitis. Warm packs are usually ordered to cover the entire extremity and seem to have a beneficial effect, although their exact therapeutic action is not fully understood. Heating pads permanently set on "low" are best for keeping the packs at a consistently safe temperature.

There is no medical agreement as to whether or not the limb should be elevated; therefore the nurse should be certain that she understands the doctor's wishes. Some physicians believe that the danger of an embolus being released is greater if the limb is elevated, while others believe that elevation is essential for clearing of the vascular congestion and prevention of further edema. Physicians also differ in regard to the amount of activity the patient should have. Some believe that the clot is sufficiently adherent to the vein wall to make its release unlikely and that moving about helps to improve general circulation and to prevent further congestion of blood in the veins. Others believe that complete immobilization is necessary to prevent a part of the thrombus from breaking away and becoming an embolus.

The patient who has thrombophlebitis of large and deep vessels should usually be kept quiet. He should not cough vigorously, strain at defecation, or take deep breaths. Care must be taken that the patient is not frightened by these restraints, and the nurse should not hesitate to seek the doctor's help in explaining to the patient why precautions are necessary. Sudden coughing, respiratory difficulty, hemoptysis, and signs of shock must be reported at once since they may be signs of *pulmonary embolism.*

Heparin and Dicumarol are used for patients who have thrombophlebitis and sometimes patients must remain on prophylactic doses of Dicumarol for an indefinite period to prevent recurrences of the disease. Vasodilating drugs are given to combat the arterial vessel spasm which occurs at the site of a venous thrombosis and to improve general circulation and speed up absorption of the thrombus.

The period of immobilization depends entirely upon the response of the patient to treatment. Following thrombophlebitis in a lower limb severe enough to require hospitalization or bed rest, the patient is usually required to wear an elastic stocking when walking. *Elastic stockings* are also often ordered for those who have superficial thrombophlebitis which tends to recur. The elastic stocking, preferably accurately fitted to the patient's measurements, must be obtained before the patient gets up. Stockings of various lengths and sizes are stocked by some large department stores. Some clinics have samples and forms so that the patient may be measured and may then order a stocking which fits. The most satisfactory length is one inch below the bend of the knee joint. The patient must be taught how to put on the stocking. It should be rolled on evenly before he gets out of bed in the morning. Once during the day it should be removed for a few moments and the skin very gently stroked and powdered as necessary. The stocking need not be worn during sleeping hours.

Elastic bandages may be used instead of an elastic stocking, but they are more conspicuous and are difficult to apply evenly. They may be used for short periods following surgery and when lifting heavy objects or standing still. If a bandage has been ordered for continuous use, it should be applied before the patient gets out of bed in the morning. The bandage is applied to the entire foot, usually including the heel, and extends to just below the knee or up to the groin, depending on the doctor's order. It should be smooth and snug but must not be so tight that it interferes with circulation. After a month to six weeks, if the patient is progressing favorably, the stocking may be removed for one-half to one hour and the results noted. If there is no evidence of edema or discomfort, the stocking or bandage may be finally removed completely, although it usually takes months for this to be accomplished. Many patients wear the stockings indefinitely if their work necessitates standing for long periods of time or sitting with the knees bent. Two stockings or bandages are necessary for each affected limb so that they can be laundered as necessary.

Swimming and wading in water are among the best activities for prevention of recurrences of thrombophlebitis of the lower extremities and are highly recommended for patients with other venous diseases as well. Water, which is denser than air, exerts a smooth even pressure on the skin, and wading is especially beneficial because the greater pressure (the deeper water) surrounds the distal portion of the extremity and helps in the return flow of venous blood.

Lymphedema

Lymphedema may be of unknown cause (primary) or may be due to infection or other disease to small veins and lymph vessels. This relatively rare condition is seen most often in young women. It is believed that primary lymphedema is due to congenital underdevelopment in the lymph vesesls. Symptoms often appear at the time of puberty. They begin with mild swelling on the dorsum of the foot, usually at the end of the day, and this gradually extends to involve the entire limb. Lymphedema is aggravated by prolonged standing, pregnancy, obesity, warm weather, and the menstrual period. Exaggerated forms of this disease are known as *elephantiasis.*

One of the greatest problems in this condition is the emotional reaction of patients to the disfigurement. The patient often attributes difficulties encountered in working in her chosen field or social rebuffs to her disfigurement and tends to become withdrawn and depressed. The emphasis upon women's legs in our culture adds to her difficulties. One leg only may be involved, and in fairly mild cases this accentuates the abnormality.

The treatment of lymphedema is not too satisfactory. Present recommended treatment is conservative, making use of basic physiologic principles. Many of the conservative measures recommended for all patients with venous disease apply. Gravity can be assisted by elevating the limb, and the patient may be advised to sleep with the foot of the bed elevated four to eight inches. Constricting clothing should not be worn. Elastic stockings, moderate consistent exercise, and avoidance of foods that increase thirst and predispose to edema are helpful. Very light massage in the direction of the lymph flow is recommended.[11] Pneumatic cuffs or sleeves that help to exert a steady gentle massage are being tried and appear to be helpful, although no spectacular reports have been made. There is no cure for this condition, and the patient needs help and encouragement in learning to live with an exasperating chronic condition. Surgical removal of lymph nodes and vessels is sometimes tried. This procedure has been found beneficial for some patients with lymphedema due to filariasis or infection with a tropical organism which blocks the lymph channels.

Varicose veins

Varicose veins occur more often than any other abnormality of the veins; at least 10 per cent of our total population is affected. The highest incidence is in the third, fourth, and fifth decades of life.[16] There are several definite factors which predispose to the development of varicosities. Among them are hereditary weakness of the vein walls and prolonged standing, which places strain on the valves because muscle action is not helping to return the blood. Man's upright position further aggravates this, and poor posture with sagging of abdominal organs causes additional pressure. Pregnancy and abdominal tumors which cause pressure on the large veins of the lower abdomen and interfere with good venous drainage predispose to the development of varicose veins. Chronic systemic disease, such as heart disease and liver cirrhosis, may interfere with good return of blood to the heart and contribute to varicosities. Infections and trauma to the veins with resultant thrombophlebitis may lead to varicose veins, since the valves are destroyed as the acute inflammation subsides.

Signs and symptoms. Varicosities of superficial veins are often quite apparent through the skin even before they cause symptoms. They appear as darkened, tortuous, raised blood vessels that become more prominent when the patient stands and when he assumes positions which cause congestion, such as sitting with the knees crossed. Sometimes the sclerosed valves can be seen as nodular protrusions; the varicosity is more pronounced just above the valve, which has become ineffective. The patient may have pain, fatigue, feeling of heaviness in the legs, muscular cramps, and emotional reactions of discouragement and depression. Discomfort is worse during hot weather and when the patient goes to higher altitudes; it is greatly increased by prolonged standing.

The simplest test for varicose veins is known as the *Trendelenburg test.* The patient lies down with the leg raised until the vein empties completely; he then rises and the vein is observed as it fills. A normal vein fills from below, whereas in a varicose vein the opposite is true.

Medical treatment and nursing care. Mild discomfort from varicose veins may be treated conservatively by advising the patient to elevate his feet for a few minutes at regular two to three hour intervals throughout the day, to avoid constrictions about the legs, to avoid standing, and to wear an elastic stocking or elastic bandage. Improvement in posture sometimes helps to prevent further development of the varicosities, and the patient may be advised by his physician to lose weight.

Sclerosing solutions have been used for years in the treatment of varicose veins, and medical authorities differ in their convictions as to whether they should be tried for a long period before surgery is done or whether early surgery will free the patient of discomfort and control the condition more quickly and efficiently. These solutions cause an irritation within the vein with formation of a thrombus, and as the inflammation subsides the lumen of the vein is usually obliterated. Results are not always uniformly good. Sometimes recanalization occurs through the thrombus and scar tissue, and the symptoms may then return. Sclerosing solutions are often used to treat varicosities in small veins after a ligation of larger veins has been done. Since sclerosing solutions cause a thrombus to form, there is always some danger of a clot being released into the general circulation.

Sodium morrhuate and sodium tetradecyl sulfate (Sotradecol) are solutions often used. Both of these cause severe generalized reactions in sensitive persons. Epinephrine and antihistaminic drugs such as Benadryl are kept ready for immediate injection if signs of reaction such as hives and marked pruritus occur. Occasionally severe reactions that require the intravenous injection of epinephrine and the administration of oxygen and cardiac stimulants such as caffeine sodium benzoate occur. The injection of sclerosing solutions is usually done in the clinic or in the doctor's office. The nurse must take the responsibility for seeing that emergency equipment is on hand and for preventing other accidents to patients. Many patients are elderly and some tend to become faint when standing for the treatment. Footstools can be equipped with side attachments and handle bars on which the patient may lean for comfort and security. The site of injection is covered with a small dressing. The patient is urged not to scratch the skin over the site of injection since this might lead to an infected excoriation and eventual ulceration. The greatest care also must be taken not to bruise or otherwise traumatize the veins since this, too, may lead to ulceration.

Stasis of blood in tissues around

marked varicosities, particularly when deep veins are also involved, leads to replacement of normal tissue with fibrous tissue which is firm to the touch and colored with pigment from extravasated blood cells. This condition often causes severe pruritus and general discomfort in the limb; it is called *stasis dermatitis.* Ulcers occur easily when stasis dermatitis has developed, and these are difficult to control. Ligation of varicosed veins is usually necessary, since the ulcer will not heal while marked varicosities persist in the vessels above it. Besides the general measures already mentioned for any ulcers of vascular origin, treatment of *varicose ulcers* include grafting of skin to cover the wound and pressure bandages. Success in grafting depends partly on whether or not the arterial supply is also affected; healing is usually slow in these ulcers because of poor circulation to the fibrotic tissue surrounding them.

Gelatin paste bandages applied to the entire lower limb, and known as "boots," are widely used in the treatment of varicose ulcers. This dressing, or boot, provides constant even pressure which supports the superficial veins, protects the ulcer from injury and infection, and fosters healing. *Unna's paste boot* is the best known; it contains zinc oxide, glycerin, gelatin, and water and must be melted before it is ready for application. It is applied with a brush, usually four layers of 3- to 4-inch bandage being alternated with layers of the paste. Many variations of this boot are now available in which 3- to 4-inch bandage comes already impregnated with the paste, sealed in a special airtight wrapping, and ready for immediate use. These save time and obviate the danger of burning the patient when melted paste is used.

Before a paste bandage is applied, the patient rests for one-half hour with the feet elevated. Hair on the legs should be shaved, and a small dry sterile dressing is placed over the ulcer; adhesive tape should not be used to hold this in place since it is irritating to the skin. While the patient is resting with the feet elevated, the nurse should learn whether or not he has been able to follow the doctor's instructions in regard to diet, rest, and exercise and discover any particular problems he may have that may need referral to the social worker or the doctor. The boot is evenly applied beginning with the instep and ending two inches below the knee (see Figure 31). Fifteen to twenty minutes are required for the paste to set and the boot is then dusted with talcum powder and may be covered with a Surgitube dressing, although a stocking or sock may be worn directly over the boot. Boots are usually changed about every ten days to two weeks, depending upon the condition of the patient and the amount of drainage from the ulcer.

Ligation and stripping of veins. Surgical treatment for varicosities consists of ligation of the vein above the varicosity and removal of the varicosed vein distal to the ligation, provided, of course, that the deep veins are able to return the venous blood satisfactorily. The great saphenous vein is ligated close to the femoral junction if possible, and the great and small saphenous veins are then stripped out through small incisions at the groin, above and below the knee, and at the ankle. Sterile dressings are used to cover the wounds, and an elastic bandage, extending from the foot to the groin, is firmly applied.

Ligation and stripping are usually done under general anesthesia since the procedure is very tiresome and painful. To prevent the development of thrombosis in other veins, the patient usually walks about on the day of the operation and at frequent intervals during his remaining two or three days in the hospital. Usually the foot of the bed is elevated on blocks for the first twenty-four hours to help in venous return of blood unless the patient is elderly and also has arterial insufficiency. Moving, walking, and bending are extremely difficult for the patient, and he may have more pain and discomfort following this surgical procedure than following much more serious surgery. Although the operation is

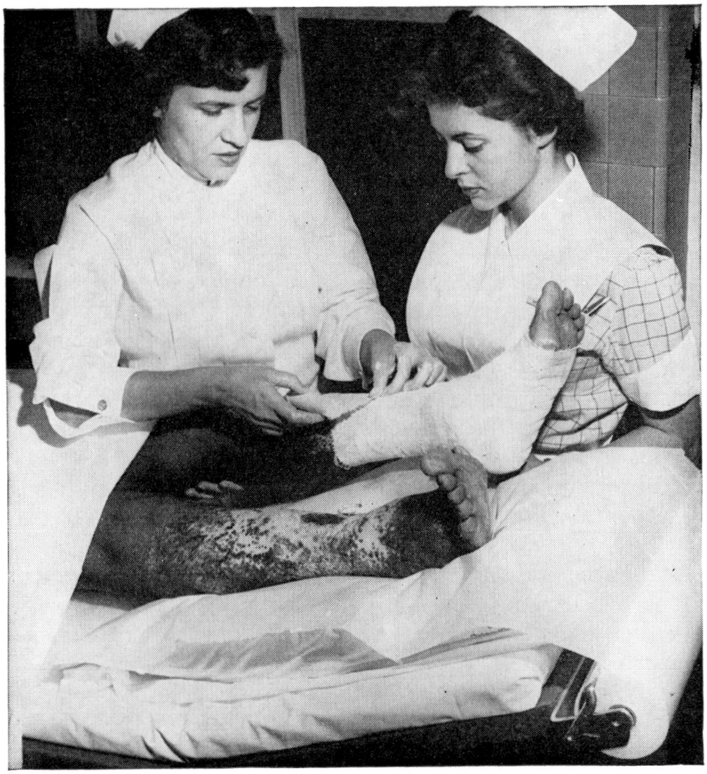

Figure 31

The zinc oxide bandage can be applied easily to the ambulatory patient in the clinic. Note the skin discoloration around the leg ulcer.

considered a relatively minor one and the patient is out of bed almost at once, nursing care is important. The patient should be assisted when he walks on the first day and thereafter if he is receiving analgesic drugs such as meperidine hydrochloride (Demerol). He should have encouragement and assistance as needed. The elastic bandage and the dressings should be checked, since they may become loosened with walking and the wounds may be exposed; hemorrhage may also occur. If hemorrhage does occur, the leg should be elevated, pressure should be applied over the wound, and the doctor should be notified. Since the patient has difficulty in handling himself because of the firm binding around his knees, he must be protected from accidents. When analgesic drugs have been ordered they should be given for the first twenty-four to forty-eight hours.

Patients who have had an operation for varicose veins should know that the condition may recur since large superficial collateral vessels may develop and in turn become varicosed. The patient should take the general precautions of any patient with varicosities since the operation cures his acute symptoms but does not remove his tendency to have varicose veins. Weight reduction, posture improvement, avoidance of pressure on blood vessels, and elevation of the lower limbs should be practiced postoperatively exactly as is recommended for the patient with mild varicosities who is receiving conservative treatment only. A booklet, *Varicose Veins,* which is useful in teaching patients who have this condition can be obtained from the American Heart Association.

Aneurysm

An aneurysm is an abnormal enlargement of an artery at some point in its course. It may be caused by a congenital anomaly or weakness in the vessel wall, it may follow trauma, or it may be caused by disease such as syphilis which often attacks the aorta or by degenerative disease such as arteriosclerosis. By means of angiograms (arteriograms) and other diagnostic procedures, aneurysms in such locations as the aorta can now be clearly identified. The treatment for aneurysms usually is surgical; treatment and care differ somewhat depending on the location of the aneurysm.

Aneurysm within the abdominal cavity. Aneurysms may occur anywhere in the ascending or the descending aorta or in the upper iliac arteries which lie within the abdominal cavity. Previously, attempts were made to support the bulging vessel with fascia or other substances or to toughen its wall by thrombosis formation following stimulation with electric current. In recent years grafts have been widely used. Grafts of human arteries (taken from young, healthy adults and carefully preserved) or plastic material (carefully selected to match the normal vessel in size) are used. The plastic graft material which resembles a firm thick nylon mesh attaches readily where it is sutured to the vessel and becomes quickly lined with endothelial cells.

If the aneurysm is above the renal arteries, hypothermia and/or the heart-lung machine must be used. Preoperative and postoperative care are exactly the same as that described for the patient having heart surgery (see Chapter 18).

If the aneurysm is below the renal arteries, hypothermia and the heart-lung machine are not necessary because arterial flow to the lower extremities can be interrupted safely for the time needed to complete the operation.[20] Postoperative nursing care for patients having this operation includes constant nursing observation for several hours with recording of blood pressure, apical-radial, posterior tibial, and dorsalis pedis pulses, and respirations every fifteen minutes until they are stabilized and then every hour for at least twenty-four hours. Skin over the dorsalis pedis pulse may be marked with ink before the operation so that its location can be easily determined postoperatively. Initial spasm may cause this pulse to be absent upon the patient's return from the operating room, but if this continues it may indicate a thrombosis beyond the graft and loss of arterial blood to the limb.

The patient usually is placed flat in bed and sharp flexion of the hip is avoided because it causes pressure on the femoral artery. Flexion of the knee is also avoided because it causes pressure on the popliteal artery. The patient can be gently moved from side to side and should dorsiflex and extend his feet at regular intervals to prevent congestion of venous blood in the lower legs. Because the incision is a long one and pain may be pronounced, the patient is able to breathe more deeply, cough productively, and move more easily if a firm abdominal binder is used and if he is instructed to support his abdomen as he coughs or moves. Often the nurse must help with this. Narcotics are given fairly liberally for pain during the first few days postoperatively.

Since some handling of the viscera must occur during surgery of the aorta, postoperative distention is sometimes a problem. Aspiration of flatus from the stomach may be necessary in which case a stomach tube is passed and food, fluid, and electrolytes must be supplied intravenously.

The patient must be watched for low back pain which may indicate hemorrhage or thrombosis at the site of the graft. Pain and cramping in the legs are significant since they may indicate that a clot has formed beyond the graft and floated on to occlude an artery in the extremity. The signs of peripheral arterial occlusion (such as pain, coldness, whiteness, or numbness of all or part of an extremity) must be watched for.

On about the fourth postoperative day, the patient usually is permitted out of bed for a short time and often he may leave the hospital in about two weeks.

Aneurysm in the extremity. Occasionally an artery and a vein are congenitally joined or become joined following trauma, with the result that the part of the limb beyond the aneurysm is deprived of an adequate supply of arterial blood, and various signs of poor blood supply such as atrophy, cyanosis, trophic changes, or even gangrene may occur. Sometimes, when the aneurysm is superficial, the pulsating enlargement may be felt and an audible sound can be heard with each pulsation. This is called a *bruit.* If the aneurysm is in an artery, the bruit is intermittent; when there is an arteriovenous aneurysm or a fistula between an artery and a vein, the bruit may be constant and may resemble a purring sound.

The preferred treatment of a peripheral aneurysm is surgical removal without destroying the pathway of the main vessel. Sometimes this is not possible. If the fistula cannot be closed or a portion of the aneurysm removed, the vessel may be ligated if this is compatible with life of tissues distal to the lesion. Arterial and plastic grafts can also be used in larger blood vessels of the extremities either to replace portions of the artery that contain the aneurysm or to bypass the abnormality. Bypassing is done by grafting a replacement to the portion of artery involved by attaching it proximally and distally but without removing the involved portion. In addition to general postoperative care, the patient who has had this surgical procedure may be treated with any or all of the medications and other means described in this chapter to augment circulation when arterial supply is limited or when thrombosis threatens.

Embolus

An *embolectomy* is the surgical removal of a lodged embolus forming a clot within an artery. This operation is quite difficult, and results are unpredictable in that thrombosis is likely to occur following the trauma to the vessel, even if the obstructing embolus has been successfully removed.

The signs of sudden lodging or formation of a large embolus in an artery are dramatic. There is severe pain at the site of the thrombus formation Fainting, nausea, vomiting, and signs of pronounced shock may appear. Almost immediately signs may be noted in the extremity. Whiteness, coldness, blotching, tingling, and numbness of areas supplied by the vessel are common. Cyanosis, followed by even greater darkening and gangrene, occurs if the blood supply is completely obstructed and collateral circulation is inadequate.

An embolectomy is usually done within a few hours of the onset of acute symptoms of lodging of the embolus; sometimes operation must be attempted within an hour if the limb is to be saved. Surgical procedures that may be done include opening the vessel and removing the clot *(embolectomy),* removal of the clot and also removal of adherent substances and part of the lining of the vessel *(endarterectomy),* arterial resection with removal of the clot and the adherent diseased artery surrounding it with subsequent grafting, and bypassing the diseased portion of the vessel with a graft as is sometimes done for an aneurysm. Vasodilating drugs are given to improve the collateral circulation, warmth is applied to the body, and a sympathetic block of the lumbar ganglia may be done in an attempt to produce vasodilation of other vessels. Heparin and Dicumarol may be given to help prevent further thrombus formation. The patient who has an acute embolic obstruction of a large artery needs constant nursing supervision. Pain is severe and fear is pronounced.

Occasionally very large clots form slowly in the descending aorta at its bifurcation into the iliac arteries. With this "*saddle embolus,*" symptoms may not occur so suddenly but life is threatened.

Anticoagulants are given and surgery may be done to remove the clot. Nursing care is similar to that needed by the patient who has had surgery for an aneurysm. Blood pressure must be carefully recorded preoperatively so that suitable comparisons can be made postoperatively. It is important that the blood pressure not vary too much from what it was preoperatively since doing so would predispose to thrombus formation. A complication that must be carefully watched for postoperatively is hemorrhage. Small arteries that may have been useless while the embolus was in the artery may not bleed freely at operation and may therefore be missed in tying bleeding vessels. These may resume normal function after the operation and cause hemorrhage.

SPECIAL SURGICAL PROCEDURES

Sympathectomy

Although there is not full agreement as to the value of a sympathectomy for vasospasm, the operation is done frequently, and the nurse should understand the nursing care involved. Occasionally the operation is done as an emergency when there is severe spasm from poisons such as ergot, when a limb has been frozen, or when an arterial embolism has lodged in a major vessel supplying the limb. Usually, however, before a sympathectomy is performed the ganglia are injected with procaine to determine whether or not the treatment will be of value for the particular patient.

A lumbar sympathectomy is accomplished by making a small incision in the lower lateral aspect of the abdomen. The peritoneal cavity is not opened, but the ganglia supplying the lumbar region are removed and their fibers cut. After a lumbar sympathectomy the patient should be placed on his side. Blood pressure must be taken every fifteen minutes until it is stable. Pulse rate and respiratory rate are also checked, and the patient is watched closely for signs of shock. Distention may be marked after a lumbar sympathectomy, and Prostigmin is often given for this; 0.5 mg. (1/120 grain) is given every four to six hours for three doses. A rectal tube may be used to relieve distention. Hourly turning should be insisted upon, and deep breathing should be encouraged.

Following a lumbar sympathectomy the patient is not plagued with the dizziness and other symptoms which may follow operation on the higher ganglia of the sympathetic chain. He may notice a new feeling of warmth in his feet and legs. Very occasionally this causes slight discomfort and a feeling of fullness which is relieved by wearing an elastic stocking.

Amputations

While amputations may be necessary as a result of sarcoma and infections such as gas bacillus infection, the majority are necessitated by arteriosclerosis and by trauma. It is believed that amputations will increase each year because of the longer life span and the consequent increase in the number of elderly people in whom cardiovascular disease is likely to develop and because of increased motor car accidents.

An amputation is a serious operation that is usually done as a lifesaving measure although occasionally a deformed leg is amputated because it is believed that the patient can walk better with a prosthesis than with a deformed limb that is not amenable to corrective surgery. Only lower limb amputations are considered here. (See the selected reading list at the end of this chapter for articles dealing with arm amputation and hip disarticulation.)

Emotional reaction to amputation

Because of severe emotional reaction to the idea of an amputation, the news that amputation is necessary is usually withheld from the patient for as long as possible. Very occasionally a patient with severe pain such as occurs in thromboangiitis obliterans may welcome an amputation; however, to most patients the thought of losing a limb is almost intolerable.

Emotional reactions of distress are normal and to be expected. In ancient times the human body with perfect symmetry was glorified, as reflected in the remarkable sculpture which remains. In some ancient cultures only the physically perfect could perform certain religious rites since it was believed that only the physically perfect should appear before God. Even though one's personal faith may emphasize beauty of the spirit rather than of the body, some feeling of rejection at marring of the body is probably felt by each of us. This must be faced by the patient who must have an amputation.

Loss of the power of locomotion means loss of the power of flight, and this is one of the instinctive means of self-preservation. It may be for this reason that loss of a leg depresses the patient more than loss of an arm, even though the latter is a much greater handicap. Something about the loss of power to move about at will casts a shadow on the patient's spirit that can be relieved only by the most thoughtful and sensitive care. Even the patient who has suffered for a long time with a chronic disease that has hampered his freedom of motion feels the anticipated loss very keenly. Perhaps this is because there is such finality in an amputation. As long as the limb is there—imperfect though it may be—the patient usually retains the hope that normal or near-normal function will be restored. If amputation is necessary because of an accident, the suddenness of the changes in the patient's picture of himself may produce real shock.

Other emotional reactions are more tangible and more easily understood. The handicap is obvious (or at least the patient believes that it is), and he fears that he will be pitied. To the wage earner, father, and husband, an amputation may mean that he must learn a new occupation or that he may lose his place as head of his household. To the older person, it may mean dependence upon children or upon the community.

Emotional reactions to an amputation have an enormous effect on the patient's rehabilitation. Such reactions depend on his emotional make-up and his response to other life crises, as well as on circumstances leading to the amputation and the care he receives. The most perfect surgical operation and the best-fitting prosthesis are useless if the patient remains a complete invalid and a burden to himself, his family, and the community. The nurse must think of the long-range plans for the patient from the time that she learns that an amputation is necessary. It is at this time, when emotional reactions to the amputation and the idea of using a prosthesis are forming, that she can make her greatest contribution to the patient's rehabilitation, by helping him to realize that his problems are not insurmountable and by watching him carefully for responses that may indicate need for care by various members of the health team.

In the past, teaching the patient to walk with a prosthesis often was left to the limb maker. Although the limb maker can teach the patient a great deal about the new limb and its effective use, learning to walk with an artificial limb is usually a complicated procedure that requires instruction by a skilled physical therapist. It is the responsibility of nurses working with the surgeon, the social worker, the physical therapist, and other members of the professional health team to see that the patient gets continuous care, teaching, and encouragement until he is able to manage on his own. Members of the patient's family can often be called upon for help. They are usually told of the amputation before the patient, or at the same time, so that they can help him accept the news. When the patient does know that an amputation is necessary, he often benefits from a visit from someone who has undergone the same operation and has made a full recovery. With the right mental outlook, most patients can return as functioning and useful members of society. The percentage is, of course, lower among the aged many of whom have other disabilities such as cardiac disease and osteoarthritis which slow their progress in learning to manage themselves independently.

The amputation

The surgeon endeavors to remove all diseased tissue yet leave a stump that permits satisfactory use of a prosthesis. There is not full agreement among surgeons and limb makers as to the correct levels for amputations for best use of the stump. Most agree, however, that an amputation below the knee should be in the middle third of the leg, and that thigh amputations should be in the lower third of the thigh. Each inch of bone that must be removed from the femur above the lower third decreases the function of the limb. Two and one-half inches above the knee is often considered the optimum level from the standpoint of fitting the prosthesis.

Below-the-knee amputations are best for wearing a prosthesis and permit a more natural gait than thigh amputations because knee function remains. Unfortunately, many patients with arterial disease require amputations above the knee because the poor circulation extends far up the limb.

For the best function of the limb, the stump should be long enough to permit sufficient leverage to move the artificial limb but not long enough to interfere with the movement of the joint distal to the amputation. The end of the bone should be covered with skin, subcutaneous tissue, and muscle which is not adherent to the bone end; the stump should be healthy and firm, without creases, folds, and flabby parts. The stump should be painless, with no nerve endings remaining in the scar, and the scar should not fall over the weight-bearing end of the bone. The stump should have a smooth conical contour and should be freely movable by the patient in any normal range of motion.

There are two types of amputations. One, the guillotine or circular amputation, is done when there has been serious trauma, when gas bacilli are present in the wound, or when there is moist gangrene (gangrene with infection). The blood vessels and nerves are ligated, but the wound is left open. This is a relatively simple and quick operation which can be done on patients who are quite poor operative risks. The disadvantage of this amputation is that usually another operation is necessary before the patient can be fitted with a prosthesis. Since the wound is not sutured, there may be muscle and skin retraction which makes the fitting of a prosthesis difficult or impossible. Healing is slow after a guillotine operation and may require weeks or months unless a secondary closure operation is done.

The flap type of amputation is by far the more satisfactory if it can be done. The wound usually heals completely within two weeks. In arterial disease it has been found that, if possible, surgery should be delayed until demarcation sets in so that healthy tissue can be more accurately identified.

Preoperative care. If the operation is not an emergency one, the patient is told what to expect before and following the operation. The doctor explains the operation to him and usually mentions phantom limb sensation. He is also told whether it is expected that traction will be used. The nurse tells the patient that he will be turned or asked to turn and move about almost immediately following the operation, and she explains why he must be asked to lie on his abdomen. If the condition of the diseased limb permits, she may teach him to do push-up exercises while lying on his abdomen. Simply by using his arms to raise his chest from the bed and repeating this several times at regular intervals daily, the patient can improve substantially the muscle tone and muscle strength of his arms and shoulders.

The choice of anesthetic depends on the surgeon and the condition of the patient. An amputation can be done while the patient is under spinal anesthesia, although this is very distressing to the patient since the sawing of bone can be heard despite large doses of sedation. Refrigeration anesthesia has been widely used, although general anesthesia (intravenous and inhalation) is the most frequently used. An intravenous infusion is usually started before the patient goes to the operating room or is started in the operating room before surgery begins so that fluid can be replenished immediately if signs of shock or hemorrhage occur.

Postoperative care. When the patient returns from the operating room or the recovery room, vital signs should be checked and signs of hemorrhage from the stump should be watched for. A heavy tourniquet is always kept fastened to the foot of the bed so that it may be applied immediately if sudden, severe hemorrhage should occur. If the patient is sent to the operating room in his bed, the tourniquet should be attached to it. The nurse must know how to apply the tourniquet and if sudden hemorrhage occurs she does not wait for a doctor's order to use it. Drainage from the wound should be watched for; if there is bright red drainage, an outline of the stain should be marked on the outside of the dressing with pencil so the rate of drainage can be followed closely. Usually the stump is elevated on a rubber-covered pillow when the patient returns from the operating room, and it is left in this position for twelve to twenty-four hours. This lessens edema and bleeding or serous oozing from the wound. However, the pillow must be removed after twenty-four hours at the most to prevent hip and knee contractures. When a guillotine operation has been done, the patient usually returns to his room with traction applied to the stump. Wide bands of adhesive tape are placed on the skin above the wound, a spreader is used, and traction is applied to prevent retraction of skin and muscle away from the line of operation. Traction pulleys at the foot of the bed may be placed toward the center so that the patient can turn onto his abdomen, or a Thomas splint may be used so that the patient can be moved more easily and can be out of bed without the traction being released. (See Chapter 36 for care of the patient in traction.)

If the amputation is below the knee, the stump may be firmly bandaged on a padded board to prevent contracture at the knee joint. When this is done, the nurse must check the padding carefully, since muscle spasm resulting in the limb being pulled against the board may be so great that a pressure sore is produced. If spasm seems severe, a piece of sponge rubber can sometimes be slipped between the bandaged stump end and the padded board for additional protection. Sometimes the surgeon removes the limb from the board for part of the day.

Exercises. Unless there is a medical order to the contrary, the patient who has had a lower limb amputation should turn on his abdomen for a short time the day following operation, and thereafter he should lie on the abdomen for some time at least twice each day. When in this position, he can practice the push-up exercises he started before the operation. The patient who has a limb in traction can also turn with assistance. If the amputation has been done below the knee, the patient can begin at once to hyperextend the thigh and leg. This strengthens muscles in preparation for walking. If the amputation is above the knee, a medical order should be obtained before the patient hyperextends the thigh, since this exercise might possibly cause strain on the suture line. Lying on the back and lifting the stump and buttocks off the bed helps to develop the abdominal muscles which are necessary in stabilizing the pelvis when the patient stoops or bends.

When the patient is permitted out of bed, the nurse should begin to teach him self-care activities such as getting out of a chair. To preserve his center of gravity and balance, the patient should keep his good leg well under him before he shifts his weight, as when rising from a chair. If a physical therapist is available the nurse should consult him regarding exercise.

The patient who has had an amputation because of vascular disease must be reminded to take particular care of his re-

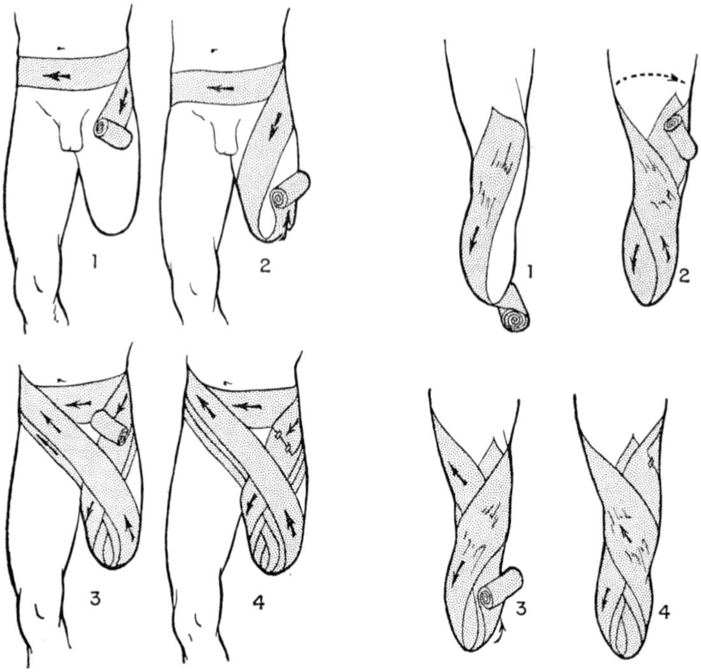

Figure 32

The four sketches on the left side of the diagram illustrate the correct method for bandaging a mid-thigh amputation stump. Note that the bandage must be anchored around the patient's waist. The four sketches on the right side of the diagram illustrate the correct method for bandaging a mid-calf amputation stump. Note that the bandage need not be anchored about the waist.

maining foot and leg. Exercises and other measures to keep the arterial supply as good as possible must be carried on while the patient is in the hospital, and he must be urged to follow his doctor's instructions carefully when he leaves the hospital.

Care of the stump. If a prosthesis is to be worn comfortably, a healthy stump is necessary. Teaching the patient how to care for his stump is a nursing responsibility which may be carried out both in the hospital and in the patient's home. The length of hospitalization depends on the kind of operation, the patient's general condition, and his home circumstances. He may be discharged from the hospital within a few weeks and yet may not be fitted satisfactorily for a limb for from six weeks to six months.

When the wound is completely healed, the patient is taught to wash the stump daily and to massage the skin gently, directing the motion toward the suture line. He may be instructed to push forcefully over the bone to toughen the limb for weight-bearing. Sometimes this is begun by placing a pillow on a footstool, chair, or high stool (depending upon the site of operation) and by having the patient bear some weight on the stump while steadying himself on the bed or against the wall.

There should be no tenderness, redness, or other signs of skin irritation or abrasion at the end of the stump. The skin and underlying tissues should be firm and without flabbiness and should be without tautness over the bony end of the limb. If there is a tendency to flabbiness, the stump may be bandaged firmly during both the day and night. Some patients are taught to do this for themselves; however, they need careful instruction and supervision. (See Figure 32.) The bandage must not be tight enough to cause pain or numbness from hampered circulation; if it is too loose it will defeat its purpose. If the patient is unable to apply a firm bandage, a member of his family may help him with this. The bandage should be removed and reapplied twice daily, and the skin should be washed, dried, powdered, and exposed to the air for a short time before the bandage is reapplied. The patient should have at least two bandages so that one may be washed daily; these should not be stretched while drying.

The patient should have several pairs of stump socks of the right size. These should be made of cotton and wool and should be washed daily after use and dried over a dryer or a mold to prevent shrinkage. Usually the patient wears out about one sock a month when he begins to use a prosthesis. They should not be mended because this may cause irritation to the stump.

When the prosthesis is used, the patient should continue the routine care of the stump, including bathing, massage, and inspection. Most surgeons advise their patients not to soak the stump because this may cause maceration of the skin, although it should be washed daily. Alcohol or mild skin creams can be used, depending on the natural condition of the skin. If the weather is warm and the skin perspires freely, the limb should be removed from the socket, bathed, exposed to the air for a short time, and then powdered at least once during the day. The patient who works may take an extra stump sock with him so that he can change during the day in hot weather. To prevent tension on the sock as the limb is placed in the socket, a string may be attached to the end of the sock and brought through a hole that is usually left in the prosthesis below the level of the stump. The patient should be instructed to report calluses or any abnormalities on the stump to his doctor at once.

Phantom limb sensation. Phantom limb is an unpleasant complication which sometimes follows an amputation and which is difficult to treat. It may be only a sensation of the limb being in its normal position and may disappear if the patient looks at the stump and recalls that the limb has been amputated. *Phantom limb pain* also occurs. The patient may have the sensation, for example, that something is burning the foot, that his toes are being stepped upon, and the like. Phantom limb pain may disappear of its own accord, or it may lessen for a time and then recur with severity. When it is really troublesome to the patient, the nerve endings may be injected with alcohol to give temporary relief. Occasionally, when pain persists, an operation is done for removal of the nerve ends which may have developed to form a tuft on a weight-bearing part of the stump. A few patients are troubled with phantom limb pain for an indefinite time following amputation, and this may interfere seriously with their rehabilitation. Reamputation is sometimes considered, but even this may not always bring relief since the same sensations may be experienced at the end of the new stump.

Crutch-walking. Teaching the patient who has had an amputation to walk with crutches, with crutches and prosthesis, and then with prosthesis alone is a complicated task that lies within the responsibility of physical medicine. The nurse, however, has a responsibility to prepare the patient for the use of crutches and should know the essentials of their use and something about the gaits that the patient will use.

Preparation for the use of crutches should begin before the operation by teaching the patient to lie on his abdomen and do push-up exercises. Further preparation includes prevention of contractures and deformities that will interfere with use of crutches and with use of a prosthesis. Contracture at the hip, which follows letting the patient lie with the head of the bed elevated for weeks at a time, is an example. Every patient should lie on his abdomen for some part of the day so that extension at the hip joint prevents contracture of that joint. Contracture of the knee joint can also occur and interfere with the use of crutches and prosthesis. The nurse must not become so occupied with the affected limb that she neglects the good leg and foot if the amputation involves only one limb. Supervision of regular exercises to strengthen leg muscles and care that drop foot and pronation deformities do not occur are part of good nursing. The patient should have a firm board or block of wood at the foot of the bed against which he can push and thereby get essential active exercise.

The patient needs exercise to strengthen the triceps, which is a muscle used to extend the elbow and is therefore most important in the satisfactory use of crutches. When lying on his back, he can hold bags of sand or other weights on his palms and straighten out his elbows. Use of an overbed trapeze bar is helpful in that it enables the patient to handle himself much more independently than would otherwise be possible. Its use, however, strengthens primarily the biceps muscle, which is less essential in crutch-walking than is the triceps. Another exercise for strengthening the triceps muscles is to have the patient sit up on the edge of the bed with his feet in a chair and, while pressing his palms against the mattress, lift his hips off the bed. This provides good exercise in extension of the elbow and helps the patient become accustomed to resting his weight on his hands rather than on the axillae.

Crutches should be measured for each patient. One method is to have the patient lie on his back with his arms at his sides. The measure is taken from the axilla to a point six inches out from the side of the heel; this is the length of the crutch minus three fourths of an inch for the crutch tips. Another method is to measure from two inches below the level of the axilla to the base of the heel. Still another method is to subtract sixteen inches from the patient's total height. Even with careful measurement, alterations may have to be made after the crutches are used. Posture, for example, may change, and this may alter the needed length. The crutch should not cause pressure on the axilla, and the patient is taught not to rest his weight on the axillary bars for more than a few minutes at a time. To do so causes pressure on the radial nerve and this can lead to severe and sometimes permanent "crutch paralysis." The patient is taught that weight should be borne on the palms of the hands.

Before the patient attempts to walk with crutches, he should be assisted out of bed and should stand by the bed to get the feel of normal balance. A walker or parallel bars can also be used for this. At this time he begins to practice good standing posture, with head up, chest up, abdomen in, pelvis tilted inward, a 5-degree angle in the knee joint, and the foot straight. Practice in front of a mirror is very helpful. The patient is encouraged not to look down at his foot, the crutch, or the prosthesis.

In all crutch-walking, the patient is taught to concentrate on a normal rhythmic gait. The first gait that he will use is the swing-to or swing-through gait that requires no carefully guided instruction, provided the patient knows how to bear his weight and has been taught to check posture, balance, and rhythm. In this gait the amputated limb and the crutches both advance either to or beyond the level of the normal limb and are followed by the normal leg. This is a simple fast gait which gives little leg exercise but is useful for rapid maneuvers such as are needed in crossing streets. The patient may use this gait when he begins to walk with a prosthesis, in which case both crutches and the prosthesis move forward, followed by the normal leg. From this he may progress to one crutch and then to a cane, which should be abandoned eventually. The crutch or cane should be held in the hand on the side *opposite* the prosthesis since, as the patient normally walks, the arm on the opposite side of the body alternately swings forward. Holding the cane or crutch on the same side as the prosthesis results in an awkward unrhythmic gait.

When the patient with double amputations has been fitted with prostheses, he may be taught the four-point gait, and it is to be expected that he will learn to manage himself much more slowly than if only one limb were gone. Patients with amputations above the knee also take much longer to learn to walk and otherwise manage their movements. The four-point gait is taught to the count of four and is as follows: left crutch, right foot, right crutch, left foot. Some patients with bilateral amputations must always use this gait (which is also widely used by those with involved neuromuscular disabilities and poor balance). It is a safe gait because the patient always has three points of contact with the ground at any time. Most patients progress to the two-point gait, in which the foot and opposite crutch move together and then the prosthesis and the opposite crutch. It is often taught to the count of two as follows: left crutch and right foot (one) and right crutch and left foot (two). The two-point gait produces a much faster gait and is easier to maintain in a rhythmic pattern than the four-point gait. It is important for the nurse to know which gait the physical therapist is teaching the patient so that she may remind him if, upon leaving the physical therapy department, he reverts to a swing-to gait, for example.

The prosthesis. The doctor prescribes the type of prosthesis that is best for the patient and usually refers him to a limb maker. After the limb is made the patient returns to the clinic, hospital department of physical medicine, doctor's office, or rehabilitation center to learn the best use of the artificial limb. The public health nurse, particularly if she is also trained in physical therapy, often gives care and supervision to the patient in his home.

Most prostheses are made of well-seasoned willow wood, although some are made of metal (Durallumin and aluminum) and fiber materials. Metal prostheses can be lighter in weight than wooden ones, but they tend to be noisy. The type of prosthesis is selected for the individual patient. Usually the below-the-knee prosthesis weighs about five pounds and the mid-thigh prosthesis about seven and one-half pounds, although the weight of the prosthesis is adapted to the size and weight of the patient and the kind of work he does.

The prosthesis has a socket or "bucket" into which the limb fits. In the past, leather was the material most widely used for this, but plastic materials and wood are now widely used since they are lighter and easier to keep clean and odorless. The stump should fit snugly into the socket, and no more than two socks should be needed for a comfortable fit. If more are needed, it means that the stump has shrunk and the prosthesis needs adjusting. Shrinking may continue for as long as ten years and is usually greater after amputation of the foreleg than after amputation of the thigh. Suction cups are now quite generally used to hold the stump in the socket and obviate wearing a heavy laced belt about the waist, although all patients with lower limb prostheses wear some kind of waistband and those with thigh amputations also wear a shoulder strap attachment to the waistband. The patient is advised to keep his shoulders straight and not permit the one on which the strap is worn to sag. He needs constant encouragement to use the prosthesis, particularly in the beginning when he is adjusting to all features of the device. He should start to use the prosthesis at once. Most doctors prefer that the patient not use a "peg leg" or other temporary device since this may spoil his gait for use of an artificial limb.

The nurse should learn whether or not the patient is really using his prosthesis when at home. If he is not, she should learn the reason and report this to the doctor. Often she can help make the arrangements for more instruction. It is important that there be no delay, because the longer the patient puts off using the prosthesis, the less likely he is to use it satisfactorily. If crutches are used for too long and if the patient depends on other forms of getting about, such as a wheel chair, he may have real difficulty in developing a normal rhythmic gait.

Care of the prosthesis should be reviewed with the patient. He should be taught to fasten the cuff above the stump from the bottom up, even though this may seem more difficult at first. The cuff should be snug but not uncomfortable. He should keep his shoes in good repair, should wear rubber heels, and should replace broken shoestrings at once. If the limb has a joint, he should keep this free from lint and dust, should oil the joints and locks every few weeks, and should keep screws tightened, yet make no adjustments. If the cuff is leather, care should be taken that the stump sock is long enough to protect it from perspiration, and it should be rubbed with saddle soap at least weekly. The inside of the stump socket should be washed frequently to ensure cleanliness.

The patient should be told that his artificial limb is a tool and that it will be most useful to him when he has mastered its use. With good care it will last him from three to ten years. Its value will depend on how well he can learn to balance himself, how much muscle strength he develops, and how smooth and rhythmic a gait he learns. Above all, its value will depend on his attitude toward the challenge that its use presents.

Long-term care. Most patients who have an amputation must remain under medical supervision for a long time. If possible, a public health nurse should visit the patient's home before he leaves the hospital so that she can help the family make any structural changes necessary for facilitating the patient's ambulation. If it should happen that a patient is equipped with an artificial limb but is not taught how to use it, the community nurse should initiate steps toward his rehabilitation. Occasionally the limb fitter believes that the hospital clinic personnel is taking responsibility for teaching the patient to walk and the doctor or the hospital clinic personnel believe that the limb fitter is doing this. It is safe to assume that any patient with an amputation needs medical and nursing care and supervision long after the wound has healed. He may become discouraged and, after months of what appears to be a good adjustment, may lay the limb aside and return to a wheel chair or crutches. Sometimes he reports that it is not comfortable and that he is reluctant to go back to the limb fitter because of costs. If this is so, the nurse can help to find agencies in the community that can give appropriate assistance. It may be, however, that this statement is made by the patient to conceal a much more important and deep-seated rejection of his difficulties. This, of course, is a much more difficult problem and should be reported to the doctor, who will decide what steps should be taken.

The National Rehabilitation Council has facilities to help amputees; they provide financial assistance, medical aid, job-placement services and counseling. There are many rehabilitation centers in the United States, but most of these are located in the larger cities. The division of vocational rehabilitation of the department of education in every state is, however, available to all patients. Most communities, counties, and states have voluntary programs which are designed to help the physically handicapped, including the amputee. The nurse should turn to her local health department for information on the resources available to her own community. Three excellent pamphlets are available: *Handbook for the Leg Amputee,** *A Guide for the Arm Amputee,*† and *Industrial Amputee Rehabilitation.*‡

---

*V. A. Pamphlet 10-37, Washington D. C., 1951, U. S. Government Printing Office.

†V. A. Pamphlet 10-38, Washington D. C., 1952, U. S. Government Printing Office.

‡Published by Liberty Mutual Insurance Co., Boston.

REFERENCES AND SELECTED READINGS*

1 Allen, Edgar V., Barker, Nelson W., and Hines, Edgar A. Jr.: Peripheral Vascular Diseases, ed 2, Philadelphia, 1955, W. B. Saunders Co.
2 *Alpenfels, Ethel J.: The Anthropology and Social Significance of the Human Hand, Artificial Limbs **2**:4-21, May 1955.
3 Barnes, Gilbert H.: Skin Health and Stump Hygiene, Artificial Limbs **3**:4-9, Spring 1956.
4 *Cannon, Jack A., and Quint, Jeanne C.: Endarterectomy and Nursing the Patient With Endarterectomy, Am. J. Nursing **58**:1996-1998, July 1958.
5 Cecil, Russell L., and Loeb, Robert F. (editors): A Textbook of Medicine, ed. 10, Philadelphia, 1959, W. B. Saunders Co.
6 Cliffton, Eugene E., and others: Symposium on Fibrolysin, Am. J. Cardiology **6**:367-563, Aug. 1960.
7 Davis, Loyal (editor): Christopher's Textbook of Surgery, ed. 6, Philadelphia, 1956, W. B. Saunders Co.
8 De Takats, Geza: Vascular Surgery, Philadelphia, 1959, W. B. Saunders Co.
9 Dembo, Tamara, Leviton, Gloria, and Wright, Beatrice: Adjustment to Misfortune—A Problem of Social-Psychologic Rehabilitation, Artificial Limbs **3**:4-6, Autumn 1956.
10 Fletcher, Anthony P., and Sherry, Sol: Thrombolytic (Fibrinolytic) Therapy for Coronary Heart Disease, Circulation **22**:619-626, Oct. 1960.
11 Foley, William T.: The Medical Management of Lymphedema, Mod. Concepts Cardiovas. Dis. **24**:255-257, Jan. 1955.
12 Foley, William T., and Wright, Irving S.: Medical Management of Arterial Occlusion and Thrombophlebitis, Mod. Concepts Cardiovas. Dis. **22**:162-165, Feb. 1953.
13 Goodman, Louis S., and Gilman, Alfred: The Pharmacological Basis of Therapeutics, ed. 2, New York, 1955, The Macmillan Co.

*References preceded by an asterisk indicate material particularly well suited for student reading.

14 Gottlieb, Marvin S., and others: Some Experiences With Prosthetic Problems of Upper Extremity Amputees, Artificial Limbs **4**:4-40, Spring 1957.
15 Kessler, Henry H.: Rehabilitation of the Physically Handicapped (revised), New York, 1953, Columbia University Press.
16 *Krause, G. Lynn, and Vetter, Frances C.: Varicose Veins—Diagnosis and Treatment and Nursing Care, Am. J. Nursing **53**:70-72, Jan. 1953.
17 Krug, Elsie E.: Pharmacology in Nursing, ed. 8, St. Louis, 1960, The C. V. Mosby Co.
18 Levy, S. William: The Skin Problems of the Lower Extremity Amputee, Artificial Limbs **3**:20-35, Spring 1956.
19 *Marple, Charles D., and McIntyre, Marie J.: Anticoagulant Therapy—Medical Aspects and Nursing Care, Am. J. Nursing **56**:875-879, July 1956.
20 *Martin, Dorothy M., Case, Flossie G., and Miller, Arthur C.: Nursing Care of the Patient With an Abdominal Aortic Aneurysm, Am. J. Nursing **59**:60-62, Jan. 1959.
21 Meakins, Jonathan Campbell: The Practice of Medicine, ed. 6, St. Louis, 1956, The C. V. Mosby Co.
22 Moskoff, Mary Elizabeth, and Sloane, Jane: Nursing Care for the Amputee, Am. J. Nursing **50**:550-555, Sept. 1950.
23 Newton, Kathleen: Geriatric Nursing, ed. 3, St. Louis, 1960, The C. V. Mosby Co.
24 Olmstead, Lois: Crutch Walking, Am. J. Nursing **45**:28-35, Jan. 1945.
25 *Sensenig, David M., and Morson, Betty J.: Buerger's Disease, Am. J. Nursing **57**:337-340, March 1957.
26 *Smith, Lester A.: An Orthotist, Prosthetist—What Are They? Nursing Outlook **7**:34-35, Jan. 1959.
27 Wright, Irving Sherwood: Vascular Disease in Clinical Practice, ed. 2, Chicago, 1952, Year Book Publishers, Inc.
28 *Young, Eleanor, and Barnes, William: Hemipelvectomy, Am. J. Nursing **58**:361-364, March 1958.

The patient with a blood dyscrasia

Chapter 20

Study questions for review

1 What are the normal constituents of blood? Where are blood cells formed; how are they destroyed? What is the normal red blood cell count for men? for women?
2 Trace the successive processes that occur when blood clots. List the nursing responsibilities in preparing for and assisting with a blood transfusion. What observations should the nurse make while blood is being given?
3 From your understanding of physiology, explain why the patient who is anemic may have dyspnea and cyanosis.
4 Find out the price of vitamin B_{12} from your local druggist or from your hospital pharmacy. How must this drug be given?

This chapter will include only a few of the more important aspects of nursing care for those with blood dyscrasias and diseases of the blood-forming organs. Since detailed discussion of blood transfusions and nursing problems related to the taking and giving of blood can be found in fundamentals of nursing texts, they will not be included here.

DIAGNOSTIC TESTS AND PROCEDURES

Of the many tests that may be done to help determine the patient's exact blood disease, the simplest and perhaps the most significant are the red blood cell count, platelet count, examination of white blood cells, hemoglobin determination, and the bleeding and clotting times. Blood for these tests is obtained from the patient's finger or ear lobe. Other tests, such as prothrombin time determination, require blood from a vein. Because most patients with a blood dyscrasia have a tendency to bleed abnormally, prolonged bleeding from the puncture site or bleeding into surrounding tissues may occur. The nurse should inspect the site of venipuncture frequently to see that clotting does occur. Since frequent examinations of the blood are required to determine the patient's progress and are used as a guide for treatment, the patient with a blood dyscrasia should understand why they are necessary. Having blood samples taken is an unpleasant procedure, particularly when many have to be obtained. The nurse can help to see that the veins are entered as few times as possible by properly preparing the patient for the test and having the bottles and other equipment available, by checking the amount of blood to be withdrawn, by labeling the bottles correctly, and by having all the blood samples taken at one time.

Capillary fragility test. This simple test helps to determine the status of small capillaries which become fragile and rupture easily in certain blood disorders. The test is also known as the *Rumpel-Leede phenomenon.* A blood pressure cuff is placed on the patient's arm and inflated, and pressure about midway between systolic and diastolic pressure is maintained for fifteen minutes. When the skin is examined five minutes after removing the cuff, only one or two petechiae per square inch will normally be found. If the platelet count is low, numerous petechiae may appear. This test is painless, but it should be explained to the patient lest he become overly concerned with the results. It usually helps to tell him that every person will respond to this test with the appearance of some petechiae.

Sternal puncture. A sternal puncture or sternal bone marrow biopsy procedure is done to obtain a sample of the cells active in blood cell production. It may be done when leukemia, aplastic anemia, sickle cell anemia, or a number of other conditions are suspected. Most institutions require that signed permission from the patient be obtained before this procedure is done. The procedure is upsetting to some patients who fear that it will be painful and who dread the insertion of a needle "so near the heart." Actually, there is danger of puncturing the pericardium during this procedure, particularly if the sternum is abnormally thin. It is important that the patient be as relaxed and composed as possible; if he expresses extreme fear or apprehension, the nurse should report this to the doctor since he may then order a sedative.

A sternal puncture is usually done in the treatment room, although it may be done in the patient's room if he is critically ill. The patient lies on his back, and a small pillow may be placed lengthwise under the thoracic spine to bring the sternum forward. The skin is cleansed and prepared with an antiseptic solution and the area is anesthetized with procaine. A few minutes are allowed for this to take effect on the periosteum before the sternal needle (a short, stout needle with a protecting hub to prevent its being inserted too far) is inserted and tapped gently with a small mallet until the center of the bone is entered. The stylet is then withdrawn, a dry 5 or 10 ml. syringe is attached, and a small amount of fluid is aspirated; at this time the patient may have a feeling of mild pain or discomfort. The specimen is deposited immediately into a specimen bottle containing sodium oxalate, and several direct smears are made. The patient may have slight soreness over the puncture site for several days, but this should not cause real discomfort unless the sternum is inadvertently disturbed by contact.

GENERAL NURSING CARE

Chronicity of disease. With the exception of a few conditions such as nutritional anemia and fulminating leukemia, diseases of the blood and blood-forming organs are chronic. Patients with these diseases are seldom cured and knowledge of this colors their attitude toward treatment and may alter their efforts in carrying on from day to day. Each patient is individual in his response to knowledge that he has a chronic disease. Some patients become depressed, discouraged, and resigned to invalidism while others show magnificent courage in overcoming their problems and living productively from day to day.

The nurse can help the patient by listening to him when he becomes discouraged, giving him attention and care as needed, helping him determine realistic goals, discussing the need for and encouraging him to continue medical care and treatment, maintaining a positive attitude about his progress and prognosis, and contributing to patient and family planning so that, within his limitations, he may remain a productive and contributing member of society. Individual family members may also turn to the nurse and may be in need of much the same help as the patient.

Acuity of the disease. When the patient suffers from an acute blood disease such as acute leukemia and has only a short life expectancy, the nurse's role is one of support for both the patient and the family. The family will need help in understanding the nature of the disease and in accepting the diagnosis. They will need encouragement, reassurance, and strengthening of faith in the medical care being given. Present treatment increases the length of life, controls symptoms, and may restore the patient to apparent health for periods of time. When the patient is to be at home during a remission, the nurse instructs the family in the care needed so that the patient will be protected from infection and injury but permitted to live as normally as possible. While the patient is hospitalized, the nurse should be aware of the concern of the patient's family and should try to give them necessary help by listening, observing, and answering questions. The patient is likely to be irritable, discouraged, and apprehensive. The nurse should accept his reaction and understand his need for the love and attention of his family.

Fatigue. Most patients with diseases of the blood and the blood-forming organs suffer from fatigue that may be almost overwhelming. The patient may go to the doctor because he is "tired of being tired." Chronic fatigue adds to discouragement and influences the patient's emotional reaction to his symptoms.

Fatigue may be caused in part by a low red blood cell count and a low hemoglobin level since insufficient oxygen is being carried to the tissues. Insufficient blood supply may cause fainting, which is fairly common among those who have severe anemia and which may lead to serious accidents. Some patients who do not really faint complain of feeling "lightheaded"; this combined with general fatigue, also predisposes to accidents. Frequent short rest periods, lying flat without a pillow, increase arterial supply to the brain and may help to prevent this.

Fatigue may be lessened by specific medications and treatments such as transfusions. The nurse should question the ambulatory patient to be certain he is taking the medications as prescribed. Fatigue may also lessen with better nutrition, and this should be emphasized to the patient. The patient should be encouraged to discuss the problem of fatigue frankly with his doctor; the ambulatory patient may feel that this complaint will appear trivial to the busy doctor and may therefore fail to mention it.

Temperature, pulse, and respirations. These three classic signs of sickness or health are particularly important when the patient has disease of the blood or the blood-forming organs. Temperature, pulse, and respirations are taken with such regularity and become so routine in hospitals that the tendency may be to regard them as not too important. This is unfortunate since probably few complicated tests give as useful clues to the patient's progress as do these simple ones. If the temperature, pulse, and respirations are taken and recorded by auxiliary nursing personnel, the nurse has a responsibility to see that their findings are accurate and that they are correctly recorded.

Increases in pulse rate and respiratory rate are common in anemia, regardless of its cause. The heart beats faster in an effort to send the limited number of red blood cells more quickly on their way to the tissues or the lungs. The lungs work harder in response to the great need of the limited blood cells for oxygen. Increase in respiratory rate may also be a sign that disease such as Hodgkin's disease or leukemia is causing pressure on the bronchi or the trachea, with resultant respiratory distress. Episodes of high temperature that last for several days and then disappear for several weeks, only to recur, are characteristic of Hodgkin's disease and of some forms of leukemia. Finally, increase in these vital signs may mean that the patient—whose resistance to superimposed infection is very poor—may be developing an infection of some kind.

Hemorrhage. Bleeding from various body orifices is common in those who have blood dyscrasias. The nurse should be particularly alert for signs of bleeding from anywhere in the body. Stools should be examined at regular intervals for signs of fresh blood or for the tarry appearance characteristic of bleeding high in the gastrointestinal tract. The doctor often orders examination of stools for occult or hidden blood, since it is possible for patients to lose small amounts of blood regularly from the intestinal tract and to become severely anemic without frank blood or tarry stools giving any warning. Red meat is usually restricted for twenty-four to forty-eight hours before the stool sample is collected, and this must be explained to the patient.

Urine should be noted for evidence of blood. Bright blood in the urine is seldom missed even by the patient, but smoky urine caused by "old blood" may go unnoticed.

The patient should be protected from trauma that may cause bleeding into the tissues. The ambulatory patient is cautioned to avoid bumps and similar injuries. He should not, for example, walk in the dark. If the patient is critically ill and is disoriented, his finger nails should be cut short to prevent scratching the skin, and side rails should be used to prevent the possibility of falling out of bed. Tight clothing should not be worn; for example, the patient's gown should be left untied at the neck if he is inclined to be restless.

Bleeding from the mouth and gums is common in patients with blood dyscrasias. Sometimes awareness that gums bleed excessively after brushing the teeth is the first sign to the patient that anything is wrong. Mouth care for patients with advanced blood disease such as leukemia becomes a major nursing problem. The lips may become cracked and bleed easily, and mouth odor follows the accumulation of old blood in the mouth. The patient is often reluctant to have care given for fear that it may start fresh bleeding. Petrolatum or a similar preparation should be applied to the lips. Solid preparations that have a pleasing taste and odor may be softened slightly by warming them to facilitate gentle application with an applicator. A weak solution of hydrogen peroxide (1 per cent) seems particularly effective in cleansing old blood from the mouth. Sodium perborate is sometimes used provided a doctor's order has been secured permitting its use. Carbonated beverages are sometimes a pleasant means of softening crusts of blood and exudate in the mouth; if the patient tires of sweet fluids, plain carbonated water may be tried. Boric acid solution and zinc peroxide have been found effective for some patients. Toothbrushes should never be used. The teeth and gums should be carefully swabbed with large, soft cotton applicators. Flavored mouthwashes can be tried. Many patients like aromatic solutions such as Dobell's solution. Peppermint flavoring can also be used in solutions to cleanse the mouth. If the patient is alert and can be relied upon not to inhale the solutions, oil solutions which can be sprayed into the mouth with an atomizer help to protect bleeding or oozing surfaces. Mineral oil flavored wtih peppermint, oil of cloves, or menthol may make the patient's mouth feel better. The nose needs the same kind of meticulous care as the mouth. Small wicks of cotton soaked in mineral oil are usually better than nose drops since they remain longer and seldom drain into the posterior nasopharynx. These wicks are sometimes placed in the nostrils alternately, or else very small ones may be used against oozing surfaces in the nares, permitting breathing through the nostrils.

Diet. Almost all patients with disease of the blood or the blood-forming organs should have a diet high in protein, minerals (especially iron), and vitamins. If there is gastrointestinal bleeding and if the mucous membrane of the mouth is irritated, foods containing roughage should be avoided. Hemorrhage of the gums and of mucous membrane anywhere along the gastrointestinal tract can follow the ingestion of rough food such as whole kernels of corn. Hot foods should also be avoided because the thin, irritated mucous membrane of the mouth is easily burned. Highly spiced foods are not given because they may cause irritation.

Seeing that the patient eats enough is a real nursing challenge in many instances. The patient may be too tired or too discouraged to be interested in food, he may have a poor appetite, and he may have anorexia or even nausea from the constant presence of blood in his mouth. Companionship during meals, small attractive servings of foods that he likes, and mouth care before meals often help to improve his appetite. The ambulatory patient or his family are often interested in suggestions for planning high protein meals that are palatable yet within their means and for including enough vitamins yet avoiding high roughage foods.

The patient's environment. The patient with anemia is almost always cold. Extra covers should be provided so that windows can be opened without danger of chilling. The general environment of the patient's room should be kept quiet and free from disturbance. If the patient is critically or terminally ill, his family should be considered in giving care. If he is in a hospital, close relatives may appreciate opportunities to help in giving care; if he is at home, they may welcome assistance from the public health nurse so that they may continue to participate in care and prevent the need for hospitalization. Sometimes relatives may be overcome by their own feeling and want to avoid sight of such things as bleeding or the patient's growing helplessness; the nurse must accept this reaction as normal for some persons.

ANEMIA AND THE ANEMIAS

Anemia is an extremely common condition in which there is a decrease in the number of circluating red blood cells below normal limits and a low hemoglobin content. Asthenia, fatigue, and pallor are the classic signs of anemia. Its main causes are loss of blood, faulty blood cell production, and excessive destruction of red blood cells.

Anemias due to excessive blood loss

Anemia resulting from frank hemorrhage such as may follow trauma, childbirth, surgery, or administration of drugs such as Dicumarol is usually apparent. It presents relatively simple medical problems provided that not too much blood is lost and the cause of hemorrhage can be corrected. The adult of average build has approximately 6,000 ml. of blood in the total circulating blood system. Usually he can lose 500 ml. without serious or lasting effects. If the loss reaches 1,000 ml. or more, serious consequences may result, and one to two months may be required for the volume to return to normal. Care of the patient who suffers from hemorrhage is discussed in Chapter 14.

The body has remarkable adaptive powers and may adjust fairly well to a marked decrease in red blood cells and hemoglobin provided the condition develops gradually. The total red cell count may even drop to almost half its normal figure of between 4½ and 5 million without the patient experiencing the usual symptoms to a noticeable extent. Another example of the body's adaptive capacity is the increase in red blood cells which occurs when a person moves from a low to a high altitude (more cells are needed to carry oxygen from the rarefied atmosphere).

Chronic, unrecognized blood loss can also cause anemia. It may occur in the presence of an unsuspected gastrointestinal malignancy, a slowly bleeding peptic ulcer, or hemorrhoids that bleed without the patient's awareness. When blood loss is continuous and moderate in amount, the bone marrow may be able to keep up with the losses by increasing its production of red blood cells if enough protein and iron are supplied in food. Eventually, however, if the cause of chronic blood loss is not found and corrected, the bone marrow usually cannot keep pace with the loss, and symptoms of anemia appear.

Anemias due to defective blood production

There are several reasons for defective and inadequate red blood cell production. A diet deficient in protein and iron (raw materials from which blood cells are manufactured) and poor absorption of food from the gastrointestinal tract can lead to anemia. Lack of production of substances within the body which are essential in blood cell formation, such as the intrinsic factor secreted by the stomach, may cause anemia. The bone marrow's capacity for manufacturing red blood cells may be depressed by toxic chemicals such as benzol and the sulfonamides, by toxins from infection, by aplasia of unknown cause, and by hyperactivity of white blood cell production, which occurs in leukemia.

Nutritional anemia. Nutritional anemia is common and may sometimes be due to lack of knowledge of the foods necessary for building normal blood cells, lack of money to purchase essential foods, and fads or notions about diet. Occasionally a nutritional anemia follows lengthy adherence to a special diet for a condition such as an allergy. To manufacture red blood cells, foods containing the extrinsic principle must be ingested and absorbed, so that it may react with the intrinsic factor which is secreted by the stomach. The actual nature of the extrinsic factor is unknown, but it is present in meat, eggs, yeast, and whole grain cereals. Nutritional anemia should be entirely preventable in a country such as ours. The nurse can help in prevention by teaching the importance of good nutrition. Emphasis should be upon the essentials of good nutrition and upon a wide selection of foods. When nutritional anemia has occurred, it is necessary for the patient to have more than the usual amounts of protein, minerals, and vitamins.

Extra iron is also usually given; the simple form of ferrous sulfate is as effective as more elaborate trade preparations. Since iron tablets may cause irritation of the empty stomach, they are given after meals. The patient who is given iron should be told that the stools will be black lest he worry about bleeding from the gastrointestinal tract. Iron may be given intramuscularly. By this route the drug is more completely absorbed than when taken orally. An iron preparation widely used for intramuscular injection is Inferon.

Pernicious anemia. Pernicious anemia was first described by Thomas Addison in London in 1885, and the term addisonian anemia is still sometimes used. In this disease a substance called the *intrinsic factor*, normally produced by the stomach mucosa, is lacking. In normal function the intrinsic factor reacts with the *extrinsic factor* (found in food) to produce an *erythrocyte-maturing factor* which is essential to proper red blood cell formation. Without the intrinsic factor the red blood cells become abnormal. They may be large (macrocytic), contain more hemoglobin than usual (hyperchromic), and assume peculiar shapes and sizes (anisocytosis and poikilocytosis). A diet high in protein and iron does not correct this, since the basic defect is not in the raw materials provided.

Pernicious anemia usually occurs after the age of 40 years. More people are affected in the temperate zones than in the far northern or southern hemispheres. In the United States the incidence is higher in the northern sections of the country than in the south. There appears to be a hereditary influence in the development of pernicious anemia; several members of the same family may have the disease. Many patients with pernicious anemia have characteristics in common; many are of the Nordic race and have broad faces, blond hair which grays early, and wide-set blue eyes.

Pernicious anemia develops slowly. Fatigue is a common symptom, but it comes on so slowly that the patient selddom remembers its beginning. There may be anorexia and symptoms of poor digestion, yet little weight loss. Gastric analysis reveals an absence of free hydrochloric acid in the stomach secretions *(achlorhydria)*. The tongue becomes smooth, and the patient may notice soreness, burning, or other signs of irritation in the mouth. These may disappear, only to reappear after a few weeks or months. There is usually a characteristic waxy pallor which, as the disease progresses untreated, will turn to a light lemon yellow, with moderate jaundice noticeable in the sclera. Dyspnea and palpitation also occur.

Pernicious anemia affects the nervous system. Irritability and depression are signs of the disease, and occasionally the patient even develops a psychosis which usually responds almost immediately to treatment for the anemia. As neurologic involvement develops, there may be numbness, tingling, or a burning sensation in the hands and feet. Some patients have signs of peripheral neuritis with decreased or lost sense of vibration in the feet and legs. Sense of position becomes disturbed, and eventually there is incoordination. Some patients complain of a sensation of constricting bands around the lower limbs and the trunk. It is estimated that approximately 80 per cent of those with pernicious anemia have some neurologic involvement by the time they seek medical care. In those with advanced disease the rectal and urinary sphincters may function poorly. Although patients with far-advanced and permanent neurologic damage are now seldom seen in the

United States, some patients still have neurologic symptoms for months before they seek medical advice. When the nurse sees a patient with signs of pernicious anemia who feels that his symptoms are not serious, she should encourage him to seek medical aid at once.

There is no cure for pernicious anemia since at the present time, there is no way to help the stomach lining regain its capacity to produce the intrinsic factor. Fortunately, however, quite satisfactory treatment can be given by supplying essentials which the body cannot provide. The patient may now live out his life with no serious increase in symptoms provided he continues treatment. Liver extract is specific for the disease, since it contains the erythrocyte-maturing (erythropoietic) factor. Either the crude or the purified extract may be used. Liver extract is administered intramuscularly in units. Usually the patient is given at least 15 units upon confirmation of the diagnosis; then 5 to 10 units are given every day or every other day for a week, followed by a maintenance dose of approximately 10 units per week. As he improves, the maintenance dose may be spaced so that injections are necessary only at biweekly or monthly intervals. Vitamin B_{12} is now widely used in the treatment of pernicious anemia. Research indicates that "Vitamin B_{12} (cyanocobalamine) is the therapeutically active substance in pernicious anemia and that liver extracts are potent only by virtue of their cyanocobalamine content."[3] The preparation of vitamin B_{12} is extremely potent, and daily intramuscular injections of as little as 1 μg will cause production of normal blood cells. Vitamin B_{12} is marketed in 5 and 10 ml. vials and in four different strengths; each milliliter may contain 10, 15, 30, or 50 μg. An initial dose of 30 μg is given and is repeated every day or every other day for ten doses. Dosage is then usually reduced to 15 to 30 μg once or twice a week, and after a few weeks the patient can often be maintained on a dosage of 40 to 60 μg every other week. Sometimes adequate treatment is maintained with injections given as infrequently as every six months.

Folic acid is used in the treatment of pernicious anemia; for reasons not understood, it enables the body to produce red blood cells of normal appearance. However, it is seldom used because it does not prevent the development of neurologic involvement in pernicious anemia. Desiccated hog stomach (Ventriculin) can also be used in the treatment of pernicious anemia since it contains the intrinsic factor. Since the discovery of vitamin B_{12}, however, it is seldom used.

Nursing care for the patient with pernicious anemia depends on the symptoms present at the time of treatment. Irritability, impatience, and apprehension should be expected and should be dealt with by showing the patient particular attention and by giving medications and other treatments on time and with as little confusion as possible. The patient may need extra warmth, special mouth care, and a carefully selected diet until severe symptoms subside. However, with present treatment the more superficial symptoms usually disappear within one or two weeks. Neurologic symptoms may be much more persistent and may even be partially irreversible despite intensive treatment with liver extract, vitamin B_{12}, and physical therapy. Since the patient may be discouraged when he finds that the neurologic symptoms do not disappear as quickly as the others, he may need encouragement. In the presence of permanent nerve damage, patience and persistence are tremendous assets to the patient in learning to manage himself effectively.

The prospect of needing intramuscular injections at weekly or biweekly intervals. for the rest of one's life is not a happy one. The nurse can help the patient in his adjustment to this by her skill in giving injections quickly and as painlessly as possible. She may remind him that, although injections must certainly be continued, he may need them less often when symptoms completely subside. A review should be made of the daily food intake of every patient who has pernicious anemia to be certain that he understands the essentials of a good diet. Cost may be a problem in the selection of suitable foods. This may be particularly so since liver extract and vitamin B_{12} are expensive, and some of the money that the patient has previously budgeted for food may be needed for their purchase. Usually the patient with pernicious anemia benefits from having a public health nurse visit his home to help teach him or a member of his family to give the injections and to help plan low-cost nutritious meals. The patient with residual neurologic involvement also needs help in learning safe and relatively simple methods of getting about without assistance. If a cane or a crutch is necessary, the patient needs encouragement in accepting this aid which he may feel is conspicuous.

Aplastic anemia

Aplastic anemia is characterized by aplasia, depression, or cessation of activity of all blood-producing elements. There is a decrease in white blood cells (leukopenia), a decrease in platelets (thrombopenia), and a decrease in formation of red blood cells. The disease may be idiopathic, occurring, for example, in more than one child in a family. It may follow exposure to chemical agents or ingestion of certain drugs. Benzol, arsenicals, gold compounds, mustard gas, Atabrine, hair dyes, insecticides, streptomycin, and chloramphenicol are among the substances known to have been responsible for the development of aplastic anemia.

Symptoms of aplastic anemia may appear suddenly but usually develop gradually over a period of weeks and months. They include pallor, weakness, dyspnea, anorexia, headache, fever, and bleeding of the mucous membranes, often first noticed in the mouth or the nose. Treatment consists of removing causative toxic agents if they are known and of giving transfusions to raise the hemoglobin level and to supply platelets so that bleeding may be controlled. Liver, iron, and vitamin B_{12} are not effective. Antibiotics may be given to prevent and control secondary infection. The mortality rate from aplastic anemia is high, and almost all patients with the disease die; occasionally, recovery occurs when the causative agent is found and removed. Nursing care of the patient with aplastic anemia includes all the measures mentioned in the first part of this chapter.

Hemolytic anemia

In hemolytic anemia there is abnormal destruction of red blood cells. Cells are destroyed at such a rate that the bone marrow is unable to make up the losses. Hemolytic anemia can be due to an inherited condition or an acquired one. Acquired hemolytic anemia can be caused by burns, snake venom, fava beans, and drugs which are derivatives of benzene and toluene, certain heavy metals, or quinine. Bacterial toxins from such microorganisms as the streptococcus, plasmodium, Welch's bacillus, and viruses can also cause hemolytic anemia. Marked hyperpyrexia can cause hemolysis of blood cells. Secondary hemolytic anemia can result from abnormalities in the spleen which cause it to destroy red blood cells excessively. The treatment for this is splenectomy, which will be discussed later in this chapter under hemorrhagic diseases.

An acute episode of hemolytic anemia, with rapid destruction of red blood cells, usually causes chills and fever, headache, irritability, precordial spasm, and pain. There may be abdominal pain with nausea, vomiting, and diarrhea. Urinary output may be diminished. Shock and prostration may occur, and jaundice follows the destruction of red blood cells. In chronic forms of the disease there are varying degrees of weakness, pallor, dyspnea, and palpitation. Stones may form in the biliary tract.

Sickle cell anemia is one of the chronic types of hemolytic anemia which is inherited and occurs chiefly in Negroes. The red blood cells are characteristically shaped like sickles. This condition causes other bodily changes, including thickening of the skull bones and thinning of the long bones, with retardation of growth when it develops before growth is attained. Other symptoms are varied and may include chronic leg ulcers, cardiac failure, and symptoms of an acute inflammation of the abdomen. Drowsiness, stupor, headaches, irritability, and convulsions can also occur. The mortality from this disease is high since there is no specific treatment. Treatment includes transfusions, sedation, oxygen, analgesics, and physical therapy. Frequently, packed red cells (a concentrated transfusion) are given since there is no decrease in circulating plasma in this disease.

THE LEUKEMIAS AND HODGKIN'S DISEASE

Leukemia

Leukemia is a disease of the blood-forming tissues characterized by an extensive and abnormal production of mature and immature forms of white blood cells (myelocytes, lymphocytes, monocytes) which appear in the blood stream, bone marrow, spleen, liver, and lymph nodes. Anemia is usually also present and is thought to be due to the diminished production of erythrocytes in the bone marrow as the tissue forming abnormal leukocytes increase and spread throughout the marrow. Leukemia is a progressive malignant disease and for statistical purposes is now classified with cancer. It has increased in frequency and now accounts for over 11,000 deaths annually. The cause of leukemia is unknown. Acute leukemia is one form of the disease which has a short fulminating course, usually of less than a year. Chronic leukemia usually has an expected duration of several years.

Acute leukemia. Acute leukemia—whether it is lymphatic or myelocytic is often difficult to determine—usually occurs in persons under 25 years of age. Its highest incidence is in children under the age of 4. It has an abrupt onset; symptoms include pallor, extreme fatigue, upper respiratory infection, fever, and bleeding from the mucous membrane of the mouth, nose, or other body orifices. The total number of leukocytes in the various types is most often between 15,000 and 30,000 or less, although occasionally they may go much higher.[1] At the onset they may fall below 8,000 and may be as low as 2,000 to 3,000 per cubic millimeter or less. A severe anemia almost always develops with the red blood count falling as low as 1 million per cubic millimeter, and the platelet count is also markedly reduced. The lymph nodes, spleen, and liver are usually enlarged but less so than in chronic leukemia.

Treatment consists of blood transfusions given repeatedly to maintain the red blood cell count and the hemoglobin and the platelet count at normal levels. Antibiotics to control infection and drugs such as corticosteroids (ACTH and cortisone) are given to control the fever and to attempt curtailment of the abnormal activity within the bone marrow. Since folic acid is necessary for cell growth, drugs which inhibit its formation (Aminopterin) and drugs which are antagonistic to its action (6-mercaptopurine) also may produce remissions.

The course is rapidly progressive and, while there may be a remission, death caused by hemorrhage, general debility, or infection usually occurs within a period of months.

Chronic lymphatic leukemia. Chronic lymphatic leukemia usually occurs in those over 45 years of age. The onset is insidious, and the patient may complain of pallor and fatigue and may notice a painless lump in the neck, axilla, or groin. The lymph nodes, liver, and spleen are enlarged. The total white blood cell count is increased to between 30,000 to 100,000 per cubic millimeter with 60 to 90 per cent of these cells resembling normal small lymphocytes. The basal metabolic rate is usually increased, perhaps as a result of the increased consumption of oxygen by the leukemic cells and the accelerated rate of destruction of these cells. Abnormal bleeding usually occurs only during acute exacerbations of the disease and in the terminal phase. Average length of life after appearance of symptoms is three to five years, but some patients live eight years or more.

Treatment consists of x-ray therapy, administration of radioactive phosphorus, blood transfusions, antibiotics, folic acid antagonists, chlorambucil, and corticosteroids. If there has been no active bleeding, packed red cells are often given in preference to whole blood.

Chronic granulocytic leukemia. Chronic granulocytic leukemia occurs most often in persons between 35 and 45 years of age. The onset is insidious, and usually marked changes in the white blood cells have occurred before the patient has any specific complaint. Initial symptoms are usually weakness, pallor, palpitation, and dyspnea. Fever and chills often occur. There is marked enlargement of the spleen and liver, pronounced anemia, and increase in metabolic rate. Complications occur in a variety of body organs as they become infiltrated with leukocytes. An abnormal tendency to bleed occurs during acute exacerbations and immediately preceding death. The average length of life is approximately three to five years after onset of the disease.

Treatment consists of x-ray therapy, and the administration of radioactive phosphorus, 6-mercaptopurine, blood transfusions, antibiotics, and corticosteroids. Dimethanesulfonoxybutane (Myleran) and triethylenemelamine (TEM) are also sometimes used.

Hodgkin's disease

Hodgkin's disease produces painless enlargement of the lymph nodes. The first nodes to be involved usually are those in the cervical region followed by the axillary nodes and those in the inguinal region. There is no known cause for this disease, but it is believed to be caused by an infection or a neoplastic process. Highest incidence is in young adults, men are affected more often than women. The clinical findings vary from mild lymph node enlargement without other symptoms to generalized disease with severe symptoms including fever, excessive diaphoresis, anemia, anorexia, and weight loss. Twenty-five per cent of patients with Hodgkin's disease have skin conditions such as pruritus.[5] Changes in the blood count are not significant though leukocytosis or anemia may occur. Markedly enlarged nodes can cause severe symptoms from pressure. For example, respiration may be severely hampered by enlarged nodes in the mediastinum and neck. The average length of life is three to five years, although some patients with a benign type of the disease live longer. Death is usually caused by pressure of the enlarged lymph nodes on the bronchi and mediastinum.

Since it appears to produce the longest remissions and the best relief of symptoms, x-ray therapy is thought to be the treatment of choice. Nitrogen mustard given intravenously is sometimes used as an adjunct to x-ray therapy. To prevent this highly irritating substance from coming into contact with linings of blood vessels, it is injected into the tubing of an infusion that is running well. Because the drug causes local skin reactions also, rubber gloves should be worn during its preparation and administration, and the skin should be washed thoroughly after any contact with the drug. Since nitrogen mustard causes nausea and vomiting within a few hours of injection, administration should be carefully planned so that height of reaction does not coincide with meal hours. Other treatment includes administration of corticosteroids, chlorambucil, antibiotics, and transfusions of whole blood or packed red cells when necessary.

HEMORRHAGIC DISEASES

Purpura

In purpura there is extravasation of blood into the tissues, under the skin, and through the mucous membranes. In the skin, areas of hemorrhage may be small (petechiae) or large and "black and blue" (ecchymosis). Purpura may occur with many acute and chronic illnesses. In these cases the bleeding and clotting times are normal. For example, dark areas of hemorrhage into the skin are characteristic of a severe fulminating form of meningitis which swept Europe in the sixteenth century and produced the "black death" so vividly described in medical annals of that time. Some forms of purpura occur with vitamin C deficiency (scurvy), and one form of purpura, with actual abnormality in the blood, occurs with liver disease and failure to utilize vitamin K. The treatment for secondary purpura is obviously to remove the cause if this is possible.

There is no known cause for idiopathic purpura. It can occur when platelet count is normal, and the main anomaly appears to be in the permeability of the capillaries. This condition is more common in children than in adults. It may be associated with joint symptoms (Schönlein's disease) or with acute abdominal symptoms (Henoch's purpura).

When purpura is caused by a lack of platelets, it is called *thrombopenic* or *thrombocytopenic purpura.* This is usually a disease of young people. Usually the spleen enlarges and actively destroys platelets before their useful life is over. Immature red blood cells (reticulocytes) appear in the blood stream in response to the excessive loss. The treatment for this condition is a splenectomy. If the spleen is markedly enlarged, irradiation may be given to decrease its activity and make it less vascular to lessen danger of severe hemorrhage at operation.

Splenectomy is usually done during the fall and winter. Since the platelets normally decrease in number during hot weather, operation during the summer is avoided when possible. Preparation for a splenectomy is similar to that for other major abdominal surgery. Usually a transfusion is given a very short time before operation. The bleeding and clotting times are recorded, and the patient's blood is typed and crossmatched preparatory to giving additional transfusions if necessary.

Following a splenectomy the patient must be observed very carefully for signs of internal hemorrhage. As a rule he gets out of bed a day or two postoperatively to prevent thrombosis. If thrombosis does occur, its treatment is difficult because anticoagulants are considered contraindicated. Care must be taken that the patient does not bruise or otherwise injure himself when he first gets out of bed. A general diet high in iron and protein is given as soon as it can be tolerated. The patient with purpura and resultant anemia from blood loss responds very quickly to a diet high in protein and iron, together with supplementary iron.

Occasionally the patient is not cured by a splenectomy. The abdominal lymph nodes may take over the activities of the spleen which has been removed and may destroy platelets prematurely. If this happens, irradiation to the lymph nodes is sometimes given. The patient should be advised to continue under medical supervision for an indefinite time and to report any signs of bleeding to his doctor at once.

Hemophilia

Hemophilia is a hereditary hemorrhagic disease which is transmitted to the male by the female through a recessive sex-linked characteristic. In this disease the coagulation time is prolonged and bleeding can occur at any time. The platelet count, however, is normal. Hemophilia is largely a disease of children, since only one third of patients with this condition reach the age of 30 years.

The patient with hemophilia must learn to avoid trauma of all kinds. The slightest bump will cause bruising with bleeding into the tissues. Bleeding into joints is common, requiring immobilization of the affected joint; repeated injuries cause bone destruction and deformity. The gums bleed easily, and any hemorrhage is stopped with extreme difficulty. Care must be taken in the use of pins, nail files, scissors, and even toothbrushes. Since such care in ordinary activities is necessary, the patient and his family have serious psychologic handicaps, particularly since it is the active growing child who is affected. Since repeated episodes of bleeding are wearing and frightening, the child may become sensitive and retiring or may attempt to defy his handicap. Social activities need to be planned to meet the patient's special needs. Minor medical problems that go almost unnoticed in the average household assume major proportions. For example, a simple tooth extraction requires hospitalization and transfusions.

Treatment consists of treating bleeding as it occurs. Local application of fibrin foam and thrombin helps to stop external bleeding. When giving an injection, particular care must be taken to use a small needle and to apply pressure at the site of injection and to inspect it for bleeding frequently for some time thereafter. The patient should have a diet high in iron. One of nature's compensations for this condition is a remarkable capacity to regenerate red blood cells when bleeding has caused their loss. The patient who has hemophilia should carry a card on his person which includes his name, his blood type, his doctor's name, and the fact that he has hemophilia, so that medical treatment will not be delayed if he should accidentally sustain injury and lose consciousness.

POLYCYTHEMIA VERA

In polycythemia vera there is excessive production of red blood cells, the count often being between 7 and 12 million. The hemoglobin is increased, and the patient characteristically has a reddish-purple complexion, with reddening of the hands and feet. Headache, weakness, dyspnea, itching, and lacrimation may be other complaints. There may be bleeding from the skin and from the mucous membranes. This disease usually occurs in persons over 50 years of age, and the average age at death is approximately 60 years. Death is usually from thrombosis.

Phlebotomy is the main treatment, and it may be necessary every six months or oftener. Radioactive phosphorus and triethylenemelamine (TEM) sometimes achieve remissions. The patient should have a diet low in iron, and the nurse can help him with the selection of foods. Other nursing care during an exacerbation consists of supportive care, with special attention to hemorrhage.

AGRANULOCYTOSIS

Agranulocytosis is a disease in which production of white blood cells is depressed, and the total white blood cells may be reduced to between 200 and 500 per milliliter. Exposure to drugs, chemicals, and physical agents about the home can cause the disease. Sulfonamides, barbiturates, coal-tar analgesics, Pyribenzamine, thiouracil, chloramphenicol, and heavy metals such as gold are examples. The nurse has a real part in the prevention of this disease. In the community she has frequent opportunity to advise against use of medications not therapeutically prescribed. In the hospital as well as in the home she must constantly be aware of the possible toxic effects of various drugs. Many times good nursing care can reduce the period of necessary treatment with drugs. Also she must be constantly alert for toxic signs of the drugs she administers.

Treatment consists of removing the offending agent. Sometimes the cause is difficult to determine and careful history is essential. With such a low white blood cell count, precautions must be taken to control infections. The first signs of the disease may be the onset of an acute infection with chills, fever, sore throat, and prostration. There may be enlargement of cervical lymph nodes. Infection may occur anywhere in the body. The mortality in agranulocytosis is high, although antibiotics have been found extremely helpful in controlling the infection until the cause can be found and removed. Transfusions of fresh whole blood are often given.

REFERENCES AND SELECTED READINGS*

1 Cecil, Russell L., and Loeb, Robert F. (editors): A Textbook of Medicine, ed. 10, Philadelphia, 1959, W. B. Saunders Co.

2 Faddis, Margene O., and Hayman, Joseph: Care of the Medical Patient, ed. 1, New York, 1952, McGraw-Hill Book Co., Inc.

---

*References preceded by an asterisk indicate material particularly well suited for student reading.

3 Goodman, Louis, and Gilman, Alfred: The Pharmacological Basis of Therapeutics, ed. 2, New York, 1955, The Macmillan Co.
4 *Hartman, John R., and Bolduc, Rose A.: Hemophilia: Medical Care and Nursing Care, Am J. Nursing **56**:169-174, Feb. 1956.
5 *Hynes, John F., and Jonsson, Eleanor B.: Hodgkin's Disease, Am. J. Nursing **58**:371-372, March 1958.
6 MacBryde, Cyril Mitchell: Signs and Symptoms, ed. 2, Philadelphia, 1952, J. B. Lippincott Co.
7 Meakins, Jonathan Campbell: The Practice of Medicine, ed. 6, St. Louis, 1956, The C. V. Mosby Co.
8 Weintrobe, Maxwell M.: Blood Dyscrasias, Am. J. Nursing **60**:496-500, April 1960.
9 *Wilson, Henry E., and Price, Geraldine: Leukemia—Clinical Characteristics and Therapy, and Nursing Care, Am. J. Nursing **56**:601-605, May 1956.

Study questions for review

UROLOGIC EXAMINATION

1 Review the anatomy of the male and female urinary systems.
2 Review the physiology of urine formation. What are the parts of the nephron? What is the function of each part? What is the normal specific gravity of urine?
3 Review the procedure for catheterization of the urinary bladder.
4 What is the action of castor oil? licorice powder?
5 What are the untoward reactions of iodide solutions given intravenously? What are the names of intravenous preparations with iodide bases which are used as x-ray opaque substances?

THE PATIENT WITH SPECIFIC MEDICAL DISEASE OF THE URINARY SYSTEM

6 Review the chapter on electrolyte balance.
7 What foods contain potassium? What are complete protein foods?
8 What are the end products of protein catabolism?
9 What is the normal nonprotein nitrogen? blood urea nitrogen?
10 What is meant by dialysis?
11 What are the symptoms of cardiac failure? pulmonary edema? cerebral edema?
12 What is the action of 50 per cent glucose? 50 per cent magnesium sulfate?

THE PATIENT WITH A UROLOGIC DISORDER

13 Review procedures for measuring intake and output. What is the relation of output to intake in the normal person?
14 Review the physiology of voiding. What is the normal bladder capacity? At what point does one normally have the "urge to void"? What is retention of urine?
15 What is the normal capacity of the kidney pelvis?
16 Review the signs and symptoms of hemorrhage.
17 Review the general principles of patient teaching.

CARE OF THE PATIENT FOLLOWING SURGERY OF THE URINARY SYSTEM

18 What are the therapeutic action, the untoward results, and the method of administration of each of the following drugs: mandelic acid, methenamine (Urotropin), aluminum hydroxide gel, neostigmine bromide (Prostigmin), and Banthine?
19 What is an acid-ash diet? an alkaline-ash diet? a 1,300 mg. phosphorus diet?
20 How may bowel regularity be maintained? What is a paralytic ileus, and how is it treated?
21 With what large blood vessels do the renal vein and artery anastomose? At what three points are the ureters normally narrow? Which kidney is lower? What holds the kidneys in position? What is meant by the parenchyma of the kidney? The calyces? Is any portion of the urinary tract within the peritoneal cavity?
22 Locate the prostate in relation to the urethra, the bladder, and the rectum. Locate the external and internal bladder sphincters in women and in men.

The patient with disease of the urinary system

Chapter 21

Urologic examination

Urology is the study of the urinary and genital systems in the male and of the urinary system in the female. However, this chapter will be concerned only with the male and female urinary systems. The male reproductive system, with the exception of the obstructive lesions of the urethra, is considered in Chapter 22.

Whenever there is disease of any part of the urinary system, preservation or improvement of renal function is the primary objective of treatment. This is because the kidneys are the organs mainly responsible for maintenance of normal fluid and electrolyte balance and for the excretion of certain waste products (see Chapter 6). Without kidney function, life can continue for only a few days. Some substances such as plasma proteins (albumin, globulin, and fibrinogen) and red and white blood cells are not normally filtered through the glomerular capillary walls; their presence in the urine is, therefore, indicative of kidney damage and disturbance of kidney function. Dyes which can be filtered by the glomeruli and excreted by the tubules can be used to help determine the efficiency of kidney function. Some of these are phenolsulfonphthalein, indigo carmine, methylene blue, and iodide preparations such as Urokon.

The complex processes of kidney function take place in the million or more nephrons located in the cortex and medulla of the kidney. The urine is excreted into the kidney pelvis at a pressure of about 50 to 60 mm. Hg and passes by peristaltic action along the ureters to the collecting reservoir, the bladder, which has a lower pressure. Although the pelves, ureters, bladder, and urethra serve merely as the drainage and reservoir system, any obstruction or infection in these ultimately causes damage to the kidneys. When the pressure below the kidney becomes equal to or greater than that within the kidney, the efficiency of the system is lessened and damage to the nephrons can occur.

UROLOGIC DIAGNOSTIC PROCEDURES

Since kidney function is a prerequisite for life, it is fortunate that diseases in the urinary system can be diagnosed with an unusually high degree of accuracy. The urologic examination usually begins with a complete medical history and physical examination, including pelvic and rectal examinations. Thorough examination is important because urinary symptoms may be secondary to other systemic disorders; the nurse may have to interpret for the patient the need for these procedures. She may do this as she prepares him for the examinations and as she assists the doctor.

The examinations and tests mentioned in this section are commonly done to assist in the diagnosis of many different urologic conditions. Examinations used in diagnosing specific problems will be discussed with each disorder.

Examination of urine

Urinalysis. A voided urine specimen is usually examined first. While a normal specimen usually indicates that there is no urinary tract infection or kidney disease, an abnormal one does not necessarily indicate disease. For example, blood in a woman's specimen may be due to menstruation; albumin in a man's specimen may be due to prostatic fluid, and pus cells may have come from an adjacent area of infection and not from the urinary tract. When a voided specimen contains abnormal constituents, a *catheterized* specimen of urine is usually examined. Since a catheterized specimen consists of urine that has passed through the kidneys, the ureters, and the bladder, further examination of specimens collected by means of catheters placed into each of the ureters may be necessary to locate the trouble more definitely.

Abnormal constituents in the urine give important clues in diagnosis. Sugar may indicate diabetes mellitus. Acetone may be found in the urine of those with diabetes mellitus, but it may also be present in ketosis resulting from other conditions such as starvation. Plasma proteins such as albumin, globulin, or fibrinogen are suggestive of disorders involving the glomeruli. Because the size of the protein molecule determines the ease with which it passes through the damaged membrane, albumin, having the smallest molecule, is the protein found most often in the urine (albuminuria). Hemoglobin in the urine

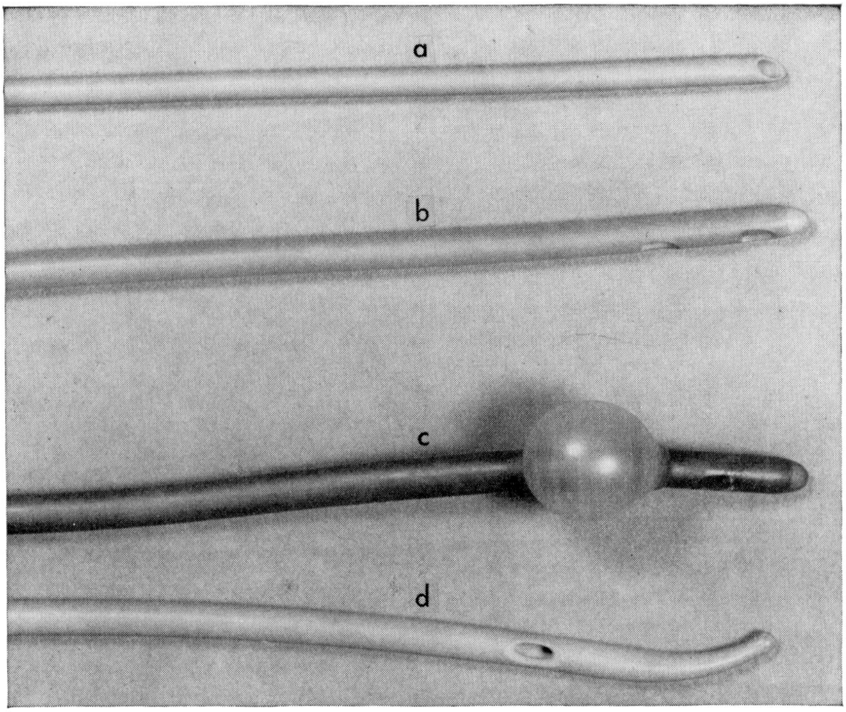

Figure 33

Urethral catheters: *a,* whistle-tip catheter; *b,* many-eyed Robinson catheter; *c,* Foley catheter; *d,* Coudé catheter.

(hemoglobinuria) is caused by lysis of red blood cells and may occur in the bladder because of strongly acid urine or in the circulatory system because of acute hemolytic anemia or a transfusion reaction from incompatible blood. Blood cells and frank blood in the urine are indicative of damage somewhere within the system.

Any abnormality in the specific gravity (below 1.003 or above 1.030) is usually due to inability of the kidney tubules to be selective in reabsorption and excretion. For example, a marked decrease in specific gravity is found in diabetes insipidus due to a deficiency of posterior pituitary hormone which influences tubular water absorption.

Multiple glass test. Occasionally it is helpful to have separate specimens from one voiding to determine if the abnormality is in the urethra, the bladder, or the prostate. The patient is asked to void about 100 ml. into the first container; this gives urethral "washings." Then he voids 100 ml. into a second container; this gives the kidney and bladder "washings." If, in the male patient, prostatic "washings" are desired, the best results are obtained when the doctor gently massages the prostate immediately after the second voiding. The patient then finishes emptying the bladder, and this third specimen will contain prostatic secretions.

Residual urine. The doctor may order a catheterization to determine if the patient has residual urine in the bladder. Normally, following voiding, the bladder will contain less than 15 ml. of urine; if larger quantities are allowed to remain, they cause stagnation of urine, with resultant infection and possible bladder stone formation. When the residual urine decreases to 50 ml. or less in a patient who is being catheterized because of incomplete emptying of the bladder, it is considered an indication that function is returning to normal and catheterization usually is discontinued. Before a residual urine determination is done, the patient should empty the bladder completely *immediately* before the catheterization. If there is a delay, additional urine will be excreted from the kidneys, thus giving an inaccurate result. It is best to explain the procedure to the patient and then leave him for a few moments since he is likely to void if left alone. It is important to stress that the bladder should be completely emptied because patients with urethral obstruction tend to void only enough at a time to relieve the pressure; with additional concentration, the patient can often empty his bladder quite completely. If, upon catheterizing the patient, the doctor finds that there is residual urine, the amount should be measured and recorded. The urine should be saved as a catheterized specimen; this will obviate having to catheterize the patient again if a sterile specimen is needed.

To evaluate the size and strength of the urinary stream and to estimate the difficulty that the patient has in voiding, the doctor may wish to observe the male patient void. Since this observation is more meaningful if the patient does not know that he is being watched, he may be given a basin to use rather than a urinal, and the screen or door may be left slightly ajar.

Calibration of the urethra. When a catheterization is done, the doctor needs to know the size of catheter since this may help him in ruling out significant strictures of the urethra. A size 14 to 20 Fr. soft rubber catheter is commonly used for women and a size 16 to 25 Fr. for men (French is the scale used to graduate catheters: 1 Fr. equals ⅓ mm. in diameter). A *coudé* or soft, red rubber, *curve-tipped* catheter is often used for male catheterizations because it is easily inserted into the curved male urethra. A *whistle-tip* or a *many-eyed* Robinson catheter may also be used. If, however, the doctor suspects that the patient has a large amount of residual urine, he usually uses a Foley catheter, which may be left in the bladder and attached to drainage equipment. (See Figure 33.)

Female catheterization. When the doctor is to catheterize a woman, the nurse should drape the patient for the procedure (see texts on fundamentals of nursing). She should remain with the patient and should encourage her to take deep breaths which will relax the vesicle sphincters and make the procedure less uncomfortable.

Male catheterization. When a man is to be catheterized, the nurse should place a bath blanket from the chest to the knees, fanfolding the bedclothes back to the knees. A protective pad should be placed under the thighs. The nurse should provide the doctor with a tray containing the following sterile equipment in addition to equipment for cleansing: a towel for draping the patient's thighs, a 4 by 8 inch gauze sponge with which to grasp the penis, a forceps with which to handle the catheter, and two well-lubricated catheters. A culture tube and a basin in which to collect the urine should also be available. When the patient and the equipment are ready, the nurse leaves the patient with the doctor. When the procedure is finished, she returns to see that he is comfortable and to take care of the specimen and the equipment.

Insertion of a Foley catheter. If a Foley or self-retaining catheter with an inflatable balloon is used, the doctor will need a bulb syringe, a basin, and irrigating solution such as sterile physiologic solution of sodium chloride so that he may irrigate the catheter to determine if it is correctly placed. A syringe (5 to 30 ml., depending upon the size of the balloon) with a catheter adapter is needed to inflate the balloon. (See Figure 34.) Usually a 30 ml. balloon is used. It is best to use black silk to tie off the inflation tube because a metal clamp may be accidentally released and may cause irritation or pressure on surrounding tissues. Self-sealing catheters (Gilbert) which can be inflated by using a syringe and a 22-gauge needle

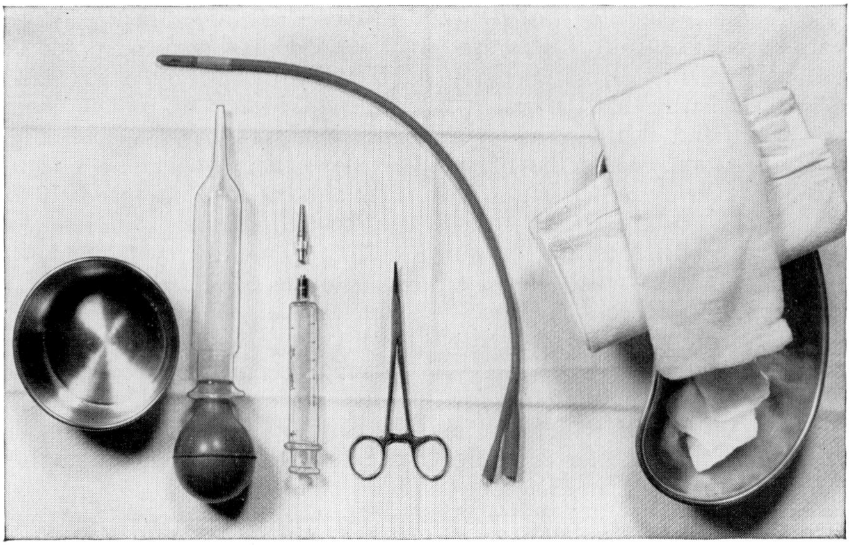

Figure 34

Setup for inserting a Foley catheter in a male patient.

are now available. If a retention catheter is to be left in place, the nurse should ask the doctor the type of drainage he plans to use and should have this ready to be connected when the catheterization is completed.

Occasionally, the doctor may need to use a metal catheter director to pass a catheter into the bladder. This director should be well lubricated so that it will slip out easily from the catheter following insertion in the bladder. A nurse should never use a metal catheter director because when such a hard piece of equipment is used there is danger of perforating the urethra or the bladder.

Urine culture. When infection appears to be present in the urinary system, a urine culture is often ordered. A 5 to 10 ml. specimen of urine is collected in a sterile tube under aseptic conditions. This is sent to the laboratory, where any organisms present are allowed to grow in culture media and then identified microscopically. This information guides the doctor not only in making the diagnosis but also in ordering drug therapy.

If a urine specimen for culture is to be obtained from a woman, she frequently is catheterized because it is difficult to prevent contamination of a voided specimen. After a catheter is passed, allow a small amount of urine to drain into the waste basin. Then collect 5 to 10 ml. directly into the culture tube, taking care not to touch the rim or the inside of the tube with the catheter or with the hands. If a cotton plug is used as a stopper, the tube should be kept upright to prevent moistening the cotton. At the conclusion of the procedure, the patient should be left in a comfortable position and the equipment removed. Prepare the specimen for delivery to the laboratory by labeling the tube with the patient's name, the date, and the cavity from which the urine has been obtained. Cultures are sometimes ordered on urine taken from the kidney pelves during ureteral catheterizations or when ureterostomy or nephrostomy tubes are in place.

The collection of a voided specimen for culture is becoming quite common since, even in women, bacterial infection of the urinary tract frequently follows catheterization although it may not become evident for several weeks. In order to collect a sterile specimen, the nurse should first cleanse the genital area thoroughly with soap and water; then, wearing a sterile glove, she should separate the labia in such a way that the urinary meatus is exposed and cleanse it as for a regular catheterization. While the nurse (or the patient wearing a sterile glove) continues to hold the labia well separated, the patient voids. After the stream of urine has started, the nurse places a sterile container so as to collect a specimen. The specimen is then cared for as for any urine culture.

When a urine culture is requested for a male patient, a voided specimen is usually used unless a catheter is being passed for some other reason. This is because of the danger of infecting the male reproductive tract during catheterization. (See Chapter 8.) The penis should be well cleansed with a cotton pledget saturated with a mild antiseptic such as benzalkonium chloride 1:1000; slight friction is used, and special attention should be given to the meatus. The patient is then asked to void 50 to 100 ml., which is discarded. This decreases the possibility of contaminating the specimen with organisms present in the urethra. The patient then voids 10 to 15 ml. into a sterile pitcher. Pour this urine into the culture tube and proceed as for the female patient. This procedure is usually done by a male member of the nursing team or by the patient himself if he can collect the specimen with the necessary aseptic precautions.

Renal function tests

If anything in the general examination or the urinalysis is suggestive of renal damage, the doctor will probably order a number of renal function tests. Since the concentration of urea in the body is regulated primarily by the rate at which the kidney excretes urea, the level of urea in the blood is a good index of renal function. When renal function is impaired, there is an elevation in the blood urea level. Either a blood urea nitrogen (BUN) or a blood nonprotein nitrogen (NPN) may be done. In either case, it is important that the patient have no food or fluid containing protein for six hours before the blood is obtained. Since urea is an end product of protein metabolism, only a fasting blood specimen gives an accurate index to kidney function. The normal blood urea nitrogen is 10 to 20 mg. per cent; the normal nonprotein nitrogen is 25 to 40 mg. per cent. The nurse needs to note the blood urea levels of patients who have kidney damage; if the level is high, the patient may have convulsions or may become confused or disoriented. Accidents and injury should be prevented by close observation and by having padded side rails and a mouth gag ready for immediate use.

Phenolsulfonphthalein test. Since phenolsulfonphthalein (a red dye) is a substance which the normal kidney excretes completely, it is used to determine kidney function. If the blood urea nitrogen is normal, a phenolsulfonphathalein test (PSP test) may still be done to estimate the amount of obstruction below the kidney which may be delaying the emptying of the kidney pelvis.

It is helpful for the nurse to know how this test is done in the laboratory so that she will be more aware of how to prevent inaccurate results when obtaining specimens. Water is added to each specimen until it has a volume of 1,000 ml.; the specimen is then alkalinized by adding sodium hydroxide since the dye is not visible in acid urine. Then the color of each specimen is compared to a standard on a colorimeter to determine the amount of dye excreted in each specimen. The injection of more or less than 1 ml. of dye will cause inaccuracies because 1 ml. of phenolsulfonphthalein is the basis for the color indicator. Blood in the urine will make the test inaccurate; Pyridium, a urinary antiseptic which gives urine a red color, will also cause inaccuracies.

The test is as follows: the patient voids, and this sample of urine is discarded after being inspected for any red discoloration. Then the patient is given an intravenous injection of exactly 1 ml. of phenolsulfonphthalein dye. Special care must be taken that the dye does not infiltrate the tissues; if it does, the test must be delayed for twenty-four hours. The patient is urged to drink several glasses of water or other fluid before the dye is injected and during the test. He may eat if he wishes. Specimens consisting of all the urine the patient can void are collected exactly 15 minutes, 30 minutes, 1 hour, and 2 hours after the injection of the dye. Occasionally the patient is unable to void at the desired time, but urination can usually be promoted by forcing fluids. If the patient is known to have residual urine in the bladder after voiding, a catheter may be passed before the dye is injected. If, during the test, the nurse becomes aware that the urinary output is inadequate in comparison to the fluid intake, the patient may be catheterized to assure accurate results. Specimens are then obtained at the desired times by unclamping the catheter and draining the accumulated urine. Each specimen must be carefully labeled with the exact time of collection. The label on the first specimen should indicate the time the dye was injected. Normally the dye will begin to appear in the bladder three to six minutes after injection, with 15 to 20 per cent of it appearing in the first specimen and 80 per cent being excreted within two hours.

The patient who is not acutely ill can usually collect his own specimens for a phenolsulfonphthalein test if he is given a watch, properly labeled bottles, and careful instruction. The nurse must make certain that he does this correctly and that he will send for her if he is unable to collect any one of the specimens at the appointed time.

Urea clearance test. The urea clearance test measures the efficiency of the glomerular filtration of plasma. Normally, 55 to 75 ml. of plasma are cleared of urea per minute. Since some urea is reabsorbed, it is important that the total specimen of urine be sent to the laboratory so that the rate of urine flow can be determined. If an accurate result is to be obtained in the laboratory, the urine flow must be at least 2 ml. per minute. Therefore, most laboratories ask that the patient drink 2 glasses of water when the "discard specimen" is obtained and 2 more after voiding for the first urine specimen. The patient should fast until after the blood sample is taken. One hour after obtaining the "discard specimen," the patient is asked to void again, emptying his bladder completely. This entire voiding is collected and labeled as the first specimen. The exact time that the "discard specimen" and this specimen were collected should be indicated. Then a blood sample is taken for blood urea nitrogen determination. An hour later, a second urine specimen is obtained, and all the specimens, carefully identified, are sent to the laboratory. If the patient is unable to void normally and to empty his bladder completely, catheterized specimens should be collected. If the test has been accurate, the blood urea will be elevated and the urine urea decreased in patients with poor kidney function, while the reverse will be true if there is no disease. The two urine specimens should give comparable results.

Urine concentration and dilution tests. When kidney damage has occurred, one of the first functions to be lost is the ability of the renal tubules to concentrate and to dilute urine. If body waste excretion is normal and fluids are restricted for a relatively long period of time or if large amounts of body fluids are lost by other routes such as perspiration, respiration, diarrhea, vomiting, or hemorrhage, larger than normal amounts of the plasma fluid will be reabsorbed through the tubules, causing a concentrated urine. When large amounts of fluid are taken into the body, the normal kidney will excrete larger amounts, causing the urine to be more dilute than usual. When damage is severe, the specific gravity of the urine is said to be "fixed," meaning that no matter what the fluid intake is, the specific gravity of the urine will be that of the plasma without its protein (that part filtered through the glomeruli into the tubules), or about 1.010

to 1.012.[2] A fixed low specific gravity, therefore, is indicative of serious kidney disease.

The ability of the kidney to concentrate urine may be measured by several tests. The *Fishberg concentration test* is commonly used. The patient eats his usual evening meal and is instructed to take no more food or fluids until after the completion of the test the next morning. Urine specimens are collected at 6 A.M., 7 A.M., and 8 A.M. Morning specimens are collected because a normal kidney concentrates urine during the night at approximately twice the rate it does during waking hours.

The *Addis concentration test* is much more vigorous in the dehydration of the patient. It gives a more sensitive measurement, but if the patient's nonprotein nitrogen determination is high, it is used with caution because of the danger of precipitating a serious electrolyte imbalance. Fluids are markedly restricted for twenty-four hours; the amount allowed varies with the laboratory making the test. During the last twelve hours of the test all urine is saved.

The *Mosenthal concentration test* is a twenty-four hour test in which neither food nor fluids are restricted. Total urinary output from 7 P.M. to 7 A.M. is saved, and then separate specimens are collected at two hour intervals through 7 P.M.

The *Fishberg dilution test* is used to determine the ability of the kidney to dilute urine. It may be done at any time of day, but the patient should remain inactive during the test. He should completely empty the bladder at the beginning of the test and drink 1,200 ml. of fluid within one-half hour. Urine specimens are then collected every half hour for three hours. A person with normal hydration and normal kidney function will excrete almost the total 1,200 ml. in the three hour period, and the urine will have a specific gravity of about 1.022.[1] Since most patients will have difficulty in drinking 1,200 ml. of fluid in a half hour period, it sometimes helps if water is mixed with fruit juice to make a weak fruit ade. Each specimen should include all urine voided and should be sent to the laboratory; the label on the specimen should include the exact time of each voiding.

Collecting urine specimens

When collecting urine excreted over a specified period of time, the collection should be started at the appointed time by having the patient empty the bladder and discarding this urine. It should be completed by having the patient empty his bladder at the designated time and by including this urine in the specimen. It is important for the patient to understand that all urine must be saved. He should be instructed to void into a separate receptacle before defecation lest part of the specimen be lost. Toluene is usually added to the specimen until a film forms over the surface; this prevents bacterial growth which may alter the composition of the urine. Sometimes formaldehyde is also used as a preservative. The specimen should be kept in a refrigerator. One should always check to find out how much of the specimen the laboratory needs. If only a sample of the twenty-four hour urine output is needed, mix the total specimen well before taking the sample and record on the label the total amount of urine voided in the allotted period.

When a test involves the collection of total urine output, it is important that the urine be collected from all available sources if more than the normal one exists. For instance, the patient may void normally yet have a nephrostomy tube from which urine drains. Specimens from each source should be collected in separate containers, since this may help determine the function of each kidney. Urine from a cystostomy tube and a urethral catheter may, however, be combined in the same specimen because both come from the bladder.

Intravenous pyelography

An intravenous pyelogram is usually ordered when kidney or urinary tract disease is suspected. In this test, the roentgenogram shows the kidney shadows and the filling of the kidney pelves, and it outlines the ureters and the bladder. Before the test is scheduled, an attempt is made to learn whether or not the patient is sensitive to iodine, because the radiopaque medium which is injected intravenously contains iodine; serious and even fatal reactions have occurred in sensitive persons. A history of allergy or of serious kidney or liver damage may also be contraindications to the use of radiopaque substances. The patient should be prepared initially for this examination by an explanation of the procedure, its purpose, and the reasons for the physical preparation. He is usually instructed to omit food and fluids from 12 o'clock the night before until after the examination is completed, because this produces a better concentration of the radiopaque medium in the urinary tract and a clearer roentgenogram.

Since the kidneys lie retroperitoneally, it is important that the bowel be empty of gas and fecal material which may cause shadows on the film. Many physicians order 12 ml. (1 tablespoon) of licorice powder dissolved in water or milk or 30 ml. (1 ounce) of castor oil to be given about 6 P.M. the evening before the test is to be made. Castor oil is made more palatable if it is mixed with a citrus fruit juice and if a few milliliters of sodium bicarbonate are stirred in immediately before offering it to the patient. Some patients prefer to suck on a section of orange or lemon immediately after taking castor oil. If the patient has evidence of peptic ulcers, colitis, a colostomy, a ureterosigmoidal transplant, or extreme debility, these relatively vigorous cathartics are contraindicated. Therefore, before giving the medication, the nurse should know something about the physical condition of the patient and should bring to the doctor's attention any order for a cathartic which she believes is contraindicated. The patient who has received a cathartic should not be given sedation to induce sleep, and he should be told where to find the call light and the bathroom or bedpan. If he is elderly or debilitated, he must be urged to call for the assistance of the nurse to go to the bathroom. Patients can become quite weak from drastic catharsis, and this may lead to accidents. Occasionally if the cathartic has been ineffectual or if it is contraindicated for some reason, enemas may be given. The enema must be given early in the morning to allow time for excretion of the fluid absorbed during the enema and for expulsion of flatus. The very elderly patient usually has difficulty emptying the bowel completely following an enema; for this reason enemas are sometimes given the evening before. The nurse should determine and record the effectiveness of efforts to evacuate the bowel, reporting ineffective results. If the patient has received barium prior to an intravenous pyelogram, the bowel must be especially well emptied because any residual barium may obscure the kidney picture. Usually, however, this problem is prevented by careful scheduling of the tests so that those for kidney function precede barium swallows, gastrointestinal series, or barium enemas.

The patient is placed on an x-ray table, usually in a lithotomy position. Sometimes he is placed on a full-length table and a large plastic ball is strapped firmly on the abdomen to prevent dye from passing freely down the ureters until after the roentgenogram of the kidneys has been taken. If a lithotomy position is used, all the precautions discussed under placing a patient in position for a vaginal examination should be taken. (See Chapter 22.) A roentgenogram of the abdominal area (a flat plate) is taken first. This gives information as to the size, shape, and position of the kidneys and reveals radiopaque stones anywhere along the urinary system.

Several radiopaque preparations are used for intravenous pyelogram examinations. All of them contain iodine and all may cause serious reactions in persons sensitive to the drug in this form. Urokon and Diodrast are preparations widely used at the present time. The nurse never,

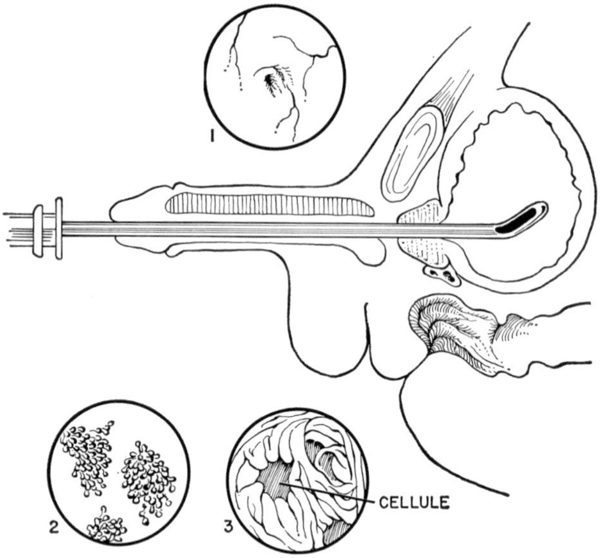

Figure 35

Schematic diagram of a cystoscope inserted for examination of the bladder. *1,* Appearance of a normal ureteral orifice as seen through the cystoscope. *2,* Appearance of papillomas of the bladder as seen through the cystoscope. *3,* Appearance of a trabeculated bladder as seen through the cystoscope. Note the formation of cellules.

under any circumstances, injects the substance herself. The patient should know that he may have a feeling of warmth, a flushing of the face, and a salty taste in the mouth as the doctor slowly injects the drug intravenously. This usually lasts only a few minutes and is often relieved by taking deep breaths. The nurse should then watch for any signs of respiratory difficulty, sudden diaphoresis and claminess, and urticaria, any of which may indicate an untoward reaction to the contrast medium. If the patient complains of numbness or tingling of any part of the body, of palpitation, or of any other unusual sensation, he must be attended constantly, and the doctor must be immediately summoned. Pyribenzamine, Benadryl, Adrenalin, and oxygen should be available for immediate use if necessary.

Roentgenograms are usually taken seven and fifteen minutes after the drug is injected. If poor renal function is suspected, films may also be taken one and two hours later. When delayed films are necessary, the patient must either be returned to his bed or protected from discomfort on the table. A soft bath blanket should be placed under him, and he should be assisted in changing position at fifteen mintue intervals.

Fluids should be forced for twenty-four hours following an intravenous pyelogram to help eliminate any remaining drug and to compensate for the slight dehydration preceding the test.

Cystoscopy and retrograde studies

A cystoscopy is the examination of the inside of the bladder through a metal instrument called a *cystoscope.* (See Figure 35.) The instrument is constructed with illumination, enabling the examiner to see the interior of the bladder.

A cystoscopic examination is indicated for all patients who have, or have had, hematuria because, although blood in the urine may be due to other causes, it is one of the earliest signs of malignant growths anywhere along the urinary system. The examination may be done as part of an intensive diagnostic study, or it may be done as an emergency diagnostic measure. By doing an immediate cystoscopy the doctor may locate a point of hemorrhage in the prostate, the bladder, or the upper urinary tracts which might otherwise escape detection because such hemorrhages frequently stop spontaneously for a time. If the examination of only the urethra and prostate appear necessary, a shorter instrument known as an *endoscope* is used.

Nursing attention before and during a cystoscopic examination can contribute greatly to its success and to lessening the patient's discomfort. The patient should know just what he will experience in the cystoscopy room; he may not have any idea of what to expect and may be reluctant to ask the doctor. The nurse should give thorough explanations before the procedure is begun, and she should remain with the patient during the procedure, giving him reassurance and encouragement. This helps him to relax and decreases discomfort, much of which is due to contraction or spasm of the vesical sphincters. Most hospitals require a signed permit before this procedure is done.

Fluids are usually forced for several hours before the patient goes to the cystoscopy room. This ensures a continuous flow of urine in case urine specimens are to be collected from the kidneys. If an anesthetic is to be given, fluids may be given intravenously. A sedative such as phenobarbital and a narcotic such as morphine or Demerol may be given about a half hour prior to the examination. A local anesthetic such as procaine (usually 4 per cent) may be instilled into the urethra immediately prior to the insertion of the cystoscope. If the patient is very apprehensive or if much manipulation is anticipated, a general anesthetic may be given to avoid sudden vigorous movement during the examination which might cause trauma to the urethra or even perforation of the bladder.

Clothing must be removed and a hospital gown and lithotomy boots used. The patient is placed in a lithotomy position on the cystoscopy table and is draped in such a manner that only the perineum is exposed. In placing the patient in position, care must be taken that pressure is not exerted upon the popliteal spaces, since such pressure might cause circulatory embarrassment and lead to thrombosis in blood vessels. Because of arthritis and related disorders, some elderly patients are unable to rest comfortably in the stirrups. It may be necessary to use slings in place of the stirrups and to place extra pillows under the patient's head and shoulders. If prolonged time on the table is necessary, the patient's legs should be removed from the stirrups at intervals and flexed and extended a few times.

If the patient is emotionally prepared and relatively comfortable, he should be able to relax enough so that the cystoscope can be passed with little pain, provided there is no obstruction in the urethra. Deep breathing will sometimes help the patient relax. The passing of the instrument will be followed immediately by a strong desire to void. This is because of the pressure of the instrument against the internal sphincter and because the bladder is filled with distilled water during the examination to distend its walls and thus make visualization more effective.

When the trouble is not located in the bladder, urethral catheters (nylon, radiopaque, calibrated, and size 4 or 6 Fr.) are passed through the cystoscope and inserted into the ureteral opening in the bladder, up the ureter, and into the kidney pelvis (see Figure 36). This procedure is known as a *ureteral catheterization* and may involve one or both of the ureters. Specimens obtained directly from the kidneys are examined microscopically and for concentration of urea. Urine obtained in this manner may be cultured and studied for tubercle bacilli, cancer cells, and other abnormal constituents. Kidney function tests may be carried out by injecting indigo carmine (a blue dye) or phenolsul-

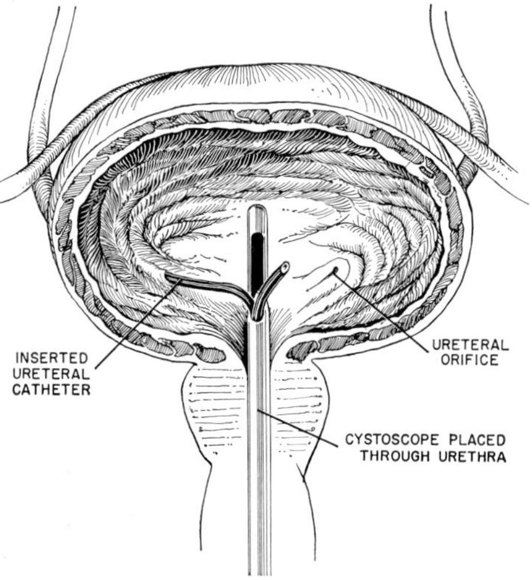

Figure 36

Schematic drawing of ureteral catheterization through the cystoscope. Note the ureteral catheter inserted into the right orifice. The left ureteral catheter is ready to be inserted.

fonphthalein (a red dye) intravenously and timing the appearance of the dye from each kidney. With normal function, the dye will appear from each side in three to six minutes.

Ureteral catheters may be inserted and left in place even though the cystoscope is withdrawn. They are frequently left in place prior to gynecologic or extensive lower colon surgery in which there may be danger of accidentally injuring an unrecognized ureter. They may also be left in place to provide better kidney drainage in certain conditions; for example, when a stone is lodged in the ureter.

A sharp x-ray outline of the kidney and the ureters is obtained by injecting 4 to 8 ml. of radiopaque substance such as Urokon or Skiodan gently up each ureteral catheter after urine specimens have been collected. While the solution is being injected, the patient may feel slight discomfort in the kidney region, but pain should not be experienced unless too much of the solution has been injected, causing overdistention of the kidney pelvis. As the doctor withdraws the catheters and the cystoscope, he again injects the contrast medium (1 to 2 ml.) which fills the ureters and immediately has another roentgenogram made which will show the outline of the ureters. This examination is known as a *retrograde pyelogram.*

When a retrograde examination is to be made, the patient is usually urged to drink large amounts of fluid prior to the test so that specimens can be obtained easily. Solid food is usually withheld because apprehension may cause the patient to feel nauseated. Cathartics and enemas may be ordered as for an intravenous pyelogram.

After any cystoscopic procedure, the nurse should observe the patient's urinary output. The urine may be pink-tinged, but more extensive bleeding should be reported to the doctor. If dyes have been used, the patient should be told that the urine will be an unusual color. The patient may have a "full" sensation and a feeling of burning in the bladder; he may also have low back pain. Mild analgesics such as acetylsalicylic acid and codeine sulfate may be prescribed for discomfort, but usually the greatest relief is obtained from warm tub baths, which produce relaxation and relieve muscle tension. If the patient feels chilly, a heating pad or hot-water bottle applied over the bladder region or to the lower back may be used. Fluids should be forced to dilute the urine and thereby lessen irritation to the mucous membrane linings of the urinary tract. Fluids should be offered at hourly intervals for at least four hours.

Sharp abdominal pain should be reported to the doctor, and analgesic drugs should be withheld until he has examined the patient because the bladder or ureters may have been accidentally perforated, causing peritonitis. Chills and marked elevation of temperature may follow cystoscopic procedures. These are thought to be caused by a general systemic reaction to the foreign substances introduced, the instrumentation, and the pain. The patient should remain in bed for a few hours following these procedures and should be asked to notify the nurse if he has any sensation of chilling. Chilling and elevation of temperature usually respond within a short time to extra warmth and to warm fluids by mouth.

Care should be taken that the patient, especially an elderly one, does not stand or walk alone immediately after the procedure, since blood which has drained from the legs while he was in the lithotomy position flows back into the vessels of the feet and legs as he stands up. Accidents due to dizziness and fainting can occur from the sudden change in distribution of blood, which reduces the blood supply to the brain.

Examinations of the urinary system are often done on an ambulatory basis either in a clinic or in a doctor's office. Even though a period of rest in the clinic is encouraged, the patient should be advised to bring someone with him who can be certain that he gets home safely. If food has been withheld before the examination, the patient should have something to eat before leaving for home. He or his relatives should be given printed instructions both for the preparation for examinations and for care at the conclusion of the tests. These should be used as a supplement to verbal instructions, since the latter must often be given as the patient is preparing to leave the clinic and after he has had sedation.

The nurse needs to be especially aware of her function as an intermediary between the patient and the urologist, since the patient is often reluctant to discuss with the specialist matters that he would mention freely to his family doctor.

The patient with nonoperative disease of the urinary system

Unfortunately some diseases of the urinary system cannot be helped by surgery. These nonoperative diseases, particularly of the kidney, cause many deaths each year in all age groups.

RENAL FAILURE

Since many disorders of the urinary system, as well as some general systemic diseases, result in impairment of kidney function and in consequent renal failure, renal failure will be discussed before specific diseases of the urinary system are considered.

Development and progress of renal failure

Renal failure, which is also referred to as *renal insufficiency* or *renal suppression,* is a serious derangement of kidney function in which the kidneys are unable to carry out normal excretion of waste products and other essential functions (see Chapter 6). When a patient shows signs of renal failure, he is said to have *uremia.*

There are many signs and symptoms of renal insufficiency and impending uremia. A common symptom is *oliguria,* or decrease in normal urinary output. Output of urine, however, may be normal or even increased in quantity, yet the waste products contained therein may be below normal; this results in a low specific gravity of the urine. Occasionally there may be *anuria,* or no urinary output at all. Repeated examinations of the blood may show a gradual increase in the nonprotein nitrogen content. Sometimes the nonprotein nitrogen level becomes markedly elevated before any other symptoms occur. In the diseased kidneys' effort to carry on normal functions, water and electrolyte balance also becomes upset.

The patient with renal insufficiency usually has a marked pallor, and he may be either edematous or dehydrated, depending upon whether salt and water are being retained or lost. Edema is often first noticed as puffiness about the eyes, fullness in the lower abdomen and lower trunk, and "pitting edema" of the ankles. "Pitting edema" refers to a soft fullness in which pressure on the edematous area causes a depression that slowly returns to normal.

Waste products in the form of urea and salt crystals (uremic frost) may appear as a white, powdery substance on the skin. This may not be noticed at first, although the patient may complain of pruritus or itching of the skin. Later the "frost" may become clearly visible, especially on those patients who have unusually dark skins. Halitosis is usually pronounced, the tongue is coated, and the patient may have a generalized body odor which is suggestive of urine.

Early signs of renal failure may be caused by edema resulting from salt and water retention. These signs may include headache, blurred vision, dizziness, irritability, and slowing of mental processes. The headache, dimness of vision, and spots before the eyes may be due to retinal hemorrhages caused by the hypertension which commonly accompanies kidney failure. Projectile vomiting and convulsions may occur later and are caused by cerebral edema.

Electrolyte imbalance may lead to acidosis, with nausea, vomiting, thirst, and air hunger. Calcium metabolism is often altered, and calcium may be excreted by the failing kidney in abnormally large amounts. Its depletion may cause muscle twitching, irritability, tetany, and convulsions. Potassium retention is one of the most serious problems, since potassium intoxication causes increasing generalized weakness, cardiac failure, and pulmonary edema. Some patients remain mentally alert for a surprisingly long time when the extent of electrolyte imbalance is considered but, if kidney function is not restored, irritability, drowsiness, and coma eventually occur.

A fairly common accompaniment of renal failure is ulceration of the entire gastrointestinal tract. Blood may be found in the feces, and the mucous membranes of the mouth frequently bleed. This blood loss causes a marked anemia. In the patient with uremia, it is not unusual for death to be immediately preceded by convulsions and the vomiting of blood (hematemesis).

The rapidity of onset may give a clue to the nature of the patient's difficulty and to his prognosis. If the renal failure is acute, it is usually due to *lower nephron nephrosis;* this will terminate either in death or in return to normal renal function within two or three weeks. In lower nephron nephrosis the ascending loop of Henle and the distal tubules are damaged. If the renal failure is slow in onset, it is usually caused by damage to the glomeruli and the proximal tubules; it is usually secondary to a chronic disease, such as chronic glomerulonephritis, chronic pyelonephritis, nephrosclerosis, malignant hypertension, or collagen disease. The prognosis in renal failure due to chronic disease is poor.

Renal failure and uremia *may be due to primary damage to the nephrons.* The damage may be caused by infection of the kidneys, mechanical obstruction of both ureters or renal pelves, polycystic kidneys, poisons such as mushrooms, bichloride of mercury, and carbon tetrachloride, or allergic reactions to transfusions and to drugs such as the sulfonamides. Necrosis of the renal tissues *may be secondary to a decrease in the blood supply to the kidneys.* Emboli or thrombi in renal arteries or veins may prevent flow of blood to the nephrons. There may be an insufficient blood supply passing through the kidneys due to severe dehydration, loss of blood, circulatory collapse secondary to such things as anesthesia or toxemia of pregnancy, or shock resulting from internal fluid loss and unusual distribution of body fluids following burns and severe tissue trauma.

The prognosis in renal insufficiency depends on the underlying cause. If the primary cause can be removed, as is often possible in lower nephron nephrosis, the renal insufficiency is reversible in about 80 per cent of the patients.[11] If the primary disease is irreversible, as is chronic glomerulonephritis, the onset of uremia may indicate that death is imminent, although remission may occur and may be prolonged by avoidance of infections, overactivity, obesity, and any other conditions that increase the work load of the damaged kidneys.

Treatment and nursing care in acute renal failure

Acute renal failure can sometimes be prevented. Federal legislation controls the distribution to the layman of drugs which may damage the kidneys. If drugs, such as streptomycin, that may have an untoward effect on kidneys are prescribed, kidney function should be evaluated periodically. Careful observation of the blood pressure should be made during and immediately after surgery and, if it is low, treatment should be instituted to prevent its falling to levels that markedly decrease the blood flow through the kidneys. Immediate restoration of fluids to patients who have sustained serious accidental blood loss also decreases the likelihood of renal damage. Patients with streptococcal infections should have medical attention, since this type of infection always precedes acute glomerulonephritis. The removal of obstructions of the urinary tract which cause pressure on the nephrons also helps to prevent acute renal failure. Details concerning the prevention and treatment of these conditions that may be complicated by renal failure are discussed more fully in other sections of this chapter.

There are two main objectives in the medical management of patients with acute renal failure. First, the primary cause is treated in an attempt to prevent further kidney damage—obstructions are relieved, fluid and blood losses are replaced when there is shock, hemorrhage, or dehydration, and antidotes for poisons and injurious drugs are given when possible. Second, an effort is made to maintain the fluid and electrolyte balance as close to normal as possible and to decrease the work of the kidneys so that the injured tissues may regenerate. The following discussion is concerned only with maintaining the patient until the primary cause is removed and the kidney has had time to return to normal.

The nurse should report early signs of renal insufficiency since early treatment for fluid and electrolyte imbalance may minimize the renal damage. Changes in the urinary output are significant. Any decrease in the urinary output below 500 ml. a day should be reported at once, since it is known that, even if the patient fasts and goes without water, the normal kidneys will excrete at least that amount of urine a day.[11] Unless excessive amounts of fluid are being lost through other routes, the urinary output per day for a normal person should approximate the fluid intake. If excessive amounts of fluid are being lost through other routes, such as the lungs and skin, normal urine will appear concentrated and have a high specific gravity.

When the kidneys fail to excrete an adequate amount of urine, fluids are usually limited to 800 to 1,000 ml. a day plus enough extra fluids to replace those lost through routes other than the urinary system.[11] If larger amounts of fluid are given, cardiac failure may occur, since the kidneys are unable to excrete the excess fluid. Salt intake also is limited to no more than the amount that is lost daily so that large amounts will not be retained in the body and thus cause retention of fluid in the tissues.[11] Since thirst is a common complaint, fluids by mouth should be judiciously spaced throughout the twenty-four hour period. Frequent mouth care will help to prevent drying of the mucous membranes and will add to comfort. This is especially important if the patient is vomiting or is unable to drink. All intake by mouth and other routes and all output from the kidney and other routes, such as vomiting, must be carefully measured and recorded because this information helps the doctor determine how much fluid the patient should have. Signs of sodium and other electrolyte depletion should be reported to the doctor at once. (See Chapter 6.)

To decrease the work of the kidneys, it may be considered desirable to decrease protein catabolism, by limiting protein foods. Food intake may be limited to carbohydrates and moderate amounts of fat; many foods high in carbohydrate, including fruit juices, may be restricted to lower the intake of potassium. If the patient is nauseated, he may receive carbohydrates by intravenous infusion. If he can take fluids by mouth or by tube into the stomach, sugar and water mixed with melted butter may be given in small amounts; tube feedings may be prepared with peanut oil and dextrose. Since this diet it not palatable, it should always be served on attractive trays in a pleasant environment to those taking it by mouth. Since the feeding may leave an unpleasant sensation in the mouth, mouth care should be given after each meal. If the patient can tolerate hard candy, "sour balls" can be given; they counteract the sweet, yet greasy, mouth sensation of which the patient complains, and they also increase the carbohydrate intake without adding potassium. Ginger ale is often permissible and acceptable to the patient. Ginger ale is especially helpful in alleviating the morning nausea and headache which are characteristic of uremia.

Insulin is occasionally given with concentrated glucose in an effort to help the liver to store glycogen, since in this storage process potassium is removed from the blood stream, decreasing the possibility of potassium intoxication.[11] When insulin is being used, the patient must be observed carefully for signs of insulin shock, which are apprehension, cold clammy skin, tremor, rapid pulse, feeling of faintness, and loss of consciousness.

Any infection increases protein catabolism, increases the work load of the kidneys, and speeds the onset of uremia. It is important to protect the patient with renal failure from infection. Chilling must be prevented by careful ventilation of the room, with avoidance of drafts. Doctors, nurses, members of the patient's family, and others who have upper respiratory infections should not go near the patient. Occasionally the patient is placed in a single room, and visitors are often restricted as an additional protection. If there are surgical wounds to be cared for, special attention should be given to aseptic technique; contamination of wounds from such sources as feces, urine, and flies should be prevented. Penicillin often is given to prevent infection or to control spread of existing infection.

The patient must be observed carefully for signs of respiratory and cardiac complications. To prevent hypostatic pneumonia, he should be turned from side to side and encouraged to take deep breaths at two hour intervals. Since cardiac failure and pulmonary edema due to potassium intoxication are common complications, the nurse should be alert for tachycardia and auricular fibrillation. If these signs appear, sodium intake is further decreased and digitalis may be ordered. Mercurial diuretics are contraindicated because they may cause further kidney damage and may lead to sodium depletion since the diseased kidneys already may be hampered in their ability to reabsorb sodium salts.[11] Loss of body fluids following the administration of mercurials is caused by the temporary inhibition of tubular reabsorption. (See Chapter 20 for discussion of these drugs in treatment of cardiac failure and pulmonary edema.)

Muscular twitching anywhere in the body should be reported to the doctor at once. The nurse may be asked to grasp the patient's wrist, constrict the circulation for a few minutes, and notice whether or not the hand goes into a position of palmar flexion due to tetany (Trousseau's sign), or she may be asked to tap the patient's face lightly over the facial nerve just below the temple and notice if the facial muscles twitch (Chvostek's sign). If either reaction occurs, the doctor is notified at once. Calcium gluconate and calcium chloride are usually kept readily available so that either may be given intravenously if convulsions resulting from decreased ionized blood calcium occur or threaten.

If the patient shows any signs of increased intracranial pressure due to cerebral edema or any signs of tetany, padded side rails should be placed on the bed and a mouth gag kept at the bedside (see Chapter 34 for signs of increased intracranial pressure). Fifty milliliters of 50 per cent glucose, a hypertonic solution, are usually given intravenously if convulsions are caused by cerebral edema. Fifty per cent solution of magnesium sulfate also may be given intramuscularly or rectally. The patient with cerebral edema is usually irritable and may become irrational. He may become upset if he feels confined; therefore, even though the side rails must be padded, the bed should be placed so that he can see about the room. If he is so confused or irrational that his behavior is unpredictable, he should not be left alone; sometimes family members are glad to stay with him. If it is impossible to have the patient constantly attended, it is sometimes helpful to use a drawsheet restraint (with the diagonally twirled sheet placed loosely over the chest and anchored to the side rails) or a Posey belt, which will serve to remind the forgetful patient where he is and thus prevent injury if he attempts to get out of bed. Persuasion, long explanations, and arguments with the patient should be avoided since they only upset him. The nurse who has a calm voice, a calm manner, and a positive approach can usually help him. If he objects to a treatment, it is better to delay it for a short time. If he continues to resist essential treatment, however, the doctor must be notified. Loud noises and bright lights tend to increase irritability, and the number of persons entering the room, as well as frequent changes of nursing personnel, disturb the patient.

Special treatment for potassium intoxication. If potassium intoxication occurs, the patient may be treated by dialysis in an attempt to provide an emergency substitution for the action of normal renal tissue. Dialysis is now frequently used to remove excess amounts of salicylates, barbiturates, and bromides from the blood stream following accidental or intentional overdoses of these drugs. At the present time three methods are being used: the artificial kidney, peritoneal lavage, and intestinal catharsis.

Artificial kidney. The artificial kidney is a complex mechanism which might be described as an external kidney. The patient's arterial blood is shunted into the artificial kidney via tubing. Here, it circulates through special cellophane tubing which resembles capillary walls in permeability and which is surrounded by a solution of approximately the same electrolyte composition as that of normal extracellular fluid, allowing for the elimination by dialysis of moderate amounts of body waste products such as urea and potassium. The blood is then returned to the venous circulation. Heparin is used to prevent blood clotting, and requires that the patient be watched closely for signs of hemorrhage. The danger of hemorrhage makes the use of an artificial kidney impossible for most postoperative patients. Dialysis by means of the artificial kidney is limited in usefulness by the need for constant attendance by a trained team of doctors, nurses, and laboratory technicians during the entire time that the kidney is being used.

Peritoneal lavage. Peritoneal lavage requires that two incisions be made into the peritoneal cavity. Through tubing placed into the upper incision, large volumes of sterile solution similar to that used in the artificial kidney, combined with antibiotics, are directed continuously into the peritoneal cavity. Body wastes pass out with the solution through the drainage tube placed in the lower incision. Peritoneal lavage can be used only for one or two days because there is danger of peritonitis and because such large amounts of irrigating solution are difficult and costly to provide. This method, therefore, is used relatively infrequently.

Intestinal catharsis. Intestinal catharsis is the safest method of dialysis. Sodium or ammonium cation exchange resins which will absorb potassium and carry it out by way of the intestines are given either by mouth or, if the patient is likely to vomit, as a retention enema. Usually 50 Gm. of the powder (dissolved in a small amount of water) are given in divided doses.[11] A cathartic such as citrate of magnesia and a cleansing enema or a colonic irrigation are given daily to ensure the elimination of potassium from the bowel and thereby prevent its reabsorption in the lower intestine.

Intestinal catharsis may make an already weak patient weaker, so special consideration must be given to measures that will conserve his strength. He must be given support while sitting on the bedpan, there must be provision for lengthy and undisturbed rest periods, and he must be given assistance with eating and general hygiene. Daily blood and urine specimens will be collected for determinations of sodium and potassium levels.

The patient convalescing following acute renal failure. If the patient can be maintained during the crucial period of acute renal failure, diuresis will usually occur during the second week of kidney failure, and function will gradually return to normal over a period of weeks. As recovery occurs, the fluid intake is increased to equal the output. It is important to watch for signs of dehydration due to sodium depletion or for signs of sodium retention (edema) during this period because the sodium-water balance may be quite unstable. Until renal function returns to normal, a high-caloric, low-protein diet, with plenty of fluids should be continued and only moderate activity allowed.

Since a period of convalescence is necessary following acute renal failure, arrangements may need to be made for care in a nursing home or in a convalescent home. If the patient cannot be cared for in his own home, the social service worker should be consulted early in the patient's convalescence in the hospital to help the family make appropriate arrangements. Even if care is feasible at home, financial assistance may be needed, particularly if the patient happens to be the family wage earner. Many families need help in budget planning and in food selection so that needed foods can be afforded when the patient is at home. Homemaking service may make it possible for members of the family to prepare proper meals and otherwise care for the patient in his own home. The patient must be consulted in all plans for his convalescent care. If a nursing home or convalescent home is to be used, the nursing staffs of such a facility should be informed of the particular nursing needs and problems of the patient; the interagency referral form commonly used in referral of patients to public health nurses in community nursing agencies can be used for this.

CHRONIC UREMIA

In chronic uremia the treatment is designed to maintain physiology as close to normal as possible in order to keep the patient relatively comfortable for as long as he lives.

Provided the urinary output does not decrease or edema does not increase, fluids are forced since the kidney has a lessened ability to concentrate solids and more fluid is required to excrete wastes. If there is edema, however, fluids must be restricted. An accurate record of the intake and output should be kept, and fluids should be forced only to the point at which a positive balance of intake and output is maintained.

Since the patient usually has severe anorexia, many physicians feel that he should have any food that appeals to him. While an attempt is made to give him a well-balanced diet, unusual combinations of foods that do not appeal to him should not be forced. Salt should not be used in excess, but neither must it be limited unless there is edema. Some doctors, however, believe that the diet should be low in salt and low in protein since this may lessen tax on the limited kidney reserve. Salt substitutes containing potassium are contraindicated for patients with kidney disease because the kidney is often unable to eliminate potassium normally. Vinegar, lemon, brown sugar, minced parsley, mint, rum, cloves, cinnamon, and salt-free tomato juice are a few suggested flavorings which may make unsalted foods more palatable.[12] Often the patient can tolerate fruit juices and carbonated beverages when other foods are rejected. Foods prepared in his own home are often more acceptable to him than hospital meals.

Relatives should be encouraged to bring foods to the very ill patient in the hospital provided that they are able to do so and know what seasonings must be avoided. If the gastrointestinal tract becomes ulcerated, bland foods and fluids may have to be given.

Nursing measures for counteracting thirst and making the diet acceptable are the same as those mentioned for the patient with acute renal failure. Mouth care is extremely important for the patient with chronic uremia, since mouth sores, once developed, are almost impossible to cure. Mineral oil is an acceptable protective lubricant unless the patient is comatose, in which case he is likely to aspirate the oily fluid into the lungs. A water-soluble lubricant with a vegetable base, such as K-Y lubricating jelly is preferable for the unconscious patient. Hydrogen peroxide is helpful in removing caked blood from the mouth and the nose.

Severe anemia, which is common in chronic uremia and contributes to the patient's general weakness, is best treated by blood transfusions. Hematinic drugs appear to be of little value.[11] If blood cells are hemolyzing, corticosteroids may be given.[14] Acidosis is usually not treated unless hyperventilation of the lungs becomes distressing. If the patient can take aluminum hydroxide by mouth, this decreases the absorption of phosphates in the gastrointestinal tract and helps alleviate symptoms. The phosphate combines with the aluminum to form aluminum phosphate, which is eliminated through the bowel. Sodium bicarbonate may also be given by mouth to combat acidosis. When oral medications cannot be tolerated, intravenous solutions such as 1/6 molar lactate may be given.[11]

Since waste products are not being eliminated adequately through the kidneys it is important that the bowels be kept open and that the skin be bathed frequently so that these routes of excretion function adequately. More urea and sodium are excreted through the skin than normally, and itching may occur. The best treatment for this is to bathe the itching skin areas with a weak vinegar solution (2 tablespoons to 1 pint of water) which dissolves the urate crystals.

If there is edema, it is important to provide the best possible lymph and venous drainage. This may be accomplished by stimulating the circulation with either active or passive exercises and by elevating the edematous areas to encourage gravity drainage of lymph and venous blood. If the eyelids are puffy, the head should be elevated. In edema of the arms or legs the parts should be supported slightly above the heart level with pillows. Edematous tissues require meticulous hygienic care and frequent change in position to help prevent pressure sores which heal slowly and become infected easily.

The patient who has chronic uremia easily contracts systemic infection; preventive nursing measures for this are the same as for the patient with acute renal failure. The complications of chronic uremia are the same as those of acute renal failure. The treatment, however, is never so vigorous. Tetany, convulsions, cardiac failure, and pulmonary edema are managed in the same way, but it is useless to employ dialysis.

The patient should be kept active and occupied within the limits of his strength for as long as possible. Since he usually has failing vision, safety measures similar to those needed for patients with eye conditions should be employed. The patient may enjoy being read to or listening to the radio. If he cannot see, the nurse should read his mail to him and keep him informed of headlines in the daily papers since this helps to keep him in contact with the world around him. Although vision is poor, he may be able to feed himself for some time; the nurse or a member of the patient's family should prepare the food and tactfully indicate the foods being served and their placement on the tray. Later the patient may need to be fed by others, and ultimately tube feeding may be required.

Giving emotional support to the family is probably one of the most important duties of the nurse in caring for patients with both acute and chronic uremia. The patient requires many treatments which may alarm the family even more than they do the patient. A brief, simple explanation of the reasons for things that are done may prevent anxiety which often is transmitted from the family to the patient. If the family wishes to participate in care, there is much that they can do to help maintain a pleasant, safe, calm environment for the patient. However, they must understand the need for this and must be helped to plan appropriately. Often both the patient and the family appreciate visits from their spiritual adviser. By her interest and attitudes during this period the nurse can do a great deal to help the family accept the patient's ultimate death if this is inevitable. When the patient becomes comatose, additional care will be required. (See Chapter 9 for care of the unconscious patient.)

NEPHRITIS

Nephritis, or Bright's disease, is a general term sometimes used to describe noninfectious inflammatory and degenerative diseases affecting the nephrons of the kidney. Under this classification are such diseases as acute glomerulonephritis, subacute and chronic glomerulonephritis, and nephrosclerosis.

Acute glomerulonephritis

Acute glomerulonephritis is a disease seen usually in children or young adults, and it occurs twice as often in males as in females. Although the cause is unknown, the patient with this disease usually gives a history of a recent upper respiratory infection, such as tonsillitis, laryngitis, sinusitis, common cold, or "grippe," or has recently recovered from scarlet fever or chickenpox. Hemolytic streptococci either have been the causative organisms or have caused complications in each instance. The organisms, however, are not present in the kidneys when glomerulonephritis occurs.

Because of the association between acute glomerulonephritis and streptococcal infections, early treatment of the latter with antibiotics, especially penicillin, seems advisable as a prophylactic measure. Potential foci of infection, such as diseased tonsils, may be removed after the acute infection has subsided.

The onset of acute glomerulonephritis may be either sudden or insidious. The patient may not present a classic picture with all the common symptoms but may have only one or two of the common symptoms.

If the onset is insidious, the patient may complain of weakness, pallor, and anorexia, followed by hematuria, puffiness of the face (especially about the eyes), headache, and decreased urine volume. Hypertension may be present. Nausea, vomiting, a low-grade fever, and nocturia are common. If the disease is of the acute or fulminating type, the patient suddenly develops generalized edema, visual blurring, marked hypertension, and nitrogen retention. The condition may rapidly progress to uremia and result in death.

Laboratory findings in glomerulonephritis vary widely, but albumin, casts, and red and white blood cells are almost always present in the urine. The blood urea nitrogen is usually only slightly elevated. The phenolsulfonphthalein test may show almost the same amount of dye present in each specimen because of the low filtration rate. The specific gravity of the urine is often high because of the low filtration rate in the kidney, the continuing normal reabsorptive function of the distal tubules, and the retention of fluid in the tissues.[9]

Treatment of glomerulonephritis consists of supportive measures. Bed rest is essential. Since the period of bed rest may be long and the patient does not usually feel ill, the nurse needs to help him understand why bed rest is necessary. She should make arrangements to keep him occupied and relatively content during waking hours. The patient is allowed to begin progressive ambulation when the blood sedimentation rate and the blood pressure have returned to normal levels. If ambulation causes any increase in albuminuria or hematuria, the patient must again be placed on complete bed rest for a time. This may cause the patient to become discouraged, depressed, and hostile to treatment; he should be encouraged to discuss his feelings, and it should be explained to him that return to complete bed rest is not too unusual an occurrence. The room should be kept at a constant temperature to avoid his becoming chilled; if he is in a cool room or is ambulatory, warm pajamas and bedsocks should be used for additional warmth. Exposure to upper respiratory infections should be avoided, since even a mild infection such as the common cold may reactivate the kidney disease.

Diet restrictions depend on the symptoms; effort is made to give the kidneys rest. If there is edema, salt is restricted; if there is anuria or oliguria, fluids, protein, and potassium are restricted, and carbohydrate is forced in the same manner as for the patient with lower nephron nephrosis. As improvement occurs, the diet is changed to a low-protein one (50 to 60 Gm. of protein daily). This should consist mainly of complete protein foods which should be divided equally among the three usual meals to ensure their maximum utilization. If this diet is tolerated and improvement continues, a normal diet is ordered.[11]

The nurse should be alert for signs of complications such as cardiac failure, pulmonary edema, or increased intracranial pressure. Since cerebral edema may develop within a few hours, the patient with any elevation of blood pressure should have his blood pressure and pulse checked at least twice a day and preferably every four hours.

Acute glomerulonephritis is usually self-limiting, with complete recovery occurring within a few days to a year. Only about 5 per cent of patients with this condition die, and the deaths are usually due to complications.[11] A few patients with acute glomerulonephritis may develop the chronic form of the disease. However, the severity of the symptoms, provided death from complications can be prevented, seems to have little relationship to the prognosis. A patient with a rather mild case of acute glomerulonephritis may develop chronic glomerulonephritis, while the patient who is acutely ill and has severe hypertension may recover completely and have no recurrences.[11]

Subacute and latent glomerulonephritis

When complete recovery from acute glomerulonephritis has not occurred in from six to eight weeks, the disease is termed subacute. In this stage, recurrent streptococcal infections often produce acute exacerbations. If symptoms continue up to or beyond a year, the disease is termed chronic. When no symptoms are present but albumin and cylindrical casts continue to be present in the urine, the term latent nephritis is used.

During the subacute and latent stages of nephritis, the patient may continue his normal activities. He should, however, avoid fatigue. Upper respiratory infections should be prevented, if possible, and all infections deserve early medical attention. Diet is not restricted, but fluid intake should be kept high. The rules of good general health should be stressed in an effort to prevent exacerbation of the nephritis. Since the patient usually feels well, he often needs to be convinced of the need to follow the prescribed regimen and to return for routine medical follow-up. Examinations are usually done at least annually and may include many kidney function tests and studies of the blood to determine the status of the disease. If symptoms occur at any time, the patient should be advised to seek immediate medical attention even though he may have been thoroughly examined only a short time previously.

Chronic glomerulonephritis

Although chronic glomerulonephritis may follow the acute disease, the majority of patients with this disease give no history of acute glomerulonephritis. Various symptoms, none of which are usually acute, may bring the patient to the doctor. He may notice the slow onset of dependent edema which comes and goes. He may complain of headache, especially in the morning; this is usually associated with hypertension. Hypertension may also cause dyspnea upon exertion. Blurred vision may lead the patient to consult an ophthalmologist, who may be the first to suspect chronic nephritis as he observes the changes in the retinas of the eyes. Nocturia is a common complaint since the kidneys are unable to concentrate efficiently and must work overtime and eliminate more fluid to excrete sufficient waste products. Occasionally chronic nephritis is discovered during a routine physical examination because of the presence of albuminuria, or it may be discovered by the school nurse who observes marked visual change and lassitude in a student. Weakness, lassitude, and weight loss are common but nonspecific symptoms of chronic nephritis.

Early in the disease, urinalysis shows the presence of albumin, cylindrical casts, and blood in microscopic amounts. At this stage, kidney function tests may be normal, but the ability of the kidneys to concentrate will gradually decrease as the glomeruli become fibrotic. Finally, when only a few glomeruli are left to function, the tubules begin to degenerate, so that reabsorption and excretion are decreased, there will be less albuminuria, cylinduria, and hematuria, and the specific gravity will become "fixed." At this time the nonprotein nitrogen in the blood increases.

The course of chronic glomerulonephritis is unpredictable, but it ultimately terminates in death. Some patients with rather marked decrease in kidney function and hypertension may be able to lead a normal life for years, whereas others with identical symptoms may progress quickly to uremia and death.

With any exacerbation of hematuria, hypertension, and edema, the patient is put to bed, and the treatment is similar to that for acute glomerulonephritis. If sleeplessness, irritability, and headache become distressing, sedatives are ordered. Chloral hydrate and bromides are usually the most effective. The patient should be urged to take rest periods during the day and avoid excessive emotional and physical exertion. Obese patients usually are placed on reducing diets. The treatment is basically that used for hypertension associated with cardiac disease. (See Chapter 18.)

Since large amounts of albumin may be lost in the urine, the serum protein level becomes lower than normal, and this may lead to generalized edema. This is known as the *nephrotic syndrome.* Bed rest tends to decrease the edema. In this condition diet is important. Salt is limited to that found in natural foods. If the doctor believes that an attempt should be made to replace serum protein losses in the urine, he may order a diet high in protein (100 to 125 Gm. daily). A low-protein diet (50 to 60 Gm. daily) is ordered by doctors who believe that restriction of protein will cause less burden to the damaged kidneys. To provide a high-protein, low-sodium diet, some of the protein will have to be supplied as low-sodium, high-protein beverages such as Protinal and Lonalac.[12]

It is unwise for the patient with chronic glomerulonephritis to become pregnant since toxemia or abortion may occur. Some patients have no difficulties during pregnancy, but others may develop a severe toxemia and must have labor induced prematurely. The patient who has had nephritis of any kind must be urged to see a physician if she plans to become pregnant, to report at once if pregnancy occurs, and to follow the physician's instructions carefully during pregnancy.

As chronic glomerulonephritis continues into the later stages, the complications are the same as those described for chronic uremia. It is wise to encourage the family of the patient whose condition seems to be progressing rapidly to begin to make arrangements for terminal care. The social worker in the hospital or in the public health agency can often help the family make suitable plans.

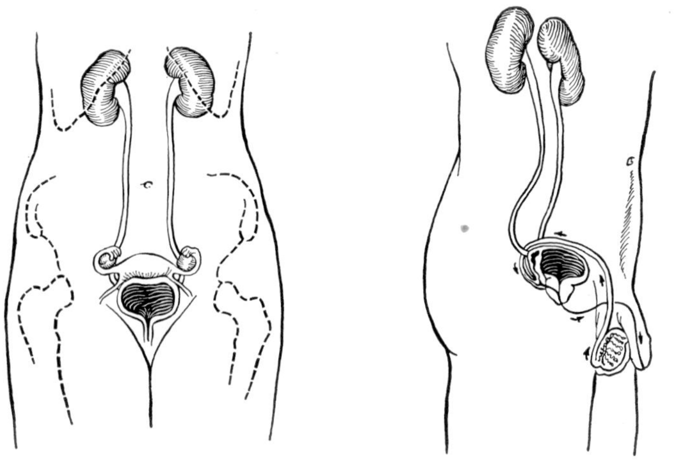

Figure 37

Diagram of the female and the male genitourinary tracts and reproductive systems. The arrows indicate the route by which seminal fluid passes from the testes to the urethra.

Nephrosclerosis

Ten per cent of patients with hypertensive vascular disease die from renal insufficiency and uremia because the blood supply to the kidneys is gradually decreased by narrowing of the renal blood vessels.[11] Patients with this condition, nephrosclerosis, may have signs and symptoms similar to those of the patient with chronic glomerulonephritis and to those of the patient with hypertensive cardiac disease. (See Chapter 18.)

The patient with operative urologic disease

The patient with urologic disease who must have surgery has many problems. The nurse who understands these problems can give the patient better care.

PSYCHOSOCIAL AND CULTURAL ASPECTS

Fear and embarrassment are common in the patient with a urologic disorder and may be expressed in a variety of ways. For example, the patient may become depressed and withdrawn, he may seem extremely aggressive and perhaps even immodest, or he may show his anxiety by repeatedly asking the same questions.

Although most laymen have only a vague understanding of the anatomy and physiology of the urinary system, they do know that the kidneys are necessary for life. When a diagnosis of kidney disease is made, they become frightened. Diseases which make voiding difficult not only cause discomfort, but also lead to worry. Men are often fearful that disease or surgery involving the genitourinary system may decrease sexual ability. This is very threatening to a man of any age. There is also a great fear of cancer. Patients with benign disease of the urinary system have been known to commit suicide because they were unable to believe the condition was nonmalignant.

The patient is often too embarrassed to ask the questions that concern him. A man frequently is inhibited by cultural and emotional patterns in his discussion of sex. This may make it difficult for him to question the doctor as well as the nurse. Careful explanations of the procedures to be done will help to allay many fears. In order for these explanations to be effective, the patient often needs some instruction in the anatomy and physiology of the genitourinary system; simple diagrams are helpful (see Figure 37). Such instruction not only helps to overcome fear of the unknown, but it also helps to make the genitourinary system a less "unmentionable" subject since the patient learns the necessary anatomic terms with which to ask questions.

Many patients hospitalized because of urologic conditions are in the geriatric age group; prostatic hypertrophy, a disease of aging men, is one of the most common problems treated by the urologist. Because most of these elderly patients will have one or more other chronic diseases in addition to the acute urologic condition, the nurse should be alert for exacerbations of such common chronic ailments as cardiac decompensation, diabetes mellitus, emphysema, and arthritis.

SPECIFIC ASPECTS OF NURSING THE PATIENT WITH DISEASE OF THE URINARY SYSTEM

The maintenance of an adequate urinary output and of an adequate fluid intake might be considered a specific urologic nursing measure, since obstruction and infection of the urinary system are the most common disorders treated by the urologist. Usually both conditions are present, and the treatment is based primarily upon removal of the obstruction. Often this must be accomplished, at least temporarily, by placing a catheter into the urinary system above the obstruction to allow for maximum drainage. If the obstruction does not resolve spontaneously, surgical removal will be required. Occasionally a permanent means of diverting urinary drainage must be provided.

Maintenance of the drainage system

Catheters are usually allowed to drain by gravity. In order to drain a closed cavity by gravity, air must be accessible in the drainage system. Since there is less danger of infection and since better drainage is provided when the tubing is not immersed in the drainage, it is preferable to use a system in which the tube is attached to a bottle cap which has an air outlet (see Figure 41). Such a system of drainage also decreases odor. With the increasing incidence of staphylococcal infections, either this system or clamping the catheter with periodic opening for drainage is advocated.[21]

The lumen of the connectors and the tubing should be comparable to that of the catheter. The inner bore for any tube draining urine should be at least 3/4 mm. in diameter.

Improperly cleansed catheters, glass connectors, drainage tubing, or connectors at the bottle caps may cause partial obstruction of the lumen. To keep catheters and drainage systems in good condition, immediately after use they should be soaked in cold water to which a detergent such as Solvental has been added. Next, warm water and soap should be forced through the lumens with a syringe; then 5 per cent acetic acid (full strength white vinegar) (to dissolve urate crystals) and hydrogen peroxide (to remove any old blood) should be forced through. The glass connectors can be cleaned easily with a small tube brush, and benzene or ether can be used to remove adhesive from the outside of the tubes. After a final thorough rinsing in cold water, the catheters and tubing are ready for sterilization.

When a white sediment begins to encrust a glass connector, or when a tube rubbed between the fingers feels "sandy," the equipment should be changed. Usually the catheter will also need changing at this time. Ordinarily, tubing will need to be changed only once a week. If the bottles are cleansed and boiled daily, however, there will be less odor.

If thick-walled latex tubing is used, obstruction of drainage due to kinking can be reduced. Care should be taken not to obstruct the lumen when attaching

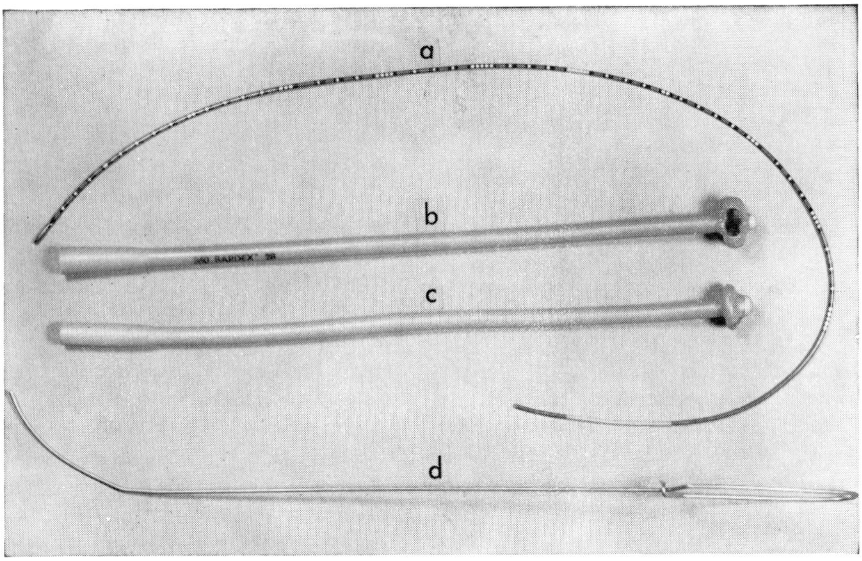

Figure 38

a, b, and *c,* Catheters used to drain the kidney pelvis: *a,* ureteral catheter; *b,* Malecot or bat-winged catheter; *c,* Pezzer or mushroom catheter. *d,* Stylet used to insert Malecot and Pezzer catheters.

the drainage tubing to the bed. A large paper clamp is convenient to use and is unlikely to squeeze or kink the tubing (see Figure 41). Tubes are frequently clamped off by the weight of a patient lying on them. To prevent this and also to lessen the danger of decubiti, it is best to run drainage tubing over the thigh. However, if this causes kinking, the tubing should be run under the knee or directly to the foot of the bed, where it will not be under any body part. Special care must be taken that nephrostomy and ureterostomy tubes are not kinked when the patient is on his side.

To provide complete drainage of a cavity by gravity, the tubing must run directly from the level of the cavity to the drainage receptacle with no loops of tubing below the level of the drainage bottle. Clipping the tubing to the bed and coiling the excess length on the bed help to prevent accidental decompression or partial emptying of the bladder.

The use of an "up bottle" (a small drainage receptacle which can be attached to the gown or to the thigh) provides for a system of straight drainage for the ambulatory patient. A flat eight-ounce bottle attached to the gown with tape and a safety pin works satisfactorily as an "up bottle"; plastic leg urinals now on the market are also useful (see Figures 9 and 43). Patients should be cautioned not to fasten the "up bottle" so high that the catheter or tubing is kinked or must drain against gravity. "Up bottles" and leg urinals do not provide adequate drainage for the patient who is in bed because no gravity is provided.

Principles of catheter care

The nurse should know *why a catheter has been inserted* and *what cavity it is draining.* If the ureter is obstructed or partially obstructed, a catheter must be placed directly into the kidney pelvis to assure adequate drainage. If there is complete obstruction of the ureter, a *nephrostomy tube,* usually a Pezzer (mushroom) or Malecot (bat-winged) catheter (see Figure 38), may be inserted through the

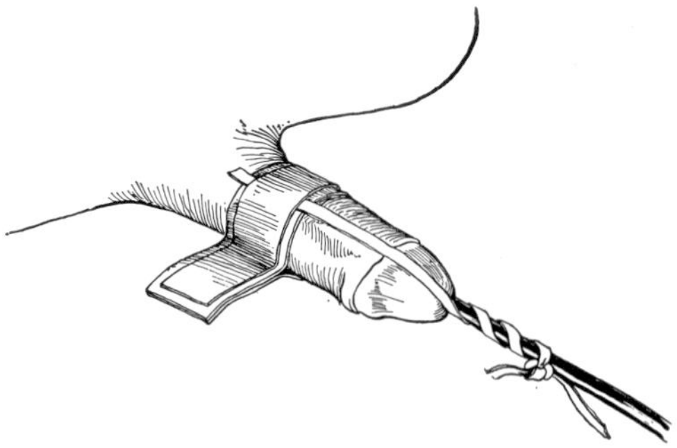

Figure 39

A method of securing a straight catheter used as an indwelling catheter in a male patient.

substance of the kidney into the kidney pelvis, from a surgical wound made laterally and posteriorly in the kidney region. A *pyelostomy tube* is placed directly into the pelvis—it is not passed through the cortex and medulla. The kidney may also be drained by a *ureterostomy tube* (a whistle-tip or many-eyed Robinson catheter) which is passed through a surgical opening into the ureter made through an incision in the upper outer quadrant of the abdomen. The catheter is passed up the ureter to the kidney pelvis. The kidney pelvis may be drained by a *ureteral catheter* which is passed by means of a cystoscope to the bladder and up the ureter to the kidney pelvis (see Figure 36). A catheter that is directly draining a kidney must *never* be clamped for even a very short period since the normal kidney pelvis has a capacity of only 5 to 8 ml. If the patient has two functioning kidneys but only one is being drained by a ureteral catheter, there will also be a collection of urine in the bladder. The output from each kidney—that obtained from the ureteral catheter and that coming directly from the bladder—should be recorded separately.

If there is obstruction below the bladder, constant drainage is necessary to preserve kidney function because the back pressure produced by inadequate emptying of the urinary system will ultimately damage the nephrons. The most common means of draining the bladder is through the *urethral catheter*. Usually a self-retaining type such as a Foley or Gilbert catheter is used. Sometimes a coudé, many-eyed Robinson, or a filiform catheter will be used as an indwelling catheter for male patients since a straight catheter can be adequately anchored to the penis (see Figure 39). The method of anchoring is as follows: (1) Cut 2 strips of adhesive tape 1½ by 4 inches; (2) cut 2 pieces of twill tape 12 inches long; (3) shave the penis and apply tincture of benzoin to the mid-shaft; (4) apply one strip of the 1½ by 4 inch adhesive tape, bringing the edges together beyond the penis; this permits easy removal and allows for expansion in case of penile erection; (5) place one end of each piece of twill tape over the adhesive tape on either side of the penis and apply the second strip of adhesive to hold the tapes in place; (6) wind the two pieces of twill tape in alternate directions around the catheter and tie them securely near its tip.

Occasionally, the male patient may have a perineal urethrostomy (a new opening into the urethra from the perineum made to bypass an obstruction below the prostatic urethra). In this case the urethral catheter may be brought through the perineum (see Figure 49). When the urethra is completely obstructed or when there is danger of infection of the male genital system because of extended intubation, *cystostomy drainage* may be necessary. A catheter (usually a Malecot or Pezzer) is placed into the bladder through a suprapubic incision. Sometimes postoperatively the bladder will be drained by both a cystostomy tube and a urethral catheter. If so, each catheter will not necessarily drain equal amounts, but both should be kept open, and the total output should be measured and should be adequate.

Since the purpose of using a catheter in any patient with disease of the urinary system is to provide better drainage of the urinary system, catheters should never be left clamped nor allowed to become completely or partially plugged. Also, in case of accidental removal, they should be promptly reinserted. It is important that catheters be adequately anchored to prevent accidental dislodgment. Self-retaining urethral catheters rarely need further anchoring.

Cystostomy, nephrostomy, and ureterostomy tubes should have two points of anchorage since the openings made for the insertion of these tubes are essentially fistulas which rapidly decrease in size upon removal of the catheter. As soon as a half hour after removal it is often impossible to reinsert a catheter of the same size. If the catheter is inserted during an operation, it usually is sutured in place. In that case, only the two-flap adhesive anchorage is necessary (see page 349). If the tube is not sutured in place, a piece of adhesive tape should be placed around the catheter, leaving a tab to pin to the dressing. When the patient has no dressing, the catheter can be gently curved (taking care not to kink it) and attached to the abdomen at two points by two-flap adhesive anchorage.

Catheters must be checked frequently. To check a catheter for patency, disconnect the drainage tubing at the catheter and allow the urine in the tubing to drain. Then reconnect the catheter to the tubing and hold the glass connector at a slight elevation so that the urine will be draining against gravity, running uphill to fill the glass connector. If, under these conditions, urine appears in the connector within a minute or two, the catheter is draining adequately.

If there is little drainage, one should make sure that the patient is not dehydrated. Drainage often will start within half an hour after the patient is given two or three glasses of water. The drainage system, starting with the drainage bottle and working back to the catheter, should be systematically checked to be sure that it is not obstructed at any point. A catheter or the drainage tubing may be blocked by a blood clot or a plug of mucus which sometimes may be dislodged by gently "milking" the tubing. If drainage remains poor, the catheter should be irrigated. The doctor often leaves an order to irrigate the catheter if necessary. If there is no order, or if irrigation is not successful, the doctor should be called. No catheter should be allowed to drain inadequately for more than an hour.

The color of urinary drainage should be checked and recorded. An accurate check of the color can be made only at the glass connector distal to the catheter, since the urine in the drainage bottle is a collection of several hours. One should be alert for any indication of hemorrhage, report it immediately, and take added precautions to prevent stoppage of the catheter drainage. If there is any hematuria, further bleeding must be watched for, and it may be necessary to change the catheter within fifteen to twenty minutes. Purulent and dirty-appearing urine suggests infection; cloudy urine, albuminuria; smoky urine, hemoglobinuria. Certain foods and drugs may also cause color and odor changes in urine. The consumption of excessive amount of beets may cause the urine to be red temporarily; Pyridium, a urinary antiseptic, also turns the urine red; asparagus may cause the urine to appear cloudy and to smell musty. Mucous shreds and small pieces of tissue may also appear in urine.

While the catheter is being checked the surrounding skin should be inspected for dryness and cleanliness. Occasionally, following a traumatic urethral intubation, there may be marked edema of the foreskin; this should be reported to the doctor immediately. It is usually treated by sitz baths or by cold applications to the penis.

Inspection of the catheter and genital area will be less upsetting to the patient if it is done in a matter-of-fact, efficient manner and without undue exposure. He should be told why the inspection is being made. If there is a man on the nursing team, it is usually preferable that he cleanse the genital area of the male patient.

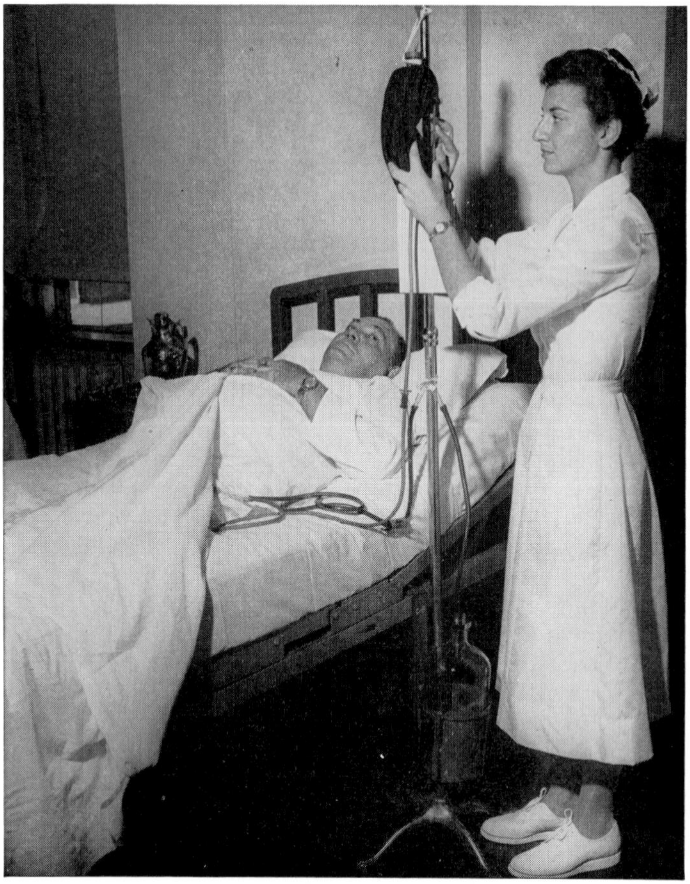

Figure 40

The nurse is checking the amount of fluid left in a Kelly flask. Note the setup for intermittent irrigation and that the catheter is attached to high decompression drainage. The Kelly flask is covered because silver nitrate solution, which turns black if exposed to light, is being used.

Principles of catheter irrigation

If adequate fluids are being given and if there is no hematuria with clots, it is unusual for a catheter to need irrigation. The safest and most effective means of irrigating the urinary system is by "internal irrigation" (fluids by mouth or parenterally).

When tubes are irrigated, one should realize that the purpose of the procedure is to maintain patency of the tube and to prevent obstruction, not to lavage the organ which the tube drains. Vigorous irrigation of the kidney and bladder will almost certainly damage these structures and spread infection, resulting in pain, hematuria, chills, fever, and even abscess formation. Gentleness is mandatory.

If a catheter is to be irrigated, one needs to consider the size of the cavity into which the fluid is being instilled. The kidney pelvis should never be irrigated with more than 8 to 10 ml. of fluid; the fluid should be instilled gently and allowed to drain back by gravity. Most pa-

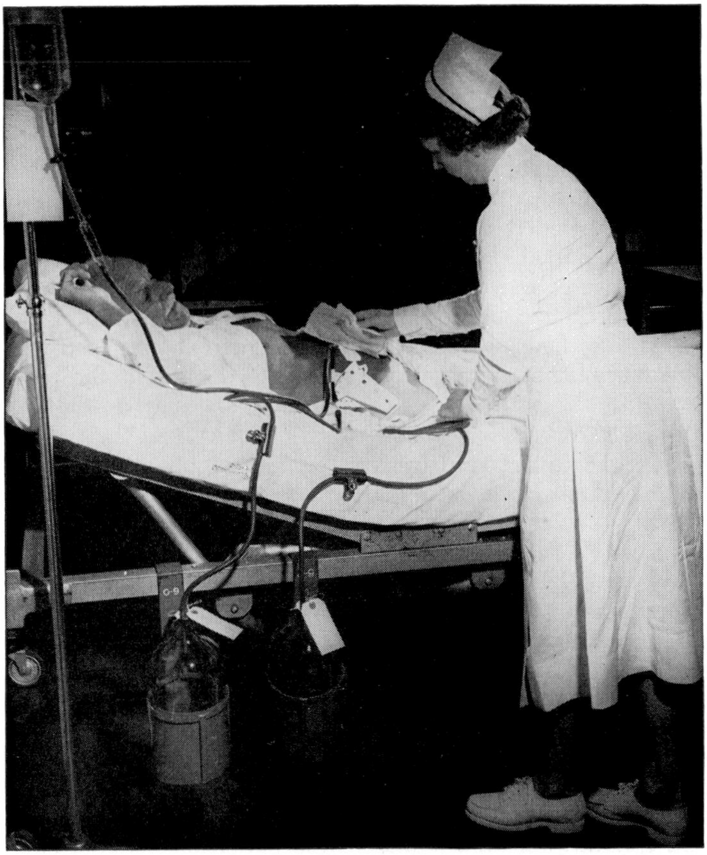

Figure 41

The nurse is checking the drainage from the suprapubic tube and the Foley catheter. Note that she checks the glass connection proximal to the catheters. This setup is for continuous irrigation of the bladder. The card for recording the amount of irrigating fluid used is readily available on the pole. The drainage bottles are labeled according to which contains urine draining from the suprapubic tube and which contains urine draining from the urethral catheter. Note that the drainage tubing has no loops between the mattress and the drainage bottles.

tients will tolerate 75 to 100 ml. of fluid in the bladder, but one should never use more fluid than a patient can tolerate without pain. Irrigations are carried out until the returns are clear. If fluid flows in readily but fails to return, there probably is a clot acting as a valve over the eye of the catheter. In this situation, do not continue to add fluid but try to dislodge the clot by "milking" the tubing. If this is unsuccessful, the doctor should be called. He may use a suction-syringe to evacuate the clots. (The Toomey syringe is the type often used.) A nurse should not use a suction syringe because the mucous membrane lining of the bladder can be damaged if too much pressure is exerted.

Sterile normal saline solution is usually used to irrigate catheters because its clearness makes observation of the return flow easy. Also, it is isotonic, and it has a hemostatic property which is useful if there is bleeding.

If the urethral catheter needs frequent irrigation, it may be practical to set up *intermittent irrigation.* This is simply an adaptation of the method of irrigation in which a syringe and a basin of solution are used. The reservoir flask holds the irrigating solution, and the tubing from the flask to the catheter allows the solution to flow through the catheter upon release of the inflow clamp provided the drainage tubing has been clamped (see Figure 40). This method obviates the danger of contamination and breakage of an irrigation set left at the bedside; it also makes using a new set for each irrigation unnecessary.

If intermittent irrigation is used, an accurate record of the amount of fluid used for irrigating must be kept since the solution returns into the drainage bottle. The amount of irrigating fluid used must be subtracted from the total drainage each time the drainage bottle is emptied so that the urinary output may be accurately recorded. This method of irrigation is not safe for kidney irrigations because the inflow cannot be regulated carefully enough to allow only 8 to 10 ml. of fluid to be instilled at a time.

If the catheter provides for both inflow of irrigating fluid and outflow of drainage, such as a three-way Foley catheter does, or if the patient has both a cystostomy tube and a urethral catheter in place the doctor may order *constant irrigation.* The equipment is identical to that used for intermittent irrigation except that a dripometer is placed below the Kelly flask (see Figure 41). The rate of the drip may be increased or decreased as necessary to keep the catheter draining well. When using this method, it is also necessary to provide accurate recording of urinary output, for the drainage will be made up of both urine and irrigating solution. Sometimes irrigation with 5 per cent glucose in water is ordered. This is because some absorption takes place when an irrigation is constant, and the doctor may not wish normal saline solution to be absorbed. Glucose is a good substitute since it also has a hemostatic effect.

Care of the patient after removal of a catheter

A great deal has been said about caring for patients with catheters in place, but the nurse also needs to be aware of the urinary output of patients from whom catheters have been removed. The man with an enlarged prostate or the patient who has recently had a catheter removed may be asked to record the *time* and *amount* of each voiding for several days. The nurse should instruct the patient in how to do this; if the patient is confined to bed, she may do the recording herself. She should note the results at least every four to eight hours.

For a few hours after a catheter is removed, the patient may have some dribbling because the sphincters have been dilated. This usually can be controlled if he is taught to do perineal exercises (see Chapter 8). Continued dribbling should be reported to the doctor since it may indicate that a vesical sphincter has been damaged. It is important to find out if the incontinence is complete (constant dribbling) or if it is only "on urgency" since such information guides planning for the patient's rehabilitation. Another pertinent observation is whether the patient is incontinent in all positions (lying, sitting, or standing). If the major problem is muscle weakness, he will probably have the least difficulty with control when in a prone position and the most while walking. A patient who is having difficulty regaining normal urinary control should limit his fluids after 6 P.M. so that sleep will not be disturbed unduly.

No patient who has an adequate fluid intake should go longer than eight hours without voiding. If the patient has a small bladder capacity, such as may be present after a bladder resection, check to see that he is voiding more frequently. It is not unusual for the patient to need the catheter replaced since it is impossible to know how much edema is present around the bladder neck until after the catheter has been removed.

The color and consistency of the urine should be noted. Some patients develop a

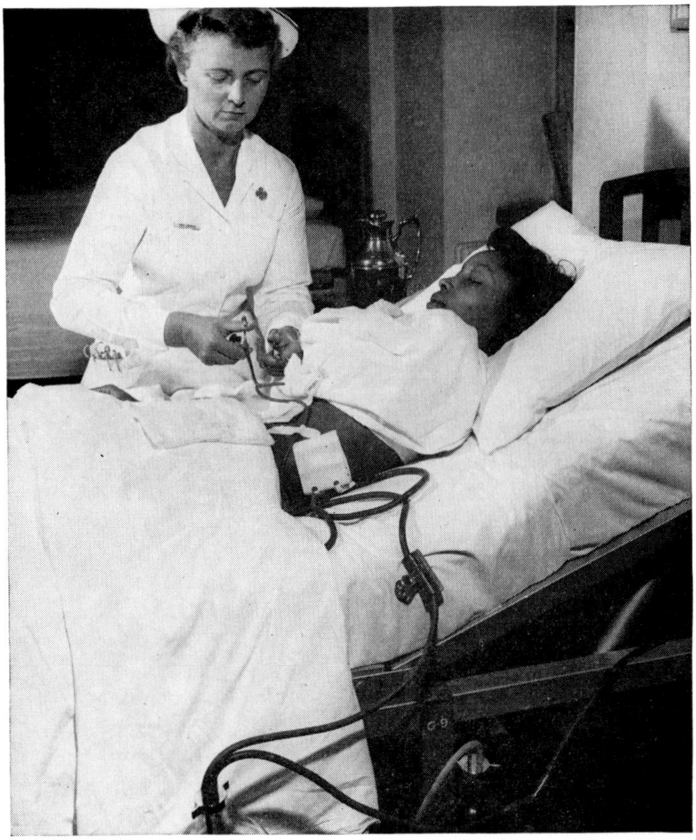

Figure 42

The nurse is incorporating a sterile catheter attached to "bubble" suction drainage into a gauze dressing. This will collect urine draining from a ureterolithotomy incision. Note that the catheter is anchored to the skin with two flaps of adhesive tape, that the drainage tubing is attached to the bedclothes with a clamp, and that the excess tubing is coiled on the mattress.

cystitis (infection of the bladder) which is caused by incomplete emptying of the bladder. The urine may appear cloudy or even purulent. It is not unusual for some hematuria to occur from eight to fourteen days after urologic surgery, especially if bleeding has been controlled during surgery by fulguration (electric dessication), which is followed by a period of sloughing in which the dead tissue breaks away from the healing wound. If hemorrhage occurs, the doctor should be informed because it is sometimes necessary to use some kind of hemostasis to prevent a serious secondary hemorrhage.

The relationship of fluid intake to urinary output

The nurse not only must keep a careful record of the patient's total fluid intake and urinary output, but also must study the record critically in relation to the expected ratio of intake to output. A well-hydrated person who is not losing fluid by other routes will normally excrete amounts of urine almost equal to his fluid intake. Any marked decrease in this ratio is indicative of kidney failure (suppression). However, one should be certain that decreased output is not caused by retention of urine in the bladder.

Unless the patient's cardiac or kidney status contraindicates forcing fluids, all patients with urologic disorders of any type should drink between 2,500 and 3,000 ml. of fluid a day. Not only does this serve to irrigate the urinary system, but it also prevents waste materials from passing through the system in concentrated form, predisposing to the formation of calculi. This advice should not only be given during the acute stage of the illness, but should also be included in the health-teaching plan.

Care of the patient requiring urologic surgery

Emotional support. The basic needs of patients requiring urologic surgery are the same as those of any other surgical patient. However, since urologic surgery may necessitate mutilation of normal anatomy, the patient may have to adjust to the problem of "being different," such as having to adjust to a new route of urine excretion. The male patient may be made sterile, impotent, or both by some operative procedures. If a radical operative procedure is contemplated, the doctor usually discusses the implications in detail with the patient and his family. Many doctors feel that the patient should make the final decision to undergo such an operation. While attempting to reach a decision, the patient often is very depressed; if he accepts surgery, he usually has a second period of depression about the time active rehabilitation begins.

During these stages there is little that the nurse can do except to give moral support by providing for privacy, allowing extra family visits if these seem to help the patient, caring for his physical needs, and answering or channeling to appropriate persons the questions raised by either the patient or his family. The patient also is often helped by talking with his spiritual adviser, with understanding members of the family, and with patients who have made good adjustments following similar surgical procedures. The nurse should be alert for changes in mood or behavior that might indicate the need for psychiatric guidance.

Hemorrhage. Hemorrhage may follow such operative procedures as transurethral prostatectomy, suprapubic prostatectomy, nephrolithotomy (complete kidney split), and nephrectomy. If drainage tubes are used, the bleeding may be visible. After surgery involving the urinary system, urine is usually dark red to pink, but it should not be bright red or viscid or contain clots. The wounds often normally drain copious amounts of light red urine. Bright red blood on dressings indicates hemorrhage. Following surgery on the kidney, the nurse should look along the posterior edge of the dressing for blood draining over the sacral area. If the patient has a suprapubic incision, blood may be noted along the side of the dressing and in the inguinal region. The classic symptoms of hemorrhage, including pallor, skin claminess, and apprehension will usually be present. The blood pressure drops and the pulse becomes rapid and thready. Since such a patient frequently has hypertension, the blood pressure may be relatively high but still represent a marked drop for the individual. If hemorrhage occurs, the doctor should be called at once. If the bleeding is external, a pressure dressing should be applied over the incision while awaiting the doctor's arrival. The patient should be placed flat in bed and equipment obtained to place him in the position used for shock. Patients bleeding from the prostate frequently are not placed in a Trendelenburg position since control of bleeding depends on keeping the bladder empty so that it does not become overdistended and cause further bleeding by exerting pressure on the prostatic fossa. Head-low position is not conducive to good drainage of the bladder by gravity. If the patient is lying in a pool of blood, slip some absorbent material under him; this will make him less apprehensive and more comforta-

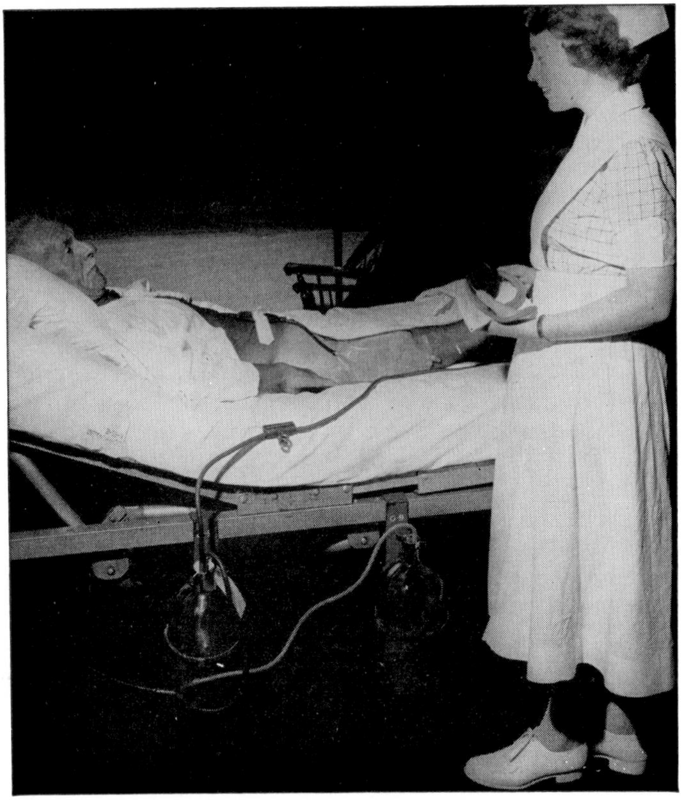

Figure 43

The nurse has just removed the suction cup from a draining suprapubic wound and has placed a drainer attached to a plastic leg bag over the fistula. The patient is now ready to get up. Note that the suction cup was connected to "bubble" suction drainage.

ble. Dressing materials and material for intravenous therapy should be at the bedside. If the patient has a catheter in place, materials for irrigation should be prepared; in addition, a suction syringe, several liter bottles of sterile physiologic saline solution and several large waste basins should be available.

Dressings. Since urine drains from many urologic incisions, the nurse working with a urologic patient is more likely to have an order to change postoperative dressings as necessary than is the case when she cares for other surgical patients. Montgomery straps are often used to hold these dressings in place. It is not necessary nor is it good practice to allow dressings to become saturated with urinary drainage. Not only is the patient made very uncomfortable, but frequently he is unable to rest and the skin becomes irritated and there is an unpleasant odor.

There are many ways to prevent the patient from lying in wet dressings. If the wound must be kept sterile, incorporate a small, sterile many-eyed Robinson catheter inside a sterile 4 by 8 inch dressing and place it with the eyes directly over the drainage site. Fasten the catheter and gauze in place with a strip of adhesive tape, and attach end of catheter to a suction apparatus. (See Figure 42.) Any suction used to drain closed cavities or pulling against a mucous membrane or the skin surface should be limited to a specific, constant negative pressure; 2 inches of negative pressure are commonly ordered. This is often accomplished by placing a bottle containing water between the source of suction and the drainage apparatus. One arm of tubing from the suction apparatus is attached to a tube emersed a specified number of inches, dependent on the amount of suction desired, under the water; the other arm is attached to the drainage bottle as is the drainage tubing from the catheter. Since the water bubbles when the apparatus works properly, this is often called *"bubble" suction.* (See Figure 42.) This method not only keeps the patient dry, but also permits the amount of drainage to be recorded. The patient may be out of bed but only within range of the suction.

Suprapubic wounds may sometimes be kept dry by the use of a piece of equipment known as a *suction cup* (see Figure 43). A suction cup can be used only after the sutures have been removed. Before applying it, protect the skin around the area with tincture of benzoin and then place the cup so that the drainage spout is uppermost over the fistula. Be careful not to cover the air outlet in the top of the cup, since the increased suction that this produces may cause the skin under the cup to be blistered. Securely fasten the cup in place by a wide strip of adhesive tape, Montgomery straps pulled snugly together, or skin cement applied to the edges of the cup. Attach the cup to "bubble" suction. If the patient is to be out of bed or if gravity drainage is needed, a drainer cup may be substituted for the suction cup. This differs from the suction cup in that it has no collecting tube around the inner edge and will cause blistering of the skin if attached to suction drainage; it must only be used with gravity drainage. (See Figure 43.)

If the urethral catheter is still in place and there is leakage from the suprapubic wound, the catheter should be checked to make sure that it is draining and is properly placed. The urethral catheter should provide for draining of urine, and the suprapubic wound should be dry.

Another method sometimes used to drain urine from an abnormal opening is the application of a large-sized ureterostomy cup over the fistula, attaching it to straight drainage (see ureterostomy care in this chapter).

Disposable *plastic ileostomy bags* may be secured over the fistula with skin paste. Since the opening in these bags can be cut to the appropriate size, the skin can be completely protected from urine. The bag may be emptied as necessary and no dressings are required. This method often works well following ureterolithotomy when the drain is still in place.

In still another method, a 12-inch square of rubber dam is used. An opening large enough to fit around the draining wound is cut in the center and the rubber dam pasted to the skin area immediately surrounding the fistula. Dressings are then placed over the drainage site, with the rubber dam folded over them in envelope style. (See Figure 44.) Montgomery straps will be needed to hold such a dressing in place. If this method is used, dressings still require frequent changing; although the patient may be dry externally, the urinary drainage lies in a pool over the incision. Unless the dressings are frequently changed, the wound will become infected from organisms growing in the stagnant urine. Patients can usually be taught to change their own dressings when necessary.

None of the methods described always work well with every patient. The nurse must study the type of wound, the placement of the incision, and the contour of the surrounding tissue to determine the most satisfactory method for the particular patient.

Frequently, in changing a urologic dressing, a catheter must also be irrigated. If the wound opens into the same cavity drained by the catheter, the same sterile field may be used for the irrigation and the dressing. Each kidney and the bladder are considered separate cavi-

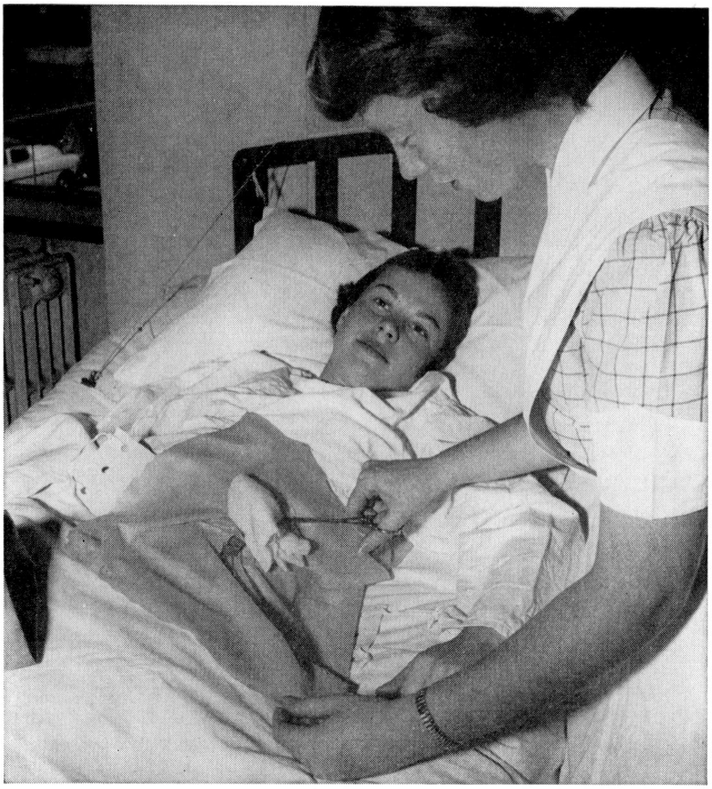

Figure 44

The student nurse is changing the dressing over a drain which is inserted into a ureterolithotomy wound. Rubber dam has been pasted to the skin around the drain so that urine will not run over the skin.

ties, and care must be taken not to cause cross-contamination. Irrigation should be done before redressing the wound since some fluid may seep out through the incision around the catheter.

HOME-CARE PLANNING FOR THE PATIENT WITH URINARY DRAINAGE

In many types of urologic conditions, patients will be discharged from the hospital with catheters still in place in the bladder or kidneys. This may be only a temporary arrangement (for a short period postoperatively or preparatory to further surgery), or it may be a permanent arrangement. The doctor usually wants the patient or a member of his family to be taught to care for the catheter. *The nurse in the hospital should plan the teaching program* so that the patient, under supervision and using his own equipment, will be able to assume complete care of the catheter before discharge. It is wise to ask a public health nurse to visit the patient at home to supervise his technique at least once more and to answer any questions. The patient who knows he will have at least one visit from the nurse is usually less apprehensive about going home. A written routine on the home care of catheters, such as the following, is helpful to the patient as well as to the nurse who does the teaching and the supervising.

HOME CARE OF CATHETERS*

(Ureterostomy [single and bilateral]; Nephrostomy [single and bilateral]; Urethral; Cystostomy)

You are being sent home with your catheters in place because your doctor believes you can continue to get well just as easily at home if you take care of them yourself. It is important that you keep your tubes clean and draining properly at all times. It will take only about a half hour to prepare your equipment and irrigate your catheters if you follow our directions. Your catheters should be irrigated ——— times daily. You may plan the time to fit your schedule. (This procedure is adaptable to single and bilateral catheters by crossing out the phrases in parentheses [below] that do not pertain.)

Equipment needed for irrigating

1 Pot 10 inches in diameter with a handle and a cover
(2 pieces of string 18 inches long)
(4 pieces of string 18 inches long)
2 (Small glass Asepto syringe and rubber bulb)
(2 small glass Asepto syringes and rubber bulbs)
3 (Small jar, such as a mayonnaise jar)
(2 small jars)
4 Small pan for waste fluid
5 Package of absorbent cotton
6 Bottle of 70 per cent alcohol
7 Irrigating solution—if doctor does not order special kind, use boiled water

Equipment needed for changing adhesive strips

(This equipment is not needed by patient with urethral catheter.)

1 Can of ether or benzene
2 Bottle of tincture of benzoin
3 Q-tips or cotton-tipped applicators
4 ½-inch adhesive tape

Equipment needed for drainage

1 Six glass or plastic Y connectors
2 Eight straight glass or plastic connectors needed if using 2 urinals or 2 night bottles
3 Three feet of latex rubber tubing; 6 feet needed if 2 night bottles used
4 Large jar with screw top—make 2 holes in cover with a punch-type can opener
5 Rubber or plastic leg bag or urinal with 2 leg straps
6 Vinegar
7 Small tube brush

*Adapted from the New York Hospital—Visiting Nurse Service of New York Agreement, 1957.

Procedure for irrigating

1 Fit (bulb) (bulbs) into (syringe) (syringes). Tie (string) (strings) around (neck of syringe) (neck of each syringe). Place in pot, winding string around handle of pot. Tie (string) (strings) around (neck of jar) (neck of each jar) and place in pot, winding string around handle.
2 Fill pot with water until all equipment is completely under water and place on stove to boil.
3 Cover and let boil for 10 minutes after water starts to bubble.
4 Remove from stove, leave covered, and do *not* pour water off. Place pot in larger pan containing cold water or iced water to cool before using. You may feel less rushed if you can plan to start cooling process ½ to 1 hour before you wish to irrigate.
5 When equipment is ready for use, seat yourself comfortably within easy reach of all equipment. It is easiest to have a small table to put it on.
6 Pull up 1 glass jar from pot by its string. If you irrigate with water, leave water in jar. If you irrigate with a special solution, pour water out of jar into waste basin or sink and pour special solution into jar and place jar on table.
7 Pull up 1 syringe from pot by its string. Holding syringe over waste basin or sink, press on bulb to drain water out of it. Place syringe in glass jar.
8 Prepare first catheter to be irrigated by removing it from connection to leg bag. Wipe end of catheter with small piece of cotton saturated with 70% alcohol. Discard cotton in waste basin.
9 Remove syringe from jar. Press on bulb with your thumb and, still holding the bulb pressed down, place tip of syringe back into irrigating solution. Release pressure on bulb and syringe will fill. Holding catheter steady with your left hand, fit tip of springe snugly into it. Be careful not to touch tip of syringe against your hand. Press fluid gently into catheter.
Note: If catheter is in your kidney, do not use more than half a syringe full of fluid at a time.
10 Before releasing your thumb from bulb, remove syringe from catheter and allow fluid to drain from catheter into waste basin.
11 Repeat Steps 9 and 10 at least three times or until returns look clear.
12 Reattach catheter to urinal and place syringes and jar to one side.

13 If you have another catheter, repeat Steps 6 to 12.

Aftercare of equipment

1 Empty waste basin into toilet.
2 Wash all equipment with soap and water, rinse, dry thoroughly, and put away.

Procedure for changing adhesive strips

This procedure is not done by patient with urethral catheter.

1 This is done only when adhesive is loosened or soiled.
2 Cut 2 pieces of 1½-inch adhesive tape 4 inches long; round 4 corners to prevent it from curling.
3 Holding catheter in place by putting your fingers close to opening in skin from which it comes out, remove top adhesive flap; then remove flap from skin.
4 Cleanse skin and catheter with ether to remove old adhesive marks.
Note: ETHER IS INFLAMMABLE! DO NOT SMOKE OR BE NEAR AN OPEN FLAME SUCH AS PILOT LIGHT ON A GAS STOVE WHILE USING IT!
5 Wash skin with soap and water. Rinse and dry thoroughly. If necessary, shave skin.
6 Paint skin area and catheter where tape is to be reapplied with tincture of benzoin, and allow to dry thoroughly.
7 Apply 1 piece of tape on skin above catheter since it will stay clean longer in this position. Place catheter against this tape and put second piece of tape over catheter. Run your finger along tape-covered catheter in order to secure it.
8 A piece of cleansing tissue held with a narrow strip of tape may be placed over area where catheter enters skin to protect your clothes from any mucous drainage.

Procedure for securing urinal to leg

Secure the urinal to your leg with leg straps. To give better support to the bag, take a piece of adhesive tape 1½ × 4 inches, make a one-inch tab and, after fastening a large safety pin through it, put the tape on your leg about one inch above the top of the bag. Paint the skin under the tape with tincture of benzoin. Open the pin and fasten through the loop of the bag. If you prefer, the bag can be suspended from a belt placed around your waist.

Emptying leg bag

1 Standing over toilet, turn screw on bottom of leg bag one-half turn.
2 Allow leg bag to drain and retighten.

Preparation for sleep

1 Remove urinal and day tubing and wash thoroughly with soap and water.
2 Soak urinal and tubing in vinegar solution, 4 tablespoons to 1 pint of water, for 15 minutes.
3 Run tube brush through connectors and into top of urinal
4 Rinse with cold water.
5 Hang up to dry and air overnight.
6 Attach your catheter to 3-foot tubing which drains into large bottle at side of your bed.
Alternate method for Step 6: You may take a clean rubber urinal and pin it by loop at top to side of mattress, attaching about 2 feet of tubing between it and your cup.
Note: When you lie down, your drainage apparatus must be at level lower than tube or you will have pain because your kidneys cannot drain properly. You may also have leakage.

Care of night equipment

Daily:

1 Wash bottle or urinal and all tubing thoroughly with soap and water.
2 Soak for 15 minutes in vinegar solution.
3 Rinse with cold water.

Twice a week:

1 Boil tubing and bottle for 10 minutes. (This will control odors and ensure cleanliness.)

Suggestions

1 Drink 3 quarts of fluid a day, since this will provide continuous irrigation. If you are perspiring excessively, you should drink more.
2 You may take a shower with your tubes in place unless you have a dressing. Simply plan to replace adhesive as soon as you are dry.
3 Change location of tapes frequently to prevent irritation of your skin. If your skin becomes sore, lie under a heat lamp for 20 minutes. Use a bridge lamp or a gooseneck lamp with a 60-watt bulb. Place it two feet above your abdomen. DO NOT USE A SUN LAMP!
4 If you leak around tube or if it stops draining:
   a Check to see that all tubing and connections are clean. Crystals should not form in it if you care for it as outlined each day.
   b Check to see that no part of tubing or bag is kinked.

c Be sure that you always have your drainage container at a level lower than opening from which tube comes.

d Be sure leg bag is closed tightly. You may need a new washer in bottom.

e Irrigate catheter.

f If you have checked all possible causes and still have trouble, return to clinic or your private doctor.

5 If tube accidentally comes out, you should make arrangements to have it reinserted as soon as possible, for opening will begin to close up. It should be changed at least every month.

6 If you are going away on a trip, you will need to remember to pack equipment for caring for your tube and night drainage equipment. If you will not have access to a stove, you will need to take along a small hot plate or several cans of Sterno.

7 In some instances it may be easier for you to boil equipment at night. If you leave equipment tightly covered, you may use it in the morning, but do not leave it more than 12 hours.

8 If you follow directions for caring for equipment, there should be no problem of odor.

9 If you have back pain, fever, or any other unusual symptoms, contact your doctor.

10 To protect your mattress in case of leakage, plastic material such as a shower curtain, pillowcase, or oilcloth used only for this purpose may be placed under your sheet. Occasionally, if you are restless, you may kink a tube by lying on it and this might cause a slight leak. Some people prefer to use plastic-lined pants which can be obtained in any large department store.

11 Where to obtain the equipment you use: ______________________

(This information must be prepared for each individual patient, depending on location, ability to pay, community resources, etc.)

Care of the patient following surgery of the urinary system

A variety of conditions affecting the urinary system may necessitate medical therapy and/or surgery. A specific kind of care is required following each treatment.

ACUTE OBSTRUCTION AND INFECTION OF THE URINARY SYSTEM

Obstruction and infection of the urinary tract are the most common causes of renal failure. Rarely is one condition seen without the other. If obstruction is the primary problem, residual urine will form, and this is a good culture medium for bacterial growth. If infection is the primary condition, it frequently causes edema and inflammation, resulting in scarring, which leads to obstruction.

Whenever obstruction occurs at any point along the urinary system, the tubal system above the obstruction becomes dilated. No matter what has caused the obstruction and/or the infection, the symptoms are the same.

Hydronephrosis

Obstruction of the upper urinary tract eventually causes hydronephrosis, or dilatation of the kidney pelvis. Common symptoms of hydronephrosis are pain, nausea, vomiting, local tenderness, spasm of the abdominal muscles, and a mass in the kidney region. The patient may, however, have no symptoms. The pain is caused by the stretching of tissues and by hyperperistalsis. Since the amount of pain is proportionate to the rate of stretching, a slowly developing hydronephrosis may cause only a dull flank pain, while a sudden blockage of the ureter, such as may occur from a stone, causes a severe stabbing (colicky) pain in the flank or abdomen. The pain may radiate to the genitalia and thigh and is caused by the increased peristaltic action of the smooth muscle of the ureter in an effort to dislodge the obstruction and force urine past it. Narcotics with an antispasmodic action, such as morphine, and antispasmodic drugs, such as a Banthine derivative, are usually used to relieve severe colicky pain.

The nausea and vomiting frequently associated with acute ureteral obstruction are caused by a reflex reaction to the pain and will usually be relieved as soon as pain is relieved. A markedly dilated kidney, however, may press on the stomach, causing continued gastrointestinal symptoms. If the kidney function has been seriously impaired, nausea and vomiting may be symptoms of impending uremia.

When the upper urinary tract becomes infected, the usual symptoms are fever, malaise, costovertebral angle tenderness, pyuria, and leukocytosis. The onset is often heralded by a chill. If the infected kidney is completely obstructed, no pus or bacteria may be found in the bladder urine.

When obstruction occurs, the treatment consists of re-establishing adequate drainage from the urinary system. This may be temporarily accomplished by placing a catheter above the point of obstruction. Sometimes surgery must be performed to insert a catheter (for example, nephrostomy). Later, definitive treatment is dependent upon the cause. The infection is treated with antibiotics, chemotherapy, fluids, and rest. Urinary antiseptics such as Urotropin and the mandelates may also be given. For these drugs to be effective, the urine must be made acid in reaction; sodium acid phosphatase by mouth and an acid-ash diet may be ordered to achieve this.

The patient is frequently acutely ill, but if he has acute colic, he may not be able to remain in bed until the pain has been relieved. It is not unusual to see a patient with acute renal colic walking the floor, "doubled-up," and vomiting. After narcotics have been given, such a patient must be protected from injury due to dizziness. As the pain eases, the patient can usually be made relatively comfortable in bed. As soon as the nausea subsides, large amounts of fluids should be urged.

Pyelonephritis

An inflammation of the kidney pelvis is known as *pyelitis*. This condition rarely exists alone; the infection most often has invaded the parenchyma of the kidney, causing an *acute pyelonephritis*. The causative organisms are commonly *Escherichia coli* or streptococci, which may be blood borne or introduced from the outside.

About 1 per cent of pregnant women develop an acute pyelonephritis,[50] probably due to the physiologic stasis of urine in the upper urinary system caused by the pregnancy. This stasis of urine provides a good medium for growth of any organisms that may be present.

If the patient with acute pyelonephritis is treated promptly with antibiotics, fluids, rest, and drainage (if necessary), the prognosis is good. If treatment is inadequate, acute pyelonephritis progresses to chronic pyelonephritis. Patients with chronic pyelonephritis have repeated exacerbations, and each attack causes further kidney damage until the patient eventually succumbs to kidney failure.

Other kidney infections

Blood-borne infections of the kidney frequently cause a *perinephritic abscess* or a carbuncle. The perinephritic abscess forms in the soft tissue of the kidney. The patient may have symptoms of obstruction dependent upon the location of the abscess, but he frequently has fever, chills, flank tenderness, malaise, and leukocytosis. Treatment consists of incision and drainage, antibiotics, fluids, and rest. Following a flank incision, nursing care will be the same as that for any patient having kidney surgery.

A *carbuncle* is an inflammation of soft tissue. It occurs in the cortex of the kidney. Treatment usually consists of the administration of antibiotics, but incision and drainage may be required.

Ureteral constriction

Hydronephrosis may be caused by ureteral constriction. The constriction may be due to trauma, but is often caused by a congenital anomaly. Often symptoms will not appear for years; the constriction, however, finally increases and causes an acute obstruction. In a child or adult with undiagnosed recurrent attacks of acute pyelonephritis, the possi-

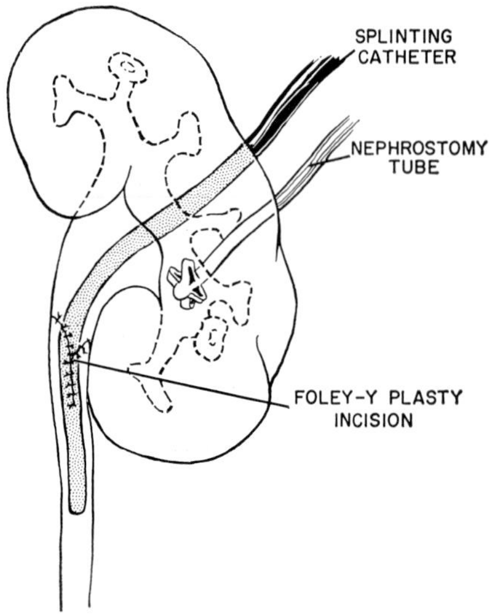

Figure 45

Schematic drawing showing placement of a splinting catheter after repair of a ureteropelvic stricture. Note the use of a nephrostomy tube for drainage of urine during healing of the anastomosis.

bility of a congenital lesion is always considered.

A plastic repair of the ureter must be done to relieve ureteral strictures. A flank or suprapubic incision is made, dependent on the location of the stricture. If a ureteropelvic stricture has been repaired, the patient will return from the operating room with a nephrostomy tube in place and a splinting catheter in the ureter (see Figure 45). He will require the routine care given any patient having kidney surgery plus the special considerations mentioned here.

The splinting catheter is usually a small, red-rubber catheter which extends into the ureter to a point below the anastomosis; it is brought out through the wound beside the nephrostomy tube. The splinting catheter should not drain; it is in place to keep the ureter open as the anastomosis heals. If it drains, it is likely that the nephrostomy tube is partially blocked or that the splinting catheter is displaced into the kidney pelvis. The splinting catheter is incorporated into the dressing, not attached to drainage, and it is not removed until two or three weeks postoperatively.

The nephrostomy tube may be left in place for several months; many patients go home with it in place and return later for its removal (for instruction for home care of catheters see page 348). Before it is removed, evidence of ureteral patency is desirable. This may be obtained by several methods. The patient may be taken to the x-ray department and radiopaque dye run by gravity into the nephrostomy tube. If the ureter is patent, the dye will pass through into the bladder, and the roentgenograms will give evidence of the size of the lumen.

A *burette test* may be ordered. In this test the nephrostomy tube is attached to a calibrated burette, placed so that the center is at kidney level, and filled with a solution of methylene blue dye to a level equal to kidney pressure. This is done by the doctor. The patient remains flat in bed during this test, which may last from four to twenty-four hours. A burette reading is taken every hour. Notation should be made of the activity of the patient at the time of the reading, since any activity that causes increased intra-abdominal pressure, such as turning, coughing, and straining, will give an elevated reading. If the ureter is patent and the patient is quiet, the reading will not fluctuate from the original reading by more than 3 to 5 cm. (1 to 2 inches). If the ureter is still obstructed, the urine will become stagnant in the kidney pelvis, causing increased pressure; the burette readings will progressively increase, and the urine will be forced out through the top of the burette. If pressure increases, the test should be immediately discontinued and the nephrostomy tube reattached to straight drainage equipment. Otherwise, infection is likely to occur. Before the nephrostomy tube is finally removed, it is usually clamped off for a day or two. If fever or back pain occurs, the catheter will be reattached to drainage apparatus.

If the stricture is at the ureterovesical juncture, the surgery is done through the bladder; the ureter is resected and then reimplanted into the bladder. The splinting catheter may then be brought out through the urethra or through the ureterostomy onto the abdominal wall. This catheter is used for drainage and as a splint. The patient may or may not have a cystostomy incision with urinary drainage through a cystostomy tube.

If the strictures are bilateral, as is often true in patients with congenital lesions, bilateral nephrostomies are performed, and later the ureters are resected and reimplanted into the bladder. In this case, if the nephrostomy tubes are correctly placed and patent, the splinting catheters should not drain urine.

Nephroptosis

Since the kidneys are not anchored in place by ligaments but are kept in normal position by blood vessels, the fatty pads surrounding them, and the pressure of the abdominal organs, they may drop slightly under certain circumstances, such as when a patient has lost a considerable amount of weight. This is known as nephroptosis, commonly called "dropped kidney" or "floating kidney" by the layman. The right kidney which normally is lower than the left, is most frequently affected. The liver, a very large organ, lies directly above the right kidney.

Nephroptosis rarely causes severe symptoms. The patient may have a "dragging ache" in the flank which is usually relieved by bed rest. Occasionally the doctor suggests that the patient sleep in the Trendelenburg position. This may be accomplished at home by placing six-inch blocks under the foot of the bed; if higher elevation is desired, the footboard can be placed on the seat of a sturdy straight chair. A kidney belt may be ordered. This should be applied before arising in the morning and fastened from the bottom up since its purpose is to help hold the kidneys in normal position. A high-calorie diet is ordered if the condition follows weight loss; additional weight helps to replace the fatty pads around the kidneys.

Conservative treatment is usually effective, but occasionally the kidney drops enough to cause the ureter to become kinked and impairs the flow of urine. If this happens, *nephropexy* is done. This is a procedure in which the kidney is sutured to the adjacent structures in order to straighten the ureter and provide adequate kidney drainage. The patient is usually kept either flat in bed or in the Trendelenburg position for two weeks to prevent tension on the sutures until healing is well underway. The nursing care is similar to that given any patient undergoing surgery of the kidney.

Renal calculi

Although the cause of renal calculi is not completely understood, stasis of urine is known to predispose to stone formation. Especially may this be true if there is associated infection which makes the urine markedly alkaline, because calcium phosphate, a common element in stones, is relatively insoluble in alkaline urine. In order for stones to form, there must be some nucleus; this may be pus, blood, devitalized tissue, crystals, tumors, or a foreign body such as a catheter.

Some elements such as cystine and uric acid are insoluble in acid urine. A diet that is deficient in vitamin A also predisposes to stones; this deficiency, however, is rather rare among people in the United States.

Patients with fractures or other bedridden patients who cannot move about freely are prone to stone formation. This probably is due to the excessive amount of calcium released from the bones in such patients and to positional stasis of urine in the lower calyces of the kidneys. Prophylactically, these patients should be mobilized early or at least turned from side to side in bed every one to two hours. If a patient is unable to walk, he should be placed in a wheel chair or, if necessary, on a stretcher twice a day for an hour or two. If his legs are immobilized, he should be encouraged to exercise his arms. The use of a trapeze does more than just help the patient move himself; it also helps to prevent formation of renal calculi.

Hyperthyroidism and gout are metabolic diseases which result in hyperexcretion of calcium and uric acid, respectively. These substances are excreted through the kidney and may form stones.

Since there is a very high incidence of recurrence of renal calculi, the immediate problem must not only be treated, but the reason for stone formation must also be discovered, if possible, and treated. Therefore, intensive diagnostic studies may be done after the removal of stones.

The patient usually seeks medical care because of symptoms of obstruction and/or infection. He may have gross hematuria due to trauma from the jagged stone, although hematuria from stones is more often microscopic. Sometimes he complains of frequency and urgency—symptoms of cystitis; the bladder infection is probably a direct extension of an infection behind the stone. Any or all of these symptoms may occur. Often a stone is "silent," causing no symptoms for years; this is true especially of large kidney stones.

Diagnostic procedures. The diagnosis of calculi is made from the history and by intravenous pyelography. Sometimes a cystoscopic examination is done and a ureteral catheter with wax applied to the tip may be passed. This procedure is done if there is any suspicion that the defect in the ureter is a tumor rather than a stone; a stone will scratch the wax.

If it is impossible to pass a catheter beyond the stone and a retrograde pyelogram is needed, a perforated bulb tip may be placed on the ureteral catheter to block the ureter, and the pressure thus created forces some of the dye beyond the stone. This procedure is known as a *Woodruff pyelogram.*

Stones are usually sent for laboratory study to determine their composition. The results serve as a guide in further search for the cause and in determining suitable prophylactic treatment.

Twenty-four hour urine specimens may be analyzed for their chemical content. Blood uric acid levels are done if gout is suspected; calcium and phosphorus blood levels and the *Sulkowitch test,* to determine the calcium content of the urine (a single urine specimen), may be ordered if hyperparathyroidism is suspected. Infections and obstructive lesions are looked for.

Medical and nursing care. Ninety per cent of renal calculi pass out through the urethra spontaneously.[50] All patients with relatively small stones therefore should have the urine strained. Urine can be strained easily by using two opened 4 by 8 inch gauze sponges over a funnel. The urine from each voiding should be strained, and one needs to watch closely for the stone, because it may be no bigger than the head of a pin, and the patient may not realize it has passed. Stones larger than 1 cm. in diameter are rarely passed.

If there is no infection and if there is not a complete obstruction, the stone may be left in the ureter for several weeks. The patient is usually allowed to continue work and the stone is closely observed by x-ray examination. A person who is up and about is more likely to pass a stone than is one in bed; therefore, after an acute attack of colic, the patient should be urged to move about actively. Fluids should be taken freely.

Patients frequently have two or three attacks of acute pain before the stone passes. This is probably because the stone gets lodged at a narrow point in the ureter, causing temporary obstruction; the ureters are normally narrower at the ureteropelvic and ureterovesical junctions and at the point where they pass over the iliac crest into the pelvis. If the stone is to pass along the ureter by peristaltic action, the patient must expect some pain. He should determine his tolerance to pain and anticipate when he needs medication to prevent colic.

If the stone fails to pass, one or two

ureteral catheters may be passed through a cystoscope up the ureter and left in place for twenty-four hours. The catheters dilate the ureter, and when they are removed they may pull the stone down into the bladder.

If the patient shows signs of infection, an attempt is made to pass a ureteral catheter past the stone into the kidney pelvis. If such an attempt is successful, the catheter is left as a drain, since pyelonephritis will quickly follow if adequate urinary drainage is not re-established.

Ureteral catheters may be most effectively attached to drainage equipment without encroaching on the catheter lumen by punching a small hole in the rubber top of a medicine dropper and threading the catheter through it. To make the hole, use a large red-hot needle or a pin; hot metal permanently perforates rubber. The medicine dropper top is then attached to the glass connector of the drainage tubing. If there is a catheter in each ureter, consult the doctor to determine which is right and which is left; label the catheters with adhesive tape. Check ureteral catheters frequently to see that they are draining. If the urine is purulent, the catheters may become obstructed. If there is no order for irrigation or if a patency cannot be re-established by irrigation, the doctor should be notified at once. Patients with uretheral catheters should be kept in bed and in a low Fowler's position to prevent dislodgment of the catheters.

If the stone has passed to the lower third of the ureter, it can somtimes be removed by *manipulation.* Special catheters with corkscrew tips, expanding baskets, and loops are passed through the cystoscope and an attempt is made to "snare" the stone. This procedure is done under anesthesia, and the patient knows that if the manipulation is unsuccessful, he may have surgery immediately. The aftercare of a patient in whom manipulation has been carried out is the same as that following cystoscopy. Any signs suggestive of peritonitis or a decreased urinary output should be carefully watched for, since the ureter may possibly be perforated during manipulation. A roentgenogram is taken immediately preceding surgery, since the stone may have moved and it is desirable to make the incision into the ureter directly over the stone. The operation for removal of a stone from the ureter is a *ureterolithotomy.* If the stone is in the lower third of the ureter, a rectus incision is made; if it is in the upper two thirds, a flank approach is used. If the patient has a ureteral stricture which causes stones to form, a plastic operation to relieve the stricture may be done as part of the operation.

Removal of a stone through or from the pelvis of the kidney is known as a *pyelolithotomy;* removal of a stone through the parenchyma is a *nephrolithotomy.* (See Figure 46.) Occasionally the kidney may have to be split from end to end (a kidney split) to remove the stone; patients in whom such a split is done may have severe hemorrhage following surgery.

Nursing the patient who has a ureteral incision. The patient who has had a ureterolithotomy through the rectus incision needs the routine postoperative care given any patient undergoing abdominal surgery. The incision, however, will drain large amounts of urine for two or three weeks postoperatively since the ureter usually is not closed with sutures for fear this will cause strictures to form. A tissue drain is placed proximal to the ureteral incision and may be left in place for a week or more. (For special nursing measures that should be used to care for the draining urinary fistula see page 345.) Occasionally a ureteral catheter will be left in place for several days.

If the ureter has been approached through a flank incision, nursing includes the general care given any patient with kidney surgery and care of the urinary fistula.

Nursing the patient with a flank (kidney) incision. Whenever there has been a flank incision, there are special nursing responsibilities. Because the incision is directly below the diaphragm, deep breathing is painful and the patient is reluctant

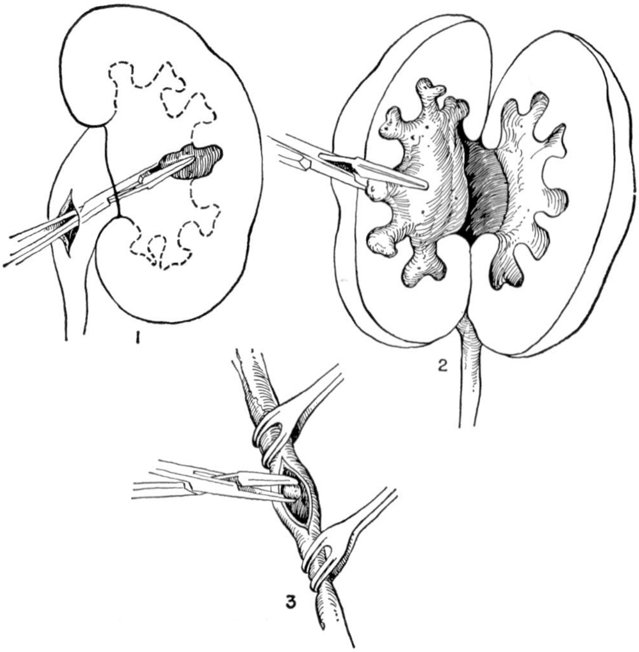

Figure 46

Diagram showing location and methods of removing renal calculi from the upper urinary tract. *1,* A pyelolithotomy; removal of stone through the kidney pelvis. *2,* A nephrolithotomy; removal of stone from the kidney parenchyma (kidney split). *3,* A ureterolithotomy; removal of stone from the ureter.

to take deep breaths or to move about. He tends to splint his chest and, therefore, is likely to develop atelectasis or hypostatic pneumonia. He needs adequate medication for pain; usually he will need a narcotic every four hours for twenty-four to forty-eight hours after surgery; after this time it may be slowly tapered off. After the patient has been given enough medication to relieve pain and mechanical support has been given to the incision, he should be encouraged to expand the rib cage fully and to cough at least every two hours. He should turn from side to side while he is in bed, and he should be encouraged to get up as soon as ordered. Most patients will be more comfortable turning themselves. After kidney surgery the patient can turn to either side unless he has a nephrostomy tube in place. Even then, he can be tilted to the affected side, with pillows placed at his back for support; it must be ascertained that the tube is not kinked and that there is no traction upon it.

Following surgery on the kidney, most patients have some abdominal distention since there is considerable pressure on the stomach and intestinal tract during surgery. Patients who have had ureteral colic prior to surgery frequently develop paralytic ileus postoperatively; this may be related to the reflex gastrointestinal symptoms caused by the pain. Because of the problem of abdominal distention following kidney surgery, the patient is often given no food or fluids by mouth for twenty-four to forty-eight hours postoperatively. He may have a gastric tube passed prophylactically. Fluids by mouth should be started slowly, and the nurse should watch for signs of distention. It is preferable to give warm fluids; iced fluids, citrus fruit juice, and milk should be omitted. By the fourth postoperative day most patients tolerate a regular diet. Fluids should be forced to 3,000 ml. (3 quarts) a day and the patient instructed regarding the desirability of continuing this throughout his life.

If distention occurs, a rectal tube and heating pad may be ordered. Prostigmin and carminative enemas may also be ordered. If Prostigmin is given, a rectal tube should be left in place for twenty minutes after its administration. As a prophylactic measure, the patient should be turned, since this tends to help push the gas along the bowel from loop to loop.

Hemorrhage may be a sequel of kidney surgery. It occurs more often when the parenchyma of the kidney has been incised since this is highly vascular (see page 344 for a discussion of hemorrhage in urologic surgery). The bleeding may occur on the day of surgery, or it may occur eight to twelve days postoperatively, during the period when tissue sloughing normally occurs in healing. Because of the possibility of hemorrhage, some doctors put the patient who has had extensive surgery of the parenchyma back to bed for three or four days after the eighth postoperative day. The nurse should closely observe the patient during this period for any signs of hemorrhage.

Following surgery on the kidney, the patient frequently will have a nephrostomy or pyelostomy tube inserted. He may have a moderate amount of urinary drainage on his dressing, but if the catheter drains adequately, this problem should be minor.

Prophylaxis and home care. Since urinary calculi are likely to recur or to develop following surgery on the kidney, patients should understand the importance of following prescribed prophylactic measures. A patient who has had any kidney pathology should force fluids for the remainder of his life. It is unwise for him to consume excess amounts of high calcium foods, although adequate nutrition should be maintained. He should avoid upper respiratory infections and any other infections; if he develops an infection, he should force fluids, take extra rest, and seek medical attention at the first sign of complications. Toxins from infections are eliminated through the kidneys. He should return to his doctor regularly for physical examinations as recommended.

Special medications and diets designed to eliminate conditions conducive to the formation of stones may be prescribed. If elements found in the stone settle out readily in acid urine, an alkaline-ash diet may be prescribed and an alkalinizing medication such as sodium bicarbonate or potassium citrate given. If the stone forms in alkaline urine, an acid-ash diet may be ordered and an acidifying drug such as sodium acid phosphatase given.

Recently, the Shorr regimen has shown beneficial results in the prevention of phosphatic calculi. A diet containing only 1,300 mg. of phosphorus daily is prescribed, and 40 ml. of aluminum hydroxide gel are taken after meals and at bedtime. The aluminum combines with the excess phosphorus, causing it to be excreted through the bowel instead of through the kidney, thus decreasing the possibility of stone formation. Patients who must have a catheter left in place for long periods of time may be placed on this regimen prophylactically.

No special diet is easy to continue indefinitely. The nurse, who is aware of the patient's diet prescription, can often help the patient fit the foods into menus or adjust the ingredients to his cultural diet pattern and his food preferences. If the patient must take a lunch or eat in restaurants, he may need guidance in selecting appropriate foods. Many patients on special diets feel that they cannot eat at friends' homes; on these occasions the patient may safely eat sparingly of those foods served that he does not usually eat. He should discuss with his doctor the amount of leeway he may take on such occasions.

Aluminum hydroxide gel tends to constipate some persons. Usually this tendency can be counteracted by eating more raw fruits and vegetables or drinking a glass of prune juice each morning. If not, a mild cathartic such as milk of magnesia may be taken at bedtime. Patients should be advised not to take mineral oil routinely since it may decrease absorption of vitamin A. Since the patient usually discontinues the regimen because of constipation, the nurse should anticipate this and tell him that bowel regularity can often be maintained by drinking plenty of fluids, eating fresh fruits and vegetables which will add bulk to the diet, and defecating at a regular time each day.

Cysts and tumors of the kidney

Masses in the kidney may represent cysts or tumors. Either may eventually result in obstruction.

A *solitary cyst of the kidney* may usually be differentiated from a tumor by x-ray examination. The solitary cyst may be aspirated with a needle, or it may be surgically decapsulated. Fluid from a cyst is usually sent for cytologic examination since some cysts are secondary to malignancies.

Polycystic disease is a familial disease characterized by multiple cysts of both kidneys. The cysts press on the parenchyma and cause the patient to die from renal failure. There is no specific treatment, and the patient usually dies between 20 and 30 years of age.

Tumors of the kidney are usually malignant. They grow insidiously, producing no symptoms for a long time, and finally the patient seeks medical care because of hematuria, dragging back pain, or weight loss. Unfortunately, the hematuria is often intermittent, lessening the patient's concern and causing procrastination in seeking medical care. Any patient with hematuria should always have a complete urologic examination, since it is only by immediate investigation of the first signs of hematuria that there is any hope of early cure.

A small tumor in the parenchyma may not be apparent in a routine pyelogram; therefore a special technique which gives pictures of sections of the kidney may be used. This is known by various names: *tomography, laminography, planigraphy, stratigraphy,* or *body section radiography.* The patient is placed on an x-ray table and a circulation time study is done to guide the timing of the serial roentgenograms. A radiopaque dye such as Urokon, with Decholin added, is then given intravenously. The patient is instructed to indicate the moment that he tastes the Decholin, and the films are then taken. Physical preparation of the patient is the same as that for an intravenous pyelogram. He should be instructed to expect the same sensations when the dye is given, and he should be observed for the same drug reactions. Since the regulation of the time interval is dependent upon the patient's cooperation, the nurse should carefully explain the procedure so that the patient will understand his role.

If a series of "metastatic" roentgenograms show no signs of metastasis and there is good function of the unaffected kidney, the diseased kidney is removed; this operation is called a *nephrectomy.*

The nursing care following nephrectomy is similar to that of any patient who has had kidney surgery. The patient usually has less distention than patients who do not have the kidney removed. There should be only a minimal amount of serosanguineous drainage on the dressing. Since the renal vessels, which are normally short, are often involved in the tumor mass, the patient should be carefully observed for signs of internal hemorrhage. If a suture should slip, death from exsanguination will occur quickly.

Following surgery for a malignant tumor, the patient is usually given a course of x-ray therapy. He will not necessarily be hospitalized during this time.

Benign prostatic hypertrophy

Benign prostatic hypertrophy (prostatism) is a common urologic disease. Sixty-five per cent of all men over 50 years of age have some symptoms of prostatic enlargement; 20 per cent of these require operation.[50] The cause is unknown. The prostrate is an encapsulated gland weighing about 25 Gm. It encircles the urethra directly below the bladder; as it hypertrophies, it impinges upon the bladder outlet.

Although the patient's main complaint is inability to void, destruction of renal function is the most serious consequence of this disease. The patient first notices that the urinary stream is smaller and more difficult to start as the urethra becomes partially obstructed by the adenomatous growth. As time goes on he may develop frequency, urgency, and burning on urination. These are symptoms of cystitis, caused by incomplete emptying of the bladder over a time. Stagnant urine is held in trabeculations or cellules; this is caused by sagging of the atonic mucous membrane between overworked hypertrophied muscle bands in the bladder. The patient complains of increasing frequency as the bladder fails to empty completely at each voiding and, therefore, more quickly refills to the amount that causes the urge to void (usually 250 to 500 ml.). Nocturia is used as a good index of frequency since it is unusual to awaken frequently to void.

The earlier the treatment is instituted, the greater the likelihood of an uncomplicated course; therefore, if any of the problems just mentioned come to the nurse's attention, she should recommend immediate urologic examination. Sometimes, even though there is little obstruction of the lower urinary system, the prostatic growth obstructs the ureters, causing symptoms of kidney failure, which prompt the patient to see a doctor.

Management of acute retention. It is not uncommon for men with prostatic disease to be admitted to the hospital with acute retention of urine (inability to void). This occurs especially after drinking alcoholic beverages and after being exposed to cold. If the patient has acute retention, a urethral catheter will be inserted. When the residual urine is more than 1,000 to 1,500 ml., the catheter may be connected to a decompression drainage apparatus, since sudden emptying of an overdistended bladder may cause loss of bladder muscle tone.

Decompression drainage is an arrangement which encourages bladder muscles to maintain their tone since the urine must flow against gravity and the bladder does not empty completely. If the mechanical pressure caused by a markedly distended bladder is suddenly released from the large abdominal vessels and bladder mucosal capillaries, the patient may faint or develop hematuria. As blood rushes to fill the vessels, the blood supply to the brain is momentarily depleted, causing dizziness and faintness. The hematuria is caused by the rupture of some of the capillaries.

The decompression may be high (5 to 8 inches above bladder level), medium (3 to 5 inches above bladder level), or low (at bladder level). A Y tube is attached to a standard at the desired level. The tubing from the catheter is connected to one arm of the Y and the tubing to the drainage bottle is connected to another arm; the third arm of the Y tube is left open as an air outlet (see Figure 40). Since changing the position of the bed, such as raising the bed to a high Fowler's position for meals, changes the bladder level of the patient, the Y tube must be adjusted accordingly.

The catheter will usually be attached to the high decompression drainage apparatus first and the level then lowered an inch at a time (usually every hour) until low decompression is reached. It may be then attached to straight drainage equipment.

Preoperative preparation (medical and nursing). Not all patients require catheter drainage prior to prostatic surgery. The results of the residual urine and kidney function tests are used to determine the need. If no catheter is used, the patient should measure and record the time and amount of each voiding for from twenty-four to forty-eight hours; such a record gives a fairly accurate picture of the severity of his difficulties.

If a catheter is inserted, it should be connected to drainage at all times since the purpose is to provide an empty bladder, which in turn provides for better emptying of the kidney pelves. Some patients will have so much kidney damage that a cystostomy tube is inserted, and they are sent home with this in place for several months before prostatic surgery can be performed.

The usual diagnostic procedures are a blood urea nitrogen or blood nonprotein nitrogen test, an intravenous pyelogram, a residual urine test, cystoscopy, and occasionally a urethrogram. (A *urethrogram* is a roentgenogram of the urethra. There is no special preparation. A radiopaque dye of jelly consistency is injected into the urethra and a roentgenogram is taken.) A fasting blood sugar determination is usually taken since diabetes mellitus is common in the age group affected by prostatic hypertrophy. An electrocardiogram and a roentgenogram of the chest are taken.

In caring for patients with prostatic disease, the nurse should apply principles of geriatric nursing. Elderly patients may need smaller doses of narcotics than younger ones, and sometimes no narcotic is given preoperatively; they often have a low tolerance to sedatives, narcotics, and anesthetics and in some instances are less sensitive to pain.

Surgical treatment. In treating benign prostatic hypertrophy the capsule of the prostrate is left intact, while the adenomatous soft tissue is removed by one of four surgical routes: transurethral, suprapubic, retropubic, or perineal.

A transurethral resection of the prostate is done when the major enlargement is in the medium lobe, directly surrounding the urethra. There must be a relatively small amount of hypertrophied tissue so that undue bleeding will not occur and so that the patient will not be under anesthesia for too long since removal by this method is time-consuming. The surgeon needs special training to use this technique.

A resectoscope (an instrument similar to a cystoscope but equipped with a cutting and cauterization loop attached to electric current) is passed through the urethra. The bladder is kept filled with fluid (5 per cent glucose in water) to decrease the possibility of accidentally perforating it and to make visualization possible. The patient is grounded against electric shocks by a lubricated lead plate placed under his hips. Tiny pieces of tissue are cut away, the bleeding points are sealed by cauterization, and the bladder is irrigated to control hemorrhage (see Figure 47). A transurethral prostatectomy is usually performed under general anesthesia, but occasionally a spinal anesthetic is used.

Following a transurethral resection of the prostate, a large Foley catheter (24 Fr.) with a 30 ml. inflation bag is inserted into the urethra. After the retention bag of the catheter has been inflated, the catheter is pulled down so that the bag rests in the prostatic fossa and provides hemostasis. The bag puts pressure on the internal sphincter of the bladder, giving the patient a continual feeling of having to void and causing bladder muscles to contract. This causes painful contraction of the bladder muscle which is called "bladder spasm."

The nurse should discuss the physiology of the "need to void" with the patient preoperatively. He will be less upset by the occurrence of spasms if he understands that this is expected. He can be told that the catheter is placed so that it gives the same sensation as a full bladder but that, since the bladder is empty and the urine is being continuously drained out by the catheter, he will have severe pain if he tries to void around the catheter; this causes the bladder muscle to contract and the bladder mucosa to be irritated by the catheter. Drinking plenty of fluids helps since it ensures constant passage of fluid over the bladder mucosa; this decreases irritation. Narcotics should be given to the patient as ordered since they lessen the pain, but do not decrease the contraction of the bladder muscle. A Banthine derivative is sometimes given, but its effectiveness in decreasing the contractions is unproved. As the nerve

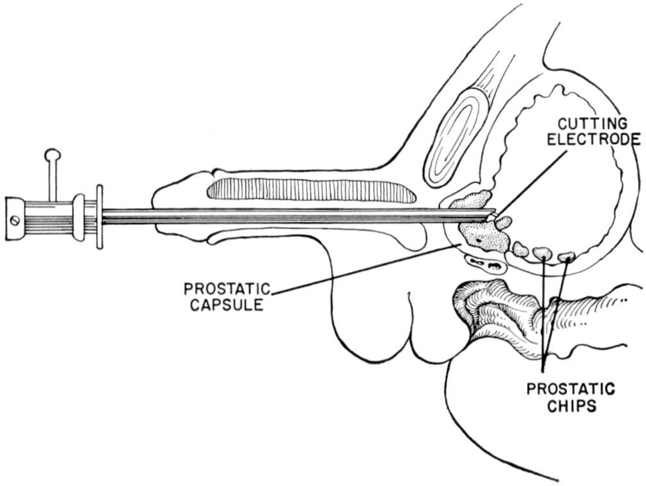

Figure 47

Diagram of a transurethral section of the prostate by means of the resectoscope. Note the cutting and cauterizing loop of the instrument, the enlarged prostate surrounding the urethra, and the tiny pieces of prostate tissue which have been cut away.

endings become fatigued, the frequency and severity of the spasms will decrease; the length of time required for this to occur varies. Most patients have less spasm by the end of twenty-four to forty-eight hours.

Sometimes the catheter is attached to medium or high decompression drainage. The purpose of decompression drainage after a prostatectomy is to provide hemostasis by maintaining the constant presence of urine at the bladder neck. The fluid level also tends to decrease the severity of bladder spasms since the muscles do not contract down on an empty bladder. Although some urine in the bladder provides hemostasis, a full bladder tends to put pressure on the outside of the prostatic fossa and "milk" the bleeding vessels. For this reason the catheter must be kept open. The patient should not strain to have a bowel movement because this may cause prostatic hemorrhage. The laxative, citrate of magnesia, usually is given three days postoperatively. Enemas are not given, nor are rectal tubes and rectal thermometers used for about a week postoperatively, since they may exert pressure on the resected prostatic capsule and might even cause perforation or hemorrhage. Hemorrhage is a fairly common and a serious complication.

Since the bladder occasionally is accidentally perforated during surgery, symptoms of abdominal or pelvic pain or inadequate urinary output should be reported to the doctor. In this case, narcotics should be withheld until the patient has been examined.

The catheter may be removed from four to seven days after a transurethral prostatectomy, depending upon the extent of the resection. If the patient has been taking a Banthine derivative, this should be discontinued at least twenty-four hours before removal of the catheter, or the bladder muscle may fail to contract effectively.

Following removal of the catheter, the patient should measure and record the time and amount of each voiding. The nurse should ascertain if he has any incontinence. Since the external sphincter of the bladder lies directly below the prostate and the internal sphincter directly above it, damage to one or both sphincters occasionally is a complication of this kind of surgery. The patient may not be able to void upon removal of the catheter because of urethral edema; if this is the case, the catheter may be reinserted for another day or two.

About two weeks after a transurethral prostatectomy the patient may have a severe hemorrhage as desiccated tissue is sloughed. He usually is at home by this time; therefore, before discharge, he should be told to contact his doctor at once if any bleeding occurs. Irrigation with 1:10,000 silver nitrate solution or reinsertion of a Foley catheter for a day or two usually controls the bleeding. Occasionally, it is necessary to cauterize the bleeding points.

The patient should not exercise vigorously or do any heavy lifting for about three weeks after discharge from the hospital. If he becomes constipated, a mild cathartic should be taken to obviate straining. Fluids should be forced for at least three weeks after discharge. After healing is complete, dilatation of the urethra may be necessary because urethral mucosa in the prostatic area is destroyed by the operation and strictures may have formed with healing.

A *suprapubic prostatectomy* is the most rapidly performed surgical procedure for removal of the prostate gland, and is, therefore, elected for patients who are poor operative risks or who have very large adenomatous prostates that extend into the bladder. A low midline incision is made directly over the bladder; the bladder is opened; and, through an incision into the urethral mucosa, the adenomatous prostatic tissue is enucleated (see Figure 48).

Following a suprapubic prostatectomy, the patient may have various types of drainage and measures for hemostasis. There will be, however, some type of hemostatic agent in the prostatic fossa (a hemostatic bag, Foley catheter, gauze packing, or oxidized cellulose packing). There will also be some provision for urinary drainage. This may be a Foley catheter and a cystostomy tube, only a Foley catheter with tissue drains into the cystostomy wound, or only a cystostomy tube. If the latter is used, the prostatic fossa is packed or a hemostatic bag is used. Hemostatic bags may be inflated to 75 or 100 ml. and may be placed on traction to ensure constant steady pressure. This is accomplished by placing a padded wire frame (known as a bird cage) between the patient's thighs and tying the catheter to it. Traction is only used for a few hours, and part of the fluid from the bag is removed after four to six hours to prevent damage to the sphincters. Since so much pressure is placed on the internal sphincters, patients usually have severe bladder spasm and require narcotics for pain.

Hemorrhage is a common complication of suprapubic prostatectomy; the precautions are the same as those taken following transurethral prostatectomy. Since there is usually some oozing of blood from the prostatic fossa, continuous or intermittent bladder irrigations may be ordered (see page 342 for procedure).

If the gauze packing or a hemostatic bag has been used, it is usually removed in the operating room with the patient under anesthesia. Following its removal, a many-eyed Robinson catheter is usually inserted into the urethra to ensure drainage.

The urinary fistula made by the suprapubic incision heals slowly. It is likely to drain large amounts of urine even while the catheters are in place, and it usually takes from two to four weeks to heal completely (see page 345 for suggested techniques to use in keeping the patient dry). Cystostomy wounds easily become infected; *Bacillus pyocyaneus* often is the causative organism. Such infection can be recognized by the light bluish-green drainage it causes. It is treated by irrigations and packing with 1/4 per cent acetic acid. Infections with other organisms are treated with antibiotic drugs. The cystostomy tube is usually removed three or four days postoperatively, but the urethral

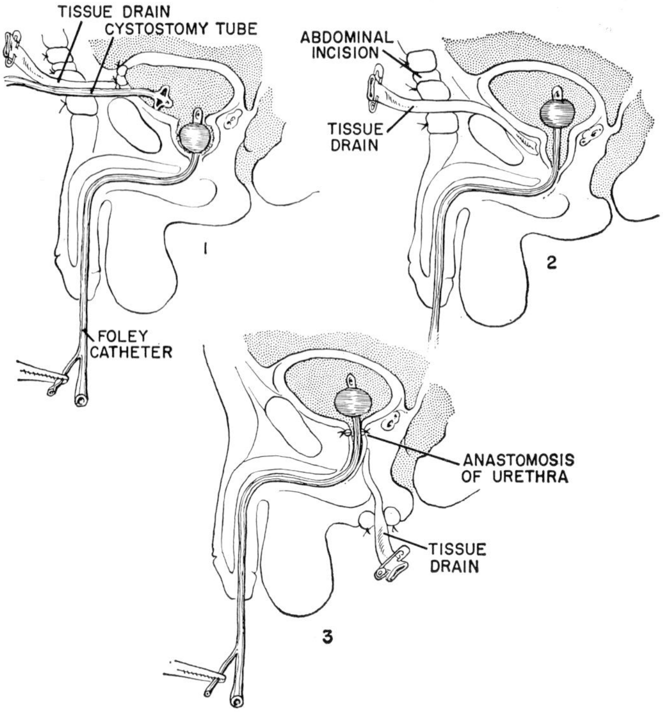

Figure 48

Diagram of three methods for surgical removal of the prostate gland. *1,* Suprapubic prostatectomy. Note placement of the tissue drain, the cystostomy tube, and an inflated Foley catheter in the prostatic fossa. *2,* Retropubic prostatectomy. Note the intact bladder, the placement of tissue drain, and the retention catheter. *3,* Radical perineal prostatectomy. Note the placement of the tissue drain in the incision between the scrotum and the rectum and the anastomosis of the urethra made necessary by the excision of the prostate and its capsule.

catheter cannot be removed until the suprapubic wound is well healed. When the urethral catheter has been removed, the nursing care of the patient is the same as that for a patient who has had a transurethral resection of the prostate. One should check to be sure that the suprapubic wound does not reopen and drain urine. If it does, the urethral catheter will have to be reinserted. If oxidized cellulose gauze has been used, the urine may have a blackish discoloration caused by disintegration of the gauze.

The instructions for home care are the same as those after a transurethral operation except that the patient is less likely to have hemorrhage.

In a *retropubic prostatectomy* a lower midline, abdominal incision is made but the bladder is not opened. It is retracted and the prostatic adenoma is removed through an incision into the anterior prostatic capsule (see Figure 48).

The sphincters are not likely to be damaged by this operation, and there is no urinary fistula. A large Foley catheter is inserted postoperatively, but there is usually less bleeding following this operation since bleeding vessels can be more easily located and cauterized when this approach is used. Since less pressure is needed for hemostasis, the patient has only mild bladder spasms, and on removal of the catheter he rarely has difficulty voiding. Straining to defecate is discouraged just as in other prostatic surgery.

There should be no urinary drainage on the abdominal dressing. Deep wound infection and plevic abscesses sometimes occur; the first symptom is usually fever. Such infection may appear after the patient has been discharged. The patient is usually hospitalized only a week. During his convalescence he should take the same precautions previously suggested for patients who have had other types of prostatectomy operations.

The adenomatous tissue of the prostate can also be enucleated through a perineal incision. This is a *perineal prostatectomy.* The incision is made between the scrotum and the rectum; the posterior capsule of the prostate is incised and the adenoma removed.

Preoperative and postoperative care following perineal prostatectomy is similar to that given a patient having a radical perineal prostatectomy. (See Chapter 22.) The patient, however, will not be impotent, and he is less likely to have urinary incontinence after a simple perineal prostatectomy. Convalescent care is the same as for patients who have had other types of prostatectomies.

Urethral strictures

Scar formation following trauma, operations, or infections of the urethra may cause interference with the urinary output, and surgery must be performed to reopen the passage through the urethra or to divert the urinary stream. This is usually done by one of three techniques; internal urethrotomy, external urethrotomy, or a plastic repair of the urethra.

An *internal urethrotomy* consists of cutting through the strictured mucosa, which is reached through the urethra by means of a urethrotome, and then leaving a large-sized retention catheter in place for approximately three weeks or until the urethral mucosa has healed (see Figure 49).

An *external urethrotomy* consists of making a permanent opening into the urethra from the perineum between the scrotum and the anus. This can be done only when the strictures are below the external sphincter of the bladder or the patient will have urinary incontinence (see Figure 49).

A *bladder mucosal graft* is a plastic procedure used to rebuild the urethra from the strictured area to the tip of the penis. A cystostomy tube is used to deflect the urine from the operative site until it is fully healed; this may be several months. Occasionally a temporary urethrotomy is performed instead of a cystostomy. A splinting catheter is left in the urethra for about three weeks or until the mucosal graft is healed (see Figure 49).

Bladder diverticula and bladder calculi

A bladder diverticulum is a large herniated sac of bladder mucosa which has sagged between the hypertrophied muscle fibers. Diverticula are usually seen in men and are often secondary to prostatic obstruction and resultant pressure within the bladder. Since the diverticulum holds stagnant urine, infection often occurs. Calculi also form in an obstructed and infected bladder even when there is no diverticulum. Diverticula are excised surgically and the bladder wall repaired. The care is the same as that for a patient having a segmental bladder resection.

Bladder stones may be removed through a suprapubic incision, or they may be crushed with a lithotrite (stone crusher) which is passed transurethrally. The procedure is known as a *litholapaxy.*

Following bladder stone removal, the bladder may be irrigated (intermittently or constantly) with an acid solution such as magnesium and sodium citrate (G solution) to counteract the alkalinity due to the infection and to help wash out the remaining particles of stone. If there has been a suprapubic incision, the care of the incision is similar to that following a suprapubic prostatectomy.

Cystitis

Cystitis is an inflammation of the bladder mucosa. It is often secondary to infection or obstruction elsewhere in the urinary tract. As a primary condition, it is

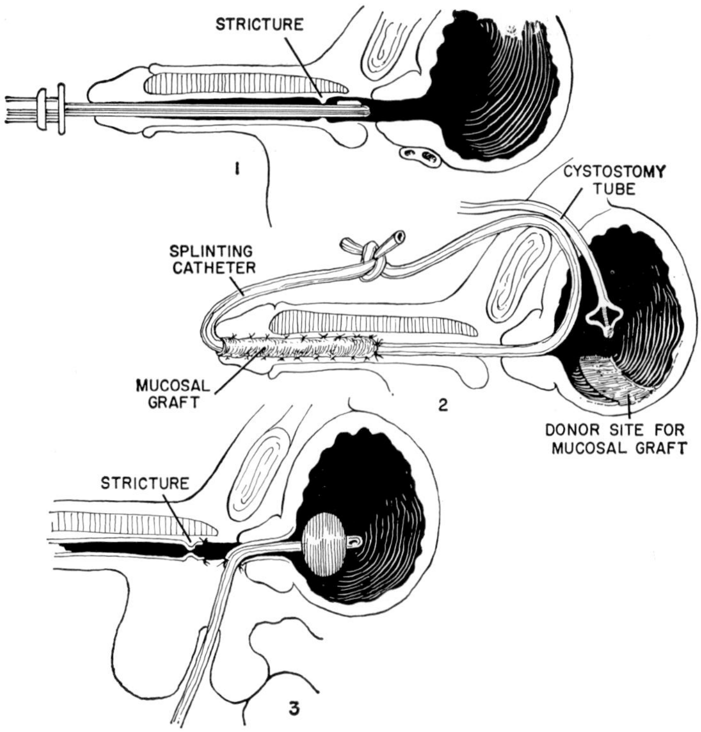

Figure 49

1, Schematic drawing showing passage of a urethrotome in treatment of stricture of the male urethra (internal urethrotomy). *2,* Schematic drawing of plastic reconstruction of the urethra with a splinting catheter in place. Drainage of urine during healing of the graft is through the cystostomy tube. Note the donor site in the bladder. *3,* Schematic drawing of a retention catheter in the bladder following a perineal (external) urethrotomy. Note the urethral stricture below the external sphincter of the bladder.

seen more frequently in women than in men and is usually associated with a nonspecific urethritis. It is sometimes caused by vaginal trauma and contamination of the urethra with organisms in the vagina and rectum. A urine culture, however, is often sterile. Frequency and urgency are the usual symptoms, but hematuria may occur.

A patient with an acute attack of cystitis is treated with antibiotics, chemotherapy, and fluids. Hot sitz baths give relief, and tincture of hyoscyamus, an antispasmodic drug, and potassium citrate, a urinary alkalinizer, may be prescribed. Cystitis frequently becomes chronic. If this happens, the urethra may be dilated to open the ducts of the periurethral glands and allow them to drain. Dilatation is followed by the instillation of 20 to 30 ml. of 1:10,000 silver nitrate solution. Improvement of general health and the eradication of vaginal infections may help the patient to overcome the chronic infection. The patient should continue to take large amounts of fluid.

Tuberculosis of the urinary system

The bladder is often called the "sounding board" for infection elsewhere in the urinary tract. Although painless, gross hematuria may be the symptom that brings the patient to the doctor. The first symptoms of tuberculosis of the kidney frequently are urgency, frequency, and dysuria.

Urinalysis may reveal a pyogenic infection. This is secondary to the tuberculosis and often is recurrent. Eventually, continuing infection leads to a more extensive examination in which a search for tubercle bacilli is made. Twenty-four hour or single urine specimens are sent to the laboratory for the determination of the presence of acid-fast bacilli. Single urine specimens should be the first-voided morning specimen since more organisms are likely to be present in a concentrated specimen; tubercle bacilli often are difficult to locate in a urine specimen. Pyelograms may reveal "ragged" calyces indicative of tuberculosis. A history of pulmonary tuberculosis or close contact with someone with tuberculosis is usually revealed in the history of the patient with tuberculosis of the urinary system.

Tuberculosis of the urinary system is secondary to pulmonary tuberculosis. The pulmonary lesion, however, may have been minimal so that it was never diagnosed. The organisms reach the kidney through the blood stream, but there may be no symptoms until several years after development of the original lesion. The disease is usually seen in patients between 20 and 40 years of age and is more common in men than in women.

Since the pulmonary lesion usually is not active at the time of the kidney involvement, the isolation techniques used for the patient with pulmonary tuberculosis may not be necessary. Patients are taught to wash their hands thoroughly with soap and water after any contact with urine or the genitalia. If there is a draining wound or lesion, soiled dressings should be wrapped in paper and disposed of immediately. Instruments should be washed thoroughly with soap and water and boiled or autoclaved immediately after use. Linen contaminated with urine or drainage should be sent to the laundry in marked bags so that necessary precautions may be taken. The patient should not have sexual intercourse while there are tubercle bacilli in the urine because it is possible to spread the disease to others by this means.

If the disease is unilateral, a nephrectomy usually is done. Preceding the operation the patient is given short courses of antitubercular drug therapy (streptomycin, para-aminosalicylic acid [PAS], and isoniazid) in various combinations; following surgery, drug therapy is continued—sometimes for as long as two years. If the disease is bilateral, an extensive course (eight months to one year) of antituberculosis drug therapy is given in conjunction with sanatorium care (see Chapter 23 for medical treatment of pulmonary tuberculosis). If home conditions warrant, the patient may be on rest therapy at home. A public health nurse may give the streptomycin, or a member of the family may be taught to administer it.

The nurse should guide patients and their families in planning for rest. Opportunity should be made for patients to talk about their worries. With the prospect of a long period of forced rest, they may face financial problems which seem insurmountable. The social worker may need to plan with the patient, his family, and other social agencies to provide assistance. Both the patient and his family may dread the anticipated hours of boredom. An occupational therapist can give helpful suggestions as to acceptable diversional activities which may help to pass the long days, weeks, and months; sometimes such activity may even be gainful occupation. If there is no occupational therapist, the nurse should plan activities with the patient; she can often call upon talented volunteer workers to assist. The activity should be light and should not require extensive arm movement. If the patient is to stay at home, he may be alone during the day, and plans may need to be worked out to provide for meals. Patients may worry about giving tuberculosis to others or fear that they can never safely have sexual intercourse again. Time should be spent explaining and answering questions about the disease, its communicability, and the probable rehabilitation course. Patients who are going into a sanitorium often are afraid that they will contract pulmonary tuberculosis. It is a relief to them to learn something about the probably daily routines in this type of hospital and to learn that they will be with patients who have inactive lesions and who will be no more contagious than they are. Mental rest and acceptance are essential if physical rest is to be effectual.

TUMORS OF THE URINARY BLADDER

All hematuria should be investigated. Although it occurs in many nonmalignant urinary diseases, painless hematuria is the first symptom in about 60 per cent of all vesical tumors.[50] It is usually intermittent; because of this, patients may fail to seek treatment. Hematuria may not be an early symptom of a tumor. Cystitis may be a symptom of a bladder tumor since the tumor may act as a foreign body in the bladder. Renal failure due to obstruction of the ureters sometimes causes the patient to seek medical care. Vesicovaginal fistulas may be the acute problem. The last two conditions are indicative of a poor prognosis because usually the tumor has infiltrated widely.

Medical treatment and nursing care

Most bladder tumors start as *benign papillomas* or as *leukoplakia.* Although these conditions may be successfully treated by early fulguration, a new tumor may appear as long as five years later.[50] Any patient who has had a papilloma removed should have a cystoscopic examination every six months since further symptoms may not appear until a new papilloma has become a far advanced tumor. This prophylaxis may seem unnecessary and unacceptable to some patients since cystoscopy may seem "an ordeal." The necessity for this procedure should be fully explained by the doctor and the explanation reinforced by the nurse. Emphasis can be placed on how fortunate the patient is to know about his disease so that early treatment, the only successful treatment of bladder tumors, can be instituted if necessary. If he had never had symptoms from the papilloma, a cancer might have been far advanced prior to diagnosis.

Carcinoma of the bladder is diagnosed by cystoscopy and biopsy. The treatment is dependent upon the size of the lesion and the depth of the tissue involvement. Small tumors with minimal tissue layer involvement may be adequately treated with *transurethral fulguration.* The patient may or may not have a Foley catheter in place after surgery. The urine may be pink-tinged, but gross bleeding is unusual. Burning on urination may be relieved by forcing fluids and applying heat to the bladder region by means of a heating pad or sitz bath. The patient is discharged within a day or two after surgery.

Sometimes *radon seeds* are implanted around the base of a tumor. This is usually done through a suprapubic incision; the tumor is also fulgurated. The radon is sealed in gold or platinum encasings which do not have to be removed. Following surgery, the patient may have a cystostomy tube in place, but more often he will have only a uretheral catheter. He usually has rather severe cystitis caused by the radiation. Treatment consists of sedatives, antispasmodic drugs, fluids, and local heat. For the first two or three days, while the radon is radioactive, the nurse should avoid excessive exposure when caring for the patient (see Chapter 16). When the cystostomy wound has healed, the urethral catheter is removed, and the patient is then discharged within a day or two.

Surgical procedures

Segmental resection of the bladder. If the tumor involves the dome of the bladder, a segmental resection of the bladder may be done. Over half of the bladder may be resected, and although the patient may have a capacity of no more than 60 ml. immediately postoperatively, the elastic tissue of the bladder will regenerate so that the patient is able to retain from 200 to 400 ml. of urine within several months.

The decreased size of the bladder, however, is of major importance in the postoperative period. The patient will return from surgery with both a cystostomy tube and a urethral catheter in place. Two catheters are used to obviate the possibility of obstruction of drainage, since it would take only a very short time for the bladder to become distended and there would be danger of disrupting the vesical suture line. One or both of the catheters may be drained by "bubble" suction (see Figure 43). Since the bladder capacity is markedly limited, the catheters usually cause severe bladder spasm. The urethral catheter is not removed until three weeks postoperatively. Sometimes, if the cystostomy wound is not completely healed, the catheter will have to be left in place longer.

As soon as the urethral catheter is removed, the patient becomes acutely aware of the small capacity of the bladder; he usually will need to void at least every twenty minutes. He needs to be reassured that the bladder capacity will gradually increase. Meantime, he should be urged to force fluids to 3,000 ml., but he should be given advice on how to space the fluids in such a way that he is not a "prisoner in the bathroom." This may be done by taking large quantities of fluids at a time, limiting fluids for several hours before he plans to go out, and taking no fluids after 6 P.M.

Cystectomy. A cystectomy, or complete removal of the bladder, is done only when the disease seems curable. Complete removal of the bladder requires permanent urinary diversion. This may be accomplished by various methods. The ureters may be transplanted into the intact bowel *(ureterointestinal anastomosis)*; a sigmoidal colostomy may be performed to divert the fecal stream, and the ureters transplanted into an *anal bladder*. A section of the ileum may be resected, maintaining the blood supply and suturing the ileum closed at one end; the other end is brought to the skin as an ileostomy, the intestine is reanastomosed, and the ureters are transplanted into the *ileo-bladder*. The ureters also may be opened directly onto the abdomen *(ureterostomies)*.

The patient whose ureters are transplanted into the bowel is usually happier socially, but hydronephrosis and kidney infection frequently occur. The kidney may empty poorly because the rectum normally has a higher pressure than the bladder due to fecal contents and peristalis. As the ureters and kidney pelves dilate, bowel flora easily start an infection. The intestinal tract also has absorptive powers, and waste products in the urine may be reabsorbed, upsetting the electrolyte balance of the body. For these reasons, it is better physiologically to transplant the ureters onto the skin of the abdomen. When this procedure is done, however, the patient has two permanently draining fistulas. These must be cared for by some type of drainage system, and the patient who is thus encumbered finds this embarrassing, aggravating, and an almost impossible adjustment to make. With constant psychologic support and encouragement, however, most patients adjust in some manner and accept the tubes as the "price they pay for their lives." Some lead relatively happy and productive lives for several years.

Immediately after the cystectomy the patient is usually acutely ill. Since not only the bladder but also large amounts of surrounding tissue are removed (the male patient also has a radical perineal prostatectomy), the patient may have a circulatory disturbance; this may be surgical shock, thrombosis, or cardiac decompensation. There is a horizontal abdominal incision extending from one side of the abdomen to the other, and there is a perineal incision. The abdominal wound is held by wire retention sutures. The patient is kept on "nothing by mouth" for several days and has a gastric tube in place. The nursing care is the same as that given any patient after major abdominal surgery plus the routine care for a perineal wound. (See Chapter 22.)

Ureterointestinal anastomosis. The ureters may be transplanted before the cystectomy or at the same operation. If the ureters are transplanted into the bowel, the patient is given a bowel preparation (cathartics, enemas, Sulfathalidine or neomycin, and a clear liquid diet) for three days preoperatively. After giving about 500 ml. of the enema, the nurse should ask the patient to retain the fluid for as long a period as possible. This gives evidence of anal sphincter control and helps the patient to begin, preoperatively, to adjust to fluid in the bowel.

Postoperatively, a large rectal tube (30 Fr.) is left in the rectum to drain the urine. It is secured in the gluteal fold with a double-flap adhesive tape anchorage. If it becomes obstructed, the doctor should change it, since there is danger of perforating the closely resected rectal tissues for the first four or five days. A sterile tube is used, and it is inserted only four inches since the anastomosis is about six inches above the anus. Because of its local anesthetic effect, ethyl aminobenzoate ointment is used to lubricate the tube. The urinary output should be carefully measured and recorded; the patients may be anuric for as long as twenty-four hours postoperatively. The rectal tube is not removed until the tenth postoperative day. It may be removed, however, for the patient to defecate and then be reinserted. A low-residue diet is usually ordered until the tube is removed. When the tube is first removed, the patient usually has diarrhea-like bowel movements; therefore, the tube is replaced for several nights to prevent loss of sleep. As the bowel adjusts to being a reservoir for urine, the stool will be soft, but the patient will be able to tell when he needs to void and when he needs to defecate. He will be able to retain about 200 ml. of urine.

The patient needs specific instructions prior to discharge. He should void (rectally) every two to four hours to minimize the reabsorption of waste products and to improve kidney emptying. He should report any nausea, vomiting, diarrhea, or lethargy to the doctor; these symptoms are suggestive of electrolyte imbalance, and alkalinizing or acidfying drugs may be prescribed. He should not be given enemas or strong cathartics such as castor oil or licorice powder because the increased peristalsis in the lower bowel may force contaminated urine up the ureters. Milk of magnesia may be given if a cathartic is necessary. If the patient is ever readmitted to a hospital, he should tell the hospital personnel that he voids through the rectum. He may eat a regular diet, but he should drink 3,000 ml. of fluid daily.

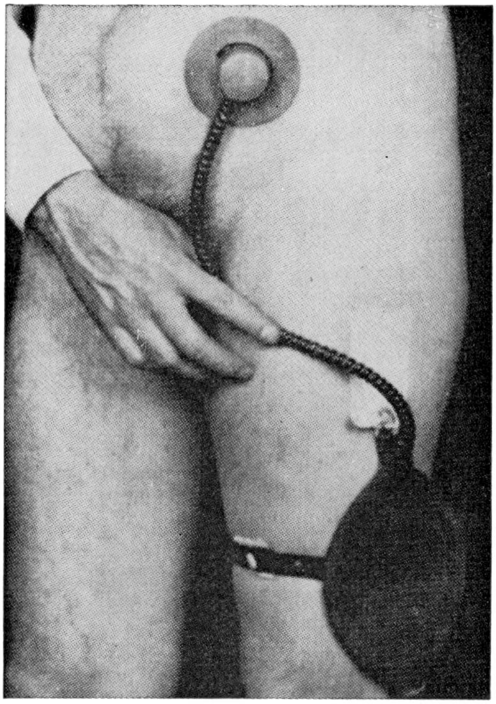

Figure 50

The ureterostomy cup. Note that the tube is protected from kinking by the plastic coil. The tab of adhesive tape gives additional support to the rubber leg urinal. (From Trafton, Howard M., and Kaufman, Manuel: Care of Cutaneous Ureterostomy; A New Apparatus, J. Urol. **58**:159, 1947.)

Ileo-bladder. If the ureters are transplanted into an ileostomy, an ileostomy bag is used to collect the drainage (see Chapter 26 for rehabilitative instructions). Symptoms of electrolyte imbalance frequently occur after this procedure.

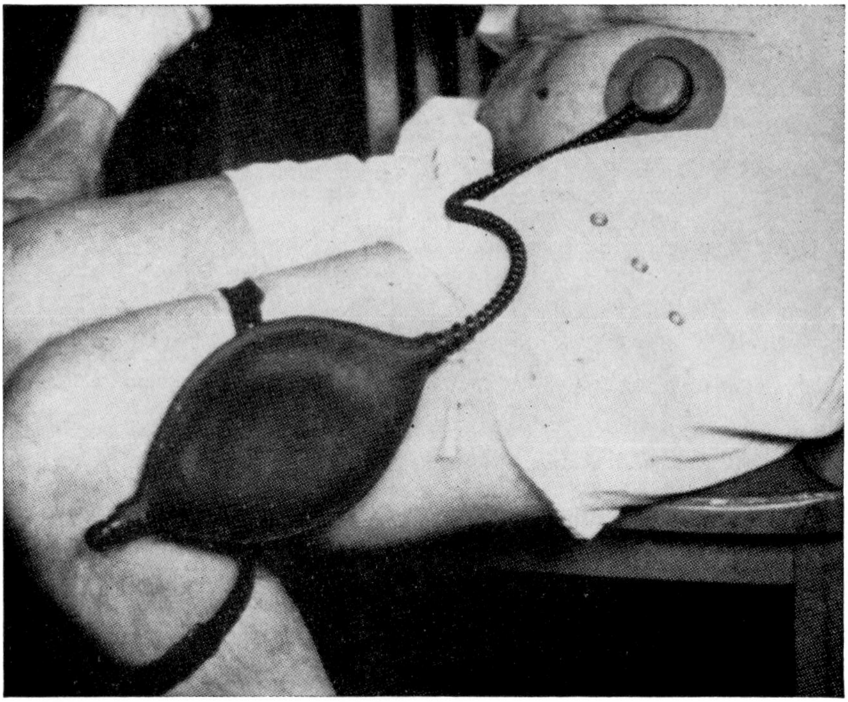

Figure 51

The position of cutaneous ureterostomy apparatus with the patient in a sitting position. Note that the leg urinal is attached by straps around both the thigh and the calf and that there is no kinking of the tubing or tension on it. (From Trafton, Howard M., and Kaufman, Manuel: Care of Cutaneous Ureterostomy; A New Apparatus, J. Urol. **58**:159, 1947).

Cutaneous ureterostomy. When the ureters have been transplanted to the abdominal wall, the patient will have soft rubber urethral catheters in place for three weeks or until the retention sutures are removed from the abdominal wound. During the first five days, the ureteral buds (mucosal linings of the ureters which are sutured to the abdominal wall to hold the ureters permanently open) are kept moistened with a sterile normal saline compress to promote healing. The saline must be applied every hour. This is easily done by placing a piece of sterile 2 by 2 inch gauze over the bud and covering it with a piece of sterile cellophane; to wet the gauze, lift a corner of the cellophane and direct the sterile saline solution onto the gauze with an Asepto syringe.

If the ureteral buds form, the patient can use ureterostomy cups instead of catheters for drainage. Singer cups are the type commonly used (see Figures 50 and 51). The cups are applied to the skin with skin paste and may require changing only every two or three days. The technique for applying the cup is not difficult, but it does take practice. With guidance, the patient can often apply it himself after the first time. When it is first applied, make sure that there is adequate drainage from the kidney; if the patient complains of any back pain, remove the cup at once and have a catheter reinserted immediately. Sometimes the obstruction to drainage is caused by an angulation of the ureter or by temporary ureteral edema. If the ureter angulates or if there are no buds, the kidney will have to be drained permanently with a catheter.

A written routine on home care of ureterostomies with cups, such as the following, is helpful to the patient.

HOME CARE OF URETEROSTOMIES WITH SINGER CUPS*

You are being sent home with cups because your doctor believes they will be more convenient for you than catheters. It is very important that you follow this plan of care to keep the bud and skin in good condition.

Equipment needed for changing cup

1 Ureterostomy cup with tubing coil
2 Skin cement
3 Rubber leg-bag or urinal with 2 straps
4 Cotton-tipped applicators
5 Tincture of benzoin
6 Can of cement solvent
7 Absorbent cotton
8 Small tube brush
9 Clean soft rags or cheesecloth
10 Paper bag for waste
11 Vinegar

Other equipment needed

1 Six glass or plastic Y connectors
2 Eight straight glass or plastic connectors, if 2 urinals or 2 night bottles used
3 Three feet of latex rubber tubing 6 feet long, if 2 night bottles used
4 Large glass jar with a screw top; make 2 holes in cover with a punch-type can opener

Routine procedure

1 Collect all equipment on a tray and go to bathroom.
2 While running bath water, sit near tub and with small cloth saturated with ether, rub along upper edge of cuff until it begins to separate from skin.
Note: ETHER IS INFLAMMABLE! DO NOT SMOKE OR BE NEAR AN OPEN FLAME SUCH AS PILOT LIGHT ON STOVE WHILE USING ETHER!
3 Grasp loosened edge of cuff and gently pull away from skin, continuing to apply ether-saturated cloth until cup is completely separated from skin.
4 Clean remaining cement from skin with ether-saturated cloth.
Note: If you have 2 sets of cups, you may prefer to do Steps 5 and 6 after you have replaced clean cups.
5 Wash cup thoroughly with soap and warm water. Soak it in vinegar solution (4 tablespoons of vinegar to 1 pint of water) for 15 minutes. Run tube brush through connectors. Rinse with cold water. Dry cups thoroughly, wipe cup off with ether if it is to be used immediately to assure dryness. *This step should be done each time cup is changed.*
6 Cement does not need to be cleaned from cup each time cup is changed but only when cement is about 1/8 inch thick. Then, most of it can be easily peeled off with your fingers. Remove remainder with cement solvent.
7 Get into bathtub with water at waist level and bathe thoroughly. Do not rush this bath which is not only for cleansing but also for soothing ureteral openings. It is preferable to take a tub bath rather than a shower because it is more soothing to the buds.
8 After stepping out of tub and drying yourself completely, you are ready to reapply cups. If your skin or bud is irritated, however, you should first lie under a heat lamp for 20 minutes. Use a bridge or a gooseneck lamp with a 60-watt bulb. Place it 2 feet above your abdomen. DO NOT USE A SUN LAMP.
9 Secure urinal to your leg with leg straps. It is only necessary to wear 1 urinal, but some people are more comfortable with 2. To give better support to bag, take a piece of adhesive tape 1½ by 4 inches and, after fastening a large safety pin through it, put it on your leg about 1 inch above the bag. Paint skin under tape with tincture of benzoin. Fasten pin through loop on bag. If you prefer, the bag can be suspended from a belt placed around your waist.
10 Place cup over ureterostomy with ureteral opening in center of opening of cup.
11 Holding cup in position, dip a cotton-tipped applicator in tincture of benzoin and trace outline of cup on skin.
12 Removing cup, place a tightly rolled ball of absorbent cotton over ureteral opening. You will need to have about 6 of these ready for use.
Note: If at any time during following steps cotton becomes wet, change quickly to a dry piece. Any urine running over skin will cause your cup to leak.
13 Holding cotton in place, once again thoroughly wash and dry skin around bud in order to remove any urine.
14 With tincture of benzoin paint area within circle that you traced on your skin.

*Adapted from procedure used at The New York Hospital.

15 Be sure cup is dry and then apply a continuous stream of cement to cup and smooth it with your finger or a small brush. Set cup aside.

16 Apply a continuous stream of cement to painted area of skin, and getting into a position so that the abdomen is as free from wrinkled skin as possible, smooth this paste with your finger or a brush.

Note: In applying cement, use long strokes rather than dabbing. Try not to go back over areas already covered, for this tends to pull the cement off.

17 Keeping in position as above, take a deep breath and hold it to make your abdomen firm. Immediately place lower cuff of cup, with outlet in position to attach to urinal, on benzoin line and press firmly. Remove cotton and bring upper part of cup into position. Hold it securely for about 2 minutes.

18 Attach outlet of cup to leg-bag.

Note: Should cup start to leak at any time, with a cotton-tipped applicator dry loosened area under cuff and try to patch it by putting cement on with an applicator. If unsuccessful, remove cup and reapply.

Emptying leg-bag

1 Standing over toilet, turn screw on bottom one-half turn.

2 Allow to drain and retighten.

Preparation for sleep

1 Remove urinal and day tubing and wash thoroughly with soap and water.

2 Soak urinal and tubing in vinegar solution for 15 minutes.

3 Run tube brush through connectors and into top of urinal.

4 Rinse with cold water.

5 Hang up to dry and air overnight.

6 Attach your drainage appliance to tubing with an air outlet. Allow it to drain into a large bottle at side of your bed. Cut 3 feet of tubing so that 1 foot goes to the bottle and 2 feet to you. Air vent is needed to prevent swelling of ureteral bud and to provide better drainage.

Alternate method for step 6: Take a clean rubber urinal and pin it by loop at top to side of your mattress. Attach about 2 feet of tubing between it and your cup.

Note: When you lie down, your drainage apparatus must be at a level lower than tube or you will have pain because your kidney cannot drain properly and you will have leakage around cup.

Care of night equipment

Daily:

1 Wash bottle or urinal and all tubing thoroughly with soap and water.

2 Soak for 15 minutes in vinegar solution.

3 Rinse with cold water.

Twice a week:

1 Boil the tubing and bottle for 10 minutes. (Controls odor and ensures cleanliness.)

Suggestions

1 It is easier to change your cup after you have not had any fluids for 3 or 4 hours since there will be less urine flowing. However you must still plan to drink between 2 and 3 quarts of fluid a day.

2 If your cup leaks:

a Review your method of changing it carefully. You may not be getting skin cleaned and dried properly.

b Check to see that all tubing and connections are clean. Crystals should not form in it if you care for it each day as outlined.

c Check to see that no part of tubing or bag is kinked.

d Be sure that you always have your drainage container at a level lower than opening of ureters.

e Be sure leg-bag is closed tightly. You may need a new washer in bottom.

f If all above have been checked and you still have trouble, return to clinic or to your personal physician.

3 If your skin becomes reddened and sore:

a Increase length of time you are spending in your daily tub bath.

b Use heat lamp 20 minutes each time cup is taken off (see Step 3 of the routine procedure).

c Do not be afraid to reapply cup for oxide in cement has healing properties as does pressure of cup.

d Some people find it helps to remove the cup applied with cement for several nights and to apply a Whitfield cup which is held in place with an inflated cuff and a belt, not by cement.

e If these methods are not satisfactory or if the skin is oozing, return to clinic or your private doctor. A catheter will probably be inserted for several days until the skin heals.

4 If bud swells or becomes irritated:

a Be sure that you are changing your cup every day and soaking in a tub of warm water 15 minutes.

b Use heat lamp.

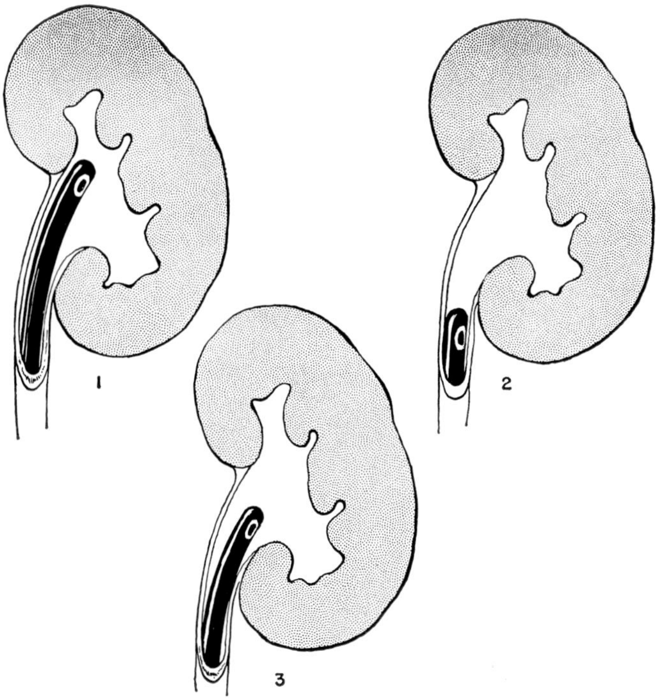

Figure 52

Schematic diagram to show correct position of ureteral catheter in kidney pelvis. *1,* It is inserted only far enough to obtain urine, *2,* pulled back to the point at which drainage of urine ceases, and then, *3,* reinserted 2.54 (1 inch). In the final position, urine should drain freely, leaving none in any portion of the kidney pelvis.

c Be sure you are using drainage with an air outlet at night.

d You might try placing a No. 20 hypodermic needle into tubing (place with hub uppermost) to provide an air outlet during day.

e If bud is so swollen that cup irritates it, plastic postoperative ileostomy appliances may be used. Cut opening in these large enough to prevent pressure on bud. Use skin cement in applying. Close bottom of bag with a rubber band. You must empty it about every 2 hours, or weight will pull bag off. Wear this for several days, or until swelling subsides.

f If there is no improvement, return to clinic or see your personal physician.

5 Sports, including swimming:

a If doctor does not limit your activity for some reason, your ureterostomies should not keep you from participating in any activity.

b If you wish to go swimming, you may wear plastic ileostomy appliances.

c If you do not wear a tight bathing suit, no one will notice these appliances.

6 Most people carry a tube of cement and several applicators in their pocket or bag at all times. They seldom need to use these, but it is reassuring to them. Wearing a girdle or a surgical belt over cups may make you feel more secure also.

7 If you are going away on a trip, you will need to remember to pack a supply of equipment to change cups and your night drainage equipment.

8 If you follow directions for caring for equipment, there should be no problem of odor.

9 If you have back pain or any other unusual symptoms, return to clinic, call your personal physician, or go to a hospital emergency room.

10 Protect your bed with a full-length piece of plastic because you may accidentally kink the tubing while you are asleep and cause a leak in the system.

If there are no ureteral buds or if the kidneys do not drain properly when using ureterostomy cups, the patient must wear ureteral catheters (see Figure 52). Patients are taught to irrigate these each day (see page 348). Most patients return to the doctor to have their catheters changed every two to four weeks; some are taught to change their own. Latex rubber, many-eyed Robinson catheters, or whistle-tip catheters usually give the best drainage and cause the least trauma to the uretheral tissues. The catheters are anchored to the skin with adhesive tape and are attached by tubing to a drainage receptacle.

If the patient is to change his own catheters, he should change one catheter each day while he is in the hospital to get the needed practice. This procedure should not be taught until he has mastered the procedure for irrigation. It is helpful to review the anatomic placement of the catheters with the patient, using diagrams. The doctor or a nurse specialist should give the first instruction. The nurse who is to do the follow-up teaching should be present. Referral to a public health nurse should be made for additional supervision.

A written routine on the changing of ureterostomy catheters, such as the following, is helpful to the patient.

CHANGING OF URETEROSTOMY CATHETERS*

For your convenience the doctor is going to have you learn how to change your own catheters. This should be done only once a week unless catheter is not draining properly.

Equipment needed to change 2 catheters

1 All equipment used for irrigation of catheters.
2 Clean marked catheters (same size as ones to be removed)
3 Two pairs of forceps with a 15-inch string tied to each handle

Procedure

1 Prepare and assemble equipment exactly as for irrigation.
2 Place all equipment in pot, winding strings around handle of pot. Catheters do not need a string attached since you can pick them out with forceps.
3 Boil and cool equipment in same manner as for irrigation.
4 Cut 4 pieces of adhesive tape 1½ by 4 inches and round corners.
5 Prepare your irrigation materials so as to be ready to irrigate. Leave forceps and catheters in pan. All equipment should be within convenient reach.
6 Loosen old tape from skin around 1 catheter. Do not remove catheter.
7 Cleanse skin with ether, wash with soap and water, and dry. Apply tincture of benzoin to skin, and allow this to dry. Apply first piece of adhesive.
Note: ETHER IS INFLAMMABLE! DO NOT SMOKE OR BE NEAR AN OPEN FLAME SUCH AS PILOT LIGHT OF STOVE WHILE USING IT!
8 Remove old catheter, putting it in basin for drainage returns. Pick up 1 pair of forceps by string. Gather string into palm of your hand. Grasping catheter with forceps about ½ inch from end that will go into ureter, pull it out of pot. Grasp irrigating end of catheter, about 2 inches from end, in your left hand.
Note: Do not lock forceps. Hold them gently closed around catheter.
9 Hold your left hand high so that catheter will not touch your skin. Position yourself in a sitting or semireclining position, whichever seems easier for you. Insert tip of catheter into opening of ureter. As you take deep breaths and blow them out, push catheter in with forceps. If you feel an obstruction, take another breath and catheter will probably slide in. If you cannot get catheter in easily, stop and notify hospital doctor or your personal physician.
Note: Be sure to gradually lower your left hand as you insert catheter so as to allow a slack section to push into ureter.
10 Insert catheter up to mark. (This will originally be determined in hospital, and you should mark this point on each new catheter with colored fingernail polish.) Most people will find that catheter drains and irrigates best when it is inserted about 7 or 8 inches, but this will be individually determined and may be different on each side.

*Adapted from procedure used at The New York Hospital.

11 Put the forceps aside. DO NOT RETURN IT TO PAN.
12 Gently curving catheter, place it against first piece of tape. Place second piece over catheter and first tape. Run your fingers along tape-covered catheter in order to secure it.
13 Irrigate as usual. If catheter is properly placed, it will irrigate easily—fluid going in by gravity and returning steadily. If you pinch it off momentarily, with about half a syringe full of irrigating fluid injected, a steady flow should return as you release it.
14 Put aside all equipment used for this catheter.
15 Repeat Steps 6 to 13 on other side. (If a catheter must be changed other than weekly, you will probably only need equipment for changing one side.)

Aftercare of catheters

1 Remove adhesive from catheter with ether.
2 Wash it with soap and warm water, and then soak it in vinegar solution (4 tablespoons of vinegar to 1 pint of water) for 15 minutes. Rinse with cold water. Use syringe to flush each of these solutions through catheter.
3 Hang catheter up to dry and air.

TRAUMA TO THE URINARY TRACT

The urinary tract may be seriously damaged by external trauma. If the pelvis has been fractured, one should observe the patient for any signs of a perforated bladder or urethra. There may be no urinary output; the urine may be bloody; or there may be symptoms of peritonitis. When the lower urinary tract is injured, provision must be made for urinary drainage at once; a cystostomy frequently is performed. Reparative surgery is undertaken when the patient's condition warrants it.

The kidney may be contused, torn, or completely ruptured by an external blow. Since spontaneous healing may occur, the patient is closely observed, and surgical intervention is usually necessary only if the kidney has been ruptured or if severe hemorrhage follows.

REFERENCES AND SELECTED READINGS*

Urologic examination

1 Brown, Amy Frances: Medical Nursing, ed. 3, Philadelphia, 1957, W. B. Saunders Co.
2 Cecil, Russell L., and Loeb, Robert F. (editors): Textbook of Medicine, ed. 10, Philadelphia, 1959, W. B. Saunders Co.
3 Fuerst, Elinor V., and Wolff, LuVerne: Fundamentals of Nursing, ed. 2, Philadelphia, 1959, J. B. Lippincott Co.
4 Guze, Lucien B., and Beeson, Paul B.: Observations on the Reliability and Safety of Bladder Catheterizations for Bacteriologic Study of Urine, New England J. Med. **255**:474-475, Sept. 6, 1956.
5 *Lenkowski, Michael F.: Catheterization of the Male Patient, Am. J. Nursing **51**:401-403, June 1951.
6 *Marshall, Victor: Textbook of Urology, New York, 1956, Hoeber-Harper.
7 Marshall, Victor F.: The Diagnosis of Genitourinary Neoplasms, New York, 1949, American Cancer Society, Inc.
8 McDonald, Harold P., and Upchurch, Wilborn, E.: Twenty-Five Years of Progress in Intravenous Urography, Am. Surgeon **21**:989-995, Oct. 1955.

The patient with specific medical disease of the urinary system

9 Brown, Amy Frances: Medical Nursing, ed. 3, Philadelphia, 1957, W. B. Saunders Co.
10 Catlow, Charles E.: The Treatment of Acute Traumatic Renal Insufficiency, J. Urol. **73**:913-920, June 1955.
11 Cecil, Russell L., and Loeb, Robert F. (editors): Textbook of Medicine, ed. 10, Philadelphia, 1959, W. B. Saunders Co.
12 Cooper, Lenna F., Barber, Edith M., Mitchell, Helen S., and Rynbergen, Hendericka, J.: Nutrition in Health and Disease, ed. 13, Philadelphia, 1958, J. B. Lippincott Co.
13 Corcoran, A. C.: Renal Failure, Am. J. Nursing **56**:768-770, June 1956.
14 *Danowski, T. S., and Mateer, F. M.: Therapy of Acute and Chronic Glomerulonephritis, J. Chron. Dis. **5**:122-137, Jan. 1957.
15 Editorial: Intermittent Lavage, Lancet **2**:551, Oct. 10, 1959.
16 *Keitzer, Walter A.: Treatment of Uremia, J. Urol. **73**:921-928, June 1955.
17 Kolff, W. J.: Experiences in the Treatment of

*References preceded by an asterisk indicate material particularly well suited for student reading.

Surgical Patients Having Anuria and Uremia, Surg. Gynec. & Obst. **101**:563-576, Nov. 1955.
18 *Maclean, M. Moira, and others: Hemodialysis and the Artificial Kidney, Am. J. Nursing **58**:1672-1675, Dec. 1958.
19 Meakins, Jonathan Campbell: The Practice of Medicine, ed. 6, St. Louis, 1956, The C. V. Mosby Co.
20 *Twiss, Mary R., and Maxwell, Morton H.: Peritoneal Dialysis, Am. J. Nursing **59**:1560-1563, Nov. 1959.

The patient with a urologic disorder

21 Adams, Ralph: Prevention of Infections in Hospitals, Am. J. Nursing **58**:344-348, March, 1959.
22 *Anthony, Catherine Parker: What Makes Fluids Flow, Am. J. Nursing **56**:1256-1258, Oct. 1956.
23 *Chute, Richard: Preoperative and Postoperative Care of Aged Patients Undergoing Urological Surgery, J.A.M.A. **148**:184-187, Jan. 19, 1952.
24 Kass, Edward H., and Sossen, Harold S.: Prevention of Infection of Urinary Tract in Presence of Indwelling Catheters, J.A.M.A. **169**:1181-1183, March 14, 1959.
25 Lowsley, Oswald Swinney, and Kirwin, Thomas Joseph: Urology for Nurses, ed. 2, Philadelphia, 1948, J. B. Lippincott Co.
26 Newton, Kathleen: Geriatric Nursing, ed. 3, St. Louis, 1960, The C. V. Mosby Co.
27 Sholtis, Lillian: Nursing the Elderly Surgical Patient, Am. J. Nursing **51**:726-728, Dec. 1951.

Care of the patient following surgery of the urinary system

28 *A Cancer Source Book For Nurses, New York, 1950, American Cancer Society, Inc.
29 *Ansell, Julian S., and Taufic, Marjorie R.: Nephrectomy and Nephrostomy, and Nursing the Patient After Nephrectomy, Am. J. Nursing **58**:1394-1398, Oct. 1958.
30 Baker, William J., and Firfer, Raymond: A Study of Drainage Tubes After Suprapubic Prostatectomy, J. Urol. **73**:849-851, May 1955.
31 *Barnes, Roger W., and Purdey, Angus H.: Prostatic Tumors, Am. J. Nursing **56**:982-987, Aug. 1956.
32 Beneventi, Francis: Retropubic Prostatectomy, J. Internat. Coll. Surg. **21**:559-572, May 1954.
33 Burkland, Carl E., and Rosenberg, Milton: Survey of Urolithiasis in United States, J. Urol. **73**:198-207, Feb. 1955.
34 Campbell, Meredith: Ureterosigmoidostomy: Its Advances During the Past Twenty-Five Years, Am. Surgeon **21**:663-673, July 1955.
35 Campbell, Meredith: Urology, vols. 1-3, Philadelphia, 1954, W. B. Saunders Co.
36 Cancer of the Bladder, Cancer Bull. **7**:22-25, March-April 1955.
37 Cordonnier, Justin J.: Urinary Diversion, A.M.A. Arch Surg. **71**:818-827, Dec. 1955.
38 *Creevy, D. Donald, and Tollefson, Dorothy M.: Ileac Diversion of the Urine and Nursing Care of the Patient with Ileac Diversion of the Urine, Am. J. Nursing **59**:530-536, April 1959.
39 Dean, Archie L.: Treatment of Tuberculosis of Genito-urinary Organs by Drugs, J. Urol. **73**:599-608, March 1955.
40 de Vries, John K.: Permanent Diversion of Urinary Stream, J. Urol. **73**:217-225, Feb. 1955.
41 Emmett, John L.: Experience With Implantation of Radon Seeds for Bladder Tumors: Comparison of Results With Other Forms of Treatment, J. Urol. **73**:502-514, March 1955.
42 *Hand, John R.: Infections of the Urinary Tract, Am. J. Nursing **57**:1008-1010, Aug. 1957.
43 *Heckel, Norris J.: Kidney Stones—Their Etiology and Treatment, Am. J. Nursing **55**:194-197, Feb. 1955.
44 *Herbst, William P.: Factors Involved in the Management of Prostatic Obstruction, J.A.M.A. **157**:579-580, Feb. 12, 1955.
45 *Jackson, Arlene Ferris: Cancer of the Bladder, Am. J. Nursing **58**:249-250, Feb. 1958.
46 *Lattimer, John K.: Renal Tuberculosis, Tuberc. Abst., June 1955.
47 Leadbetter, W. F., and Clarke, B. G.: 5 Years' Experience With Uretero-enterostomy by "Combined" Technique, J. Urol. **73**:67-82, Jan. 1955.
48 *Littlepage, Sylvia: Genito-urinary Injuries—Nursing Care, Am. J. Nursing **55**:973-974, Aug. 1955.
49 Maluf, N. S. R.: Further Studies on Absorption Through the Human Bladder, J. Urol. **73**:830-835, May 1955.
50 *Marshall, Victor: Textbook of Urology, New York, 1956, Hoeber-Harper.
51 *Millsap, J. G., and Hayes, B.: Retropubic Prostatectomy, Am. J. Nursing **50**:435-438, July 1950.
52 Nelson, O. A.: Indications for and Results in Retropubic Prostatectomy, Surg. Gynec. & Obst. **101**:80-84, July 1955.
53 *Nicolai, Charles H.: An Improved Recepta-

cle for Patients With Ileal Bladders, J. Urol. **74**:254, Aug. 1955.
54 *Nursing Division, Memorial Center: Home Care for the Patient After Urological Surgery, Am. J. Nursing **55**:741, June 1955.
55 Paull, David P., and Hodges, Clarence V.: The Rectosigmoid Colon as a Bladder Substitute, J. Urol. **74**:360-367, Sept. 1955.
56 *Peck, Mordant E., and Newland, D. E.: Substitute for Urinary Bladder, J.A.M.A. **150**:177-182, Sept. 20, 1952.
57 *Roen, Philip: Atlas of Genito-urinary Surgery, New York, 1952, Appleton-Century-Crofts, Inc.
58 Smith, Gilbert I., and Hinman, Frank: The Rectal Bladder (Colostomy With Ureterosigmoidostomy): Experimental and Clinical Aspects, J. Urol. **74**:354-359, Sept. 1955.
59 Spellman, Robert M., and Marshall, Victor, F.: Aluminum Gel Dietary Prophylaxis After Extensive Nephrolithotomy, J. Urol. **73**:660-662, April 1955.
60 Spellman, Robert, and Swanwick, Mary: The Management of Cutaneous Ureterostomies, Am. J. Nursing **55**:800-803, July 1955.
61 *Spence, Harry: Genito-urinary Injuries, Am. J. Nursing **55**:970-973, Aug. 1955.
62 Stockwell, Lloyd: Suprapubic Prostatectomy, A Restatement of Principles, J. Urol. **60**:128-132, July 1948.
63 Weinbrem, M.: A Manual of Tomography, Springfield, Ill., 1947, Charles C Thomas, Publisher.
64 *Whitmore, Willet F., and Bongart, Theodore: A Device for the Management of Cutaneous Ureterostomy, J. Urol. **74**:603-606, Nov. 1955.

The patient with disease of the reproductive system

Chapter 22

Study questions for review

1 Review the anatomy of the male and female reproductive systems.
2 Review the menstrual cycle. During which period does ovulation occur? What is the relationship of estrone and progesterone to the cycle?
3 Review the methods of draping a patient for a pelvic examination and of assisting the physician with this examiantion.
4 What physical, hormonal, and psychologic changes occur at puberty in girls? in boys?
5 List the male hormones. What physiologic changes do they stimulate? List the female hormones. What physiologic changes do they stimulate?
6 Review the following basic nursing procedures: catheterization, insertion of retention catheters, use of T-binder and methods of securing perineal dressings, measurement of drainage and care of drainage equipment, use of cold applications.
7 What are the main purposes of a douche? Review the procedure. What solutions are most often used?
8 What are the purposes of using heat lamps and sitz baths? What is the physiologic principle for these therapeutic actions? Review both procedures.

Nursing related to health education, common diagnostic tests, and procedures

The nurse's role in general health education and prevention of disease and in helping with diagnostic measures will be discussed before nursing care of the patient with disease.

HEALTH EDUCATION

People, especially women, often turn to nurses with questions and problems related to the reproductive system. The nurse must, therefore, have a sound knowledge of the normal system and its function. She should also be able to recognize deviations from normal so that she may guide the patient to medical care when this is needed.

Preparation for puberty

Sex education. The nurse is in a position not only to answer parents' questions regarding themselves, but also to advise them of the importance of sex education for their children and of how and what to teach. Often parents want to teach their children, but they do not know how to proceed. They should themselves understand the anatomy and physiology of the reproductive system. Sex education is usually simple for parents who are prepared to give frank answers as the child grows and asks questions. For young children, lengthy explanations are not necessary; the child needs only a direct answer to his specific questions.

The nurse should critically evaluate articles in daily papers and popular magazines so that she may guide parents in the use of the information they offer. Often she can be helpful in suggesting books that the parents may read in anticipation of their children's questions or that they may make available to their children. There are many pamphlets and books on sex education, but only a few can be mentioned here. Most state departments of health supply useful material.

*How to Tell Your Child About Sex** is helpful to parents in answering typical questions. *The Gift of Life*† is an excellent booklet to put into the hands of children. *A Girl Grows Up*‡ is highly recommended for teen-age girls. *Attaining Manhood*§ is good for the adolescent boy. Three books» on reproduction that are written for various age levels are as follows: *The Story of Life*, for boys and girls about 10 years old; *How Life Goes On and On*, for high school girls; and *The Age of Romance*, for college girls. *The Wonder of Life*¶, by a pediatrician and a teacher, explains sex and reproduction frankly for the preadolescent boy and girl. Especially recommended for Roman Catholics is *Parents, Children and the Facts of Life*.#

Menstruation. Many women ask questions regarding menstruation. Their understanding may have been limited by no instruction except that passed to them by friends or misinformation given to them by their parents who are unfamiliar with physiologic functions. On the other hand, the nurse may find women who know about the entire menstrual cycle yet have difficulty in accepting it as a normal periodic process. Again the nurse can be helpful to parents in preparing them to teach facts about the menstrual cycle to their children.

Instruction concerning menstruation should precede the menarche. Menstruation is a normal process and should be treated as such. The "period" or the "monthly period" are sensible and accurate terms to use. The psychologic implications of "being sick" and "having the curse" are poor. The girl should know how menstrual flow comes about, what its purpose is, and any special care that she should give herself during this time. She will probably have little discomfort if she has adequate rest, maintains good posture, eats a balanced diet, and participates in regular, moderate exercise. There may be slight discomfort in the lower back, legs, and pelvis, particularly on the day of the onset, and a slight tendency to fatigue. Some adolescent girls are concerned about circles which appear under their eyes during menstruation and which they fear are obvious; additional rest will usually control these. Girls should know that breast changes may occur either preceding the period or at various times throughout the monthly cycle; in some instances, rather marked tenderness and enlargement of the breasts occur. Mild mood swings also occur in the normal menstrual period and should be understood and accepted, but too many allowances should not be made for them.

Normally there is a loss of from 150 to 300 ml. of blood during the period, which usually lasts from three to five days.[7] The average person probably needs approximately a dozen napkins for the entire period. Tampons are acceptable for adult use, but they should be changed frequently during the height of flow. If the string should break and the tampon cannot be removed, a doctor should be consulted within a few hours. Tampons left in place too long may cause cervical irritation and infection.

There is considerable individual variation in speed of onset and duration of menstrual flow. Some irregularity is usual in the first few months and continues indefinitely in some women. It is not unusual for the pattern of the menstrual cycle to be upset by such things as changes in climate, changes in working hours which necessitate a change in the total life pattern, emotional upsets, and acute or chronic illness. Any of these may

---

*Hymes, James L.: Public Affairs Pamphlet, No. 149, New York, 1949, Public Affairs Committee, Inc.

†Prepared by the New York State Office of Public Health Education, Albany, 1951, New York State Department of Health.

‡Fedder, Ruth: ed. 2, New York, 1948, McGraw-Hill Book Co., Inc.

§Corner, George: ed 2, New York, 1952, Harper & Brothers.

»Published by the American Medical Association, Chicago, Ill.

¶Levine, Milton I., and Seligman, Jean H.: New York, 1940, Simon & Schuster, Inc.

#Sattler, Henry V.: Garden City, New York, 1956, Image Books.

temporarily upset the nerve centers in the hypothalamus, thus causing a change in the rate and timing of the secretion of the pituitary hormone which maintains the normal menstrual cycle. An early menstrual period or absence of the period is not significant if it occurs only one month, but if either condition continues, a gynecologist should be consulted. Girls should be advised to report any marked change in amount or duration of flow as well as marked irregularity. During menstruation a bath should be taken at least once daily; while a warm tub bath often allays any slight pelvic discomfort, showers are preferable during this period from the esthetic standpoint. It is well to avoid cold baths and showers, particularly if there is a tendency to discomfort. Many women, however, use tampons and go swimming during their period with no ill effects.

Regarding marriage

It is advisable for engaged couples to have complete physical examinations prior to marriage, including a serologic test for syphilis (now compulsory in all but two states). Women should have a pelvic examination; at this time a tight hymenal ring which could make intercourse difficult can be dilated or incised, provided this is psychologically and culturally acceptable to both the woman and her prospective husband.

Prior to marriage the couple should talk freely with their doctor, religious adviser, and particularly with each other concerning the physical, psychologic, and religious implications of sex. It is important that cultural differences be considered, and any questions or differences regarding intercourse and size and spacing of the prospective family should be discussed at this time. *Married Love** and *Marriage Manual*† are books often suggested for reading either shortly prior to or immediately following marriage. Roman Catholic engaged couples are encouraged to read *Beginning Your Marriage** and *The Catholic Marriage Manual.*†

Married women often ask nurses about intercourse. Tremendous variation exists in the sexual activity of married couples. With adequate knowledge, patience, and understanding, a husband and wife can usually work out a plan that is satisfactory to both. Frequency of intercourse may vary from one or more times a day to once a month or less; the frequency normally drops considerably after the first year or two of marriage.

From 25 to 50 per cent of married couples have some difficulty in intercourse because of emotional maladjustment. This often is due to worry or guilt feelings related to the sexual act or to inability to meet cultural standards for satisfactory intercourse. This condition is called frigidity in the woman and impotence in the man. The couple should be urged to discuss these problems frankly with their doctor and spiritual advisor since reassurance and additional sexual education may relieve the situation. A few persons may need psychiatric treatment.

Married couples should understand the menstrual cycle and should know the times during the cycle when fertilization is most likely to occur. For most normal women who have a regular cycle of twenty-eight days, the period of ovulation falls between the fourteenth and sixteenth day after the beginning of the previous menstrual period. If couples have a reasonable cause for using the rhythm method of family planning, physicians usually instruct them to avoid intercourse three days before and three days after ovulation. However, ovulation may not be regular, and fertilization has been known to occur on any day of the monthly cycle.

Absence of menstruation (amenorrhea) in the recently married woman who is

*Stopes, Marie C.: ed. 24, New York, 1939, G. P. Putnam's Sons.

†Stone, Hannah M., and Stone, Abraham: New York, 1952, Simon & Schuster, Inc.

*Cana Conference of Chicago, Chicago, 1957, Distributed by Delaney Publications, Oak Park, Ill.

†Kelly, George A.: New York, 1958, Random House.

having intercourse regularly is usually indicative of pregnancy. Regardless of the cause of amenorrhea, medical advice should be sought at once.

Some women may have a slight vaginal discharge following intercourse. If this is irritating, a douche with plain water or with a tablespoon of white vinegar to a quart of water may be taken from one to three hours after intercourse. For marked discharge not alleviated by this means, medical advice should be sought. Normally, douches are not needed for cleanliness, and it is inadvisable to take a douche routinely. However, some normal women have a troublesome odor, especially in warm weather and following the menstrual period, and this can be relieved by an occasional warm water or vinegar douche.

The reproductive system in later life

The *climacteric* or "change of life" is frequently misunderstood by both men and women. The nurse should assist them with facts to help allay fears and give supportive encouragement if the patient has actually reached this time of life.

The climacteric begins to take place in the female with the end of the active childbearing period. This is usually between 44 and 47 years of age. If it occurs before 42 or after 48 years of age, it may be normal, but medical consultation is recommended because disease may be the cause. The climacteric, which usually lasts from one year to eighteen months, is a period in which there is a gradual decline in ovarian function. It ends with the cessation of menstruation, or the *menopause*. During this time the menstrual periods usually are normal except that the interval between them becomes increasingly longer and the flow may decrease in amount.

Vasomotor reactions often occur due to the lack of production of ovarian hormones, and the woman may complain of hot flashes and excessive perspiration, headaches, nervousness, heart palpitation and sleeplessness. Depression and other psychologic reactions such as feelings of futility or uselessness may appear. These severe reactions are more likely to occur in women who expect the climacteric to be difficult or in those who have a history of being emotionally unstable. Unfortunately, the climacteric often comes at the very time when children are moving away from home and emancipating themselves. This in itself may make the mother feel that the better part of her life is over. Keeping busy, developing new interests, and recognizing her emotional reactions as an expected adjustment to a new hormonal environment help the woman to maintain a normal outlook. Most women's symptoms are relieved by a sedative such as phenobarbital. Thyroid extract may be given to alleviate the vasomotor reactions,[7] and occasionally hormones are prescribed to relieve marked depression until such time as adjustment can be made. Usually estrogens are given; androgen therapy is also effective, but the masculinizing side effects make it less desirable. The use of estrogen is limited, however, because there is some suspicion that it may contribute to endometrial adenocarcinoma. More important, however, is the fact that estrogen therapy prolongs the menopause. Thus vaginal bleeding may not be viewed with suspicion and malignancy may progress unchecked. Many doctors feel that if estrogen therapy is used, vaginal smears should be taken to regulate the dosage at a level insufficient to cause bleeding. In order to do this, the therapy usually must be interrupted for about ten days every three to four weeks. This is an ideal period to observe the patient for progress in adjustment to the climacteric.[8] It is not unusual for patients on estrogen therapy to develop tender breasts.[8]

Men may also have a climacteric; however, it is usually less severe and occurs at a much older age, or it may never occur. At this time, men also suffer from feelings of depression and uselessness as the sexual drive diminishes. They, too, frequently have vasomotor instability. These changes may tempt some men to be promiscuous in an effort to prove to themselves that the aging process has not affected their virility.[5]

It is an erroneous assumption that sexual activity must end with the climacteric; the frequency simply is decreased. Many women have a capacity to enjoy normal intercourse up to 65 years of age and even beyond. This may be true even when the actual cessation of menstruation has occurred at a relatively early age. Men, too, often continue a fairly active sexual life after many signs of normal aging, such as hypertrophy of the prostate, have taken place.[5]

Women may have pain with intercourse (dyspareunia) after the menopause because of shrinkage or adhesions of the vaginal canal due to tissue atrophy. This condition is occasionally treated surgically by a plastic repair of the vagina, but usually hormones are given. Treatment is determined by the physician after reviewing the wishes and living pattern of the patient.[8] A low-grade vaginal infection may also follow atrophy of the cells lining the vagina. This sometimes responds to vinegar douches, but if it continues to be troublesome, hormones may be prescribed.[8] The older woman with such an infection should be advised to bathe frequently in a tub of warm water and to soak for fifteen to twenty minutes at each bath.

With the onset of the climacteric, the predisposition to cancer of the sex organs, which are at this time undergoing involutional changes, seems to increase for both sexes. After the age of 35 years, every woman, married or single, should have a yearly pelvic examination, including a cytologic smear of cervical secretions, since this is the best way to diagnose early cancer of the female reproductive system. Women who have had children are more prone to cancer of the cervix than single women, but cancer of any part of the reproductive system is quite common in all women. Since cancer of the cervix has an unusually good prognosis if diagnosed and treated early, any delay in diagnosis by failure to have regular examinations is deplorable.

After the age of 40 years, the male prostate also becomes unusually prone to carcinoma. Every man over 40 years of age should have a yearly rectal examination, since by this simple means many carcinomas of the prostate may be diagnosed early enough for satisfactory treatment.

EXAMINATION OF THE REPRODUCTIVE TRACT

Both men and women often put off medical examinations of the reproductive system, since this type of examination arouses intense emotional reactions in both sexes. Fear, embarrassment, and cultural background play an important part in this emotional distress. In our culture, people frequently are afraid that their anxieties concerning carcinoma, venereal disease, sterility, or the climacteric will be verified. Many people are embarrassed to discuss problems concerning their sexual life, such as inability to perform in the culturally accepted pattern during intercourse. Many are embarrassed by the necessary exposure of the external genitalia during the medical examination. A person may also be fearful that some condition will be discovered that will require surgery which will result in sterility. The nurse who is sensitive to the many thoughts and fears that may trouble the patient will be better prepared to help him accept the necessary medical examination.

It often reassures patients to know that medical information will be given only to the doctor and that this information goes no farther. They should know that complete, frank answers to the doctor's questions will help considerably in determining the cause of any difficulty and in planning suitable treatment. Patients should be encouraged to discuss with the doctor any other related problems that may be of concern to them but about which the doctor may fail to ask specifically. The woman should be prepared for the questions she will be asked. If she is told that before the doctor examines her he will probably ask her all about her monthly periods and about her pregnancies and deliveries, she is given a chance to think through her answers under less pressure and thus give more accurate information.

It is necessary to explain to the patient the procedures that will be performed during the examination, what he or she will be expected to do, and what the doctor will do. For example, if there is any likelihood that a cramping discomfort will be felt (as will occur if *anything* is introduced into the cervical canal), this should be explained to the patient. A calm, thoughtful, interested, yet matter-of-fact, manner often helps put patients at ease. The nurse should, however, appraise each patient and adjust her approach accordingly; some patients, particularly girls who are very fearful, may need either a much more personalized or, perhaps, a more detached approach. It is important for a woman to know that the nurse will be present during the examination and for a man to know that, after the nurse has made the necessary preparations for his examination, he will be left alone with the doctor.

Examination and diagnostic measures used for female patients

Pelvic examination. This is a relatively simple examination; however, if the patient is extremely unstable and unable to relax sufficiently for satisfactory palpation or if any undue pain is anticipated, it may occasionally be done under anesthesia. The following equipment is needed:

- Several specula (various sizes)
- Rubber gloves (correct size for the doctor) and talcum powder
- Lubricating jelly (water soluble, vegetable base)
- Applicators
- Cotton balls

In addition the physician may request the following:

- Uterine tenaculum forceps
- Sponge forceps
- Biopsy forceps
- Cautery unit with cautery tips

Good light is important for a pelvic examination. Probably the best lighting is obtained with a head mirror. Gooseneck lights are also frequently used.

The woman should know that the examination may be somewhat uncomfortable; it should not be painful unless disease makes it so. She can help most in making the examination effective and brief by relaxing as completely as possible; breathing through the mouth often helps to relax the abdominal muscles. She should be assured that her modesty will be maintained; while on the table she will be draped, the door will be kept closed, and the nurse will be present during the entire procedure. Ambulatory patients should always be told what clothing must be removed, since panties or girdles interfere with the examination, waste time, and cause unnecessary embarrassment for both the patient and the doctor. The patient should void immediately prior to the examination since an empty bladder makes palpation easier, eliminates any possible distortion in the position of the pelvic organs caused by a full bladder, and obviates the danger of incontinence during the examination. The urine specimen should be saved.

Several positions may be used (see Figure 53); the doctor will indicate the one in which he wishes the patient placed. The nurse should check to see that the patient does not have arthritis or any other condition that may limit position or movement and will interfere with her assuming the desired position. Some positions, such as the knee-chest position, are uncomfortable and embarrassing for patients of almost any age or physical condition. As the nurse places the patient in the position desired, she should explain why the position is necessary for an adequate examination.

1. *Dorsal recumbent position (also known as lithotomy position) (Figure 53).* The lower leaf of the examining table should be dropped before the patient gets onto the table, since dropping it may be frightening to her after her feet have been placed in the stirrups.

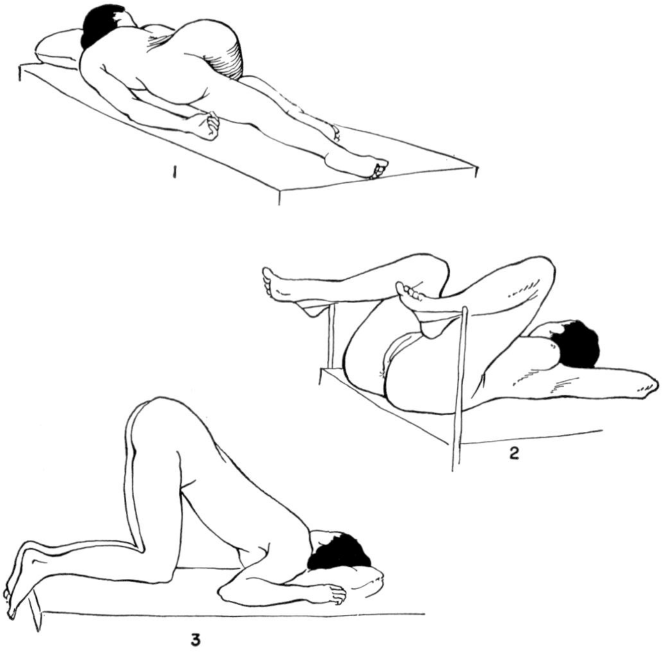

Figure 53

This diagram shows the various positions that can be assumed for examination of the rectum and the vagina. *1,* Sims' (lateral) position; note position of the left arm and right leg. *2,* Lithotomy position; note position of the buttocks on the edge of the examining table and support of feet. *3,* Knee-chest (genupectoral) position; note placement of the shoulders and head.

There should be a footstool handy, and the patient should be guided to step up on the stool, turn, sit down on the edge of the table, and then lie back. It is better to place both legs in the stirrups at the same time; this must be done gently to prevent muscle strain; this is essential if the patient is anesthetized. Metal stirrups are the most satisfactory; however, if they are being used, the patient should wear her shoes because the heels help to hold the feet in the stirrups. Care must be taken to see that there is no pressure on the legs when sling stirrups are used, since nerve damage can occur. The buttocks need to be moved down so that they are even with the end of the table. The nurse should see that the pillow under the head is pulled down at the same time to assure comfort for the patient. The patient is then draped in such a manner that only the perineum is exposed. The triangular drape is most often used since it provides a flap which can be brought down for protection if a few moments should intervene between draping and examination.

If this examination must be done in bed, the patient is placed across the bed with her feet resting on the seats of two straight chairs. This method can be used in the home if necessary.

2. *Sims' position (used also for rectal examination) (Figure 53).* For this position the patient is placed on her left side, with her left arm and hand placed behind her; the left thigh should be at an acute angle with the body, and the right knee should be flexed upon the abdomen. She should be draped so as to expose only the perineum.

3. *Knee-chest position (Figure 53).* After dropping the lower end of the examining table, have the patient get on her hands and knees on the table. The buttocks will be uppermost, and the thighs should be at right angles to the trunk; the chest and the head rest on the table, and the head is turned to one side; the arms are raised over the head, and the knees should be apart; the feet should extend over the lower edge of the table to prevent pressure on the toes. Drape so as to expose only the perineum.

If this examination must be done in bed, place the patient crosswise on the bed.

The pelvic examination consists first of inspection of the external genitalia for signs of inflammation, bleeding, discharge, swelling, erosions, or other local skin changes. The speculum examination may be omitted if the patient is a virgin, or a very small speculum may be used. Using the speculum, the doctor examines the vaginal walls and can actually see the cervix, thus making it possible to note any unusual signs, such as alteration in the normal size or color, tears, erosion, or bleeding. The nurse should see that the light is adjusted so that the vaginal canal and cervix are well illuminated. If no other light is available, the nurse may hold a flashlight to provide suitable lighting. A digital examination then follows; for this the doctor will need gloves and lubricating jelly. Placing one or two fingers in the vagina, he palpates the abdomen with his other hand. He concludes with a rectal examination, using one finger. (See Figure 54.) By digital examination he can usually detect abnormalities in the placement, contour, motility, and tissue consistency of the base of the bladder and the uterus and its adjacent structures, including the ovaries, the fallopian tubes, and the rectum.

Responsibilities of the nurse during the examination include being present during the entire procedure for the protection of both the patient and the doctor, encouraging the patient to relax, and assisting the doctor as necessary. Additional equipment that may be needed should be available in the room so that she will not have to leave the patient unattended. This equipment will depend upon the doctor and the patient, but may often include materials for taking and preserving smears for cytologic study, packing for use following biopsy, and tampons.

Following the examination, the nurse should quickly remove any lubricating jelly or discharge that may be on the genitalia and should assist the patient from the table, taking both legs out of the stirrups simultaneously. In elderly patients, unnatural positions, such as knee-chest and lithotomy, may alter the normal circulation of blood sufficiently to cause faintness. Extreme care must be taken not to leave these patients sitting on the table; with the aid of a footstool, the nurse should assist them from the table and help them to a chair where they may wish to rest for a moment before beginning to dress. If necessary, the nurse may help the patient to dress, and during this time or later she may explain any statements made by the doctor which are not clear to the patient. She tells the patient that after she is dressed the doctor will wish to talk to her again.

Equipment should be rinsed with cold water, washed well with soap and water, rinsed, and sterilized. The linen on the table should be changed. Often a rubber square covered with a treatment towel or paper napkins is placed under the buttocks to prevent gross contamination of the linen; the rubber square must be thoroughly washed with soap and water if it has become moistened. The nurse should form the habit of washing her hands thoroughly after handling of used equipment and should be especially careful to keep her contaminated hands away from her eyes and face to prevent infection with organisms such as the gonococcus.

After the patient has completed her interview with the doctor, the nurse is responsible for follow-up teaching as necessary. This may include further explanation

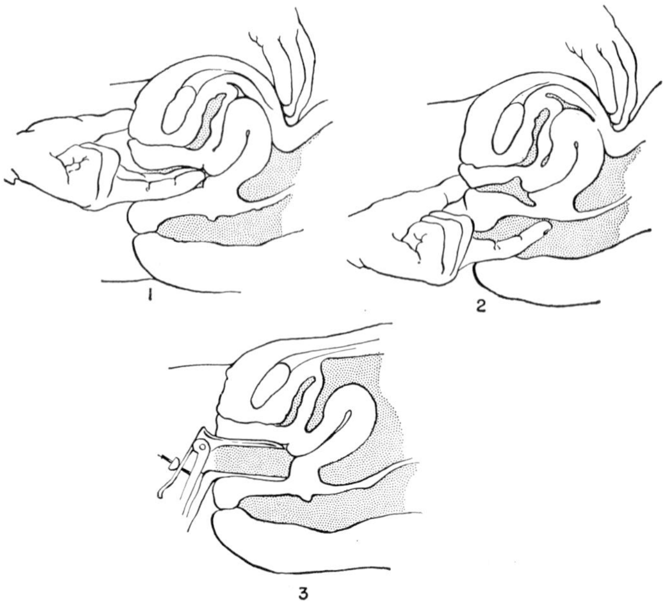

Figure 54

Schematic drawing showing method of pelvic examination. *1,* Digital examination of the vagina with abdominal palpation to determine size and position of the uterus. *2,* Digital rectal examination with abdominal palpation. *3,* Examination of the vagina and cervix using a bivalve vaginal speculum.

of information or orders given by the doctor such as the technique of douching, general health education, time and importance of her next appointment, and any referrals to a special department or doctor.

Cervical biopsy and cautery. Sometimes the doctor wishes to send a piece of cervical tissue to the laboratory for pathologic examination. The biopsy procedure will usually be scheduled for a week after the end of the menstrual period, since the cervix is more vascular immediately before and after menstruation. The patient should know what is to be done and why. She should know that there may be momentary discomfort, but that no actual pain will be felt because the cervix does not contain pain fibers. If a cautery is to be used, she should be told that a small lubricated sheet of lead will be placed against the skin under the lumbar area as a safety device for grounding electrical charges and that there will be slight bleeding which will be controlled by a tampon or packing that will be inserted by the doctor.

In addition to the equipment needed for a pelvic examination, the nurse should have the following available:

- Biopsy forceps
- Uterine tenaculum forceps
- Specimen bottle containing 10 per cent formalin or, if specimen can be delivered to pathology laboratory immediately following procedure, wet saline sponge and waxed paper may be used (specimens should be labeled with patient's name, date, source of specimen, and doctor's name)
- Cautery unit and cautery tips
- Gauze packing or tampon

Following the procedure, the nurse should be certain that the patient understands the doctor's instructions; sometimes the main points are written out for her. Instructions will vary but the usual management includes the following:

1. Rest more than usual for the next twenty-four hours. Avoid lifting and marked exertion.

2. Leave the tampon or packing in place as long as the doctor advises (usually eight to twenty-four hours).

3. Report to the hospital or doctor's office if bleeding is excessive. (Usually more than occurs during a normal menses is considered excessive.)

4. Do not use an internal douche or have sexual relations until the next visit to the doctor unless he has given you specific instructions as to when intercourse can be safely resumed.

5. If cauterization has been done, an unpleasant and somewhat profuse discharge may appear four to five days following the treatment; a warm bath several times each day will help make this less unpleasant.

The doctor may suggest a douche if there is a vaginal discharge. Usually vinegar (2 tablespoons of white vinegar to 2 quarts of water) is ordered. The nurse should make sure that the patient knows how to take a douche: the temperature should be 40° C. (105° F.) unless otherwise ordered; most doctors prefer that the patients take the douche while lying in the bathtub rather than while sitting on the toilet seat; a bath should be taken first to avoid introduction of contamination; the douche tip should be inserted upward and backward and moved about to prevent fluid being forced into the mouth of the cervix and to ensure flushing of the posterior fornix. If a medicated or hot douche is to be taken, the labia should be held together for a few moments to allow the vagina to fill up and thus benefit all areas. Douches prescribed to provide local heat should be continued for about a half hour. Petroleum jelly may be used to prevent burning the sensitive tissues of the labia. Following douching, the tub should be well cleaned with soap and warm water.

Cytologic test for cancer (Papanicolaou smear test). This examination may be used in diagnosing cancer of any organ or other part of the body from which exfoliating (normal sloughing) cells can be obtained for study. It was first used, however, by gynecologists; in diagnosing cancer of the female reproductive system, results have been found to be 96 to 98 per cent accurate.[31] Results are classified as positive, negative, or questionable.[31] This test is also used to screen patients needing further examination as well as to measure the effectiveness of radiation and surgical treatment. The test is based on the simple fact that tumor cells, as well as normal cells, of such structures as the fallopian tubes, the uterus, and the vagina exfoliate and pass into the cervical and vaginal secretions. By aspirating these secretions and making smears, lesions of the cervix and of the lining of the fallopian tubes and the uterus may be detected in their early stages. Malignant lesions in the ovary and in the outer structures, such as the outer layers of the uterus, do not, of course, exfoliate cells that are available for study in this manner. This test is extremely valuable in leading the doctor to suspect cancer of the cervix while there is yet no visible or palpable evidence of tumor growth. Cancer of the cervix, one of the most common forms of cancer in women, may thus be treated much earlier than was previously possible, and the rate of cure is relatively high. The patient should understand, however, that the smear test is not necessarily conclusive and that biopsy or even operation may be necessary to verify the diagnosis.

Smears for cytologic study may be taken from the vagina or, under sterile precautions, from within the cervix. Many patients are familiar with the vaginal smear test from descriptions given in popular magazines. The test is not done if profuse bleeding has occurred or if cauterization or curettage has been done within two weeks of the examination. The test will not be accurate if the patient has taken a douche within two hours of the examination, since the desired cells may have been washed away. This test is not painful, and some patients are taught

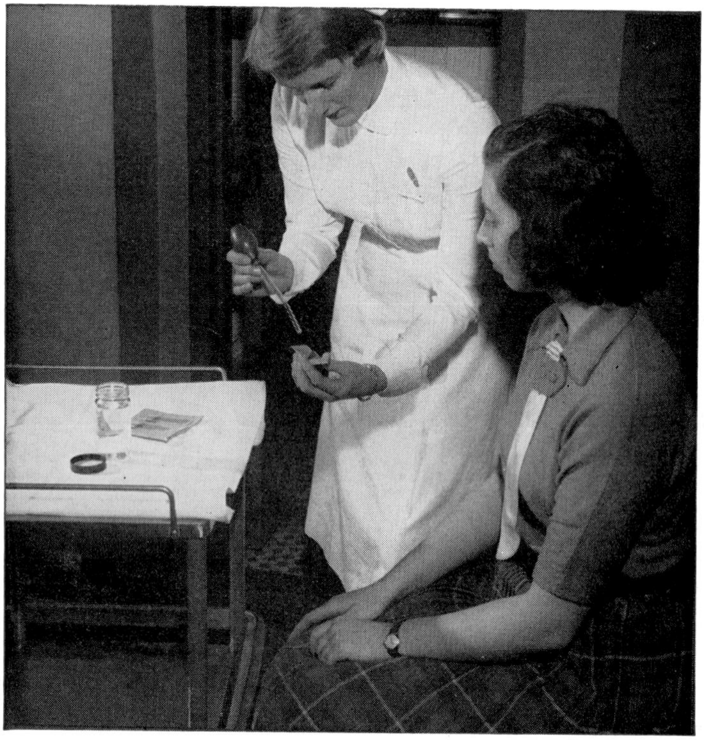

Figure 55

The nurse shows the patient how to fix the slide after taking a vaginal smear; a necessary procedure if the patient must make daily smears at home.

to take smears themselves daily, especially when the doctor is interested in determining the pattern of endometrial growth in women with sterility problems or in those having estrogen therapy. (See Figure 55.) Bathing should not precede the taking of such smears.

The equipment needed for taking a vaginal cytologic smear includes a vaginal pipette with a rubber bulb, an applicator for obtaining secretions from the external mouth of the cervix, a spatula for scraping around the cervix in order to obtain cells loosened but not yet exfoliated, slides, a widemouthed bottle containing equal parts of 95 per cent alcohol and ether, and appropriate labels and laboratory slips.

With the patient in lithotomy position, the doctor will take the smears before he begins the vaginal examination. Dry, clean, unlubricated equipment is used and the label on the slide is checked to be sure that it contains the name of the patient, the date, and the source of the specimen. After air is expressed from the bulb of the vaginal pipette, the pipette is inserted with an upward and backward motion so that the specimen will be obtained from the posterior fornix, which is most likely to contain cells from the fallopian tubes, the cervix, and the vagina. A specimen of the secretion is aspirated and the pipette is withdrawn. The secretion is then expressed thinly and evenly on the prepared slide, and the slide is placed in the solution of ether and alcohol. The secretion must not be permitted to become dry, since the cells will be distorted in appearance if this occurs. Patients who take their own smears often do the aspiration while standing with one foot on a low stool or chair.

If the equipment must be sterilized with moist sterilization and if it is needed for use before it has thoroughly dried, it should be rinsed in equal parts of 95 per cent alcohol and ether to hasten drying.

Obtaining an endocervical smear is a sterile procedure which is done only by the doctor. The preparation is the same as for a vaginal smear except that a sterile metal cannula (laryngeal cannula) with a bulb or syringe attached is needed. The patient may have some discomfort due to the dilation of the cervical canal, but there should be no real pain. There may be some cramping pain from uterine contractions after the procedure; usually heat applied to the lower abdomen and the administration of acetylsalicylic acid will give complete relief.

Tests for pregnancy. There are two tests for pregnancy. In the *Friedman test* the blood serum of the patient is injected into a white rabbit; maturation of its ovaries occurs if the test is positive. In the *Aschheim-Zondek test* the patient's urine is injected in a mouse; again, maturation of the ovaries occurs if the test is positive. The urine specimen should be the first voiding in the morning, since this urine is likely to be more concentrated. In men the Aschheim-Zondek test is used to diagnose a type of testicular tumor in which chorionic gonadotropin, the substance normally produced by pregnant women, is present in the urine.

Dilatation and curettage. Dilatation of the cervix and curettage (scraping) of the endometrial lining of the uterus are minor surgical procedures usually done at the same time either to diagnose disease of the uterus or to correct excessive and prolonged bleeding. Occasionally dilatation of the cervix alone is done to treat dysmenorrhea or to treat sterility caused by stricture or stenosis of the cervical canal. Since the procedure is carried out under general anesthesia, the patient needs physical and emotional preparation and care similar to that given any patient undergoing general anesthesia. In addition, the patient should be told preoperatively that the pubic and perineal area will be shaved, that a nurse will be present with her during the entire procedure, and that she will not be exposed any more than during a pelvic examination. Sometimes the perineal shave and entire preparation is done in the operating room after the patient has been put to sleep and placed in the lithotomy position. If this procedure is followed, the patient should know what is planned; otherwise she may worry because the preparation is not done in her room or be upset when she awakens from anesthesia to find that it has been done. As in all surgery involving the perineum and lower abdomen, the lower bowel and bladder must be empty so that they will not interfere with the operation or be damaged.

At the conclusion of the operation, packing is placed in the cervical canal and vagina, and a sterile pad is placed over the perineum. When the patient returns to her room, the nurse should check the pad for any excessive bleeding every fifteen minutes for two hours and then every one to two hours for eight hours. Usually the pad is only slightly stained; any excessive bleeding should be reported to the doctor. For the comfort of the patient, the pad should be anchored with a sanitary belt and changed as necessary. Sterile perineal pads are used until the packing is removed, usually within 24 hours after operation.

The packing in the cervical canal may cause cramping similar to moderately severe menstrual cramps, since a dilated cervical canal stimulates uterine contractions. Usually codeine sulfate and acteylsalicylic acid are ordered to relieve this and are given every four hours for the first twenty-four to forty-eight hours as necessary. Any really severe abdominal pain that is not relieved by analgesics should be reported at once; a very uncommon but serious complication of curettage is accidental perforation of the uterus during the procedure, with resultant peritonitis.

Voiding may be difficult following a dilatation and curettage because of the pressure of the packing against the urethra or because of local trauma and irritation from the procedure. Usually, however, the patient is permitted to be up almost as soon as she reacts from the anesthetic, and she can void if permitted to use a commode. Any packing that extends beyond the vagina should be kept dry during voiding if this is possible, and the patient should be instructed to protect the vaginal orifice from fecal infection by cleansing with a backward motion.

Patients often go home the day after a dilatation and curettage. They can resume most of their normal daily activities, increasing the amount of activity daily for a week. Vigorous exercise such as horseback riding, tennis, and dancing are usually advised against since these activities may tend to increase pelvic congestion. The patient should abstain from sexual intercourse until her return visit to the doctor, at which time he will advise her as to when intercourse may safely be resumed. The menstrual cycle usually is not upset by a dilatation and curettage, but a vaginal discharge may appear during the healing period. The doctor will usually prescribe a vinegar douche for this.

Examination and diagnostic measures used for male patients

Examination of the male genitalia. Physical examination of the reproductive system in the male consists of careful inspection and palpation of the scrotum, noting skin lesions, differences in size and contour of the scrotum, and any evidence of swelling. Transillumination of the scrotum is done to detect absence of testicles and any unusual density of the structures contained within the scrotal sac. By means of a rectal examination, the doctor can detect enlargement, and general consistency of the prostate (see Figure 56) and any nodules in the adjacent tissues. The penis, foreskin, and meatus are inspected for signs of lesions or other abnormalities. By means of cystoscopic examination the doctor can detect prostatic encroachment on the urethra and observe the condition of the urethral and bladder mucosa. This is not a part of routine examination, however. X-ray visualization and catheterization of the seminal vesicles to obtain specimens are also sometimes done.

The nurse should see that the patient is draped and that he understands what the doctor will do and what will be expected of him, such as giving a specimen of urine and breathing deeply to make palpation easier for the doctor. He should not empty his bladder immediately before examination because the doctor may, by watching him void, be able to identify signs of possible urethral obstruction. Necessary equipment is prepared and the nurse then leaves the patient alone with the doctor.

After the examination, the male patient may have questions to ask the nurse. If he is to have special examinations or treatments later, the nurse is responsible for explaining the preparation and the procedure to him. (See Chapter 21 for preparation for cystoscopic procedures and aftercare.)

Prostatic smears. If cancer or tuberculosis of the prostate is suspected, a prostatic smear may be desired. The doctor first massages the prostate via the rectum; the next voided urine specimen is collected in an appropriate container (a sterile bottle for acid-fast [tubercle] bacilli; a bottle containing alcohol 95 per cent for Papanicolaou or cytologic examination) and sent to the laboratory.

Testicular and prostatic biopsies. Testicular and prostatic biopsies may be obtained either by aspiration of cells through a needle or by obtaining a specimen of tissue through a surgical incision. Both of these procedures are carried out under sterile conditions using local or general anesthesia. If a general anesthetic is to be used, the preoperative and postoperative care is similar to that given any surgical patient. The incision used to obtain a testicular biopsy is a small one in the scrotum, usually about one inch in

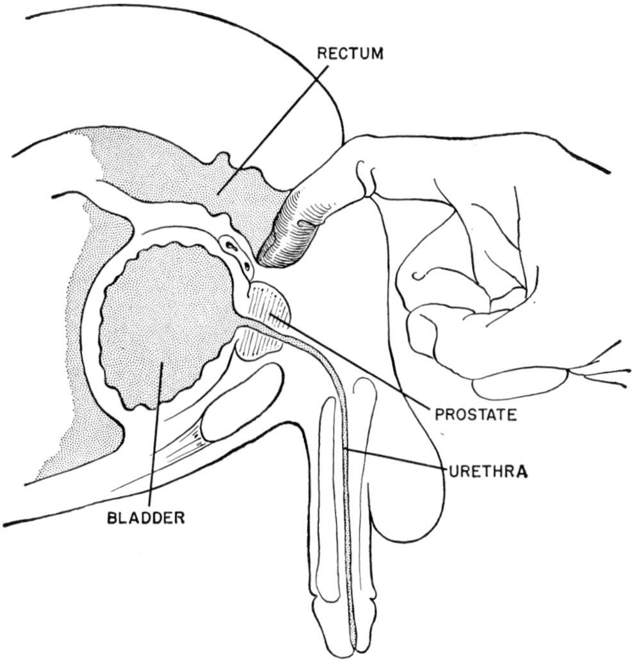

Figure 56

Digital examination to determine the size and consistency of the prostate gland. Note location of the gland in relation to other structures.

length. The only dressing is usually a sterile 4 by 8 inch gauze sponge inside a firm scrotal support. The patient may go home the evening of the operation, returning to have the sutures removed or to be prepared for further treatment if the biopsy shows that this is necessary.

To obtain a prostatic biopsy, a small incision is made in the perineum between the anus and the scrotum. The dressing is usually held in place by a two-tailed binder. The patient must be instructed to be careful not to contaminate the incision while cleansing himself following defecation. If the incision is accidentally contaminated, the area should be carefully cleansed; irrigation of the perineum by pouring sterile water over it or by washing with sterile benzalkonium chloride (Zephiran) sponges is sometimes done routinely following defecation. A heat lamp with a 60-watt bulb placed twelve inches from the perineum is often used two or three times a day to encourage healing. The patient must be in a position in which the scrotum is elevated so that the heat strikes the incision. This is best accomplished by allowing the scrotum to rest on a wide piece of adhesive tape extending from thigh to thigh. Occasionally an exaggerated Sims' position gives satisfactory wound exposure. When the sutures have been removed, sitz baths are used instead of the lamp treatment, and these add a great deal to the general comfort of the patient. Usually following a prostatic biopsy the patient remains in the hospital until the laboratory findings are reported. A patient who has a needle aspiration biopsy will not usually require hospitalization and has no dressings.

Frequently patients, both men and women, show signs of anxiety and depression following diagnostic procedures which necessitate waiting for pathologic reports. The nurse should reassure them by emphasizing their intelligence in seeking medical advice and, without undue discussion, should let them know that results of the examination will be available soon.

Evaluation of infertility problems

The problem of infertility among married couples is of major medical and social concern. Goldzieher[12] says that one out of every seven couples in the United States is unwillingly childless. Forty-five per cent of the time the problem rests with the wife and 20 per cent of the time with the husband; 30 per cent of the time both partners are responsible.[22] It was many years before the husband was considered as a possible cause of sterility. However, it is now recognized that over one-half million men in the United States are responsible for barren marriages.[22] Thus both the husband and wife should be urged to seek medical attention.

Evaluation of male fertility. Some doctors prefer to carry out a complete examination of the husband first, as this is more easily accomplished. Following a thorough physical examination, the first special test will be *multiple semen examinations* to determine the presence, number, maturity, and motility of the sperm. The husband should bring the specimen immediately to the doctor. The date of the last emission and the time of this specimen should be recorded. If sperm are not present in the semen, it may indicate a stricture somewhere along the vas deferens or absence of sperm production.

A *biopsy of the testicle* will show sperm production if the absence of sperm (azoospermia, is due to stricture of the tubal systems above the testes. Occasionally strictures may be repaired by a plastic surgery procedure (vasoepididymal anastomosis), but the results are often poor. Bilateral cryptorchism or undescended testicle, even though corrected, may be the cause of sterility because of failure of the testicles to develop their sperm-producing function. This is particularly true if the correction is not done before puberty. Men sometimes will have no further sperm production following orchitis as a complication of mumps or following x-ray exposure of the testicles. A lack of vitamins A and E in the diet may also cause some atrophy of the spermatogenic tissue.

When the husband is completely aspermatic, conception is impossible and the couple should consider adoption of children if they really want a family. If the sperm count and the motility rate of the sperm cells are low, the doctor usually prescribes thyroid extract and vitamins and treats any low-grade infections. It is important for the patient to eat a well-balanced diet, to maintain normal weight, to obtain adequate rest, and to participate in moderate exercise (preferably outdoors). The doctor will suggest that the couple have frequent intercourse during the fertile period (fourteen to sixteen days after the beginning of the menstrual period); several days of continence should be practiced just prior to this period. If these methods are unsuccessful, the injection of several drops of the husband's semen into the upper portion of the cervical canal may produce a pregnancy.

Evaluation of female fertility. The wife should also have a thorough physical examination, including a pelvic examination. In addition, a systematic check should be made of each organ influencing the reproductive system.

In order for the ovum to be fertilized, the vagina, cervix, and uterus must be completely patent and have mucosal secretions that are not hostile to the sperm. The Huhner test and vaginal and endometrial smears give this necessary information.

In the *Huhner test* the doctor aspirates cervical secretions within one hour after intercourse and examines them for the presence and viability of the sperm cells. The woman should be instructed not to void, douche, or bathe between intercourse and the examination; she should put a perineal pad in place and go immediately to the doctor's office. If the sperm are being killed by the secretions, vaginal smears are examined and an appropriate antibiotic may be given to change the flora in the woman's vagina and cervix, timing its administration so that the secretions are least noxious to the sperm at the time of ovulation. If the secretions are too acid or too alkaline, medicated douches may be ordered. If the sperm cells do not reach the uterus, dilatation of the cervix may be tried.

The ovary must be producing ova, estrogen, and progesterone in order for an ovum to be fertilized and implanted in the uterus. *Endometrial biopsy* and *vaginal smears* taken premenstrually give some of this information, but a *complete endocrine work-up,* including a basal metabolic rate and twenty-four hour urine studies, may also be indicated. As an indication of pituitary gland function, the urine studies will determine the amount of gonadotropin in the urine. A low basal metabolism or under par general health may prevent an otherwise normal woman from conceiving. Thyroid extract therapy, regulated by periodic basal metabolic rate determinations, is sometimes advocated. Vitamins C and E and extra rest may also be prescribed.

If the wife has an irregular menstrual cycle, it is important that she keep a temperature chart for several months to help the doctor determine her exact period of ovulation. The temperature will usually be lower at ovulation (the time at which conception most likely will take place) and then will rise abruptly as the corpus luteum begins to produce progesterone. It will drop to a lower level again a day or two before the start of the menstrual period. The temperature should be taken rectally before arising each morning. The temperature chart should be interpreted by the doctor since there may be individual variations.

If the ovum is to reach the uterus, the fallopian tubes must be mechanically patent and not in spasm. The *Rubin test* will provide the doctor with information concerning patency of the tubes. In this test the patient is prepared as for a pelvic examination, and then compressed air is forced into the uterus under sterile conditions. If the fallopian tubes are open, the doctor will be able to hear free air in the peritoneum on auscultation; the patient will feel pain under the scapula on the same side as the patent tube. If considerable pressure is required to force air into the tubes, there may be spasticity or partial stricture. Roentgenograms of the uterus and fallopian tubes (hysterograms) may be taken by forcing a radiopaque substance through the uterus into the tubes. This examination is usually not carried out more than seven days after the end of the menstrual period, since ovulation may be taking place.

The patient should prepare for these tests by taking a laxative the night before the examination and an enema in the morning so that distention of the bowel will not obstruct the fallopian tubes and so that the roentgenograms will not be distorted by gas shadows in the intestine. Soluble phenobarbital is usually given before this examination since there will be some discomfort; low abdominal pain, cramping, nausea, vomiting, and faintness are common. After the examination is over, the patient usually has "gas pains"; these may be relieved by lying with the head lower than the feet for one or two hours, since this position allows the gas to rise into the lower pelvis. Since the x-ray medium may stain the patient's clothing, she should wear a perineal pad for several hours.

Tubal strictures may be the result of acute or chronic infections involving the fallopian tubes; although they sometimes can be repaired by plastic surgery, the results are successful in only 5 per cent of the cases.[8] Tubal insufflation is often therapeutic in itself, opening the fallopian tube(s) enough to allow the free passage of the fertilized ovum into the uterus.

A displaced uterus may occasionally be the only known cause of the infertility. Treatment for this usually consists of pelvic exercises (see dysmenorrhea) and/or the use of a pessary.

The couple should not be disappointed

if, even with medical treatment, pregnancy does not occur immediately, since many normal couples must wait many months before pregnancy occurs.

Often no physical cause for sterility can be found in either the husband or the wife. Pregnancy has been known to occur after years of childless marriage, perhaps because the couple begin to accept their situation and thus become more relaxed. Many couples will benefit simply from reassurance of normalcy. Others may need marriage counseling or psychiatric help to gain insight into psychologic and emotional problems that may be preventing conception. Sterility problems always deserve medical consultation in order to correct deficiencies and to clarify the problem.

Nursing related to disease of the female reproductive system

Advances in medical science have made it possible to treat effectively many diseases of the female reproductive system, but for optimum benefit from treatment an early diagnosis is essential. As the layman becomes better informed about normal reproductive functions throughout life, he or she should be able to recognize and report symptoms indicative of early disease. Since the nurse is often the first member of the health team consulted about symptoms related to the reproductive system, she needs to know those for which she may safely suggest conservative hygienic measures and those for which she should guide the patient to seek medical advice. If disease is found, she may also play an important part in helping patients accept the prescribed treatment as well as in providing nursing care which is coordinated with the efforts of other disciplines to return the patient to a normal productive life.

COMMON GYNECOLOGIC DISORDERS

Abnormal menses

Dysmenorrhea. Thirty-five per cent of all women complain of some pain with menstruation.[60] This is known as dysmenorrhea. Industrial studies have shown dysmenorrhea to be one of the most important causes of absenteeism among working women, resulting in an average loss of two or more days a month for many employees.[45] The nurse frequently is asked for practical suggestions to relieve dysmenorrhea. She should first determine if the period is in any way abnormal. If it is not, she may suggest rest in bed for an hour or two, application of heat to the lower abdomen, and the use of a mild analgesic such as acetylsalicylic acid in moderate doses. She should advise against repeated use of large amounts of analgesics such as acetylsalicylic acid which is widely used by the laity without medical prescription. Reading something interesting while resting may bring faster relief. A person who is busy, either mentally or physically, doing something she enjoys is less likely to notice discomfort. These measures will suffice in most instances, but anyone with further difficulty or consistent dysmenorrhea should be urged to seek medical attention. There are many causes which are not obvious, and curative treatment can only be given when the cause of the difficulty is known.

When the patient visits the doctor, a pelvic examination is usually performed, and health practices are analyzed. Congestion of blood in the pelvic cavity or intrapelvic pressure resulting from constipation, a full bladder, or a tumor often causes menstrual pain. Frequently no definite cause can be determined, and the patient may be urged to try such health measures as securing adequate rest, improving posture, participating in moderate exercise, eating a nonconstipating diet, and taking warm, rather than cool, baths during the menstrual period. An English physician found that, following health education, approximately 70 per cent of his

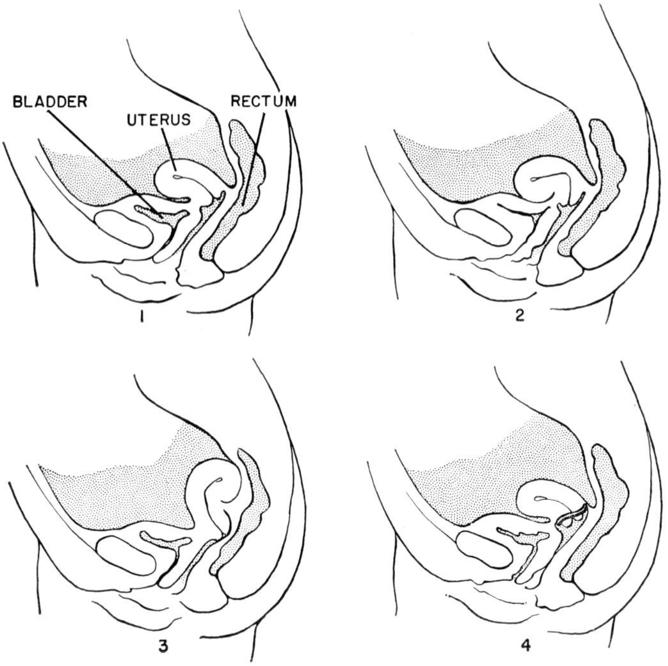

Figure 57

Diagram showing normal and abnormal positions of the uterus. *1,* Normal anatomic position of the uterus in relation to adjacent structures. *2,* Anterior displacement of the uterus. *3,* Retroversion or backward displacement of the uterus. *4,* Normal anatomic position of the uterus maintained by use of a rubber S-shaped pessary.

patients had less dysmenorrhea.[60] The nurse, who by her own attitude shows that she considers menstruation to be a normal function and who augments the patient's understanding of normal sexual functions by giving explanations whenever possible, may help some women make a better adjustment to the menstrual cycle.

If premenstrual fluid retention causes slight swelling of the abdomen and ankles, headache, and noticeable mood swings, eating a low-salt diet and limiting fluid intake during the week prior to the onset of menstruation may help. The patient in whom these difficulties are marked should consult a gynecologist since they may be due to hormonal dysfunction. Tenderness of the breasts, either immediately preceding the onset of menstruation or at any other time during the cycle, is due to hormonal influences and should be reported to the physician if it is at all marked or troublesome. For marked fluid retention the doctor may order a salt-free diet, and occasionally ammonium chloride is prescribed. The chloride unites with the sodium in the extracellular fluid to form sodium chloride, which is excreted by the kidneys, carrying with it the excess fluid. This treatment is usually only necessary for the two weeks prior to menstruation.

Although displacement of the uterus may cause dysmenorrhea, many women with known displacements have no difficulty. Some patients with displacement complain of chronic backache, pelvic pressure, easy fatigue, and leukorrhea in addition to painful menstruation.

Common kinds of displacement are *anteflexion, retroflexion, and retroversion* of the uterus caused by congenitally weak uterine ligaments, adhesions following infections or surgery in the pelvic region, or the strain of pregnancy on the ligaments. A space-filling lesion in this region, or even a full bladder or rectum, may also displace the uterus enough to cause symptoms. Normally the body of the uterus flexes forward at a 45-degree angle at the cervix. In retroflexion this angle is increased; in anteflexion it is decreased. In retroversion the whole uterus is tipped backward. (See Figure 57.)

If the displacement is not due to some coexistent pelvic disease, various pelvic exercises may be recommended by the doctor in an attempt to return the uterus to a normal position. These exercises, employing the principles of gravity, stretch or strengthen the uterine ligaments. Some exercises used are knee-chest exercises, the monkey trot,[42] lying on the abdomen two hours a day, and premenstrual exercises.[49] Corrective exercises for poor posture may also be prescribed.

In doing *knee-chest exercises,* the patient is instructed to assume a knee-chest position (see Figure 53) and to separate the labia to allow air to enter the vagina, since this helps to further normal position of the uterus. This position should be maintained for five minutes two or three times a day.

In doing the *monkey trot,* the patient is instructed to walk about the house on her hands and feet, keeping the knees straight. This should be done for five minutes two or three times a day.

Premenstrual exercises should be done once a day in the week prior to menstruation and three times a day during menstruation. The patient is instructed to stand with her feet together, knees straight, elbow raised to shoulder level, with her left forearm resting against a wall. While keeping her feet flat on the floor and without bending her knees, she should touch the wall with her left hip three times. This exercise should be repeated with the right forearm resting against the wall. She should then stand facing the wall with both forearms raised to shoulder level resting against it. The pelvis should be tilted slightly forward. Keeping her feet flat on the floor, she should tilt the pelvis forward until the lower abdomen touches the wall. This should be repeated three times.

The nurse may be responsible for teaching the patient how to do prescribed exercises. The patient should begin exercising gradually; for example, knee-chest position should be maintained only one minute the first time, two minutes the second time, with gradual progression up to five minutes. Results from a program of exercising will not be immediately noticed; the patient should be told this and should be encouraged to exercise regularly over a period of months. Performance of exercises should be reviewed each time the nurse sees the patient.

If the uterus can be manually replaced in a normal position, a *Smith-Hodges pessary* may be inserted for a trial period to learn whether malposition causes the dysmenorrhea (see Figure 57). The pessary is an appliance introduced into the vagina for the purpose of supporting the uterus in normal position. Sometimes, after the removal of a pessary, the uterus will remain in normal position. If, after about a six-month trial, the uterus still returns to its displaced position after removal of the pessary and if the pessary has relieved the symptoms, the ligaments may be shortened surgically through an abdominal incision. While the pessary is in place, the patient should be instructed to take a daily cleansing douche with warm tap water. The pessary is usually changed every three to six weeks. If it is left in place indefinitely, it may cause erosion of the cervix and become adherent to the mucosa.

A stricture of the cervical canal may cause dysmenorrhea. If so, dilatation of the cervical canal may relieve the discomfort. Dysmenorrhea may be due to endocrine disorders, or it may be a manifestation of an allergic reaction. Extensive metabolic and allergic diagnostic tests are done only when there seems to be no other possible cause. In some instances psychiatric therapy may be needed to attempt to relieve symptoms. The nurse may be helpful in making this treatment acceptable to the patient.

If dysmenorrhea is incapacitating and unrelieved by conservative therapy, a *presacral neurectomy* may be performed. In this procedure the pain fibers from the uterus are surgically interrupted through an abdominal incision. If a pregnant woman has had this operation, she will not feel uterine contractions during labor and contractions must be carefully palpated to prevent precipitate birth of the baby.

Amenorrhea. Amenorrhea is the absence of menstruation. Before the seriousness of this symptom can be ascertained, one needs to know if there has ever been menstruation and if there has been any recent change in the normal life pattern or in the general state of health of the person. It is not unusual for a woman to miss one period, especially if she is adjusting to a change in her life pattern such as working nights instead of days, going from a hot climate to a cold one, adjusting to married life, or if she has had an acute illness. If menses continue to be absent, however, medical consultation should be advised.

The most common cause of amenorrhea, aside from the menopause, is pregnancy. Some women, however, continue to menstruate during the first months of pregnancy. Menses are also usually absent at least until six weeks after delivery of the baby, and sometimes throughout the period of lactation. If a girl is over 14 years of age and has not started to menstruate, she should be examined by a gynecologist to rule out a congenital deformity such as imperforate hymen or absence of the vagina, uterus, or ovaries. If there is no apparent cause for the failure to menstruate regularly, endocrine studies may be done. Sometimes thyroxin and female hormones need to be supplemented. Nutritional anemia, wasting chronic illness such as tuberculosis, and psychogenic factors such as fear of pregnancy or desire for pregnancy may cause amenorrhea. A certain type of ovarian tumor (arrhenoblastoma) also causes amenorrhea.

Abnormal menstruation. Abnormal bleeding from the vagina requires immediate medical attention. There are two types: *menorrhagia,* or prolonged profuse menstrual flow during the regular period, and *metrorrhagia,* or bleeding between periods. Metrorrhagia may be only a slight spotting to be significant.

Menorrhagia in an adolescent girl may be due to a blood dyscrasia or to an endocrine disturbance; this is called functional bleeding. Menorrhagia in adult women is likely to be a symptom of an ovarian tumor, a uterine myoma, or pelvic inflammatory disease.

Metrorrhagia may be a symptom of many disorders such as benign or malignant uterine tumors; pelvic inflammatory disease; abnormal conditions of pregnancy such as a threatened abortion, ectopic pregnancy, or hydatid mole; blood dyscrasias; senile vaginitis; and bleeding at ovulation caused by the withdrawal of estrone. If there is no delay in seeking medical examination, metrorrhagia should not cause undue anxiety since its cause may not be serious. However, the cause, not the symptom, must be treated, and the nurse has a responsibility to help disseminate this information to all women. Early diagnosis and treatment increase the possibility of cure even when the cause is a malignancy.

Vaginal infection

Many women complain of leukorrhea, a white vaginal discharge. It is normal to have a slight white vaginal discharge the month prior to the menarche and then monthly around the period of ovulation and just prior to the onset of menstruation. Ordinarily the vagina is protected from infection by its acid secretion and by the presence of Döderlein's bacilli. Occasionally, if the invading organisms are very virulent or if the resistance of the person is lowered by malnutrition, aging, disease, or emotional disturbances, a vaginitis may develop. Profuse discharge, yellow discharge, and mucoid discharge are abnormal and are signs of vaginitis, inflammation, or infection. Urethritis usually occurs simultaneously because the mucous membranes of the vagina and urethra are contiguous. The discharge may be irritating and cause redness, edema, burning, and itching; the burning and pruritus may be aggravated by voiding and by defecation.

Vaginal jellies and vaginal suppositories are frequently prescribed for patients with vaginitis; the nurse will need to instruct the patient in the procedures for their use. Vaginal jelly is dispensed in a tube to which is attached an applicator. This is inserted into the vagina in a manner similar to the way a pipette is inserted when obtaining a vaginal smear. The medication is then expressed into the vagina and the applicator is withdrawn. A vaginal suppository should be lubricated with a vegetable fat, inserted into the vagina, and left in place. It is dissolved by body heat, and the medication is absorbed through the vaginal mucosa.

Simple vaginitis. Simple vaginitis is caused by contamination of the vagina with organisms from the rectum such as *Escherichia coli* or with other common pyogenic organisms such as staphylococci and streptococci. The organisms are usually introduced from outside sources such as clothing or a douche nozzle. Simple vaginitis is treated with warm douches of a weak acid solution such as vinegar (1 tablespoon to 1 quart of water). This increases the acidity of the bacterial environment within the vagina. To help control the infection, beta-lactose, a sugar which stimulates the growth of Döderlein's bacilli, may be given orally, and sulfonamide cream may be prescribed as an intravaginal application. The sulfonamide cream should be applied after douching. Sitz baths, taken two or three times a day to help relieve local irritation, and thorough gentle cleansing of the perineum with water after voiding and defecating are recommended.

Trichomonas vaginitis. Trichomonas vaginitis is one of the most common forms of vaginal infection and is often found in combination with other infecting organisms. A protozoan called the *Trichomonas vaginalis* is probably the causative agent. The disease is diagnosed by examining a drop of vaginal secretion microscopically. When this test is to be made, a dry speculum should be offered the doctor; the slide should be dry and warm, and as soon as the drop of vaginal secretion is placed on the slide, a drop or two of normal saline solution should be added.

The general treatment for trichomonas vaginitis is similar to that for simple vaginitis. Specific treatment consists of the local use of suppositories, powders, or jellies containing antibiotic drugs, sulfonamides, or carbarsone, which is an arsenical preparation effective against protozoans. Carbarsone is usually prescribed as a vaginal suppository—one every day for twelve days. It should be inserted intravaginally at bedtime, and no more than one douche should be taken during the period of treatment. Trichomonas sometimes attack the cervix, bladder, or rectum. If the cervix is involved, the infected portion may need to be surgically removed (conization of the cervix). When the bladder is infected, instillations of mild silver protein (Argyrol) or sulfonamide solutions are used, and carbarsone suppositories may be used to clear up persistent rectal involvement. Sunshine, rest, good nutrition, and treatment of any focal infections may help to improve the patient's general resistance. Trichomonas vaginitis often resists treatment and may persist for months and years despite extensive treatment. It is discouraging and distressing to the patient; if she is to be encouraged to continue the treatment and not "shop around" in her effort to be cured, she needs to be treated with much patience and understanding.

Monilial vaginitis. Monilial vaginitis is a fungus infection commonly seen in patients with uncontrolled diabetes mellitus because the fungi thrive on sugar. A white membrane appears in the vagina, and there is a very irritating, watery discharge mixed with white cheesy particles. If the infection is due to untreated diabetes mellitus, it usually responds to better control of the blood sugar level. Local treatment consists of painting the vagina three times weekly with 5 per cent aqueous gentian violet and the nightly instillation of propionate compound. Douches should not be taken during the period of treatment. Since this drug stains clothing, a perineal pad should be provided for the patient who has been treated with gentian violet. Monilial infection is sometimes resistant to treatment and tends to recur just when it is believed that treatment has been successful. Total recovery may be aided by attention to the improvement of general health.

Senile vaginitis. Senile vaginitis (atrophic) is caused by the invasion of the thin, atrophied, postmenopausal vaginal mucosa by pyogenic bacteria. The main symptom is an irritating vaginal discharge which is sometimes accompanied by pruritus and burning. The treatment is the same as that for simple vaginitis. In an effort to improve the general resistance of the tissues, vitamin A, vitamin B, and vitamin E are often given. Estrogenic hormones, given by mouth or applied locally as ointment, will help to restore the epithelium to normal. These hormones are seldom used, however, because they alter normal involutional changes, and there is some suggestive evidence that they may contribute to the development of cancer of the reproductive system.

Perineal pruritus

Perineal pruritus is not always associated with a vaginal discharge. In older women whose diet is inadequate in butter, milk, and yellow vegetables, the lack of vitamin A may cause perineal itching. Patients with uncontrolled diabetes mellitus may complain of severe itching of the perineum due to local irritation from the high concentration of sugar in the urine. When there is perineal itching, the possibility of pediculosis pubis is considered. Allergies, cancer of the vulva, scabies, and superficial skin infections such as *tinea cruris* (a fungus infection) may also cause perineal itching without any abnormal discharge.

Venereal diseases

These diseases are discussed under Lesions of the External Genitalia (see page 424).

Cervicitis

Cervical erosion. Cervical erosion is the mildest form of cervicitis. A small, reddened, irritated area appears about the external mouth of the cervix. It occurs in both married and single women, and the cause is obscure. Inflammation of the cervix may be due to an acute pyogenic infection such as sometimes follows abortion and childbirth, or it may be due to lodging of the gonococcus in a cervical erosion or laceration. This is known as *acute cervicitis;* if inadequately treated, it may become chronic.

In untreated cervicitis the local tissues are constantly irritated, and there is some evidence that this irritation predisposes to cancer. Since leukorrhea, the only sympom of cervicitis, does not appear unless there is severe irritation, the presence of unrecognized cervicitis must be determined by pelvic examination, including visualization of the cervix. If the practice of returning to the doctor for a careful examination six weeks after the birth of every baby were adhered to, much chronic cervicitis could be prevented. The cervix is frequently lacerated as it stretches and thins out to allow the baby to pass through the birth canal, and the torn surfaces do not always heal properly. At the examination made six weeks following delivery, improperly healed lacerations of the cervix can be cauterized so that the everted portion of the mucosa is turned back into the cervical canal. This is a minor procedure which can be done in the doctor's office or the clinic, and it will prevent a chronic inflammatory process from ensuing. Cervical erosions are often discovered during routine pelvic examinations. A biopsy is taken, and the erosion is then cauterized with silver nitrate.

Acute cervicitis can usually be adequately treated with hot douches and the local application of antibiotics. Antibiotics also may be given both orally and parenterally.

In chronic cervicitis the infection has extended deep into the tissues, and the patient must be hospitalized for at least one day for *conization* of the cervix. This is the removal of a cone-shaped portion of the cervix containing the infected tissue. The nursing care is the same as that required after a dilatation and curettage; in addition, hemorrhage which may occur from the operative site is treated by such means as packing the vagina, raising the foot of the bed, and keeping the patient absolutely quiet for several hours; very occasionally the patient must be returned to the operating room for resuturing or cauterization of the site of hemorrhage. Untreated chronic cervical infections eventually may extend into the uterine cavity and into the pelvic cavity, causing endometritis (inflammation of the uterine lining) and pelvic inflammatory disease.

Pelvic inflammatory disease

Pelvic inflammatory disease is an inflammatory process outside the uterus which may include the fallopian tubes, the ovaries, pelvic peritoneum, pelvic veins, or pelvic connective tissue. Inflammation of the fallopian tube is known as *salpingitis,* and inflammation of the ovary is known as *oophoritis.*

Pathogenic organisms causing pelvic inflammatory disease are usually introduced from the outside and pass up the cervical canal into the uterus. They seem to cause little trouble in the uterus but pass into the pelvis either through thrombosed uterine veins or through the lymphatics of the uterine wall; here they cause an inflammation. Tubercle bacilli may also cause the disease but these organisms are usually blood borne from the lungs. Although any pathogenic organism can cause a generalized peritonitis and death, the infection more frequently is localized, causing abscess formation and adhesions of the pelvic viscera. An abscess of the cul-de-sac of Douglas is common; in this location the abscess may rupture spontaneously into the vagina or may require surgical incision through the vagina for drainage.

Signs and symptoms of pelvic inflammatory disease may include severe abdominal and pelvic pain, malaise, nausea and vomiting, and elevation of temperature, with leukocytosis. Often there is a foul-smelling purulent vaginal discharge. The patient is usually hospitalized and placed on bed rest in a mid-Fowler's position to provide dependent drainage so that abscesses will not form high in the abdomen, where they might rupture and cause generalized peritonitis. The sulfonamide and antibiotic drugs are almost always given. Heat applied to the abdomen, either a hot-water bottle or an electric heating pad, or a hot vaginal douche to be taken twice a day may be ordered. Heat improves circulation to the involved parts, and thereby allays the discomfort caused by stasis of blood and enhances the effectiveness of the body's natural defenses—leukocytes. If there is a vaginal discharge, tampons should not be used, since the drainage may be coming from the vaginal wall and a tampon would obstruct it. The nurse should instruct the patient and ancillary personnel who may be giving the nursing care to report any change in the amount, appearance, or odor of vaginal discharge. If the patient is ambulatory, she should be advised that she should not have sexual intercourse during the acute stage of the disease.

Pelvic inflammatory disease becomes chronic unless it is quite vigorously treated at its onset. Chronic pelvic discomfort, disturbances of menstruation, constipation, and periodic exacerbation of acute symptoms sometimes occur. Occasionally the patient may be considered neurotic because of the repeated and nonspecific nature of her complaints. The most serious of the complications of pelvic inflammatory disease is *sterility,* which is caused by strictures of the fallopian tubes. Strictures of the salpinges may cause an *ectopic pregnancy,* since the fertilized egg may not be able to reach the uterus even though the smaller sperm has been able to pass the stricture and produce conception. Adhesions form as a result of chronic inflammation, and the ovaries, fallopian tubes, and uterus may have to be compeltely removed.

Pelvic inflammatory disease frequently is a complication of acute infectious processes such as gonorrhea, puerperal infection, tuberculosis, and pelvic peritonitis. Prevention or early and adequate treatment of the original infection should decrease the incidence of this problem.

Gonorrhea. Before the discovery of sulfonamides and penicillin, the gonococcus was the most common organism causing pelvic inflammatory disease. This organism typically invades the pelvis through the fallopian tubes. Pus forms in the tubes, and adhesions seal off the ends. Sterility is a common complication. With early recognition and treatment of gonorrhea, these problems have been greatly reduced (see Chapter 17).

Puerperal infection. Pelvic infection caused by staphylococci or streptococci is usually a sequela to a puerperal infection—a uterine infection following interruption of pregnancy or a normal delivery. The organisms extend into the pelvis through the fallopian tubes, the lymphatics in the uterine wall, or thrombosed uterine veins. With improved obstetric care, puerperal infection now occurs most frequently in women who have had criminally induced abortions. Puerperal infections may occur, however, if the membranes have been ruptured for several days before delivery, if the removal of the placenta has been incomplete, or if clots or edema has prevented normal drainage from the uterus following delivery. When the baby is delivered at home or in a car, where it is impossible to use aseptic technique, there is increased danger of infection. If the cervical and uterine canals have been contaminated or if any symptoms of infection appear after a delivery, antibiotics are given. If pieces of the placenta have been retained, a dilatation and curettage of the uterus will be performed, because the retained tissue not only causes continued bleeding, but also serves as a culture medium. Cramping uterine pains, continued vaginal bleeding, or scanty normal uterine drainage (lochia) following delivery should be noted and reported so that appropriate treatment may be started if necessary.

Tuberculosis. Tuberculosis of the female reproductive system most frequently involves the fallopian tubes, but may also involve the uterus, ovaries, and pelvic peritoneum. It is secondary to a lesion in the lungs. The tubercle bacilli reach the pelvis through the blood stream but rarely cause symptoms in the pelvis until eight to ten years following occurrence of the primary lesion. Often the pulmonary lesion was minimal and was never diagnosed.

The symptoms are those of acute pelvic inflammatory disease plus the general malaise, weight loss, afternoon temperature elevation, and night sweats which are typical symptoms of tuberculosis. Since the lung lesion is usually inactive, isolation is not necessary. The precautions used for patients with tuberculosis of the urinary system should be followed since the vaginal discharge may contain live tubercle bacilli. (See Chapter 21.)

The treatment is that given for pulmonary tuberculosis—rest and antituberculosis drug therapy. Sexual intercourse is prohibited. If treatment is ineffectual, the affected pelvic structures may be removed surgically.

Other causes. The rupture of any adjacent structure may spill organisms into the pelvic cavity, producing secondary inflammation; e.g., when the appendix perforates, pelvic peritonitis usually follows.

Abortions

An abortion is the expulsion of, or removal of, a fetus before it is viable, or before twenty-eight weeks of fetal life. The term miscarriage is used by the laity to indicate spontaneous abortion without human interference and is used occasionally by the medical profession to indicate a pregnancy lost in the second trimester (late abortion). The term abortion is commonly used if the fetus weighs under 1,000 Gm.; the infant weighing more than that amount is usually viable, and the term *premature labor* is used.

There are several kinds of abortions. A *threatened abortion* is one in which there is a bloody vaginal discharge and sometimes uterine contractions. In this condition the cervix does not dilate, and immediate bed rest and conservative treatment can often prevent abortion. An *inevitable abortion* is one which occurs despite conservative treatment of early signs. A *complete abortion* is one in which the fetus and all the surrounding tissues are passed, while in an *incomplete abortion* some of the products of conception remain in the uterus. A *missed abortion* is one in which the fetus dies (usually early in pregnancy) but is not expelled for as long as two months thereafter.

A *spontaneous abortion* is one that occurs naturally with no known specific cause. It may be due to intrinsic factors, such as a defective ovum or sperm or an improperly placed placenta, or it may be due to extrinsic factors, such as hormonal imbalance, or chronic debilitating disease such as tuberculosis. *Habitual abortion* is the repeated abortion of successive pregnancies with no known cause. Many kinds of treatment have been tried for this: bed rest during the entire pregnancy, thyroid extract, stilbestrol and progesterone in an attempt to prevent sloughing of the endometrium, and psychotherapy. None of these are really satisfactory, although hormones appear to have helped in some cases.

A *therapeutic abortion* is one performed by a physician when serious maternal disease threatens the mother's life. Usually more than one physician is called in for consultation before decision is reached to perform this procedure. The patient's husband is always consulted before a therapeutic abortion is considered, and often the spiritual adviser must also be consulted. For details of the convictions of certain religious groups on this subject, the nurse should consult special references. The Roman Catholic viewpoint, for example, is available in material on medical ethics.[56]

A *criminal abortion* is the illegal destruction of the products of conception by the patients or by others. Figures on the frequency of this procedure vary and cannot be accurate since most criminal abortions are performed secretly. It is estimated, however, that between 100,000 and 500,000 such operations are performed annually.[72] Criminal abortions are responsible for a large number of maternal deaths each year since they are almost always performed by unskilled persons. Infections often follow criminal abortions and caused many deaths each year before the use of antibiotics. Some women still die because they hesitate to seek competent medical care when complications of a criminal abortion occur. Some fatalities have been due to the ingestion of huge doses of drugs in an effort to induce abortion; others have been due to trauma, such as perforation of the uterus by crude instruments in unskilled hands. The nurse is often in a situation in which she can stress to women that there is no safe way to induce an abortion and that there are no drugs that can be taken to safely dislodge a fetus normally implanted in the uterus. If asked for information on birth control, the nurse can suggest that the patient ask her physician.

The nurse can often encourage the patient to continue with her pregnancy. If the patient is unmarried she should direct her to agencies especially equipped to help her. Many of our larger cities, for example, have local branches of the Florence Crittenton League which serves unmarried mothers. The Salvation Army maintains facilities for care of pregnant women in many cities. Local health departments or their equivalents are usually able to provide information about available resources. The nurse must, in all instances, avoid planning with the unmarried pregnant woman for the disposition of her unborn child; she should refer such a matter to the doctor and to reliable social agencies.

The patient who enters the hospital with a history of *threatened, partial,* or *complete abortion* is put on bed rest. If abortion is inevitable or if partial expulsion of the products of conception has occurred before the patient was admitted, drugs such as Prostigmin and ergot may be given to stimulate the uterus to expel its remaining contents. The patient should not go to the bathroom but should use a bedpan; auxiliary nursing personnel should be instructed to save all bedpan contents since pieces of placental tissue and even a fetus may be passed unknowingly by the patient while she is having a bowel movement. If a fetus is over five months, papers recording a stillbirth should be filed with the Bureau of Vital Statistics. Antibiotics are usually ordered to combat infection. The patient's temperature should be carefully taken and recorded. Pain in the abdomen is also reported at once.

Surgical treatment. If tissue is retained following an abortion, a procedure known as *evacuation of retained secundae* (ERS) must be performed. This is similar to a dilatation and curettage, and the preoperative and postoperative nursing care is the same.

General nursing care. The patient who has had an illegal abortion presents a difficult nursing and medical care problem because she seldom gives the doctor a correct story of her condition and the treatment she has received; occasionally the nurse who is particularly skillful in gaining the patient's confidence may get information that is helpful to the doctor.

The patient who has had an abortion needs understanding and thoughtful nursing care. Regardless of the cause of the abortion or the circumstances surrounding it, the patient usually has a severe emotional reaction. She may, for example, have lost the fetus after years of attempting to become pregnant, or she may have experienced another of a series of abortions when she desperately wants a child and is approaching the age limit for future pregnancies. While the patient who has had a criminal abortion may experience a feeling of relief from knowing that she is no longer pregnant, she almost invariably suffers from guilt and often from grief as a result of the death of the fetus and of a realization of her life situation that led to abortion. The patient may talk about her feelings if the nurse gives the impression that she has time and is willing to listen and if her attitude suggests that she will not judge the patient. The nurse may be able to plan with the patient for ways to get the help she needs through a social worker, a spiritual advisor, or other resources.

Ectopic pregnancy

An ectopic pregnancy is one in which the fertilized ovum becomes embedded outside the body of the uterus. Since it is almost always located in the fallopian tube, the term *tubal pregnancy* is often used.

This condition occurs most often in women who have a narrowed fallopian tube due to either inflammation or a congenital stricture. The sperm may be small enough to pass through the stricture, but the larger fertilized ovum may be unable to do so; it may then attach itself to the tubal wall and develop into an embryo. As the embryo grows, the fallopian tube stretches and finally ruptures. This rupture usually occurs within the first six weeks of pregnancy. The patient experiences a sudden severe pain on one side of the abdomen and has a history of amenorrhea and often of suspected pregnancy. She may go into shock quickly after the onset of pain because of massive hemorrhage into the peritoneal cavity.

Emergency treatment for shock and hemorrhage is given. Early treatment of a ruptured ectopic pregnancy is imperative to prevent death. Immediately upon diagnosis the patient is prepared for a salpingectomy. If there has been serious bleeding preoperatively, the postoperative course may be complicated by peritonitis.

The nursing care combines the aspects of emergency treatment of a patient who has sustained a severe hemorrhage, general care of a patient who has had major abdominal surgery and who may have peritonitis, and care of a woman whose pregnancy has been prematurely terminated. The patient needs reassurance regarding future pregnancies. She needs to understand that since ova are produced from alternate ovaries, she still has a good chance to become pregnant and have a normal pregnancy.

Hydatidiform mole

A hydatidiform mole is a tumor mass of fetal cells in the uterus that masquerades as a pregnancy. The uterus rapidly increases in size, and the ovaries also increase in size because of enlargement of the ovarian follicles. The hormonal balance is upset and usually causes uterine bleeding. Hydatidiform mole is usually a benign condition and is relieved by curettage of the uterus to remove the abnormal growth. If all tissue is not removed, however, there is some suspicion that cancer may develop either in the uterus or elsewhere in the body because the cells may get into the blood stream. Since some spontaneous abortions actually may be the expulsion of hydatidiform moles, all aborted tissue should be sent for pathologic examination. Persons with hydatidiform moles are followed medically with periodic Aschheim-Zondek tests; if cancer develops this test will become positive.

Uterine displacement due to relaxation of the pelvic musculature

Downward displacement of the uterus is due to a relaxation of the muscles of the pelvic floor. This usually results from unrepaired lacerations due to childbirth. With better obstetric care, use of episiotomies to prevent tearing of the pelvic muscles, and immediate repair of all tears, fewer women should require vaginal wall repairs late in life than is now the case. Apparently relaxation may also be caused by a congenital weakness of the muscles of the pelvis because it occasionally occurs in women who have had no children.

As the uterus begins to drop, the vaginal walls become relaxed, and a fold of vaginal mucosa may protrude outside the vaginal orifice. This is known as a *colpocele.* With the relaxation of the vaginal walls, the bladder may herniate into the vagina (a *cystocele*) or the rectal wall may herniate into the vagina (a *rectocele*). (See Figure 58.) Both conditions may occur simultaneously.

A sign of relaxation of the pelvic musculature is a dragging pain in the back and in the pelvis. This is made worse by standing on the feet or by walking. The patient who has a cystocele may complain of urinary incontinence accompanying activity that increases intra-abdominal pressure such as coughing, laughing, walking, or lifting. The cystocele may become so pronounced that the bladder must be pushed back into place by holding the finger against the anterior vaginal wall. If the patient has a rectocele, she may complain of constipation and resultant hemorrhoids.

Older women may have suffered from these conditions for years, yet may not have sought medical attention. They may remember that their mothers had a similar condition and think that it is to be expected in women who have borne children. Since they are not incapacitated, some decide not to spend money to have reparative surgery that they know is available. Some delay seeking treatment because they dread surgery.

Displacements of the uterus may cause complications such as cervical ulceration and infection, cystitis, and hemorrhoids. Each of these conditions may require treatment.

Vaginal repair. Cystoceles and rectoceles are treated by plastic operations designed to tighten the vaginal wall. The operation is done through the vagina. The repair for a cystocele is called an *anterior colporrhaphy;* that for a rectocele, a *posterior colporrhaphy.* Old tears of the pelvic floor may also need to be repaired; such repair is called a *perineorrhaphy.*

The patient should have routine preoperative preparation, and a cleansing

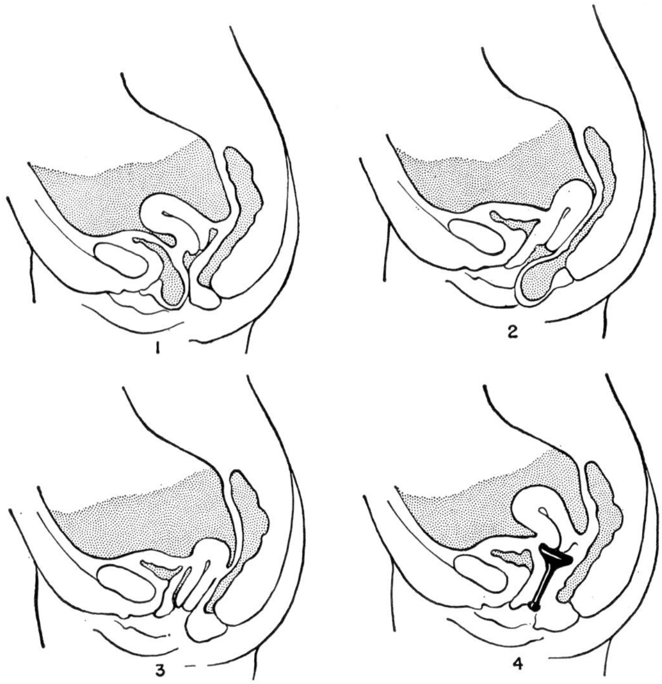

Figure 58

Abnormalities of the vagina. *1,* Cystocele—downward displacement of the bladder toward the vaginal orifice. *2,* Rectocele—pouching of the posterior wall of the vagina by the rectum. *3,* Prolapse of uterus into the vaginal canal. *4,* Stem pessary in place to maintain normal anatomic position of the uterus.

douche is frequently ordered the morning of surgery. When vaginal plastic surgery is done, postoperative nursing care includes prevention of pressure on the vaginal suture line and prevention of wound infection. Perineal dressings are seldom used. *Perineal care* is given at least twice a day and after each defecation. Sterile cotton balls moistened with benzalkonium chloride, bichloride of mercury, or normal saline solution may be used, or the patient may be placed on a douche pan and the solution poured over the perineum. Cleansing is always done away from the vagina toward the rectum so that fecal contamination is avoided. A heat lamp may be used for one hour two or three times a day to encourage healing of the perineum. The heat lamp should be used after perineal care to help dry the area and thereby prevent sloughing of tissue. If the patient complains of perineal discomfort, an ice pack applied locally helps to reduce swelling and gives relief; a rubber glove, filled with ice, firmly tied and covered, makes an adaptable pack. When sutures have been removed, sitz baths are usually ordered. Beginning on the tenth postoperative day, most doctors prescribe a daily vaginal douche with normal saline solution. Occasionally douches are ordered during the immediate postoperative period. Sterile equipment and sterile solution should then be used; the douche nozzle should be very gently inserted and very carefully rotated.

After discharge the patient who has had a vaginal repair should continue to take a daily douche and a daily tub bath. The doctor also usually orders mineral oil to be taken each night. When she returns to the clinic or to the doctor's office, she is told when to discontinue the douches and the mineral oil. The doctor also tells her when it is safe for her to resume sexual intercourse. Patients who have had vaginal repair procedures, like other patients having gynecologic surgery, need to avoid jarring activities and heavy lifting for at least six weeks postoperatively.

If a posterior colporrhaphy is scheduled, a cathartic may be given approximately twenty-four hours before surgery, and several enemas are given preoperatively to help assure an empty bowel at the time of surgery and immediately thereafter. Up to twenty-four hours preoperatively the patient may be permitted only clear liquids by mouth to further reduce bowel contents. Postoperatively the patient may be kept flat in bed or in a low Fowler's position to prevent increased intra-abdominal pressure. Special attention must be given to exercise for the patient's legs, to having her turn frequently, and to having her cough deeply. For five days only liquids are permitted by mouth, and camphorated tincture of opium (paregoric) is also given to inhibit bowel function. At the end of this time mineral oil is given each night, and an oil retention enema is given the morning after the first laxative is given. Only a soft rectal tube and small amounts of oil (200 ml.) should be used; the nurse should discourage straining to produce a bowel movement. Enemas for relieving flatus and for cleansing the bowel are not given until at least a week postoperatively.

After an anterior colporrhaphy an indwelling catheter is usually left in the bladder for about four days. The catheter should keep the bladder completely empty. If a catheter is not used and if the patient is taking sufficient fluids, voiding should be checked at least every four hours; no more than 150 ml. of urine should be allowed to accumulate in the bladder. It is usually very difficult to catheterize a patient following a vaginal repair since the urethral orifice may be distorted and edematous. Having the patient take deep breaths may help in locating the orifice because it dilates slightly with each breath. A soft rubber catheter should be used. The patient is usually allowed out of bed immediately after surgery. A regular diet is given, and mineral oil is taken each night to lessen need to strain on defecation.

Sometimes a vaginal plastic procedure does not relieve the *stress incontinence* caused by a cystocele and by general relaxation of the pelvic floor. When this happens the ligaments about the bladder neck may be shortened in such a way that the bladder drops less easily into the vagina. The degree of incontinence may be tested by filling the bladder and then having the patient cough or strain while standing over some protection on the floor. With the patient in a lithotomy position, the doctor also usually fills the bladder with normal saline solution and then supports the bladder neck with a finger or with a clamp in the vagina to test the effectiveness of the bladder with this support. If the patient can cough and strain down without being incontinent, she is considered a good candidate for the operation. The surgery is done through a suprapubic incision, and it is usually combined with further vaginal repair. A ureteral catheter is left in place, and the nursing care is similar to that following a vaginal repair.

Prolapse of the uterus. Prolapse of the uterus, or *procidentia uteri,* is a marked downward displacement of the uterus. The severity of the displacement is designated as first, second, or third degree. In a first-degree prolapse the cervix is still within the vagina; in a second-degree prolapse the cervix protrudes from the vaginal orifice; in a third-degree prolapse the entire uterus, suspended by its stretched ligaments, hangs below the vaginal orifice. In both second-degree and third-degree prolapses, the cervix becomes irritated from clothing, the circulation becomes impaired, and ulceration often follows.

The usual treatment for a uterine prolapse is hysterectomy. This may sometimes be done by the vaginal route. If any operation is contraindicated because of the age or general condition of the patient, a *Gellhorn* or *stem pessary* may be inserted to hold the uterus up in the pelvis. A string should be attached to the pessary, and after its insertion the patient should be instructed to pin the string to her underclothing. This type of pessary occasionally becomes displaced and might cause the patient embarrassment.

Vaginal fistulas

Ureterovaginal fistulas complicate gynecologic treatment rather frequently. In treating cancer of the cervix, either by radiation or panhysterectomy, the blood supply to the ureter sometimes is impaired. The ureteral wall sloughs, and a fistula opens from the ureter to the vagina. This causes a constant drip of urine through the vagina. A ureterovaginal fistula usually heals spontaneously after a period of time. If it does not, repair procedures may be attempted, or the ureter may have to be transplanted to the bowel or to the skin through an abdominal opening. (See Chapter 21.)

Vesicovaginal fistulas, or fistulas between the bladder and the vagina, may follow radiation of the cervix, gynecologic surgery, or trauma during delivery. It is impossible to perform surgery to repair the fistula until the inflammation and induration have subsided; this may take three to four months. A suprapubic incision is made into the bladder, the fistula tract is dissected out, and the defect from the bladder to the vagina is closed by primary closure or by using a graft from the bladder mucosal wall.

Postoperatively the patient usually has both a suprapubic tube and a urethral catheter in place to drain the bladder. These tubes are sometimes attached to a "bubble" suction drainage apparatus in order to assure that the bladder is kept empty (see Chapter 21). Bladder drainage is maintained for about three weeks or until the wound is completely healed. The catheters should not be irrigated unless it is absolutely necessary, and only very gentle pressure should be used when irrigating them. Signs of urinary drainage from the vagina should be noted. There is normally a small amount of serosanguineous drainage from the vagina for a few days postoperatively. Vaginal douches may be ordered and should be given very carefully. The patient is kept on bed rest for several days and then she is usually allowed to sit at the side of the bed. She must remain in her room and beside her bed if "bubble" suction is being used. Such confinement is tiring since she is not acutely uncomfortable. Visitors, television, radio, reading materials, and a variety of occupational therapy activities may help her to pass the time satisfactorily.

The results of repair operations for fistulas are not always successful. The patient must sometimes have several operations, and each successive hospitalization increases her anxiety about the outcome of surgery and lessens her reserve in accepting the discomforts and inconveniences entailed. All possible nursing measures should be taken to prevent infection and to be certain that free drainage of urine is assured. Obstruction of drainage tubes may place pressure against the newly repaired vesicovaginal wall and cause healing tissue to break down, resulting in return of the fistula.

Rectovaginal fistulas are less common than vesicovaginal fistulas but are equally, if not more, distressing to the patient. They may be due to the same causes as vesicovaginal fistulas. Surgical repair is usually done through the rectum; it may not be satisfactory, and operations may have to be repeated. The nursing care is similar to that needed by patients following surgery for other types of rectal fistulas; in addition, the patient will need sympathetic understanding and encouragement since the emotional reactions are much more severe. The constant escape of flatus and fecal material through the vagina is particularly distressing to the patient, especially so because rectovaginal fistulas are quite resistant to satisfactory surgical treatment.

The dribble of fecal material into the vagina may be temporarily lessened by

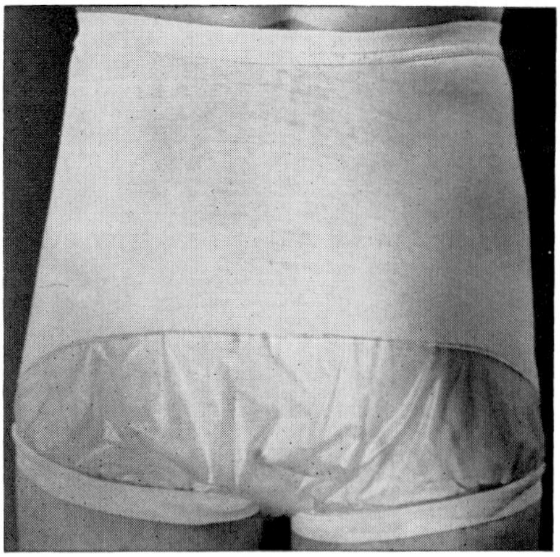

Figure 59

Pantie with plastic reinforcement of the crotch. This usually gives adequate protection to the woman with stress incontinence. (Courtesy Ferguson Manufacturing Co., Grand Rapids, Mich.)

giving a high enema, and the patient who is at home is encouraged to do this before going out. A soft rubber catheter should be used and should be directed carefully on the side of the rectum opposite the fistula. The catheter must go beyond the fistulous opening or else the fluid will return through the vagina and no benefit will be derived from the treatment. After surgery this procedure is, of course, never permitted until healing is complete; it may be used while the patient is awaiting another operation. While a constipating diet will temporarily prevent fecal material from going into the vagina, it eventually will cause pressure and may aggravate the condition and increase the size of the fistula. The patient, therefore, must be advised against restricting diet and fluids in an effort to control bowel movements.

Most patients with vesicovaginal and rectovaginal fistulas tend to become withdrawn. Occasionally, however, a patient becomes immune to the odors, and this presents a serious problem to her family. It puts a strain on family relationships at a time when the patient is desperately in need of approval and acceptance. The nurse should consult the doctor before discussing this matter with the patient. Often it is better for the doctor or nurse to bring the problem to the patient's attention than to have it mentioned by a member of the family. The nurse must then help the patient to devise means of caring for herself so that she can be assured that she is free of odor. Chlorine solution (for example, 1 teaspoonful of Clorox to 1 quart of water) makes a satisfactory deodorizing douche, and this solution is also excellent for external perineal irrigation. Sitz baths and thorough cleansing of the surrounding skin with mild soap and water are helpful. Deodorizing powders such as sodium borate can be used. Rubber pants can be worn for protection. Some large department stores now stock rubber pants for women that button at the side to avoid bulkiness (Figure 59). Rubber aprons also protect the patient from the embarrassment of soiling clothing or furniture when she is seated. Care is time-consuming and must be repeated at regular intervals to ensure cleanliness. The patient needs encouragement from the medical and nursing staff, and she needs assurance that they understand her problem. When fistulas persist, married couples have special problems which require patience and understanding. They should be encouraged to plan together a recreational and activity schedule that will help to minimize tensions until normal sexual relations can be resumed.

Tumors

Among American women, cancer of the reproductive system ranks as the second cause of death from malignant disease. It has been determined that about 70 per cent of the 33,000 women in whom a diagnosis of cancer of the cervix or body of the uterus is made each year could be cured. However, because of delay in seeking medical examination, only about 30 per cent of the lesions are discovered at a stage in which they are curable.[61]

Cancer of the cervix. The most common cancer of the female reproductive

Table 7 Cancer of the cervix

<table>
<tr><th>Classification</th><th>Involvement</th><th>Diagnosis</th><th>Treatment</th><th>Prognosis</th></tr>
<tr><td>Stage 0</td><td>Limited to mucosa of cervix with no erosion</td><td>Nonvisible; Papanicolaou smear followed by cervical biopsy which shows noninvasive cancer cells</td><td>Radium or radioactive cobalt therapy or simple hysterectomy</td><td>Curable</td></tr>
<tr><td>Stage 1</td><td>Growth confined to cervix</td><td rowspan="3">Pelvic examination reveals ulcerated growth of cervix</td><td rowspan="2">Panhysterectomy (removal of ovaries, tubes, uterus with cervix, and parametrial tissues with all regional nodes)
or
Intracavitary radium in uterus and vagina preceded or followed by x-ray therapy or radioactive cobalt therapy
or
Any combination of radical surgery, radium, radioactive cobalt therapy, or x-ray therapy</td><td>Curable, but only 10% of patients seen at this stage</td></tr>
<tr><td>Stage 2</td><td>Growth has spread to vagina or parametrium but has not reached pelvic wall</td><td>Curable, but only 30% of patients seen at this time</td></tr>
<tr><td>Stage 3</td><td>Growth has reached pelvic wall at one point so that no operation can effect its complete removal</td><td>Radium and/or pelvic evisceration (block dissection of pelvic tissue including bladder and/or rectum if indicated)
and/or
X-ray therapy or radioactive cobalt</td><td>About 40% of patients first seen at this stage; estimated 26% "5-year cure rate"*</td></tr>
<tr><td>Stage 4</td><td>Growth has invaded bladder or rectovaginal system; may have extended above pelvic brim, filling pelvis (frozen pelvis) or it may have given rise to metastasis in liver or lung</td><td>Same as above; metastatic x-ray series (lungs, spine, skull, long bones)</td><td>Same as Stage 3 if there is no evidence of distant metastasis; otherwise radium, radioactive cobalt, or x-ray therapy, supportive care</td><td>About 20% of patients first seen at this stage; estimated 5% "5-year cure rate"*</td></tr>
</table>

*A Cancer Source Book for Nurses, New York, 1950, American Cancer Society, Inc., p. 68.

system is cancer of the cervix; about 25,000 cases are diagnosed annually.[61] It usually occurs in women who have had children and who are between 30 and 50 years of age. Since 10 per cent occur in women who have not had children,[33] all women over 35 years of age should have a complete pelvic examination, including a Papanicolaou smear test, at least once a year and should seek medical attention for abnormal menses or for any abnormal vaginal bleeding or discharge.

In 1929, the Cancer Committee of the League of Nations developed for statistical study an international classification for cancer of the cervix. This classification originally ranged from Stages 1 to 4; however since the discovery of the Papanicolaou smear technique, Stage 0 has been added (see Table 7).

As shown in Table 7, the amount of tissue involved at the time of diagnosis and treatment greatly influences the prognosis. Probably one of the greatest responsibilities of the nurse is to encourage every woman over 35 years of age to have a yearly pelvic examination and to be aware of the warning signs of cancer of the cervix. If there is early diagnosis, the prognosis is excellent because the preclinical stage (Stage 0) of cancer frequently exists five to ten years before the visible Stage 1 lesion appears.[33] In the early stages the symptoms are a slight watery vaginal discharge, lengthening of the menstrual period, or occasional spotting of blood between periods. Spotting is often noticed following intercourse, after taking a douche, after defecating, or after heavy lifting.

If treatment is not instituted, the disease will advance progressively, with the vaginal discharge becoming dark, bloody, and foul smelling, due to infection and necrosis of tissue. Bladder or rectal symptoms such as fistulas or symptoms of pressure may appear. As lymph glands anterior to the sacrum become involved, back and leg pains occur from pressure on the nerves. Emaciation, anemia, and irregular fever, secondary to the local infection and tissue necrosis, may then follow. The woman with untreated cancer of the cervix has a life expectancy of from two to four years following the appearance of the cervical lesion. Death usually is caused by obstruction of the ureters, with resultant renal failure, by pelvic peritonitis, by urinary system infection, or by massive uterine hemorrhage.

Cancer of the fundus uteri. Eight thousand cases of cancer of the fundus uteri (body of the uterus) are diagnosed each year in the United States, most of them in women of their early sixties.[33] Fifty per cent of all postmenopausal bleeding is due to this.[33] If the irregular vaginal bleeding is heeded and medical attention is sought, there is a good chance of cure because malignant tumors of the body of the uterus grow slowly and metastases occur late. Since these tumors often arise from a polyp, anyone who has *uterine polyps* or who has had polyps removed from the uterus should have periodic pelvic examinations.

Cancer of the fundus may be treated by panhysterectomy or by irradiation therapy (intrauterine radium and deep x-ray therapy to the pelvis). Often, even if surgery is contemplated, intrauterine irradiation is used preoperatively to shrink the tumor and to decrease the amount of local infection so that the operation will be safer and more easily performed. Since tumors of the fundus of the uterus occur late in life, the surgical course is frequently complicated by other conditions commonly seen in geriatric patients, such as hypertension, diabetes mellitus, poor circulation, and malnutrition.

Fibroid tumors of the uterus. About 40 per cent of all women between 25 and 40 years of age develop myomas or fibroid tumors of the uterus.[42] These tumors are more prevalent in Negro women and in women who have not had children. They are benign lesions and very rarely become malignant. With the advent of the menopause, they tend to disappear spontaneously because their growth is stimulated by ovarian hormones.

Menorrhagia is the most common symptom of myomas. If the tumor is very large, it may cause pelvic circulatory congestion and may press on surrounding viscera; the patient may complain of low abdominal pressure, backache, constipation, or dysmenorrhea. If a ureter is compressed by the tumor, there may be signs and symptoms of ureteral obstruction. Sometimes the pedicle on which a myoma is growing becomes twisted, and this causes severe pain. Large tumors growing into the opening of the fallopian tubes may cause sterility; those in the body of the uterus may cause spontaneous abortions; and those near the cervical opening may make the delivery of a baby difficult.

The treatment of fibroid tumors depends upon the symptoms and the age of the patient and upon whether she wants more children and how near she is to the menopause. If the symptoms are not severe, the patient may simply need close medical supervision. If the tumor is near the surface of the uterus, a *myomectomy* (surgical removal of the tumor) may be performed. This operation leaves the muscle walls of the uterus relatively intact. If there is severe bleeding or obstruction, a *hysterectomy* (surgical removal of the uterus) is usually necessary. Occasionally, if surgery is contraindicated or if the patient is approaching the menopause, x-ray therapy or radiation is used to reduce the size of the tumor and to stop vaginal bleeding.

Cancer of the ovary. Although about 80 per cent of all ovarian tumors are benign, most gynecologists believe that all patients suspected of having tumors of the ovary should have an exploratory abdominal operation.[33] This is because malignant tumors of the ovary usually give no symptoms until local metastasis occurs and there is ascites from increased pressure within the portal system, edema of the legs from pressure on veins passing through the pelvic cavity, or pain in the back or the legs from pressure on nerves, or until there are symptoms of distant metastasis. The silent onset and growth of ovarian tumors almost surely doom the patient in whom diagnosis is not made prior to onset of symptoms. The only effective means of assuring early diagnosis is a pelvic examination every six months, including careful ovarian palpation, and surgical exploration of any questionable ovarian growth. If possible, the ovary and the tumor are completely removed at operation. If the tumor is malignant, the operation often is followed by deep x-ray therapy.

Benign tumors of the ovary. Benign tumors of the ovary may cause changes in the secondary sex characteristics. One type produces marked feminizing characteristics, precocious menstruation, resumption of menstruation after the menopause, or prolongation of the menopause. Another type causes development of male characteristics, such as voice changes, male distribution of hair on the face and body, flattening of the breasts, and cessation of menstruation. Symptoms can be relieved by surgical removal of the tumor.

Ovarian cysts. The most common ovarian growth is a cyst of the graafian follicle or corpus luteum; this usually reabsorbs spontaneously. There are, however, other types of ovarian cysts arising from various types of tissue. Some are partly solid, such as the *dermoid cyst,* which may contain skin, hair, teeth, and bone. Others grow very large and cause distortion of the abdomen. Ovarian cysts are surgically removed; this usually includes an *oophorectomy* (removal of the ovary).

Sometimes an ovarian cyst twists on the pedicle which carries its blood supply. This causes sudden, sharp pain and shock. An emergency oophorectomy is done since without blood supply the tissues rapidly become necrotic.

Endometrial cysts. Endometrial or chocolate cysts of the ovary are of very serious consequence. The cysts are lined with endometrium similar to that lining the uterus. With the monthly hormone cycle, these patches of endometrium, as well as the endometrial lining of the uterus, menstruate. Since the blood cannot drain to the outside, the cysts become filled with the blood and eventually rupture and seed endometrial tissue through the pelvis.

Endometriosis. The widespread growth of endometrial tissue throughout the pelvis is known as endometriosis. As the tissue bleeds into the pelvis each month, it causes such severe adhesion formation that the pelvic organs may become fused together. The patient has recurrent pain and fullness in the lower abdomen beginning and ending with the menstrual period and may become a chronic invalid.

If the woman is young and wants to have children, the treatment for endometriosis is usually as conservative as possible. Pregnancy is beneficial because the hormone cycle is interrupted. If a young married woman has endometriosis, the couple is usually advised to have their family without delay since sterility due to adhesions frequently occurs. When the involvement is severe, a *panhysterectomy* (removal of the uterus with the cervix, the tubes, and ovaries) may be necessary to remove the diseased tissue and the ovarian hormones. Removal of the ovaries prevents further bleeding of endometrial implants that cannot be removed. The menopause cures this condition, and removal of the ovaries produces a surgical menopause. The menopausal symptoms may be quite severe for some time, but they are seldom treated with female hormones; sedative drugs are usually used.

Cancer of the vulva. Cancer of the vulva is seen most often in women over 60 years of age who have *chronic leukoplakia of the vulva.* The skin appears white and thickened, itches, and is easily fissured. In women approaching 60 years of age some doctors recommend a *vulvectomy,* or surgical excision of the vulva, to prevent the development of cancer. If cancer is already present, the treatment is also vulvectomy; however, in addition, *bilateral inguinal node dissection* may be done, and deep x-ray therapy may be used. If there is no node involvement, 50 per cent of those with cancer of the vulva can be cured.[33] Patients with cancer of the vulva are often poor operative risks because of concurrent medical conditions related to age.

Kraurosis vulvae. Another condition seen in older women, kraurosis vulvae, causes a shrinking of the skin of the vulva. The skin is shiny and thin and itches severely. Kraurosis vulvae is not a precancerous condition, but it sometimes requires surgery because adhesions may interfere with voiding and with sexual intercourse. Occasionally female hormones are given, and local injections of alcohol may be tried to relieve the pruritus.

Nursing the patient having a vulvectomy and inguinal node dissection

The patient who had a vulvectomy has some special nursing needs in addition to routine preoperative and postoperative care. Preoperatively she is given enemas, and postoperatively she is given a low-residue diet. These measures obviate the need for straining to defecate and help prevent contamination of the vulval wound. A Foley catheter usually is used to provide urinary drainage. When the catheter is removed, the patient may be unable to void due to difficulty in relaxing the perineum; sitz baths may help.

The vulval wound is frequently left exposed, but if a dressing is used, it should be held in place with a T-binder. The wound is cleansed twice a day with solutions such as peroxide, normal saline solution, benzalkonium chloride, or other antiseptic solutions. Following this, a heat lamp is used to dry the area. The heat also improves local circulation, thus stimulating healing. If the inguinal nodes have been dissected, a heat lamp may also be directed to the groins. After all the sutures are removed, hot sitz baths may be substituted for the heat lamp.

Large amounts of tissue are removed from the vulva and the groins during the operation, and the sutures are usually quite taut. This leads to severe discomfort, and the patient will usually need analgesic medication at frequent intervals during the two or three weeks before sutures can be removed. Following an inguinal node dissection, pillows need to be arranged to prevent undue pulling on the taut inguinal sutures when the patient moves. If the patient is lying on her side, she will be more comfortable if her upper leg is supported by a pillow. If she is lying on her back, a low Fowler's position puts less tension on the sutures. The wounds heal slowly, and the patient may become quite discouraged. Diversional occupations and socializing with other patients may help to keep the patient from thinking too much about herself and help her to pass the time. Privacy should be assured, and women should be encouraged to express their feelings concerning this disfiguring surgery. Some women feel that their femininity has been irreparably damaged or that this may really end their sexual life. By the time the patient is discharged, the wounds are usually healed and the convalescence will be similar to that following any surgical procedure. After several weeks, sexual intercourse, for the married patient, can usually be resumed.

Nursing the patient receiving radium therapy

Radium is used to treat cancer of the cervix and cancer of the body of the uterus because of the accessibility of the cervix and body of the uterus. Radium gives off three types of rays—alpha, beta, and gamma; the gamma rays are the ones used for treatment. Since the alpha and beta rays cause sloughing, the normal tissue must be protected from them. The glass capsules in which the radioactive substances are sealed stop the alpha rays, and the adjacent tissue is protected from beta rays by two means: (1) the incorporation of the glass capsules inside brass, platinum, or silver capsules covered by rubber and (2) the use of "distance screening," which means keeping normal tissues away from the radioactive rays. This is accomplished by giving the patient a cleansing enema prior to the instillation of the radioactive substance, by keeping her on a low-residue diet to prevent distention of the bowel, by constantly draining the bladder with a catheter, and by placing gauze packing in the vagina to push both the rectum and the bladder away from the area being irradiated. To prevent any displacement of the radioactive substance, the patient is kept flat in bed and is only allowed to turn from side to side. A roentgenogram is taken after the radium is inserted to determine its exact location.

Radium may be placed in various types of applicators. However the colpostat and intrauterine applicators are most commonly used. (See Figure 60.) The amount of radioactive substance used and the number of hours it is left in place are determined by the amount of radiation needed to kill the young less stable cancer cells without damaging normal cells. Radium must be removed at exactly the indicated time, and the nurse is often responsible for reminding the doctor to do this. If possible the time of insertion should be planned so that removal will be at a convenient hour, e.g., not in the middle of the night or during visiting hours.

Care must be taken that no radium is displaced or lost. Sutures or strings attached to the applicators should be anchored to the thigh with adhesive tape. Before bedpans are emptied and before linen is placed in hampers, they should be carefully inspected. If radioactive substance accidentally is expelled, it must be handled at arm's length with a sponge forceps, and it should be held above the waist to prevent irradiation of the ovaries or testicles of workers. It should be put in a covered metal container, well labeled, in an isolated part of the patient's unit until the lead-lined radon cart is obtained. The doctor must, of course, be notified at once if radioactive substance is accidentally expelled. (See Chapter 16 for further discussion of the handling of radium.)

Since the presence of *anything* in the cervix stimulates uterine contractions, the patient who has a colpostat or intrauterine applicator in place may have severe uterine contractions as a result of dilatation of the cervix. The patient should know that this will occur. Often a narcotic is given at

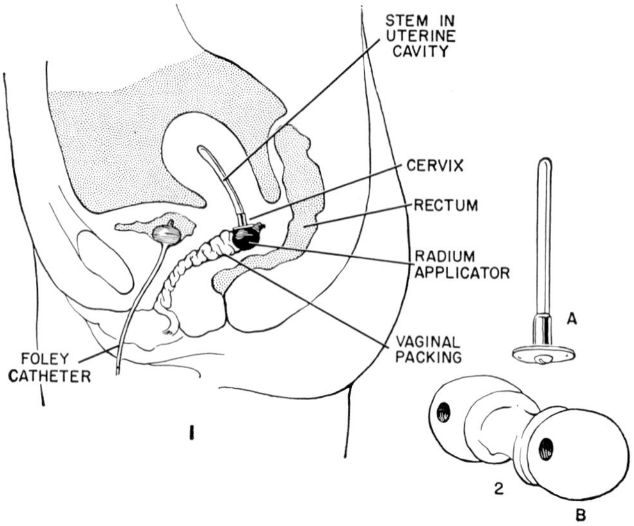

Figure 60

1, Radium applicator in place in the uterus. Note that a Foley catheter is used to decompress the bladder and the vaginal packing. *2, A,* Intrauterine applicator; *B,* colpostat.

regular intervals while the applicator is in place. There will be foul-smelling vaginal discharge from destruction of cells. Good perineal care is essential, and it must be remembered that since the patient must lie on her back, she cannot do this herself. A deodorizer is helpful.

Patients may develop radiation sickness, with nausea and vomiting, diarrhea, malaise, and fever. This is a systemic reaction to the breakdown and reabsorption of cell proteins. (See Chapter 16 for further discussion.) Camphorated tincture of opium (paregoric) helps relieve the diarrhea; if it is severe, a cornstarch enema (1 tablespoonful of cornstarch to 250 ml. of lukewarm water) may be ordered. Oil retention enemas are also sometimes given. The patient is urged to drink at least 3,000 ml. of fluid a day to help relieve any irritation of the urinary system.

Since the woman who is receiving radiation treatment usually either knows or suspects the diagnosis, she is likely to be depressed. While she is in bed, the nurse should plan to spend some time talking with her. If the nurse is not actually giving physical care to the patient, however, she should stand at a distance of at least four feet to prevent unnecessary exposure to radioactive rays. If she explains to the patient that this precaution is necessary because nurses are in frequent contact with radioactive material, and if she really takes time to talk to her while remaining at a safe distance, the patient usually will not feel neglected. Close members of the family should be encouraged to visit.

When the radioactive applicators are to be removed, the following equipment is needed: a lead-lined radon carrier, sterile gloves, two sterile long-handled forceps and two bowls—one containing soap and water and a gauze sponge and the other containing peroxide and a gauze sponge. As the applicators are removed by the doctor, they should be washed in peroxide and then in soap and water before being returned to the carrier. The loaded applicators should be handled only with long-handled forceps. Rubber gloves should be used, and the material should be kept above waist level.

Following the removal of the applicators, the catheter is removed, a cleansing enema is given, and the patient is allowed out of bed. Vaginal discharge will continue for some time. The patient may need to take douches for as long as the odor and vaginal discharge persist; usually douches are ordered twice a day. The patient who is returning home needs detailed instruction in how to give herself douches after this treatment and what solutions to use. Some vaginal bleeding may occur for from one to three months after irradiation of the cervix or body of the uterus. If the rectal irritation persists, the patient who is at home should report this to the doctor; emollient enemas may be prescribed to be taken at home. The patient is usually discharged from the hospital within a day or two after the applicators are removed but may return for another course of radiation.

Complications to watch for following radiation of the uterus are vesicovaginal fistulas, rectovaginal fistulas, ureterovaginal fistulas, cystitis, phlebitis, and hemorrhage. Each is due to irritation and destruction of adjacent tissue either by the x-rays or by extension of the disease process. The patient is urged to report even minor symptoms or complaints to her doctor.

If the patient is treated by x-ray therapy for a lesion of the reproductive system, the care is the same as that given a patient receiving this treatment elsewhere in the body. However, one important point should be emphasized: the patient should always void immediately before the treatment to prevent damage to the bladder.

Nursing the patient who must have all or part of the female reproductive system removed

Surgery such as a bilateral oophorectomy or a hysterectomy upsets most women emotionally. All women worry about the effect it will have on their feminity and wonder about possible changes in secondary sex characteristics. Young women may feel bitterly disappointed because they can no longer have children. Some women worry about gaining weight, although weight gain is more often due to overeating than to hormone changes. It is true that the childbearing function will be terminated, but the vagina is intact so that several weeks following surgery married women can resume normal sexual intercourse.

Older patients are usually less upset by the prospects of surgery of this kind than are those who have not reached the menopause. Postoperatively, however, almost all patients feel weepy and "blue" for several days. This apparently is due to a change in hormonal balance and to psychologic reaction. The patient often is unable to explain why she is depressed and crying. During this period, she needs understanding and sympathetic care since she may appear somewhat unreasonable at times. Families need to be helped to accept these unusual responses calmly, and a husband may need to reassure the patient repeatedly of his love and affection.

If a hysterectomy is to be performed, the preoperative physical preparation is the same as that for any other abdominal surgery, except that the perineum is completely shaved. A vaginal douche may be given. Postoperatively the patient has an abdominal dressing and wears a perineal pad. If a vaginal hysterectomy is performed, there will be no abdominal incision, but sterile perineal pads will need frequent changing. The dressings should be observed for any sign of bleeding every fifteen minutes for two hours and then at least every hour for eight hours; there is normally a moderate amount of serosanguineous drainage. The perineal pad should be held in place with a T-binder, and some doctors prefer that a snug scultetus binder be applied to the abdomen, especially if there has been a *radical hysterectomy* (removal of the ovaries, tubes, uterus with the cervix, and

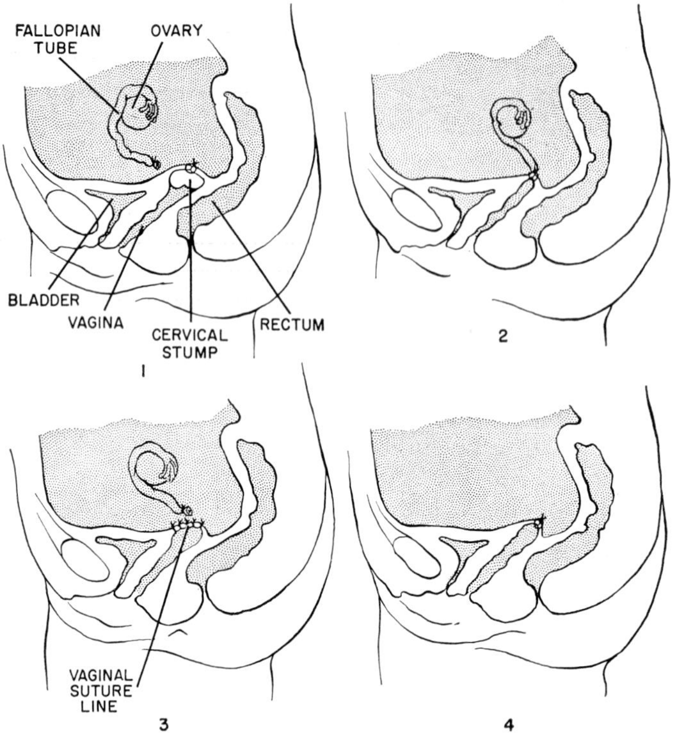

Figure 61

1, Cross section of a subtotal hysterectomy. Note that the cervical stump, fallopian tubes and ovaries remain. *2,* Cross section showing total hysterectomy. Note that the fallopian tubes and ovaries remain. *3,* Cross section showing a vaginal hysterectomy. Note that the fallopian tubes and overies remain. *4,* Cross section showing a panhysterectomy. Note that the uterus, fallopian tubes, and ovaries are completely removed.

parametrial tissue) and extensive node dissection. (See Figure 61.)

Following a hysterectomy, especially one in which there has been extensive node and parametrial resection, the bladder may be temporarily atonic as a result of nerve trauma. A Foley catheter is used to maintain constant drainage of the bladder. If no catheter is used and if the patient is unable to void within eight hours, she is usually catheterized. The catheter (if used) is removed on the third or fourth postoperative day, and the patient is catheterized for residual urine every six to eight hours until less than 100 ml. of residual urine is obtained for three consecutive times. This procedure is usually routinely ordered for patients having pelvic surgery.

Abdominal distention frequently complicates a hysterectomy. It is caused by nerve damage or by sudden release of pressure on the intestines such as occurs on removal of a large myoma. Some doctors insert a stomach tube prophylactically following surgery, and most doctors restrict food and fluids by mouth for from twenty-four to forty-eight hours. There is usually an order for a rectal tube and for a heating pad to the abdomen to be used as necessary. If the surgery has been extensive, a soft rectal tube should be selected to prevent trauma to the bowel. A carminative enema is usually given on the second or third day postoperatively. When peristalsis returns, the patient is started slowly on fluids. Many physicians restrict fruit juices and milk in an attempt to prevent flatus. A regular diet is usually tolerated by the fourth postoperative day.

There may be interference with circulation during hysterectomy, and thrombophlebitis of the vessels of the pelvis and upper thigh is a rather common complication. The patient should never rest with the knees bent or with the thighs sharply flexed. Many doctors request that the knee gatch not be used and that the bed not be raised at the head to more than a mid-Fowler's position. The patient should exercise her feet and legs every hour, and she should move about in bed, turning from her side to her back and to a partial face-lying position. A pillow can be used to support the abdominal wound. The head of the bed should be put completely flat for a short time every two hours. These precautions help prevent stasis of blood in the pelvic vessels. If the patient has varicosities, the doctor may order elevation of the legs for a few minutes every two or three hours to permit blood to drain from the legs. Ace bandages may be ordered to be applied from the toes to the groin. These should be reapplied twice a day to assure a snug, even pressure. The patient often is permitted out of bed the day following the operation. Other nursing care is the same as that following any abdominal surgery. Special attention should be given to any complaint of low back pain or to lessened urinary output since it is possible that a ureter could have been accidentally ligated. Very occasionally, the ureter, the bladder, or the rectum is traumatized.

The patient should know what surgery has been done, what changes in herself she should expect, and what care she needs when she leaves the hospital. If a *total hysterectomy* has been done, she will not menstruate. A *subtotal hysterectomy,* however, permits menses to continue, since a portion of the uterus with its endometrial lining is left. She should not have sexual intercourse until told by the doctor that it may be safely resumed. Most patients are more comfortable if they wear a girdle. Heavy lifting should be avoided for about two months. Jarring activities such as riding over rough roads, walking swiftly, and dancing tend to cause congestion of blood in the pelvis and should be avoided for several months. Other physical activity which does not cause strain, such as swimming, may be engaged in since it is helpful both for the physical and mental well-being of the patient.

The patient who has a *unilateral salpingectomy* (removal of one fallopian tube) or a *unilateral oophorectomy* usually requires postoperative nursing care similar to that given any patient having abdominal surgery. If the surgery is done to remove a large ovarian cyst, however, the patient may have considerable abdominal distention due to the sudden release of pressure on the intestines; the care is similar to that given for distention following a hysterectomy. If the surgery is done to remove a tumor which has caused changes in sex characteristics, the patient is usually quite sensitive and needs much understanding and encouragement from the nurse. She may shun others prior to surgery, and it is wise to let her have privacy if she so desires. She may be reassured following surgery that the abnormal sexual changes will gradually disappear. If the patient seems to withdraw from contact with others the nurse should spend extra time with her provided she seems receptive to the nurse's interest.

The patient who has a *bilateral oophorectomy* or *radiation treatment of the ovaries* has specific problems. Although immediate preoperative and postoperative nursing needs are no different from those needed by the patient with other abdominal surgery, she will have an emotional reaction to being sterile that will need consideration; the extent of this reaction depends upon her age, whether or not she already has or wants children, and her emotional make-up. She also will have symptoms of the climacteric. When the menopause is artificially induced, the symptoms are often more severe than in the normal climacteric; therefore, at least a portion of an ovary is left unless this is detrimental to the patient's prognosis. Estrogens relieve the symptoms and may be given to most patients unless surgery has been done for a malignancy. The period of adjustment after a bilateral oophorectomy is long and is often trying not only for the patient but also for her family.

A bilateral oophorectomy may be done primarily to remove the estrogen supply. This procedure is now used quite frequently in conjunction with radical mastectomy for cancer of the breast.

Nursing care for the patient who has a *pelvic exenteration* (all reproductive organs and adjacent tissue removed) includes the care given the patient having a hysterectomy, the care given the patient having an abdominal perineal resection of the bowel, and the care given the patient having a cystectomy with transplantation of the ureters to the skin, since this operation includes a radical hysterectomy, pelvic node dissection, cystectomy, vaginectomy, and a rectal resection. This surgery requires unusual physical, social, and emotional adjustments on the part of the patient. The patient will have undergone extensive surgery which temporarily upsets the circulation and causes hormonal and electrolyte imbalance; both urine and feces must pass from the body through new openings in the abdominal wall; the patient cannot contemplate having children and cannot have sexual intercourse; and she will have symptoms of the menopause. Until she is able to accept her situation realistically, her rehabilitation will progress very slowly. This acceptance cannot be forced upon the patient, but she must be encouraged gradually to resume self-care. She will undoubtedly have recurring periods of depression and discouragement. She should be helped to express her feelings and be given ample time and consideration by the nurse in order to do this. The family should understand what the surgery will entail, and they, too, need encouragement. Acceptance of the situation by the patient's husband is a very important factor in giving her the reassurance and courage necessary to face her future. The knowledge that other patients have been depressed and that this is expected helps some patients through periods when life seems futile. The nurse needs to be a good listener. She must seek help from the patient's family, the social worker, the doctor, and the patient's spiritual adviser as she thinks necessary. The family needs guidance in accepting the patient's moods and in giving her moral support. They, too, may need to talk to persons outside the family.

Nursing the patient with incurable disease of the female reproductive system

The patient with incurable disease of the female reproductive system frequently has a lingering terminal illness. Most cancers of the female reproductive system do not metastasize to vital areas, such as the liver; by direct spread they eventually cause death from carcinomatosis and from kidney failure that results from obstruction of both ureters by the tumor.

The nursing management is the same as that for any patient with a terminal illness, but there are some special things that help to make the patient more comfortable. Frequent changes of position help relieve abdominal and pelvic pressure. Alternate hot and cold applications to the abdomen may bring some relief from pain. Often the use of these measures and the prescription of mild analgesics such as acetylsalicylic acid keep the patient comfortable for an indeterminate period of time. Use of narcotics is delayed as long as possible. However, now that synthetic narcotics are available, it is possible to change from one to another and thus lessen danger of addiction or of too much dependence on one drug. Most physicians believe that the patient should receive analgesics for severe pain and should be kept relatively comfortable. A chordotomy for relief from pain is sometimes necessary. (See Chapter 34.)

The vaginal discharge is usually profuse and has a foul odor. This is upsetting to the patient, her family, and her friends.

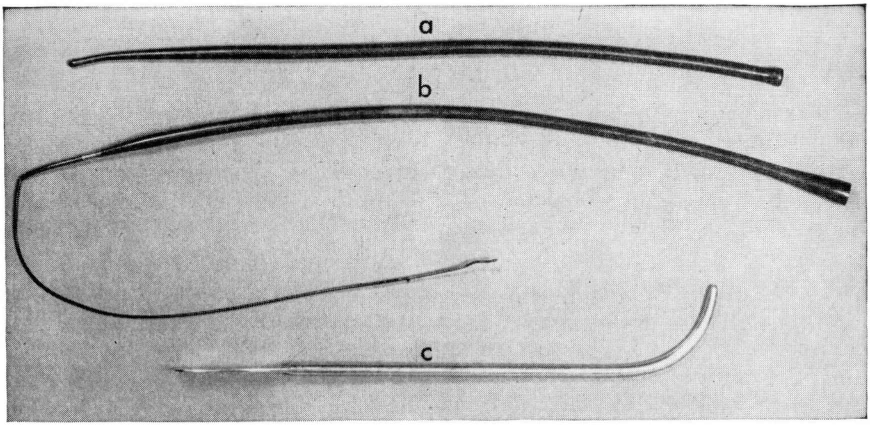

Figure 62

a, Bougie for urethral dilatation. *b,* Filiform. Note the long, fine, flexible tip. *c,* Metal sound for urethral dilatation.

The most effective means of decreasing the odor is to give the patient perineal care every four hours and to give a cleansing douche at least twice daily. Copious amounts of water should be used. Solutions containing chlorine are useful in destroying odors, and aromatic trade preparations added to the water may make the patient feel cleaner and more acceptable.

Meticulous care must be given to the skin since the patient is usually emaciated and may develop pitting edema. If the patient has ascites, she may rest better if the head of the bed is elevated. (For further discussion of the care of the terminally ill cancer patient see Chapter 16.)

Nursing related to disease of the male reproductive system

The nurse must be particularly aware of the reactions and feelings of male patients who have disease of the reproductive system. She should not hesitate to ask the doctor to discuss with the patient any problems that can best be handled by him.

Infections

Nonspecific pyogenic organisms, as well as specific organisms such as gonococci and tubercle bacilli, may cause stubborn infections of the male reproductive system. Urethritis, prostatitis, seminal vesiculitis, and epididymitis are the most common infections. Infections of the reproductive system may also be blood or lymph borne.

Men should not be catheterized unless it is absolutely necessary. Because of the length and curvature of the male urethra, some trauma to the urethral mucosa is likely to accompany catheterization or the passage of instruments such as a cystoscope. This trauma makes the area susceptible to bacterial attack. Since the urethra is not sterile, infection ensues and readily passes into the prostatic urethra. Every means should be used to help them void normally; they are often allowed to stand to void even when they are to be on bed rest otherwise. Fluids should be given liberally following passage of instruments through the urethra. (See Figure 62.)

Nonspecific urethritis. Nonspecific urethritis is an inflammation of the urethra caused by such organisms as staphylococci, *Escherichia coli,* Pseudomonas, and streptococci. Although the symptoms and complications are essentially the same as those of gonorrheal urethritis, this infection is rarely caused by sexual contact. The patient complains of urgency, frequency, and burning on urination. There may be a purulent urethral discharge. (See Chapter 17 for discussion of gonorrheal urethritis.)

Treatment of nonspecific urethritis consists of antibiotics and chemotherapy, hot sitz baths, and increased fluid intake. To drain periurethral glands, the urethra may be dilated with sounds. Dilatation is followed by the instillation of a mild antiseptic such as 1:10,000 silver nitrate solution. Physical rest, improvement of general health, and decreased sexual activity are usually suggested. Nonspecific urethritis is difficult to eliminate and may become a chronic problem which ultimately results in chronic prostatitis.

Prostatitis. The patient with prostatitis usually has acute symptoms of urinary obstruction; he suddenly has difficulty in voiding, perineal tenderness and pain, and elevation of temperature. Treatment is usually conservative; i.e., antibiotics and chemotherapy, forcing fluids, physical rest, and local application of heat by sitz baths and/or low rectal irrigations.

Before giving a *rectal irrigation,* the patient should have a cleansing enema. Then, using a Y connector on the rectal tube, tap water is allowed to flow alternately in and out of the rectum. Using 2,000 ml. of water 46° C. (115° F.) and inserting the tube only three to four inches into the rectum heat will be concentrated in the area of the prostate.

Prompt treatment of prostatitis may obviate the need for an indwelling catheter. Occasionally *prostatic abscesses* complicate the clinical course. These may have to be drained surgically. Recurrent episodes of acute prostatitis may cause fibrotic tissue to form, and a prostatectomy may be necessary to relieve the resultant obstruction. (See Chapter 21.)

Epididymitis. Epididymitis, one of the most common infections of the male reproductive system, may be caused by any pyogenic organism, but it frequently is a complication of gonorrhea or of tuberculosis of the urinary system. The patient complains of severe tenderness, pain, and swelling of the scrotum, which is hot to the touch. His temperature may be markedly elevated, and he has general malaise. He often walks with a charactertistic "duck waddle" in an attempt to protect the affected part. It is by this sign that the observant nurse may first detect difficulty in the patient who is too embarrassed to describe his trouble. The patient with a tuberculous infection frequently develops a *scrotal fistula.*

The patient with epididymitis is usually put to bed and the scrotum elevated either on towel rolls or with adhesive strapping. Ice is used to help reduce the swelling and to relieve the pain and discomfort. Heat is usually contraindicated because the normal temperature of the scrotal contents is below normal body temperature, and excessive exposure to heat may cause destruction of sperm cells. If an icecap is used, it should be placed under the scrotum and should be removed for short intervals every hour to prevent ice burns. Antibiotic therapy is given; at least three quarts of fluid should be taken daily. When the patient is allowed out of bed, he should wear a scrotal support.

Patients with *tuberculous epididymitis* are placed on a tuberculosis regimen (see Chapters 21 and 23). If they have a draining fistula, contamination of others with the drainage must be prevented.

Since bilateral epididymitis usually causes *sterility,* special attention is given to the prevention of this infection. Untreated epididymitis leads rather rapidly to necrosis of testicular tissue and septicemia because the blood supply is obstructed by the swelling. Men in whom a catheter is necessary for bladder drainage over a long period of time will usually require a cystotomy so urine can be drained directly from the bladder through a cystostomy tube.

An older patient who must have surgery of the prostate that will require leaving a urethral catheter in place for a long time may be advised to first have a *bilateral vasectomy* to prevent any infection descending via the vas deferens to the epididymis. Since this procedure sterilizes the patient, it is not done on a young man. Permission must be granted by the patient. The vasectomies are done through two very small incisions in the scrotum or in the groins. Often the operation is done prior to any cystoscopic examination. Local anesthesia is used. Postoperatively the patient should still be watched for symptoms of epididymitis, since the organisms may have invaded the epididymis prior to the vasectomy. Prevention of epididymitis is discussed also in Chapter 8.

Phimosis. Phimosis is a condition in which the opening of the prepuce is too small to allow it to be retracted behind the glans penis. It may be congenital or acquired. In the adult it is frequently associated with the edema and inflammation caused by *balanitis,* an infection of the glans penis. It is treated by *circumcision*—the surgical excision of the prepuce.

Following *circumcision,* the patient may have a petroleum jelly gauze dressing over the penis. The patient is usually taught to change the dressing which must be changed after each voiding. Excessive bleeding may occur; therefore a pressure dressing may be used. This dressing may elevate the penis, but it usually can be removed by the time the patient needs to void. It should be replaced by a petroleum jelly dressing. The patient should be given petroleum jelly dressings to use at home until the wound is well healed. Frequently adults are given an estrogen preparation for several days postoperatively to prevent penile erections.

In *paraphimosis,* the foreskin cannot be reduced after it has been retracted behind the glans, and the penis is constricted. This condition is frequently associated with an infection of the glans. The prepuce usually can be forcefully reduced, and then a circumcision is done to prevent recurrence and to provide for easier eradication of the infection in the glans penis.

Orchitis. An infection of the testicle is known as orchitis. It may be caused by pyogenic bacteria, the gonococci, or the tubercle bacilli, or it may be a complication of mumps contracted after puberty. Although the latter occurs in a relatively small percentage of the cases, it usually causes sterility. Any boy or man who is exposed to mumps after puberty should receive gamma globulin immediately unless he has already had the disease. If there is any doubt, the vaccine should be given. Although the vaccine may not prevent mumps, the disease is likely to be less severe.

The symptoms and the treatment of orchitis are the same as those of epididymitis. Stilbestrol and cortisone, as well as antibiotics, may be given.

Scrotal and testicular enlargement

Immediate medical attention should be sought for any swelling of the scrotum or the testicles within it. Scrotal enlargements should be diagnosed—not treated symptomatically with suspensories which give relief and encourage procrastination.

Hydrocele. A painless swelling of the scrotum may be due to a condition known as hydrocele. This is a benign collection of fluid within the tunica vaginalis, and the cause is usually unknown. Occasionally it is treated by aspirating the fluid and injecting a sclerosing drug such as urea hydrochloride into the scrotal sac, but excision of the tunica vaginalis (hydrocelectomy) is the preferred treatment. Postoperatively a pressure dressing is applied on the scrotum, which is elevated. The patient should be observed carefully for any symptoms of hemorrhage; bleeding may not be external. The patient needs a scrotal support when he is up and about, and may still require one after he is discharged from the hospital. He should have two scrotal suspensories since they should be washed each day. Immediately after operation or following an infection, most patients require an extra large suspensory or perhaps a jockey strap.

Testicular neoplasm. Cancer of the testicle is usually painless, but it may be accompanied by an aching or dragging sensation in the groin and by swelling of the testicle. The swelling is frequently first discovered by the patient following trauma, but it usually is not caused by the trauma. Testicular swelling should always make one suspicious of neoplasm of the testicle. This condition is usually seen in men between 25 and 35 years of age, but it causes only about 1 per cent of the deaths from malignant growths in men.[33]

An *undescended testicle* is much more likely to become malignant than one that is in the scrotum at birth or descends shortly thereafter. This is an important reason for encouraging parents to consent to surgical intervention to bring down a testicle of a young boy. This does not decrease the possibility of a neoplasm, but the testicle is located in a position where it may be examined carefully and regularly.

Men with suspicious testicular swelling are asked to collect a first-voided morning urine specimen. This is sent for an Aschheim-Zondek test, the same test used to detect pregnancy in women. One type of testicular tumor, the one with the poorest prognosis, gives a positive Aschheim-Zondek reaction. For all types of testicular tumors, the testicle is surgically removed (orchiectomy) and the adjacent area is explored for metastatic node involvement. The prognosis is poor since there is often widespread metastasis before the initial lesion is discovered.

The patient with cancer of the testicle is usually given a course of x-ray therapy, and a *radical node dissection* may be done. This dissection may be unilateral or bilateral and a thoracoabdominal incision is used.

Following a radical node dissection, there is danger of hemorrhage. Active movement may be contraindicated since nodes may have been resected from around many large abdominal vessels, but gentle passive turning and leg and arm movement are essential to prevent postoperative pneumonia and thrombosis. Deep breathing should be encouraged at hourly intervals. A turning sheet and a chest support are usually helpful. The patient is extremely uncomfortable and needs frequent and large doses of narcotics and sedative drugs.

When a radical node dissection is done, the patient may be placed in a Trendelenburg position for two weeks to allow the kidney to become fixed in place, since frequently all the fatty tissue supporting it must be removed. The patient may need to be fed and bathed during this period. He may have difficulty voiding in this position; for defecation, permission from the doctor may have to be obtained to lower the foot of the bed. Occupational and diversional therapy should be provided. Since many patients find it impossible even to read in the Trendelenburg position, they may appreciate being read to, having the use of books that can be projected on the ceiling, or having access to talking books used for the blind.

Since x-ray therapy is begun the day after surgery, the patient may develop radiation sickness during his hospital stay.

Patients and their families are extremely upset by the diagnosis of neoplasm of the testicle. The doctor frequently is quite frank with the family and with the patient because he believes the man needs to be able to make necessary arrangements to provide for his family. The patient's prognosis may be measured in only months or in several years. Some patients are openly depressed; others seem to be "taking it too well." The nurse should listen carefully to both the patient and his family and, if it is indicated, suggest that help be obtained from others, such as the social worker or spiritual adviser. A psychiatric consultant may be able to help the nurse give realistic support to the patient and his family.

Spermatocele. A spermatocele is a nontender cystic mass containing sperm; it is attached to the epididymis. Because excision may cause sterility, the man is usually advised to wear a scrotal support to prevent undue discomfort until after he has a family. Large masses may then be excised.

Varicocele. A varicocele is a dilatation of the spermatic vein and is commonly seen on the left side only, probably because the left spermatic vein is much longer than the right. A varicocele on the right side only is suggestive of an abdominal tumor. The use of a scrotal support is usually all that is necessary to relieve any dragging sensation, but the spermatic vein may be ligated.

Torsion of the testicle. Torsion of the testicle or kinking of the spermatic artery causes severe pain, tenderness, and swelling of the testicle. It often follows activity that puts a sudden pull on the cremasteric muscle such as may occur from jumping into cold water. Operative intervention may be indicated and must be done within a few hours in order to maintain fertility because the blood supply to the testicle is interrupted.

Cancer of the prostate

On autopsy examination, from 15 to 20 per cent of all men past 50 years of age have been found to have microscopic carcinoma of the prostate. Although many of these men did not have clinical symptoms, it is known that the incidence of clinical cancer of the prostate increases with increasing age. With an increase in life expectancy, the incidence of cancer of of the prostate probably will increase.[79]

Cancer of the prostate is most often diagnosed when the patient seeks medical advice because of symptoms of prostatic obstruction or because of "sciatica" or low back, hip, and leg pains. Cancer of the prostate frequently occurs with benign prostatic hypertrophy with obstruction, or the cancer itself may be so far advanced as to cause obstruction. Back and leg pains usually indicate bony metastasis.

Since cancer of the prostate which causes obstruction of the urethra or back and leg pains may be too far advanced for curative treatment, one can readily understand the need for men past 40 years of age to have routine rectal examinations. Most carcinomas of the prostate are adjacent to the rectal wall and thus can be detected by rectal examination.

It is usually the lesions that are detected prior to symptoms that can be cured. A biopsy should be taken of suspicious masses (see page 390 for a discussion of prostatic biopsies).

An elevated acid phosphatase blood level is indicative of cancer of the prostate, but, since the acid phosphatase produced by prostatic cancer is not absorbed by the blood until the lesion has extended beyond the prostatic capsule, it is not a useful technique for early diagnosis.

In patients in whom a diagnosis is made prior to local extension of the cancer or metastasis, a *radical resection of the prostate* usually is curative. The entire prostate, including the capsule and the adjacent tissue, is removed. The remaining urethra is then anastomosed to the bladder neck. Since the internal and external sphincters of the bladder lie in close approximation to the prostate, it is not unusual for the patient to have urinary incontinence following this type of surgery. He also will be both impotent and sterile. The perineal approach is most often used, but the procedure may be accomplished by the retropubic route. (See Figure 48.)

The patient returns from surgery with a urethral catheter in place. A large amount of urinary drainage on the dressing for a number of hours is not unusual. This should rapidly decrease, however. There should not be the amount of bleeding which follows other prostatic surgery and, since the catheter is not being used for hemostasis, the patient usually has little bladder spasm. The catheter is used both for urinary drainage and as a splint for the urethral anastomosis; therefore, care should be taken that it does not become dislodged or blocked. The catheter is usually left in place for two or three weeks.

If the patient is to have a perineal approach in surgery, he is given a bowel preparation, which includes enemas, cathartics, and phthalylsulfathiazole (Sulfathalidine) or neomycin preoperatively and only clear fluids the day before surgery to prevent fecal contamination of the operative site. Postoperatively, he may be kept on "nothing by mouth," clear liquids, or a low-residue diet until wound healing is well advanced. He may also be given camphorated tincture of opium to inhibit bowel action.

The care of the perineal wound is the same as that following a perineal biopsy except that healing is usually slower. If there has been a retropubic surgical approach, the wound and possible wound complications are the same as for a retropubic prostatectomy (see Chapter 21).

Since perineal surgery causes relaxation of the perineal musculature, the patient may suddenly have fecal incontinence. This is disturbing to the patient and sometimes can be avoided by starting perineal exercises within a day or two after surgery. Control of the rectal sphincter usually returns readily. Perineal exercises should be continued since they also strengthen the bladder sphincters. Unless the bladder sphincters have been permanently damaged, the patient who has practiced perineal exercises will regain urinary control more readily on removal of the catheter. (See Chapter 8 for perineal exercises.)

The patient is often very depressed after surgery, because he suddenly realizes the implications of being impotent and perhaps permanently incontinent. He usually has been told by the doctor before the operation that these are possible consequences, but he has not fully comprehended their meaning. He needs to be encouraged, and provision should be made to keep him dry so that he will feel able to be up and to socialize with others without fear of having "an accident."

When cancer of the prostate is inoperable, the *Huggins treatment* may be used. This is based on the elimination of androgens by removal of the testicles and/or the giving of estrogenic hormones. Occasionally it is necessary to resect the prostate to relieve obstruction. This is most often done transurethrally (see Chapter 21).

In the Huggins treatment, the estrogen given is usually stilbestrol 5 mg. (1/12 grain) a day for one to two weeks. The dosage is then reduced to 1 mg. (1/60 grain) a day. This frequently will relieve the pain and sometimes will decrease obstruction sufficiently to obviate the need for a prostatectomy. Stilbestrol causes engorgement and tenderness of the male breasts. It may also cause nausea. Severe side effects should be reported to the doctor so that the dosage or type of estrogenic preparation may be adjusted.

When symptoms begin to recur, or if the patient is very uncomfortable and needs immediate relief when the diagnosis is first made, a *bilateral orchiectomy (castration)* is done. This is a minor operative procedure and is often done under local anesthesia. The patient's permission must be obtained; if he is married, he is usually urged to discuss the operation with his wife. This surgery eliminates the testicular source of male hormones and seems to cause regression or at least slows the cancer growth. Relief from conservative treatment is quite dramatic in many patients. This relief lasts an average of ten months, and then the patient's condition will usually deteriorate rapidly.

Lesions of the external genitalia

Any lesion on the external genitalia requires medical attention, and no ulcer of the genitalia should be treated by the patient before seeing the doctor lest the diagnosis be obscured. Although lesions are present in a wide variety of conditions, they should always be considered infectious until proved otherwise, since each of the veneral diseases, with the exception of gonorrhea, produces a genital lesion or ulceration.

Chancroid. Chancroid is a veneral disease seen in both men and women and is caused by *Ducrey's bacillus.* It is characterized by a raised lesion on the external genitalia one to five days after the contact. This lesion becomes a pustule and then develops into a painful ulcer, with extensive local inflammation and spread. It is treated locally with sulfathiazole powder and systemically with chloramphenicol or chlortetracycline.

Granuloma inguinale. Granuloma inguinale is a veneral disease caused by the *Donovan bodies.* It is seen most often in the Negro, and it is common in the southern United States. There is a gradual superficial painless ulceration and granulation of the vulva in women and of the glans penis in men. This ulceration extends to the inguinal region in both men and women. It is treated with streptomycin, chloramphenicol, or stibophen (Fuadin) and antimony preparation.

Lymphogranuloma venereum. Lymphogranuloma venereum is a veneral disease caused by a filtrable virus carried via the lymph stream. It is diagnosed by a positive *Frei test* (blood test). At any time from six to sixty days after contact the inguinal nodes in the man and the perirectal nodes in the woman become very swollen and tender, and they may ulcerate. These nodes are known as *buboes.* Rectal strictures and fistulas and urethral strictures develop. There may be complete destruction of the bladder or bowel sphincter muscles, with resultant incontinence. If there is interference with lymph channels, elephantiasis or a hard lymphatic swelling of the lower trunk and legs which completely distorts their size and shape may also develop and may make walking about impossible. Until the advent of chlortetracycline, the treatment was unsatisfactory.

For a discussion of syphilitic lesions, see Chapter 17. Men may also have pruritus similar to that which occurs in women.

Cancer of the penis. Carcinoma of the glans penis is rather rare. It is practically never seen in men who have been circumcised as children; this is a good reason for circumcising male babies. The lesion may originate as a local irritation which itches and has a slight purulent discharge due to secondary infection. It may be only a scaly patchlike area, or it may be an ulcerating sore that will not heal. Metastasis is usually to the inguinal and femoral nodes. The treatment is *penile amputation.* If the amputation must be complete, a permanent *perineal urethrostomy* must be done to provide urinary drainage (see Chapter 21). If there is any nodular involvement, bilateral inguinal node dissections are done. The nursing care is similar to that described for the woman with a radical inguinal node dissection (see page 412 of this chapter). The surgery is psychologically traumatizing to the man; he is impotent, his body form is mutilated, he must sit to void, and he may know or suspect that he has cancer. He is usually quite depressed and is reticent to express his feelings. He should be assured privacy when he voids since he will have to use a bedpan or sit to void; this in itself is a tremendous adjustment. Psychiatric assistance may be needed.

If the course of cancer of the glans penis is not checked, severe lymphedema of the legs occurs, and there is extensive local spread of the ulcerating lesion. Death may be caused by hemorrhage following erosion of the femoral vessels.

REFERENCES AND SELECTED READINGS*

Nursing related to health education, common diagnostic tests, and procedures

1 Bain, Katherine: What Makes a Good Adoption? Am. J. Nursing **57**:306-308, March 1957.

2 Bernard, Jessie, and Jensen, Deborah: Sociology, ed. 4, St. Louis, 1954, The C. V. Mosby Co.

3 Bruehl, Frances Sabina, and Lesh, Ruth Ellis: The Nurse in a Gynecologist's Office, Am. J. Nursing **55**:187-192, Feb. 1955.

4 *Carson, Ruth: So You Want to Adopt a Baby, Public Affairs Pamphlet No. 173, New York, 1951, Public Affairs Committee, Inc.

5 Cecil, Russell L., and Loeb, Robert F.: A Textbook of Medicine, ed. 10, Philadelphia, 1959, W. B. Saunders Co.

---

*References preceded by an asterisk indicate material particularly well suited for student reading.

6 *Clark, Charles: When Patients Ask You About Sex, Am. J. Nursing **53**:73-76, Jan. 1953.
7 Crossen, Robert James, and Campbell, Ann Jones: Gynecologic Nursing, ed. 4, St. Louis, 1951, The C. V. Mosby Co.
8 Curtis, Arthur H., and Huffman, John W.: A Textbook of Gynecology, ed. 6, Philadelphia, 1950, W. B. Saunders Co.
9 *DeSchweinitz, Karl: Growing Up, New York, 1943, The Macmillan Co.
10 *Diagnosis of Cancer of the Prostate, Cancer Bull. **7**:2-4, Jan.-Feb. 1955.
11 Dickinson, Robert Latou: Tampons as Menstrual Guards, J.A.M.A. **128**:490-494, June 16, 1945.
12 Goldzieher, Joseph W.: Progress in Female Endocrinology, Am. J. Nursing **55**:831-833, July 1955.
13 *Harmer, Bertha, and Henderson, Virginia: Textbook of the Principles and Practice of Nursing, ed. 5, New York, 1955, The Macmillan Co., pp. 896-904.
14 *Hymes, James L.: How to Tell Your Child About Sex, Public Affairs Pamphlet No. 149, New York, 1949, Public Affairs Committee, Inc.
15 Karnaky, Karl John: Normal Physiological Douches, Am. J. Surg. **69**:107-115, July 1945.
16 *Kroger, W. S., and Freed, S. C.: Psychosomatic Aspects of Sterility, Am. J. Obst. & Gynec. **59**:867-873, April 1950.
17 MacLeod, John: The Present Status of Human Male Infertility, Am. J. Obst. & Gynec. **69**:1256-1264, June 1955.
18 McDonald, Harold P., Upchurch, Wilborn E., and Sturdevant, Clinton E.: Perineal Biopsy Combined With Radical Retropubic Prostatectomy for Early Carcinoma of the Prostate, J. Urol. **73**:575-579, March 1955.
19 McFadden, Charles J.: Medical Ethics, ed. 2, Philadelphia, 1949, F. A. Davis Co.
20 Malone, Alice: The Nurse in a Fertility Clinic, Am. J. Nursing **57**:348-350, March 1957.
21 *Marshall, Victor: The Diagnosis of Genitourinary Neoplasms, New York, 1949, The American Cancer Society, Inc.
22 Marshall, Victor: Textbook of Urology, New York, 1956, Hoeber-Harper.
23 Meaker, Samuel Raynor: A Doctor Talks to Women, New York, 1954, Simon & Schuster, Inc.
24 *Oed, Minnie K.: Helping the Bewildered Adolescent, Am. J. Nursing **50**:298-301, May 1950.
25 *Pearson, Jed W.: The Physician's Role in Premarriage Counselling, Am. J. Obst. & Gynec. **71**:363-367, Feb. 1956.
26 *Scott, Roger B.: Common Problems in Geriatric Gynecology, Am. J. Nursing **58**:1275-1277, Sept. 1958.
27 Simmons, Fred A.: The Treatment of Male Infertility, Fertil. & Steril. **1**:193-198, May 1950.
28 *Stone, Abraham: Infertility, Am. J. Nursing **47**:606-608, Sept. 1947.
29 Stone, Abraham, and Ward, Mildred E.: Factors Responsible for Pregnancy in 500 Infertility Cases, Fertil. & Steril. **7**:1-12, Jan.-Feb. 1956.
30 Titchener, James L., and others: Problems of Delay in Seeking Surgical Care, J.A.M.A. **160**:1187-1193, April 7, 1956.
31 Walker, Elizabeth: Cytological Test for Cancer, Am. J. Nursing **49**:43-45, Jan. 1949.
32 We Grow Up, Circular No. 102, State of Illinois, 1949, Department of Public Health.

Nursing related to disease of the female reproductive system

33 *A Cancer Source Book For Nurses, New York, 1950, American Cancer Society, Inc. pp. 64-70, 93-97.
34 Anderson, Mary Helen, and Reich, Walter J.: Dysmenorrhea, Am. J. Nursing **49**:220-221, April 1949.
35 *Baer, Joseph L.: Carcinoma of the Reproductive Organs in Women, Am. J. Nursing **49**:78-80, Feb. 1949.
36 Barnett, Margaret, and Myers, Nancy E.: Nursing Care of Women With Carcinoma of the Reproductive Organs, Am. J. Nursing **49**:80-82, Feb. 1949.
37 Bowes, Kenneth (editor): Modern Trends in Obstetrics and Gynecology, New York, 1950, Paul B. Hoeber, Inc.
38 *Bruehl, Frances Sabina, and Leah, Ruth Ellis: The Nurse in a Gynecologist's Office, Am. J. Nursing **55**:187-192, Feb. 1955.
39 Colvin, E. D., and others: Salvage Possibilities in Threatened Abortion, Am. J. Obst. & Gynec. **59**:1208-1222, June 1950.
40 Counsellor, Virgil S.: Methods and Techniques for Correction of Stress Incontinence, J.A.M.A. **145**:27-30, May 5, 1951.
41 Crossen, Robert James: Diseases of Women, ed. 10, St. Louis, 1953, The C. V. Mosby Co.
42 Crossen, Robert James, and Campbell, Ann Jones: Gynecologic Nursing, ed. 5, St. Louis, 1956, The C. V. Mosby Co.
43 Curtis, Arthur H., and Huffman, John W.:

A Textbook of Gynecology, ed. 6, Philadelphia, 1950, W. B. Saunders Co.
44 Daut, Richard V.: Urological Conditions in Women, Am. J. Nursing **50**:479-484, Aug. 1950.
45 Dick, A. C., Billig, H. E., and Macy, H. N.: Menstrual Exercises, Indust. Med. **12**:588-590, Sept. 1943.
46 Dorgan, Lewis T., and Carter, John J.: Vaginal Hysterectomy, Am. J. Obst. & Gynec. **69**:320-332, Feb. 1955.
47 *Green, Thomas: Urinary Stress Incontinence in Women, Am. J. Nursing **57**:598-600, May 1957.
48 Hahn, George A.: Carcinoma of the Cervical Stump With Special Reference to Delay in Therapy, Am. J. Obst. & Gynec. **71**:413-420, Feb. 1956.
49 Haman, John O.: Exercises in Dysmenorrhea, Am. J. Obst. & Gynec. **49**:755-761, June 1945.
50 Harmer, Bertha, and Henderson, Virginia: Textbook of the Principles and Practice of Nursing, ed. 5, New York, 1955, The Macmillan Co.
51 *Hofmeister, Frederick J., Reck, Robert P., and Anderson, Nancy Jane: Vulvectomy—Surgical Treatment and Nursing Care, Am. J. Nursing **60**:666-676, May 1960.
52 Holloway, Howard J.: Injury to the Urinary Tract as a Complication of Gynecological Surgery, Am. J. Obst. & Gynec. **60**:30-40, July 1950.
53 *Kegal, A.: Physiologic Therapy for Urinary Stress Incontinence, J.A.M.A. **146**:915-917, July 7, 1951.
54 *Manfredonia, Genevieve: Radiation Therapy for Cancer of the Cervix, Am. J. Nursing **59**:513-515, April 1959.
55 *Miller, Norman F., and Avery, Hazel: Gynecology and Gynecologic Nursing, ed. 4, Philadelphia, 1959, W. B. Saunders Co.
56 McFadden, Charles J.: Medical Ethics, ed. 2, Philadelphia, 1949, F. A. Davis Co.
57 McFadyen, E. H.: The Retroverted Uterus in Private Practice, Am. J. Obst. & Gynec. **69**:256-258, Feb. 1955.
58 McLaughlin, Eileen: Nursing Care in Hysterectomy, Am. J. Nursing **50**:295-298, May 1950.
59 *Morton, Joseph H.: Premenstrual Tension, Am. J. Obst. & Gynec. **60**:343-352, Aug. 1950.
60 *Novak, Emil, and Novak, Edmund R.: Textbook of Gynecology, ed. 5, Baltimore, 1956, Williams & Wilkins Co.
61 Pfizer Spectrum 4, June 15, 1956.
62 *Prentiss, R. H., and Mulleniz, R. B.: Management of Ureteral Injuries in Pelvic Surgery, J.A.M.A. **145**:1244-1248, April 21, 1951.
63 Ranney, Brooks: Endometriosis, Am. J. Nursing **52**:1465-1467, Dec. 1952.
64 Sargent, James: Vesico-vaginal Fistula: An Effective Technique of Repair, J. Urol. **73**:520-524, March 1955.
65 *Schafer, George: Treatment of Female Genital Tuberculosis, Am. J. Obst. & Gynec. **69**:1333-1341, June 1955.
66 *Schauffler, Goodrich C., and Foster, Jean: Irregular Menstrual Bleeding in Adolescence, Am. J. Nursing **54**:1472-1475, Dec. 1954.
67 Scheffey, Lewis, and Lang, W.: Adequate Measures in the Diagnosis of Uterine Cancer, S. Clin. North America **32**:1729-1743, Dec. 1952.
68 *Scott, Roger B.: Common Problems in Geriatric Gynecology, Am. J. Nursing **58**:1275-1277, Sept. 1958.
69 *Te Linde, Richard W.: Hysterectomy, Am. J. Nursing **50**:293-295, May 1950.
70 Williams, Robert H.: Textbook of Endocrinology, ed. 2, Philadelphia, 1955, W. B. Saunders Co.
71 Wishard, William Niles: Surgical Injuries of the Ureters and the Bladder, J. Urol. **73**:1009-1014, June 1955.
72 Zabriskie, Louise, and Eastman, Nicholson J.: Nurses' Handbook of Obstetrics, ed. 9, revised, Philadelphia, 1952, J. B. Lippincott Co.

Nursing related to disease of the male reproductive system

73 *Carroll, G., and Brennan, R.: Endocrine Therapy in Carcinoma of the Prostate, J.A.M.A. **157**:580-583, Feb. 12, 1955.
74 Colby, Fletcher: Essential Urology, Baltimore, 1950, Williams & Wilkins Co.
75 Davis, Edward, and Lee, LeRoy W.: Progress in Perineal Prostatectomy: Results in 2050 Consecutive Patients, J. Urol. **73**:142-154, Jan. 1955.
76 Ferguson, L. Kraeer, and Sholtis, Lillian A.: Eliason's Surgical Nursing, ed. 11, Philadelphia, 1959, J. B. Lippincott Co.
77 Hinman, F., Jr.: Optimum Time for Orchiopexy in Cryptorchidism, Fertil. & Steril. **6**:206-214, May-June 1955.
78 Marshall, Victor F.: Textbook of Urology, New York, 1956, Hoeber-Harper.
79 *Marshall, Victor F.: The Diagnosis of Genito-urinary Neoplasms, New York, 1949, American Cancer Society, Inc.

80 McCrea, Lowrain, E.: Clinical Urology, ed. 2, Philadelphia, 1948, F. A. Davis Co.
81 Melicow, M. M.: Classification of Tumors of the Testis: A Clinical and Pathological Study Based on 105 Primary and 13 Secondary Cases in Adults, and 3 Primary and 4 Secondary Cases in Children, J. Urol. 73:547-574, March 1955.
82 Staubitz, William J., Lent, Melbourne H., and Oberkircher, Oscar J.: Carcinoma of the Penis, Cancer 8:371-378, March-April 1955.
83 *Van Schoick, M. R., and Huggins, C.: Carcinoma of the Prostate, Am. J. Nursing 48:427-429, July 1948.

The patient with pulmonary disease

Chapter 23

Study questions for review

1 Review the anatomy and physiology of the lungs and diaphragm. How does lack of function in the diaphragm affect respiration and lung disease?
2 Which muscles can be used as accessory muscles in breathing? What is meant by maximal, minimal, and residual air?
3 Explain the exchange of oxygen and carbon dioxide in normal respiration. What is the normal respiratory rate? What is the normal carbon dioxide level in the blood stream? How does carbon dioxide content affect respiration and general body function?
4 Review the drugs which facilitate the raising of sputum.
5 How many diseases can you name which begin with symptoms of the common cold? What is the best treatment for the common cold?

THE PATIENT WITH RESPIRATORY DISEASE

The list of respiratory illnesses is long. The nurse often will encounter the common cold. Others that she will see quite frequently include pneumonia, bronchitis, tuberculosis, bronchiectasis, lung abscess, spontaneous pneumothorax, empyema, asthma, emphysema, and carcinoma.

The nurse needs to understand the particular characteristics of each of these diseases, yet she should realize that most respiratory diseases cause common symptoms. For example, the common cold may be acute and brief in comparison to asthma, yet the patient with a cold may temporarily experience some of the same feelings as does the patient with asthma when easy, effortless breathing is hampered. The constant irritation of coughing can be much the same for a patient with pneumonia as for one with tuberculosis. The cough, the "tickle" in the throat, the constant need to clear the throat, and the need to expectorate frequently can be tiresome and wearing. The unpleasant odor of sputum and the residual taste in the mouth when sputum is raised can cause nausea and subsequent lack of appetite. Lack of sleep is a common complaint in respiratory disease because the patient may be unable to breathe freely or may be constantly beseiged with coughing. Chest pain may cause discomfort, and the patient may hesitate to breathe deeply because he anticipates pain. All of these problems demand special nursing care. Thus, in the care of any patient with respiratory illness, the nurse needs to observe the patient particularly for problems related to breathing, coughing, raising sputum, chest pain, nose and throat irritation, eating, and sleeping.

General nursing care

Difficulties in breathing. The patient with respiratory disease has difficulty in breathing; this difficulty may be very slight or severe. There may be obstruction to the free passage of air somewhere in the respiratory tract, or the normal functioning capacity of the respiratory system may be lowered because of damage to lung tissues. The patient may have both of these difficulties. When this is so, more effort is required for breathing, and the patient is more aware of breathing. He has dyspnea, which has been defined by Meakins as "the consciousness of the necessity for respiratory effort." This is a tiring and unpleasant sensation. With increased difficulty in getting air, most patients become apprehensive and even panicky. A nurse who understands this can be a great comfort to the patient since the presence of another person helps the patient to control fear and thus eases his efforts in breathing.

Position. The most comfortable position for more relaxed breathing is a semi-upright or upright sitting position. In these positions the lungs and respiratory muscles are not cramped and thus are not working against resistance. A pillow placed lengthwise at the patient's back will support him and will keep the thorax thrust slightly forward, allowing freer use of the diaphragm and therefore deeper breathing. For those patients who must be upright, the overbed table with a pillow on top can be used as a support and a resting place for the head and arms. If the patient has marked breathing difficulty and is not sufficiently alert or is very alert and fearful, side rails should be used for additional security. The patient may also use them to pull himself up into a higher sitting position.

Ventilation. Proper ventilation and temperature of the room will aid the patient in easier breathing. Patients may have preferences as to room temperature and amount of fresh air, and the nurse should respect these. In general, most patients breathe more easily if the air is cool; warm air tends to increase efforts to breathe.

For those patients with nose, throat, and bronchial irritation, warm moist air produced by a *vaporizer* may be beneficial. A vaporizer can be used to humidify the air throughout the room, or it can be put in close proximity to the patient so that he can inhale the steam as it is released. The large electrically operated vaporizers used in hospitals serve to moisten the air in the entire room. Water flowing from a gallon-sized jar is heated to form steam which is then directed out through a long flexible spout. Inhalations of plain steam or of an aromatic medication such as tincture of benzoin or menthol are often ordered.

If the patient is at home, the nurse can help him and his family to improvise equipment for inhalations and for proper humidity. An empty coffee can or a shallow pie tin can be filled with water and placed on an electric plate in the patient's room to increase humidity. If the inhalation is to be directed, an ordinary steam kettle or a kettle with a longer improvised paper spout may be used. The paper needs to be changed frequently. A few drops of menthol or oil of eucalyptus can be put into the water. Benzoin will cause corrosion in the kettle and this is exceedingly difficult to remove. The kettle and electric plate should be placed a safe distance from the patient's face so that he can breathe the medicated steam, yet not be burned by accidentally tipping the kettle or by touching the hot plate. After the twenty-five to thirty minute treatment, equipment should be removed from the bedside.

Small electric vaporizers can be purchased at most local drug stores. They usually consist of a pint-sized jar with a heating element extending into the jar. The jar should be filled with ordinary tap water and a pinch of salt added to hasten heating. The top of the jar holds a small, removable perforated cup, to which is attached a small metal spout. Cotton saturated with medication is placed inside the cup and the small metal spout fitted over the cup. As the water boils, the medicated steam is directed out through the small spout. Jars for the set are usually replaceable and inexpensive.

If breathing is so difficult that the patient cannot get enough oxygen from the air, it may be necessary to give additional oxygen. Cyanosis is not always present, and increased pulse rate is often the first detectable sign of oxygen shortage. The nurse, therefore, should keep a close check on the patient's pulse rate as well as his color and the character and the rate of respirations. Oxygen may be administered by tent, by nasal catheter, or by mask; the method used depends on the patient, his need, and the concentration of oxygen necessary. If oxygen is not readily available, increasing the amount of fresh air may help. The nurse should be familiar with operation of the various devices used to administer oxygen and should check frequently to note whether they are operating properly. (For details of nursing care of patients receiving oxygen, see textbooks on fundamentals of nursing.)

When the patient is having difficulty in the exchange of inspired and expired air, oxygen or sometimes compressed air may be given under *positive pressure*. Positive-pressure masks and the Bennett respirator are most often used. In an emergency, mouth-to-mouth breathing may be used. (See Chapter 15.) If the patient's greatest difficulty is exhalation and if inspiration becomes slower and deeper, there is danger of carbon dioxide narcosis and oxygen should *not* be given. The nurse must notify the doctor at once if this occurs.

Continued uncorrected difficulty in breathing may cause an excess of carbon dioxide or a deficiency of carbon dioxide in the blood stream. The former is due to incomplete exhalation and causes respiratory acidosis; the latter is due to hyperventilation and causes respiratory alkalosis. (See Chapter 6.)

Coughing. Two of the most troublesome symptoms of respiratory disease are the increase in mucous secretions as a result of inflamed mucous membranes and the stimulation of cough due to irritation of the respiratory tract. If coughing is productive, the patient should be encouraged to cough since this keeps air passages clear and allows sufficient oxygen to reach the alveoli. Changing the patient's position will help to prevent pooling of secretions in the lungs and will stimulate coughing. The patient should be instructed to breathe as deeply as possible to loosen secretions and stimulate productive coughing. If he cannot cough forcefully enough to raise sputum and if his respirations are very shallow or sound very moist he is often given a medication to thin the secretions. This is often given as an aerosol treatment so that the medication is topically applied to the respiratory passages.

Many patients with obvious, noisy respirations caused by accumulated sputum hesitate to cough because they fear it will cause pain. The nurse can assist these patients by placing her hands on the front and back of the chest to give support as the patient coughs. A towel placed around the chest and held snugly as the patient coughs can also be used. Constant nonproductive coughing and hacking can lead to exhaustion.

Medications are often prescribed for coughing. The type depends on the nature of the cough and the secretions. The purposes of various cough medications are to increase secretions, to decrease secretions, to thin secretions so they can be raised and expectorated more easily, or to depress the cough reflex.

Sedative expectorants increase secretions, protect irritated membranes, and lessen the amount of coughing. Increased secretions may result in a productive cough and make paroxysms of coughing less frequent. For this purpose, ammonium chloride in wild cherry or orange syrup is often ordered, and other mixtures such as iodide solutions or ipecac syrup are sometimes used. Detergent drugs such as Alevaire which help to thin secretions and bronchiodilators such as isoproterenol hydrochloride (Isuprel) may be given with oxygen under positive pressure. Stimulating expectorants diminish secretions and promote repair and healing of the mucous membrane. Terpin hydrate is an example of these. Sometimes codeine is added to elixir of terpin hydrate to depress the cough reflex and thereby lessen irritation.

When respiratory difficulty is severe, secretions are present, yet coughing is unproductive, intratracheal suctioning and occasionally bronchoscopy are resorted to. By means of bronchoscopy, mucous plugs may be loosened or removed and intratracheal suctioning made more effective. Equipment for emergency bronchoscopy may be kept in the patient's room. When this is ordered the nurse must see that electrical outlets are adequate and that the necessary equipment is assembled in one place and ready for immediate use. (See page 437 for care of the patient during bronchoscopy.)

Postural drainage. Postural drainage may be used to assist the patient who has difficulty in raising sputum. By means of gravity, secretions flow upward in the bronchi and trachea or to the back of the throat and can be raised and expectorated more easily. A position providing gravity drainage of the lungs can be achieved in several ways, and the procedure selected usually depends on the age of the patient and his general condition, as well as the location in the lungs where secretions have accumulated. The young patient may tolerate more lowering of the head than an elderly patient whose vascular system adapts less quickly to positional change; a severely debilitated patient may need a modified procedure because of the danger of an accident. To accomplish postural drainage, the patient may lie across the bed on his abdomen with his head and chest extending over the edge of the bed. A chair or a high stool can be placed on the side of the bed so that he can support himself in this jackknife position. A small basin or wide-mouthed cup can be placed on the chair, which should be protected with newspaper.

A Gatch bed can be used for postural drainage. Most patients prefer this method because it provides more support and therefore is less taxing than being suspended over the side of the bed. The knee-gatch is raised as high as possible, and the patient lies over the bend in the bed foundation so that his head and chest are dependent. To provide something firm on which the patient can rest his arms and hands for more security and to provide a place for the sputum container, a board can be placed flat across the lower part of the bed frame in the space between the springs and the mattress.

Postural drainage achieved merely by putting blocks under the casters at the foot of the bed sometimes produces excellent results. The footboard of the bed may also be supported on the seat of a firm chair to provide a position in which the head is lowered. Tilt boards (special tables that can be raised or lowered to any angle) are sometimes used, but many doctors prefer raising the foot of the bed since this entails much less exertion for the patient.

If the nurse knows the part of the lung affected and then helps the patient assume a position which is best for draining that portion, thorough drainage usually can be achieved. For example, if the right middle lobe of the lung is affected, drainage will be best accomplished by way of the right middle bronchus. The patient should lie on his back with his body turned at approximately a 45-degree angle. The angle can be maintained by pillow supports placed under the right side from the shoulders to the hips. The foot of the bed should then be raised about twelve inches. This position can be maintained fairly comfortably by most patients for half an hour at a time. On the other hand, if the lower posterior area of the lung is affected, the jackknife position already described is most effective.

Patients having postural drainage of any kind are encouraged to breathe deeply and to cough forcefully to help dislodge thick sputum and exudate that is pooled in distended bronchioles, particularly after inactivity. Expectorant drugs and any medication to thin secretions, dilate the bronchioles, or stimulate expectoration should be given fifteen to twenty minutes before postural drainage. The patient may find that he can raise sputum upon resuming an upright position even though no drainage appeared while he was lying with his head and chest lowered.

Since some patients complain of dizziness when assuming position for postural drainage, the nurse should stay with the patient during the first few times, and she should report any persistent dizziness or unusual discomfort to the doctor. Postural drainage may be contraindicated in some patients because of heart disease, hypertension, or age. However, most patients can be taught to assume the position for postural drainage and can proceed without help. The position usually is maintained for ten minutes at first, and the period of time is gradually lengthened to fifteen or twenty or even thirty minutes as the patient becomes accustomed to the sometimes almost "upside-down" position. At first, elderly patients usually are able to tolerate the unusual position only for a few minutes. They need more assistance than most other patients during the procedure and immediately thereafter. They should be assisted to a normal position in bed and requested to lie flat for a few minutes before sitting up or getting out of bed; this helps to prevent dizziness and reduces danger of accidents.

The patient may feel nauseated because of the odor and taste of sputum; therefore, the procedure should be timed so that it comes at least forty-five minutes to an hour before meals. A short rest period following the treatment often improves the appetite. The patient needs mouth care following postural drainage, and provision should be made for this. Aromatic mouthwashes should be available for frequent use by any patient who is expectorating sputum freely.

Care of sputum. Since the causative organisms may not be known early in the respiratory disease, the nurse should use caution in the disposal of sputum and should instruct the patient to protect others. The patient who is coughing or clearing his throat forcefully should be instructed to cover his mouth and nose with several thicknesses of disposable tissues to prevent possible spread of infectious organisms. She should be calm and matter-of-fact in doing this so that the patient does not feel that he is dangerous to others or that he is shunned by them. Used tissues should be folded carefully and placed in a paper bag or flushed directly down the toilet. If a bag is used, it should be closed and preferably burned. Used tissues should be collected from the bedfast patient at frequent intervals and whoever handles the bags should wash his hands thoroughly to avoid transfer of infection to others.

If the patient has a copious amount of sputum he may be instructed in the use of a sputum cup. Waxed paper cups with lids may be used. In some hospitals the waxed paper cups are placed in metal containers. At least once daily, the inner cup should be discarded and a fresh one provided. The metal containers frequently become contaminated with sputum and therefore should be washed and boiled often. Some hospitals have a schedule for boiling them daily.

If the patient cannot care for and dispose of his own sputum, he must have assistance. Tissues may be placed in the patient's hand, and a paper bag may be placed on each side of the bed so that he does not have to turn to dispose of the soiled tissues. The bedfast patient who handles his own sputum should be offered water with which to wash his hands before meals.

Oral hygiene and appetite. The odor and taste in the mouth caused by frequent raising of sputum may seriously affect appetite and may impair nutrition. Provision should be made for oral hygiene before meals, handwashing must be encouraged, and sputum cups or other evidence of sputum must be removed before meals are served. Some patients find that a strong, clear, well-seasoned broth helps to make the mouth feel fresher and improves appetite for the rest of the meal. Other patients report that beginning a meal with acid fluids, such as grapefruit or tomato juice, improves acceptance of other food. The nurse should report food preferences to the dietitian.

Rest. Adequate rest is important in combating respiratory disease. During respiratory illness, however, normal sleep may be interrupted for a number of reasons. The patient may be plagued with frequent coughing, and breathing may be difficult. Airways may become blocked with secretions, and the patient may be awakened by the resultant increased difficulty in breathing.

The nurse should be alert for signs of what irritates the patient, precipitates cough, and therefore prevents rest. For example, too much talking, smoking, sitting in a draft or in a dry, overheated room, or laughing excessively all may predispose to coughing. Cough medications given before the hour of sleep and when rest is disturbed by coughing are often helpful. However, when the patient has noisy breathing and it is obvious that secretions are present in the respiratory tract, he should be encouraged to cough deeply and to expectorate until the airway is free of obstruction before medication is given. A suitable position in bed and changes in position also help the patient to rest more quietly. Room temperature and ventilation should be kept at what the patient feels is best for him.

Prevention of new infection. Patients with any type of respiratory disease should protect themselves against exposure to new infection. They should avoid outdoor exertion in cold weather and extremes of cold or humidity. If they must go out in cold damp weather, warm clothing should be worn; if the clothing gets wet, it should be changed immediately. Smoking should be done in moderation if at all. Undue emotional stress may also lessen the patient's resistance and increase susceptibility to additional infection.

Diagnostic examinations and related nursing care

The diagnosis of a specific respiratory illness is made after a series of tests has been done. Once a clear-cut diagnosis has been made, some tests may be repeated at intervals to determine the progress the patient has made.

Examination of sputum. Examinations of sputum are almost always done. Since the mucous membrane of the respiratory tract responds to inflammation by an increased flow of secretions which often contain the offending organisms, microscopic examination of a *smear of the sputum* often gives useful information in diagnosis. A *culture of the sputum* is often ordered also. Suitable growth media are inoculated with the sputum. Growth on media of the same organism as that identified on microscopic smears will help confirm a diagnosis. The sputum may be examined for carcinoma cells by using the Papanicolaou technique. It may also be examined grossly for color, consistency, and special constituents; clear mucoid "currant jelly" sputum is indicative of possible carcinoma of the lung; purulent blood-streaked sputum has long been considered suggestive of tuberculosis; thick tenacious sputum containing casts of bronchioles is often found in asthmatic bronchitis.

Tests to be done on sputum should be explained to the patient so that he will understand the need for obtaining a suitable specimen. He should be instructed to collect only sputum which has come from deep in the chest. Patients often expectorate saliva rather than sputum when they do not understand the need for deep coughing and for raising secretions from the lungs. They are likely to exhaust themselves unnecessarily by shallow, frequent coughing which yields no sputum suitable for study and which affords them little relief from discomfort. The first sputum raised in the morning is usually the most productive of organisms. During the night secretions accumulate in the bronchi and only a few deep coughs will bring them to the back of the throat. If the patient does not know this, upon awakening he may, almost unconsciously, cough, clear his throat, and swallow or expectorate before attempting to procure a specimen.

The patient should be supplied with a widemouthed bottle or jar for collecting the specimen, and he should be instructed to expectorate directly into the bottle to avoid contamination of the outside of the bottle. Since the sight of sputum is often objectionable to the patient, and particularly to others about him, the outside of the container should be covered with paper or other suitable covering. To prevent the possibility of contamination of the air with organisms in the sputum, a paper lid or cap should be kept over the top of the container. Usually 4 ml. of sputum are sufficient for necessary laboratory tests and examinations. Occasionally, however, all sputum collected over a twenty-four to thirty-six hour period is needed. If there is any delay in sending the specimen to the laboratory, it should be placed in the refrigerator; for example, when a total three day specimen is requested, the bottle should be changed at least daily and the used bottles should be kept refrigerated until taken to the hospital or delivered to the laboratory.

Gastric washings. If the patient raises little or no sputum, a gastric aspiration may be done. Since most patients swallow sputum when coughing in the morning and during sleep, an examination of gastric contents may reveal causative organisms. Breakfast is withheld for gastric aspiration. The procedure for passing the gastric tube is the same as that discussed in Chapter 26. Once the tube is passed, a large syringe is attached to the end and by gentle suction a specimen of stomach contents is withdrawn. The specimen is placed in a covered bottle, and the tube is withdrawn. The specimen is examined microscopically on slides, and culture media are inoculated as is done with other sputum samples. Gastric specimens may be obtained two or three days in succession, particularly if tuberculosis is suspected.

Respiratory function tests. To determine the functional capacity of the lungs, vital capacity readings and bronchospirometry may be ordered.

Vital capacity readings. Vital capacity readings are measurements of expired air and may be taken by the nurse. The patient is instructed to take as deep a breath as possible; he then expires as much of this air as possible into the mouthpiece of the vital capacity machine while the nurse records the reading. It is important that the lungs are as completely aerated as possible and that all possible air is expelled since this is indicative of the respiratory reserve.

Bronchospirometry. Bronchospirometry measures both the ventilatory efficiency and the oxygen-absorptive function of the lungs. It gives an accurate determination of the degree of respiratory impairment. For this test a double-lumen catheter may be introduced into the trachea (see discussion of bronchogram for care of the patient). A nose clip is used, and air is inhaled or exhaled through the tracheal catheter which is attached to a device that measures both the amount of air taken and exhaled. Samples of arterial blood are taken to determine the arterial oxygen and carbon dioxide tensions. This test is usually done in a special laboratory.

X-ray examination of the chest. When chest disease is suspected, a roentgenogram is almost always ordered to help identify the disease and to visualize the effects and extent of the disease process. Various types of roentgenograms may be ordered. For survey purposes a *microfilm* may be used. If this small plate indicates any abnormality, a large plate is taken. Large x-ray plates may be called an AP (anterior-posterior view). *Lateral views* may be ordered. *Stereoscopic* roentgenograms may be made as these give a three-dimensional (depth) view. When carcinoma is suspected, a *tomogram* may be ordered. This is a series of roentgenograms done in such a way as to give depth views of various sections of the lung. If the patient is acutely ill a portable x-ray machine may be brought to the patient's bedside, and the nurse assists the patient into correct position and protects him from exposure. If oxygen is being used, it must be discontinued before the roentgenogram is taken. The x-ray plate is placed in a clean pillow case and then it is placed flat on the bed. If the patient can sit up, the plate is put in place, he leans back on it, and the bed is lowered as far as can be tolerated. If he is unable to sit up, he is turned on his side, the plate is correctly placed on the bed, and he is rolled onto it.

If the patient is ambulatory or well enough to be moved, he is taken to the x-ray department in a wheel chair or on a stretcher for the procedure. He must always be accompanied, and the nurse should be certain that he is wearing an open-backed gown and has removed or will remove from his person or his gown all metal above the waist since metal restricts the passage of the x-rays and will cause a shadow on the film. Care should be taken that such articles are not misplaced or lost.

Fluoroscopic examination is often done. The patient must go to a room where the fluoroscope is installed. He may need assistance in rising to a sitting position or in remaining still during the examination; if he is in a wheel chair, he is assisted to a stool in front of the machine. The doctor wears an apron and gloves containing lead to protect him from the x-rays, and he uses plastic goggles to aid his adaptation to the dark. Fluoroscopic examination is done with the lights off, and the doctor operates the machine with a foot pedal. The patient needs a careful explanation of the procedure and should be told that he will be in darkness and that he may be asked to hold his breath for a few seconds during the examination. He should be assured that there will be no pain.

Bronchogram and bronchoscopy. Examinations by bronchogram and bronchoscopy are somewhat complicated diagnostic procedures that may be ordered. Both procedures are unpleasant and uncomfortable for the patient. A thorough explanation of what will happen and what will be expected of him during these examinations can do much to allay his anxiety. Since instruments are passed through the mouth and pharynx making the patient apprehensive about being able to breathe, he should practice breathing in and out through the nose with the mouth open. He can also practice consciously relaxing the shoulders and hands while lying on his back. Clenching the fists causes the neck muscles to tense, and this interferes with the procedure. If the patient is to have a bronchoscopic examination, he should know that the room lights will be off, that his eyes will be covered, and that a mask and gloves will be used by the doctor.

A *bronchogram* enables the doctor to visualize the bronchial tree. When the roentgenograms are taken, nonirritating radiopaque oil is injected through the trachea into the bronchi and the bronchioles. To lessen the number of bacteria introduced from the mouth into the bronchi, the patient should pay particular attention to oral hygiene on the night before and the morning of the procedure. No food or fluids are allowed for eight hours preceding the examination. Since, if the smaller bronchi contain secretions, the iodized oil will not reach them, postural drainage may be ordered for the morning the bronchogram is made. Usually he remains in postural-drainage position for about fifteen minutes, and he should breathe deeply and cough. Mouth care should follow. The patient should be asked about any loose or capped teeth or dental bridges. Dental prostheses should be removed and loose teeth should be pointed out to the doctor.

Approximately one hour before the injection of oil, the patient is given a mild sedative such as Seconal to relax him and to counteract the effect of the Pontocaine or cocaine used for local anesthesia. Usually 0.5 per cent Pontocaine or cocaine is used for this. The doctor anesthetizes the pharynx, larynx, and major bronchi immediately before the radiopaque substance is introduced. The patient should be told that this will taste bitter and that he should not swallow it but expectorate into the emesis basin or tissues provided. When the gag reflex disappears, a metal laryngeal cannula is passed into the trachea, and then a catheter is passed through the nose into the cannula and into the trachea. Iodized oil is then introduced, and the patient is tilted into various positions to distribute the oil to the bronchi and bronchioles. A series of roentgenograms is then taken. Following this procedure, postural drainage is usually ordered to help remove the oil from the lungs. No permanent damage results, however, if some of it remains for an indefinite period. Food and fluid should be withheld until the gag reflex returns. This can be tested by gently tickling the posterior pharynx with a cotton swab.

A *bronchoscopic examination* is performed by passing a bronchoscope into the trachea and bronchi. The bronchoscope is a long, slender, hollow instrument through which light can be reflected and visual examination can be made. Bronchoscopy may be done to remove a foreign body, to facilitate free air passage by removal of mucous plugs with suction, or to obtain a biopsy and samples of secretions for examination. Preparation of the patient for a bronchoscopic examination is similar to that for a bronchogram, except that postural drainage is less often ordered. In addition to a spray anesthetic, cocaine is applied locally by holding small cotton pledgets soaked in solution in the posterior fossa of the pharynx.

Following bronchoscopy, the patient is given no food or fluids until the gag reflex returns. Some doctors prefer that the patient lie flat after this procedure, while others prefer a semi-Fowler's position. The patient is awake and conscious although rather drowsy from the sedation. Rather than attempt to swallow saliva, he should be urged to lie on his side and to let mucus from the mouth flow into disposable tissues or a small emesis basin conveniently placed. He should be urged to lie quietly and not try to talk, cough, or clear his throat since these activities only increase the secretions and the desire to clear the throat. A pencil and a piece of paper should be at the bedside so that he can write if he needs to communicate. He should have his call light within easy reach, and he should be instructed to call for the nurse if he feels uncomfortable. Occasionally, severe laryngeal edema follows this procedure; this causes respiratory embarrassment and may even necessitate a tracheostomy.

The patient may be hoarse and have a sore throat for several days following a bronchoscopy. Warm fluids by mouth may relieve the soreness and sometimes warm gargles are ordered. If the discomfort is severe, acetylsalicylic acid, 0.3 Gm. (5 grains), may be dissolved in the mouth and then swallowed.

If a biopsy is taken during bronchoscopy, the patient is kept under close surveillance until clotting occurs—usually five to seven minutes. His sputum should be carefully observed for a few hours after the procedure for signs of hemorrhage. The patient should not smoke for several hours because this may cause coughing and start bleeding. Although normally the sputum may be streaked with blood for a few days after a biopsy has been taken, any excessive bleeding must be reported at once to the doctor.

DISEASE CONDITIONS

Respiratory viral infections

Viral infection is exceedingly prevalent; there are now over 90 viruses recognizable in man and many of these cause respiratory disease.[17] Some diseases may be caused by one special virus or different ones may cause the same symptoms.

If specific signs are not produced, the clinical illness is termed a common cold, virus infection, fever of unknown origin, acute respiratory illness, or the grippe. The most common specific respiratory illnesses caused by the various viruses are epidemic pleurodynia (Bornholm's disease), acute laryngotracheobronchitis, virus pneumonia, and influenza. Most adults have developed antibodies for the more common viruses and most virus infections are relatively mild. They, however, are frequently complicated by secondary bacterial infections. When a new strain such as the Asian flu virus (1958) develops, severe epidemics ensue and many people die from secondary infections such as pneumonia.

The common cold

Few persons escape having a "cold." The general population averages three colds per person each year.[6] It is estimated that the nation loses 5 billion dollars in wages and production yearly because of the common cold, and the United States Public Health Service reports that 150 million workdays are lost yearly from this cause.[30] More time is lost in industry as a result of upper respiratory infections than from any other single group of disorders.[3] Most colds occur between September and May, and women are more often affected than men. The frequency of their occurrence, the numbers of people affected, the resulting economic loss, and the possibility of a cold leading to more serious disease are reasons why colds merit serious attention.

Since persons with colds are rarely hospitalized, the nurse will encounter them at work, in public places, or in their homes. It is important for her to check the symptoms at the onset of the cold. Many other more serious diseases begin with a cold or with symptoms resembling those of the common cold. Because a cold is considered a minor but bothersome condition and because the patient has possibly had many colds, he, rather than a physician, makes the diagnosis. Helping others to respect an illness which may appear slight but which may have serious consequences is an integral part of nursing.

The common cold is caused by a filtrable virus, and it is spread rapidly, easily, and directly by droplet infection. Symptoms of a cold usually appear suddenly and the infection may be full blown within forty-eight hours. The acute inflammation usually begins in the pharynx, and there is a sensation of dryness or soreness of the throat. This is followed by nasal congestion with a thin, watery, profuse discharge and frequent sneezing. The eyes may water, the voice may become husky, breathing may be obstructed, and sense of smell and taste may diminish. Often a cough develops which is nonproductive at the beginning but becomes productive later.

The patient with a cold may have variable complaints. At times he may feel lethargic and have vague, aching pains in the back and limbs. Most adults are afebrile, but those with a tendency toward developing complications, such as persons with chronic illness and low resistance, may have a temperature elevation. The course of the cold is variable, but ordinarily it lasts from seven to fourteen days. It is difficult to determine when the cold ends and when complications appear. Laryngitis and tracheitis may be part of the cold. Tracheobronchitis is a complication usually due to secondary bacterial infection. Acute sinusitis and otitis media may follow the common cold.

Prevention. There is no known way to prevent the common cold, and there is no specific treatment. However, there are measures that help to prevent the development of a cold, help to prevent complications, and help to prevent its transfer to others. Attention to good general hygiene, with plenty of rest, an adequate diet, and sufficient exercise and fresh air, presumably help to maintain resistance to colds. The nurse should teach that the patient can go through the usual course of a common cold without difficulty if he obtains enough rest, eats a well-balanced diet, including ample fluids, maintains regular elimination of waste products, and avoids chilling and exposure. Doctors disagree on the necessity for bed rest in treatment of colds, but they agree that bed rest is needed for those who have low resistance to infection or chronic illness. Forcing fluids helps to maintain normal temperature and helps the body get rid of waste products. By varying the types of fluids, a person is often able to take more liquids than would otherwise seem possible. If the throat is sore, bland fruit juices, soft drinks, milk drinks, and water can usually be swallowed more easily than solid food. Since taste and smell may be diminished part of the time, it is important to make all drinks and foods attractive and appetizing. An elevation of temperature may mean the beginning of complications. The nurse can do much toward prevention of complications by being alert to early signs and symptoms.

Treatment. All treatment of colds is directed toward relief of symptoms and control of complications. If the patient has an elevated temperature and complains of headache and muscular aching, he should seek the advice of a physician; acetylsalicylic acid may be prescribed for mild aches and discomfort. Salicylates, however, do not influence the course of the common cold and lack specific action in this disorder.

If the patient has *nasal congestion,* the physician may recommend nose drops. Ephedrine, 0.5 to 2 per cent aqueous solution, with isotonic sodium chloride solution is used frequently. This medication shrinks swollen nasal tissues and allows for the free passage of air. Many physicians advise against the use of nose drops, maintaining that constriction of blood supply to the tissues lowers resistance. In general, oily solutions are not recommended because of the danger of the inhalation of oil droplets which might cause lipid pneumonia. The nurse should emphasize to patients and their families the importance of using only prescribed solutions and only those that are fresh. Nose drops should be prescribed by a doctor, and only the specified amount should be used; excessive use may only aggravate symptoms. Many persons prefer a medicated nasal inhaler since it can be carried easily in a pocket and is more pleasant to use. Benzedrex containing propylhexedrine is an example of one which is widely used. Prophylhexedrine is a volatile drug with minimum stimulating effect on the central nervous system.[14] Soft disposable paper tissues or old, soft, cotton handkerchiefs should be used to help prevent dryness, redness, and irritation about the nose. Some dryness can be prevented by treating the skin early in the cold with mild soothing creams, such as cold cream.

The *dryness, cough,* and *"tickling sensation"* in the throat so often associated with a cold can be relieved in a variety of ways. There are many cough drops and lozenges on the market. Lozenges relieve irritation and are pleasant to use; patients should be advised not to use them just before dozing off to sleep since they may be accidentally aspirated into the trachea during sleep. A mixture of honey and lemon may be preferred to cough medications by some patients. This mixture increases mucous secretions and thereby softens exudate and facilitates its expectoration; it also relieves the dryness which predisposes to coughing. Some people report that undiluted lemon or orange juice is helpful. A section of the fruit with the rind may be placed at the bedside for easy accessibility during the night. Hot fluids often relieve coughing. The patient may be advised to keep a small vacuum bottle of hot water or other liquid at the bedside. If cough medication has been taken, it should not be followed by water because the effect will be dissipated. Patients should keep prescribed cough medications within reach to avoid chilling from getting out of bed during the night. If the cough associated with a common cold persists or does not yield to the simple home remedies mentioned or to specific medication that may have been ordered, the patient must be urged to report to his doctor.

The nurse should emphasize to the patient with a cold the importance of avoiding spread of his cold to others. Crowded places, such as the theater, should be avoided by those with colds. The patient should particularly avoid coming into contact with and, therefore, exposing infants and young children, persons who have chronic chest disease such as bronchiectasis, those who have recently had an anesthetic, and elderly people. He should remember to cover his nose and mouth when sneezing, coughing, and clearing his throat. Frequent handwashing, covering of coughs and sneezes, and careful disposal of waste tissues are protective health measures which are advisable for everyone in everyday life, but they become increasingly important when known respiratory infection exists. Since the common cold is a communicable disease, the principles of protection of oneself, as well as the ways in which a cold can be transferred to others, should be remembered.

Pneumonia

Pneumonia can occur in any season, but it is most common during the winter and early spring. Persons of any age are susceptible. However, those with lowered resistance are most often affected. The use of anesthetics and of large doses of morphine may be contributing causes since they slow reflex action of the epiglottis, permitting aspiration of infected secretions from the upper respiratory tract. Chilling and exposure may permit organisms already present to become active. Alcoholics are particularly susceptible to pneumonia because of general malnutrition, frequent exposure to cold, and poor general health practices. Elderly persons are susceptible to pneumonia because of the slowing of reflex action of the epiglottis and because of limited expansion of the rib cage and poorer aeration of the lungs. Organisms such as pneumococci in the nasopharyngeal secretions may be carried to the distant bronchioles and to the alveoli, where they may cause an acute inflammation. Accumulation of fluid in the alveoli caused by such conditions as cardiac failure, viral infection of the lungs, trauma to the thorax, or pulmonary stasis resulting from prolonged bed rest in the same position provides an ideal medium for the growth of bacteria. Pneumonia is also a communicable respiratory illness, and it may be spread directly from person to person by droplet infection. The pneumococcus causes 95 per cent of all primary pneumonia of bacterial origin;[6] other bacterial causes of the disease are Friedländer's bacillus, tubercle bacillus, staphylococcus, and streptococcus.

Prevention. Pneumonia can often be prevented in susceptible patients by careful nursing care. Preoperative and postoperative patients, those receiving heavy sedation for any reason, alcoholics, elderly patients, chronically ill patients, those with gross limitation of movement, and those with difficulty in swallowing need frequent mouth care to help keep the mouth free of excessive bacteria. Prompt suctioning of secretions in patients who cannot cough and expectorate secretions forcibly will reduce the chances of aspiration and accumulation of fluid in the lungs. Regular, frequent turning or help in changing position will lessen the possibility of stasis. Such patients will need special attention when they are being given medication, food, or drink by mouth. An apprehensive patient with swallowing difficulties needs time in learning to swallow with expiration; he needs constant encouragement in his efforts to relax and continue his efforts to swallow safely.

Medical treatment and nursing care. The patient with pneumonia has a temperature elevation and may have shaking chills. Increased temperature and pulse are indications that body defenses are mobilized into action and additional strains on the body will be detrimental. Bed rest is a "must." The nurse can help to assure adequate rest for the patient by helping him with personal hygiene, keeping the environment generally quiet, allaying fears and apprehension, and arranging for regular rest periods during the day. If the disease is severe, the patient should move only enough to maintain good general circulation. Sometimes passive exercises are prescribed by the doctor. The patient must be told that he must not try to help; otherwise he may feel impelled to move when he does not have energy to expend in this way.

When the temperature is elevated, both fluids and salt are lost. Fluids are forced to 3,000 ml. a day, and additional salt may be given either in food or in intravenous fluids. If the patient is nauseated or otherwise unable to take sufficient fluids by mouth, infusions may be given.

Since the treatment and prognosis of

pneumonia depend upon the causative organism, the sputum is examined for type of organism and cultures are grown. Pneumonia is now classified according to offending organism rather than to anatomic location (lobar or bronchial), as was previously the practice. The type of organism determines the drug or drugs that are given. For example, pneumococcal infections are usually treated with penicillin; a mixed type of infection may be treated most effectively with streptomycin, chlortetracycline (Aureomycin), or oxytetracycline (Terramycin), as well as penicillin. Medications must be carefully given as ordered to ensure that the amount necessary to combat the infection is present in the blood stream. A sputum specimen for exaimination should be obtained *before* administration of the drug is started, and it is a nursing responsibility to help obtain this specimen as quickly as possible.

If antimicrobial therapy is instituted promptly, the temperature drops markedly in twenty-four hours, the pulse rate may become normal, and the patient may feel generally much better. When the temperature falls, the patient usually perspires profusely. He must be kept warm and protected from drafts; clothing that becomes damp with perspiration should be changed at once. The patient must be observed closely for "pseudocrisis." In this condition the temperature falls but the pulse remains elevated and the patient's general condition does not improve; the lowered temperature indicates failure of the body's resources to meet the threat of bacterial infection in an adequate way.

Because of high temperature, dehydration, and mouth breathing, the patient needs frequent mouth care. Maintenance of cleanliness of the mouth may also inhibit extension of infection to the ears. Herpetic blisters about the mouth are common and are a source of much discomfort to the patient. Tincture of benzoin can be applied, and sometimes camphor ice is beneficial; cold cream can be used to soften the crusted areas. If the nostrils are dry or are crusted with exudate, swabs moistened with water or peroxide can be used and cold cream can be applied to the external nares.

Chest pain in pneumonia is caused by inflammation of the pleura and usually is confined to the affected side. It may be severe and stabbing in nature and may be exaggerated by coughing and by deep breathing. Respirations are often described as "grunting." Close observation of the chest may show that there is limitation of movement of the affected side. The patient may use accessory muscles to aid in breathing instead of expanding the lower chest fully. The patient with severe chest pain usually needs help and encouragement in changing his position at intervals. Lying on the affected side may relieve the pain since this helps to splint the painful side of the chest. Raising the head of the bed will often make it easier for the patient to breathe, but he may need pillows to support the arms, since otherwise the weight of the arms dropping forward puts a strain on the shoulder girdle and increases fatigue. Oxygen is often used for the patient who has severe chest pain and difficulty in breathing adequately since the higher concentration of oxygen makes deep breathing less necessary for obtaining an adequate supply of oxygen. (For care of the patient receiving oxygen, see texts on fundamentals of nursing.) Occasionally pain is severe enough to require regional block of the intercostal nerves (see Chapter 13). If narcotics are used, codiene is usually the drug of choice since it is less likely to inhibit productive coughing than the stronger narcotic drugs.

Severe cough and blood-tinged or "rusty" sputum are characteristic of pneumonia. The patient must be encouraged and helped to cough deeply to produce sputum from the lungs and not expend needed energy in raising secretions from the upper trachea and posterior pharynx only. The nurse can help the patient to cough without too much pain by giving prescribed medications and by helping to splint the chest as the patient coughs.

In severe pneumonia, peristaltic action

may be affected. The nurse should report failure to have a bowel movement and any distention, rigidity, or tenderness in the upper abdominal quadrant, since these are signs of paralytic ileus. If peristalsis becomes suppressed or absent, there is respiratory distress due to elevation of the diaphragm and vomiting may occur. Enemas are seldom given because they will be retained unless siphoned off, and they may increase distention and discomfort. Insertion of a rectal tube or the administration of Prostigmin may help to relieve distention. Continuous gastric suction may be started and intravenous fluids containing electrolytes are given, since electrolyte imbalance will be made worse by removal of stomach secretions and potassium loss may contribute to the development of paralytic ileus. Peristalsis seems to be encouraged by exercise; if the patient's condition permits, sitting up in bed or even walking a little often helps. Eating solid food also appears to prevent the occurrence of paralytic ileus in some instances; for this reason, if they are able to take this kind of nourishment, some physicians order solid food for patients who are quite ill. However, the patient who has had paralytic ileus or in whom the condition has threatened should not be given foods that are gas forming.

Prevention of complications. With the advent of antibiotics and better diagnostic measures such as x-ray procedures, complications during or following pneumonia are rare in otherwise normal persons. Atelectasis, delayed resolution, lung abscess, pleural effusion, empyema, pericarditis, meningitis, and relapse are complications that were quite common in the past. Strict adherence to the prescribed medical treatment, careful, accurate observation, and sufficient time for convalescence now ensure the average patient a smooth recovery from pneumonia. However, aged persons and those with chronic illness are likely to have a longer course of convalescence, and there is a greater possibility of their developing complications. Recently there has been an increase in the incidence of staphylococcal pneumonia subsequent to influenza. Consolidation of lung tissue, pleural effusion, and empyema frequently occur soon after the onset of this type of pneumonia.

Acute bronchitis

Bronchitis can be acute or chronic. Acute bronchitis is an inflammation of the bronchi and sometimes the trachea (tracheobronchitis). It is often caused by an extension of an upper respiratory tract infection such as the common cold and is, therefore, communicable. It also may be caused by physical or chemical agents such as dust, smoke, or volatile fumes, and since 9,500 communities in the United States have an air pollution problem this is an increasing public health problem.[27]

The patient with acute bronchitis usually complains of chilliness, malaise, muscular aches, headaches, a dry scratchy throat, hoarseness, and a cough. The temperature may be elevated. The patient may be confined to bed at home or in the hospital. In either case, exposure to others should be kept to a minimum.

The treatment of acute tracheobronchitis is usually conservative in an attempt to prevent extension of infection to the smaller bronchi, the bronchioles, and the alveoli of the lungs. The patient usually is kept on bed rest and should avoid prolonged activity of any type. He should be protected from drafts, and he should take from 3,000 to 4,000 ml. of fluid daily. A simple bland diet is usually most easily eaten. Often a single dose of procaine penicillin, 300,000 units, is given intramuscularly if the patient has an elevation of temperature. If the temperature remains elevated, penicillin, 300,000 units, may be given daily, or other antibiotics such as oxytetracycline (Terramycin) may be used.

Early in the disease the patient's main complaints are the dry irritating cough and the feeling of tightness and soreness in the chest that follows coughing. The patient may get relief by the same means as those described for the common cold. Mustard plasters over the anterior chest may help to counteract local soreness (see texts on fundamentals of nursing). Cough may be relieved by cough mixtures containing potassium iodide or ammonium chloride which increase secretions. Humidifying the air eases breathing and lessens irritation. Tincture of benzoin, menthol, or oil of eucalyptus may be added to the steam vaporizer for its soothing and aromatic effect. As the disease progresses, secretions usually increase; congestion and dryness of the bronchial mucous membrane are then relieved.

Most patients need a period of convalescence following an attack of acute bronchitis. Patients usually complain of weakness and fatigability. The nurse should caution the patient to guard against overexertion, including return to work without medical approval. He should be encouraged to take extra rest, to eat a well-balanced diet, and to avoid conditions which might expose him to further infection or predispose him to possible relapse.

Chronic bronchitis

Chronic bronchitis is a recurring inflammation which involves the smaller as well as the large bronchi and usually results from other infection within the respiratory tract. Infection may be in the mouth, the sinuses, or in the terminal bronchi. In each of these instances, infected material is breathed into the bronchial tree, causing inflammation of the mucous membrane, and exudate.

Bronchial infections are more common in the winter months. Cold damp weather, variations in temperature between indoor and outdoor environment, and lack of sunshine play a part in recurrences. It is important, however, that the underlying bacteriologic cause be determined so that the lesions can be treated with specific antibiotics. The causative agent may not be specific. Any of the pyogenic organisms such as *Streptococcus hemolyticus,* Friedländer's bacillus, pneumococcus, and influenza bacillus may be associated with chronic bronchitis.

Most patients have difficulty with persistent cough, the production of sputum, and dyspnea. If the sputum is thick, medications such as potassium iodide may be given. Some patients are plagued with large amounts of sputum upon arising in the morning since inactivity causes secretions to collect in the bronchi. Postural drainage is often necessary and is particularly useful for the elderly patient who may not be able to expel secretions forcibly. Steam inhalations also soften secretions; it is often helpful for the patient to inhale steam for a few minutes before attempting to clear secretions from the bronchi. If severe dyspnea and cyanosis develop as a result of severe coughing and inability to clear the respiratory passages adequately, oxygen may be necessary. This may be given by mask; both in the hospital and in his own home, the patient may be taught to turn the oxygen on and off so that he can administer it to himself as he finds necessary. If oxygen is being used in the home, members of the family as well as the patient must be cautioned about the danger of fire from lighted matches or other flame.

The patient with chronic bronchitis is usually advised to stop smoking or to limit his use of inhaled tobacco. Good nutrition, plenty of rest, sunshine, and avoidance of dust and smoky air are usually advised. He should be protected or instructed to protect himself against extremes of cold or dampness. It may be possible for him to move to a climate where he may improve. The patient with abundant sputum may be advised to seek a dry, warm climate, while the one with little sputum may be urged to visit the seashore in a warm climate. The benefits of climatic changes, of course, are unavailable to many patients because of lack of money or for other reasons.

Tuberculosis

purulent blood-streaked sputum

Tuberculosis has affected man from the earliest times. It has even had periods of relative acceptance; it has been considered fashionable, disgraceful, and mysterious. Today there is need for better interpretation and for clearer understanding of the disease. It is still looked upon by many as being associated with un-

Table 8 Tuberculosis morbidity and mortality, primarily between 1947 and 1953, in the United States*

Year	*New cases*	*Tuberculosis deaths*†	*Case fatality (per cent)*	*Case rate*	*Death rate*‡
1947	134,946	48,064	36	94	33
1948	137,006	43,833	32	93	30
1949	134,865	39,100	29	90	26
1950	121,742	33,959	28	80	22
1951	118,491	30,863	26	77	20
1952	109,837	24,261	22	70	16
1953	106,925	19,393§	18	67	12
Change 1953/47	− 28,021 =21%	−28,671 =60%	−18	−27 =29%	−21 =64%

*From Drolet, Godias J., and Lowell, Anthony M.: Whereto Tuberculosis? The First Seven Years of the Antimicrobial Era, 1947-1953, Am. Rev. Tuberc. **72**:419-452, Oct. 1955.

†All forms.

‡Per 100,000 population.

§Provisional.

Population estimated as of 1953: United States, 159,629,000 (including Armed Forces overseas).

cleanliness and with careless living; many families hesitate to admit that tuberculosis has attacked one of their members. Fear of the disease is one of the greatest barriers to control and treatment. This fear exists among health workers as well as patients, their families, and the general public. If nurses clearly understand the disease themselves, they can do a great deal to eradicate barriers to effective control and treatment.

The changing picture of tuberculosis. Mortality from tuberculosis has decreased markedly. In 1900 there were 200 deaths per 100,000 population, and tuberculosis was in first place as the cause of death in the United States.[15] As of 1947 these figures had been reduced to 38 deaths per 100,000 population, and in 1957 there were only 8 deaths per 100,000 population.[28] Tuberculosis has now moved to tenth place as the cause of death.[28]

The number of active cases of tuberculosis, or the *tuberculosis morbidity rate,* has not declined as much as the mortality rate. In fact, while the mortality rate has decreased 33 per cent in the past 4 years, the morbidity rate has increased 22 per cent. This increase probably represents an increase in known active cases because of improved case-finding rather than a real increase in the active cases. It is estimated that there are 250,000 active cases of tuberculosis in the United States today and of these 100,000 are unrecognized and therefore untreated.[28] However, the morbidity rate bears continued close scrutiny since tuberculosis still ranks as the first cause of death from *infectious disease* in the United States. In 1947 there were 94 active cases per 100,000 population; in 1953, 67 active cases per 100,000 population. In 1957, the National Tuberculosis Association reported 150,000 known cases; this is 87.7 cases per 100,000 population.[28] There are about 9 active and another 9 inactive cases of tuberculosis for each death annually.

Tuberculin testing has revealed a marked decrease in the number of people infected with tubercle bacilli prior to the age of 20 years. Fifty years ago it was found that almost 100 per cent of the population were infected prior to the age of 20 years.[15] At the present time in the United States, only about 32 per cent of the population is infected, and in recent testing of Navy personnel less than 5 per cent reacted positively to the tuberculin test.[2]

The age of those now developing tuberculosis is also interesting. The morbidity and mortality rates are now proportionately much higher among older people, as indicated in Table 9. Older men, particularly, are increasingly affected by tuberculosis. Today, over 50 per cent of persons dying from tuberculosis are 45 years of age or older as compared to 25 per cent in 1900.[15] The increasing number of older persons in the population has contributed to these changes. Tuberculosis mortality is highest in the first year of life; it drops between the ages of 1 and 5 years, and it is lowest between the ages of 5 years and puberty.[15]

The biggest forward step during recent years in the control and treatment of tuberculosis has been improvement in treatment through discovery of antituberculosis drugs and through improved methods of surgical treatment. Improvement in living standards, better nutrition, shorter working hours, and earlier diagnosis and treatment also have contributed to the declining mortality rate. With the relatively high number of active cases, however, tuberculosis still remains a public health problem.

Prevention and control. As more is learned about the behavior of the tubercle bacillus and as new drugs are developed, medical recommendations change. To keep informed of the latest developments in case finding, prevention and treatment, the student should refer to current periodicals and to specific publications in the field of tuberculosis. One of the most valuable sources of education for the prevention and control of tuberculosis is the National Tuberculosis Association. This voluntary association was organized in 1904 as the National Association for the Study and Prevention of Tuberculosis and has grown to tremendous size. Each state has had an organization since 1917, and there are local organizations in all sections of the states. These state associations and the National Association have worked steadily in the study of tuberculosis, in the dissemination of information about the disease, and in furthering the scientific treatment of tuberculosis. By contacting her local health department, the nurse can learn about branches of this organization in her local area. The Na-

Table 9 Tuberculosis death rates and case rates per 100,000 population, by age, for 1930 and 1950 and ratio between 1920 and 1950 rates*

Age	*Death rates*			*Case rates*		
	1930	*1950*	*Ratio of 1930 to 1950 (1950 1)*	*1930*	*1950*	*Ratio of 1930 to 1950 (1950 1)*
All ages	56.0	17.6	3.2	139.6	68.5	2.0
Under 5	24.6	4.1	6.0	37.3	24.1	1.5
5–14	9.8	1.0	9.8	74.1	14.9	5.0
15–19	39.7	2.5	15.9	140.7	38.2	3.7
20–24	71.5	7.4	9.7	243.3	81.3	3.0
25–34	89.8	12.1	7.4	235.3	79.7	3.0
35–44	78.0	18.0	4.3	161.5	73.9	2.2
45–54	81.9	28.5	2.9	140.3	99.6	1.4
55–64	74.2	39.7	1.9	114.7	105.9	1.1
65–74	76.5	46.4	1.6	85.3	95.1	0.9
75 and over	73.7	46.4	1.6			

*From Bulletin of State Department of Health, Albany, N. Y., September 17, 1956.

tional Tuberculosis Association is financed through the sale of Christmas seals. By contracts with the state tuberculosis associations, both city and county associations hold annual campaigns and pay a percentage of the money raised to the state association. The state association, in turn, pays 6 per cent of the money raised in the state to the National Association. Thus, 94 per cent of all the money raised by Christmas seal sales within a state remains in the state for use by the state and local organizations.

The local organizations help to evaluate problems of tuberculosis in the community and find out what methods of control are being used. After collecting the necessary information, the local association passes it along to members of the community by means of exhibits, posters, talks, the press, films, and television. Local organizations work closely with hospitals, departments of health and of welfare, and local physicians. They give guidance to families and patients, and many local associations have sponsored x-ray examination and tuberculin-testing programs in their areas.

Case-finding has proved to be one of the most valuable methods of tuberculosis control, since early diagnosis and careful medical treatment prevent the spread of infection to others. Observation of symptoms, physical examinations, tuberculin-testing, and examination of known contacts were once the main methods of case-finding. With the advent of x-ray examination and particularly of the less expensive methods of x-ray examination in 1931, case-finding extended to the discovery of patients with early symptomless disease. Case-finding by means of mass x-ray screening began in local tuberculosis associations and in local communities. With its success, x-ray surveys spread rapidly throughout the nation. The idea of taking periodic films of seemingly healthy persons followed. Today the practice of routinely taking roentgenograms of the chests of all patients admitted to hospitals or accepted for outpatient care is growing. Over 20 per cent of all general hospitals have instituted the practice of obtaining routine screening roentgenograms on admission of patients. Many hospitals have done this in cooperation with tuberculosis associations and with state or local health departments. Twenty million patients admitted to the hospital and 50 million registered in outpatient departments are x-rayed and the results reported annually by the 5,000 general hospitals in the United States.[31] Approximately 10 per cent of all patients so examined have been found to have significant findings of chest disease. However, in the present atomic age, the hazards of repeated exposure to radiation (in the x-ray procedure) has become greater, and the practice of making x-ray examinations of large groups of apparently healthy persons is becoming less common. Pregnant women are no longer advised to have an x-ray examination of the chest unless there are definite indications that this is necessary. The United States Public Health Service now recommends that x-ray examination of the chest as a case-finding technique be limited to groups with the greatest risk of contracting the disease. In groups with a low risk, tuberculin skin-testing is advised as the first step in case finding.[28]

Tuberculin skin-testing is a widely used method of learning whether or not the patient has ever been exposed to tubercle bacilli. A negative tuberculin skin reaction usually rules out disease and also any past exposure to the infection. A positive test indicates that infection has occurred and that there has been a sensitizing reaction to the organisms.[25] It gives no indication of the activity or inactivity of disease; however, it has been shown recently that those who have more extensive local reactions are more likely to develop active tuberculosis or to have been in recent contact with someone with active disease. Usually following positive tests a roentgenogram is taken to rule out the presence of active pulmonary disease.

Two substances are used in tuberculin skin-testing: OT (old tuberculin), which is prepared from dead tubercle bacilli and contains their related impurities, and PPD (purified protein derivative), which is a highly purified product containing protein from the tubercle bacilli in a dry, stable form. PPD is made up in the desired dilution from tablets immediately before use. OT comes in liquid form, having been prepared in various dilutions each week during the culture of the living organism.

Since it gives the most accurate results, the tuberculin test most often done is the *Mantoux test,* or intracutaneous injection of either PPD or OT. A tuberculin syringe and a short (½ inch), sharp, 24 to 26 gauge needle are used. With the skin (usually the inner forearm is used) held taut, the injection of an exact amount of the PPD or OT is made into the superficial layers, and it produces a sharply raised white wheal. Weak dilutions are used first; if the reaction is negative, stronger dilutions are used. This prevents severe local reactions which might occur in highly sensitive individuals if the higher dilution were used initially. If old tuberculin is used, tests are begun with a dilution of 1:10,000 or 0.001 mg. of OT. If this test is negative, successive tests with 1:1000, 1:100, and 1:10 dilutions are made. If PPD is used, the first strength contains 0.00002 mg. of tuberculoprotein and the second strength contains 0.005 mg. Each injection dose is 0.1 ml. For broad screening and case-finding purposes, a single test using a relatively high dilution is recommended. Interpretations of the tests are made after forty-eight hours. A positive reaction may begin after twelve to twenty-four hours with an area of redness and a central area of induration, but it reaches its peak in forty-eight hours. The area of induration indicates how positive the test is; it is sometimes read as 1, 2, 3, or 4 plus. When successive dilutions are being used, it is advisable to have tests read by the same person since individual variation in interpretation cannot be prevented. If the test is negative, there may be no visible reaction or there may be slight redness with no induration.

The *Vollmer patch test* is done by applying an adhesive patch to the skin. Usually the skin over the sternum, between the scapulae, or on the forearm is used. The patch consists of two squares, one impregnated with concentrated tuberculin and one impregnated with a synthetic control medium. It is left on for forty-eight hours. It is then removed, and the reaction is read forty-eight hours after its removal. Care should be taken not to wet the patch during the first forty-eight hours.

The *Pirquet test* is made by scarring the skin by inoculation with a drop of OT. The skin over the deltoid muscle is usually used, and readings are done after forty-eight and seventy-two hours.

The *Heaf test* is made by wetting the skin on the forearm with concentrated tuberculin solution and then an instrument with six short needles arranged in a circle is used to lightly puncture the skin. The readings are done after forty-eight hours and the test is considered positive if there are four or more small red blebs. There seems to be less ulceration of local tissues and of lymph nodes using this method than there is with the Mantoux test. However, it is considered accurate in case-finding.[11]

When a diagnosis of active tuberculosis has been made or when the presence of the disease is strongly suspected, members of the patient's family and close associates are urged to have an examination. Tests and examinations that may be recommended include tuberculin skin-testing, roentgenograms of the chest, sputum examinations, and possibly gastric aspirations. The nurse has an active part in explaining to them why it is advisable to be examined and in helping to make the necessary arrangements. Depending on where they live and their particular circumstances, they may go to their doctor, to the local health department, or to a hospital clinic. Members of the family are often extremely upset and even panicky at the knowledge that the patient has tuberculosis and at the threat to others in the family. They need repeated explanation and reassurance. They should

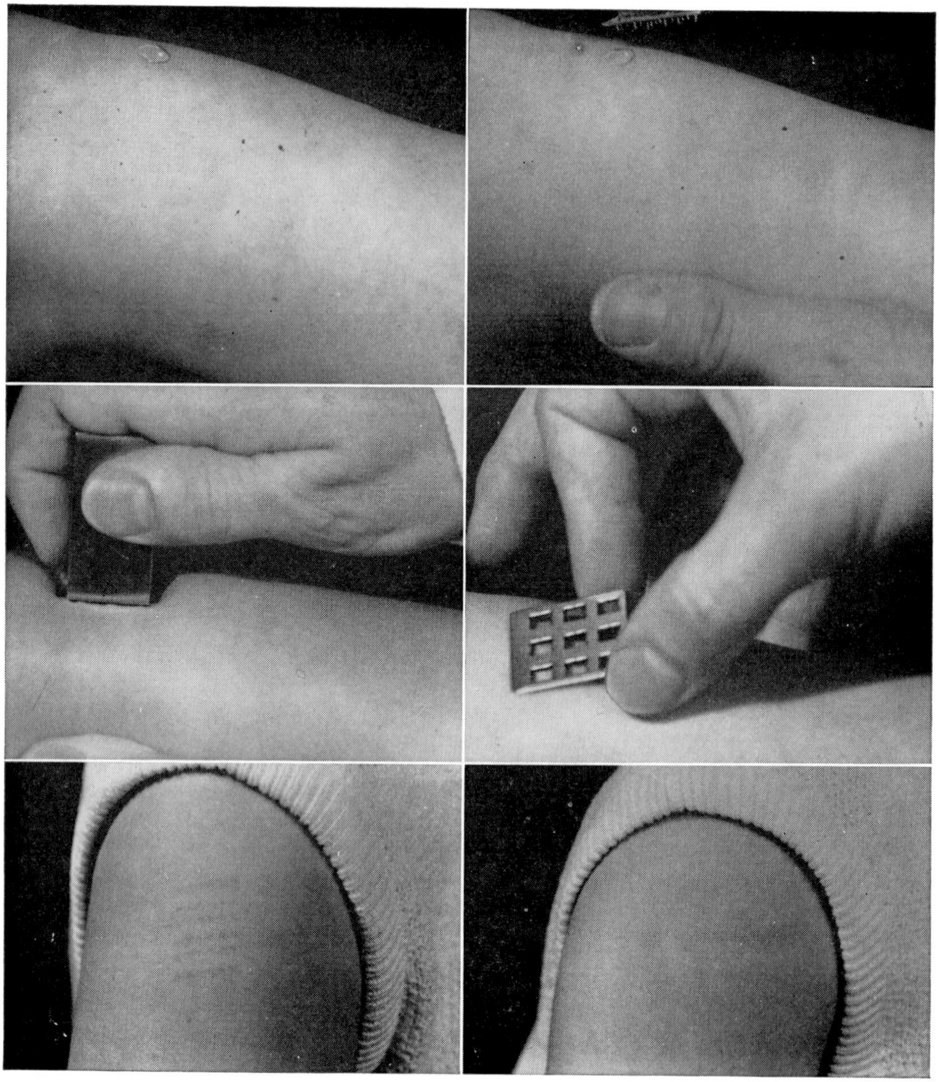

A. B. C. D. E. F.

Figure 63

Vaccination with BCG. *A,* A drop of BCG vaccine is placed on the arm. *B,* The drop of vaccine is spread by tapping with the wide end of a metal disk. *C,* The points of the metal disk are pressed through vaccine to penetrate the skin. *D,* The vaccine is redistributed by a tapping motion. *E,* The site of vaccination after thirteen days. *F,* The site of vaccination after ninety days; note absence of scar. (Courtesy Research Foundation, Chicago, Ill.)

be told, for example, when results of a chest film can be expected and where they should go to learn about the results. They should also know that some tests take more time than usual for laboratory studies of other disease; for example, that cultures grow slowly.

A specific dependable vaccine against tuberculosis has not been developed. *BCG* (Bacillus Calmette-Guérin) is one of a number of tuberculosis vaccines that have been tested. BCG is considered safe, and it is believed to give some protection against the disease. It is given to those persons who do not react positively to tuberculin-testing and who are likely to be exposed to those with active disease. It is emphasized that the vaccine should be used only as part of a complete control program, including case-finding and isolation of patients with active disease; it should never be relied upon as the only preventive measure.

BCG vaccine contains avirulent tubercle bacilli; they are alive but through many generations of growth in artificial media (attenuation) they have lost their ability to produce disease. The vaccine should be given only by those who have had careful instruction in the proper technique. A multiple puncture disk is used as shown in Figure 63. When there is a positive reaction to skin-testing with tuberculin, when acute infectious disease is present, or when there is any skin disease, BCG is not given. Possible complications following vaccination are local ulcers which occur in a relatively high percentage of those vaccinated and abscesses or suppuration of lymph nodes which occur in a small percentage.

Diagnosis and course of disease. Tuberculosis is caused by a bacillus, the *Myocobacterium tuberculosis* or tubercle bacillus. This is a gram-positive and acid-fast organism. Microscopic study of a slide prepared from the sputum of a patient with active infection reveals the organisms quite readily. The tubercle bacillus is capable of survival outside its host particularly when it is embedded in sputum or pus, but growth outside the host requires very special conditions. Carefully prepared cultures on the most favorable media grow very slowly, and several weeks are needed to obtain growth suitable for study. When organisms are widely scattered in body fluids, such as spinal fluid, gastric washings, or fluid aspirated from the pleural cavity, it may be difficult to get sufficient concentration for study by means of a stained prepared slide. A healthy guinea pig may be inoculated with the fluid, however, and if, on examination after two weeks, the animal shows signs of tuberculosis, the diagnosis is confirmed.

When the tubercle bacilli enter the air passages, they cause an inflammation in the alveoli. The natural body defenses then attempt to counteract the infection. This reaction produces a small, firm, white, nodule called the *primary tubercle*. The center of the nodule contains tubercle bacilli. Cells gather around the center, and usually the outer portion becomes fibrosed. Thus, blood vessels are compressed, nutrition of the tubercle is interfered with, and necrosis occurs at the center. The area becomes walled off by fibrotic tissue around the outside, and the center gradually becomes soft and cheesy in consistency. This latter process is known as caseation. This material may become calcified, or it may liquefy. The first infection is usually successfully overcome, and the calcified nodule is known as the *Ghon tubercle*. Subsequent infections, however, may not be so well dealt with; liquefied material may break through the containing walls and empty into the bronchus and be raised as sputum. The amount of sputum produced depends upon the extent and stage of the disease. As the patient responds to treatment, including rest, well-balanced diet, and antimicrobial drugs, the area heals by fibrosis and calcification; this healing requires months and sometimes years. Sometimes surgery is necessary to speed recovery.

Prevention of spread. Tuberculosis is spread either directly or indirectly from one individual to another. The usual way of transmission is by inhalation of droplets or dust containing tubercle bacilli. Despite the fact that many people inhale tubercle baccilli during the course of their lives, the majority of them overcome the infection and active clinical tuberculosis does not develop. The defensive forces of the body overcome the first bacterial invasion. The amount of exposure to the baccilli, the length of time exposed, the virulence of the bacilli, and the resistance of the individual all help to determine whether or not active disease will develop. Tuberculosis does not often follow the swallowing of tubercle bacilli, but one can be indirectly exposed by placing contaminated hands in the mouth, by using contaminated utensils, by contact with contaminated handkerchiefs, and the like.

The best way to protect others from active pulmonary tuberculosis is by helping the patient to understand how the disease is transmitted and how he can prevent bacilli from reaching the surrounding atmosphere and in turn, infecting those who breathe the air. The nurse should teach the patient to cover his mouth and nose when clearing his throat, sneezing, or coughing, as well as emphasize the other important points of care of sputum discussed at the beginning of this chapter. The patient should wash his hands after handling any sputum or receptacle containing sputum. It is possible for him to reinfect himself if he breathes air infected with organisms, since such organisms may invade other portions of the lungs. Helping members of the family who are to give most of the care to the patient to provide for these precautions is an important nursing responsibility.

Tubercle bacilli remain alive in dried sputum or dust in dark places for weeks or months and in moist sputum for six weeks or more. Thus moist sputum should be disposed of promptly, and rooms, furniture, and other articles should be kept as free of dust and as clean as possible. The danger to the public from indiscriminate spitting on streets and in public places by those who may have active tuberculosis is obvious. The most effective way to kill the tubercle bacillus in moist sputum is by burning; all tissues and disposable receptacles for the collection of sputum should be burned. Direct sunlight destroys the bacillus in from one to two hours. Five minutes at boiling temperature and thirty minutes at pasteurizing temperature, 61.7° C. (143° F.) kill the bacillus. Boiling is therefore the best method of caring for articles used by the patient with active infection. If boiling is impossible, then exposure to direct sunlight should be used. Ordinary chemical disinfectants take many hours to kill tubercle bacilli, since the organisms can survive the action of strong acids and alkalies that destroy most other bacteria rapidly. For example, there is no entirely safe method of disinfecting mouth thermometers after use by a patient with tubercle bacilli in his sputum. Thorough cleansing with soap and running water should be relied upon more than the action of disinfectant solutions. Handwashing is important. The nurse should emphasize the main reason for handwashing—the mechanical removal of foreign material. Hand brushes are not advised since they tend to irritate the skin and are difficult to keep clean. Disinfectant solutions are not necessary.

Many patients with active tuberculosis are cared for in their own homes; the nurse can help patients and their families to understand the communicability of tuberculosis and to take the necessary precautions. Family members and friends may be frightened at the thought of contact with the patient and with articles he has touched. On the other hand, they often point to long, intimate contact they have had with the patient without developing the disease. Careful observation of the family will help the nurse determine how much and what kind of explanations are needed regarding spread of infection. If the family is overly cautious in handling the patient's personal articles, the nurse can advise against discarding articles which may be costly to replace. In contrast, if the family is too casual in regard to spread of the disease, the nurse should emphasize more care in handling dishes and other articles as well as sputum. If possible, the patient should occupy a room alone, but he should not be strictly isolated from the rest of the family. Careful planning with the family often helps to ensure that he will not infect others, yet located so that he and his family can be as happy as possible under such circumstances. The susceptibility of babies and very small children must be emphasized in all teaching of the patient and of his family.

Acceptance of the disease. While the nurse may well be aware that the patient has tuberculosis, is the patient aware? Acceptance of a diagnosis of tuberculosis and of its many implications for the future is difficult for any one. Real acceptance may come only after months of illness and after slow, steady help and support from the family, the doctor, the social worker, and the nurse. The rate and degree of acceptance of facts and realities vary according to each patient's basic personality and his life-long pattern of behavior in stress situations. The nurse should realize that for some time after the diagnosis is made and treatment started the patient's true self may not be evident. At first the patient may seem to accept everything, and then, little by little, his behavior may reveal that he has not accepted the disease at all. For example, the patient may be pleasant and agreeable, accept suggestions readily, and follow recommended medical treatment carefully for the first month or two. But when the third or fourth month is reached, he may begin to complain about the food, he may get out of bed oftener than is recommended, he may object to taking medications, and he may make occasional sarcastic remarks. The length of time necessary for "cure" is often the most difficult problem for the patient to face. Particularly is this true if time must be spent in a hospital away from his family, job, and usual way of life.

Some patients do not have the capacity ever to accept the disease, and they may experience frustration and despair at the changes in their lives that it entails. The patient may completely "block out" all thoughts of the disease and continue as if nothing had really happened. Other patients may welcome the long period of rest and the lessening of life's responsibilities; however, as recovery progresses and they must once again face adjustment to normal life outside a hospital or sheltered care facility, they may experience fear and anxiety.

Knowledge and understanding of his disease only follows acceptance of the disease by the patient. The degree of understanding and knowledge varies with the degree of acceptance, and lack of acceptance may lead to inconsistent behavior. For example, a patient may carefully cover his mouth and nose when coughing, but he will get out of bed oftener than is recommended by the doctor; he is willing to protect others, but he fails to protect himself. Since the treatment of tuberculosis extends over a long period of time, periodic re-evaluation and follow-up are necessary.

The patient with tuberculosis, like any other person, reveals his awareness and his understanding by his behavior. To know the patient takes time, careful observation, analysis of observation, and comparison of observations with others who know him. It is easy for one nurse to interpret a patient's behavior as she sees it, but perhaps another nurse, the doctor, or the social worker will have a different interpretation based upon their observations and collective information. Conferences among staff members caring for the patient provide an excellent opportunity for all persons to discuss their observations and interpretations.

Acceptance of tuberculosis as a disease by the nurse is closely related to her ability to know and to help the patient with tuberculosis. If a nurse fears tuberculosis, she may show this in her own behavior. Most patients with tuberculosis are extremely sensitive to ways in which various health workers approach them. If the nurse is obvious about precautions in giving care, she may cause the patient to feel rejected. Her touch when giving physical care, or even when placing articles such as food trays within reach, may be clues to him as to her acceptance of him with his disease. Nurses may be fearful of the disease for various reasons. If the nurse is conscious of her fear, discussion with a more experienced person may

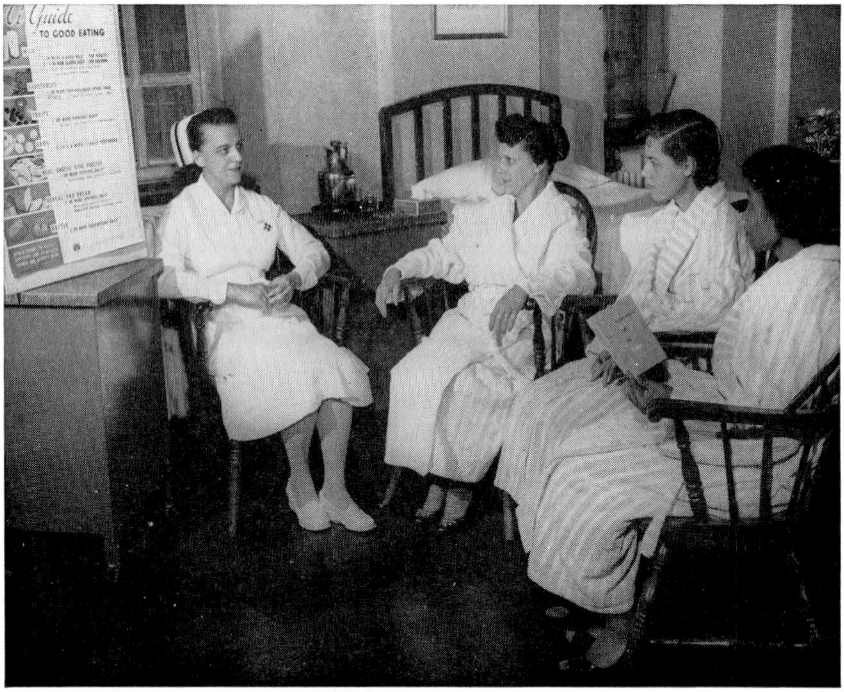

Figure 64

Some of the best opportunities for teaching occur during discussions with small groups of patients. General health principles, as well as understanding of disease, can be discussed. Here the nurse is discussing the selection of well-balanced meals.

help her to learn more about the disease, to accept it better, and, therefore, to alter her own feelings and reactions.

Many nurses feel that because recovery is slow, care of the patient with tuberculosis is very routine. Although things done for a patient may be repetitive and routine, no person is "routine." The nurse who focuses on the patient as a person will not find her work routine or monotonous. Sincere interest in the patient, interest in learning more about him, and a real desire to be helpful to him will yield wide and varied nursing experience.

Nursing care in tuberculosis. If the patient is seriously or critically ill, he will need care similar to that given any patient who is unable to do anything for himself. Probably he will be isolated, and the usual isolation techniques will need to be carried out, using special precautions in caring for sputum or drainage from any lesions, wounds, or sinuses that may contain live organisms. (For details of isolation techniques, see textbooks on fundamentals of nursing and on communicable disease.)

The majority of patients with tuberculosis are able to assume responsibility for most of their own care. Proper rest, good nutrition, administration of prescribed drugs, and attention to good body alignment are essential. The nurse's major responsibility is to teach the patient what he should do and why and to give encouragement and supervision in the simple but essential elements of good care. (See Figure 64.)

Rest must be mental as well as physical, and this presents a real challenge to the nurse and to all others. Learning why mental rest is impossible for the patient is sometimes difficult, but continued friendly interest usually leads to understanding. Loneliness, need for privacy, financial worries, concern for loved ones are only a few of the many problems that may be interfering with rest.

It is often extremely difficult for the average patient with tuberculosis who feels well and looks well to remain on bed rest. Activities that can be carried on while in bed often are useful. Sometimes when the patient is restless and resentful in bed and not really resting, the doctor decides that being up for stipulated intervals and engaging in some quiet activity during such time are better for the patient than strict bed rest.

Patients may be able to comply better with orders to rest when given adequate explanations of why it is necessary. One simple explanation which can be used is a comparison of a damaged lung with an injured finger. The more one moves the finger, the more time is required for it to heal. In the same way, the more one uses the lungs, the more time is required for their healing. Breathing rate is increased with any activity—this is obvious to all patients. Lying down allows for a slower rate of breathing. Good body alignment also aids breathing. If the patient sits or lies in a cramped position in bed, easy, relaxed breathing is hindered.

Many hospitals have classified degrees of activity for patients. The patient is placed on bed rest and in the beginning is given very little responsibility for his own care; activities are progressively increased as the patient's physical condition improves. When the patient can be out of bed, going to the bathroom is usually one of the first activities allowed. Other examples are sitting in a chair at the bedside, sitting in a solarium for a short time, or getting up for meals. Trips to the occupational therapy department usually constitute more advanced activity.

If the patient is confined to bed in a hospital or in his own home, the nurse can help to maintain his contacts with the outside world and his interest in activities outside his restricted world. Spending more time resting with little change in surroundings can be trying even to the best-adjusted patient, and it is to be expected that his horizons may narrow somewhat. If the patient must remain hospitalized for a period of time, members of the staff or the patient's family are his only contacts with the outside. Thus, in conversation, many patients turn to the nurse to learn about the latest movies, various shows, community activities, prices in stores, and the like.

Small day-by-day routine tasks and activities should be planned. The patient should be encouraged to maintain interest in his appearance and in his grooming. Manicures, shampoos, and hair styling can be done easily with groups of patients. Men patients also often welcome regular shampoos and manicures. Personal belongings tend to collect, and the patient needs help in sorting and arranging these. The nurse or anyone else she delegates to help with this should bear in mind that all personal articles are important to the patient. Rearranging and sorting should always be done with the patient present, or at least with his full permission. The patient may need to be urged to let some one "clean house"; performing this task without his permission might be compared to entering his home and rearranging it to satisfy a stranger's preference. Any patient who has a long-term illness and who is confined to bed or to limited activity for a long time values his smallest possessions in a way quite different from the person who is well and participating actively in life.

Ordinary small routine activities which every well person takes for granted can be very important to the patient on limited activity. For example, the patient who must brush his teeth in bed would appreciate having the toothbrush rinsed under running water. If he is allowed one tub bath a week, he enjoys a really clean tub and ample time to enjoy it. Supplying frequent changes of hospital pajamas or helping his family arrange for use of his own, remembering a second helping of a favorite food, and remembering radio or television programs of special interest are some of the many small ways in which the nurses can help the patient have a brighter and pleasanter day. If an organized occupational therapy department is available, the patient is encouraged to avail himself of this within his prescribed activity program. The interests of others in his projects adds to his enjoyment. Patients may enjoy telling the nurse about their projects or even teaching her some of the skills involved. When occupational therapy service is not available, the nurse can teach some simple skills to patients or arrange for them to take responsibility for small jobs such as distributing mail and taking orders for papers. Some patients who are allowed activity enjoy doing jobs.

Food and meal schedules can present many problems in the care of patients with tuberculosis. Adequate nutrition is essential to increase or to maintain natural body resistance and to help in the repair of damaged lung tissue. Some patients may have lost weight, and they may lack appetite. No matter how carefully the menus are planned and the food prepared and served, patients tire of institutional food. Members of the patient's family can help by occasionally preparing food and bringing it to the patient. This may replace the regular hospital meal, or it may be used as in-between-meal supplements. The nurse can help the patient with a poor appetite by preparing items of food in a particular way which she knows he enjoys; for example, by preparing eggs the particular way the patient prefers them. In many institutions in which patients with tuberculosis are cared for, a weekly check of weight is requested. When other outlets for their interest are restricted, some patients may be too preoccupied with food and they may gain weight. Contrary to popular opinion, some patients with tuberculosis are overweight, and reasonable dieting may be ordered. The nurse then needs to help make low-calorie foods attractive and satisfying.

Today, many patients with tuberculosis are not hospitalized. Since the newer drugs are more effective than conservative general care in controlling the communicability of the disease, some physicians feel that it is safe and better for the patient to remain at home and either visit the doctor's office or a clinic for his medication or have a public health nurse come in to give it. Many public health nurses are now administering the newer drugs to patients in their homes; the patient then usually visits the doctor's office or the hospital clinic at regular intervals.

If the patient is being treated at home, a definite schedule of activities must be arranged. Upon visiting a patient at home, the nurse may find that he is doing more than is advisable or recommended. It is particularly difficult for many persons to conform to a routine of restricted activity if they remain at home. If patients have had a period of hospitalization first, it is more likely that a daily program will have been planned with them, and the adjustment to home routine may be less difficult. The patient then understands more thoroughly the necessity for rest; he has had an opportunity to work out plans suitable for him with the medical staff, and he has developed habits which help him to get necessary rest at home. Patients at home who have not had the advantage of working closely in this way with a medical staff may find themselves adding activities one by one with little awareness that they are doing so. For example, a housewife may feel well and, seeing work to be done, may be tempted to do more than is good for her. She may add new activities daily until she is doing almost a full day's work. It is important that members of the family clearly understand the patient's rest and activity schedule so that they can help him to carry out the doctor's orders.

Men who have been used to regular working hours may feel guilty about being home during those hours. Since they are temporarily unable to support their families, they may feel that they must help with chores about the house, and they argue that some of these duties are light and will do them no harm.

Careful planning for the time when the patient leaves the hospital must start as soon as there is real evidence that this goal is within the patient's reach. His care at home should be reviewed with his family. They may wish to have a public health nurse visit their home to help them arrange for continued care. The public health nurse may continue the teaching begun in the hospital concerning menu planning for the family and rest and activity for the patient and other essentials of his care. The patient may have viewed his future with uncertainty for so long that he finds it difficult to express an interest in his future. Assistance in vocational rehabilitation is available to many patients and may include vocational retraining or counseling and guidance regarding future work. New abilities can be explored; for example, the patient may learn typing or some other gainful occupation that can be done while sitting.

Most patients who have had active tuberculosis return to work on a part-time schedule. In sheltered workshops the process of readjusting to a working and earning situation is often referred to as a "hardening process." Again, alternate periods of rest and activity are used; for example, the patient may spend twenty minutes traveling to work, rest for an hour, work for two hours, rest for an hour, return home, and rest again, or he may work two hours in the morning and two hours in the afternoon, with rest periods and mealtime separating the two work periods; gradually he works up to the usual eight-hour day.

Chemotherapy and antibiotic treatment. Regardless of whether the patient with tuberculosis is being treated at home or in the hospital, the same drugs are given. Streptomycin, para-aminosalicylic acid (PAS), and isonicotinic acid hydrazide (isoniazid) are the drugs in common use. These are used in combinations, such as streptomycin and para-aminosalicylic acid, streptomycin and isoniazid, and isoniazid and PAS. Many studies are being conducted to determine which combination is most effective.

Streptomycin is an antibiotic cultured from a fungus, the actinomycete *Streptomyces griseus.* It is now produced commercially and distributed in crystalline salt form or in solution. PAS is a chemical compound which inhibits the growth of the tubercle bacillus. PAS is usually distributed in tablet or capsule form. Isoniazid is the hydrazide of isonicotinic acid and is also distributed in tablet or capsule form.

Streptomycin is effective against the bacillus for a limited time only; after this, the bacillus develops resistance to the drug, thus making it ineffective. With the addition of PAS, the development of this resistance is lessened, although PAS given alone has little, if any, effect on the tubercle bacillus. Isoniazid is as effective as streptomycin and has certain advantages in that it can penetrate certain parts of the body such as the spinal canal and brain in much greater concentrations than can streptomycin. The tubercle bacillus, however, develops resistance to isoniazid.

The usual treatment consists of 1 Gm. of streptomycin intramuscularly twice a week and 12 Gm. of PAS by mouth daily in three doses. Usually isoniazid is not given to the patient at the beginning of the treatment but is reserved lest the bacilli become resistant to streptomycin and PAS cannot be tolerated. The usual dosage of isoniazid is 300 mg. by mouth daily in two or three doses. PAS is also given with isoniazid; the dosage is the same as when streptomycin is being given. Drug treatment is continued over a long time; the majority of physicians favor at least one to one and one-half years of treatment before the drugs are discontinued.

One of the most important points nurses can stress to patients is that they must continue drug therapy without interruption. During periods of interrupted treatment, resistant bacilli begin to appear. If this should happen, the drugs are less effective and may be completely ineffective. Interruptions may be made by the patient because he does not realize the importance of prolonged, steady treatment. Patients at home may neglect taking medications; others may leave hospitals against advice, discontinuing medication as well as failing to remain under medical supervision.

The length of drug therapy is often discouraging for the patient. The first few months may reveal little apparent improvement. Repeated intramuscular injections cause local tenderness even when the most skillful technique is used. A careful record must be kept of the site of injection, and care must be taken to give the injections in alternate thighs or buttocks. The skin should be observed closely for discoloration, and continued pain at the site of an injection should be noted. Brown discolorations with extreme tenderness may mean that a sterile abscess is forming, and the doctor should be notified at once.

Quite recently, patients remaining at home or returning home have been taught self-administration of streptomycin. The nurse teaches the patient how to give these injections and how to care for the medication and for the equipment he will need at home. Self-administration of streptomycin is, of course, never taught without the approval of the doctor. Members of the family may also be taught to give injections.

The nurse should observe the patient for, and teach him about, the side reactions to streptomycin: fever, rash, dizziness, deafness, and ringing in the ears. With the development of signs of hypersensitivity, such as fever and rash, the drug may be stopped or a reduced dose may be prescribed. Usually burning and itching are quickly relieved by giving an antihistamine drug. Vertigo (dizziness) is common in patients who receive large doses of streptomycin; it is less likely to occur if doses are small. Sometimes vertigo is accompanied by nausea and vomiting. In most instances, however, symptoms subside when the drug is discontinued, and only unusual sudden shaking of the head will produce them. Deafness is uncommon; however, when it occurs, it may be either temporary or permanent. Tinnitus, or ringing in the ears, usually disappears when the drug is discontinued.

Repeated large daily doses of PAS also cause toxic effects. These include nausea, vomiting, epigastric burning and discomfort, and diarrhea. Much of the epigastric distress can be alleviated by giving milk or an alkali such as sodium bicarbonate.

Isoniazid is a relatively nontoxic drug. The nurse should be alert, however, for signs of drowsiness, tremor, twitching of the legs, difficulty in voiding, abdominal discomfort, and flushing of the face. Occasionally patients have mild psychotic reactions to this drug.

Cycloserine, viomycin, and pyrazinamide are newer antimicrobial drugs that are being used for patients in whom the tubercle bacillus has become resistant to streptomycin and isoniazid. However, viomycin frequently seems to cause kidney damage and disturbance of the electrolyte balance. Pyrazinamide used with isoniazid is reported to be one of the most potent antitubercle combinations employed thus far.[9]

Complications and their nursing care. When caring for a patient with tuberculosis, hemorrhage and spontaneous pneumothrax are two complications for which the nurse should be alert.

Hemorrhage. The patient may mention that he has had pink-tinged sputum, or the nurse may discover that the sputum is streaked with red. She should check the color of the sputum regularly, and she should also teach the patient to do this. Some patients will not attach any significance to pinkish sputum, particularly if this is raised only upon arising or only on an occasional morning.

The patient may have a frank hemorrhage and expectorate bright red blood. Coughing may be severe since blood in the lungs and bronchi causes irritation and initiates coughing. Sometimes a patient may have hemorrhage from the lung with severe hemoptysis, yet not have had warning signs such as blood in the sputum. The patient is usually apprehensive and restless prior to hemorrhage; in the absence of other signs, however, these may go unnoticed.

The patient who is having a hemorrhage from the lungs should be kept quiet and lying flat in bed. He must be attended constantly since coughing up fresh blood is extremely frightening, and fear may interfere with rest. If the loss of blood has been severe, extra warmth may be needed and fluids may be replaced by giving an infusion. Infusions are given quite slowly so as not to increase the blood volume and consequently increase bleeding. Bed linen and clothing that has been soiled with blood should be covered or changed, since the sight of this is disturbing to the patient. Sometimes, however, changing linen on the bed must be delayed in favor of complete quiet for the patient. Mouth care should be given to remove the unpleasant taste of blood. After a few hours the patient may be permitted to hold ice chips in his mouth, and later cold fluids may be given in small amounts. If the patient is nauseated because of having swallowed blood, the doctor may order that he have "nothing by mouth"; the physical exertion of retching and vomiting may cause further bleeding.

For several days following a hemorrhage, the patient must be kept absolutely quiet, and all his personal needs must be attended to by others. During this time he must be carefully checked for signs of bleeding. Pallor, thirst, and pulse changes should be noted and reported at once. If the hemorrhage was severe, the patient remains on bed rest for several weeks. If he coughed a good deal prior to the hemorrhage, every effort is made to inhibit coughing which may cause hemorrhage to recur. Too much talking should be avoided. Since drying of the throat may cause coughing, changes in temperature and humidity should be avoided. Smoking is prohibited, and the patient should be in a room where others do not smoke. Oxygen may sometimes be given to help supply enough oxygen despite secondary anemia and limited lung excursion.

Spontaneous pneumothorax. Pneumothorax means the presence of air in the pleural cavity between the lung and the chest wall. (See Figure 65, *4*.) Normally the lung and the chest wall are in contact. Air in the pleural space reduces normal negative intrapleural pressure and causes the heart and mediastinum to shift toward the unaffected side. This hampers activity of the lung on the unaffected side and leads to severe dyspnea.

A spontaneous pneumothorax occurs without warning. The patient has a sudden sharp chest pain accompanied by dyspnea, anxiety, increased diaphoresis, weak and rapid pulse, fall in blood pressure, and cessation of normal chest movement on the affected side. When a spontaneous pneumothorax is suspected a doctor should be summoned immediately. The patient must not be left alone. He must be reassured and urged to be quiet and not to exert himself. Pneumothorax equipment or a thoracentesis set and oxygen are brought to the patient's room. Air is immediately aspirated from the affected pleural space, and the level of pressure is brought to normal. If air continues to flow into the pleural space, continuous drainage of air with closed chest drainage equipment is necessary (see page 474).

The patient who has had a spontaneous pneumothorax is usually most comfortable in a sitting position. Physical activity is kept at a minimum for at least twenty-four hours. The patient is asked to remain as quiet as possible and to avoid stretching, reaching, or moving suddenly. He should breathe normally and not hold his breath. His pulse rate and respirations must be checked frequently. Roentgenograms are always ordered to determine the amount of air in the pleural cavity and the amount of collapse of the lung, as well as the degree of mediastinal shift. When roentgenograms are taken, the patient needs help to prevent overexertion.

Extrapulmonary tuberculosis. Tuberculosis may attack other parts of the body besides the lungs. Tuberculous infection may attack the larynx, particularly if the pulmonary disease is not under control and the sputum remains positive for a long time. Constant passage over the larynx of sputum laden with tubercle bacilli may result in infection. The gastrointestinal tract may also be invaded by infection due to swallowing sputum. The tubercle bacilli may be transported by way of the blood and lymph to other parts of the body, such as the genitourinary tract, the bones and joints, and the meninges.

Patients with *laryngeal tuberculosis* usually have hoarsenes, and some have pain on swallowing. In addition to the bed rest and chemotherapy used in other tuberculosis infections, voice rest is essential. The nurse must be certain that paper and pencil are provided so that the patient can communicate with others. She must see that aides and orderlies understand the patient's restrictions and that all members of the staff anticipate his needs so that he is not tempted to speak or irritated by constantly having to write. Sometimes the patient is allowed to whisper instead of writing. If this is permitted, those in attendance must listen carefully, stay near the patient when he is communicating, and remind him not to strain in whispering. If swallowing is painful, diet modifications may be necessary.

The patient with laryngeal tuberculosis must have laryngoscopic examinations at intervals because this is the only way to learn how the lesion is progressing. Care must be taken to see that the patient receives the prescribed medication before the procedure is done. If he is reasonably relaxed, he experiences much less discomfort during this unpleasant procedure; when he returns to his room after the procedure, thoughtful care makes him dread the next examination less. (See Chapter 24 for care following laryngoscopy.)

The patient with *tuberculosis involving the gastrointestinal system* is always given a special diet. Gas-forming foods, highly spiced foods, and foods containing roughage are excluded. Foods and drinks which stimulate peristalsis to an unusual degree are restricted. Vigorous peristalsis may sometimes be prevented by having the patient take essential foods slowly. For example, drinking a full glass of orange juice quickly will often stimulate peristalsis and give the patient the sensation of needing to have a bowel movement. If the fruit juice is taken in small amounts over the course of an hour, this may be prevented. When the patient has diarrhea, camphorated tincture of opium (paregoric) is often prescribed and other medications which coat the lining of the intestine, such as bismuth subcarbonate, may be used.

The onset of symptoms of *tuberculous meningitis* usually is sudden. The patient has marked constipation, an elevation of temperature, chills, headache, convulsions, and sometimes loss of consciousness. If untreated, this disease causes death within three to six weeks. With the use of streptomycin, this disease is usually controllable. A twelve-month course of medical treatment is necessary, however, and the nurse must help to make the patient and his family realize that this is absolutely necessary. Streptomycin, isoniazid, and PAS are all given concurrently. In addition, streptomycin is given intrathecally (into the spinal canal). When this kind of tuberculosis is being treated, signs of sensitivity to drugs or toxic reactions must be watched for particularly carefully. Special attention and consideration during the administration of medication into the spinal canal makes the whole treatment more endurable for the patient. Early in the disease sedation may be needed, and before the spinal puncture is done, meperidine hydrochloride (Demerol) is often given. Habit-forming drugs, however, are given with caution to patients with disease because of the length of time involved in treatment and the consequent danger of addiction.

Since the discovery of antibiotics, better case-finding, pasteurization of milk, and tuberculin-testing of cattle, *skeletal tuberculosis* is growing less common. It is most common in children, but adults also are sometimes affected. Although tubercle bacilli may attack any bone or joint in the body, the spine, hips, and knees are most often involved. This blood-borne infection localizes in a joint, and it may invade either the synovial membrane or the bone adjacent to the joint. Whereas the bony involvement is rapid, with destruction of bone and abscess formation, disease of the synovial membrane progresses slowly. In contrast to most abscesses, tuberculous abscesses cause little increase in local skin temperature. They are therefore called "cold abscesses." The patient may have limitation of motion, muscle spasm, swelling of the joint, and atrophy of muscles above and below the joint. Deformities occur as a result of bone destruction.

Tuberculosis of the spine is called *Pott's disease,* named for Percival Pott who identified it in 1779. Although the condition is now rare in the United States, the "hunchback" deformity it causes can still be seen in some people, particularly in those who have come from other countries where standards for pasteurization of milk and tuberculin-testing of cattle are less rigid than ours. The thoracic and lumbar regions are most often affected. Patients with this disease develop abnormal curvatures of the spine and may have abscesses whose fistulas drain through the skin or which may become localized in the psoas muscle. Patients with tuberculosis of the spine are now treated with antibiotics and by immobilization. Immobilization is achieved by applying a bivalved body plaster cast, by keeping the patient on a frame in a position of hyperextension (Whitman frame), or by surgical fixation of the spine, usually using bone grafts.

In addition to the good general nursing care given any patient with tuberculosis, the nurse should give special attention to good body alignment (using proper support in moving and turning), nutrition, and skin care in the patient with tuberculosis of the bone.

Tuberculosis of the hip is usually treated by traction, which relieves pain, controls muscle spasm, and helps to prevent adduction deformity. Care of the patient receiving this treatment is similar to that of other patients in traction (see Chapter 36). Hip spica casts and other plaster casts are also used, depending upon the part of the body involved.

Tuberculosis may also involve the urinary system and the male and female reproductive systems (see Chapters 21 and 22).

Histoplasmosis

Histoplasmosis is a fungus disease which affects the lungs. Now that more has been learned about the disease it is recognized that the incidence is quite high in the United States. It is most prevalent in the rural sections of the central states. It is not communicable from man to man; organisms are transmitted to man by his inhaling spores which thrive in moist, dark, protected soil. The disease masquerades as either influenza or chronic cavitary tuberculosis. It is diagnosed by the presence of nodular infiltrations found on roentgenography and a skin reaction to the intradermal injection of histoplasmin.

Until recently there was no treatment for histoplasmosis except rest and general supportive care. Now an antibiotic, *amphotericin,* appears to be most useful in treatment. Since it must be given intravenously and causes toxic reactions, such as gastrointestinal symptoms, headache, and cough, the patient is hospitalized and closely observed during treatment. Nurses working in areas where this disease is prevalent have an important role in helping to locate sources of infection and in teaching the public to prevent inhalation of potentially infected material. Since the disease can be fatal and children appear to be particularly susceptible, the nurse should point out potential danger to rural families when it is known that the soil is contaminated.

Bronchiectasis

Bronchiectasis means dilatation of the bronchus or bronchi. When infection attacks the bronchial lining, inflammation occurs and an exudate forms. The progressive accumulation of secretions mechanically distends the bronchioles. With repeated infection, the bronchioles become permanently distended and appear saccular and cylindrical in shape. Their expulsive force is diminished, and they may remain filled with exudate. Only forceful coughing and postural drainage will empty them. Bronchiectasis may involve any part of the lung parenchyma, but it usually occurs in the dependent portions or lobules. The disease begins in young people, many patients showing symptoms by the age of 20 years. The initial contributing factor is a congenital weakness in the structure of the alveoli so that elasticity is not normal. Bronchiectasis may occur without previous pulmonary disease, but it usually follows such diseases as bronchopneumonia, lung abscess, tuberculosis, or asthma.

Symptoms of bronchiectasis vary with the severity of the condition. The patient may complain of fatigue, weakness, and loss of weight. Appetite can be affected by the fetid sputum. The condition may develop so gradually that the patient is often unable to tell when symptoms first began. Clubbing of the fingers is common, as it is in most chronic respiratory disease. The patient's chief complaint in bronchiectasis is severe coughing (brought on by changing position) which is productive of large amounts of sputum and causes dyspnea. The patient may have a paroxysm of coughing when he gets up in the morning and again when he lies down.

Treatment of bronchiectasis is not too satisfactory. Surgical removal of a portion of the lung is the only cure. Therefore, patients who have bronchiectasis that involves a large part of the lung are not amenable to surgical cure and do not have a good prognosis. The life expectancy usually is considered to be no more than twenty years. Many patients develop cardiac complications because of the extra strain on the heart caused by inability of the lungs to oxygenate the blood adequately.

Postural drainage at least twice a day helps to remove secretions and thus helps to prevent coughing. During severe episodes of coughing, the patient should not be left alone, since a large plug of thick secretion may block a large bronchiole and cause severe dyspnea and cyanosis. Occasionally, bronchoscopy must be done to remove the plug of mucus or to break adhesions which may be interfering with postural drainage by blocking passage to the main bronchi. Penicillin and other antibiotics may be used in the treatment of bronchiectasis. While these drugs do not cure the condition, they may prevent further infection and are often used prior to surgery, both by parenteral and aerosol administration. If the involvement of the lung is widespread, oxygen may be used.

Lung abscess

A lung abscess is an area of localized suppuration within the lung. It usually is caused by bacteria that reach the lung through aspiration. The infected material lodges in the small bronchi and produces inflammation. Partial obstruction of the bronchus results in the retention of secretions beyond the obstruction and the eventual necrosis of tissue. Before the advent of antibiotics and specific chemotherapy, lung abscess was a fairly frequent complication following pneumonia. When a lung abscess forms, various organisms are found. Lung abscess may follow bronchial obstruction caused by a tumor, a foreign body, or a stenosis of the bronchus. Metastatic spread of cancer cells to the lung parenchyma may also cause an abscess, and occasionally the infection appears to have been borne by the blood stream.

In recent years the incidence of lung abscess due to infection has decreased. Improved methods of administering anesthetics, better postoperative care, and early treatment of pneumonia and other respiratory infections with antibiotics are the main reasons for this decrease. Secondary lung abscess following bronchogenic carcinoma, however, has increased with the increased incidence of that disease.

Symptoms of lung abscess include cough, elevation of temperature, loss of appetite, malaise, and, if the condition is of long standing, clubbing of the fingers. Unless the abscess is walled off, so that there is no access to the bronchi, the patient usually raises sputum. There may be hemoptysis, and often the patient raises dark brown "chocolate-colored" sputum which contains both blood and pus.

The general course of the patient's illness is influenced by the kind of drainage which can be established. If the purulent material drains easily, the patient may respond well to postural drainage, antibiotic therapy, and good general supportive care. Antibiotic therapy, however, cannot cause a walled-off abscess to disappear. If surgery is necessary the portion of lung containing the abscess is removed. Small adhesions that may be interfering with drainage into the bronchi may be broken by means of a bronchoscopic procedure. Today, surgical treatment to establish drainage has become increasingly less necessary; chemical débridement is accomplished by aerosol administration of crystalline trypsin (Tryptar). Trypsin, 125 mg., is dissolved in water, 2 ml., and inhaled daily for 5 to 10 days; along with this, antibiotics are given systemically.

Empyema

Empyema means pus within a body cavity; it usually applies to the pleural cavity. Empyema occurs as a result of, or in association with, other respiratory disease, such as pneumonia, lung abscess, tuberculosis, and fungus infections of the lung, and also following thoracic surgery or chest trauma. The patient with any kind of lung infection or chest injury should be closely observed for signs of empyema, which include cough, dyspnea, unilateral chest pain, elevation of temperature, malaise, poor appetite, and unequal chest expansion. The condition may develop several weeks after an apparently minor respiratory infection. The diagnosis can usually be made from the signs and symptoms and the medical history, but it is confirmed by a roentgenogram of the chest and examination of the lungs under a fluoroscope. Sometimes a thoracentesis is done to confirm the diagnosis of fluid in the pleural space, to obtain a culture of the organisms, and to relieve the patient's respiratory symptoms. (For details of equipment needed for this treatment, see texts on fundamentals of nursing.)

If a *thoracentesis* is to be done, the procedure should be explained to the patient. It is important that he be instructed not to move suddenly when the needle is inserted lest damage to the pleura occur. Usually procaine is used to eliminate pain at the site of insertion of the needle; however, when the pleura is entered, a sensation of pain or pressure may occur. The patient must be in a sitting position, and he should be made as comfortable as possible. Sometimes leaning forward over an overbed table well padded with pillows is satisfactory since the table can be raised to support the arms and shoulders and keep them slightly elevated. Raising the arms and shoulders elevates the ribs and makes it easier for the doctor to carry out the procedure. If the patient is extremely ill, apprehensive, or debilitated, two nurses must assist with this procedure; one assists and observes the patient and the other assists the doctor. The patient's respiratory rate should be taken several times during the procedure, and he must be watched for any changes in color, for any change in his breathing, and for excessive diaphoresis. The needle and syringe should be carefully checked to see that they fit snugly since no air should be permitted to enter the pleural cavity. After the fluid is withdrawn into a 20 or 50 ml. syringe, it should be placed in a proper container and carefully labeled for microscopic examination and for culture. Following a thoracentesis the patient is watched for signs of coughing or raising blood since these might indicate that the lung was traumatized inadvertently.

After diagnosis and determination of the organisms within the pleural space, treatment is begun. If the organism is one that responds to penicillin therapy, the patient is often given 20,000 to 200,000 units of penicillin intrapleurally on alternate days for three days. A thoracentesis is done twenty-four hours after each injection to determine the activity of remaining organisms. The primary aim of treatment is to clear the infection, eliminate fluid, and promote expansion of the lung. When organisms disappear and only a small amount of fluid remains, the lung will expand to its normal size. This usually takes a few months.

During the period of intensive chemotherapy and while he has definite symptoms, the patient is kept on bed rest. He is usually more comfortable lying on his affected side since this helps to splint the chest and thus to lessen pain; a firm mattress also lessens discomfort. If he has dyspnea, the head of the bed may need to be elevated to allow for easier lung expansion. Changes in pulse rate, color, and rate of respiration are most important since sudden changes may indicate pressure on the lung.

Mobility is encouraged during convalescence, and the nurse should allow the patient opportunity to help himself in his own daily personal care. She should encourage use of the extremities on the affected side since the patient may feel activity will cause renewed pain or regression of the disease. When the infection is controlled and the pleural space is obliterated, the arm can be used for stretching and reaching without harm.

Since the discovery of the antibiotics and specific chemotherapeutic agents, surgery is seldom necessary in the treatment of empyema. Occasionally, when infection persists and adhesions form and areas become walled off, it may be necessary to resort to surgical drainage.

Asthma

Asthma is a lung disease caused by an allergic response to a substance (antigen) to which the person is sensitive. Asthma affects men and women in equal numbers, and all races are susceptible. It occurs at any age, but the type due to outside forces (extrinsic) usually appears in the first four decades of life, whereas that due to sensitivity within the body (intrinsic) usually begins in middle age. Asthma is but one of many evidences of man's sensitivity to substances in his environment and within his body. Many persons who develop asthma as adults have a history of having had eczema in early childhood; eczema is a common manifestation of allergic reaction.

Asthma may follow a hypersensitivity or allergy to certain antigens such as dusts, foods, or drugs. This is known as *extrinsic asthma* since the antigens are found in the external environment. It also may result from infections; in this case there is a specific hypersensitivity to bacteria. This is known as *intrinsic asthma,* and it may follow such chronic infections as sinusitis, tonsillitis, or adenoiditis. Many patients are affected by sensitivity to both external and internal antigens. Asthma may be acute, subacute, chronic, or constant. An acute continuous attack is called *status asthmaticus;* if emergency treatment is not given, it can cause death from heart failure.

The main symptoms of asthma are dyspnea and a wheezing sound on breathing. These symptoms may come on suddenly and be severe, or they may develop very slowly; the wheezing sound may even go unnoticed by the patient for some time. If asthma has developed during childhood or has persisted for a long time in younger persons, there is a characteristic barrel-shaped deformity of the chest, and there may be clubbing of the fingers.

Prevention. Patients can help to avoid asthmatic attacks by learning to identify the antigens to which they are sensitive and by avoiding such antigens if possible. Skin tests will determine sensitivity to external allergens. Small amounts of various allergens are injected intracutaneously on the outer surface of the upper arm. Positive reactions are indicated by the appearance of *wheals.* Allergens are usually given in series, and in some clinics the nurse may inject the substances which the doctor has chosen on the basis of the patient's symptoms, the time of occurrence, and the significant family history of allergy. Once the offending allergens have been determined, an attempt is made to slowly desensitize the patient by the injection of increasingly larger doses of the allergen at regular intervals (usually one to four weeks) over a long period of time. While the patient is becoming desensitized, he needs help in avoiding antigens to which he is sensitive. If the patient is sensitive to a certain food, he should be instructed to eliminate this food from his diet until he has had sufficient injections for desensitization. If this requires some time, he may need help in the selection of substitute foods so that nutritional deficiency does not develop.

If the patient is sensitive to an antigen such as dust, mold, spores, animal dander, feathers, insecticides, glues, or lint from fabrics, he must decide the best way to avoid the offending substances. Daily damp-dusting lessens the amount of dust in the air. New homes must sometimes be found for pets, although usually the patient goes through a long period of treatment for desensitization before he consents to this. Pillows containing feathers can be covered with plastic covers. In most instances, while the patient is receiving injections for desensitization, either the substance causing the asthmatic attacks can be eliminated or the effects can be lessened. Thus, asthma is often quite amenable to treatment provided the substances to which the patient is sensitive are found.

After asthma has become established in the patient, other factors besides the antigens to which he was originally sensitive may precipitate an acute attack. Emotional stress, changes in temperature and humidity, irritating fumes and smoke, strong odors, and physical exertion have been known to precipitate attacks in those who have the disease. The patient must often make an attempt to lessen emotional stress and to control physical exertion since these factors are less amenable to management than are specific excitants such as drugs or foods. If the underlying allergy is obscure or if it is resistant to treatment, the recognition and control of secondary factors may be the main approach to treatment.

Nursing care. There is perhaps no disease in which knowing the patient well is more important than in asthma. Since sensitivity tests can be done with only a very small fraction of the substances with which the patient is in contact, the doctor usually makes the diagnosis on the basis of a careful history. Knowing how the patient lives, how he spends his leisure time, what he eats, what type of work he does, his social contacts, and many other circumstances may give useful clues as to the cause of his trouble. Although the allergist urges patients to report seemingly trivial and insignificant details, they often hesitate to do so since they are used to reporting only physical changes within themselves. If the nurse is alert, she can often be of real help to the doctor in making the diagnosis of the cause of the allergic reaction. In conversation with the patient, for example, she may learn that a relative has just visited and brought a pet with her.

The nurse may make observations regarding emotional stresses that appear to aggravate the patient's condition. Careful observation of his relationships with members of his family may give clues to sources of emotional stress. Some patients remain in the hospital during an acute episode and return home relieved of serious symptoms. However, unless his circumstances can be improved, family relationships and general socioeconomic conditions which cause stress may send the patient back to the hospital with another attack.

Patients with chronic bronchial asthma may gain a sense of security while in the hospital and may be reluctant to return home. Asthmatic attacks can be precipitated by plans for discharge and the patient's stay thus prolonged. Patients with severe emotional insecurity may find help in psychotherapy.

The patient who has an occasional attack of asthma may complain of a sense of suffocation and pressure in the chest before acute symptoms occur. The respirations have a characteristic wheezing sound with prolonged, difficult exhalation, and increased effort is needed to inhale. When an attack starts, the patient should sit upright. He should be given something on which to lean forward, such as an over-bed table. Since during an acute attack, the patient uses the accessory muscles of respiration in his effort to get enough air, leaning forward helps him to use them more effectively. Since his only concern during an acute attack is breathing, he must be protected from falling and from other injury. He should be given medication for relief of the attack as soon as possible, and he should be constantly attended until acute symptoms subside. The attack usually ends with the patient coughing up large quantities of thick, tenacious sputum. He may become completely exhausted from increased physical effort, and he should rest quietly after the attack. He usually perspires profusely, and he may need change of clothing and special protection from chilling. Most attacks subside in one-half to one hour, although asthmatic attacks following infection may continue for days or weeks.

Patients who are severely affected with asthma and who have attacks that are difficult to control with the usual medications may develop *status asthmaticus;* in this case the symptoms of an acute attack continue. The patient is acutely ill; when he is admitted to the hospital, he needs emergency treatment. Prolonged attacks cause exhaustion, and death from heart failure may occur. Oxygen is administered by mask, and positive pressure may be used intermittently. In extreme cases, when the air passages appear completely obstructed, a mixture of helium and oxygen may be given by endotracheal tube or by mask. Helium has a high rate of diffusion and has a lighter molecular weight than oxygen so that it can be inhaled with less effort. During an acute attack, the lungs progressively distend as in emphysema, and actually acute emphysema exists. Unless relaxation of the bronchioles can be accomplished, insufficient oxygen passes through the alveolar membrane into the blood stream and the patient becomes progressively more cyanotic. Since food and fluids cannot be taken by mouth, intravenous fluids must be given. The patient needs constant observation, and he must have everything done for him. Repeated attacks of status asthmaticus cause irreversible emphysema, resulting in a permanent decrease in total breathing capacity.

Some patients have *chronic mild asthma.* Symptoms are not noticeable when the patient is at rest. However, after exertion such as laughing, singing, vigorous exercise, or emotional excitement, the patient develops dyspnea and wheezing. These attacks are controlled with medications, and patients usually can continue their usual mode of living with few modifications and no serious lung changes. They are not hospitalized, but they sometimes come to outpatient clinics for medical supervision.

Treatment. The treatment of asthma is directed toward symptomatic relief of attacks, the control of specific causative factors and the general care for maintenance of optimum health. The chief aim of various medications is to afford the patient immediate and progressive bronchial relaxation. One of the drugs often given to control mild attacks is *epinephrine,* which relaxes smooth muscles in the respiratory tract and counteracts the bronchial constriction which occurs during attacks. Epinephrine, 0.2 to 1 mg. (1/300 to 1/60 grain) in a 1:1000 solution, is given subcutaneously or intramuscularly and may be repeated every five to ten minutes for two to three doses. Frequent repeated doses can be avoided by giving epinephrine in oil, 0.4 to 3 mg. (1/150 to 1/20 grain) of a 1:500 solution, intramuscularly every six to twelve hours. This provides slower systemic absorption and prolongs the effect. Some patients who have frequent mild attacks are taught to give their own injections, or a member of the family may be taught to give the injections.

Patients with chronic bronchial asthma are maintained at home on active drug therapy and return to the doctor's office or the clinic for periodic supervision. Many patients take *ephedrine sulfate,* 25 mg. (3/8 grain), by mouth every four hours during the day. Ephedrine sulfate, like epinephrine, relaxes hypertonic muscles. The stimulating effects of ephedrine sulfate can be lessened by combining ephedrine with a mild sedative such as phenobarbital, 15 mg. (1/4 grain), taken by mouth several times a day. Many patients are treated with other drugs to dilate the bronchi; these are given by inhalation. The patient who is ambulatory will need instruction in the use of a nebulizer. (see page 467.) *Isoproterenol hydrochloride* (Isuprel), 0.5 ml. of 1:200 solution, is often used.

Theophylline ethylenediamine (aminophylline) may be given during acute attacks. The dosage is 0.25 to 0.5 Gm. (3¾ to 7½ grains) intravenously. Aminophylline suppositories, 0.5 Gm. (7½ grains), can also be given rectally every eight to twelve hours. Patients with severe attacks also are given oxygen by catheter or by mask.

Expectorants such as *potassium iodide* or *ammonium chloride* may be given to help loosen thick bronchial secretions. The dosage of potassium iodide is usually 0.6 Gm. (10 grains) by mouth three times a day after meals. Sedatives help to keep the patient quiet and to provide for better rest. However, they are used with caution to avoid depressing respiratory function and to avoid the danger of addiction. *Meperidine hydrochloride* (Demerol), 50 mg. (3/4 grain), given subcutaneously every four hours, is used in preference to morphine. *Barbiturates* such as phenobarbital, 30 mg. (1/2 grain), by mouth every four hours during the day and pentobarbital, 100 mg. (1½ grains), by mouth at night help to give the patient steady sedation. *Codeine,* 15 mg. (1/4 grain), or *elixir of terpin hydrate with codeine,* 5 ml. (1 dram) every four hours, helps to control excessive coughing, thus permitting more rest. In asthma following infection, various antibiotics such as *penicillin* and *chlortetracycline* (Aureomycin) are used, depending on the organism involved.

Pulmonary emphysema

In pulmonary emphysema the lung alveoli do not empty on expiration but remain overdistended and finally lose their ability to return to normal. The circulation of blood to the bronchioles is inadequate and tissue nutrition is poor; normal tissues atrophy and are displaced by fibrous connective tissue. In emphysema normal elasticity of the bronchioles is lost, and normal ciliary action is impaired. Thus, with thickened, less elastic tissues in the bronchioles, air passes into the alveoli but its natural forceful expulsion on expiration is lessened.

Pulmonary emphysema usually follows repeated respiratory infections which cause changes in the bronchial walls and in the alveoli. Low-grade infection and inadequate drainage of exudate result in mechanical stretching of the bronchioles. Asthma, which causes the bronchial mucosa to become edematous with subsequent obstruction of air passages, also leads to emphysema. Emphysema may also be caused by the distention of the lungs that occurs to fill space in the pleural cavity following surgery such as the removal of a lung. Occasionally this same reaction occurs following destruction of a portion of the lung from disease such as tuberculosis or silicosis.

Many elderly patients have emphysema as one of several diseases. Accurate statistics on the incidence of chronic pulmonary emphysema are not available, although the incidence is believed to be increasing. Chronic emphysema develops in middle or later life and is more common among men than women. As the disease progresses, the patient develops increasing dyspnea on exertion and chronic fatigue. Since the lungs are not being properly ventilated, the patient must be watched for drowsiness and changes in rate and depth of respirations. Not all the carbon dioxide is removed from the blood, and the amount in the circulating blood slowly builds up until the respiratory centers in the medulla are fatigued by the constant carbon dioxide stimulus. The patient's rate and depth of breathing then decrease and lethargy and eventual coma follow. This is also called *carbon dioxide narcosis.*

After a long period of diminished alveolar function, the patient's breathing under ordinary activity becomes jerky or spasmodic. In efforts to increase breathing comfort, he uses the upper intercostal muscles, and when full use of the diaphragm is diminished he uses deep abdominal breathing. The diaphragm eventually flattens in a fixed position. Thus, expiration is prolonged and difficult. Patients sometimes make a blowing sound through the mouth in an effort to force exhalation. The abdomen often protrudes because of loss of muscle tone.

Unless there is an acute attack of difficult breathing caused by overexertion, patients with emphysema remain at home and are given medical care in the doctor's office or in the clinic. There is no cure for emphysema; treatment is only supportive. Prevention of secondary infection should be stressed. Adequate nutrition, rest, and avoidance of exposure to sudden changes in temperature cannot be overemphasized. The low pulmonary reserve does not allow for the mildest of lower respiratory infection, and acute pulmonary insufficiency can result from such infection.

If the patient is in danger of developing acute pulmonary insufficiency, he frequently is placed in a respirator; this improves the exchange of air since it supplements the respiratory muscle action. Oxygen is not given since, rather than relieving the respiratory distress, it increases the amount of carbon dioxide that must be dissipated. (See Chapter 34 for care of the patient in a respirator.)

Nursing care. The nurse helps the patient and his family to plan so that he may live a fairly satisfactory life within the limitations of his disease. Daily schedules may need rearrangement so that activities are not too intensive at one time. For example, almost all patients with emphysema will have a severe bout of coughing upon arising as secretions which have accumulated during the night are raised; a period of rest should be planned following this. If the patient goes to work, he may have to arise earlier than usual to allow time for rest after the exertion of coughing. Since sudden exertion taxes the respiratory system and usually precipitates more coughing, the patient's morning schedule should be planned so that he can arise and dress slowly and eat breakfast in a leisurely manner. Means of getting to work and the daily work schedule may also need modifications to provide a fairly leisurely pace with rest periods at intervals.

Since the diaphragm becomes flattened and less active, some patients find breathing is helped by wearing an *elasticized abdominal support.* The support is often made of material similar to that used in elasticized girdles. Men may need to be persuaded to wear this kind of support but, upon trial, learn how much the support adds to comfort and accept it quite readily. Pressure from the girdle must be from below the umbilicus upward, so that the flattened diaphragm is forced up into the thorax.

Breathing exercises are helpful to some patients with emphysema. Since many of the patients are elderly and may not be able to notice an immediate improvement in their breathing, they need encouragement to maintain interest and effort in learning the exercises and in practicing them faithfully. The chief aim of exercises is to increase the force of exhalation largely by increasing motion of the diaphragm. If the patient can lie flat, he should lie flat on his back, with the knees bent, and take in a deep breath while letting his abdomen rise. In exhaling, he should contract the abdominal muscles as he forces the air out. Placing the hands on the abdomen while doing this exercise helps the patient to concentrate on breathing with the abdominal muscles. If he must be in a sitting position, the same exercise can be done. In addition, he should let the body relax completely while breathing out and should lean forward, allowing the arms to hang loose. Other simple exercises to increase forceful expiration are conscious forceful blowing out of air, hissing through the teeth, blowing into paper bags, blowing a pencil along a table top, and blowing balloons.

Positive pressure with oxygen or compressed air may be used intermittently in an attempt to dilate the bronchi and to allow for more efficient aeration of the lungs. It can be administered by mask. Positive pressure is applied during inspiration. Many newer mechanical devices are constructed so that the respiratory rate, instead of being fixed, is regulated by the patient's own rate of respiration. Thus, the necessity of adjusting his breathing rate to a mechanical device is eliminated. If the patient has symptoms of carbon dioxide retention, compressed air is usually given instead of oxygen, A nebulizer can also be used in combination with positive pressure. This is particularly helpful when the patient is too weak to inhale deeply and it is necessary that drugs reach the smallest air passages. The pressure level required to establish an increase in ventilation will vary from patient to patient. However, treatment is usually started with the low pressure of 5 mm. and is increased gradually until it is 15 to 20 mm. The positive pressure mask used to apply pressure during inspiration should not be confused with the type which applies pressure during expiration. The nurse should familiarize herself with the various types of apparatus and be certain of their management. It is possible for leaks to occur in the tubing or for connections to be loose, and thus the desired pressure will not be obtained. It is necesary for the nurse to check the apparatus each time she checks the patient's color, pulse, and respirations. A face mask which functions improperly will only be a source of additional obstruction and will increase symptoms.

Bronchodilating drugs to relieve bronchospasm are often ordered for the patient who has emphysema. Drugs may be given in a *nebulizer*, which is a mechanical device into which the desired liquid medication is placed; with the force of compressed air, the liquid is broken into very fine droplets or spray. The spray is then inhaled easily. This is known as aerosol administration. The nebulizer is usually connected to a tank of oxygen by rubber tubing. Midway in the rubber tubing connection a glass Y tube or a slightly bent glass tube with a tiny opening on one side is inserted. The oxygen is turned on after the desired medication has been placed in the nebulizer. Usually 4 to 6 liters of oxygen per minute are sufficient. The nurse should test the kind and amount of spray briefly by placing a finger over the open end of the Y tube. If a fine spray cannot be seen or felt on the hand, the equipment is not working properly.

Most patients learn to use the nebulizer themselves. The nebulizer may be attached to a tank of oxygen or a motor compressor, or a hand bulb can be used. In either instance the patient needs to learn how to breathe and when to close off the opening with his finger. The opening in the glass tube should be closed on inhalation and left open on exhalation. The patient breathes in through his mouth and exhales through his nose. Since he has dyspnea, he may wish to take several normal breaths before repeating a cycle of deep inspirations with the nebulizer. The principles of breathing with the use of the nebulizer are the same as with the use of a hand bulb. However, inspiration should begin as the bulb is compressed and the drug is converted to a spray.

Drugs often used by nebulizer are epinephrine, 1:1000, racemic epinephrine hydrochloride (Vaponefrin), and isoproterenol hydrochloride (Isuprel). Antibiotics such as penicillin are also given by nebulizer to combat infection, and they may be given alternately with a bronchodilator drug. Patients with emphysema may also be given aminophylline and ephedrine sulfate. Aminophylline may be given orally or it may be given rectally in suppositories; occasionally it is given intravenously.

Pulmonary fibrosis

Pulmonary fibrosis is extensive scarring of lung tissue with areas of calcification.

It often develops in persons whose work involves inhalation of dusts such as coal, marble, or iron over long periods of time. When it is caused by stone or marble dust it is known as *silicosis.* Pulmonary fibrosis also occurs with collagen diseases such as scleraderma, polyarteritis nodosa, and systemic lupus erythematosis. It may complicate histoplasmosis and tuberculosis in which there has been extensive bilateral involvement.

The patient with pulmonary fibrosis has respiratory embarrassment because of limited usable lung tissue. Cardiac complications may follow since heart action must be increased to make up for respiratory impairment. There is no cure and no specific treatment for pulmonary fibrosis. Breathing exercises may be prescribed in an effort to preserve, for as long as possible, the elasticity of lung tissue. The patient is cautioned to avoid strenuous exercise that will tax the respiratory and cardiac systems and, above all, to guard against exposure to upper respiratory infection.

In recent years adrenocortical steroids have been used in the treatment of pulmonary fibrosis. They appear to improve the condition especially when it follows or accompanies collagen disease. (For problems associated with the administration of these steroids see Chapter 28, page 639.)

Carcinoma

Carcinoma of the lungs may be either metastatic or primary. Metastatic tumors may follow malignancy anywhere in the body; metastasis from the prostate, uterus, thyroid, larynx, breast, and suprarenal gland is common. Metastasis to the lung may be discovered before the primary lesion is known, and sometimes the location of the primary lesion is not determined during the patient's life.

Since most new growths in the lungs arise from the bronchi, the term *bronchogenic* carcinoma is widely used. The growth of new cells produces bronchial narrowing, and eventually a cough and dyspnea develop. The symptoms produced by the new growth depend upon its size and location. If the growth is small and is located in the main bronchus, there may be a cough. On the other hand, if the growth is in a small bronchus in the periphery of the lung, it may grow to a considerable size before producing symptoms. Very often there are no early signs of the disease.

The cause of carcinoma of the lung is unknown, but it is believed that chronic irritation contributes to its development. Special occupations in which the workers are exposed to radioactive substances or to certain chemicals are felt to be of significance in the production of carcinoma of the lung. History of heavy smoking is common, and it is thought that this may be a factor contributing to the disease; this is being carefully studied at the present time.

During the past few decades there has been a startling increase in the incidence of carcinoma of the lung, which is now the most common cancer among men. In urban areas where good diagnostic facilities are available, cancer leads all other respiratory system diseases as the cause of death among white men. Carcinoma of the lung is six times as frequent among men as among women. Most people who develop the disease are over 45 years of age. Geographically, death rates are highest in the northeast and lowest in the south. Between 1944 and 1945 and 1954 and 1955 lung cancer among men 45 to 54 years of age increased from 34.3 to 59.2 per 100,000 population, and among men 55 to 64 years of age, from 75.3 to 143.6 per 100,000 population.[5] The numbers in the latter group have nearly doubled. Some of the factors believed to be involved in this increase include more accurate diagnosis and a tendency to name the lung as the primary site. The latter might occur, for example, when an autopsy permit is not granted and the primary site is not determined.

The nurse's greatest contributions in this disease are helping in the early detection of lesions in the lungs and teaching health measures which may possibly help to prevent development of lung cancer. All persons, particularly men over 40 years of age, should be urged to have an x-ray examination of the chest periodically in addition to a yearly physical examination. Close observation of patients and exploration of small, seemingly unimportant symptoms can be important in early case-finding. Attention should be given to persistent cough. Shortness of breath, unexplained fever, and loss of weight may be warning signs. As a result of various public educational media, such as campaigns, drives for funds, and mass x-ray examination, the public has become more conscious of early signs, but there is still a great need for people to learn about diagnostic tests that are available, including x-ray examinations, bronchoscopic examinations, and cytologic studies of sputum. The nurse should know of available cancer detection clinics in her community and should assist patients to secure proper medical supervision.

Time is most important in the treatment of lung cancer. If carcinoma is detected while it is still confined to a local area, immediate surgery, with removal of all or part of a lung (lobectomy or pneumonectomy), may be successful. The nursing care of the patient following surgery of the lung is discussed later in this chapter.

Radiation therapy may be used in the control of the growth of cancer of the lung when it is not possible to remove all the growth surgically and also after pneumonectomy if any doubt as to complete removal exists. If the disease is allowed to go untreated, the life expectancy is probably lessened.

Radioactive gold (Au^{198}) is sometimes left in the pleural cavity following surgery to help destroy any malignant cells that may remain in surrounding tissue or lymph nodes. Radioactive gold may also be given through a thoracentesis. (See Chapter 16 for care of patients receiving x-ray therapy or radioactive substances.)

Metastasis occurs to the mediastinal lymph nodes, to the walls of the esophagus, to the pericardium and heart, and to the opposite lung or to the cervical lymph nodes. If the patient has advanced carcinoma of the lung, marked dyspnea, with wheezing, weakness, loss of weight and of appetite, cough, and pain are the usual symptoms. All supportive nursing measures should be used to make the patient as comfortable as possible. (See Chapter 16 for details of these.)

Pulmonary embolism and pulmonary infarction

Pulmonary embolism is the lodgment of a clot or other foreign matter in a pulmonary arterial vessel, and pulmonary infarction is the hemorrhagic necrosis of a part of the lung parenchyma due to interruption of its blood supply, usually as a result of embolism.[6]

The embolism usually comes from a thrombosed vein in the pelvis or the lower extremities; its pressure may cause symptoms before any signs of venous thrombosis appear.

The size of the pulmonary artery in which the clot lodges determines the severity of symptoms and the prognosis. If the embolus is sufficiently large, immediate death may occur before any symptoms are reported by the patient. If it is less severe, the patient may complain of sudden sharp upper abdominal or thoracic pain, be dyspneic, cough violently and have hemoptysis; shock may develop rapidly. If the embolus is a small one and the area of infarction is small, the symptoms are much milder. The patient may have cough, pain in the chest, slight hemoptysis, and elevation of temperature with increase of leukocyte count in the blood. An area of dullness can be detected by the doctor upon listening to the patient's chest sounds.

If the patient survives a severe pulmonary infarction, the medical and nursing care are similar to that needed by the patient who has had an acute myocadrial infarction (see Chapter 18). If the infarction is a mild one the treatment is more conservative and resembles that provided for the patient with pneumonia. In either case an immediate attempt is made to locate the original source of the embolus and to treat the thrombosis.

The best treatment for pulmonary embolism is prevention. This is largely a *nursing responsibility.* Prevention of thrombophlebitis in patients undergoing surgery is discussed in Chapter 14. The nurse must remember, too, that thrombosis can occur easily in the patient who is being treated only for a medical condition. This is particularly true when the patient is elderly and has chronic vascular and cardiac disease. The *very same* nursing measures that are employed to prevent development of thrombophlebitis in surgical patients must be used.

THORACIC SURGERY

Intelligent nursing care of patients undergoing thoracic surgery depends upon knowledge of the anatomy and physiology of the chest, of the surgery performed, and of procedures and practices that assist the patient to recover from the operation. When endotracheal anesthesia became possible, surgery of the chest was given a great impetus. Before that time it had not been possible, except in the rarest of circumstances, to operate upon the lung without causing collapse of the good lung and death. By means of endotracheal anesthesia it is possible to keep the good lung expanded and functioning even when it is subjected to atmospheric pressure. Endotracheal anesthesia is used for surgery involving the lungs and for most chest surgery in which the pleural space is entered.

Chest surgery has also been aided by the discovery of antibiotics. Usually when chest surgery is done, antibiotics are given systemically.

Operative procedures

Lobectomy. A lobectomy, the removal of a lobe of the lung, is the most common of all lung operations. It may be done for conditions such as bronchiectasis, cysts of the lung, lung abscess, benign lung tumors, and tuberculosis. A *thoracotomy incision* is made, extending from the nipple line to almost the midline in the back. To remove the lower lobe, the seventh or eighth rib is resected; to remove the upper lobes, the third or fourth rib is resected. When the pleura is entered and the lung is exposed to atmospheric pressure, it collapses. The arteries and veins extending into the lobe are ligated and divided and the main bronchus to the lobe is resected, closed, and carefully covered with pleura to prevent the leakage of air. The affected lobe is then removed, the pleura is closed, and the other lobes are re-expanded with oxygen by the anesthesiologist. Drainage catheters are usually inserted through short incisions above and below the resected lobe; the upper catheter provides for removal of air and the lower catheter permits drainage of fluid. (See Figure 65, *3.*)

Pneumonectomy. A pneumonectomy or removal of an entire lung may be done for conditions such as cancer, lung abscess, bronchiectasis, and tuberculosis. This procedure carries a greater risk than lobectomy; the mortality rate is about 10 to 15 per cent.[35] Although the operative procedure is technically simpler than a lobectomy, the nature of the disease and the extent of lung involvement may make surgery difficult and may make the patient a poorer operative risk. A posterolateral or anterolateral thoracotomy incision (with resection of the third or fourth rib) is made. The pulmonary artery and pulmonary vein are ligated and divided, the main bronchus is resected, closed, and covered with adjacent tissue, and the phrenic nerve is crushed to allow the diaphragm to rise on the affected side and help obliterate the cavity left by removal of the lung. The incision usually is closed without drainage tubes. The cavity left by the removal of the lung is smaller than normal because of the elevation of the diaphragm on the operative side and because of the slight shifting of the mediastinum. The normal negative pressure found in the chest draws fluid into the cavity from the surrounding tissues. This fluid becomes incorporated with red and white blood cells, and eventually a cheesy material forms and fills the space prevent-

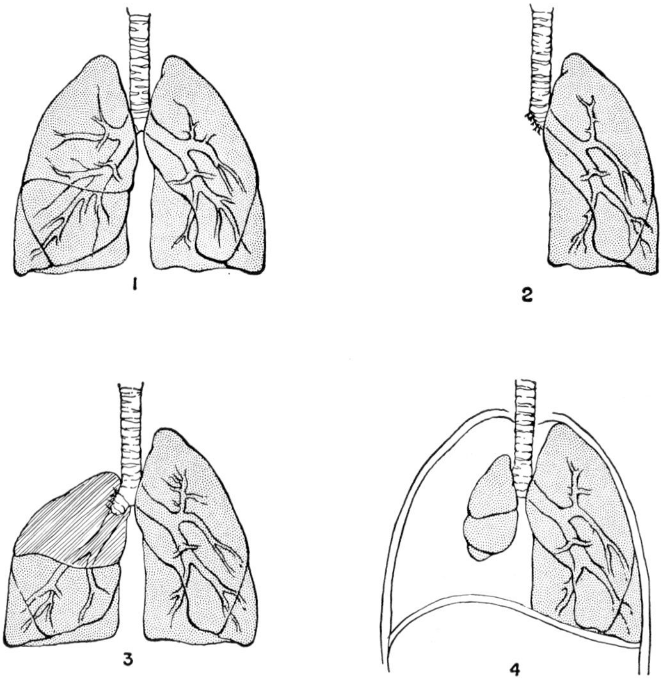

Figure 65

1, Diagram showing normal expanded lungs. *2,* Diagram showing surgical absence of the right lung following a pneumonectomy. *3,* Diagram showing surgical absence of the right upper lobe following a lobectomy. *4,* Diagram showing complete collapse of the right lung (atelectasis) due to air in the pleural cavity (pneumothorax).

ing the other lung and the heart from shifting toward the affected side. A pneumonectomy is frequently done in an attempt to cure cancer of the lung; however, since the cancer has often metastasized throughout the body before it is diagnosed, the five-year survival rate after this operation for cancer is only 5 or 6 per cent.[35] (See Figure 65, *2.*)

Segmental resection of the lung. Segmental resection or removal of a diseased part of a lobe of the lung is usually done to excise a localized bronchiectasis, lung abscess, emphysematous bleb, or a localized tuberculosis cavity that fails to heal by other methods of treatment. The success of this procedure depends on the determination of the exact part of the lobe involved. The branches of the pulmonary artery and pulmonary vein and the bronchioles to this area must be carefully located, ligated, and divided. Since it is extremely important that the correct bronchiole be resected, the anesthesiologist fills the lung with oxygen to demonstrate the collapsed area after the bronchioles have been ligated. The diseased part of the lobe is then removed. Drainage catheters are inserted below the incision, and the incision is then closed.

Thoracoplasty. An extrapleural thoracoplasty or extensive rib resection is done primarily for tuberculosis. When the ribs are removed, the chest wall becomes depressed and the underlying lung collapses, thus obliterating the cavity. When more than three or four ribs are to be removed, the operation is done in two stages; the first three ribs are removed in the first operation, and portions of the next four are removed in the second operation. Since the operation causes a deformity of the chest wall, it usually is done only when the patient is too ill to undergo a lobectomy. This surgical procedure also may be done after a pneumonectomy to decrease the size of the space to be obliterated.

Plombage. Plombage is an operative procedure used to collapse a localized portion of the lung. It is used when other means of collapse are contraindicated. A short incision is made into the chest directly over the lung cavity; a 7 to 8 cm. piece of the overlying rib is resected; the pleura is separated from the chest wall; and sterile paraffin balls or plastic ping-pong balls are packed tightly in the space created. When the healing of the lung lesion is thought to be complete, the balls may be removed. This is usually one or two years later.

Pneumolysis. Pneumolysis is the cutting of adhesions which have formed between the pleural covering of the lung and the lining of the chest wall and which are preventing collapse of the lung when air is injected into the pleural cavity for collapse therapy. The adhesions may be divided with an electric cautery through a small incision in the chest wall or with a scalpel through a thoracotomy incision. Drainage of the cavity is usually unnecessary.

Decortication. Decortication is the removal of a thick membrane that forms over the lung following empyema. This membrane constricts the lung and prevents it from expanding fully. The operation is done through a thoracotomy incision. Usually, a rib is resected and the membrane surgically removed from the lung. A catheter usually is placed in the chest cavity and attached to a closed drainage system.

Exploratory thoracotomy. An exploratory thoracotomy is an incision into the chest made to confirm a diagnosis. If cancer is suspected, a biopsy is taken, and if there has been bleeding into the pleural cavity, the lung is examined in order to locate the bleeding point. If possible, the bleeding is controlled. This operation may be done following traumatic injury in which there has been damage to the lungs or the pleura.

Pneumoperitoneum. Pneumoperitoneum is a form of collapse therapy used in treating patients with tuberculosis. A measured amount of air is injected through a needle into the abdominal peritoneum below one side of the diaphragm. The air pushes the diaphragm up on that side, compressing the lung and hindering its expansion. Following a pneumoperitoneum, the patient usually complains of abdominal distention and pain under the scapula. Until he becomes accustomed to the pressure, he should be given small meals; change of position often relieves the shoulder pain. Pneumothorax and air embolism are rare but serious immediate complications of this procedure. Spontaneous pneumothorax causes a sudden sharp pain in the chest which is followed immediately by severe dyspnea and signs of shock with marked apprehension. Treatment includes absolute quiet, reassurance, oxygen, stimulants, and immediate aspiration of air from the pleural space. *Air embolism* is accompanied by sudden signs of shock and total collapse; treatment is similar to that for any embolus and includes absolute quiet, reassurance, oxygen, and stimulants. Because the air injected is gradually absorbed, the patient who has this treatment must return regularly for "refills." The amounts of air injected and the frequency of injections vary with each patient; many patients receive more air at biweekly intervals for the first few injections and then at monthly intervals. Pneumoperitoneum is also used to treat elderly patients with hiatal hernia (see Chapter 26).

Artificial pneumothorax. Artificial pneumothorax is the injection of a measured amount of air through a needle into the pleural cavity. This compresses the lung and is used to help collapse tuberculous cavities in the lung. When the air is first injected, the patient usually complains of tightness in the chest and of dyspnea. Air embolism is also a possible complication of this treatment. Injections of air must be repeated.

Nursing care of the patient who has chest surgery

Preoperative care. If the patient who is to have chest surgery has an understanding of what is expected of him preoperatively and postoperatively, he will be less apprehensive and better able to help himself. A full explanation of all tests that will be made helps him to accept the long preoperative preparation.

In preparation for chest surgery, the patient usually has a bronchoscopic examination, gastric aspirations, roentgenograms of the chest including tomograms (special roentgenograms), and sputum examinations. He may be asked to do postural drainage several times a day and to take various medications. If he is hospitalized, drugs such as Alevaire or racemic epinephine hydrochloride (Vaponefrin) may be given by aerosol administration. Tests and treatments often are done on an outpatient basis either in a clinic or in a doctor's office. Because the patient will not be under close supervision, it is important that the clinic nurse or office nurse makes sure that the patient understands all directions and that he is able to carry out necessary procedures. Close members of his family may be called upon to help in this. When it is advisable that the patient be hospitalized for the preoperative examinations and preparation, instructions should still be given.

The operation is discussed with both the patient and his family. The surgeon discusses the type of operation, the results anticipated, the probable length of time the patient will stay in the hospital, and convalescence. It is the policy in many hospitals for the anesthesiologist to visit the patient preoperatively to evaluate his condition and to answer any questions he may have concerning the anesthetic. The nurse should tell the patient what will be done for him both preoperatively and postoperatively. The patient should be given an opportunity to ask questions, and the instructions may need to be repeated several times. The patient may receive oxygen postoperatively either by mask, catheter, or tent; he should understand that this is a routine practice for patients undergoing chest surgery and that the oxygen helps him to breathe more easily. For several days, the nurses will take his blood pressure reading, pulse rate, and respiratory rate frequently since these serve as guides in determining his progress. He should not be alarmed because these observations are being made. He should know that he will be turned and asked to cough every two hours postoperatively since this helps to bring up secretions from the lungs and prevents complications. Patients who practice coughing preoperatively usually will cough more effectively postoperatively. The nurse should instruct the patient in how to cough (see Chapter 12). In some hospitals the physical therapist instructs the patient in correct breathing and coughing and in arm and shoulder exercises. The nurse, however, must follow this up and is responsible for seeing that the patient carries out the instructions properly.

If a catheter is to be used for drainage of the chest, he can be told that this will be used to drain fluid that normally accumulates after a chest operation. He should also be told to expect to have pain for some time postoperatively because intercostal nerves are severed, but he should be told that medication can be given for this pain and that he must not let it prevent him from coughing. If he has pain on breathing deeply, he should not hesitate to ask whether medication can be given. The patient should also know that the doctor may start an infusion in a vein in the leg before he goes to the operating room; the skin is often incised and a polyethylene tube inserted into the vein to obviate the danger of infiltration of the fluid and of collapse of the vein in event of shock.

Chest drainage. Patients who are

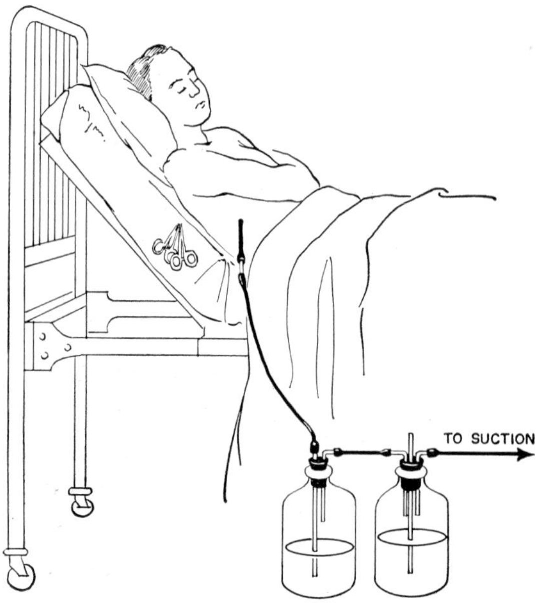

Figure 66

Schematic drawing of a chest catheter in place. The chest catheter is attached to a closed drainage system. Note that the glass tube in the drainage bottle connected to the tubing of the chest catheter is below the level of the water. The bottle to the right of the drainage bottle regulates the amount of suction transmitted to the drainage bottle, the chest catheter, and the pleural cavity. The two clamps attached to the bed are available for use when the tubing is disconnected. If two catheters are used, a Y connecting tube may be used, or both catheters may be connected to separate bottles and then attached to the control bottles.

scheduled for chest surgery rarely are given a narcotic preoperatively since it depresses respirations. A barbituarate and atropine sulfate are the usual preoperative medications used. When there is a possibility that there may be leakage of air, fluid, or blood into the chest cavity from the lung, chest wall, or any other organs or tissues that have been operated upon, a means of escape must be provided for such fluid or air to prevent impaired breathing and to prevent mediastinal shift. Catheters (drainage tubes) placed in the chest usually are placed above and below the resected area: the upper catheter allows air to escape; the lower catheter allows fluid to drain. The catheters are attached to a *closed drainage system* (underwater drainage) which prevents outside fluid or air from entering the chest cavity and causing collapse of the lung. Closed drainage is accomplished by attaching the catheter from the chest to a tube that is submerged under sterile water in a drainage bottle. If the drainage bottle is below the level of the bed, the normal negative pressure created in the pleural cavity will not be great enough to draw water up the tube on inspiration. However, sterile tubing, drainage bottles, and water should always be used lest, through some accident, the fluid is drawn back into the chest cavity. When the patient breathes out, he pushes the air and fluid from the chest cavity into the catheters, and then gravity forces them down into the drainage bottle. By coughing and breathing deeply, the patient forces the fluid out and the lung can then expand more fully. Using portable equipment, a roentgenogram is taken twenty-four to seventy-two hours postoperatively; if this shows the lung to be fully expanded and reveals no fluid level, the chest catheters are removed. When the catheters come out, the intercostal muscles contract thereby closing the openings and preventing the entrance of air into the chest cavity. As an additional precaution petroleum jelly gauze is applied immediately over the openings and is covered and taped securely with adhesive tape. The small openings heal quickly.

If the patient is not able to cough or if the drainage is such that expiration is not enough to force the fluid out the drainage tube, suction may be used on the catheter. (See Figure 66.) However, the usual type of suction machine or wall suction may create more suction than is desired so that a control bottle is placed between the drainage bottle and the suction machine to regulate the amount of suction being exerted. By filling a control bottle with water, having an air-tight system, and placing a glass tube in such a way that one end is exposed to the air and the other end is in the water, the amount of suction can be controlled. The number of centimeters the tube is submerged under the water regulates the amount of suction. If the glass tube is submerged 8 to 10 cm. (3 to 4 inches), that is the amount of suction used to draw fluid from the chest; the rest of the negative pressure (suction) escapes through the air vent.

Chest drainage is adjusted by the doctor, who determines how much sterile water should be in the bottles and how far below the water level the glass tube in the control bottle should be. The doctor may measure the drainage in the bottle and add more sterile water as necessary. In many institutions, however, this is a nursing function. If the nurse does this, she must be certain that the tube from the chest is clamped off close to the chest wall before the stopper is removed from the bottle. Care must be taken to measure drainage accurately, to use aseptic technique in handling and sterilizing the equipment, and to carry out this procedure as quickly as possible. Sometimes extra sterile bottles and tubing are available so that used equipment can be replaced immediately. When it is attached to a clean bottle, the tube must be unclamped immediately lest fluid congeal in the tube or expansion of the lung be delayed.

In caring for the patient who has a chest catheter attached to a closed drainage system, the nurse should check the equipment frequently to be sure that the system is airtight and that drainage is not obstructed by kinks, blood clots in the tubing, or other causes. When the patient is lying on his operated side, the tube should be protected from kinking or from pressure by placing towels on either side of it to make a trough or by having the patient lie with a rubber ring under the operated area. Two clamps should be kept at the bedside; if the drainage or suction system seems to be working improperly or if the drainage bottle is broken, both clamps should be placed immediately on the catheter close to the wound

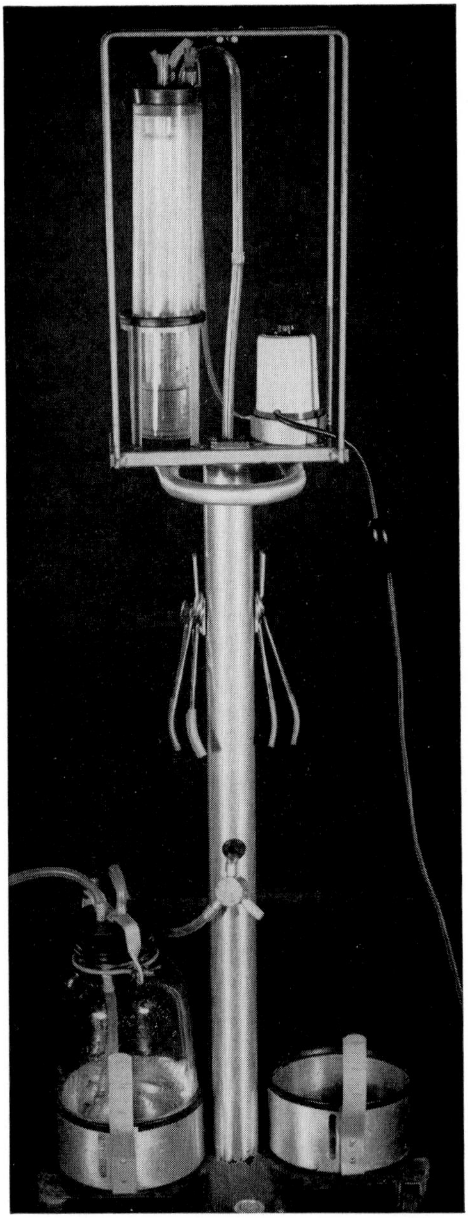

Figure 67

Commercial chest suction machines
now incorporate the principle of closed drainage.
(Courtesy General Medical
Equipment Corporation, Valley Stream, N. Y.)

dressing. The drainage bottles should never be raised above the level of the bed, since this will permit the fluid to drain back into the chest cavity. The glass tube in the control bottle must *always* be under water, the rubber tubing should be attached snugly to the glass connecting tubes, and the bottle stoppers should fit tightly to prevent air from leaking into the system. If the catheter is patent, the water will rise and fall in the glass tube in the collection bottle on inspiration and expiration. If the tubing becomes blocked or if the lung has re-expanded, this will no longer occur. If the nurse notices that the fluid in the tubing does not rise or fall with breathing, the doctor must be immediately notified since he must determine the cause. A clogged tube with drainage dammed up behind it may cause the position of the heart and the great vessels to shift. When this happens, the patient is said to have a *mediastinal shift.* The pulse becomes very rapid and "fluttery," and signs of shock will soon appear. Mediastinal shift is a serious complication and must be watched for after any type of chest surgery. It also may occur after the injection of air in collapse therapy or following trauma to the chest. A thoracentesis may be done as an emergency measure to draw air or fluid out of the pleural cavity.

Postoperative care. When the patient returns from the operating room, vital signs should be checked, oxygen administered as ordered, and the drainage tube attached to a closed drainage system. The patient should be watched for signs of shock or hemorrhage. The dressings must be observed for drainage; a moderate amount of serosanguineous drainage is expected for the first day. Dyspnea, cyanosis, or sudden sharp pain in the chest should be reported at once. These are signs of *spontaneous pneumothrax;* if this condition is not treated promptly by aspiration of air or fluid by means of a thoracentesis, a mediastinal shift may occur. When the patient has reacted from anesthesia, he should be placed in a semi-Fowler's position to facilitate breathing. Since a firm bed lessens pain, a hinged fracture board should be put under the mattress prior to surgery.

The patient should be turned at least every two hours. Many doctors believe that the patient should lie on his operated side most of the time since this lessens pain, permits better expansion of the unaffected lung, facilitates drainage, and helps to prevent spread of any possible infection to the mediastinum and the unaffected lung. Some surgeons believe that the patient should be turned on alternate sides and will specifically order this.

The patient is encouraged to cough; coughing is made easier for the patient by splinting the wound with the hands or by having the patient sit up in bed and splinting the chest with a towel or a drawsheet. (See Figure 68.) To make it easier for him to sit up, a pull rope may be placed at the foot of the bed to assist him in rising and in remaining upright for short periods.

Morphine and meperidine hydrochloride (Demerol) are usually ordered for pain. Medication for pain should be given as needed and may be required frequently during the first few postoperative days. The patient is extremely uncomfortable and will not be able to cough or turn unless he has relief from pain. In some instances the dosage of the drug is decreased so that it may be given oftener and yet not depress respirations. The tube in the chest causes pain, and the patient may attempt rapid, shallow breathing to splint the lower chest and avoid motion of the catheter.

The patient is encouraged to take fluids postoperatively, and he can progress to a general diet as soon as this is tolerated. Forcing fluids helps to keep the mucus less tenacious and thus it can be more easily expectorated. Alevaire may be given through the oxygen tent, by nebulizer, or under positive pressure to help liquefy mucous. After an inhalation of Alevaire, the patient should be encouraged to cough and bring up as much sputum as possible. Steam inhalations and inhalations of drugs such as isoproterenol hydro-

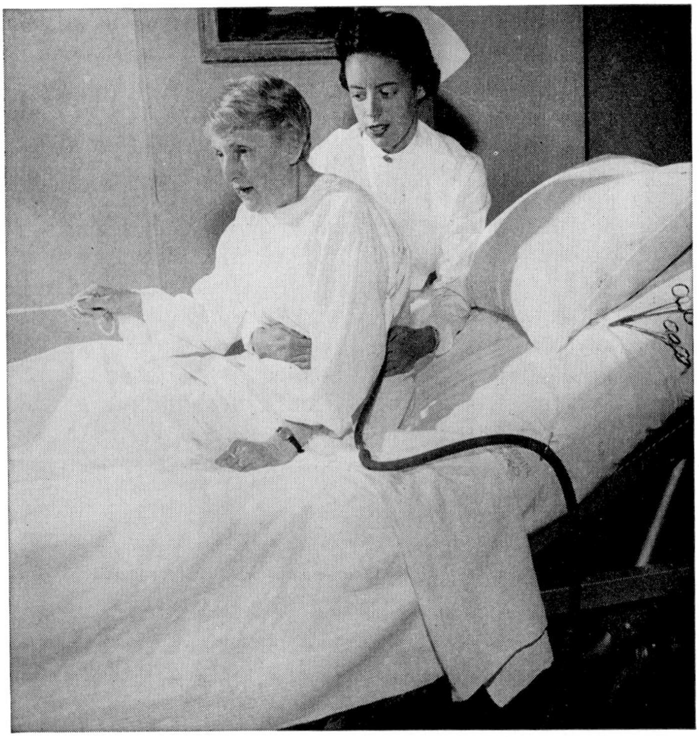

Figure 68

The nurse is splinting the chest by applying pressure; this lessens muscle pull and pain as the patient coughs.

chloride (Isuprel) or racemic epinephrine hydrochloride (Vaponefrin) also may be used.

Exercise is started early to prevent the shoulder and arm on the affected side from becoming stiff with subsequent loss of full range of motion. Passive exercise may be given for a few days after surgery. A regular program for arm and shoulder exercises should then be planned and supervised by the nurse. The patient needs encouragement doing exercises since he fears that they will increase pain; exercises can be planned for a suitable interval after analgesic medication has been given. Active movement of the arm through full range of motion should be done within a few days. It must be remembered that the patient cannot do exercises to ensure complete range of motion of the shoulder unless he is upright or lies on his abdomen; exercises such as elevating the scapula and clavicle, "hunching the shoulders," bringing the scapulas as close together as possible, and hyperextending the arm can be done only in these positions. Since lying on the abdomen may not be possible at first, these exercises should be done when the patient is sitting on the edge of the bed or when he is standing. The patient has a natural tendency to protect his operated side, and this can quickly cause stiffness, atrophy of muscles, and an awkward posture. A full length mirror helps the ambulatory patient to check his own posture.

The patient who has had extensive chest surgery usually requires a long convalescence. He may feel weak and tired for a long time. This is especially true if much of the lung has been removed and vital capacity is reduced. He is likely to complain of pain in the incision for weeks after the operation; if it is really severe, the doctor may infiltrate the nerves in the area with procaine. Some patients complain of a feeling of numbness in the area of the incision; this will eventually return to normal, and the patient is reassured by knowing this. The pain and numbness are caused by the interruption of intercostal nerves.

If the operation is for tuberculosis, the precautions used for any patient with active tuberculosis should be followed, since, although the diseased area is removed, tubercle bacilli may still be in the respiratory tract. The first few days postoperatively the patient generally is too ill to be expected to do such things as "covering his cough." The responsibility for carrying out good technique should rest with the nurse during this time. Usually the nurse wears a mask and gown which are discarded for laundering after removal.

Special care following a pneumonectomy. The nursing care of a patient following a pneumonectomy is essentially the same as that for patients having other kinds of lung surgery except that the drainage tube may not be used. Patients who have had a lung removed have a markedly lowered vital capacity, and exercise and activity should be limited to that which can be done without dyspnea. Since the body must be given time to adjust to getting along with only one lung, the patient's return to work may be delayed. If the diagnosis is cancer, radiation therapy is usually given. This may be started before the patient leaves the hospital. (See Chapter 16 for further discussion of nursing care for those receiving radiation therapy.) The patient who has had a pneumonectomy for cancer is urged to report to his doctor at once if he has hoarseness, dyspnea, pain on swallowing, or localized chest pain, since these may be signs of metastasis.

Special care following a thoracoplasty. After a thoracoplasty, early movement of the arm and shoulder is exceedingly important, since several ribs have been removed and there is a tendency for a deformity to develop which may involve the entire shoulder girdle on both sides of the body. Position in bed and postural exercises to prevent drooping of the shoulder on the unaffected side should be emphasized. Scoliosis can easily develop in those who have had a thoracoplasty without sufficient attention to posture postoperatively. A physical therapist may be able to give helpful suggestions regarding exercises that may be carried out while the patient is in the hospital. When patients return home, most of them need extra supervision either by a physical therapist or by a public health nurse who is experienced in orthopedic nursing.

CHEST TRAUMA

Fracture of the ribs. The fourth, fifth, sixth, seventh, and eighth ribs are most commonly fractured. Fractures of the ribs are caused by blows, crushing injuries, or strain caused by severe coughing or sneezing spells. If the rib is splintered or the fracture displaced, sharp fragments may penetrate the pleura and the lung. Patients with questionable rib fractures should have a roentgenogram of the chest made and should be observed carefully for signs of pneumothorax or hemothorax.

The patient with a rib fracture complains of pain at the site of the injury which increases on inspiration. The area is very tender to the touch, and the patient splints his chest and takes shallow breaths. Unless the lung has been penetrated, the usual treatment for rib fracture is strapping the chest with adhesive tape from the affected side to the unaffected side or applying a circular strapping, using an Ace bandage. A chest binder also may be used. If adhesive tape is used, the skin should be shaved and painted with tincture of benzoin to prevent blistering and other irritation. When the pain is severe and is not relieved by strapping and analgesic medications, the doctor may do a regional nerve block. This consists of infiltrating the intercostal spaces above and below the fractured rib with procaine, 1 per cent. If the lung has been penetrated, the patient may raise bright red sputum. If this occurs, an exploratory thoracotomy is usually done.

The patient who has a fractured rib is usually more comfortable in a semi-Fowler's position. After the chest is strapped, he should be encouraged to take as many deep breaths as possible. Since pain may prevent him from breathing easily enough to sleep, provision should be made for him to have medication. Because the patient with a rib fracture is often treated in the doctor's office or in the emergency room of a hospital and then discharged, his family should also be instructed about his position for comfort, medications to take, and the need for deep breathing. If the patient has difficulty breathing or develops sudden, sharp chest pain, he should call the doctor or return at once to the hospital emergency room.

Penetrating wounds of the chest. When a knife, bullet, or other foreign object has entered the chest, the major problem is not injury to the chest wall, but injury to structures within the chest cavity. Penetration of the lung can cause leakage of air from the lung into the pleural cavity (pneumothorax). Blood may also leak into the pleural cavity (hemothorax). As the air or fluid accumulates in the pleural cavity, it builds up positive pressure, which causes the lung to collapse and may even cause a mediastinal shift, thus compressing the opposite lung and the heart. The patient then has serious difficulty in breathing and may go into shock. His pulse may become weak and rapid and his skin cold and clammy, and his blood pressure falls rapidly.

Emergency treatment must be instituted to remove the air and blood from the pleural cavity before death from cardiac or respiratory failure occurs. An emergency thoracentesis is done, and a tube may be left and attached to a closed drainage system. When the patient's condition permits, the chest is opened and the injury is repaired or a section of the lung is removed.

If an open wound of the chest has been sustained, it should be covered immediately to prevent air from entering the pleural cavity and causing a pneumothorax. Several thicknesses of material may be used, and these are anchored with wide adhesive tape, or the wound edges may be taped tightly together. If an object such as a knife is still in the wound, it must never be removed until a doctor arrives. Its presence may prevent the entry of air into the pleural cavity, and its removal may cause further damage. The patient who has sustained a penetrating wound of the chest should be placed in an upright position and taken to a doctor immediately.

REFERENCES AND SELECTED READINGS*

1 *Andrews, Neil C., and MacVicar, Jean: Resection for Pulmonary Tuberculosis and The Patient With Pulmonary Resection, Am. J. Nursing **59**:962-970, July 1959.

2 Blair, Esta H. M.: Oh, for a Mask, Nursing Outlook **7**:40-42, Jan. 1959.

3 Brown, Amy Frances: Medical Nursing, ed. 3, Philadelphia, 1957, W. B. Saunders Co.

4 Brown, Elizabeth M.: The Role of Bronchoscopy in the Prevention of Postoperative Atelectasis, J.A.M.A. **165**:947-949, Oct. 26, 1951.

5 Cancer in Midlife, Statistical Bulletin, Metropolitan Life Insurance Company, **37**:1-4, June 1956.

6 Cecil, Russell, and Loeb, Robert F. (editors): A Textbook of Medicine, ed. 10, Philadelphia, 1959, W. B. Saunders Co.

7 *Creighton, Helen, and Peabody, J. Winthrop, Sr.: Inflammatory Diseases of the Pleura, Am. J. Nursing **59**:346-348, March 1959.

8 *Drolet, Godias J., and Lowell, Anthony M.: Where to Tuberculosis? The First Seven Years of the Antimicrobial Era 1947-1953, Am. Rev. Tuberc. **72**:419-452, Oct. 1955.

9 Dubois, René J. (editor): Bacterial and Mycotic Infections of Man, ed. 3, Philadelphia, 1958, J. B. Lippincott Co.

10 *Ellison, Bess M.: Nursing Care in Collapse Therapy, Am. J. Nursing **50**:473-475, Aug. 1950.

---

*References preceded by an asterisk indicate material particularly well suited for student reading.

11 *Feldman, Floyd: How to Use the Tuberculin Test, Am. J. Nursing **59**:856-857, June 1959.
12 *Furcolow, Michael L., and Rakich, Jennie H.: Histoplasmosis and Nursing Aspects of Histoplasmosis, Am. J. Nursing **59**:79-83, Jan. 1959.
13 Gold, Harry, and others: Cornell Conferences on Therapy, vol. 5, New York, 1952, The Macmillan Co.
14 Goodman, Louis S., and Gilman, Alfred: The Pharmacological Basis of Therapeutics, ed. 2, New York, 1955, The Macmillan Co.
15 Harrison, T. R., and others (editors): Principles of Internal Medicine, ed 2, New York, 1954, The Blakiston Co.
16 *Herbert, William M., and Schlesinger, Eva M.: Crushing Injuries of the Chest and Nursing the Patient with a Crushed Chest, Am. J. Nursing **59**:678-684, May 1959.
17 *Huebner, Robert J.: 70 Newly Recognized Viruses in Man, Pub. Health Rep. **74**:6-12, Jan. 1959.
18 *Jordan, William S.: Acute Upper Respiratory Infections, Am. J. Nursing **50**:39-42, Jan. 1950.
19 *Kelly, Winfield, and Poole, Hazel: Skeletal Tuberculosis, Am. J. Nursing **57**:332-336, March 1957.
20 *Kressler, Alta: Teaching Patients With Tuberculosis, Am. J. of Nursing **59**:1116-1118, Aug. 1959.
21 Krug, Elsie: Pharmacology in Nursing, ed. 8, St. Louis, 1960, The C. V. Mosby Co.
22 *Livingstone, Huberta M.: Nursing Care in Oxygen Therapy, Am. J. Nursing **57**:65-69, Jan. 1957.
23 Mass X-Ray Survey for Tuberculosis, J.A.M.A. **165**:1980, Dec. 14, 1957.
24 *McClure, Eugenia J., and Anderson, Leighton L.: Pulmonary Emphysema, Am. J. Nursing **57**:594-598, May 1957.
25 Meakins, Jonathan Campbell: The Practice of Medicine, ed. 6, St. Louis, 1956, The C. V. Mosby Co.
26 Moseley, H. F.: Textbook of Surgery, ed. 3, St. Louis, 1959, The C. V. Mosby Co.
27 National Conference on Air Pollution, Pub. Health Rep. **74**:409-427, May 1957.
28 National Tuberculosis Association Report, Pub. Health Rep. **76**:40, Jan. 1959.
29 Overhold, Richard H., and Wilson, Norma J.: Surgery in Tuberculosis, New York, 1946, The National Tuberculosis Association.
30 Plumb, Robert K.: The Common Cold—Uncommon Problem, The New York Times, June 10, 1956.
31 Porter, Alice, and Gibson, Frank: Editorial—The Admission X-Ray: A Key to TB Control, Bull. Nat. Tuberc. A. **42**:130, Oct. 1956.
32 Riley, Richard: Protective Measures—Reasonable or Ritualistic? Nursing Outlook **7**:38-39, Jan. 1959.
33 Rudy, Norman E., and Crepeau, Jacques: The Role of Intermittent Positive Pressure Breathing Postoperatively, J.A.M.A. **167**:1093-1096, June 28, 1958.
34 *Stephan, Phyllis Jean: Nebulization Under Intermittent Positive Pressure, Am. J. Nursing **57**:1158-1160, Sept. 1957.
35 Sweet, Richard H.: Thoracic Surgery, Philadelphia, 1950, W. B. Saunders Co.
36 Thomas, Mary E., and Buchanan, Margaret S.: Presurgical Conferences With the TB Patient, Am. J. Nursing **53**:944-946, Aug. 1953.
37 *Weiss, Moe: Chemotherapy and Tuberculosis, Am. J. Nursing **59**:1711-1714, Dec. 1959.
38 Wolcott, M. W., and Murphy, J. D.: The Changing Picture of Lung Abscess Therapy, Diseases of the Chest **32**:62-69, July 1957.

Study questions for review

1 Review the anatomy and the physiology of the ear, nose, sinuses, and throat. What are some specific dangers from disease of these parts?
2 What emotional reactions would probably follow the sudden inability to hear? to speak? Consider the means of communication available for those who are deaf; who cannot speak.
3 Review the procedures for throat irrigation, ear irrigation, administration of nose drops, and administration of ear drops.

The patient with ear, nose, or throat disease

Chapter 24

The purpose of this chapter is to give the nurse an understanding of the causes of ear, nose, and throat diseases and the sequence of complications so that she is better able to teach health and prevention of disease. Diagnostic procedures, treatments, and nursing care of patients with these diseases who are often treated in general hospitals are discussed briefly. For more detailed information concerning specialized care, refer to the references preceded by an asterisk at the end of this chapter and to other periodicals and special publications on this subject.

COMMON DIAGNOSTIC PROCEDURES

Visual examinations. The mucous membrane lining the antra of the nares is easily examined by using a nasal speculum, a head mirror, and a light. A cotton-tipped applicator may be needed to remove secretions. The posterior nares are usually examined at the same time as the throat. A small throat mirror, a larger laryngeal mirror, a head mirror, and a light are used for this examination, which may be referred to as an *indirect laryngoscopy*. When preparing equipment for an otolaryngeal examination, the nurse should provide a basin of boiling water or an alcohol lamp to warm the laryngeal mirror before use to prevent its becoming "foggy" and failing to reflect. The light should be bright and should be placed about nine inches to the right of, and slightly behind, the patient's head. The room should be darkened. The throat is often superficially examined with a tongue depressor and flashlight. Nose and throat cultures may be taken to determine the cause of disease, and a biopsy may be taken for pathologic study.

When a more detailed examination of the larynx is necessary than is possible with a laryngeal mirror, a *direct laryngoscopy* may be done. The throat is first anesthetized with 10 per cent cocaine. (See Chapter 26 for preparation of the patient for this examination since the preparation is similar to that for gastroscopy.) A tubular instrument with a built-in light and mirror attachment is then passed into the larynx. For this examination the patient is placed in a reclining position, with the head extending over the edge of the table and being manually supported by a doctor or a nurse. The patient may find the examination very uncomfortable even though the throat is anesthetized. Because of this, he

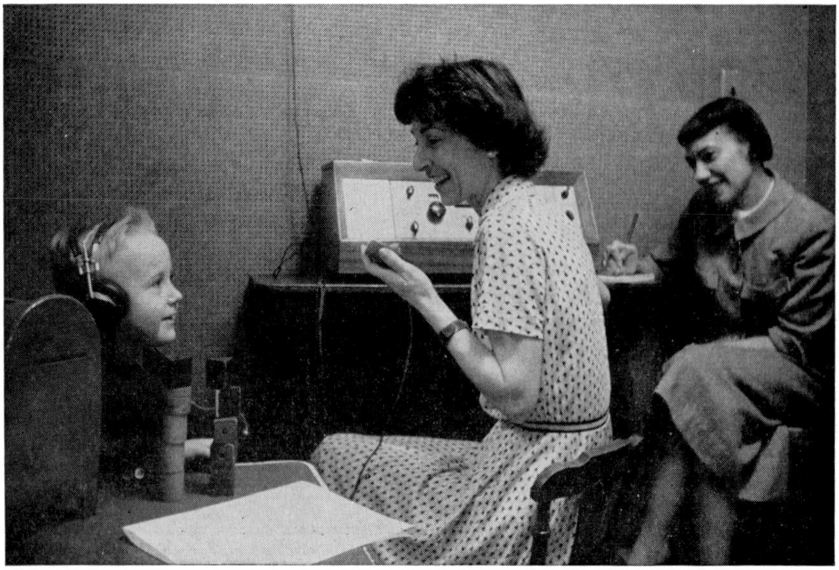

Figure 69

Testing of a child's hearing with an audiometer. Note the soundproof walls and the use of cards for the child's response. The child's mother is observing. (Courtesy New York League for the Hard of Hearing, New York, N. Y.)

is usually given a sedative such as phenobarbital sodium about an hour before the procedure is to be done.

After a laryngoscopy the patient should not eat or drink anything until the gag reflex returns. This usually takes about four hours. It can be tested by "tickling" the throat with a tongue blade or applicator. After the gag reflex returns, the patient should try first to drink water since this, if accidentally aspirated into the trachea or lungs is the least likely to cause untoward reaction.

The frontal and maxillary sinuses can be visualized by illuminating them with a flashlight in a dark room. This examination, referred to as *transillumination,* reveals fluid levels indicative of obstruction to drainage of the sinuses. Roentgenograms of the sinuses are often ordered since they help the doctor to determine if the sinuses are obstructed. No physical preparation is necessary. No contrast medium is used, since the normal sinus is filled with air which itself casts a shadow in contrast to surrounding structures.

The ears are examined with an *otoscope.* This instrument has a light attached, and with it the doctor can examine the walls of the external auditory canal and the eardrum.

Audiometric testing. Hearing may be roughly tested by having the patient tell when he hears a watch, a tuning fork, or someone whispering behind him. The patient with apparent loss of hearing needs a more detailed and accurate examination. This is done by using an audiometer.

To be accurate, audiometry must be done in a soundproof room. Group examinations such as are done in schools are helpful only in discovering children who need individual examinations. (See Figure 69.) For audiometry the patient wears earphones and is instructed to signal when he hears the tone and again when he no longer hears it. Pure tones usually are used instead of speech sounds since they are more accurate. The machine is set at plus 10 decibels (intensity), the level of normal hearing.[6] The intensity is then increased until the patient hears the tone

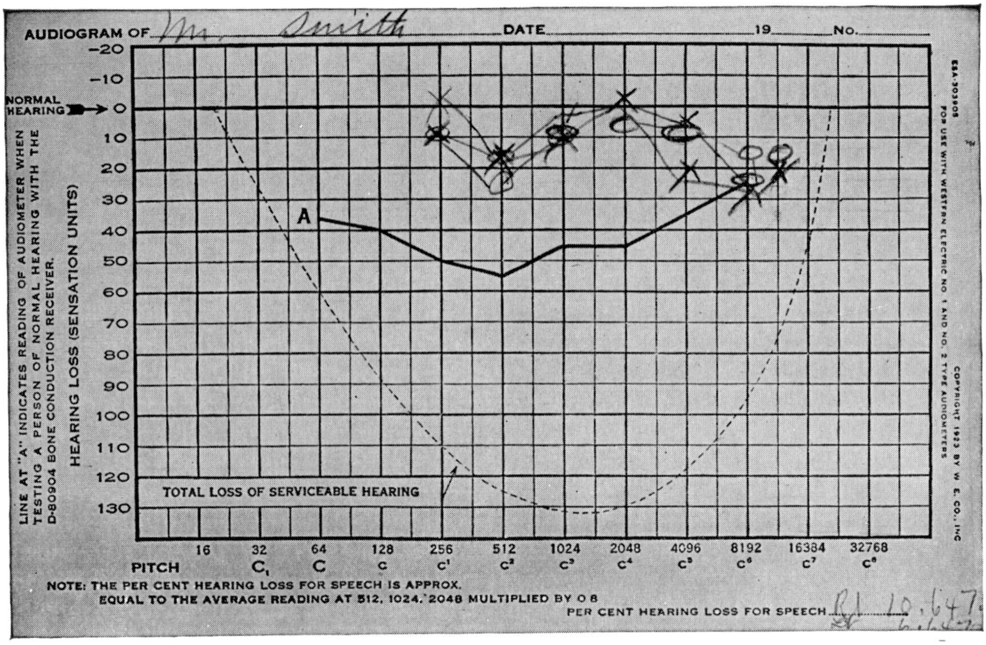

Figure 70

An audiogram. (From Parkinson, Roy H.: Eye, Ear, Nose, and Throat Manual for Nurses, St. Louis, 1959, The C. V. Mosby Co.)

and then gradually decreased to the level at which he no longer hears it. This point is charted. This is repeated using eight different frequencies ranging between approximately 250 to 10,000 cycles (pitch) per second.[22] Each ear is tested separately and is tested for both bone and air conduction. The patient who has a loss of 30 decibels (units of sound measurement) or more in the range of 500 to 2,000 cycles per second is considered to have a handicapping deafness.[15] The person with normal hearing usually hears in a range of 20 to 20,000 cycles per second, but the normal primary speech range is between 300 and 3,500 cycles per second.[15] (See Figure 70.)

Insufflation. Insufflation of the eustachian tubes may be done either to test their patency or to force them open mechanically. Air under pressure is forced through a catheter inserted through the nostril into the eustachian tube. The other nostril is held closed, and the patient is asked to keep his mouth open to prevent excessive pressure. A special rubber tube is often inserted into the external auditory canal and then attached to earpieces so that the doctor can determine whether the air passes into the middle ear. Insufflation of the eustachian tubes is likely to be quite painful, especially if the tubes are blocked. The lay person often refers to this procedure as "having his ears blown out."

INFECTIONS OF THE NOSE AND SINUSES

Infections of the nose, throat, and sinuses are among the most frequent complications of the common cold. The nurse, therefore, should be aware of the signs of these infections and of their complications.

The patient with rhinitis

Acute rhinitis. Simple acute rhinitis (coryza) is the common cold involving the mucous membrane of the nose. It is a condition which everyone probably has had at some time in his life. Swelling of the nasal mucous membranes causes obstruction to nasal breathing and results in a feeling of tightness in the head and sometimes in headache. There may be profuse mucous discharge from the nose and tearing of the eyes. Acute rhinitis rather often follows chilling, because with the constriction of the blood vessels in the nose infecting agents which are constantly present there more easily invade the mucous membranes. When the general resistance is low, infection attacks the tissues more readily. The very young are particularly susceptible.

There is no specific treatment for acute rhinitis. The treatment usually consists of rest, fluids, and the intranasal use of astringent solutions such as ephedrine sulfate, 1 per cent, or ephedrine hydrochloride, 1/4 per cent, Neo-Synephrine hydrochloride, 1/4 to 1 per cent, or naphazoline hydrochloride, 0.1 per cent (Privine). These drugs relieve the nasal congestion and may be given every four hours for several days. However, with continued use, they lose their effectiveness. In using astringent nose drops, inhalers, or sprays, the patient should sit in a chair and tip his head well backward, lie down with the head extending over the edge of the bed, or lie down and place a large pillow under the shoulders so that the head is tipped backward. He should remain in such a position for five minutes after the drops are instilled to allow the solution to reach the posterior nares. If, after ten minutes, he still has marked congestion, another drop or two of the solution may be used; the mucous membrane of the anterior nares by this time should have become constricted so that the solution may more easily reach the posterior nares. Mild antiseptics such as mild silver protein (Argyrol), 10 per cent, and soothing oily sprays containing camphor and menthol may be ordered. Since patients often instill their own nose drops or administer their own nasal sprays, they should be taught the correct method. No more than three drops or three sprays of solution should be instilled into each nostril unless more is specifically prescribed. Aqueous solutions are preferable to solutions with oil bases since they are more easily absorbed and, if they are aspirated into the lungs, are less likely to cause lipoid pneumonia. Any of the various antihistaminic drugs may be used to alleviate the symptoms. Since they usually cause drowsiness, they should not be used when driving a car or working near moving machinery. The patient should be urged to blow his nose gently and to keep both nostrils open lest infected material be forced into the sinuses or through the eustachian tube into the middle ear. He should use disposable tissues which can be discarded at once.

If the nasal discharge becomes thick and purulent, the patient should be urged to visit his doctor, since some doctors feel that sulfonamide drugs or antibiotics should be given at this stage to shorten the course of the infection and to prevent complications. People who have recurrent colds should seek medical attention because nasal deformity such as enlarged turbinated bones or a deviated septum and chronic sinusitis may cause the repeated attacks. Repeated colds eventually may lead to chronic rhinitis. (For further discussion of the common cold see Chapter 23.)

Chronic rhinitis. Chronic rhinitis is a chronic inflammation of the mucous membrane of the nose which causes a mucopurulent discharge and difficult breathing. If crusts form in the nose, the patient may be treated symptomatically with nasal irrigations. The only cure for chronic rhinitis is treatment of the basic cause. It is often due to an allergic reaction; if the patient does not respond to treatment for an infection, he usually is advised to see a specialist in allergy. (See Chapters 11 and 23 for a discussion of allergies.)

The nurse may occasionally help with nasal irrigations. The details of this procedure are described in texts on fundamentals of nursing. Care should be taken that both nostrils are open and that the pressure exerted is no greater than that produced when an irrigating can is held eight inches above the level of the nose. Excess pressure increases the danger of forcing infected material into the sinuses or the middle ear. The patient should breathe through his mouth during the procedure, and the irrigating tip should be removed from the nostril if he must sneeze or cough.

The patient with sinusitis

Acute sinusitis. Acute sinusitis is an inflammation of one or more of the sinuses. It usually follows acute rhinitis or other respiratory diseases, such as pneumonia or influenza, and is caused by infection extending through the nasal openings into the sinuses. Abscessed teeth or tooth extraction occasionally causes an acute maxillary sinusitis. Sinusitis may also be caused by allergic reaction.

The patient with acute sinusitis often complains of severe headache and of pain over the infected sinuses; this is usually constant. Maxillary sinusitis may cause pain under the eyes, while frontal sinusitis often causes pain over the eyebrows; pain from the ethmoid and sphenoid sinuses usually is referred and is felt at the top of the head. Occasionally there may be noticeable swelling over the maxillary frontal sinuses. The patient may have nausea, purulent discharge from the nose, obstruction to nasal breathing, fever, and general malaise. The throat may be sore from irritation caused by postnasal drainage.

Objectives in the care of patients with acute sinusitis are to establish drainage of the sinuses and to inactivate the infection. Sulfonamides and antibiotics are given for their specific action upon the causative organisms. Drugs which constrict the blood vessels in the mucous membrane such as phenylephrine hydrochloride (Neo-Synephrine hydrochloride), 1/4 per cent, and ephedrine sulfate, 1 per cent, may be given as nose drops or by inhalation. These drugs relieve congestion of the mucous membranes and thus improve drainage. Antibiotics and detergent preparations which loosen secretions, such as Alevaire, may be given by inhalation.

If medication is being given by atomizer or nebulizer, the adapter should be placed in one nostril and the other nostril closed. The patient then should be instructed to breathe through his nose with the mouth closed. Medication is then forced by air pressure (created with a hand bulb) through a small opening in the atomizer; such pressure breaks the large droplets of fluid into a fine mist. If a nebulizer is used, the solution is usually forced through the apparatus by a current of oxygen or compressed air.

Aspirin usually relieves the pain from sinusitis, but occasionally codeine or even morphine sulfate or Demerol may be necessary. Heat over the sinuses also gives some relief from pain; hot wet dressings or a heat lamp may be ordered. Lying in a prone position with the head down and the neck sharply flexed forward on the chest gives relief in maxillary sinusitis, since this position permits gravity to assist in draining.

If conservative measures do not cure an acute sinus infection, the maxillary and frontal sinuses may be irrigated with normal saline solution by inserting a trocar and cannula through the openings of the sinuses. Following irrigation, a sulfonamide or antibiotic solution may be instilled into the sinuses. The maxillary sinuses are the ones most often treated in this way. If it is impossible to insert the trocar and cannula through the normal opening, the nasal mucosa may be anesthetized with cocaine and the antrum (maxillary sinus) perforated with a trocar and cannula. This is known as an *antrum puncture.* The nurse should explain the procedure to the patient and should urge him to breathe through the mouth. She should remain with him while the treatment is given, since, although it is not actually painful, it causes a sensation of pressure and may produce dizziness and nausea.

Since early treatment of acute sinusitis is much more successful than treatment after the condition becomes chronic, pa-

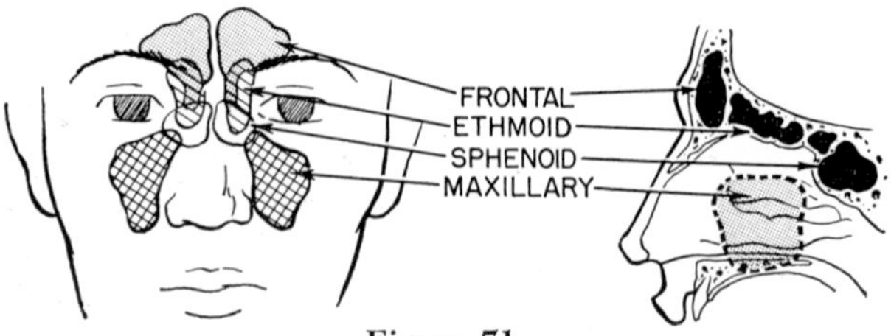

Figure 71

This schematic drawing shows the location of the sinuses.

tients with symptoms of acute sinusitis should be urged to seek medical attention at once. Chronic sinusitis is difficult to cure and may lead to further complications such as ear infections and bronchiectasis.

Operations on the sinuses. If the patient has recurrent attacks of sinusitis, it may be necessary to provide better drainage by permanently enlarging the sinus openings or by making a new opening and removing diseased mucous membrane. Surgery is usually done during the subacute stage of infection. An opening into the maxillary sinus may be made through the nostril (antrotomy) or through the mouth (Caldwell-Luc operation). The ethmoid and sphenoid sinuses may be entered through the nostril and the frontal sinus either through the nostril or through an incision under the eyebrow (see Figure 71 for location of the sinuses). Surgery through the nostril is usually done under local anesthesia.

Nursing care of the patient undergoing sinus operation. To prevent the swallowing or aspiration of bloody drainage from the nose and throat, postoperatively the patient who has had a general anesthetic should be turned well to the side. Upon recovery from the anesthesia or following local anesthesia, the patient should be in a mid-Fowler's position because this will decrease edema at the operative site. Ice compresses are usually applied over the nose or an ice bag is placed directly over the maxillary or frontal sinuses. This constricts blood vessels, decreasing oozing and edema, and relieves pain. The patient should be watched carefully for hemorrhage; excessive swallowing by the unconscious patient may indicate hemorrhage.

Gauze packing is usually inserted into the nares; consequently the patient breathes through his mouth. His lips and mouth become dry and need frequent care. Aromatic solutions are refreshing, and cold cream helps to prevent dryness of the lips. Steam inhalations often are ordered.

If the surgery is through the mouth, the patient usually is given only liquids for at least twenty-four hours and a soft diet for three or four days. Mouth care should be given before meals to improve the appetite and after eating to decrease the danger of infection at the operative site .

Fluids should be given liberally to all patients following surgery of the sinuses. Fever or complaints of tenderness or pain over the involved sinus should be reported to the doctor since they may indicate postoperative infection or inadequate drainage. Antibiotics are usually given prophylactically.

Chronic sinusitis. In chronic sinusitis the mucous membrane lining a sinus becomes thickened from prolonged irritation and infection. The patient usually has a chronic purulent nasal discharge which is sometimes referred to as *chronic nasal catarrh,* a chronic cough caused by "postnasal drip," and a chronic dull "sinus" headache which is present upon awakening and usually subsides during the day since the upright position and movements of the head help the sinus to drain.

Chronic sinusitis can seldom be cured

with antibiotics, although these drugs help to prevent additional infection. If the condition is caused by an allergy, it responds to general treatment of the allergy. If nasal deformities such as a deviated nasal septum, hypertrophied turbinated bones, or nasal polyps are obstructing the sinus openings, treatment of these conditions may give relief. Sinus irrigations and surgery to ensure better sinus drainage may be done. The best treatment, however, is prevention by urging patients with acute sinusitis to seek early medical care.

The patient with chronic sinusitis should avoid chilling, and cold, damp atmospheres. He is advised not to smoke since this further irritates the damaged mucous membranes. Air-conditioning often causes discomfort since the change from warm, moist, outside air to cool, dry, inside air aggravates the sinusitis. Improvement in general health by such means as an adequate diet high in vitamins, rest, fresh air, and sunshine helps the body to overcome this chronic condition.

The patient with nasal obstruction

Nasal polyps. Nasal polyps are growths of mucous membrane and loose connective tissue. They may be caused by irritation to mucous membranes of the nose or sinuses from an allergy or by chronic sinusitis. Since they may obstruct breathing or may bleed, nasal polyps are removed. They are excised through the nose (a polypectomy).

Deviated septum. A deviated septum means a bent nasal septum; it is often congenital in origin, or it may be the result of injury or of inadequate treatment of a fractured nose. The patient with this condition usually breathes through his mouth because the nostril is obstructed by the abnormal septum and by dry secretions. Treatment consists of removing part of the bony and cartilaginous septum (a submucous resection). The operation is done under local anesthesia through the nostril.

Hypertrophied turbinated bones. Hypertrophied turbinated bones cause nasal congestion. They are removed surgically (turbinectomy) or by cauterization. Both of these procedures are done through the nostril and local anesthetics are used.

Nursing care of the patient undergoing nasal surgery. Most nasal surgery is done under local anesthesia. The patient, however, should not be given anything by mouth for six hours preoperatively since he may become nauseated during the operation. He is given a sedative, a narcotic, and an atropine prepration preoperatively. An enema is usually ordered preoperatively because the patient is likely to swallow blood during the operation, and, if the bowel is empty, this will be evacuated more quickly.

Packing, either gauze or a tampon, is usually placed in the nose at the conclusion of the operation. If a tampon is used, the string attached to it should be securely fastened with adhesive tape so that the tampon will not slip back into the throat. Should the tampon slip into the throat the patient may have respiratory difficulty, and the nurse may have to grasp the tampon with a forceps and pull it forward through the mouth. Gauze packing occasionally extrudes from the posterior nares into the throat. If this is slight yet bothersome, it should be reported to the doctor and sedatives, if ordered, can be given. If it is obstructing breathing, the doctor is notified immediately; the packing is pulled forward through the mouth with forceps.

Following nasal surgery there is danger of hemorrhage. Blood may be evident on the external dressing that is applied under the nose, or the patient may expecotrate or vomit bright red blood. His pulse may be rapid, or he may swallow repeatedly. Some oozing on the dressing is expected, but, if it becomes excessive or if any other symptoms appear, the doctor should be notified and material for repacking the nose should be prepared. This consists of a "hemostatic" tray containing nasal tampons, gauze packing, a few small gauze sponges, a small rubber catheter, a packing forceps, tongue blades,

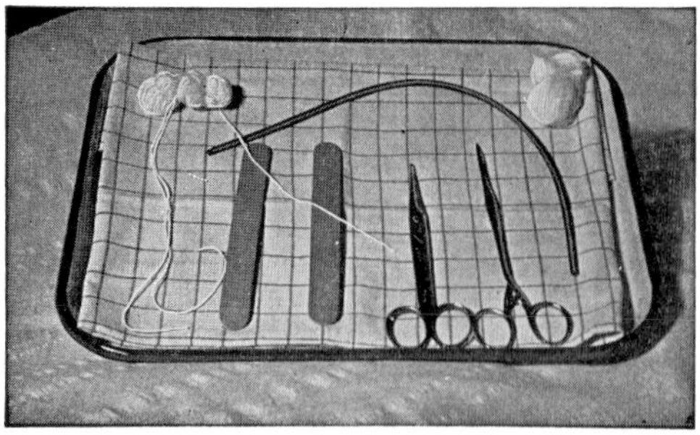

Figure 72

A nasal "hemostatic" tray. (From Parkinson, Roy H.: Eye, Ear, Nose, and Throat Manual for Nurses, St. Louis, 1959, The C. V. Mosby Co.)

and scissors (see Figure 72). A head mirror, a good light, Adrenalin (1:1000) or some other vasoconstrictor, applicators, and a nasal speculum should be available.

If the dressing under the nose becomes soiled, it may be changed as necessary. This is very important from an esthetic standpoint. Sedation and encouragement are necessary because of general discomfort and apprehension caused by having the nasal passages packed and having to breathe through the mouth. The patient can be reminded that it will soon be removed. Frequent mouth care should be given, and fluids should be given freely. Postnasal drip, the presence of old blood in the mouth, and the loss of the ability to smell lessen the patient's appetite. Because it is difficult to eat while the nose is packed, most patients prefer a liquid diet, until the packing is removed (twenty-four to forty-eight hours postoperatively), but they may have whatever food is tolerated.

After the nasal packing has been removed, the patient is asked not to blow his nose for forty-eight hours since this may start bleeding. Fever should be reported to the doctor because it may be due to infection. Since the patient has swallowed blood, the doctor may order a mild cathartic such as milk of magnesia to hasten the expulsion of old blood from the gastrointestinal tract. It is normal for the stools to be tarry for a day or two.

Following nasal surgery the patient frequently has discoloration about the eyes and should be prepared for this. To decrease local edema, he is kept in a mid-Fowler's position. Ice compresses usually are used over the nose for twenty-four hours to lessen discoloration, bleeding, and discomfort. If a bowl of ice cubes and three or four wet 4 by 4 inch gauze sponges are left within easy reach at the bedside, the patient may apply these.

Similar care is given the patient who has a plastic procedure on the nasal septum. Such a patient should know that the cosmetic result of the operation cannot be evaluated for several weeks; otherwise he may be disappointed. A protective dressing of adhesive tape or a plastic or metal mold usually is placed over the nose after a plastic procedure on the nasal septum and also after a reduction of a fractured nasal septum. If the patient has a fractured nose, however, the doctor usually removes the protective dressing daily to manually mold the broken parts. Firm healing develops about the tenth day. If a splint is used, the nurse should watch the skin about it to make sure that no pressure areas develop.

Persons who break their noses often fail to have them set, sometimes not realizing that a bone is broken. The nurse should encourage those with trauma to the nose to seek medical attention since, if not treated, a broken nose can lead to chronic sinusitis and chronic rhinitis, even though it may cause no immediate problem.

Complications of rhinitis and sinusitis

Epistaxis. Epistaxis, or nosebleed, is caused by irritation of the mucous membrane lining or by trauma to the nose. It may also be due to spontaneous rupture of small veins along the septum near the anterior nares; this frequently occurs in patients with hypertension.

Bleeding from the nose can usually be controlled at least temporarily by compressing the soft tissues of the nose between the thumb and a finger. Before pressure is applied, any clot should be removed; this may be done by gently blowing the nose. Firm pressure should be maintained for five to ten minutes, and it may be necessary for as long as half an hour. If this does not control bleeding, the help of a doctor should be sought. The anterior nares may be packed with gauze saturated in Adrenalin, 1:1000 solution, or with other hemostatic agents such as topical thrombin or Gelfoam. Ice compresses may be applied over the nose. If the bleeding still persists, the posterior nares may need to be packed in a manner similar to that used following a postoperative nasal hemorrhage. Adrenosem may be given orally or intramuscularly. The usual adult dose is 2.5 mg. (1/25 grain), and it is given every three hours until three doses have been given. To prevent recurrent hemorrhage, the patient should be warned not to blow his nose vigorously. The defective veins may later be destroyed by cauterization.

Nosebleeds may cause extreme apprehension since bleeding may be profuse, not only dripping from the nose but also running into the throat. The patient should be kept quiet and stained clothing should be removed. If he remains in an upright position with the head forward, less blood drains into the throat. A basin and tissues should be provided for expectorated blood, and the patient should be urged not to swallow blood because this may cause nausea and vomiting.

Patients who have frequent nosebleeds need a complete medical examination to determine the cause. For example, a fairly common cause is capillary fragility. Patients with this condition are encouraged to increase the vitamin C content of their diet. Fresh oranges and tomatoes are good sources of this vitamin, and usually ascorbic acid is prescribed.

Infections of the external tissues about the nose. The skin about the external nose is easily irritated during acute attacks of rhinitis or sinusitis. Furunculosis and cellulitis occasionally develop. (See Chapter 11 for detailed discussion of these conditions and of their treatment.) Infections about the nose are extremely dangerous since the venous supply from this area drains directly into the cerebral venous sinuses. Septicemia, therefore, may occur easily. If possible, infections about the nose should be avoided; however, if they do occur, medical attention should be sought. No pimple or lesion in the area should ever be squeezed or "picked"; hot packs may be used.

INFECTIONS OF THE THROAT

Acute pharyngitis

Acute pharyngitis is a mild inflammation of the pharynx. The throat appears red and feels slightly "scratchy" or painful, and the patient may have a "hacking" cough. Symptoms usually precede or occur simultaneously with the onset of acute rhinitis or acute sinusitis.

Acute pharyngitis usually is relieved by hot saline throat irrigations. If the patient is very uncomfortable, an ice collar may be applied and the doctor may prescribe acetylsalicylic acid by mouth, as a gargle, or as Aspergum; 2,000 or 3,000 ml. of fluids should be taken each day, and a liquid diet may be more easily swallowed. If temperature is elevated, the patient should remain in bed; and, even if he is ambulatory and has no fever, he should have extra rest. Occasionally sulfonamide drugs or antibiotics are prescribed prophylactically to prevent superimposed infection, particularly in those who have other disease such as rheumatic heart disease.

Acute follicular tonsillitis

Acute follicular tonsillitis is an acute inflammation of the tonsils and of their crypts. It is usually caused by streptococci or staphylococci and is more likely to occur when the patient's resistance is low. Symptoms of tonsillitis include sore throat, pain on swallowing, fever, chills, general muscle aching, and malaise. These symptoms often last for two or three days. The pharynx and the tonsils appear red, and the peritonsillar tissues are swollen; sometimes a yellowish exudate drains from crypts in the tonsils. A throat culture usually is taken to identify the offending organism.

The patient with acute tonsillitis should remain in bed and take generous amounts of fluids by mouth. Hot saline throat irrigations are usually ordered, and a sulfonamide preparation or antibiotics are usually given. Acetylsalicylic acid and sometimes codeine sulfate may be ordered for pain and discomfort. An ice collar may be applied to the neck, and, if the temperature is over 39° C. (102° F.), an alcohol sponge bath may be given. Until the temperature subsides and the sore throat improves, a liquid diet is given. This may include such foods as broths, milk drinks, bland juices, ice cream, Jell-o, custard, and Junket. After the temperature returns to normal, the patient should be kept in bed for forty-eight hours, since heart and kidney damage, chorea, and pneumonia are rather common complications of tonsillitis. Most doctors feel that patients who have recurrent attacks of tonsillitis should have a tonsillectomy. This is usually done from four to six weeks after an acute attack has subsided.

Since the patient with acute tonsillitis is usually cared for at home, the nurse should help in teaching the general public the care that is needed. The office nurse, the clinic nurse, the nurse in industry, the school nurse, and the public health nurse have many opportunities to do this.

Peritonsillar abscess

A peritonsillar abscess, or *quinsy*, may be a complication of acute follicular tonsillitis. Pain in the throat is more severe than in tonsillitis, and the patient usually is sicker. Upon examination a swelling is seen above the tonsil. The abscess sometimes ruptures spontaneously and, if this occurs, care must be taken that the patient does not aspirate the drainage; the patient's head may be lowered and suction may be used. Preferably the abscess is excised surgically. Antibiotics and hot throat irrigations are continued postoperatively, as well as other measures for the patient's comfort described under acute tonsillitis. If acute follicular tonsillitis is adequately treated, peritonsillar abscess is unlikely to occur.

Chronic enlargement of the tonsils and adenoids

Hypertrophy of the tonsils and adenoids (lymphoid structures located in the oropharynx and the nasopharynx, respectively) occurs most often in children. The child who breathes almost exclusively through his mouth should be suspected of having enlarged adenoids, since enlarged adenoids may block the nasal passages. Signs of chronic infection and enlargement of the tonsils include frequent colds and dullness of facial expression. Medical attention should be sought since chronically infected tonsils may act as foci of infection, "feeding" organisms to other parts of the body. Sometimes the child's apparent apathy and lack of attention are due to enlarged lymphoid tissue partially blocking the eustachian tubes and causing hearing impairment.

The treatment for enlarged tonsils and adenoids is surgical removal; however, most doctors do not believe that tonsils should be removed indiscriminately. Unless it is absolutely necessary, they usually prefer not to remove the tonsils until the the child is about 6 years of age. Adenoidectomies more often are done at a younger age. Some doctors prefer not to do these operations during the summer months because they believe that the operation may possibly increase susceptibility to poliomyelitis.

Tonsillectomy and adenoidectomy. About 1 million tonsillectomies are performed in the United States each year.[2] Since most of these operations are done on young children and since they often are admitted to the general hospital, the nurse needs to know something about the surgical care of a child. Hospitalization and surgery for a child who is inadequately prepared psychologically can be a very traumatic experience. The nurse who sees the parents either in the clinic or in the doctor's office and the nurse who has friends whose children are being prepared for hospitalization should be able to help the parents so that the procedure will cause as little trauma as possible.

Preparation for hospitalization should be gradual. The parents should tell the child about the hospital, why he must go there, that he will be put to sleep, and that he will wake up with a sore throat which will persist for several days. Well-written story books concerning hospitalization for tonsillectomy are available at book stores, and these may be helpful for parents. The child should know when his parents will be with him in the hospital lest he feel deserted by them. Many hospitals allow the parents to visit the child before operation, to go to the anesthesia room, to be in the room when the child returns from surgery, and to remain in his room during the first postoperative night. Other hospitals do not have adequate facilities for this. If the parents stay at the hospital, they should have a place to rest. Some hospitals have cots that can be kept under the child's bed when not in use.

The patient who is to have a tonsillectomy and adenoidectomy is often admitted to the hospital on the morning of the operation. He should have nothing to eat for six hours prior to the scheduled operation, and he must have no fever or signs of upper respiratory infection. After it has been ascertained that the patient is in good physical condition, an examination of the urine, a blood count, and tests of bleeding and clotting times are made. If any of these tests indicate an abnormality, the operation is postponed until further studies can be done. About an hour before surgery the preoperative hypodermic injection is given; it usually consists of small doses of phenobarbital sodium and scopolamine. A child is rarely given a narcotic since he tolerates this kind of analgesic poorly. The physical preparation for the adult is the same as for the child except that he is usually given a narcotic preoperatively.

Postoperatively, the patient who has had a tonsillectomy may have some dark bloody drainage from the operative area. He should, therefore, be in a position so that this drains from his mouth and is not swallowed or aspirated. If he is still unconscious, he should be propped well to the side and a waterproof protection placed under the face. If he has awakened from anesthesia or if surgery was done under local anesthesia, the patient should be placed in a "tonsil position" as follows: place a pillow under the abdomen, keep the right leg straight and the right arm at the side, acutely flex the left knee, support the forehead with a firm pillow and place an emesis basin under the mouth. (See Figure 73.) This position may be alternated from left to right, and, when the patient responds more fully, he may sit up in a mid-Fowler's position. An ice collar is applied about the throat of patients over 7 years of age to help constrict the blood vessels and thereby prevent oozing of blood and to make the patient more comfortable.

Following a tonsillectomy or an adenoidectomy, the patient should be watched carefully for signs of hemorrhage. He is urged not to cough or attempt to clear his throat since these may initiate bleeding. Efforts should be made to prevent the small child from crying lustily; if he has fully responded from anesthesia, he may be rocked. If the patient swallows frequently, hemorrhage should be suspected and the throat should be inspected since any signs of hemorrhage must be reported to the doctor at once. Vomitus containing bright red blood should be reported at once, and the specimen should be saved for the surgeon's inspection. It is especially important to watch the patient who is asleep for signs of hemorrhage, since he may swallow blood and lose a very large amount without any external evidence of bleeding. The pulse rate should be taken every fifteen minutes for the first hour and every half hour for several hours thereafter.

The nurse should have the following sterile materials ready for use in the event of hemorrhage: tongue depressors (a metal one and 2 or 3 wooden ones), a gag, suction tip, 2 tonsil hemostats, sponge forceps, scissors, 2 medicine glasses, tonsil

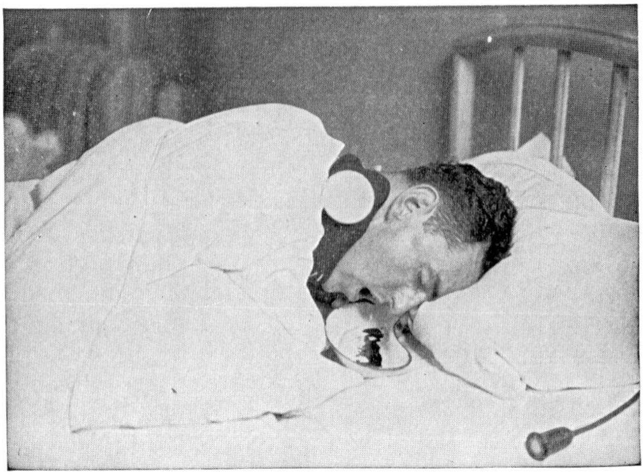

Figure 73

This patient has just returned from the operating room after having a tonsillectomy. Note the pillow under the chest and the support of the head so that there is free drainage from the mouth. (From Parkinson, Roy H.: Eye, Ear, Nose, and Throat Manual for Nurses, St. Louis, 1959, The C. V. Mosby Co.)

tampons, a small catheter, cotton balls, a needle holder, catgut and a needle, a 2 ml. syringe and hypodermic needles, 2 sterile towels, a sterile gown, and sterile gloves. This equipment should be kept ready for use on a special tray on wards which have tonsillectomy patients. A suction machine, procaine hydrochloride (1 per cent), Gelfoam, Adrenalin (1:1000), topical thrombin, sterile water, and emesis basins also should be available. The patient who is bleeding excessively often is taken to the operating room for surgical treatment to stop the hemorrhage. This may be done by ligating or by cauterizing the bleeding vessel. If sutures must be used, the patient will have more pain and discomfort than he would have following a simple tonsillectomy. He may be unable to take solid food until the sutures have been absorbed.

After a tonsillectomy, the patient is kept in bed for about twenty-four hours and is given plenty of water and bland fluids such as ginger ale, cocoa, milk, cream soups, and pear, prune, peach, or apricot juice. Ice cream, sherbet, Jell-o, custards, and Junket are also given. Ice-cold fluids are most acceptable and are frequently given; small amounts are best tolerated. The morning after surgery the patient is usually offered such foods as refined cereal and soft-cooked or poached eggs. When he goes home, he is advised to avoid citrus fruit juices, hot fluids, rough foods such as raw vegetables and crackers, and highly seasoned foods for at least a week.

If the patient is old enough to chew gum and not swallow it, he usually is given Aspergum before meals and at bedtime to relieve the pain in the throat and ears and to help keep the throat muscles supple. Pain in the ear is a common complaint postoperatively; acetylsalicylic acid by mouth may be given for this. Some doctors suggest that older children and adults gargle gently after the first postoperative day. The gargle solution is usually prepared by dissolving 0.3 Gm. (5 grains) of acetylsalicylic acid and 1/2 teaspoon of sodium bicarbonate in half a glass of water. Some of this fluid may be swallowed without harm.

Most patients are discharged from the hospital the day after surgery, but some are permitted to return home the night of the operation. If this is done, the child's parents should be instructed to watch for signs of bleeding and to report it to the doctor at once. The child is usually kept in bed for three days and indoors for one week. Adult patients may be up and about as soon as they return home but should remain indoors for three days. They may be advised by their doctor to avoid exposure to the sun, vigorous exercise, and coughing, sneezing, clearing of the throat, and vigorous blowing of the nose since these may cause bleeding. If bleeding occurs at any time, the patient should contact the doctor. Older patients may have hemorrhage between the fourth and eighth postoperative day; at this time the tough, yellow, fibrous membrane that forms over the operative site begins to break away. This accounts for the throat being more sore at this time. After this, pink granulation tissue becomes apparent, and by the end of the third postoperative week the area is covered with mucous membrane of normal appearance.

The patient or the parents of children should be given specific instructions for home care. Most hospitals and most laryngologists who do this operation in their own operative suite have these instructions written out. Acceptable foods and fluids should be outlined. The diet can be increased as tolerated but high roughage foods should be omitted for the first week. The patient should continue to drink plenty of fluids (2,000 to 3,000 ml. daily); this helps to relieve the objectionable mouth odor common after any oral surgery. If the patient fails to have a bowel movement after a day or two, a mild cathartic is usually ordered. Parents should be told that the stool may be dark or black for a day or two because blood has been swallowed at operation. A temperature of 37.5° C. to 38.5° C. (99° F. to 101° F.) may be expected for the first two or three days, and discomfort in the ears should also be expected. Persistence of temperature elevation or discomfort in the ears, however, should be reported to the doctor. The patient usually returns to the hospital clinic or to the doctor's office for a follow-up examination about one week after the operation.

The nurse may need to help some mothers plan ways to amuse the sick child. He should be allowed to play in his bed but should take a short rest in the midmorning and midafternoon. Most children like to be read to, to color, to do puzzles, and to watch selected television programs. A sick child's interest span is short, however, and one must be prepared to have various pastimes ready. Visits from other children should be restricted for the first week since they may bring upper respiratory infection to the patient.

Laryngitis

Simple acute laryngitis. Simple acute laryngitis usually accompanies a cold. It is a mild inflammation of the mucous membrane lining the larynx. It may, however, be caused by sudden changes in temperature or by irritating fumes. The patient becomes hoarse and may be unable to speak above a whisper; his throat may be sore and "scratchy," and he often has a cough. Laryngitis usually requires only symptomatic treatment. The patient should stay indoors in an even temperature and should avoid talking. Steam inhalations with aromatic vapors such as tincture of benzoin, oil of pine, and menthol may be soothing. Cough syrups or home remedies for cough such as those suggested in Chapter 23 may be tried. Smoking or being where others are smoking should be avoided.

Chronic laryngitis. Some people who use their voices excessively or who work continuously where there are irritating fumes develop a chronic laryngitis. For this, the doctor may order spraying of the throat with an astringent antiseptic solution such as hexylresorcinol (S. T. 37). To do this properly a spray tip which turns down at the end must be used so that the medication reaches the vocal cords and is not dissipated in the posterior pharynx. The patient should place the spray tip in the back of the throat with the bent portion behind the tongue. He should then take one or two deep breaths and on inhalation spray the medication. This procedure may cause temporary coughing and gagging.

INFECTIONS OF THE EAR

Catarrhal otitis media

Acute catarrhal otitis media. Acute catarrhal otitis media or acute serous otitis media is a nonpurulent inflammation of the middle ear and the eustachian tube. The patient usually complains of a sense of fullness in the ear and of decreased hearing acuity. This condition may be caused by going to high altitudes, by the exertion of excessive pressure on the middle ear such as may occur in certain industial work, or by an allergic reaction. If serum forms behind the eardrum, the preferable treatment is to incise the drum and remove the serum by suction applied to the external ear canal.

Chronic catarrhal otitis media. Occasionally a chronic nasopharyngeal infection or an allergic reaction may completely or partially obstruct the eustachian tube. This causes air in the middle ear to be absorbed and the eardrum to be drawn against the bony promontories of the middle ear. Since a low-grade infection accompanies this, the drum eventually adheres to the ossicles, interfering with their movement. This causes deafness and tinnitus (ringing in the ears).

Early and adequate treatment of nasopharyngeal infections and allergic conditions can usually prevent chronic catarrhal otitis media from developing. Any patient who complains of tinnitus or who seems to have loss of hearing should be advised to seek medical attention promptly.

Purulent otitis media

Acute purulent otitis media. Acute purulent otitis media is an acute inflammatory process in the middle ear. It most often follows the common cold or tonsillitis but may follow measles or scarlet fever. It may also be caused by contaminated water being forced into the middle ear through the eustachian tube while swimming. The offending organism is usually the streptococcus or the staphylococcus, which reaches the middle ear by way of the eustachian tube.

The patient with acute purulent otitis media complains of severe earache and inability to hear with the involved ear. He may have fever (a child's temperature may rise to 40° C. [103° F.], while the adult's may rise only slightly). Upon inspection with the otoscope, the eardrum appears red and may be bulging; if untreated, the drum will usually rupture and fluid will drain from the middle ear.

The dreaded complication of acute purulent otitis media is acute mastoid infection. To prevent this, the eardrum should be incised (myringotomy, or paracentesis) as soon as possible so that pus will not remain in the middle ear under pressure and be forced back into the mastoid cells. Antibiotics are ordered for otitis media and their use has decreased considerably the incidence of acute mastoiditis.

The nurse should urge mothers of children who complain of earache or who have fluid draining from the ears to seek medical treatment at once. Babies who are fussy, who roll their heads from side to side, or who have a persistent elevation of temperature should be taken to a doctor for examination since these may be symptoms of a middle ear infection. People should be urged to avoid swimming in uninspected pools and in stagnant water, and they should be taught to blow the nose gently, lest infected material be forced into the middle ear.

A *myringotomy* is often done in the doctor's office using nitrous oxide or a topical anesthetic. The patient or his parents should be instructed in his care. He should stay in a warm room away from drafts; if he has a fever, he should remain in bed until the temperature has been normal for forty-eight hours. He should drink large amounts of fluid and may eat anything he wishes. Acetylsalicylic acid may be prescribed to relieve pain; although when the drum is incised, pain usually disappears quickly and the patient is able to sleep soundly. Cotton should not be placed into the auditory canal because it obstructs drainage, but it can be placed loosely in the external ear; it should be replaced as soon as it becomes moist to lessen the danger of secondary infection. Plans need to be made for the patient to receive further antibiotic treatment. If an injection must be given, a public health nurse may give this in the home, or the patient may return to the hospital clinic or the doctor's office. If he goes outdoors, he should dress warmly and cover the head and ears.

If the patient has a rise in temperature, complains of headache, or becomes drowsy, irritable, or disoriented, the doctor must be notified at once. These signs may indicate that the eardrum needs to be reopened, that mastoid cells are involved, or that a brain abscess or meningitis is developing.

Chronic purulent otitis media. Chronic purulent otitis media is characterized by chronic purulent discharge from the middle ear. It is a sequela to acute otitis media and involves both the middle ear and the mastoid cells. The mastoid bone cells become thickened, and polyps may develop from the mucous membrane of the middle ear. The patient's main complaint may be deafness, occasional pain, or dizziness. If chronic purulent otitis media is permitted to progress unchecked, meningitis, brain abscess, or facial paralysis may eventually occur because the infection gradually erodes the surrounding bone.

The best treatment is prevention by early treatment of acute purulent otitis media. If the chronic condition does occur, it should be treated as soon as it is recognized. The treatment is a *radical mastoidectomy.* An incision is made either behind the ear or directly in front of it, and the mastoid cells are completely removed, converting the middle ear and the mastoid space into one cavity. If the hammer and anvil bones have not been already eroded, they and the remaining eardrum membrane are also removed. A strip of skin from the external auditory canal is laid against the bone, and it eventually becomes the new lining for the cavity. The wound is packed, and subsequent packings are done through the external ear. Healing may not be complete for three months or longer, and hearing is permanently lost in the ear.

Fortunately, a radical mastoidectomy is required much less often now than before the discovery of antibiotic drugs to treat acute infections. With continued attacks of acute infection, however, some organisms become resistant to the antibiotics.

Nursing care for the patient with a radical mastoidectomy is similar to that given the patient having a simple mastoidectomy; this is discussed under acute mastoiditis.

Acute mastoiditis

Acute mastoiditis may follow acute purulent otitis media; an abscess forms in the mastoid cells. If drainage through the middle ear becomes obstructed, the patient complains of excruciating pain over the mastoid process. This process is tender to touch and becomes swollen, pushing the external ear forward. The patient's temperature rises, and he complains of general malaise. Immediate operation may be necessary to prevent a septicemia or to save the middle ear and thus prevent permanent deafness. Through an incision behind the ear, the necrotic mastoid cells are curetted out and the middle ear is left intact (simple mastoidectomy).

Preoperative preparation for a simple mastoidectomy is similar to the routine preoperative care given any patient. If the ear aches badly, an ice bag may be used and acetylsalicylic acid may be given.

Postoperatively a tight, bulky dressing is applied which provides some hemostasis. (See Figure 74.) The dressing may be reinforced as necessary, but it is not changed by the nurse. The doctor usually changes it daily. There may be a small amount of serosanguineous drainage apparent on the dressing, but signs of bright

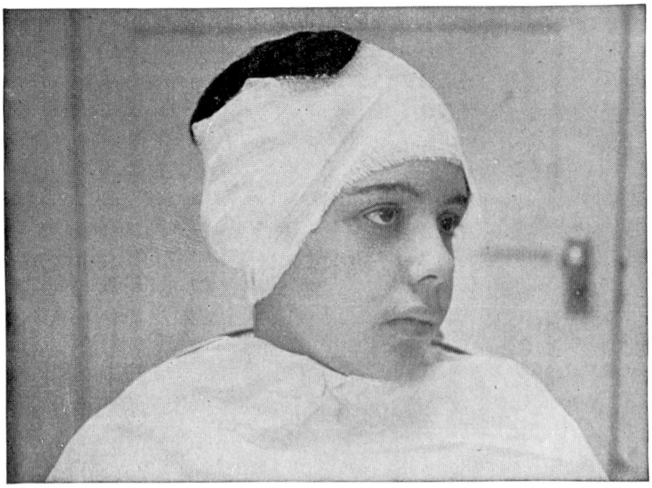

Figure 74

A mastoid dressing. (From Parkinson, Roy H.: Eye, Ear, Nose, and Throat Manual for Nurses, St. Louis, 1959, The C. V. Mosby Co.)

blood on outer dressings should be reported at once. If the tissues around the dressing become edematous, the doctor should be notified because the dressing may need to be loosened. Any signs of facial paralysis, such as inability to smile or to wrinkle the forehead, should be reported. Headache, vomiting, stiff neck, dizziness, irritability, or disorientation may forewarn of a septic thrombosis of the lateral sinus in the brain, meningitis, or brain abscess. A chronic purulent otitis media also occasionally follows this operation necessitating more radical mastoid surgery.

The patient is usually allowed out of bed within twenty-four to forty-eight hours. Fluids are forced throughout the postoperative course. The nurse should use the postoperative period to do health teaching. The patient may be prone to future hearing difficulties and should be told that help is available (see pages 498-500) if this occurs.

Labyrinthitis

Labyrinthitis is an inflammation of the inner ear. It usually is caused by infection extending from the middle ear. The patient complains of severe vertigo, nausea, vomiting and impaired hearing. If early and adequate treatment of the middle ear infection is not carried out with antibiotics and adequate drainage, meningitis may develop.

The patient who has labyrinthitis is kept in bed and given massive doses of antibiotics and at least 3,000 ml. of fluid daily. Fluids by mouth are usually retained if they are taken in small amounts and if the patient lies with his head perfectly still. If vomiting persists, fluids must be given parenterally. Since the patient is quite dizzy, side rails should be placed on the bed to prevent him from falling. (See section on nursing care of the patient with Ménière's syndrome for further nursing care.)

Furunculosis of the external auditory canal

Furuncles or boils may develop in the external ear. As is true elsewhere in the body, the cause is usually the staphylococcus. Since the skin is taut, the furuncle causes severe pain, and it may occlude the auditory canal, causing temporary deafness. Furuncles may be treated by the insertion of a cotton wick saturated with aluminum acetate solution (Burow's solution) or by incision and drainage. If the pain is not relieved, acetylsalicylic acid or codeine may be prescribed. Antibiotics may be used locally as ointments or may be given parenterally.

Fungus infections of the external auditory canal

Fungus infections of the external auditory canal are rather common. These may be treated by careful cleansing of the external auditory canal and the application of prescribed medication such as copper sulfate solution, 10 per cent; usually the ear is irrigated.

Irrigation of the ear. If the patient is to irrigate his ear at home, the nurse should teach him how to do it correctly. By sitting at a wash basin the patient may manage alone, but it may be better to have the treatment done by a responsible and informed family member. The public health nurse may give this instruction in the patient's home. The irrigation solution should be no warmer than 38° C. (100° F.); air should be expelled from the rubber bulb syringe prior to instilling solution, and the tip of the syringe should be directed either toward the roof or toward the floor of the canal but not straight inward. The canal should not be completely obstructed by the syringe since this would keep solution from flowing back and would cause pressure against the eardrum. In either irrigating the ear or instilling ear drops, the outer ear should be pulled down and out in the child to straighten the canal and it should be pulled up and back in the adult. To assure complete drainage of the irrigation fluid, the patient should lie on the affected side for several minutes; the external ear should then be dried.

Instillation of ear drops. When instilling ear drops, the dropper should not be inserted into the external auditory canal because nothing solid such as a glass medicine dropper, a hairpin, a toothpick, or a matchstick should ever be inserted into the ear lest the eardrum be accidentally perforated. Ear drops should be at room temperature; otherwise they may cause dizziness and discomfort. After the drops are inserted (usually 3 drops), the patient should remain on his nonaffected side for about five minutes so that the medication will have a chance to reach all of the affected parts. After an irrigation or after the instillation of ear drops, the external ear should be thoroughly dried to prevent skin irritation.

OTHER EAR DISORDERS

Ménière's syndrome

The cause of Ménière's syndrome is unknown. There is a dilatation of the endolymphatic channels in the cochlea due to obstruction of lymph drainage from the inner ear. Atrophy of the hearing mechanism eventually occurs. The patient is incapacitated by severe attacks of vertigo, sometimes to the extent that he is unable to cross a room without falling. He describes a sensation of dizziness, severe tinnitus (ringing in the ears), and a feeling that the room is spinning about him. During an attack, any sudden motion of the head or eyes tends to precipitate nausea and vomiting. The patient may appear withdrawn and irritable as well as acutely ill. Attacks may occur at intervals of weeks or months; they may disappear without treatment or they may continue until the patient is completely deaf in the affected ear. When the eighth nerve (acoustic) dies, symptoms cease.

Diagnosis is made from the patient's history and from the results of a caloric test made to differentiate this disease from an acoustic neurinoma. The *caloric test* consists of dripping cold water into the ear. This causes a normal patient to become dizzy, and it precipitates a severe attack in one who has Ménière's syndrome. Patients with acoustic neurinomas have no reaction to this test, although they may have other symptoms similar to those of the patient with Ménière's syndrome. Audiometry tests also are done.

The patient with Ménière's syndrome

usually is treated by an otologist unless the disease is very severe or prolonged. Then, occasionally a vestibular portion of the acoustic nerve may be divided intracranially by a neurosurgeon. In conservative treatment, vasodilating drugs such as nicotinic acid and histamine are given, and the patient may be given a low-salt diet in an attempt to improve the lymph drainage of the inner ear. Sedatives are usually necessary. Fluids may have to be given intravenously during acute and prolonged attacks.

To give the patient the support and care he needs, the nurse must first accept his behavior, which may appear somewhat negative. Even relief from surgery will not be immediate. It usually takes about two weeks for symptoms to recede. The first smile from the patient, however, is most gratifying.

Since sudden movement or jarring aggravates the vertigo, the patient usually prefers to move at his own rate and to take care of himself. If one stands directly in front of him when talking so that he does not have to turn his head or his eyes, he will experience less dizziness. Although movement increases the symptoms, the patient should be encouraged to move about in bed occasionally and to permit gentle back care to preserve good skin tone. Side rails should be on the bed at all times, and the patient should not attempt to get up and walk without assistance lest he injure himself. Because it is usually very difficult to get the patient with Ménière's syndrome to take food or fluids, efforts should be made to obtain something that he will eat or drink. Postoperatively, hearing may be lost on the operative side, but this rarely causes the patient much difficulty in adjustment.

Eczema of the external auditory canal

Eczema of the external auditory canal causes swelling. The skin itches and burns and may exude a watery discharge. The doctor may treat this condition by applying a 5 per cent solution of silver nitrate and then drying the area thoroughly and applying a 2 per cent ointment of yellow oxide of mercury.

Impacted cerumen

Impacted cerumen, or hardened wax, in the ear is a common cause of temporary deafness. This should be removed by a doctor. It is sometimes necessary to instill several drops of warm sweet oil or hydrogen peroxide into the auditory canal to soften the wax. It can then usually be removed by irrigation with a metal Pomeroy syringe. Since there is danger of perforating the ear drum, this type of ear irrigation should be done by a doctor or by a nurse specialist. If the wax still remains after irrigation, the doctor will have to remove it with a curet.

Foreign bodies in the ear

Occasionally a child inserts some object such as a pea, a bean, or a pebble into his ear; insects also sometimes get into the external auditory canal. These objects should be removed by a doctor, since there is danger of perforating the eardrum while probing for them. A few drops of warm oil inserted into the ear will allay discomfort and may float an insect out.

THE HARD-OF-HEARING PATIENT

Most hearing difficulties begin in childhood. With adequate treatment of upper respiratory infections, treatment of aching and draining ears, and care to avoid foreign objects in the ears, hearing loss often can be prevented. The nurse should be alert to every opportunity for health teaching concerning the conservation of hearing. One out of eighty people in the United States has a hearing handicap.[19]

The nurse should help to detect persons with hearing loss and to direct them to medical care since improvement in hearing often is possible. The person who seems to be inattentive or who has a strained facial expression, particularly when conversing or listening to others, may be hard of hearing. Persons with faulty articulation in speech may be deaf; their faulty articulation may result from not being able to hear themselves speak. The person who habitually fails to respond when spoken to or who makes mistakes in carrying out directions should be encouraged to have his hearing tested. The repetition of "What did you say?" or "uh huh" with a quizzical expression is often a symptom of hearing loss. Persons with marked hearing loss frequently tend to withdraw from others in an attempt to conceal their difficulty.

Unfortunately, loss of hearing has a social stigma in this country, and it may be difficult for the person with hearing loss to accept his problem. He is, however, one of the 15 million hard-of-hearing people in the United States. He should consult an ear specialist at once. The American Hearing Society, Washington, D. C., or the local office of the League for the Hard of Hearing can provide information and guidance. They have information about facilities for audiometry, clinics, and hearing rehabilitation centers in local areas.

Otosclerosis

Deafness from otosclerosis is common. The Central Bureau of Research of the American Otological Society estimates that between 10 and 12 million white persons in the United States have otosclerosis. Of this number 10 per cent have become deaf. The ossicles in the middle ear become ankylosed, resulting in a conduction deafness even though cochlear function may be normal. The cause of otosclerosis is unknown. It occurs most often in young women and is aggravated by pregnancy; the tendency to develop otosclerosis appears to be inherited.

Two kinds of surgery help some patients with otosclerosis: the *mobilization* operation and the *fenestration* operation. Since neither operation is successful in all patients and since deafness may recur later, patients are usually advised not to expect too much from an operation. Most specialists believe that operations for otosclerosis should be elective and that they should be done only after the patient has used a hearing aid and there are other clear indications for the operation.[27] Since the loss of hearing is felt so keenly, some patients find this recommendation hard to accept.

Mobilization of the stapes. Mobilization of the stapes is an operation to loosen the footplate of the stapes. It is done under local anesthesia, and the patient is often allowed to leave the hospital the day after surgery. The operation is performed through the ear canal. The ear drum is carefully dissected away from the stapes; the surgeon works through an otoscope using delicate instruments and a magnifying glass. Hearing is restored immediately upon freeing the ossicles, although dressings interfere with hearing immediately postoperatively. A dressing is placed over the ear and allowed to remain for about five days. Because vertigo occurs fairly often postoperatively, the nurse must caution the patient about the danger of accidents. Facial paresis caused by damage to the nerve by edema and occasionally damage to the labyrinth and infection also occur. Antibiotics usually are given prophylactically. If regression of hearing again occurs, the stapes may again be mobilized; regression is caused by reankylosis of the ossicles, which may cause deafness within several months. The tendency of the ossicles to again become fixed is considered a real limitation of this procedure.

Fenestration operation. In the fenestration operation a new window is made into the labyrinth in the inner ear. This allows sound vibrations to bypass the middle ear and, without bone conduction, to reach the inner ear. The operation is more extensive than a mobilization operation; some mastoid cells are removed before the new opening is made. Postoperatively, the patient may be extremely dizzy and nauseated. While these symptoms last, he is usually kept heavily sedated and flat in bed. If vertigo is severe, side rails should be used to help prevent accidents. Coughing, sneezing, and blowing the nose should be avoided. Nursing measures are similar to those described for the patient with Ménière's syndrome. The patient should lie only on the back or on the operated side so that no drainage seeps into the inner ear. He should be warned not to blow his nose since this might damage the new opening in the ear. Since the operative site is near the jaw, the patient usually has pain on chewing; this may be relieved by giving acetylsalicylic acid about half an hour before meals. Since the facial nerve may be accidentally damaged during the operation or affected by edema, the nurse should check to see that the patient can wrinkle his forehead, show his teeth, and whistle. An occasional postoperative complication is injury of the cochlea with subsequent deafness. Favorable results from this operation may not be noticeable for as long as three to six weeks postoperatively since edema may persist for that length of time.

Hearing aids

Patients who have a loss of more than 30 decibels in the range of 500 to 2,000 cycles per second in the better ear should use a hearing aid. The hearing aid is usually worn in the good ear unless the hearing loss in that ear is minimal. The patient should be directed to an otologic clinic for selection of an appropriate hearing aid. The American Speech and Hearing Association and the American Hearing Society both publish directories of acceptable aids. The American Hearing Society also publishes a monthly paper entitled *Hearing News* for those with hearing difficulty. Hearing aids are not custom made, and only minor adjustments can be made for individual patients. The type of aid used, however, depends upon the type and amount of hearing loss. If the patient is sensitive about using a hearing aid, some of the newer ones are transistor sets that are attached to eyeglasses or hairbands and are more acceptable than older models. In selecting the aid the patient is advised to consider the accessibility of service for the unit. Hearing aids cost between $75 and $225, and batteries, cords, and repairs cost approximately $30 to $75 per year.

Unfortunately, patients are often disappointed and dissatisfied with their hearing aids. They should be told that they will not hear as well as they did with normal hearing; the aid only gives them hearing in the range of 300 to 3,500 cycles per second, while the person with a normal hearing has a range of 20 to 20,000 cycles per second. The range of the hearing aid is, however, within the range of primary speech. Some patients may find that the aid only makes them aware that someone is speaking to them; they must then lip-read.

The patient should also be instructed in the care of his hearing aid. The ear mold is the only part of the apparatus that is washed. It should be washed daily in mild soap and water using a pipe cleaner to cleanse the cannula. It should be thoroughly dried before being reconnected to the receiver. The transmitter should be worn so that the microphone faces the speaker, and it should not be covered by much clothing. Men often wear it in their shirt or upper coat pocket; women may fit it into a special pocket sewed on the outside of their underclothing; children often wear it in a fabric harness placed over their undergarments. The patient who uses a hearing aid should carry an extra battery and cord at all times.

Every patient who has a hearing loss should be taught to lip-read, and while some serviceable hearing remains, he should take speech training. The American Hearing Society provides lists of available teachers throughout the United States; some local chapters offer free training courses. Textbooks for home use are also available. Most states have residential schools for the deaf child. Private schools for deaf children are also available in many localities. If the hearing loss is not acute, the child is trained to lip-read and to use a hearing aid. (See Figure 75.) He can then attend classes with children who have normal hearing.

Most persons with hearing loss can continue to be useful members of society, but it requires more than merely fitting

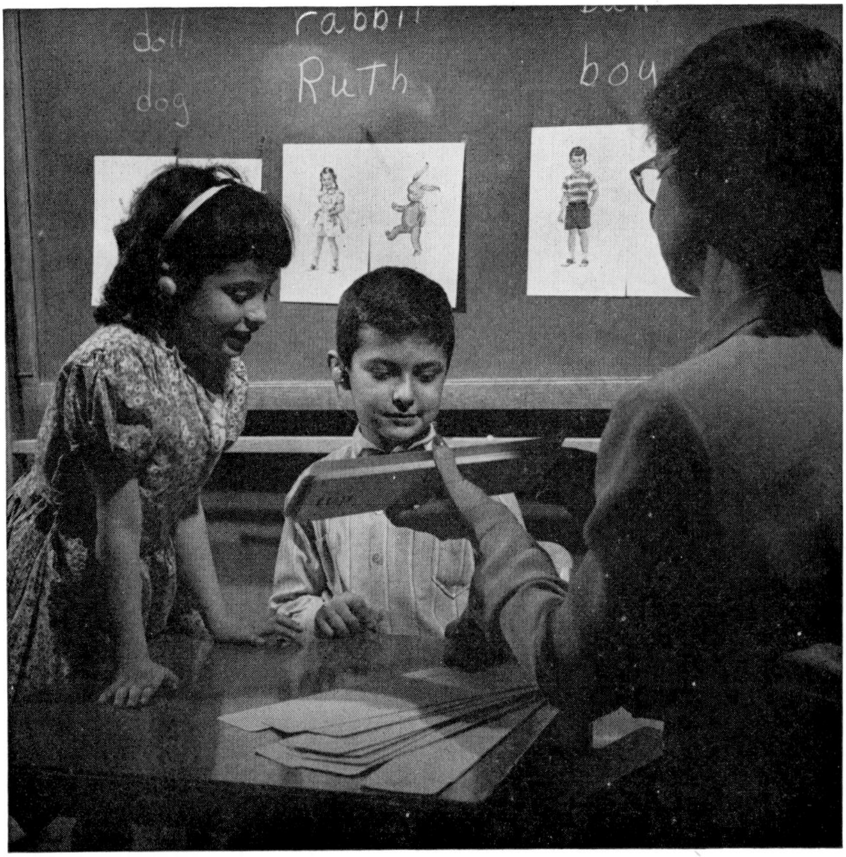

Figure 75

Children with hearing difficulties practice reading preparatory to joining classes for children with normal hearing. Note the hearing aids. (Courtesy New York League for the Hard of Hearing, New York, N. Y.)

them with hearing aids to assure this. If, however, the auditory nerve is damaged sufficiently, the patient becomes permanently deaf and hearing aids are of no help.

In working with the patient who has a hearing difficulty, the nurse should be aware of certain considerations and should teach these to others who are in contact with people who are hard of hearing. Speak in a normal voice, and tell the patient when he speaks too loudly because he cannot hear himself. This will help him to regain his normal modulation. Always talk directly to a deaf patient, making sure that the light is on your face; this helps him to lip-read. Speak clearly, but do not accentuate words. If the patient does not seem to understand what is said, express it differently; some words are difficult to "see" in lip reading. Do not smoke or cover the mouth while speaking to a person with limited hearing. If he wears a hearing aid, wait until he adjusts it before speaking. (See Figure 76.) Do not avoid conversation with a hard-of-hearing person. It has been said that to live in a silent world is much more devastating than to live in darkness, and persons with hearing loss appear, by and large, to have more emotional difficulties than those who are blind.

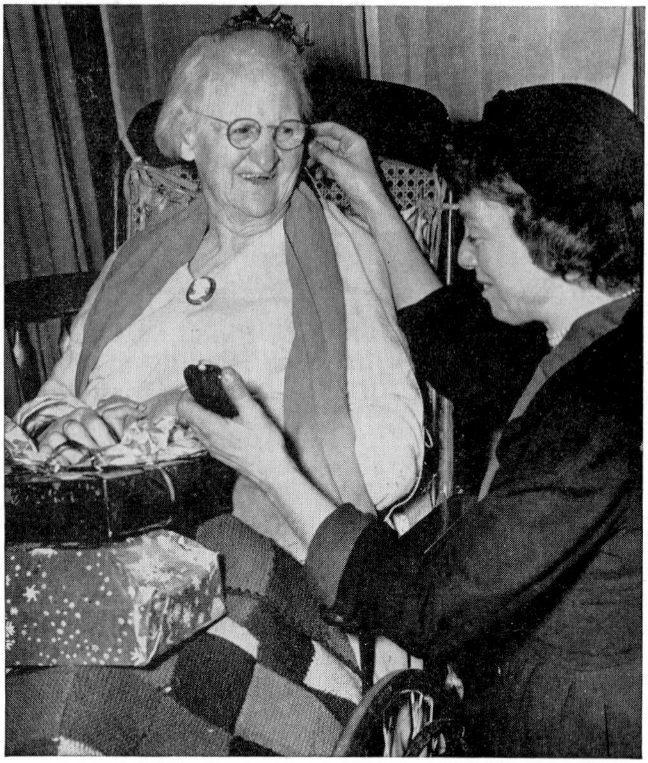

Figure 76

A nurse from New York League for the Hard of Hearing assists an elderly patient to adjust her hearing aid. (Courtesy New York League for the Hard of Hearing, New York, N. Y.)

TRACHEOTOMY AND TRACHEOSTOMY

A *tracheotomy* is an artificial opening made into the trachea to allow the patient who has obstruction above this area to breathe. It may be done as an emergency measure or it may be done prophylactically when severe edema of the larynx and throat are anticipated. If the opening is permanent (for example, following removal of the larynx), the term tracheostomy (tracheal stoma) is used. These operations may be done on patients of all ages.

If possible, it is preferable to discuss the postoperative routines with the patient before surgery so that he knows what to expect and what to do. If he knows that he will be attended constantly until he has learned to care for himself safely, he is less apprehensive. The usual hospital policy is never to leave a patient who has had a tracheostomy unattended for twenty-four to forty-eight hours postoperatively. The patient is fearful of choking, and there is real danger that this could occur. The patient should be told that he will be unable to speak and how to communicate with others by writing on a pad or a slate. Placing a bell in the unit reassures him since this makes him feel that he can attract attention as necessary. Other preoperative care is similar to that discussed in Chapter 12.

Postoperatively the patient returns to his room with a tracheotomy tube in place. This tube maintains the lumen of the fistulous opening between the skin and

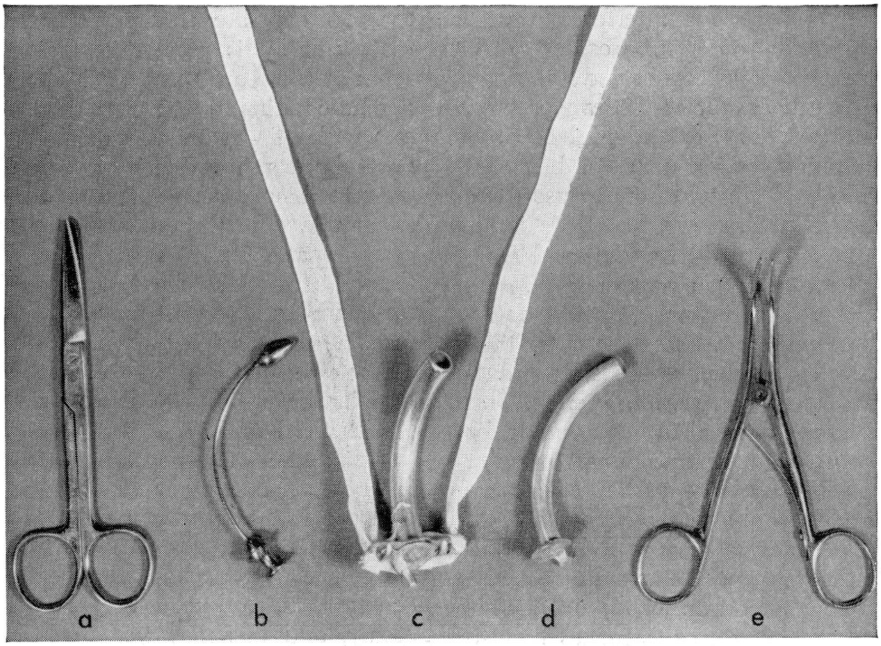

Figure 77

Material that should be kept at the bedside of a patient who has had a tracheotomy. *a,* Scissors to cut the tape if the tube becomes blocked and needs to be removed immediately. *b,* Cannula used in insertion of a tracheotomy tube. *c,* Outer portion of a tracheotomy tube with tapes for tying around the neck. *d,* Inner portion of a tracheotomy tube. *e,* Tracheotomy dilator used to keep the trachea open if the tracheotomy tube becomes blocked and must be removed.

the trachea. Since it is through this opening that the patient breathes, one of the major nursing responsibilities is to keep the tube patent and in proper position. Suction equipment is placed at the bedside, and the patient may need suction through the tube as often as every five minutes during the first few hours. The amount of mucous secretion then gradually subsides, and the patient may soon be able to go for several hours without suction being necessary. In using suction the catheter should not be inserted beyond the length of the inner cannula, and suction should be cut off as the tube is inserted. (See Chapter 13 for the correct method of using suction.) The patient is encouraged to cough; sometimes he will cough more readily if the tracheotomy tube is gently held in place since he fears that it may come out with vigorous coughing. When the patient coughs, sputum is usually expelled through the tracheotomy tube, and suction must be used immediately to help remove it. The tapes extending around the patient's neck should be securely tied with a knot to prevent the outer tube from being accidentally displaced during coughing or other exertion. If the outer tube should come out for any reason, the passageway for air is immediately obstructed. A tracheal dilator or a curved hemostat and a pair of scissors with which to cut the tape should always be conveniently placed in the patient's room, and the nurse should use the dilator to maintain an opening while she signals for assistance. (See Figure 77.)

Likelihood of serious interference with breathing if the outer tube comes out is less when the wound has healed somewhat and scar tissue has formed. However, most ambulatory patients are advised to carry a small pair of scissors and a hemostat with them and are told how to use these in an emergency.

The patient should be observed carefully for cyanosis; blueness of the lips or the nail beds, for instance, should be reported at once. Sometimes the outer tube must be changed before the air passageways can be made sufficiently clear. This is done by the doctor. An extra outer tube which is sterile and the correct size for the patient should always be kept in the room, and many hospitals require that an emergency tracheotomy set be kept available on the unit at all times.

The room should be warm, and the air should be moist since this makes breathing easier. A steam vaporizer may be placed in the room, and if more moisture is needed moist compresses made of one thickness of gauze may be placed over the tracheotomy tube.

The inner tube must be changed every three hours or oftener for the first forty-eight hours because mucus collects and partially obstructs the lumen. Unless the patient has unusual amounts of secretions, after the first forty-eight hours daily or twice daily cleansing may be sufficient. The inner tube can be changed by the nurse and should be changed as often as appears necessary (in contrast, the outer tube is changed only by the doctor). The used tube should first be placed in peroxide, 1/4 per cent, which softens the congealed secretions. Hot water is not used because it further increases coagulation of the mucus and makes it more difficult to remove; cold water, soap, pipestem cleaners, and a small tube brush are used for cleansing; silver polish helps to make the silver tube more attractive. The tube is then rinsed well and boiled for a few minutes, cooled, and reinserted. Some tracheotomy sets have two inner tubes, but in most instances only the outer tube is used while the inner one is being cared for. To expedite this procedure, a hot plate usually is placed in the patient's room so that care can be given to the inner tube without leaving the patient alone and without wasting time. Before the inner tube is reinserted, suction should be used to remove secretions that may have accumulated in the outer tube.

If a patient is to be discharged with the tube in place, he is taught to care for it and to change it himself. (See Figure 78.) He may begin to do this within a few days of the operation and is often happier being able to care for himself.

For the first few days postoperatively the patient should be watched carefully for hemorrhage either through the tube or around it. This may sometimes appear as persistent oozing or may occur suddenly when the dressing or the tube is being changed. A dressing surrounds the tracheotomy, and this may be changed when necessary. Whenever it becomes soiled, skin irritation may occur, and a soiled dressing may be esthetically disturbing to the patient and to his family. A single layer of gauze may be placed as a "curtain" over the opening to prevent powder, crumbs, or other substances from being aspirated through it.

Mouth care is especially important. The patient often has marked halitosis following this operation and may be sensitive about this. He should be encouraged to drink large amounts of water because this will contribute to good mouth hygiene and will help to thin mucous secretions. The patient who has had a simple tracheotomy may have fluids a few hours after the operation. He needs encouragement in his first efforts to swallow since he is fearful that food and fluids will "go the wrong way." This is not a serious danger, although the patient may cough when he first attempts to drink fluids. When a patient has had a recent tracheotomy the suction machine must be available and ready for immediate use at all times. Fluids are usually given parenterally during the first twenty-four hours. By the second postoperative day, the patient can drink readily and can eat most foods.

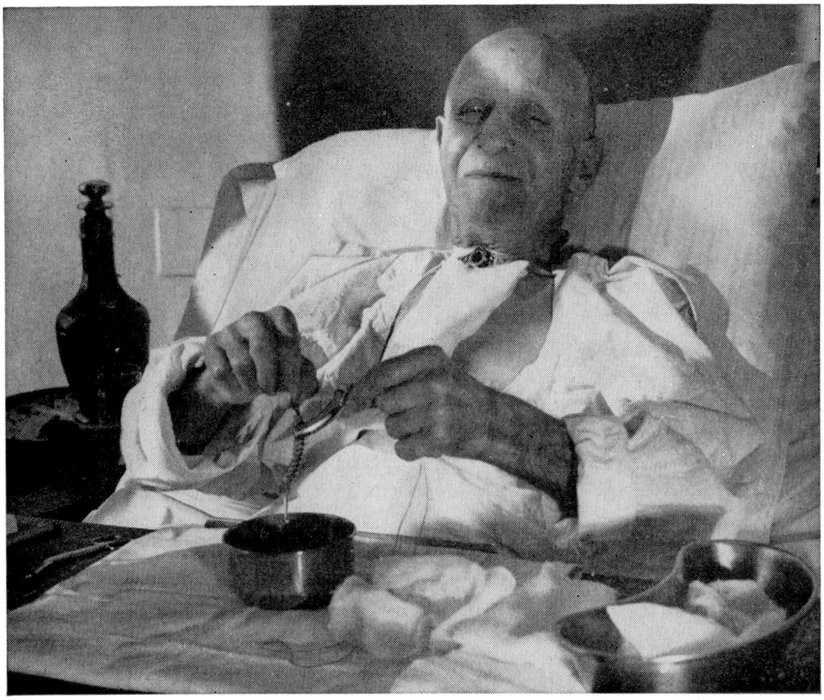

Figure 78

This 82-year-old man cares for his own tracheotomy tube. He is about to clean the inner tube with a small tube brush. (From Newton, Kathleen: Geriatric Nursing, St. Louis, 1960, The C. V. Mosby Co.)

However, foods which might be somewhat difficult to swallow, such as mashed potatoes, are usually avoided for a few days. The patient who has a permanent tracheostomy following removal of the larynx is not permitted to take anything by mouth for about a week since in this operation there are tracheal sutures that might become contaminated by food.

The tube is first partially closed with a rubber cork, and if the patient can breathe adequately, the tube may then be completely corked for a day before it is removed and the fistula allowed to heal and close. This is done only for the patient with a temporary tracheotomy because only in this case are the respiratory passages above and around the tube intact.

The patient usually is advised to avoid talking until the tracheotomy opening is occluded for increasing periods prior to removing the tube completely. With the doctor's permission, however, patients who must have the tube left open for extended periods can be taught to cover it momentarily with a finger while they speak.

Patients who go home with the tracheotomy tube still in place must be provided with necessary supplies or with instructions as to where to secure them and with knowledge of how to care for themselves. They should have suction equipment. Suction machines can be rented for home use or obtained in many communities through the local chapter of the American Cancer Society, Inc. Suction can be provided by attaching a suction hose to a water faucet; many hardware stores carry the necessary equipment for this. The amount of suction is controlled by the stream of water.

CANCER OF THE LARYNX

If treated early, cancer of the larynx is one of the most curable of all malignancies. It comprises between 3 and 5 per cent of all malignancies, and there are approximately 3,360 new cases occurring in the United States each year.[13] The early symptom, hoarseness, is easily recognized. If treatment is given when this first sign (due to the tumor preventing complete approximation of the vocal cords) appears, complete removal of cancer may be possible since metastasis occurs slowly. Late symptoms include pain in the Adam's apple which radiates to the ear, dyspnea, dysphagia, enlarged cervical lymph nodes, and cough. If ulceration develops, there may be expectoration of purulent bloodstained sputum, and frank hemorrhage may occur. Occasionally severe hemorrhage causes death.

Cancer of the larynx is ten times more common in men than in women, and it occurs most often in those past 60 years of age. There seems to be some relationship between cancer of the larynx and heavy smoking, chronic laryngitis, vocal abuse, and family predisposition to cancer. Any person who becomes progressively hoarse should be urged to seek medical attention at once. The diagnosis of cancer of the larynx is made from the history, from visual examination of the larynx with a laryngoscope, and from biopsy and microscopic study of the lesion.

Laryngofissure. If the lesion is limited to the middle or anterior portions of the vocal cord, a laryngofissure or a thyrotomy may be done. The thyroid cartilage is split, and the vocal cord and the tumor are removed. As healing takes place, the band of scar tissue becomes a vibrating surface within the larynx; this permits husky but acceptable speech. A tracheotomy tube is inserted at the time of operation but is removed when edema in the surrounding tissue subsides. For forty-eight hours postoperatively, food is usually supplied intravenously or by a stomach tube passed through the nose. The patient may then take fluids by mouth. Other care is similar to that given the patient having a simple tracheotomy. The patient who has had a laryngofissure is not permitted to use his voice until the doctor gives specific approval (usually three days postoperatively). He should then only whisper until healing is complete, after which time he adjusts quite readily to his relatively minor limitation of speech.

Complete laryngectomy. When cancer of the larynx is advanced, it is necessary to remove the larynx completely. This includes removing the thyroid cartilage, the vocal cords, and the epiglottis. The patient must have a permanent tracheostomy because the trachea no longer connects with the posterior nasopharynx. The upper portion of the trachea above the area excised is closed with sutures. Sometimes in an attempt to remove the tumor completely, a radical neck dissection is also done. (See Chapter 25 for further discussion of this.)

The patient who is to have a laryngectomy is told by the doctor that he no longer will have normal speech. He is often depressed by this news which threatens his economic, social, and emotional status, as well as his life. It helps for the patient to be visited by another patient who has made a good recovery from laryngectomy and who has undergone rehabilitation successfully. No one else can give the patient the reassurance that he can regain speech as well as a fellow patient. If no such patient is available, films* which deal with adjustment to a laryngectomy can be obtained. Local speech rehabilitation resources may be available; the local chapter of the American Cancer Society, Inc., and the local health department should be able to supply this information. Many large cities have "Lost Chord Clubs," and members are willing to visit hospitalized patients. If possible, the family, too, should learn about the method of esophageal speech that the patient will learn to use.

*Available on loan from the Cleveland Hearing and Speech Center and the American Cancer Society, Inc.

The patient and his family should know that the patient will return from surgery with a tracheostomy. They should be assured that someone will stay with the patient continuously for twenty-four to forty-eight hours. After this time he should begin to help with his own care in anticipation of leaving the hospital. Oxygen may be used for twenty-four hours since this makes breathing easier. The use of a call bell should be explained to the patient preoperatively even though he will be constantly attended, and he should be instructed to communicate by using a pencil and paper or a slate. Other preparation is similar to that for any patient about to have major surgery. Special mouth care may be given for several days preoperatively in an attempt to reduce the number of bacteria in the mouth. Sodium perborate is often ordered for this, and antibiotics may be given both preoperatively and postoperatively.

Postoperatively the patient is usually placed in a mid-Fowler's position with the head slightly flexed to prevent tension on the sutures. A stomach tube is inserted through the nose into the stomach (sometimes this is done while the patient is under anesthesia) and, when the patient has awakened from anesthesia, fluids are given through it. This tube may be left in for six or seven days; its use prevents contamination of the laryngeal suture line. Potassium iodide and ammonium chloride may be given through the tube to help liquefy secretions from the lungs and to prevent plugging of the tracheostomy opening. Alevaire is frequently given by aerosol inhalation directly into the tracheostomy opening. If intravenous fluids are to be given, care must be taken that the hand used to write is left free.

Care of the patient who has had a tracheostomy is similar to that necessary for the patient with a temporary tracheotomy. The tube is removed completely in about three to six weeks when the opening has healed and become a permanent fistula.

The patient who has a tracheostomy must take some special precautions. He must not go swimming and must be careful while bathing or taking a shower that water is not aspirated through the opening into the lungs. He is advised to wear a scarf or a shirt with a closed collar that covers the opening yet is of porous material. This helps to carry on some of the functions normally assumed by the nasal passages, such as the warming of air and the screening of dust and other irritating substances.

Speech rehabilitation may be started as soon as the tracheostomy tube has been removed. Most patients learn esophageal speech faster if they go to a special speech clinic. Speech centers such as the National Hospital for Speech Disorders in New York City and the Cleveland Hearing and Speech Center are located in various communities. The patient may need to go to a near-by city for this instruction, but usually he must remain away from home for only one or two weeks. If his emotional outlook is good, his ability to learn esophageal speech is remarkable. Patients have mastered esophageal speech in from two to six lessons.

To learn esophageal speech, the patient must first practice burping. This provides the moving column of air needed for sound, while folds of tissue at the opening of the esophagus act as the vibrating surface. The patient must learn to coordinate his articulation with the esophageal vocalization made possible by aspirating air into the esophagus. His new voice sounds are natural although somewhat hoarse; the qualities of speech provided by the use of the nasopharynx are still present, however. The patient may have digestive difficulty during the time he is learning to speak. This is due to the swallowing of air as he practices, to the unusual strain on abdominal muscles, and to nervous tension. Since he may not be hospitalized at this time and usually is away from home, he should be told that this may happen and that it should not be a cause for alarm. It abates with proficiency in speaking.

The Cleveland Hearing and Speech Center reports that about 82 per cent of those attending their clinic have returned to their original occupations and have good speech. The average patient can return to work one or two months after leaving the hospital.

Some patients have heard of the electrolarynx and the reed-type of artificial larynx. The use of these is discouraged by experts unless the patient for some reason is unable to learn esophageal speech. They are cumbersome, unsightly, and expensive, and they produce an unnatural and unpleasant voice.

REFERENCES AND SELECTED READINGS*

1 Altman, Franz: More About Mobilization, Quart. Bull. New York League for Hard of Hearing **35**:7-8, June 1957.

2 Beal, John M. (editor): Manual of Recovery Room Care, New York, 1956, The Macmillan Co.

3 *Bellam, Gwendoline: Tonsillectomy Without Fear, Am. J. Nursing **51**:244-245, April 1951.

4 Bois, Lawrence R.: Fundamentals of Otolaryngology, ed. 2, Philadelphia, 1954, W. B. Saunders Co.

5 *Conley, John J.: Tracheotomy Am. J. Nursing **52**:1078-1081, Sept. 1952.

6 Davidson, Louise E.: A Hearing Conservation Program, Am. J. Nursing **55**:582-583, May 1955.

7 Fuerst, Elinor V., and Wolff, LuVerne: Fundamentals of Nursing, ed. 2, Philadelphia, 1959, J. B. Lippincott Co.

8 *Gardner, Warren H.: Rehabilitation After Laryngectomy, Pub. Health Nursing **43**:612-615, Nov. 1951.

9 Good Hearing Must Be Protected, Washington, D. C., American Hearing Society.

10 *Greene, James S.: Speech Rehabilitation Following Laryngectomy, Am. J. Nursing **49**:153-154, March 1949.

11 *Hall, James, T., and Sadler, Julia Bland: Nursing Care in Tonsillectomy and Adenoidectomy Am. J. Nursing **47**:537-539, Aug. 1947.

12 Harmer, Bertha, and Henderson, Virginia (revised by): Textbook of the Principles and Practice of Nursing, ed. 5, New York, 1955, The Macmillan Co.

13 *Holinger, Paul H., Johnson, Kenneth C., and Mansueto, Mario D.: Cancer of the Larynx, Am. J. Nursing **57**:738-741, June 1957.

14 House, Howard P., Sheehy, James L., and Dorner, Helen: Stapes Mobilization and Teaching Patients About Stapes Mobilization, Am. J. Nursing **60**:816-820, June 1960.

15 *Markle, Donald M.: Hearing Aids, Am. J. Nursing **57**:592-593, May 1957.

16 *Martin, Hayes, and Ehrlich, Harry E.: Nursing Care Following Laryngectomy, Am. J. Nursing **49**:149-152, March 1949.

17 Mastoidectomy in the Antibiotic Area, What's New **191**:1-3, Early Winter, 1955.

18 Moore, Paul M.: General Tonsillectomy, Ann. Otol. Rhin & Laryng. **54**:494-506, June 1955.

19 *Nichols, Ruth E.: The Newly Deafened Patient, Am. J. Nursing **46**:223-224, April 1946.

20 *Osmun, Paul M.: Nosebleeds, Am. J. Nursing **56**:1411-1413, Nov. 1956.

21 *Otosclerotic Deafness by Mobilization of Stapes, What's New **191**:7-8, Early Winter, 1955.

22 Parkinson, Roy H.: Eye, Ear, Nose and Throat Manual for Nurses, ed. 7, St. Louis, 1953, The C. V. Mosby Co.

23 Putney, F. Johnson: Complications and Postoperative Care After Tracheotomy, Arch Otolaryng. **62**:272-276, Sept. 1955.

24 *Ray, Bronson S.: Ménière's Disease, Am. J. Surg. **75**:159-170, Jan. 1948.

25 Rosen, Samuel: Results of Mobilization of Fixed Stapedial Foot Plate in Otosclerosis Deafness, J.A.M.A. **161**:595-599, June 16, 1955.

26 *Rosenberger, Harry C., and Bukovina, Eleanore: Fenestration, Am. J. Nursing **47**:730-731, Nov. 1947.

27 Shambaugh, George E., Jr.: Surgery of the Ear, Philadelphia, 1959, W. B. Saunders Co.

28 Shepard, Mary Estelle: Nursing Care of Patients with Eye, Ear, Nose, and Throat Disorders, New York, 1958, The Macmillan Co.

*References preceded by an asterisk indicate material particularly well suited for student reading.

The patient with disease of the teeth and mouth

Chapter 25

Study questions for review

1 Review the anatomy of the teeth, jaws, and mouth. How are the teeth formed? To what is the tongue attached?
2 What main purpose is achieved by chewing food? What enzyme is present in saliva and what is its function?
3 Review the location and function of the thoracic duct.
4 From your notes on fundamentals of nursing review the measures that can be used to control unpleasant odors in the mouth.

This chapter will consider prevention of and nursing care in diseases of the teeth, infections, tumors, and trauma involving the mouth and closely related structures. In all of these conditions prevention is much more important than treatment and attempted cure after disease has become well established.

The mouth has special emotional significance for every individual. This may be because it is associated in infancy with food, and this in turn with sucking, warmth, love, and security. It continues to be associated throughout life with survival through the intake of food and with pleasurable sensations related to love and companionship, acceptance, and belonging. Therefore, severe emotional reactions frequently occur when treatment involving the mouth is necessary. The patient may refuse to visit his dentist, may go into complete panic when the jaws must be wired and normal eating is impossible, and may refuse to accept the fact that a lesion in the mouth is any threat to his health. An understanding of what may be some of the patient's unspoken and often unrealized fears will enable the nurse to give him better care. Patience in explaining tests and treatments often helps. Sometimes merely taking time to explain to the patient how he may be fed immediately following a mouth operation may make the difference between his acceptance or rejection of the procedure. Sometimes the patient needs time to accept the need for referral to a doctor or dentist and to accept the suggested treatment.

DISEASES OF TEETH AND CLOSELY RELATED STRUCTURES

General prevention

Dental disease is probably the most common, yet the most neglected, chronic ailment of modern man. Teaching the prevention of disease of the teeth and related structures is an important health education responsibility of nurses. Responsibilities vary depending on the needs of patients or groups of patients. They include providing public information about over-all preventive health measures such as the fluoride treatment of water, proper daily care of teeth and gums to preserve their health, care related to satisfactory use of artificial dentures, diet, general mouth health including regular visits to the dentist, and alertness to the possible significance of lesions anywhere in the mouth. It is estimated that less than 40 per cent of the population of the United States visit the dentist as often as once each year and that only about 25 per cent receive adequate dental attention.[15]

No organized teaching plan is necessary and no unit of time need be specifically set aside for dental health education. The nurse must have at her command certain facts to use throughout her day's work. Almost every patient needs to learn about care of the teeth and mouth whether he is admitted to the hospital with an acute illness or confined to his home because of a heart condition, an infection of his foot, or any other cause.

Nurses will probably be asked about some common misconceptions, and they should know the answers.[8] For example, there is no evidence that any general systemic disease is caused by decayed teeth. There is no evidence that calcium is removed from the mother's teeth during pregnancy and lactation regardless of how deficient in calcium her diet may be. There is, however, abundant evidence that a diet adequate in calcium, phosphorus, and other esssential elements during pregnancy contributes to good tooth formation in the growing fetus and that a diet rich in these substances is essential during the years of life when the permanent teeth are being formed. Calcium is deposited in the buds of the permanent teeth almost immediately after birth. A high-calcium diet after teeth have erupted probably has no effect whatever on their preservation, but local action of other foods such as carbohydrates is of tremendous importance.[9]

Dental caries. Dental caries, or cavities in the teeth, are almost universal in our society. The President's Commission, reporting in 1951, stated that 70 per cent of all children in the United States at the age of 12 years have cavities and that 85 per cent are affected by the time they reach 15 years of age. Other reports estimate that as many as 96 per cent of all children reaching school age have dental caries. Before the physical standards for the Armed Services were lowered during World War II, it was found that 8.8 per cent of all men examined failed to pass their dental examinations mainly because of dental caries and loss of teeth.

If some simple known facts were applied by all of us in daily living, the incidence of dental caries would be reduced greatly. Most important is the addition of fluoride to drinking water in the proportion of one part of fluoride to a million parts of water. This has been conclusively shown to increase the resistance of tooth enamel to bacterial action during the formative period of young children's teeth and by this means to reduce dental caries by about 60 per cent.[4] In this dilution, or even in double this concentration, repeated studies have conclusively proved that there are no harmful systemic effects.[1] It has been suggested that it may even have beneficial effects. Mottling of the teeth does occur in parts of the country where the natural water supply contains two or more parts of fluoride per million parts of water, but repeated studies have not demonstrated ill effects. It is distressing for those in the health professions to witness the long delays in protecting the teeth of the people of our nation caused by an uninformed public. At the present time, though the facts about fluoridation of water have been known for several years, many well-meaning but poorly informed citizens and citizen groups are strongly resisting efforts by health departments throughout the country to make it available to all.

Although less effective and much more expensive than fluoridation of water, local application of fluoride to the teeth of children has been found helpful. Topical application of fluoride cannot prevent cavities from progressing, but it can reduce the development of new cavities by about 40 per cent. It is recommended that all children be given this preventive treatment until such time as they are all protected from birth by fluoridation of water supplies.[9] The treatment is simple. Fluoride is painted onto the cleaned and dry teeth at weekly intervals for four treatments. This is usually recommended when the child is 3 years of age and again at the age of 7 to protect both the deciduous and the permanent teeth. It is usually repeated at 10 and 13 years of age, respectively, to protect teeth that appear after 7 years of age.

Recently it has been found that *stannous fluoride* added to a dentifrice and used regularly can reduce substantially the incidence of dental caries. It is not believed however that use of this substance can or should take the place of fluoridation of water.[18]

The elimination or drastic curtailment of refined carbohydrate foods would reduce the prevalence of dental caries. It is known with certainty that refined carbohydrates contribute to tooth decay. The refined fermentable carbohydrates such as starch, sucrose, and glucose produce an environment in which bacterial action can lead to destruction of tooth enamel. Caries may be reduced by removing the offending foods. During World War II tooth decay dropped sharply in countries where the diet was substandard and where the consumption of refined carbohydrates was severely restricted. Although the average American diet has decreased in total carbohydrate content in the last fifty years, this is largely due to a lower consumption of flour in bread. Sugar consumption has risen markedly. In 1823 the average American consumed eight pounds of sugar per year, whereas now he uses over one hundred pounds per year. The consumption of lollipops, ice cream cones, hard candies, and soft drinks which are so much a part of American culture should be curtailed and preferably eliminated. The custom of concluding a meal with a sweet dessert and/or candies contributes to tooth decay. The European custom of ending the meal with fresh fruit is an excellent one, since fresh fruit sugars and unrefined starches contain properties which inhibit bacterial enzyme action in the mouth. In fact, eating a raw apple before retiring is an excellent way to clean one's teeth.

Brushing the teeth or even rinsing the mouth with plain water immediately after ingestion of refined carbohydrate foods helps prevent decay. The times when most people brush their teeth are entirely wrong from the standpoint of prevention of dental caries. It is during the first half hour after eating refined carbohydrate that the most harm is done; immediate rinsing of the mouth with plain water is more helpful than is thorough brushing of the teeth hours afterward when the bacterial damage has been done.

Periodontal disease

Periodontal disease is the correct name for a condition which, in its advanced stages, is termed pyorrhea by the laity. It is receiving much more attention than formerly because of the recognition of the whole field of dental health as a major public health problem. The United States Public Health Service is cooperating in studies, and most states now have preventive dental health programs which include attention to other dental disease besides caries.

Periodontal disease affects the gums and bony structures surrounding the teeth and is most common after 35 years of age. After the age of 40, more people lose their teeth from this cause than from dental caries. Many factors contribute to the development of periodontal disease, among them malocclusion, accumulation of tartar, poor nutrition, poor mouth hygiene, and improper brushing of the teeth. *Malocclusion* may result in a poor bite with unequal pressure on teeth. This leads to deterioration of bony supportive structures. Removal of teeth without proper replacements permits the teeth to drift backward and alters the bite, again producing unequal pressure on working surfaces of the teeth. The pressure and irritation of tartar, a hard, irritating substance which accumulates along gum margins of the teeth, destroys the tiny tendrils holding the tooth in the socket and leads to unhealthy receding gums with lessened tooth support. (See Figure 79.) Poor nutrition, improper brushing of the teeth, and local infection further

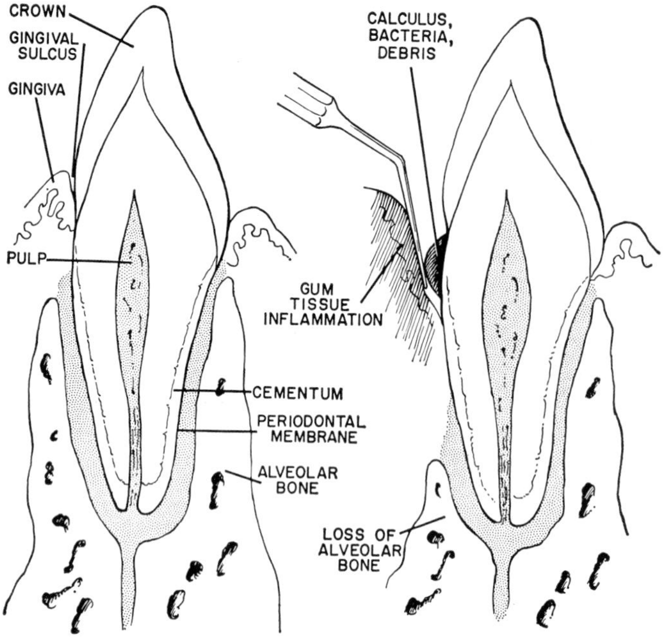

Figure 79

The diagram on the left shows a normal tooth with gum and root structures. The diagram on the right shows the presence of foreign materials between the gum margin which may lead to periodontal disease.

the destruction of gums and supportive gum structures to such a degree that they recede. The leverage of daily use then becomes too great upon the teeth, and they loosen and finally have to be removed.

The nurse must be on the alert for opportunities to direct patients so that periodontal disease may be treated early and the unfortunate results of neglect may be prevented. Many people do not know that malocclusion and space between teeth are of any significance beyond cosmetic effect and lessened efficiency in chewing. The patient may ask the nurse about what seems to him an expensive and possibly unnecessary yet recommended dental procedure. It has been found that people in their forties and beyond can benefit from improvement in equalizing their bite, eliminating space between teeth, better practice in brushing teeth, care of their gums, and regular dental inspection with prophylactic care.

General care of the teeth

The nurse is frequently asked about the kind of toothbrush to use and about general care of the teeth. There is general agreement among dental authorities that toothbrushes should be small enough to reach all tooth surfaces; usually two or three rows of bristles are recommended, depending on how much space exists between the cheek and the outer tooth surface. Bristles should be straight across the brushing surface, since tufts of bristles may traumatize the gums. Bristles should be firm but not hard; usually natural bristles are preferred to nylon. Every person should have two toothbrushes and should use them alternately, permitting each brush to dry thoroughly between uses. This helps to prevent bacterial growth and keeps the brush firmer.

Many people brush their teeth by passing the bristles quickly across the lateral surfaces of the teeth. This wears the enamel, does not clean between the teeth, and may injure the gums. The brush should be placed along the gum line with bristles toward the roots of the teeth; then with a gentle sweep, the bristles should be brought down over the gum and teeth, always using a downward or upward motion. Crosswise motion should be reserved for the top grinding surfaces of the back teeth. Brushing the teeth should remove debris from between the teeth, stimulate the gums, and yet not traumatize the delicate gingival papillae between the teeth. (See Figure 80.) Some dentists recommend a slight vibrating motion over the gums for further stimulation before each downward or upward sweep of the brush, while others recommend massage of the gums following brushing. Massage is accomplished by gentle rubbing of the gums with a finger, using very gentle pressure toward the biting surfaces of the teeth. This can be done for a few minutes two or three times a day and should include all gum surfaces. The important points to emphasize are a proper brush, correct method of brushing, and correct time of brushing (after eating).

Dentifrices and mouthwashes are not really necessary; they simply make brush-

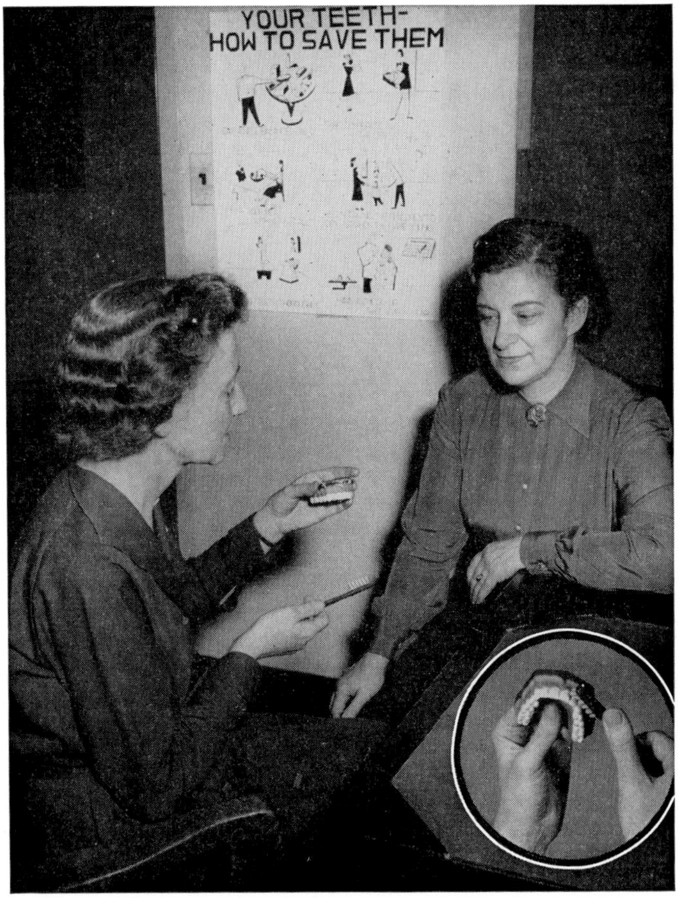

Figure 80

The correct method of brushing the teeth is reviewed with a patient. Equipment for demonstration is useful in teaching.

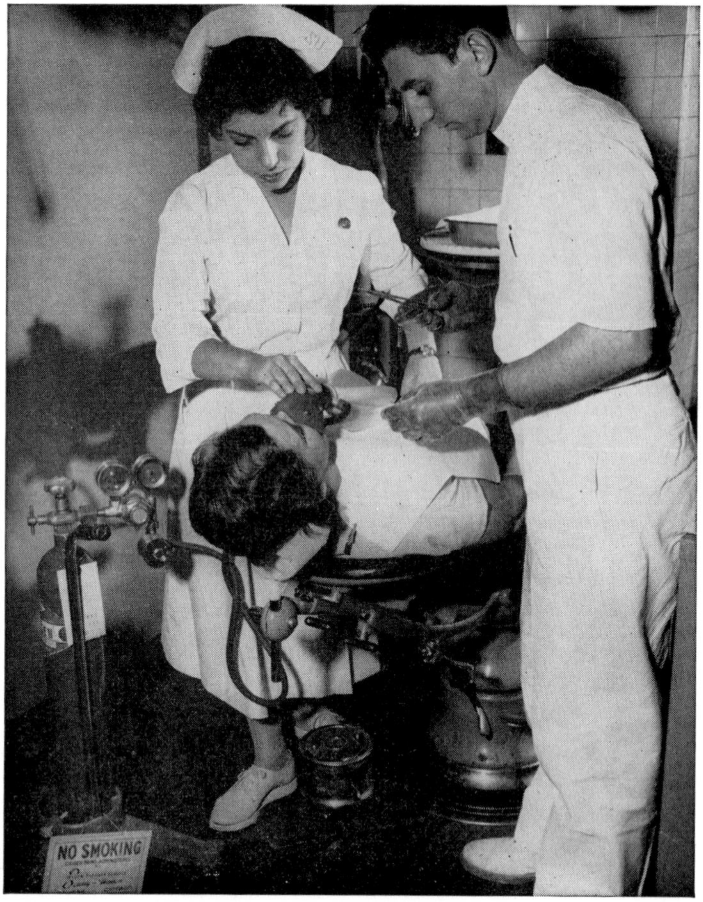

Figure 81

Emergencies that require expert nursing occur during dental treatments.

ing the teeth more pleasant. Most dentists recommend any accepted dentifrice that is preferred by the patient and suggest that salt and sodium bicarbonate are much cheaper than commercial dentifrices and equally good. It is estimated that the American public pays approximately 80 million dollars each year for mouthwashes and cleansing agents for their teeth, when sodium bicarbonate and salt flavored with peppermint would cost only a fraction of that amount. Ammoniated dentifrices and those containing penicillin and chlorophyll are subject to much inquiry at present, but so far their benefits have not been proved. Recently it has been found that a dentifrice containing stannous fluoride helps to prevent caries and its value has been officially recognized by the American Dental Association.[18]

Mouthwashes do not significantly inhibit bacterial growth in the mouth. They should not be used by the patient in an effort to treat his own mouth infection because they may be irritating to infected mouths and, if used excessively, may be harmful to natural flora in the mouth. For the most part, however, they are harmless and are acceptable additions to mouth hygiene if desired by the patient and if he can afford them. Most dentists suggest warm water and salt to rinse the mouth if occasional bleeding of the gums occurs. Sodium perborate may be irritating to gum tissues and should not be used without specific medical or dental instruction. Dental floss should not be used regularly unless it has been recommended by the dentist and instruction as to its correct use has been given. It must be gently forced between the teeth with pressure exerted toward the side of the tooth so that it will not traumatize the gingival papillae.

Nutrition is so important for patients with periodontal disease that some periodontists have their patients keep weekly food-intake charts to determine what essentials of diet may be lacking. The essentials of good nutrition should be employed. Intake should be carefully evaluated for inclusion of fresh citrus fruits and fresh vegetables, and protein food consumption should be noted since it is so important in gum healing and in gum health. The nurse may note signs of nutritional deficiency in the mouths of those who have inadequate food intake since they often have bright, spongy, gum margins that bleed easily.

Artificial dentures

Artificial dentures or dental prostheses are resisted by most people. Serious emotional reactions are manifested when the patient must give up all of his own teeth, no matter how unsatisfactory they may be. In her conversation with the patient, the nurse should stress the fact that dental prostheses need not be conspicuous, that a proper fit can be obtained in almost all instances, and that there is often cosmetic improvement. The patient must be urged to have patience in learning to use the new teeth; many elderly people become discouraged easily and are inclined to lay artificial teeth aside and then, because they are embarrassed by their appearance, avoid people.

Artificial dentures should be cleaned at least twice daily and preferably after each meal. Salt and sodium bicarbonate, a mild tasteless soap such as Ivory, or any good dentifrice can be used. Odor should not be a problem since plastic materials have largely replaced vulcanite materials which sometimes retained odors. A few drops of ammonium hydroxide or a drop of chloride household bleach, which is a good deodorant, added to the water used to wash the dentures may make the teeth feel and taste fresher. When artificial teeth are removed for cleansing, the patient should massage his gums thoroughly for a few minutes; teeth that fit snugly naturally interfere with circulation to some extent. Patients are encouraged to wear their teeth both during waking and sleeping hours since facial contours may be better preserved by this means. Dentures that fit properly should not cause discomfort as soon as the general slight discomfort associated with their newness is overcome. The patient should be advised to report any persistent pressure or irritation to his dentist, since adjustment can usually be made. Any lesion in the mouth associated with the use of dental prostheses should be reported at once since it may possibly be an early malignancy.

Very occasionally there has been so much recession and atrophy of bony structures that it is extremely difficult to fit prostheses properly. Recently a magnetic device has been perfected which can be imbedded in the palate and which, by attraction of the special dental plate, helps to hold the denture in good position.

DISEASES OF THE MOUTH AND CLOSELY RELATED STRUCTURES

The mouth, like the eyes and the skin, is an excellent barometer of general health, reflecting general disease and debility as well as good health. In any inspection of the mouth, the nurse should note the color of the mucous membrane and of the gum margins, the presence of broken or jagged teeth, deposits on the teeth, and the presence of any thickened, irregular areas. Pernicious anemia, leukemia, and vitamin deficiencies affect the mouth, and some communicable diseases, including measles and syphilis, produce lesions on the buccal mucosa. Specific disease of the mouth most often occurs when general nutrition and mouth hygiene are poor, when people neglect their teeth, when smoking is excessive, and when broken teeth irritate the tissues.

Infections of the mouth

Stomatitis. Catarrhal stomatitis is any mild inflammation of nonspecific origin affecting the mouth. It occurs most often in debilitated persons, and the treatment consists of improving the patient's general resistance and using mild alkaline mouthwashes. *Aphthous stomatitis* is the correct name for what are usually called canker sores. These small painful ulcers may appear singly or in crops; they may follow biting of the cheek or lip, or they may occur spontaneously. Some persons seem to be particularly susceptible to canker sores. Although there is no specific treatment, mild alkaline mouthwashes, better oral hygiene, and more attention to improved nutrition with increased fluid intake and cessation of smoking are beneficial. Local application of caustics is considered poor treatment since it is believed that tissue destruction is produced, and this delays healing.

Vincent's angina. *Ulceromembranous stomatitis* is commonly known as Vincent's angina. During World War I it was so common that the name "trench mouth" was acquired. It is thought to be caused by a combination of the *Bacillus fusiformis*, which resembles the spirochete of syphilis, and *Borrelia vincentii*.[3] There is some question about the communicability of this infection, since causative organisms are found in many mouths although symptoms are absent. The infection causes pain, swelling, and occasionally bleeding of the gums and produces a whitish membrane. The patient may have general lassitude and generalized pain about the jaws. If the condition is severe, antibiotics are given for Vincent's angina. Since the organisms are often harbored in pockets along the gum margins of those who have periodontal disease, dental treatment is necessary. Sodium perborate mouthwashes are often ordered. The patient may have to subsist on a liquid or soft diet for a few days; strongly acid foods, highly seasoned foods, and alcohol and smoking should be avoided.

Ludwig's angina. Infections in the mouth from the base of the teeth (alveolar abscess), the bone of the jaw, or any soft tissues may involve the cervical lymph nodes and the floor of the mouth and may lead to Ludwig's angina. Many people seem inclined to believe that mouth and throat infections are not serious, whereas they would hurry to the doctor if they had acute limb pain and suspected a fracture. Ludwig's angina was an extremely serious condition before the advent of antibiotic drugs. Once established in the soft tissues, the infection can pass rapidly between the cervical fascial sheaths and reach the mediastinum, where it can cause death. Pressure from infection and edema in the throat as the disease progresses downward can also be fatal in a short time.

Treatment for Ludwig's angina requires the immediate administration of large doses of antibiotic drugs. The doctor may order hot saline solution mouthwashes at least hourly during waking hours and hot packs applied externally if the cervical nodes are involved. Fluids are usually given intravenously. The patient must be watched closely until acute danger is over. Elevated temperature, increased pain, and swelling usually indicate extension of infection. Increased pain on swallowing and upon movement of the neck, voice changes, any difficulty in respiration or evidence of cyanosis must be reported to the doctor immediately. Surgical incision of the abscess is often done to relieve pressure and to prevent extension to the mediastinum. Occasionally a tracheostomy is necessary.

Diseases of the salivary glands

Acute infection can occur in any of the salivary glands, although the parotid gland is the one most often affected. The common name for inflammation of the parotid gland is *surgical mumps,* though the disease can occur in patients who have not undergone surgery. Surgical mumps must be distinguished from *acute communicable parotitis* (epidemic mumps). It occurs in debilitated and dehydrated patients whose mouth hygiene is poor, whose mouths have been permitted to become dry, and who have not chewed solid food regularly; elderly patients are more susceptible than younger ones. The signs are pain, swelling, absence of salivation, and sometimes purulent exudate from the duct of the gland. Antibiotic therapy is often ordered. Mouthwashes are used, and either warm or cold compresses applied externally may make the patient more comfortable.

Surgical mumps can usually be prevented by careful attention to oral hygiene, general nutrition, and fluid needs. Dental prophylactic treatment preoperatively is thought to aid prevention. Having the patient chew gum postoperatively and at other times when solid food is not permitted may prevent congestion or obstruction in the ducts of the salivary gland.

Stones may form in the ducts of the salivary glands and within the glands themselves; the submaxillary glands are most often affected. Mucous plugs may also obstruct normal salivary flow. The gland may enlarge and become tender and painful, and there may be no saliva from the duct. The possibility that the firm mass is an extension of a neoplasm into surrounding tissue must be ruled out. A radiopaque substance can be injected into the duct (sialogram), thereby visualizing the duct and sometimes the obstruction. Sometimes probing with a fine probe dislodges the obstruction, but often surgical removal is necessary. In other cases the entire gland must be removed surgically. Patients who have this condition should be advised to take larger amounts of fluid than usual and to pay particular attention to good oral hygiene.

TUMORS OF THE MOUTH

The lips, the oral cavity, and the tongue are prone to develop malignant lesions. The largest number of these are squamous cell epitheliomas which grow rapidly and metastasize to adjacent structures more quickly than do most malignant tumors of the skin. A good prognosis in treatment of malignant lesions of the mouth depends upon early diagnosis and treatment. Every nurse has a real responsibility in interpreting the possible seriousness of any mouth lesion which fails to heal within a few weeks (two to three) and in urging immediate medical care. Pain cannot be relied upon as a signal indicating need for medical attention because many advanced malignant lesions in the mouth are painless.

Repeated irritation is thought to be a factor in the development of cancer, and it may be that the mouth is particularly susceptible because of constant trauma from foods, irritation from bacteria, and irritation by the teeth. Malignant lesions of the lip often appear on the lower lip of pipe smokers at the exact location where the warm stem of the pipe frequently rests. The repeated presence of smoke in the mouth may also be a factor in the development of cancer. Cancerous lesions often occur in the inner cheek, the gums, or the palate when irritation from jagged teeth or dental plates has been allowed to persist. The tongue is a restless organ, constantly seeking out jagged edges of teeth and attempting to dislodge food that has been caught between teeth. It may be that repeated irritation from these sources is a factor in the development of cancer. Cancer of the tongue often appears on the lower surface, where there may be contact with teeth that are broken or out of normal alignment. Carcinoma of the tongue is particularly susceptible to early metastasis because of the rich blood and lymph supplies.

Leukoplakia is not a cancerous lesion, but, if allowed to remain untreated, so often becomes malignant that it is considered here. Leukoplakia begins as chalky, white, thickened patches on the tongue or buccal mucosa of heavy smokers. These patches are not readily removed. Conservative treatment includes good general mouth hygiene with use of mild alkaline mouthwashes, dental treatment if needed, and cessation of smoking. The lesions are carefully watched, and, if they do not respond to this treatment within a few weeks, they are removed by surgical excision or by cautery. Lesions that seem thickened or papillary are removed at once since they are most likely to undergo malignant degeneration.

Treatment and nursing care

The treatment for malignancies of the mouth and related structures is surgery and/or radiation, depending on the type of carcinoma, the stage of development of the lesion, and the age and general condition of the patient. In this discussion, surgery will be considered first.

Surgery. The patient who is to have surgical treatment for malignancy of the mouth needs expert and sympathetic nursing care. The public is so conscious of cancer that the possibility of spread through metastasis is well known. If it is necessary to repeat x-ray examinations or other tests, the reason should be explained to the patient so that worry may be reduced as much as possible. The patient should be prepared for each step of the proposed treatment. Before the operation, the doctor usually gives the patient as complete an explanation as is then possible. The nurse must know what the patient has been told; she must get to know the patient so that she can help judge how much he should be told. For example, some patients who are to lose teeth and part of the jaw are relieved to know something about prosthetic devices that are available; others are so overwhelmed by the prospect of the operation itself that they are far from ready to think beyond the most immediate future. Impressions are sometimes taken preoperatively to guide in making suitable prostheses following surgery.

All patients benefit from explanation of how they will be fed and how they will be able to communicate postoperatively. A pad of paper with pencil, a tiny blackboard with chalk, or a "Magic Slate" covered with plastic which makes repeated use very simple should be available. Patients who are to have extensive surgery of the mouth should be assured that they will not be left unattended immediately following the operation. If there is a possibility that a tracheostomy may be performed, they should be told about it and informed that a suction machine will be at their bedside and will be used frequently after the operation. Preoperatively the patient is usually fed a high-calorie diet, oral prophylactic treatment is often given, and antibiotics are administered. He may be out of bed for short periods the day following or soon after the operation.

The operation performed depends entirely upon the location and nature of the lesion; often if the lesion has been neglected, surgery must be extensive and may be multilating. Part or all of the lips, tongue, cheek or jaw bones, and extensive resection of cervical lymph nodes, blood vessels, and adjacent tissues on the floor of the mouth and in the neck may be removed. If there is extensive resection of cervical nodes the term *radical neck dissection* is used to describe the procedure. Usually a gastric tube is inserted through the nose and into the stomach preoperatively, through which stomach contents and flatus may be aspirated postoperatively. Later the patient may be fed through this tube. One or more drains may be used in the wound and an artificial airway will probably be in place when the patient returns from the operating room. A tracheostomy may be done if surgery has been so extensive that edema is likely to obstruct breathing or when aspiration during normal breathing is too great a danger. Massive pressure dressings are usually placed around the wound to obliterate dead spaces, help prevent edema, and splint the part. These foster healing and lessen pain.

Upon the completion of surgery, the doctor orders the position he wishes for the patient. This will probably be on the face to facilitate drainage from the mouth or else on the nonaffected side in a partial face-lying position. Occasionally the head of the bed is elevated in an effort to control edema. If a tracheostomy has been done, the nursing care will be the same as that required for all patients who have undergone this procedure (see Chapter 24). Two sets of suction equipment will be needed since different catheters must be used to remove fluid accumulations from the mouth and to suction the trachea.

The patient's breathing must be carefully watched. Any color changes, difficulty in breathing through the airway or tracheostomy tube and any changes in temperature, pulse, respiration, or blood pressure must be reported at once. The dressings are watched for signs of bleeding and constriction, which may cause edema and hamper respiration. A suction catheter is inserted through the airway, and suctioning should be done whenever there are audible signs of fluid. The artificial airway is removed by the surgeon or the anesthetist when it is believed that the patient may safely breathe without this aid.

A few hours after awakening from the anesthesia the patient is urged to sit up and cough. Coughing may be stimulated by placing the tip of the catheter used for suctioning either in the throat or, if a tracheostomy has been done, in the trachea. The nurse can help the patient feel more secure and comfortable by placing her hands firmly in a position to support his neck and the dressings over it as he coughs. The patient may be instructed to place his locked hands behind his neck, and thus support his head and neck when he moves about. Coughing must often be followed immediately by suctioning of the mouth and upper throat to remove blood and secretions. If a tracheostomy has been performed, suctioning of the bronchi will be done. If respiratory difficulty occurs, the doctor should be notified because this may be caused by displacement of packing, by edema, or by pneumothorax.

Spontaneous pneumothorax is a rare but serious complication which may result from surgical trauma about the thyroid gland. The emergency treatment may include the administration of oxygen, attempts to close the opening around the trachea into the pleural space by use of pressure dressings, and aspiration of air from the pleural space by means of an underwater drainage system (see Chapter 23). The patient must be kept absolutely quiet and is usually placed on his affected side so that the lung on the unaffected side may be helped to function at maximum efficiency.

The patient who has had throat or neck surgery usually receives antibiotics in addition to drugs for pain. Morphine and other narcotic drugs that depress respiration are used with caution, and an effort is made to limit their use by administering them only before painful procedures such as changes of dressings. Careful support of the neck and of the dressings when the patient sits up, a firm mattress, and gentleness in suctioning and in doing all other necessary procedures make medication for pain less necessary. Atropine sulfate is given with extreme caution because it seems to make secretions more tenacious and, therefore, more difficult to remove.

Dressings are usually changed by the surgeon five to seven days following the operation, although the drain may be removed earlier. Some or all of the packing and some of the sutures are removed at this time, and the massive pressure dressings are replaced by a simpler dressing that permits more freedom of movement. A rare complication is damage to the thoracic duct with a resultant *chylous fistula* and loss of body fluids, electrolytes, and protein. This condition is usually controlled by pressure dressings, although occasionally surgical correction of the fistula is necessary.

The mouth may be irrigated with sterile water, a mild alkaline mouthwash, hydrogen peroxide, normal saline solution, or a solution of sodium bicarbonate, depending on the doctor's preference. Usually sterile equipment is used even though the mouth cannot be kept sterile. Provided the patient is conscious and is turned in such a position that fluid will drain into an emesis basin, a catheter may be inserted along the side of the mouth between the cheek and the teeth and solution injected with gentle pressure. Remaining fluid and mucus may be removed with the suction apparatus. Dressings may be protected during this treatment by fitting a plastic sheet snugly over them. As soon as the patient is able to do so, he is encouraged to assist with this part of his care.

Transfusions and infusions are usually given during the operation and immediately thereafter. The patient is then fed liquids high in calories, vitamins, and protein through a tube passed into the stomach by way of the nose; 200 to 400 ml. of fluid may be given every three to four hours. The patient must be watched carefully for reaction to fluids given, since nausea and vomiting must be avoided. The sudden arrival in the stomach of fluid through a tube sometimes produces results different from those that occur when food and fluid are taken into the mouth and retained for a few moments during chewing. In addition, the act of swallowing causes some relaxation of the stomach. It is best to give a very small amount of fluid at first, to be certain that it is approximately body temperature, and to wait a few minutes before continuing with the procedure. Diarrhea sometimes occurs when patients must live on liquid foods. The patient should be prepared for this, and the doctor should be notified if the condition persists. Sometimes adjustments in the constituents of the liquid feedings help with this problem, and the dietitian may be called on for assistance. At other times a medication such as bismuth is added to the liquid food.

Swallowing is discouraged for several days since it is likely to disturb the operative area. Nasal tubes, however, can be extremely irritating to patients, even when small, thin, polyethylene tubing is used instead of rubber. As soon as the patient can safely swallow, the tube is removed. The patient then needs careful attention in his first attempts to swallow. He may feel that he is choking, may be upset if fluid comes through the tracheostomy tube, and may have severe coughing which is frightening and painful. It is extremely important that the nurse be present when swallowing is first attempted and that she be prepared to suction the trachea and bronchi at once if aspiration does occur. Only water is given until the patient has become accustomed to swallowing.

The method used to feed the patient will depend entirely upon the extent and nature of his surgery. Most patients learn to suction and to feed themselves a few days following surgery and are happier doing so. A large Asepto syringe with a catheter attached may be used, and from this the patient may progress to a feeding cup with a piece of rubber tubing attached. Through practice the patient will develop confidence in caring for himself, and he is often more adept than the nurse in placing the catheter or tube in a position where fluids can be received into the mouth and swallowed without difficulty. A mirror often helps him to do this. He needs privacy when he is experimenting with the method that is best for him. He should not be hurried and should be observed very carefully to determine how much assistance he needs. As he begins to take liquids and then soft puréed foods, he is taught to follow all meals with clear water to cleanse the mouth and foster good oral hygiene.

The patient may remain in the hospital only two or three weeks, or he may be hospitalized much longer while further stages of surgery are done or while x-ray or radium treatment is given. During this time he needs constant encouragement and careful nursing care. He must be encouraged to mingle with others and is often happier in a room with others provided there are facilities for privacy when needed. Members of the patient's family should be encouraged to visit, and they, too, should learn how the patient may take food, how he may care for himself, what prosthetic devices are available, and how speech retraining can be accomplished if extensive resection of the tongue or removal of the larynx has been necessary. Speech training is discussed in Chapter 24. Prosthetic devices cannot be fitted until healing has taken place, but pictures of others who are wearing such devices with resultant marked improvement in their appearance are often encouraging to the patient. Prostheses are individually designed to replace portions of the palate and jaw that have been resected and to make the use of dentures possible. Plastic surgery may be done to partially replace lost tissue. Meeting and talking to other patients who have had similar operations with good results and good adjustment is very helpful to the patient. The patient must be encouraged to take an interest in his personal appearance. Dribbling of saliva is sometimes a problem, and the patient may be able to learn to tilt his head at intervals in such a way that he can direct the saliva to where it can be swallowed. Men should shave as soon as this is permitted by the doctor.

Radiation. Treatment may be by implantation of radium needles that will be removed, insertion of radon seeds (small gold encasements containing radium emanations) that will be left in place permanently, use of an intraoral mold that is placed within the mouth in a carefully determined position and left for a prescribed number of hours each day and for a prescribed number of days, or deep x-ray therapy.

Whatever method of treatment is chosen should be explained fully to the patient. If radium needles are used, he must know that the needles are fastened to string that must not be pulled lest the dosage or position of radium be altered or the needle lost. He must understand that talking with the needles in place will be difficult or impossible. Radium needles must be checked several times each day; the nurse must know and must stress to the patient the importance of reporting immediately if one of them becomes dislodged. Auxiliary personnel and all others in attendance should understand the need to watch all equipment carefully for needles that have been removed or dislodged (e.g., when emptying an emesis basin) lest expensive radium be unwittingly discarded. If radium is applied with an intraoral mold, the patient must know that he will be unable to talk. He should know that any slipping or change in position of the mold will influence the dosage, so that he must report discomfort and must not attempt adjustment himself. A sling to support the chin helps to alleviate strain and discomfort in the mouth and jaw; sometimes lying down for short periods is helpful, and occasionally sedatives may be necessary. Attention to mouth hygiene, prevention of infection, and the giving of food and fluids are similar to that necessary following surgery; the medications prescribed are also similar. Suction equipment should always be ready for immediate use in the event of hemorrhage or choking.

If deep x-ray therapy is to be used for radiation of tissues in or adjacent to the mouth, it is usually necessary to remove some or all of the teeth. Since x-ray therapy causes the patient to have a sore mouth, dentures usually are not tolerated for some time. The mouth should be irrigated once an hour with a solution of 1/2 teaspoonful of sodium chloride and 1/2 teaspoonful of sodium bicarbonate to a quart of water. Some doctors order a solution of 0.3 Gm. (5 grains) acetylsalicylic acid in 2 ounces of water as a gargle which may be swallowed; this may be repeated as often as every four to six hours. Inhalation of tincture of benzoin sometimes makes the mouth and throat feel pleasanter and less dry. Mineral oil is often used for dryness of the lips and mouth. Dryness may persist for two to three months before secretory action of the mucous glands is restored. If infection occurs in the mouth, antibiotics may be given systemically. Hydrogen peroxide solution or Dobell's solution is sometimes ordered if there is sloughing, which causes fetid odor of the mouth secretions. Solutions containing chlorine are often useful when odor is a problem. A solution of 15 drops of common household bleach such as Clorox in a glass of water helps to control mouth odors and is acceptable to many patients.

Patients who have local reaction involving the mucous membrane of the mouth must have soft or liquid foods. The strange metallic taste of which they may complain may be alleviated by sour substances such as lemon candies and citrus fruit juices. Those who have had x-ray therapy involving the mouth should not smoke, for smoking is irritating to the mucous membrane. Hot and cold foods and fluids should be avoided because the injured mucous membrane is extremely sensitive to changes in temperature. A local anesthetic may be prescribed to be taken before meals when discomfort in the mouth seriously interferes with eating. Solutions of Butyn or cocaine may be used, or lozenges may be dissolved in the back of the mouth. Euphagin and Nuporals are examples of prepared lozenges that are helpful to many patients. (See Chapter 16 for further discussion of care of the patient having radium or x-ray therapy.)

Tissue necrosis and severe pain occur in advanced cancer of the mouth, either from failure in treatment or from death of tissue due to radiation. The patient is harassed by difficulty in swallowing, fear of choking, and the constant accumulation of foul-smelling secretions. The danger of severe, and even fatal, hemorrhage must always be considered. Nursing care of these patients includes the most careful and thoughtful attention to certain details; for example, secretions left in emesis basins or in suction bottles can be most upsetting to the patient. It is exceedingly difficult to get patients with advanced carcinoma of the mouth to take sufficient nourishing fluids, and the nurse can often help by finding out specifically what fluids or foods the patient likes and believes are easiest for him to take. Relatives should be permitted to prepare and bring special dishes to the hospital if the patient so desires. Most physicians prescribe analgesic drugs freely for patients whose disease has progressed beyond medical control. The patient should be observed for signs of suicidal intent. Often an important nursing responsibility is teaching a member of the family to feed, suction, and otherwise care for the patient, since many terminally ill cancer patients are happier when cared for at home by their loved ones. Relatives may learn how to care for the patient while he is in the hospital and are then often assisted in their homes by a nurse from a community nursing agency. A carefully worded referral from the nurse in the hospital to the nurse in the community helps a great deal to make the patient's adjustment from hospital to home care an easier one.

TRAUMA

Fracture of the jaw

Fracture of the jaw occurs quite frequently as a result of vehicle accidents and of men's physical encounters with each other. The treatment is usually fixation by wiring the teeth. The jaws may be held together for six to eight weeks by wire with the ends twisted between the upper and lower rows of teeth or by attaching tiny rubber bands to loops in the wiring. Rubber bands are most often used since they can be readily removed and the degree of fixation can be adjusted easily.

The patient must be prepared for the fact that he will not be able to talk or to swallow solid food. He should be assured, however, that he will be able to take sufficient food for health. Many times the patient with a fracture of the jaw can resume quite an active life during convalescence. Most patients are in the hospital a very short time or are treated on an ambulatory basis unless they have sustained other injuries.

Immediately following wiring of the jaws, the patient is watched for nausea and vomiting which may be caused by emotional trauma, blood or other swallowed material, or anesthesia. Care must be taken to prevent aspiration of vomitus. If the jaws have been wired together, a small pair of pliers should be at the bedside so that wires may be untwisted quickly if an emergency arises. A suction machine should be at the bedside. The nurse caring for the patient must have specific orders which state, among other things, the circumstances under which wires or rubber bands should be released.

Patients who have fixation by wiring for fracture need much the same care as is needed following surgery of the mouth. They must often subsist on liquids and must learn to take high-calorie fluids drawn through an aperture between their teeth. They need instruction about mouth hygiene, and they must be instructed to report any sudden swelling, pain, or other symptoms that may occur after dismissal from the hospital. Osteomyelitis is much less common now that antibiotics are given routinely, but it can occur and is more likely to do so in the unusual cases of compound fracture in which bone fragments have penetrated either the outer skin or the inside of the mouth.

Injury to soft tissue

Injuries to soft tissues within the mouth are usually caused by pressure against teeth, direct trauma from a foreign object, or protrusion of bone through the buccal mucosa following fracture of the jaw. Breaks in the skin about the mouth often accompany these injuries. Treatment consists of thorough cleansing of the wounds. Usually pHisoHex is used and is followed by sterile normal saline solution irrigation. Skin wounds are gently débrided and sutured with an extremely fine absorbable suture for best cosmetic results. Because of the vascularity of the scalp and face, infection is rare following traumatic injury to these areas.

Lacerations within the mouth are cleansed and sutured if their extent and location make this necessary. Hemorrhage must be watched for especially if total injuries necessitate extensive dressing which may hinder normal expectoration of blood and cause it to be swallowed. Edema may be pronounced following trauma to the mouth and this may interfere with respirations. Usually the head of the bed is elevated in a semi-Fowler's position to reduce circulation to the wound and thereby lessen edema. Tight dressings about the face must be carefully checked since they may contribute to development of edema and may cause headache.

Patients who have sustained penetrating wounds of the mouth are usually given antibiotics and tetanus prophylactic serum. The nurse should question the patient about a history of sensitivity to serum before treatment for prevention of tetanus is given. Mouth care and feeding of patients with these injuries present problems similar to those encountered following surgery or a fracture and have already been discussed in this chapter.

REFERENCES AND SELECTED READINGS*

1 Ast, David B., and Schlesinger, Edward R.: The Conclusion of a Ten Year Study of Water Fluoridation, Am. J. Pub. Health **46**:265-271, March 1956.

2 Brown, Amy Frances: Medical Nursing, ed. 3, Philadelphia, 1957, W. B. Saunders Co.

3 Cecil, Russell L., and Loeb, Robert F. (editors): A Textbook of Medicine, ed. 10, Philadelphia, 1959, W. B. Saunders Co.

4 Doctor—Here Are the Facts About Water Fluoridation for New York City, Form 3547, City of New York Department of Health, March 15, 1956.

5 *Hanson, Donald: The Salivary Glands, Am. J. Nursing **58**:240-241, Feb. 1958.

6 *Hayden, Mary L.: After Surgery—Rehabilitation for a Full Life, Nursing Outlook **7**:21-23, Jan. 1959.

7 *James, Arthur G., and Piatt, Barbara J.: Radical Neck Surgery, Clinical Considerations and Nursing Care, Am. J. Nursing **53**:930-934, Aug. 1953.

8 *Kesel, Robert G., and Streebny, Leo M.: Periodontal Diseases, Am. J. Nursing **55**:174-175, Feb. 1955.

9 *Kesel, Robert G., and Streebny, Leo M.: Toothbrushing, Am. J. Nursing **57**:186-188, Feb. 1957.

*References preceded by an asterisk indicate material particularly well suited for student reading.

10 Knutson, John W.: Fluoridation—Where Are We Today? Am. J. Nursing **60**:196-198, Feb. 1960.

11 National Cancer Institute, Federal Security Agency and New York Department of Health: Cancer Nursing, 1955, New York Department of Health.

12 *Phair, W. Philip: Are You Up to Date on Dental Health? Am. J. Nursing **53**:183-186, Feb. 1953.

13 President's Commission: Building America's Health Needs, vol. I, Washington, D. C., 1951, U. S. Government Printing Office.

14 Rovelstad, Gordon H.: Dental Care in a Children's Hospital, Hospitals **24**:47-50, June 1950.

15 Shafer, K. N., Simpson, D. H., and Sullivan, F. G.: The Nurse in a Dental Clinic, Am. J. Nursing **55**:460-462, April 1955.

16 Special Committee on Hospital Clinic Services: Better Hospital Care for the Ambulant Patient, Harrisburg, 1946, The Hospital Association of Pennsylvania.

17 Stafford, Edward S., and Diller, Doris: A Textbook of Surgery for Nurses, ed. 2, Philadelphia, 1954, W. B. Saunders Co.

18 Stannous Fluoride Blocks Tooth Decay, Chemical and Engineering News **38**:40-41, Aug. 1, 1960.

19 *Stark, Richard B., and Henderson, Lilian M.: Facial Injuries—Surgical Treatment and Nursing Care of Patients With Facial Injuries, Am. J. Nursing **57**:450-456, April 1957.

20 *Volker, Joseph F.: Dental Caries Can Be Prevented, Am. J. Nursing **50**:97-99, Feb. 1950.

21 Yahraes, Herbert: Your Teeth—How to Save Them, Public Affairs Pamphlet No. 147, 1949, New York, Public Affairs Committee, Inc.

The patient with disease of the gastrointestinal system

Chapter 26

Study questions for review

1 Review the anatomy and physiology of the gastrointestinal system. What are some factors that stimulate gastric motility?
2 What enzymes are present in the small bowel, and what is their action on normal skin?
3 How can electrolyte balance be affected by excessive vomiting and by persistent diarrhea?
4 In your hospital what distinction is made between a liquid, a soft, and a general diet? What foods would you exclude in a low-residue diet?
5 Review the drugs that are used to control motility of the gastrointestinal tract.

Common diagnostic tests and procedures

Complaints of gastrointestinal disturbances are common and numerous. At some time in their lives, most persons experience stomach upsets and diarrhea. These may accompany other disorders such as the "grippe," follow dietary indiscretions, or occur with emotional upsets. While these conditions are temporarily exhausting and uncomfortable, they are generally of short duration and may not even require medical attention. However, nausea, vomiting, or diarrhea which is severe and causes pain or is chronic and incapacitating should be reported to a doctor. Unfortunately, some diseases of the gastrointestinal system do not produce symptoms until the disease has progressed so far that medical treatment cannot cure it. Cancer of the gastrointestinal tract, for instance, may give no signs until far advanced.

There are many laboratory tests and examinations available to help establish the presence or absence of disease in the gastrointestinal system. Some tests are done only to help establish a diagnosis when definite symptoms of disease occur, while others are advocated as part of a yearly physical examination for persons over 40 years of age in an attempt to detect early signs of disease such as cancer.

The common diagnostic tests and examinations used to help diagnose disease of the gastrointestinal system will be considered in this discussion. Since removal of gastric and intestinal contents may be required in the treatment of patients with many kinds of gastrointestinal disorders, they also will be discussed before nursing care for specific diseases is considered.

The doctor writes an order for each test and examination; the nurse is usually responsible for scheduling the test and for instruction and physical preparation of the patient. When many x-ray examinations are ordered for a patient they should be scheduled in the following order so that the best results can be obtained with a minimum of delay: intravenous pyelogram, gallbladder series, barium enema, and gastrointestinal series. Since the tests are expensive, time consuming, and often exhausting, it is important that the patient be properly instructed and prepared so that the examinations will not have to be repeated.

X-RAY EXAMINATIONS

Barium enema. A series of roentgenograms taken after a barium enema has been given is used to demonstrate the presence of polyps, tumors, and other lesions of the large intestine and to reveal any abnormal anatomy or malfunction of the bowel. As the barium is instilled through a rectal tube, the roentgenologist, using a fluoroscope, observes its passage into the large intestine. The patient is asked to retain the barium while roentgenograms of the intestines are taken. He is then asked to expel the barium, and another film is taken to see if any pockets of barium are retained.

The preparation for a barium enema includes an explanation to the patient of the x-ray procedure, of the importance of retaining the barium during the examination, and of the need for preparatory enemas. For the barium to clearly outline the lumen of the bowel, the bowel must be empty; this is best accomplished by giving enemas until the returns are clear. The nurse should find out from the doctor what he considers the maximum number of enemas; usually no more than three are given. Repeated enemas exhaust the patient and irritate the anus and and the rectal mucosa. Because of this, some doctors feel that one small enema containing a hypertonic salt solution such as disodium phosphate or monosodium phosphate is adequate. These enemas are now prepared commercially in disposable units. Food and fluids are not restricted for these x-ray examinations.

Barium that is retained in the bowel becomes hard and difficult to expel. To ensure complete evacuation of the barium from the intestinal tract after this procedure, many physicians order an oil retention enema followed by cleansing enemas.

Since the patient is usually exhausted after a barium enema and the subsequent cleansing enemas, he should have rest. Petroleum jelly or, if ordered, a local analgesic ointment such as Nupercaine may be applied to the anus to alleviate discomfort. If the patient is not too tired, a warm bath may also be soothing.

Gastrointestinal series. A gastrointestinal series consists of several roentgenograms of the stomach and intestinal tract used to detect tumors or ulceration of the stomach and duodenum and to reveal any abnormal anatomy or malposition of these organs. As the patient swallows barium (a radiopaque substance), the roentgenologist makes a fluoroscopic examination, and then he takes roentgenograms of the stomach and duodenum. Since the barium tastes like chalk, it is often flavored to make it more palatable. After the patient has drunk the barium, he is asked to assume various positions on the x-ray table and the table may be tilted so that the barium will outline the stomach wall and flow by gravity into the intestinal loops as the doctor watches through the fluoroscope and takes the roentgenograms. Six hours after the initial films are taken, more roentgenograms are taken to see how much of the barium remains in the stomach. Barium will have passed through a normal-functioning stomach and pylorus during this time.

In preparation for a gastrointestinal series the nurse should explain the procedure to the patient and tell him that he must not take food or fluids for from six to eight hours before the examination. The presence of food in the stomach prevents the barium from outlining all of the stomach wall, and the roentgenograms will be inconclusive and misleading. If the patient eats, the x-ray examination should be postponed until the next day. The patient can be assured that the test will not cause discomfort and that he may eat as soon as the nurse is notified by the x-ray department that the series is completed; however, this may mean that breakfast is omitted and lunch delayed. After a gastrointestinal series, a cathartic is usually ordered to speed the elimination of barium from the intestines. Retained barium may become hard and cause obstruction in the intestine or an impaction in the rectum.

ENDOSCOPY

Esophagoscopy and gastroscopy. Esophagoscopy and gastroscopy are procedures done to visualize the esophageal and gastric mucosa. By these means, a disease process may be located and inspected, and a specimen of tissue may be obtained for microscopic study. Complete visualization of the stomach is not possible because it contains three blind spots: the fundus, the pylorus, and the greater curvature opposite the cardia. A negative esophagoscopy, therefore, is usually more significant than a negative gastroscopy. Roentgenograms of the stomach and the esophagus are taken prior to these examinations since an obstruction of the esophagus might make passing an instrument dangerous.

Although these procedures are not actually painful, patients find them extremely exhausting and uncomfortable. The nurse should explain the examination to the patient in simple terms, emphasizing that if he carefully follows the doctor's instructions and lies quietly during the passing of the instrument, he can help make the procedure a short and successful one. Food and fluids are withheld for from six to eight hours before the examination so that the patient does not regurgitate as the tubular instrument is passed through the mouth into the esophagus and so that the lining of the stomach is visible. Occasionally an esophagoscopy or a gastroscopy must be performed as an emergency measure to remove a foreign object such as a bone or a pin. In this case, the stomach cannot be emptied, but suction should be available for use to prevent aspiration of regurgitated food or fluid. Eyeglasses and dentures should be removed to prevent their being broken, and the woman patient's hair should be wrapped in a turban to keep it out of the way and to prevent it from getting soiled. The patient should void before the examination to prevent discomfort or embarrassment. Pajama bottoms should be worn to prevent inadvertent exposure during the procedure. The patient's written permission is obtained before this examination is done.

The patient is given sedatives one-half to one hour before the examination to lessen apprehension and to make him less aware of the passage of the instrument. The premedication also decreases the possibility of toxic effects from the local anesthetic. A narcotic such as meperidine hydrochloride (Demerol) and a barbiturate such as soluble phenobarbital usually are used for sedation. To decrease secretions, atropine sulfate is usually given. The patient should be carefully observed for possible reactions to these drugs, and he should be protected from injury while under their influence. Before the examination begins, the doctor explains the procedure to the patient and tries to gain his full understanding and cooperation. The patient's posterior pharynx is then sprayed with cocaine or Pontocaine to inactivate the gag reflex and to lessen local reaction to the instrument. In order to prevent the aspiration of medication, the patient is asked to hold his breath while the posterior pharynx is sprayed and not to swallow saliva but to expectorate it into an emesis basin that is provided. The nurse should watch the patient for any toxic reactions to the anesthetic; an emergency tray containing barbiturates should be readily available. (See Chapter 13 for the toxic reactions to cocaine and Pontocaine.) When the gag reflex has disappeared (usually within five to ten minutes), the patient assumes a dorsal recumbent position on the treatment table. For an esophageal examination his head and shoulders extend over the edge of the table, and for the passage of a gastroscope he lies on his side. The nurse supports the patient's head, and he is told again how important it is to remain perfectly still while the instrument is passed. Sudden movement at this time might cause the instrument to perforate the esophagus. Children and patients whose behavior is unpredictable should be firmly restrained if this procedure is attempted without the use of a general anesthetic. The procedure usually takes about five to ten minutes, and during this time the nurse should encourage the patient, assuring him that he is all right and that the procedure will be completed shortly. If tissue is removed for pathologic examination, it should be placed immediately into a specimen bottle and correctly labeled.

When the examination is finished, the patient is instructed not to eat or drink until the gag reflex returns. This usually takes about four hours. In the hospital the doctor or the nurse tests for the return of the gag reflex by gently tickling the back of the throat with a cotton swab or a tongue depressor. If the patient is allowed to go home, he may be told to stick his finger into his throat to see if he gags before he attempts to eat or drink. If there is any possibility that the esophagus may have been perforated, or if a biopsy has been taken, the doctor orders sterile water only for the first twenty-four hours and the patient must remain in the hospital overnight.

Following an esophagoscopy or a gastroscopy, the patient may be hoarse and may complain of a sore throat. These symptoms should disappear within a few days. The patient should be told of this because he will not notice discomfort until the anesthesia wears off. Warm saline solution gargles may give some relief. Acetylsalicylic acid, 0.3 Gm. (5 grains), often is ordered to be dissolved in the mouth and then swallowed slowly. These procedures are exhausting to the patient, and provision should be made for him to rest when they are completed.

Anoscopy, proctoscopy, and sigmoidoscopy. Anoscopy, proctoscopy, and sigmoidoscopy are procedures performed to visualize the mucosa of the anus, rectum, and sigmoid. Tumors, polyps, or ulcerations may be discovered, examined, and biopsied. An anoscopy is an examination of the anus; a proctoscopy, an examination of the anus and rectum; and a sigmoidoscopy, an examination of the anus, rectum, and sigmoid. Most often, a sigmoidoscopy is done, and this examination is routinely performed before rectal surgery and as part of the physical examination of patients who complain of chronic constipation or diarrhea or have any other indications of lower intestinal disease such as bleeding.

The preparation for endoscopic examination of the bowel varies in different hospitals and clinics, but the patient should always receive an explanation of the procedure and of the preparation to be carried out. Usually he is instructed to eat a light evening meal without fresh fruits or vegetables, fried foods, meat, or cereal. On the morning of the examination soapsuds enemas may be given until the return is clear, or a small hypertonic salt solution enema may be ordered instead. If the enemas are to be taken at home by the patient, the nurse should be certain that he knows how to carry out this procedure correctly and that he has suitable equipment. Visualization of the bowel mucosa is impossible unless all the fecal material is evacuated. Enema fluid should also be completely expelled before the examination is done since it, too, will obstruct visualization. Cathartics are seldom used in preparation for this examination because they may cause downward flow of material from the upper bowel when the test is being done. A light breakfast is usually permitted on the day of the scheduled test.

The nurse collects the necessary equipment for a sigmoidoscopy and checks the sigmoidoscope to see that it is functioning properly. Since the examination is upsetting to most patients, all possible preparations should be made before the patient is brought to the examining room to ensure a smooth-running and rapid procedure. The instrument must be checked to see that all the parts are functioning; the electric light bulb should be tested by attaching the instrument cord to the battery or to the electrical outlet. Besides the instrument, a draping sheet, rectal gloves, lubricant, cotton swabs (12 inches in length), an emesis basin, toilet tissue, bip 498 in Fundamentals

opsy forceps, a suction machine with suction tip, and a paper bag for waste are required.

Before the examination begins, the doctor again explains the procedure to the patient. It is preferable for the patient to assume a knee-chest position, and he is draped so that only the rectum is exposed. Because it may be difficult for an elderly or a very ill patient to assume or maintain a knee-chest position, a side-lying position (Sims) occasionally may be used. (For complete description of these two positions, see Chapter 22.) The nurse should assist the patient in maintaining the correct position. She should encourage him to remain still, to relax as much as possible, and to take deep breaths. She should also watch him carefully, lest he become faint and fall from the table. Since the lights are turned off during the examination, it is sometimes difficult to note the patient's color; if any doubt exists about his condition, his pulse rate should be taken.

The doctor usually first examines the rectum with his gloved finger. He then inserts the lubricated instrument. After the instrument has been passed into the rectum, the solid, round-tipped inner portion (obturator) is removed. The intensity of light is then adjusted with the rheostat so that adequate light is reflected on the mucosa. If the sigmoidoscope is being used, the instrument is advanced slowly through the bowel for about 25 cm. (10 inches). The patient feels the instrument entering the rectum and sigmoid; he is uncomfortable but does not usually have real pain. Air is sometimes pumped into the bowel through the sigmoidoscope to distend the lumen of the bowel, thus permitting better visualization. This may cause severe "gas pains." If small amounts of fluid or stool are still present in the bowel, they are removed with the cotton swabs and by suctioning. A proctoscopic procedure and maintenance of a knee-chest position usually tires the patient. As soon as the instrument has been removed and the excess lubricant removed from about the anus, he should be assisted to his bed and permitted to rest. The patient who is examined in the clinic is advised to rest for half an hour and should have some food or fluid before he leaves. This is particularly important for the elderly patient.

OTHER DIAGNOSTIC TESTS

Gastric analysis (with histamine). Examination of the fasting contents of the stomach is helpful in establishing a diagnosis of gastric disease. For example, an excessive amount of gastric secretions containing food ingested the night before suggests pyloric obstruction. An absence of free hydrochloric acid in the stomach contents may indicate the presence of gastric malignancy or pernicious anemia, while increased amounts of free hydrochloric acid suggest a peptic ulcer.

To obtain fasting stomach secretions, a gastric tube must be passed. The procedure must be explained to the patient, and food and fluids are withheld from six to eight hours before the test is to be done. The nurse assembles the equipment needed for the procedure, and at this time she gives the patient any additional information about the test that he needs.

If the patient is sitting up with his head hyperextended, the tube is passed more easily. This position can be maintained if the head of the bed is raised and if the pillows are arranged so that they are under the patient's shoulders, allowing his head to be supported on the mattress in hyperextension. The procedure may also be done with the patient seated in a chair. The nurse should make sure that the chair will fully support the patient so that he does not become tired and uncomfortable or unsteady if he leans backward. As the physician reviews the procedure with the patient, the nurse draws the screens about the patient's bed and covers his gown with a protective plastic sheet or towel. He should be provided with an emesis basin and paper tissues. A plastic or rubber gastric tube (No. 12, 14, or 16) is used. The tip of the tube is lubricated, and the physician inserts it through either nostril or through the mouth; then he gently passes it into the posterior pharynx. The patient is asked to swallow hard and repeatedly, and he may be given sips of water as the doctor quickly advances the tube into the stomach. A syringe with an adapter is then fitted onto the end of the tube, and all the stomach contents are aspirated and placed in a specimen bottle. The doctor may want to test the reaction of the aspirated secretions by using litmus paper; blue litmus paper turns pink in the presence of acid. The gastric tube is then secured to the nose and to the forehead with adhesive tape. Care should be taken that the tube does not pull or press against the nostril or cross in front of the eye. The end of the tube is closed with a clamp or with an elastic band to prevent leaking. Most patients are inclined to hold themselves very rigid while the tube is in the stomach, and they may be afraid to move. They should be made as comfortable as possible.

After the fasting specimen has been collected, histamine phosphate, 0.5 mg., is given subcutaneously. This drug stimulates gastric secretions, and it causes vasodilation of the capillaries and arterioles. When histamine is given to a patient who has a peptic ulcer, there is a definite increase in the total output of gastric secretions and an increase in the amount of free hydrochloric acid in the stomach. The patient should be told that the drug may make him feel flushed and warm but that the sensation will pass quickly. Occasionally a patient may be sensitive to histamine, and he may go into shock because of marked dilatation of the peripheral blood vessels. If this occurs, Adrenalin usually is given. After the histamine injection has been given, the stomach contents are aspirated every ten to twenty minutes until three or more specimens of gastric secretions have been obtained. These are placed in correctly labeled bottles and sent to the laboratory for study.

When the test is completed the tube is clamped and quickly withdrawn. The nurse may be asked to do this. The patient should be given paper tissues because he usually has secretions in his eyes, nose, and throat. Mouth care should then be given, and, if the hospitalized patient is not nauseated, breakfast may be served.

If the patient is not hospitalized, this test often is done in the doctor's office or in the clinic, and the nurse often does the entire procedure. If she is to be responsible for this, she must be very certain that she has an order to give Adrenalin at once if the patient has a reaction to histamine.

Tubeless gastric analysis. This procedure is thought to be useful as a screening technique for detection of gastric achlorhydria. The test will indicate the presence or absence of free hydrochloric acid but cannot be used to determine the *amount* of free hydrochloric acid if it is present. Quantitative analysis must be done through aspiration of stomach contents. The patient is given 2 Gm. (120 grains) of a cation exchange resin containing 90 mg. of azure A with 240 ml. of water by mouth on an empty stomach. If there is free hydrochloric acid in the stomach, upon the introduction of this resin a substance will be released in the stomach which will be absorbed from the small intestine and excreted by the kidneys; the urine will be blue. If there is no free hydrochloric acid in the stomach there is no such reaction. or lime green

Insulin tolerance test. An insulin tolerance test is another test used to evaluate the secreting action of the gastric mucosa. The test is carried out in the same way as a gastric analysis, except that instead of histamine a specified amount of regular insulin is given intravenously. The drop in blood sugar produced by the insulin stimulates the vagus nerve, and the flow of gastric secretions may be increased. A normal stomach responds only slightly to stimulation of the vagus nerve, and there will be no significant increase in the gastric secretions. In the patient with a peptic ulcer, however, there will be a marked increase in the total gastric output and in the amount of free hydrochloric acid. The insulin tolerance test may be used to determine the success of a resection of the vagus nerve in decreasing the hyperactivity of the stomach. It is, therefore, often done before and after this operation. In the event symptoms of insulin shock appear, orange juice should be available, as well as glucose for intravenous injection.

Papanicolaou balloon studies. These studies are done specifically when cancer of the stomach is suspected. A special gastric tube with a balloon covered by a meshlike material attached to its tip is passed into the stomach, and the balloon is then inflated. Any cells or bits of tissue that attach to the net covering of the balloon as it is moved about in the stomach are collected after the tube is removed and sent to the laboratory where they are examined for presence of malignant cells.

Stool examination. Gross, microscopic, chemical, and bacterial examinations of the stool supply information that is helpful in establishing a diagnosis of gastrointestinal disease. Stools that are abnormal in color, odor, amount, consistency, and number are significant. Abnormal stools should be accurately described and a specimen saved for examination by the doctor. The doctor may order further laboratory studies to be done. Stool examinations are required for the complete evaluation of all patients with gastrointestinal complaints.

The nurse is responsible for seeing that specimens are collected. If the patient is ambulatory, she may ask him to obtain the specimen, giving him a specimen box and a spatula with which to collect the specimen. Otherwise, the specimen should be collected by the nursing personnel. The nurse should be familiar with and also acquaint her staff with any special techniques that are required to preserve stools for special examinations. For example, a specimen to be examined for amebas must be kept warm and taken immediately to the laboratory for examination. It can be kept warm by placing the specimen box in a pan of warm water or on a hot-water bottle. If an enema must be given to collect a stool specimen, it is important that plain tap water or normal saline solution be used, since soaps or hypertonic solutions may change the consistency of the stool and alter its abnormal contents. If the stool is to be examined for occult (hidden) blood, red meat is eliminated from the diet for twenty-four hours before the specimen is collected; the reason for this should be explained to the patient.

GASTRIC AND INTESTINAL DECOMPRESSION

Decompression of the stomach. Decompression or emptying of the stomach is accomplished by attaching a suction apparatus to the gastric tube. This procedure is used to drain stomach contents. It may be used after gastric surgery to prevent distention of the stomach due to postoperative edema around the suture line. It may also be used to prevent and to treat postoperative vomiting and distention caused by the lessening of peristalsis following anesthesia or following manipulation of the viscera during surgery. In pyloric obstruction it is used to relieve dilatation of the stomach, and in gastric hemorrhage it may be used so that the blood loss can be accurately measured and replaced. When a gastric tube is to be used to keep the stomach deflated postoperatively, it usually is inserted before the patient goes to the operating room, since it is easier to pass at that time.

The length of time that the tube remains in the stomach depends on the reason for its use and the doctor's opinion about the physiologic effects of intubation on electrolyte balance and the psychologic effects upon the patient. It may be left until normal peristalsis returns postoperatively (about forty-eight to seventy-two hours); it may be removed soon after surgery and reinserted only if distention or vomiting occur; or it may be removed and reinserted once or twice a day to aspirate the stomach. When the gastric tube is used in the treatment of pyloric or intestinal obstruction, it usually is left in place until the obstruction is relieved. The gastric tube used in conjunction with gastric or esophageal surgery is carefully placed by the surgeon during the operation so that it does not intrude upon the suture line. The nurse should never maneuver this tube; if there is some question about its position or function, the surgeon should be consulted. If the tube is inadvertently removed or pulled out by the patient, the doctor may decide not to reinsert it because of the danger of perforating or otherwise injuring the anastomosis.

The need for continuous intubation should be explained to both the patient and his family. If the purpose of the tube is not fully understood, its use causes apprehension and fear. Acceptance by the patient usually facilitates passage of the tube, and there is less possibility that he will pull it out. The presence of the tube in the nasopharynx soon causes local discomfort, and the patient may complain of a lump in his throat, difficulty in swallowing, a sore throat, hoarseness, earache, or irritation of the nostril. He may also expectorate and blow his nose often because the irritation of the tube causes an increase in mucous secretions. Many patients report that discomfort from the tube far exceeds that from the incision. The nurse can help to lessen this discomfort. The tube should be secured so that there is no pressure against the nostril. Excess secretions from around the nares should be removed, and a water-soluble lubricant such as K-Y jelly should be applied to the tube and to the nostril to prevent crusting of secretions. When the tube is in the nostril, the patient tends to breathe through his mouth, and his lips and tongue may become dry and cracked. Frequent mouth rinses and the application of petroleum jelly or cold cream to the lips help prevent this. Fluids usually are restricted, but the patient may be permitted to chew gum to increase salivation or to suck small pieces of ice. Warm saline solution gargles may relieve dryness and soreness of the throat, and the physician may order steam inhalations or throat lozenges. He also may spray the throat with a local anesthetic such as Pontocaine. Frequent changing of the patient's position helps to relieve pressure from the tube on any one area in the throat. The patient often is inclined to be tense and rigid when the tube is in place. The nurse should assist him with turning and physical care, showing him how much activity is possible without displacing the tube. Sedative medication, if ordered, should be given to the patient who is seriously disturbed by the tube.

Gastric tubes usually are attached to a suction apparatus to provide drainage, since the contents must flow against gravity. The nurse should understand how the suction apparatus functions. Before the gastric tube is attached, the nurse checks the suction apparatus to be sure that it is working properly. Various types of apparatus may be used; regardless of the type, if, after it has been assembled and turned on, it will draw up water from a container, it can be assumed that it is working properly. The tubing from the suction apparatus is then connected by a connecting tube to the gastric tube, permitting observation of the fluid being removed from the stomach. A clamp or pin should be used to support the weight of the excess drainage tubing so that tension is not placed on the gastric tube. Sufficient tubing should be attached so that the patient can turn freely, and the pin or clamp used to secure the tubing to the bed should be placed so as not to obstruct the drainage or inhibit movement of the patient.

Mechanical failure of the suction apparatus or blockage of the drainage tubing or of the gastric tube itself may stop the suction, impeding drainage and causing distention, discomfort, and sometimes vomiting. The apparatus should be checked frequently to obviate this possibility. The physician may wish the gastric tube irrigated with small amounts (30 ml.) of normal saline solution at specified intervals to keep the lumen of the tube open and free from plugs of mucus or clots of blood. After the fluid is inserted into the tube, it should be aspirated, if possible. The amount of fluid inserted and withdrawn from the tube should be accurately recorded. Fluid that is instilled but not immediately withdrawn will be removed by suction, and, if the irrigating fluid is not taken into consideration, the measurement of the total gastric drainage will be inaccurate. If the fluid does not flow easily into the tube or if it does not return at irrigation, the physician should be consulted.

When continuous gastric suction is used, the gastric secretions collected in the drainage bottle should be measured every twenty-four hours, since the total amount of fluid and the electrolytes lost through drainage must be replaced by intravenous infusions. It is the responsibility of the nurse to see that the drainage is collected and measured and that there is a record of all fluid intake and output.

Decompression of the intestinal tract. Decompression or deflation of the intestinal tract can be accomplished by attaching an intestinal tube to a suction apparatus. This procedure is used to drain fluids and gas which accumulate above the mechanical intestinal obstruction, to deflate the intestines during paralytic ileus, and to deflate the bowel before or after intestinal surgery.

The tubes most often used for intestinal decompression are the Miller-Abbott tube and the Cantor tube. The length of these tubes permits their passage through the entire intestinal tract. There is a small balloon on the tip of each, which, when inflated with air or injected with mercury, acts like a bolus of food. This balloon stimulates peristalsis, which advances it along the intestinal tract. If peristalsis is absent, the weight of the mercury in the balloon will usually carry it forward.

The choice of tube depends on the preference of the physician. The Miller-Abbott tube is a tube within a tube. One tube leads to the balloon and the other to the "eyes" along its course, permitting drainage of intestinal contents and irrigation. The end of the tube extending from the patient's mouth or nostril contains a metal adapter with two openings—one for drainage of secretions and the other for inflating the balloon. (See Figure 82.) In irrigating this tube, the nurse must be careful that the correct opening is used; it is the one marked "suction." The other opening is for use by the doctor for inflating or deflating the balloon; it should be clamped off and labeled "do not touch."

The Cantor tube is a single tube. It has only one opening which is used for both irrigation and for drainage. Before the tube is inserted, the balloon is injected with mercury with a needle and syringe. The needle opening is so small that the globules of mercury cannot escape through it. The mercury can be pushed about so that the balloon is elongated for easy insertion.

Intestinal tubes are passed in the manner described under gastric analysis. The addition of the balloon on the tip of the tube makes its insertion through the nose most uncomfortable for the patient. The tube can be mechanically inserted only into the stomach; the passage along the remainder of the gastrointestinal tract is dependent upon gravity and peristalsis. After the tube reaches the stomach, its passage through the pylorus and into the duodenum can be facilitated in many ways. The mercury in the balloon helps propel the tube through the intestines. Position and activity aid in its passage. After passage of the tube, the patient is usually encouraged to lie on his right side for two hours, on his back in a Fowler's position for two hours, and then on his left side for two hours. Passage of the tube through the pylorus is usually ascertained by x-ray or fluoroscopic examination. After the tube has passed the pylorus, the patient may be encouraged to walk about to increase peristalsis and to speed the advancement of the tube through the intestines with the help of gravity. During this time the doctor or the nurse advances the tube 7 to 10 cm. (3 to 4 inches) through the nose or mouth at specified intervals. The intestinal tube should not be secured to the face until it has reached the desired point in the intestines, since taping the tube will pre-

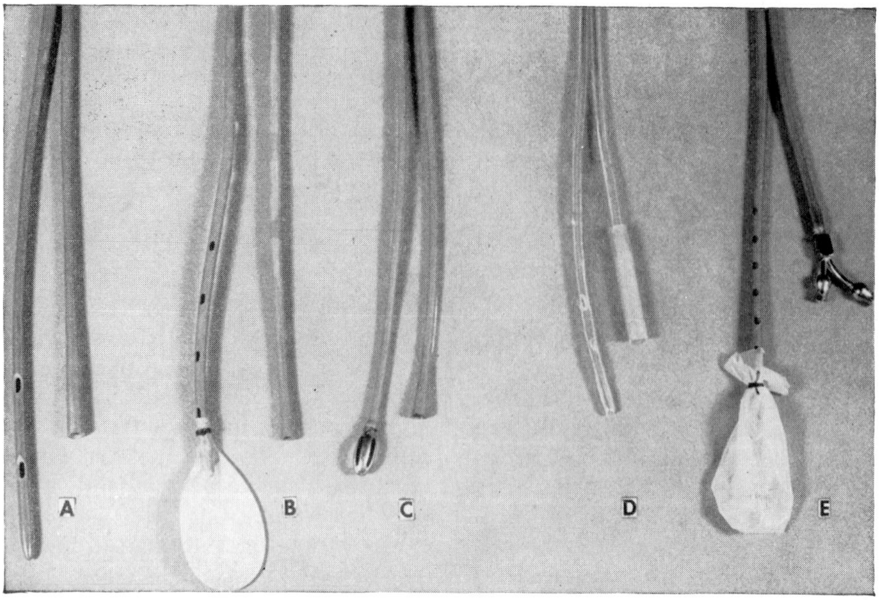

Figure 82

This picture shows the tips and the ends to be attached to suction for the various types of tubes used for gastrointestinal intubation. *A,* Rubber stomach tube. *B,* Cantor tube. *C,* Rehfuss tube for duodenal drainage. *D,* Plastic gastric tube. *E,* Miller-Abbott tube.

vent it from advancing with peristalsis. Excess tubing should be coiled on the bed.

Decompression is accomplished by attaching a suction apparatus to the tube either as the tube advances or after it has reached the obstructed portion of the bowel. Drainage should be measured every twenty-four hours, and the fluid and electrolytes lost are replaced by the parenteral route. If the tip of the tube is far down in the intestine and if the patient is not vomiting, the doctor may allow him to eat light foods such as soups, custards, Jell-o, or milk since they can be absorbed in the upper part of the small intestine. The doctor may wish the tube irrigated at intervals with normal saline solution or tap water to check its patency. Because the fluid has a longer distance to travel than that used in irrigating a gastric tube, it is difficult to aspirate the solution used. The nurse should record the amount instilled into the tube; if she is able to aspirate the fluid, this also should be recorded.

The intestinal tube is usually left in the intestine longer than the gastric tube remains in the stomach. It is often left in for from four to six days after intestinal surgery, depending upon the amount of edema around the anastomosis and the return of peristalsis. In most cases of intestinal obstruction, it must be left in for from seven to ten days, but this depends upon the disease and the patient's response to treatment. Nasal and pharyngeal discomfort usually is pronounced, and the nursing measures described under gastric intubation should be employed. Signs of the return of peristalsis and the reduction of edema, such as the passage of gas by rectum or a spontaneous bowel movement, should be reported to the physician since they usually indicate that the tube is no longer needed.

The intestinal tube is always removed gradually, several centimeters at a time.

Some resistance may be felt as it is withdrawn because of the pull against peristalsis. The patient may feel a tugging sensation and become nauseated. When the tip of the tube reaches the posterior nasopharynx, it is brought out through the mouth so that the balloon and mercury can be removed. The tube is then pulled through the nose. Since the tube usually has a fecal odor and may cause nausea, the patient should be given mouth care as soon as it is removed. For several days after removal of an intestinal tube, the patient's throat may be sore and he may be hoarse. Gargles, lozenges, and steam inhalations should be continued until these symptoms subside.

Occasionally the balloon of an intestinal tube may extrude from the anus. If this occurs, the upper end of the tube is usually cut off and the tube removed through the rectum. This is usually done slowly with the help of peristaltic action.

The patient with disease of the upper gastrointestinal system

The following discussion considers the more common diseases of the upper gastrointestinal system as well as specific medical treatment and related nursing care.

ESOPHAGEAL DISORDERS

Achalasia (cardiospasm)

Achalasia of the esophagus is a condition in which there is a narrowing of the muscular layer of the lower end of the esophagus, causing the portion of the esophagus above the constriction to be dilated and its muscular walls to be hypertrophied. The dilated area becomes atonic, and esophageal peristalsis may be absent so that little or no food can pass into the stomach. While varying degrees of the condition exist, in extreme cases the esophagus above the constriction may hold a quart or more of fluid. The cause of this disease is unknown, but it is the direct result of complete disruption of the normal neuromuscular mechanism of the esophagus. Anxiety and tension seem to aggravate the symptoms and bring on exacerbations. It may occur at any age, but it causes most distress among adults.

The patient may first complain of substernal fullness following the hasty ingestion of bulky or cold foods. Later he may have to make a determined, conscious effort to pass food beyond the constricted area. As the condition progresses, vomiting occurs. The older patient may aspirate stagnant esophageal contents into the trachea or bronchi during sleep, and atelectasis or pneumonia may develop. The diagnosis is confirmed by roentgenograms taken as the patient swallows barium and by esophagoscopy.

If the constriction is not severe, the patient usually is advised to eat a bland diet, avoiding bulky foods. Meals should be eaten slowly, and drinking fluids with meals helps the food to pass through the narrowed opening. Frequent changes of position during eating may also help. The patient should sleep with his head elevated to avoid the possibility of aspiration of esophageal residue.

If food will not pass through the opening, the periodic passage of a *bougie* (a flexible silk-woven dilator) through the constricted area may be necessary. If this must be done daily, the doctor teaches the patient to pass it himself. The bougie is lubricated with a water-soluble substance such as K-Y jelly and then passed through the mouth into the esophagus. Surgery for achalasia consists of making a longitudinal incision in the outer muscle layer of the esophagus at the site of the stricture, thus permitting the mucosa to expand so that food can pass more easily (esophagomyotomy). The surgery is usually done through an upper abdominal midline incision. Postoperatively, the nursing care is the same as the routine care given any patient who has had abdominal surgery. Only the outer layers of the esophagus have been incised so that there is no danger of esophageal leakage contaminating the mediastinum.

Esophageal diverticula

A *pulsion diverticulum* is the bulging of the esophageal mucosa and submucosa through a weakened portion of the muscular layer of the esophagus. It is most often located at the pharyngoesophageal junction or in the lower end of the thoracic esophagus. As food is ingested, some of it may pass into the diverticulum; after a sufficient amount has accumulated in the pocket, it overflows into the esophagus and is regurgitated. There is always danger that some of the regurgitated material may be aspirated into the trachea and lungs. The patient may complain of pain on swallowing, of gurgling noises in the area, and of a cough due to tracheal irritation. He usually has a foul odor of the breath caused by decomposition of food in the diverticulum. This can be alleviated somewhat by frequent brushing of the teeth and the use of aromatic mouthwashes.

If the symptoms become severe, surgery is performed. Through a supraclavicular incision for a pharyngoesophageal diverticulum and through a transthoracic incision for a lower esophageal diverticulum, the herniated sac is excised and the resultant esophageal opening closed. These procedures are well tolerated, and the administration of antibiotics makes postoperative infections rare. If a supraclavicular approach has been used, fluids are usually permitted as soon as nausea subsides, and a bland diet is given soon afterward. If a transthoracic approach is used, chest drainage may be used, and the patient usually is not allowed to take fluids for several days.

A *traction diverticulum* is a lateral outpocketing of the esophagus caused by an inflammatory process (usually tubercular lymphadenitis) in the mediastinum and the esophageal wall. As healing occurs, scar tissue may cause the wall of the esophagus to become adherent to an adjacent lymph node, forming a diverticulum. This process usually occurs at the middle third of the esophagus. These diverticula do not produce symptoms and rarely require treatment.

Chemical burns

Destruction of the mucosa of the esophagus following the deliberate or accidental swallowing of caustic materials such as lye may cause serious strictures since the mucosa heals with scar tissue. Often these strictures are so severe that no food can pass into the stomach. The patient has excruciating pain after swallowing the caustic, and he usually goes into shock. Immediate neutralization of the swallowed fluid should be attempted, and treatment for pain and shock is begun at once. Unfortunately many of the patients are small children who suffer from the effects of such an accident for the remainder of their lives. (For details concerning prevention and emergency treatment, see Chapter 15.)

Although the patient may be able to swallow fluid for a while after the accident, strictures develop as healing occurs. Careful attempts are made to dilate the stricture by passing bougies; usually this is done under the fluoroscope so that danger of causing damage which would result in further stricture is lessened.[24] If the destruction of the esophageal mucosa is extensive, a *gastrostomy* (permanent opening into the stomach) may be performed. Braided silk thread is then inserted through the esophagus into the stomach and brought out the gastrostomy opening. The two ends of the thread are tied together to form a complete loop, and the thread is used for pulling bougies or beads through the esophagus to dilate it and to prevent complete closure of the lumen. Such treatment may be necessary for months after the ingestion of the caustics. Care of the patient with a gastrostomy is discussed later.

Tumors

The most common obstructive lesion of the esophagus is carcinoma. Malignancies of the esophagus account for 27,000

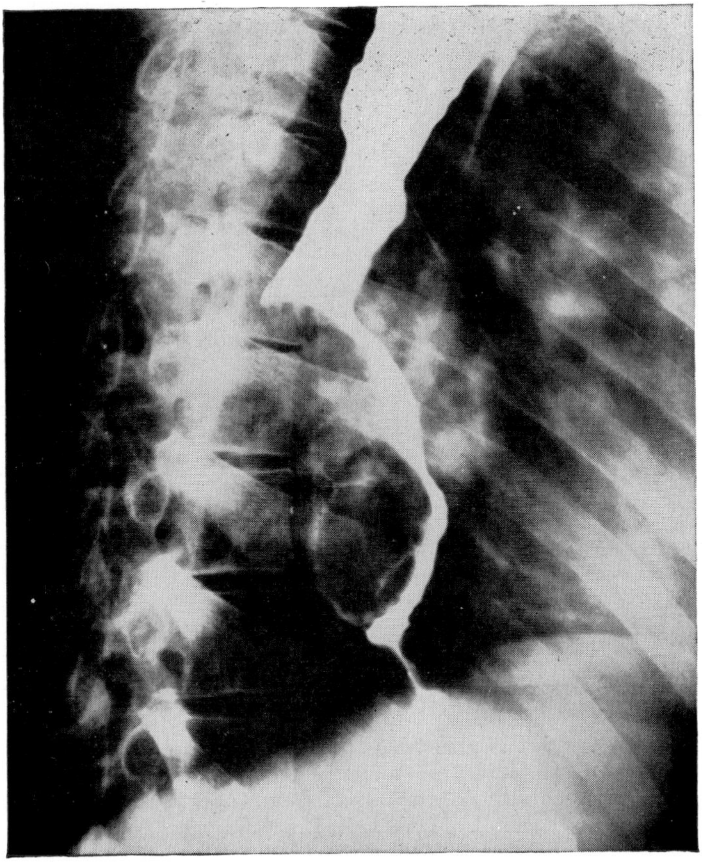

Figure 83

This roentgenogram, taken after the patient has swallowed barium, shows the location of a lesion in the esophagus as it approaches the stomach.

deaths each year.[11] The tumor may develop in any portion of the esophagus, but it is most common in the middle third.

The only possible hope for successful treatment lies in very early diagnosis and surgical treatment. The nurse should urge any patient who has difficulty in swallowing, no matter how trivial it may seem, to seek medical advice at once. This applies particularly to those over 40 years of age since cancer of the esophagus occurs more often in those in middle and later life than in younger persons.

The patient who has cancer of the esophagus initially complains only of mild and intermittent dysphagia. Gradually he finds it extremely difficult to swallow solid food, and by the time he seeks medical attention he often has resorted to strained foods and liquids. He may regurgitate after eating and has gradual weight loss. Pain in the back may indicate that the growth has extended into surrounding structures. Unfortunately, even if the patient reports to a doctor when the first symptoms appear, the disease is often already well established, has metastasized, and is incurable. Diagnosis is made by roentgenograms of the esophagus taken as the patient swallows barium (see Figure 83) and by esophagoscopy.

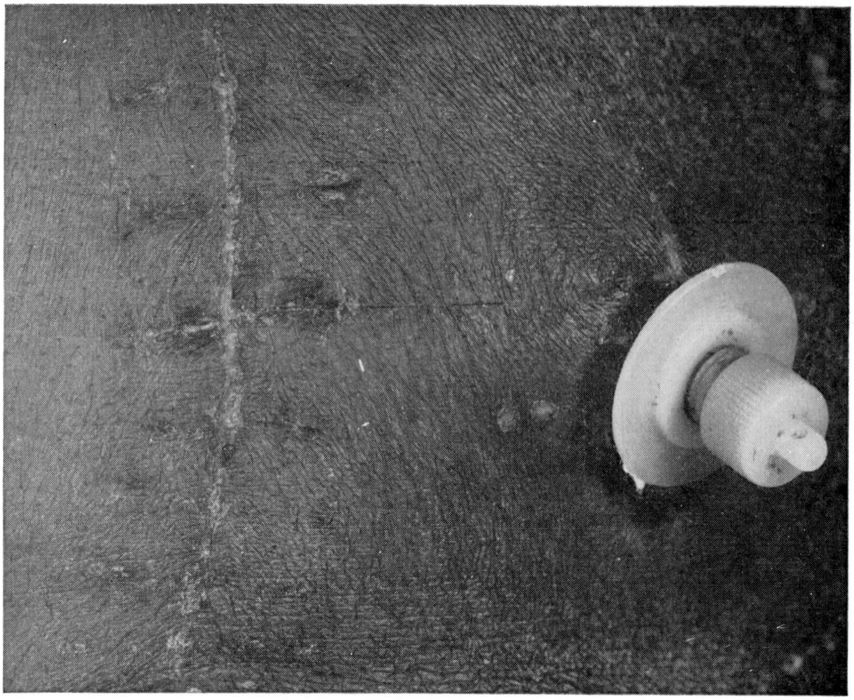

Figure 84

The Barnes-Redo button is sutured into the gastrostomy opening.
The cap can be unscrewed easily for tube feedings. (Courtesy Dr. William Barnes and Dr. Frank Redo, The New York Hospital-Cornell Medical Center, New York, N. Y.)

Treatment for cancer of the esophagus is surgical. If the lesion has been diagnosed too late and cannot be entirely removed, surgery may be palliative to permit the patient to eat normally or to provide artificial means of getting food to the stomach. If possible, an *esophagectomy* is done; the tumor is widely excised and the adjacent lymph nodes are dissected. This is done though a thoracoabdominal incision, and, as in other surgery in which the chest cavity is entered, endotracheal anesthesia is used. The anastomosis of the free end of the esophagus after resection requires bringing the stomach up into the thoracic cavity. If the growth is located in the lower third of the esophagus, a portion of the cardiac end of the stomach may be removed because of its anatomic proximity to the lesion; this procedure also requires bringing the stomach up into the chest cavity and is called an *esophagogastrostomy*. A more recent procedure involves removal of the esophageal lesion and anastomosis of the jejunum to the proximal esophageal segment. The jejunum is brought to the proximal portion of the esophagus through a tunnel which is easily made in the loose tissue lying just beneath the sternum.

If the patient cannot tolerate major surgery, a *gastrostomy* may be performed. This is usually done under local anesthesia. An opening is made into the stomach through a small upper left abdominal incision. The anterior wall of the stomach is exposed, drawn forward, and sutured to the anterior abdominal wall about the incision; this prevents stomach contents from entering the abdominal cavity. A small incision is then made into the stomach and a No. 20 or No. 22 Fr.

catheter is inserted into it. The opening is sutured tightly around the catheter so that leakage of stomach contents cannot occur. Food can then be introduced directly into the stomach. Instead of a catheter a special button (Barnes-Redo) may be sutured into the opening (see Figure 84). When feedings are to be given, the cap of the button is removed and a catheter is introduced.

Nursing care of the patient having an esophagectomy or an esophagogastrostomy

Preoperative care. Because the nutritional status of most patients with esophageal cancer is poor, an attempt is made preoperatively to restore normal nutrition and to re-establish normal fluid and electrolyte balance. Fluids, electrolytes, and vitamins usually are prescribed to be given intravenously. An accurate record of the intake and output should be kept since this information is important in ordering fluids to be given parenterally. If food and fluids can be taken by mouth, they should be high in protein and in total calories. Occasionally a temporary gastrostomy may be done to supply food preoperatively; it is closed a few weeks after the esophageal resection if this operation has been successful in re-establishing a communication between the esophagus and the stomach.

The patient with esophageal cancer requires special skin care to prevent decubiti. Protection of bony prominences, frequent massage of dependent parts of the body, and frequent change of position are necessary. Because of weakness, malaise, and depression, the patient may forget to change position as often as necessary unless he is reminded to do so. Since the breath may be foul, special mouth care should be given. The patient may be raising a mixture of pus, blood, and decomposed food. He must be assured privacy when he is attempting to clear his throat and particularly when he is attempting to get food and fluids past the obstruction. The emesis basins should be changed often and a cover should be provided. Mouthwashes, including Dobell's solution, hydrogen peroxide (1 per cent), and solutions containing chlorine such as Clorox, are useful in controlling odors and in making the mouth feel fresher. Mouthwashes should be offered the patient before he attempts to take food. They should be varied from time to time unless the patient has one he prefers. Sometimes the flavor of the solution becomes identified with the unpleasant throat secretions and becomes almost as distasteful as the secretions.

Preoperative teaching should include instructions for the patient about chest drainage, coughing and turning after the operation, postoperative exercises, restriction of fluids by mouth, oxygen, frequent observation of his pulse, blood pressure and color, intravenous injections, and the tube he will have through his nose into his stomach. This teaching is described in detail in the chapters concerned with preoperative care of the general surgical patient and the patient undergoing chest surgery (Chapters 12 and 23). The stomach tube is usually inserted immediately preoperatively provided the esophagus is not completely obstructed.

Postoperative care. The immediate postoperative care for the patient who has had esophageal surgery centers about the maintenance of an airway, observation for circulatory or respiratory difficulties, protection from injury, care of the chest drainage system, and care of the stomach tube (as described earlier in this chapter).

Small amounts of bright red blood may drain from the stomach tube for a short time (six to twelve hours); the color of the drainage should then become greenish-yellow. Because esophageal tissue is very friable and because the anastomosis may be under tension, the tube is usually left in until complete healing of the esophageal anastomosis has occurred. If the tube is removed, fluids by mouth are not permitted for several days. Intravenous fluids are given to meet fluid, electrolyte, and caloric needs. When fluids are permitted by mouth, a small amount of water (30 to 60 ml.) is given hourly, and the patient is observed for signs of leakage of fluid into the mediastinum. Signs and symptoms of such a complication are a rise in temperature and difficulty in breathing. If no untoward symptoms occur, feedings are introduced and gradually increased until the patient is receiving several small meals of bland food daily. If the stomach has been brought up into the chest cavity, the patient may complain of a feeling of fullness in the chest after eating or he may have some breathing difficulty. If this happens, serving smaller more frequent meals may help.

When the cardia of the stomach has been removed, some patients complain of nausea and vomiting. This is usually caused by irritation of the esophageal mucosa by the gastric juices. After this operation (resection of lower esophagus and cardia of stomach), the gastric secretions can readily flow into the esophagus when the patient lies flat; he should be advised to elevate his head and shoulders on pillows when he lies down.

Resumption of activity must be gradual. Since surgery for cancer of the esophagus is extensive, the patient may require several months of convalescence. In addition, since the malignant lesion is seldom completely removed, only a small percentage of patients live more than five years after the operation, and many are chronic invalids during that time. The doctor usually informs the family of the patient's prognosis, and sometimes the patient is also told. Both the patient and his family should be told of the need for close medical supervision. Upper respiratory infections should be carefully avoided and medical help sought at once if signs of even minor indisposition occur. Usually it is advised that the patient and his family be referred to the social service department while the patient is in the hospital; this establishes a relationship which may be useful to the family at a later time when institutional care may become necessary.

Many patients with cancer of the esophagus receive terminal care at home and are cared for by a public health nurse and by members of the family under the nurse's supervision. The patient and his family should always be asked if they would like to have a nurse visit the patient in his home; occasionally the nurse also helps the family to prepare for the patient's return home. The nurse who goes into the home can often give helpful suggestions regarding the preparation of suitable food, care of the mouth, rest, and prevention of accidents. (See Chapter 16 for care of the terminally ill cancer patient and Chapter 4 for description of home-care programs.)

Some patients with cancer of the esophagus are not found to be suitable candidates for esophageal surgery. Their skin care, mouth care, and nutrition are similar to that described for the patient having surgery.

Nursing care of the patient who has a gastrostomy

It is usually very hard for the patient to accept the need for gastrostomy. This is probably partly because of the deep psychologic significance of food and of eating. After a long period of vomiting, discomfort, and inability to eat, however, the patient may become so debilitated that both he and his family are willing for the operation to be done.

After a gastrostomy the catheter is secured to the abdominal wall by a suture or adhesive tape to prevent its slipping out. A clamp is applied to the end of the catheter to prevent leakage of gastric secretions onto the skin. A small dressing covers the incision, and there should be very little bloody drainage postoperatively.

The skin around the gastrostomy should be inspected frequently, since, if there is leakage of gastric secretions around the tube, the skin will become irritated and excoriated from the action of the digestive enzymes. The skin should be kept clean with frequent use of soap and water, dry, and a protective ointment such as zinc oxide and a dressing of oiled silk and gauze may be applied around the tube (see Figure 44). After from ten days to two weeks the tube may be removed and reinserted only for feedings. The patient is taught to do this himself. The tube is kept clean by washing it with soap and water after each feeding. It is inserted 10 to 15 cm. (4 to 6 inches). To prevent leakage of secretions onto the skin between feedings, a finger cot plugged with cotton may be inserted into the opening. The finger cot must be attached to the skin with adhesive tape to prevent its being drawn into the stomach. Special buttons are also available to use as a plug for the opening (see Figure 84). There is less likelihood of leakage if the patient lies flat for a short time after the feeding and if the feedings are not too large.

Soon after the operation, fluid nourishment may be given through the catheter. The initial feeding, consisting of a small amount of tap water or glucose in water, is usually given by the surgeon. Fluids are given every four hours at first. If there is no leakage of fluid around the tube and if the patient appears to tolerate the clear fluids, foods may be added until a full diet is eventually given through the tube. The tube feeding should be warmed to room or body temperature before it is given and diluted if it is too thick. The feeding should be given with screens drawn about the patient for privacy if he does not occupy a single room. A funnel or glass syringe is used to introduce the liquid into the catheter. Before the feeding is given, a small amount of water should be introduced through the tube to make sure it is patent. The fluid should flow in by gravity. Sometimes a small amount of pressure from the bulb of the Asepto or barrel of the glass syringe is necessary to pass thicker fluids through the tube. The usual amount of each feeding is 200 to 500 ml. and should take ten to fifteen minutes to flow through the tube. If the patient feels "full" or nauseated, feedings may be decreased in amount and their frequency increased. A small amount of water is instilled to cleanse the tube at the end of the feeding.

The feedings may be a special formula or regular food blended so that it will pass through the tube. The use of regular foods helps maintain the patient's nutritional needs, prevents diarrhea that often accompanies the use of specially prepared tube feedings that are high in fat, and makes it easier for the patient and his family to prepare his food at home. Food that is normally cooked should be cooked until it is soft and the juices from cooking should be included since they contain essential vitamins and minerals. Solid and liquid foods are blended into a mixture with a food blender, fork, potato masher, or egg beater and are strained. Water should be given through the tube between feedings so that approximately 2,500 to 3,500 ml. are received daily. If diarrhea occurs from the feedings, camphorated tincture of opium (paregoric) may be ordered and given with the feeding.

The patient should see, smell, taste, and chew small amounts of food before taking his feeding since this will stimulate the flow of gastric secretions and may give him some of the satisfaction of normal eating. It is sometimes recommended that the patient chew his food normally and then deposit it into a funnel attached to the gastrostomy tube. If he can accept this sensible although somewhat unesthetic procedure, it is unquestionably beneficial because saliva is mixed with the food. The teeth and mouth also maintain better health when this is done. Privacy must, of course, be assured the patient who takes his meals in this way.

If the patient is not upset by sitting down to meals with his family when he cannot eat, he should be encouraged to do so since this socializing usually helps his digestion and is good for his morale.

The psychologic trauma of not being able to eat normally is usually severe. The patient may become depressed, and he needs a great deal of encouragement. Most patients, however, as they become proficient in feeding themselves, gradually accept this method of obtaining nourishment as inevitable and adjust remarkably well.

Both the patient and his family should learn how to care for the skin and the tube and how to prepare the liquid meals as well as how to insert the tube and instill the nourishment through it. They should be told of the need for close medical supervision, and they should be encouraged to consult the doctor, the nurse, or the dietitian when problems arise. It may be desirable for a public health nurse to visit the patient at home to supervise the initial preparation of food and giving of the feeding and to answer any other questions in regard to the patient's care.

GASTRIC DISORDERS

Gastritis

Gastritis is an inflammation of the gastric mucosa and is the most common pathologic condition of the stomach. It may be acute or chronic.

Acute gastritis follows the ingestion of large amounts of alcohol, of food contaminated with *Staphylococcus aureus,* and of certain drugs. The gastric mucosa is red and congested, and sometimes there is white purulent exudate from the inflamed surfaces and evidence of abrasion. The patient complains of epigastric discomfort, nausea, vomiting, and diarrhea. While the disease is of short duration, the patient is usually weakened and occasionally prostrated because of the loss of fluids and the exertion of vomiting and wretching. In severe cases parenteral fluids may be given. Medications that decrease peristalsis such as methantheline bromide (Banthine) and camphorated tincture of opium (paregoric) may be prescribed. Bismuth preparations may also be given to coat the irritated intestinal mucosa if diarrhea is severe. When food can be tolerated, tea, toast, Jell-o, and similar bland foods are given until a regular diet can be tolerated.

Chronic gastritis is diagnosed only after tests and examinations have eliminated the possibility of other gastric diseases. The patient usually gives a history of prolonged dietary indiscretions such as eating large amounts of very hot spicy foods or drinking alcoholic beverages excessively. Symptoms may range from chronic gastric distress to massive gastric hemorrhage. The mucosa of the stomach may be red and edematous and may be covered with thin gray or green patches, and the gastric blood vessels may be visible through the mucosa. The patient is placed on a bland diet, given antacids such as Gelusil, and instructed to avoid foods and situations which have brought on symptoms in the past.

Peptic ulcer

A peptic ulcer is a loss of tissue caused by the digestive action of the gastric juices on the mucosa of the distal esophagus, the stomach, the duodenum, or the jejunum (following gastroenterostomy). It is estimated that one out of every ten persons has suffered from this condition at some time in his life.[10] The incidence of peptic ulcers has increased all over the world since 1900.[10] At the present time in the United States 10,000 persons die from the complications of peptic ulcers each year.[11] Men are four times more likely to have peptic ulcers than are women. While a peptic ulcer can occur at any age, it occurs more often in young adults and in middle-aged persons than in the very young or the aged.

The cause of peptic ulcer is not known, but it is believed that there are three factors which greatly influence its development: a source of irritation, such as an increase of hydrochloric acid with a decrease of alkaline mucus secreted by the surface cells; a breakdown of the local tissue resistance and defense mechanisms; and the influences of heredity, hormones, and personality. The hormones appear to have some effect on ulcer formation since ulcers are more prevalent in men than in women. Patients who have received long courses of corticotrophin or cortisone therapy have developed peptic ulcers, and it is thought that adrenal hyperfunction plays some part in ulcer formation. There is a tendency for ulcers to run in families. It has been demonstrated that emotional factors influence the function of the stomach and cause changes in the gastric mucosa. Persons who are under continuous pressure and who are nervous,

anastomosis - joint of two organs

tense, and unhappy may develop peptic ulcers.

Acute ulcers are usually superficial, and they occur following infections, neurologic trauma, or stress. They usually heal, but they may bleed, perforate, or become chronic.

A chronic peptic ulcer is a deep crater with sharp edges and a "clean" base. It involves both the mucosa and the submucosa. If the ulcer penetrates the stomach wall and becomes adherent to an adjacent organ or structure without communication with the abdominal cavity, these structures may become the base of the ulcer.

Peptic ulcers are described as gastric or duodenal, depending upon their location. An ulcer of the jejunum occurring near the site of anastomosis is termed a marginal ulcer. Eighty-five per cent of all gastric ulcers occur on the lesser curvature of the stomach.[11] Such ulcers tend to be larger and deeper than duodenal ulcers and they have a tendency to undergo malignant changes.

Duodenal ulcers are not so well defined as gastric ulcers, but the pathology is the same. The diameter is usually 2 to 10 mm. in contrast to 5 to 25 mm. for gastric ulcers, and the depth is usually 2 to 6 mm. in contrast to 10 to 20 mm. for gastric ulcers.[10] Most of them (95 per cent) occur on the first 3 cm. of the duodenum, either on its anterior or posterior wall.[11]

The patient who has a peptic ulcer usually complains of pain which is characteristic in its nature, intensity, radiation, location, and periodicity. The attacks of pain often occur in the spring and the fall, last for a few weeks, and then disappear. Each succeeding attack is more severe and more prolonged than the preceding one. The pain is described as gnawing, aching, or burning. It is usually located in the upper abdomen, near the midline, and it is confined to a small area. However, it may radiate around the costal border or through to the back. Pain from a duodenal ulcer is usually located in the right epigastric area, while that from a gastric ulcer is usually located in the left epigastric area. Pain usually starts one or two hours after eating, when the stomach begins to empty, and it may disappear spontaneously or after the ingestion of food or upon ingestion of an antacid medication such as Gelusil. If the ulcer is severe, it may cause pain at night. Although pain is felt at the site of the existing lesion, it is known that normal stomach mucosa does not have pain sensation. It is thought, therefore, that the inflamed mucosa around the ulcer must be sensitive to the gastric secretions because inflammation lowers the pain threshhold.[10] Eructation is common in peptic ulcer but differs from that occurring in gallbladder disease in that it occurs more often when the stomach is empty and does not follow the ingestion of fatty foods. If edema around the lesion obstructs the pylorus, gastric retention, with dilatation of the stomach, nausea, and vomiting, may occur. This, however, is not a common symptom of peptic ulcer.

The diagnosis of peptic ulcer is made from the patient's history, a gastrointestinal series, a gastric analysis, gastroscopy, and stool examinations for occult (hidden) blood.

Treatment is directed toward relief of symptoms, healing of the ulcer, and prevention of recurrence. The majority of peptic ulcers heal under medical treatment. Surgery is used in the treatment of complications; occasionally it is used when malignant degeneration is feared in chronic gastric ulcers of long standing.

Medical treatment and nursing care. Good ulcer management consists of rest and sedation, a bland diet, restriction of irritating substances such as coffee, alcohol, and tobacco, the use of antacids and anticholinergic medications, and an attempt to relieve undesirable emotional stimuli by medical counseling or psychotherapy. When the defect is covered with normal mucosa, the ulcer is considered healed. This may occur in a few weeks, or it may require months.

Rest. Because complete mental and physical rest are necessary for healing of a peptic ulcer, the patient is usually removed from the home environment if it is believed that this aggravates his condition. Hospitalization for a few weeks is usually recommended provided the financial burden does not increase the patient's worries. It may take the combined efforts of the physician, the nurse, the family, and the social worker to help the patient understand the need for complete rest and to secure his cooperation in achieving this. The patient should be on bed rest and in a section of the ward removed from activity and disturbing noise. Usually he is permitted visitors and is allowed to participate in activities which keep him interested and occupied but which do not involve physical or mental effort (such as playing games with other patients or watching television). The nurse can gain the confidence of the patient by giving thoughtful, intelligent nursing care, by explaining procedures, and by promptly attending to his needs. Although the patient may appear outwardly calm, his emotional make-up may make him react strongly to the slightest unfavorable stimulus. Foresight on the part of the nurse will prevent incidents from occurring which aggravate the patient. Nursing care that provides a regular, smooth routine is best for the patient. Feedings, medications, and treatments should be given at correctly spaced intervals and on time. Noise, rush, confusion, and impatience on the part of members of the staff should be avoided. The nurse should plan to spend time listening to the patient in an attempt to get clues to problems that should be relayed to the doctor.

When symptoms of peptic ulcer are severe and acute, large doses of sedatives such as phenobarbital and the tranquilizers may be given to help the patient rest. These may make him so drowsy that close supervision will be necessary to prevent circulatory and respiratory complications. He should be turned from side to side occasionally and encouraged to move his legs and arms and to take several deep breaths every one or two hours. Side rails should be placed on the bed of a heavily sedated patient to prevent falling and injury. The patient's skin should be inspected frequently for rashes that might indicate a toxic reaction to barbiturates.

Diet. The acid combining power of food proteins neutralizes the free hydrochloric acid secreted by the stomach. The ulcer then theoretically will heal since it is no longer constantly irritated by the gastric juices. The initial diet consists of the hourly ingestion of 90 ml. of milk and 90 ml. of cream; this combination supplies protein, and the fat in the cream slows passage from the stomach. Vitamins are usually ordered to make up for the vitamin deficiencies of this diet. Gradually small meals of cereal, soft-cooked eggs, white toast, creamed soups, and other bland foods are added until three meals are substituted for some of the liquid nourishment. The milk and cream mixture should still be taken between meals, however, and whenever necessary during the night. The patient should avoid foods which stimulate the flow of hydrochloric acid such as meat extracts, coffee, and tea, irritating foods such as raw fruits or vegetables, and chemical irritants such as spices.

Since the feedings are an essential part of the patient's treatment, the nurse must see that they are taken as prescribed. If the patient objects to the taste of milk and cream or tires of the sameness of his diet, small amounts of strawberry, malt, maple, or other flavoring may be added to the mixture. If the patient is acutely ill or has received much sedation, the responsibility for the hourly feedings must be assumed entirely by the nursing staff. If the patient is reliable and capable, a pitcher of milk and cream mixture may be left at his bedside so that he can take his own feedings. When this is done, it is important that the nurse not forget about the patient. The patient with a peptic ulcer needs attention as much as he needs food, and he benefits from a kindly inquiry from the nurse as to whether or not he has taken the feeding, whether there is enough of the mixture in the pitcher, and whether or not it is sufficiently cool. Many patients find that the feedings give them relief from discomfort and therefore anticipate a quick cure with such treatment. They are most upset if feedings are delayed. Since much of the patient's time is spent thinking about himself and his treatment and about the implications of his illness for his family, it is understandable that he becomes irritable when the schedule is not carefully adhered to.

It may be necessary to administer the milk and cream and the antacids by a continuous drip tube feeding so that the gastric secretions will be continuously neutralized. This type of feeding is also better for the patient who needs to be kept very quiet since it obviates disturbing him every half hour; this is particularly important during night hours. The gastric tube is passed in the manner described earlier in this chapter. A Kelly flask or an infusion bottle containing the milk and cream mixture and the antacids is connected by rubber or plastic tubing to the gastric tube. A screw clamp regulates the flow of solution through the tube. A prescribed amount of fluid is usually allowed to run into the stomach over a twenty-four hour period. This should include enough water to supply the patient's daily needs. To prevent the milk and cream from becoming sour, the nurse should keep only a small amount of the mixture in the bottle at any one time. The flask should be changed at least twice a day and should be washed and boiled before re-use.

Drugs. Drugs that are given to lower the acidity of the gastric secretions include calcium carbonate, magnesium carbonate, magnesium oxide, aluminum hydroxide gel (Amphojel), and magnesium trisilicate. These drugs reduce gastric acidity by physical absorption or by chemical neutralization. They are poorly absorbed from the stomach and, therefore, do not alter the pH of the blood or interfere with normal acid-base balance. When they are prescribed in the initial stages of treatment for an ulcer, they are given hourly. Because milk and cream is also given, a schedule is usually set up in which the milk and cream are given every hour on the hour and the antacids every hour on the half hour. In order to maintain this schedule, it is important that the patient be well instructed so that he can assume some responsibility for this regimen under close nursing supervision.

Since sodium bicarbonate is readily absorbed from the intestine into the blood stream, patients should be advised against taking this when gastric pain occurs. If large quantities are taken, the acid-base balance of the blood will be upset. Also, the reaction of sodium bicarbonate and hydrochloric acid forms carbon dioxide, and this may increase distress by causing distention.

Drugs used to decrease gastric motility are tincture of belladonna and propantheline bromide (Pro-Banthine). Tincture of belladonna has little effect upon the amount and character of gastric secretions, but it does decrease gastrointestinal motility, muscle tone, and peristalsis. Some relatively new antispasmodic drugs are Bentyl, Dactil, and Donnatal. Pro-Banthine decreases gastrointestinal motility, and it also diminishes the volume of gastric secretion. Patients receiving these drugs usually complain of a dry mouth. Pro-Banthine may also cause blurring of vision and urinary retention. The nurse should check the urinary output of patients receiving this drug, and untoward signs should be reported to the doctor. Other anticholinergic drugs are Antrenyl, Elorine, and Pathilon. These drugs are usually ordered to be given intramuscularly.

Patients who are on milk and cream diets or who are receiving drugs such as Amphojel and anticholinergic drugs often become constipated. The doctor may order a mild cathartic, but no cathartic should be taken without a doctor's order since it may increase gastrointestinal motility when this is undesirable.

Health teaching. To prevent exacerbations of an ulcer, the patient must learn to avoid those foods and those situations which tend to reactivate the ulcer. The doctor usually tries to ascertain what problems or pressures exist in the patient's home life or at work that bring about attacks of ulcer pain. If the patient cannot be removed from this environmental influence, he is encouraged to accept or to react less violently to the stress situation. He is encouraged to allow time for periods of rest and relaxation in his daily schedule. Occasionally the doctor may advise the patient to have psychotherapy so that he may understand his problems better and thus be more able to cope with them.

The patient should practice moderation in diet, work, and play. He should be aware that he has had an ulcer and that excesses may cause the ulcer to become reactivated.

The planning, preparation, and serving of food should be thoroughly discussed with the patient and his family, and cultural and religious preferences should be considered. Highly seasoned foods, very hot or cold food, fried foods, raw fruits and vegetables, coffee, and alcohol should be avoided. The patient should learn to eat slowly in a quiet environment, and he should try to avoid situations which cause emotional disturbance before and during meals. It is usually necessary for him to remain on a bland diet for at least a year. It is common for him to want to resume his former eating pattern as soon as pain disappears, but he should know that this may cause an immediate return of symptoms. The patient's work sometimes makes the selection of suitable meals difficult. If the selection of food is limited, the patient can take milk and cream with him in a vacuum bottle to supplement the limited selection. If the patient becomes emotionally upset by situations at work or at home, he should learn to eat a bland diet and to drink milk and cream between meals. This may prevent a serious exacerbation of the ulcer.

There seems to be a relationship between smoking and irritation of a peptic ulcer. Since this is so, most doctors believe that the patient who has a peptic ulcer should give up smoking permanently. This is often very difficult for the patient to do since often his life and work situation, as well as his personality make-up, is such that a change of this sort is a major one. The patient needs constant encouragement and understanding when he is endeavoring to give up smoking if the habit is well established.

For the successful treatment of an ulcer and the prevention of future exacerbations, the doctor must have the complete confidence of the patient. The nurse can often help to augment the patient's confidence in his doctor and in the prescribed treatment. She can also learn about doubts and worries of the patient and report these to the doctor so that reassurance or explanation may be given as needed. If every consideration is given to adjusting the prescribed regimen to fit the patient's physical, economic, and social pattern, he will be better able to follow the treatment. When plans are being made by the health team for the patient's discharge from the hospital, the patient and his family should be included. In this way existing problems can be discussed realistically in relation to future care.

The patient who has had a peptic ulcer must remain under medical supervision for about a year. He may have periodic x-ray examinations of the stomach to evaluate the healing of the ulcer. After that time, if healing is complete, he should be advised to report to his doctor at once if symptoms reappear since peptic ulcers can recur after the patient has enjoyed several years of good health.

Complications requiring surgery. When a peptic ulcer perforates and causes peritonitis, is unrelieved by medical treatment, is chronic and possibly precancerous, causes pyloric obstruction, or erodes a blood vessel causing severe hemorrhage, surgery is necessary. In some instances surgery is done as an emergency measure, but often it is elective.

Perforation. Acute perforation of a peptic ulcer is a surgical emergency and accounts for 65 to 85 per cent of the deaths from peptic ulcers.[10] After the perforation occurs, gastric contents pour into the peritoneal cavity, causing peritonitis. Both gastric and duodenal ulcers may perforate.

The patient who has a perforated ulcer has symptoms similar to those occurring when any abdominal organ or other part of the gastrointestinal tract perforates. He is seized with a sudden sharp pain that spreads quickly over the abdomen. Characteristically he bends over with pain; if in bed, he draws up his knees to prevent pull on the abdominal wall. He is reluctant to move, holds himself tense, and protests against having his abdomen touched. Upon palpation, the abdomen is found to be boardlike and very tender. The patient usually perspires profusely, and his facial expression is one of agony and apprehension. Since his breathing is rapid and shallow to prevent pull on abdominal muscles, he may be cyanotic. The temperature is usually elevated but may be normal or subnormal; the pulse is usually rapid and weak. A positive diagnosis is made by making a roentgenogram of the abdomen with the patient standing. If the ulcer has perforated, air under the diaphragm is visible on the film.

Any perforation of the alimentary tract should be closed surgically as soon as possible. The longer the perforation exists, allowing the irritating (and infected) gastrointestinal secretions to pour into the abdominal cavity, the higher the mortality rate becomes.[10]

Before operation for a perforated ulcer, a gastric tube is passed into the stomach and attached to a continuous suction apparatus to drain the gastric secretions. Parenteral fluids are given to maintain fluid balance, and antibiotics are administered. The patient is kept in a low Fowler's position so that the gastric contents that have escaped will collect in the pelvic cavity and will be more accessible surgically.

The operation used to close a perforation consists of suturing the hole and reinforcing the area with an omental graft; it is known as a *plicating* operation. The gastric contents that have escaped into the peritoneal cavity are aspirated by suction during the operation. A solution containing antibiotics may be placed in the abdominal cavity before the wound is closed.

Routine postoperative care is carried out as described in Chapter 14. As soon as the patient recovers from anesthesia, however, he is returned to a low Fowler's position. Large doses of antibiotics are given, and the gastric tube is left in place until peristalsis returns. Fluids are given parenterally, and antibiotics are often added to these. Drainage from the gastric tube is greenish-yellow, and there is usually no blood present. Nursing care for patients with gastric tubes in place is discussed earlier in this chapter.

Postoperatively the patient should be watched carefully for signs of continuing peritonitis and for abscess formation. Elevation of temperature, respiratory distress, continued abdominal pain, and signs of paralytic ileus, such as distention and the inability to pass flatus or stool, should be reported to the doctor. The doctor may also perform periodic rectal examinations to determine the presence of pelvic masses caused by abscess formation. Such an abscess may need to be incised and drained. The nurse should explain to the patient why the rectal examinations are necessary. (A full discussion of the complications of peritonitis is given later in this chapter.)

When the stomach tube is removed, the patient is given small amounts (30 to 60 ml.) of clear fluid by mouth each hour. If this is well tolerated, he is usually given 90 ml. of milk and cream every hour and, after two or three days, a bland diet with in-between feedings of milk and cream. Most patients are discharged from the hospital on a medical regimen for ulcers. The nurse should review this regimen carefully with the patient who has never had this treatment and with the patient who previously has been on this regimen.

Chronic peptic ulcers. Chronic peptic ulcers often require surgery. Even under medical treatment some keep recurring. Others do not respond to medical treatment and cause the patient so much pain that he is unable to work, sleep, or eat. These intractable chronic ulcers usually

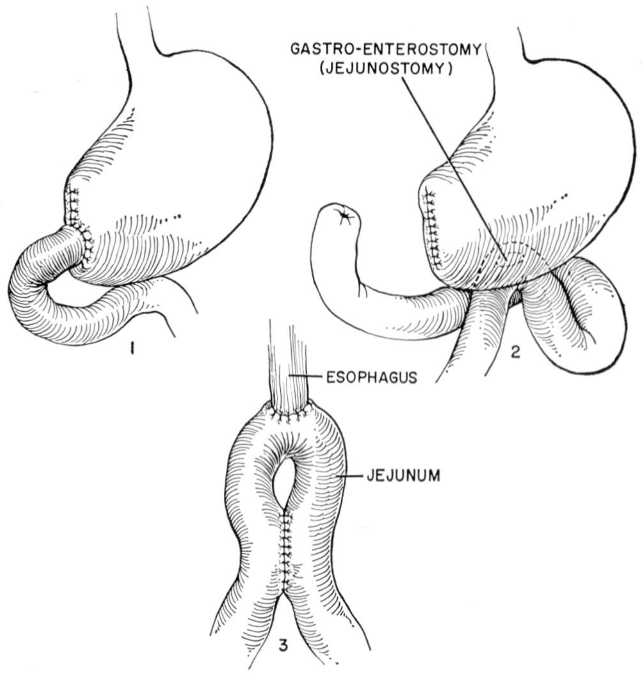

Figure 85

Types of gastric resections and anastomoses. *1,* Gastric resection with anastomosis of the remaining segment of the stomach with the duodenum (Billroth I). *2,* Gastric resection with closure of the duodenum and anastomosis of the remaining segment of the stomach to the jejunum (Billroth II). *3,* Total gastrectomy with anastomosis of the esophagus to the jejunum. The duodenum has been closed.

occur in the middle-aged or older patient. Surgery is also indicated in gastric ulcers that do not respond to medical treatment quite rapidly since 10 to 20 per cent of them become cancerous if allowed to persist.[11]

The surgical treatment most often used in the treatment of both chronic duodenal and chronic gastric ulcers is the *Billroth II operation.* This operation consists of the removal of the lower one half to two thirds of the stomach (*subtotal gastrectomy*). The duodenal stump is closed, and the remaining segment of the stomach is anastomosed to a loop of jejunum (gastroenterostomy). Following this operation, gastric contents pass directly from the stomach to the jejunum (see Figure 85). By this type of gastric resection the ulcer is removed, and the amount of acid secretions from the gastric mucosa is reduced. Since the distal end of the duodenum still connects with the jejunum, bile now flows from it to the jejunum to mix with the food.

The gastric resection known as the *Billroth I operation* is used mainly for the removal of chronic gastric ulcers and gastric carcinomas. In this operation the lower one half to two thirds of the stomach is resected, and the remaining segment of the stomach is anastomosed to the duodenum. (See Figure 85.)

If a patient is too old or in too poor physical condition to tolerate more radical surgery for treatment of the ulcer, the jejunum may be pulled up and anastomosed with the stomach. A new opening for food to escape from the stomach is thus made between the stomach and the jejunum without removal of a portion of the stomach (gastroenterostomy). Gastric surgery is usually done through a right rectus, right subcostal, or bilateral subcostal incision.

After a Billroth II procedure, the *"dumping syndrome"* sometimes occurs. After eating, the patient complains of weakness, faintness, palpitations of the heart, and diaphoresis. The symptoms are thought to be caused by the rapid, uncontrolled emptying of large amounts of food through the gastroenterostomy opening into the jejunum. This mechanism raises the concentration of the jejunal contents so that fluid from the circulating blood is drawn into the jejunum, thereby lowering the blood volume. This probably causes the cardiovascular symptoms that occur soon after eating. Fear of these symptoms makes the patient reluctant to eat, and he may lose weight. He should be advised to avoid foods that are or can become concentrated fluids such as milk or milk shakes (proteins) and carbohydrates such as heavily sweetened cereals and sweet desserts. Carbohydrates are rapidly dissolved into a concentrated solution. The patient should lie down after eating, should eat frequent, small, dry meals and should avoid drinking fluid for two or three hours after meals. The "dumping syndrome" occurs in only a few patients, but it may be a serious postoperative complication that severely hampers the patient in his work and in many other experiences of normal living.

The general preoperative and postoperative nursing care of patients having gastric surgery is described on page 552.

Pyloric obstruction. Pyloric obstruction may be caused by edema of tissues around an ulcer or by scar tissue from a healed ulcer located near the pylorus. Patients with this complication have projectile vomiting which may or may not be preceded by nausea. A positive diagnosis is made by a gastrointestinal x-ray examination. If the obstruction is thought to be due to edema about the pylorus, medical treatment is given. A gastric tube is inserted into the stomach, and a continuous drip tube feeding of milk and cream or of a protein hydrolysate solution such as Aminosol is given to neutralize the stomach secretions and to permit the inflammation to subside. A prescribed amount of the solution is permitted to run into the stomach over an eight hour period. The feeding is then discontinued for about fifteen to thirty minutes and the stomach contents are aspirated to determine how much of the feeding has not passed through the pylorus. If the patient does not vomit during the eight hour feeding period, and if the gastric retention becomes less in each eight hour period, it is usually assumed that the stenosis is temporary and that it will continue to respond to medical treatment. Antacids may be added to the tube feeding. Propantheline bromide (Pro-Banthine) and sedatives may be given by injection, and if the patient is vomiting or is unable to absorb oral feeding, fluids may be given parenterally.

If the obstruction does not respond to medical treatment, surgery is necessary. The operation performed is usually the Billroth II as described under chronic peptic ulcers. A gastroenterostomy (without the removal of part of the stomach) and vagotomy may be the treatment of choice for the very elderly person who cannot tolerate more extensive surgery or for the very young patient whose nutrition suffers irreparably from removal of large amounts of the stomach. A simple gastroenterostomy has been described under chronic peptic ulcer.

A *vagotomy* is performed by dividing the vagus nerve branch to the stomach 6 to 7 cm. above the junction of the esophagus and the stomach.[11] By eliminating cerebral stimuli to the stomach, the motility of the stomach muscle and the volume of gastric secretions are lessened. Theoretically, this should help the ulcer to heal more readily. Patients in whom a vagotomy has been performed, however, often complain of fullness after meals, belching of foul-smelling gas, abdominal distention, intestinal flatus, and diarrhea.

These symptoms are caused by the atonic stomach becoming dilated and emptying slowly. When the vagotomy is done with a gastroenterostomy, symptoms of gastric stasis and dilatation are not so outstanding since food can pass more readily into the jejunum than it can through the pylorus into the duodenum.

Hemorrhage. Peptic ulcers cause bleeding in 20 to 25 per cent of all those who have the disease.[10] If the ulcer has perforated a major blood vessel, the patient may have a severe hemorrhage, vomiting large amounts of blood and passing tarry stools. Vomiting of blood usually occurs with a gastric ulcer, while tarry stools are more common from a bleeding duodenal ulcer. Both symptoms may be present in either condition. The patient may also complain of feeling faint, dizzy, and thirsty. He may become dyspenic, apprehensive, and restless as the blood volume is reduced, the blood pressure drops, the pulse rate increases, and signs of shock become apparent. The systemic signs of hemorrhage may appear before (or without) hematemesis and before passage of blood or tarry stools.

The patient with a bleeding ulcer is placed on bed rest, and is usually given a sedative such as phenobarbital sodium to alleviate restlessness and apprehension. Morphine sulfate may be used since this aids rest and also helps to slow down intestinal peristalsis. The doctor usually orders that the blood pressure, pulse rate, and respirations be checked and recorded frequently (as often as every fifteen minutes when acute bleeding is suspected). Blood transfusions are often given to raise the blood volume; these are given slowly to avoid increasing the blood pressure and thereby increasing the bleeding.

If the patient is not vomiting and only a small amount of blood is being passed by rectum, he usually is given milk and cream every hour, and antacids are prescribed. A full bland diet may be ordered because it maintains nutrition, neutralizes gastric acidity, hampers absorption of the formed clot, and slows peristalsis. If the patient is vomiting blood, however, he is given "nothing by mouth." All bloody vomitus should be measured and described. The doctor may wish it saved for his inspection. A gastric tube may be passed and attached to a suction apparatus to collect the blood so that it can be more accurately measured and replaced by transfusion while the fluid and electrolyte balance are maintained by infusions. The patient who is vomiting blood will need special mouth care. A weak solution of hydrogen peroxide may be used to more easily remove blood from the tongue and the teeth and gums.

The number of tarry (black or currant jelly-like) stools should also be recorded, and they may be saved for laboratory examination. Since the patient may be alarmed at the sight of the blood, all evidence of bleeding should be quickly removed from the bedside, and the linen should be changed as needed without disturbing the patient any more than necessary. Two nurses should change the linen so that the patient is not tempted to move or otherwise help with the procedure. The patient should be told that he is receiving blood transfusions to replace the blood he has lost and that rest and quiet will help stop the bleeding. The sedative or narcotic should be given regularly to allay anxiety and apprehension. If large doses of sedative and narcotic drugs are given, attention must be taken to turn the patient at intervals and to encourage him to breath deeply to prevent the possibility of respiratory congestion.

If massive hemorrhage occurs, a gastric resection is usually done as soon as the blood volume is raised to a level at which surgery can be safely performed. The portion of the stomach containing the ulcer is removed; this usually is followed by a Billroth II operation as described for chronic peptic ulcers.

The general principles of nursing a patient after gastric surgery that are discussed later are applicable. The drainage from the stomach tube is usually dark red for about six to twelve hours after surgery. It should turn greenish-yellow within twenty-four hours. The patient may continue to pass tarry stools for several days postoperatively, but this is usually because the blood from the hemorrhage before operation has not yet passed completely through the gastrointestinal tract.

Cancer

Cancer of the stomach is responsible for approximately 25,000 to 35,000 deaths every year in this country, and it accounts for about 10 per cent of all deaths from cancer.[11] It is found more often after the age of 45 years and is more common in men than in women. Although the incidence of gastric cancer is increasing, this is thought to be due to the increased life span. There is no known cause for this disease, but it is believed that heredity is a factor in its development and that chronic gastritis and chronic gastric ulcer may be precursors of cancer of the stomach.

Cancer may develop in any part of the stomach but is found most often in the distal third. It may spread directly through the stomach wall into adjacent tissues, to the lymphatics, to the regional lymph nodes of the stomach, to the esophagus, to the spleen, and to the pancreas or through the blood stream to the bones. Regional lymph node involvement is found in about 60 to 70 per cent of all patients operated upon.[11]

Unfortunately, the patient with cancer of the stomach usually has no symptoms until the growth spreads to adjacent organs. Symptoms may occur only after the disease has become incurable. Vague and persistent symptoms of gastric distress, flatulence, loss of appetite, nausea, gradual weight loss, and loss of strength may be the only complaints of the patient. These vague symptoms should never be ignored. If the nurse hears of anyone with them, she should encourage him to seek immediate medical advice; however, since such symptoms are not necessarily symptoms of cancer, the patient should not be unduly frightened. Pain does not appear usually until late in the disease, and the absence of this symptom is often the reason for the patient's delay in seeking medical help. If the disease progresses untreated, marked cachexia develops, and eventually a palpable mass can often be felt in the region of the stomach.

A positive diagnosis of gastric carcinoma is usually made by means of a gastrointestinal series. The tumor may not be evident in its early stages, and the x-ray examinations may have to be repeated at intervals. An absence of free hydrochloric acid in stomach secretions obtained by gastric aspiration is suggestive of a gastric neoplasm. When other examinations are negative, cytologic studies (balloon used for collection of a specimen) may demonstrate the presence of malignant cells in the stomach. Occult blood is frequently found in the stools.

The operative treatment for cancer of the stomach is either a subtotal gastrectomy (usually a Billroth I) or a total gastrectomy. Whichever procedure is used the spleen usually is also removed because of the common occurrence of metastasis to the lymph nodes of this organ. The subtotal gastrectomy is described under chronic peptic ulcer. When the cancer is spread diffusely throughout the stomach, when it extends high in the lesser curvature, or when it arises in the cardia, a *total gastrectomy* is done. This operation is performed through a thoracoabdominal incision. The entire stomach is removed, and then continuity of the gastrointestinal tract is re-established by anastomosis of a loop of the jejunum to the esophagus (see Figure 85). This procedure is never done when signs of metastasis to other abdominal organs such as the liver are evident. A palliative resection of the stomach is usually done for patients who have cancer of the stomach with metastases.

The nursing care of a patient who has had a total gastrectomy differs in some ways from that of patients undergoing other types of gastric surgery. Since the chest cavity must be entered, the patient will have a catheter for chest drainage, and the nursing care will be that of the patient who has had chest surgery. (See Chapter 23.) There is little or no drainage from the stomach tube because there is no longer any reservoir in which secretions may collect and no stomach mucosa left to secrete. When normal peristalsis returns, the patient is given clear fluids hourly, and, if after two or three days, there is no evidence of leakage through the anastomosis, the diet is increased to several small meals (usually six) of bland foods a day. An elevation of temperature or dyspnea should make one suspect leakage from the anastomosis, and all oral intake should be stopped until the doctor has been consulted.

Following a total gastrectomy, the maintenance of good nutrition is difficult because the patient can no longer eat regular meals and because the food that is taken is poorly digested and, therefore, poorly absorbed from the intestines. Since the patient also becomes anemic, ferrous sulfate is often prescribed. Patients who have had a total gastrectomy rarely regain their strength; most of them are semi-invalids as long as they live. Survival rate for gastric cancer is unusual beyond five years because of early and extensive metastasis. X-ray therapy is sometimes used and may slow the progress of the disease although it does not cure the cancer. The gastrointestinal side effects of x-ray therapy limit its usefulness in treating cancer in this part of the body.

Nursing care of patients having gastric surgery

During the preoperative period all patients who are to have gastric surgery undergo extensive diagnostic studies. If the patient is to have surgery for an ulcer, he is maintained on a medical regimen during the preoperative period. The nursing responsibilities related to caring for patients undergoing diagnostic procedures have already been described. Specific nursing responsibilities related to caring for patients with intestinal obstruction and with gastrointestinal hemorrhage are discussed in the appropriate sections. The general preoperative instructions and preparation are those given any patient preceding major surgery (see Chapter 12). Special instructions for the nursing care of patients in whom a chest approach is used are discussed in Chapter 23.

Routine postoperative nursing care is given as described in Chapter 14. Because the incision is made in the upper abdomen, the patient is inclined to breathe shallowly to limit pain in the incision. The prescribed medications for pain should be given as necessary, and special attention should be given to encouraging the patient to breathe deeply and to cough productively. The patient with a high, abdominal, midline incision is usually more comfortable in a modified Fowler's position. The drainage from the stomach tube after gastric surgery usually contains some blood for the first twelve hours, but bright red blood, large amounts of blood, or excessive bloody drainage should be watched for and reported to the surgeon at once if it occurs. While the stomach tube is used, and until peristalsis resumes, fluids by mouth are restricted. Mouth care, therefore, is needed frequently to keep the mucous membranes of the throat and mouth moist and clean. Until the gastric tube is removed and until the patient is able to drink enough nutritious fluids, fluids are given parenterally. The average patient is given about 3,500 ml. of fluids intravenously each day (2,500 ml. for his normal body needs plus enough to replace fluids lost through the gastric drainage and vomitus). It is important that gastric drainage and urinary output be accurately measured and recorded. Vitamins are usually prescribed until the patient is eating a full, well-balanced diet. Fluids by mouth are usually restricted for about twelve to twenty-four hours after the stomach tube is removed. The patient is then given 30 ml. of water every hour the first day, 60 ml. every hour the second day, and 90 ml. every hour the third day. If this is well tolerated, small amounts of bland food are then added until the patient is able to eat six small meals a day and to drink 120 ml. of fluid every hour between meals. This dietary regimen, however, usually must be adapted to the individual patient since some patients tolerate increasing amounts of food and fluids better than others. Regurgitation after meals may be due to eating too fast, eating too much, or to postoperative edema about the suture line which prevents the food from passing into the intestines. If regurgitation occurs, the patient should be encouraged to eat more slowly and the size of the meals should be decreased temporarily. If the gastric retention continues, it is probably caused by edema about the suture line, and food and fluids by mouth usually are discontinued for a time. A stomach tube may be passed and attached to a suction apparatus, and fluids may be administered parenterally until the edema subsides.

After most gastric surgery, drainage on the dressings is minimal. If a total gastrectomy is performed, however, drains are usually inserted from the site of the anastomosis, and there may be serosanguineous drainage. The patient usually gets out of bed the day after surgery, and his activity is progressively increased thereafter.

The patient is usually discharged from the hospital two or three weeks after surgery. Before discharge, a gastrointestinal series is often done to observe the functioning of the gastroenterostomy. The patient still may be eating six small meals a day, or he may be permitted to eat three meals of bland food. He should be advised to eat slowly and to decrease the size of the meals if he is uncomfortable after eating. The remaining stomach gradually is able to accept larger amounts of food and fluids. Within six months to a year, the patient is usually able to eat three normal meals. He requires about three months to convalesce before he regains his strength and is able to resume full activity. After discharge, he needs medical supervision and should be advised to keep appointments either in his doctor's office or in the hospital clinic. During these visits the nurse can help to determine the patient's understanding of his condition. He may need to discuss problems about his diet with the dietitian.

The patient with disease of the lower gastrointestinal system

Many disease conditions affect the lower gastrointestinal system. Only some of the more common ones and the related nursing care will be discussed here.

APPENDICITIS

In the United States, there are still about 2,600 deaths a year from appendicitis.[12] If symptoms had not been neglected or if the patient had not been given a cathartic, some of these might have been prevented. It is important, therefore, that the nurse continue to help teach the public that symptoms of right lower quadrant or periumbilical pain accompanied by loss of appetite, elevation of temperature, and possibly nausea, vomiting, and diarrhea should be reported to a physician. Patients with these symptoms should not be treated at home by local heat, enemas, or cathartics.

Appendicitis is an inflammatory lesion of the vermiform appendix. It is more common among men, and it occurs most frequently between the ages of 10 and 30 years. It may occur at any age, however. While there is no known cause of the disease, mechanical factors such as occlusion of the lumen of the appendix by hardened pieces of stool (fecaliths), by foreign objects, or by kinking of the appendix may impair the circulation and lower resistance to organisms in the system such as the colon bacillus or the streptococcus. A small part of the appendix may be edematous, inflamed, or necrotic, or the entire appendix may be so involved. An abscess may develop in the appendiceal wall or in the periappendicular tissue. The serious danger in this disorder is that the appendix will rupture and cause a generalized peritonitis.

The typical symptoms of acute appendicitis are pain about the umbilicus and throughout the abdomen (which relatively quickly becomes localized at a point known as *McBurney's point,* exactly halfway between the umbilicus and the crest of the right ilium), nausea, anorexia, and often vomiting. Acute appendicitis is remarkable for the suddenness of its onset; the patient may have felt quite well an hour or two before the onset of severe pain. The temperature is usually moderately elevated and there is moderate leukocytosis. These symptoms are present in about 60 per cent of all patients with acute appendicitis.[11] Other patients have less well-defined local symptoms because of the location of the appendix. It may be retrocecal, or it may lie adjacent to the ureter. If the patient has questionable symptoms, a urinalysis and an intravenous pyelogram may be made to rule out an acute pyelitis or a ureteral stone. There are many other diseases that produce symptoms similar to appendicitis, and they sometimes need to be ruled out before a positive diagnosis can be made. Some of these are acute salpingitis, regional ileitis, mesenteric lymphadenitis, and biliary colic. The older patient with acute appendicitis may experience only dull pain; healthy children who develop appendicitis may have only slight abdominal pain, although they usually vomit. The abdominal omentum is not well developed in children; thus, if the appendix perforates, peritonitis can easily develop because the infection cannot be walled off so easily. It is recommended, therefore, that the ill child who refuses food and who vomits be taken to a physician for diagnosis and treatment. He should *never* be given a cathartic for these complaints.

Medical treatment and nursing care

When appendicitis is suspected, the patient usually is hospitalized at once and placed on bed rest for observation and the necessary diagnostic procedures that must be done. Since an operation may be done shortly after admission, the patient is not given anything by mouth while reports of the blood count are awaited. Parenteral fluids may be given during this time. Narcotics are not given until the cause of the pain has been determined. Sometimes an ice bag to the abdomen is ordered to help relieve pain. Enemas are not given unless ordered by the doctor. If an enema is ordered, tap water should be used, the rectal tube should be inserted only 3 or 4 inches, and the container should be held low while a small amount of fluid is instilled. These precautions are taken so that only the lower bowel is stimulated. A rectal examination is done to help establish the diagnosis. If the patient is not prepared for this examination by an explanation as to why it is necessary, he may be upset by the procedure.

An appendectomy is usually scheduled as an emergency operation. The patient is given a general or a local anesthetic and the appendix is removed through a small incision over McBurney's point or through a right rectus incision. Unless drains are used, the incision heals with no drainage. Drains are used when an abscess is discovered, when the appendix has ruptured and peritonitis has developed, and sometimes when the appendix appears edematous and ready to rupture and is surrounded by clear fluid.

Bowel function is usually normal soon after surgery; nausea and vomiting disappear with surgical treatment, and the patient is permitted food as tolerated. Convalescence is usually short. The patient gets out of bed the day after surgery and may resume normal activity within two to four weeks.

MECKEL'S DIVERTICULUM

Meckel's diverticulum is a fibrous tube or cord about 50 cm. (20 inches), above the ileocecal valve. It is the remnant of a duct used in fetal life and is found in about 2 per cent of the population.[38] In postnatal life the duct may connect to the abdominal wall or to the umbilicus, it may hang down loosely in the intestinal lumen, or its tip may become attached at some point in the peritoneal cavity, forming a band and causing intestinal obstruction.

The diverticulum can become inflamed, causing symptoms similar to those of appendicitis. The diagnosis is usually made at operation, and at this time the diseased diverticulum and the involved intestine are resected. The bowel is then anastomosed. The preoperative care is dependent upon the symptoms, but it is likely to be the same as that necessary for patients with intestinal obstruction or appendicitis. Postoperatively the nursing care is that required for any patient who has had a bowel resection (see page 570).

MESENTERIC VASCULAR OCCLUSION

Mesenteric vascular occlusion is common, occurring frequently in patients with extensive arteriosclerosis or serious heart disease. Often the patient is elderly. It also may occur in patients who are recovering from recent abdominal surgery. Thrombosis of the mesenteric vein may occur as a complication of cirrhosis of the liver, following splenectomy, or as a result of an extension of a thrombophlebitic process in the ileocolic veins. The superior mesenteric arteries usually are occluded.

The blood supply to the lower part of the jejunum and ileum usually is interrupted by a mesenteric vascular occlusion. The walls of the intestine become thickened and edematous, then reddened, and finally black and gangrenous. The patient complains of an acute onset of sharp abdominal pain, nausea, and vomiting. He has disturbed bowel function and may pass blood from the rectum or may have no bowel action. The white blood cell count is elevated. The patient goes into shock quickly and may be in shock when first seen by a doctor even when the condition is reported at the onset of symptoms. The patient is hospitalized at once and nothing is given by mouth, a stomach tube is inserted and attached to a suction apparatus, and parenteral fluids may be started. The treatment is always immediate surgery before the dead tissue can cause peritonitis and before symptoms of obstruction become overwhelming. The gangrenous bowel and its attached mesentery are removed and the remaining sections of the bowel are anastomosed.

The preoperative and postoperative care of patients having a bowel resection is described later in this chapter. The patient who has a resection for vascular occlusion usually is given heparin and Dicumarol to prevent further clot formation. This treatment not only requires close medical supervision, but also careful nursing supervision as discussed in Chapter 19. The patient may also be given antispasmodic drugs such as papaverine hydrochloride. He is very ill both preoperatively and postoperatively and needs constant nursing care. Close relatives usually are permitted to visit, and provisions should be made for their comfort, particularly during night hours. The mortality rate from mesenteric vascular occlusion is high.

REGIONAL ILEITIS

Regional ileitis is a nonspecific inflammation of the distal loops of the small intestine. Most frequently it involves the terminal ileum and is characterized by continuous, cobblestone-like ulcerations along the mucosa, a thickening of the intestinal wall, and the formation of scar tissue. The disease usually occurs between the ages of 20 and 30 years. Its cause is unknown. The inflammation begins in the ileocecal valve and extends upward for 15 to 30 cm. (6 to 12 inches). It may then skip whole areas of intestinal mucosa and reappear higher in the ileum toward the jejunum. The ulcers are likely to perforate and form fistulas which connect with the abdominal wall or with any hollow viscus such as the colon, sigmoid, bladder, or vagina. Scar tissue may form as the ulcers heal and may cause strictures and result in intestinal obstruction.

The patient with an acute regional ileitis usually complains of severe abdominal pain or cramps localized in the right lower quadrant. He has moderate fever and mild diarrhea. The abdomen usually is rigid and tender, and the white blood cell count is elevated. Often the disease is diagnosed as acute appendicitis, but when the patient is operated upon, he is found to have a normal appendix but an inflamed ileum. If this is so, the incision is closed without further surgery being done.

Chronic regional ileitis is characterized by a long history of diarrhea, abdominal pain, loss of weight, anemia, fistula formation, and, finally, intestinal obstruction. The diarrhea consists of three or four semisolid stools containing mucus, pus, and sometimes undigested food. Bowel movements are accompanied by abdominal cramps. A mass sometimes can be felt in the area of the appendix or cecum.

The treatment for both acute and chronic ileitis is essentially medical. The patient is given a bland diet, together with vitamins to help maintain good nutrition. Transfusions and iron compounds such as ferrous sulfate may be necessary to treat anemia. Codeine sulfate or camphorated tincture of opium (paregoric) may be given to control diarrhea. Intestinal antibiotics such as phthalylsulfathiazole (Sulfathalidine), streptomycin, and chloramphenicol (Chloromycetin) are often given.

If intestinal obstruction occurs or if there are fistulas, surgery is necessary. The diseased bowel may be resected and the remaining segments anastomosed, or it may be left and a "short-circuiting" operation performed. This operation consists of dividing the ileum, closing the distal portion with sutures, and anastomosing the proximal portion to the transverse colon (ileotransverse colostomy). If the diseased bowel is adherent to the surrounding organs and tissues, the ileotransverse colostomy may be preferable. The inflammation is treated with antibiotics.

ULCERATIVE COLITIS

Ulcerative colitis is an inflammatory disease of the colon. While its cause is unknown, it is thought to be the result of either an infectious process or a psychogenic disturbance. Neither of these causes, however, has been proved conclusively. Many patients with this disease have personality disorders, and they often are perfectionistic, sensitive, frustrated, and dependent people.

Ulcerative colitis may occur at any age in either sex, but it is found most often between the ages of 20 and 30 years. The disease varies in severity, and the patient may be symptom-free between periods of acute distress. A severe attack may be brought on by an acute infection or by an emotional upset.

In the early stages of ulcerative colitis only the rectum or rectosigmoid is affected. The rectal mucosa is friable and hyperemic and contains many superficial bleeding points. As the disease progresses, advancing up the colon, the bowel mucosa becomes edematous and thickened. The superficial bleeding points gradually enlarge and become ulcerated; the ulcers may bleed or perforate, causing abscess formation or peritonitis. The edematous mucosa may undergo changes and form pseudopolyps which may become cancerous. The continuous healing process with formation of scar tissue between the frequent relapses may cause the colon to lose its normal elasticity and its distensible and compressible characteristics. It becomes thickened, normal mucosa is replaced by scar tissue, and it becomes rigid and pipelike. The diagnosis is based on the patient's history and symptoms, on results obtained from barium enemas, proctoscopic and sigmoidoscopic examinations, and on failure to find any causative organisms in the stools.

The main symptom of an acute attack of ulcerative colitis is diarrhea; the patient may pass as many as fifteen to twenty or more liquid stools a day. These contain blood, mucus, and pus. Abdominal cramps may or may not occur before the bowel movement. The patient has loss of appetite and low-grade fever and occasionally becomes nauseated and vomits. As these symptoms persist, the patient becomes weak, dehydrated, debilitated, and cachectic. Ulcerative colitis is a serious disease with a fairly high mortality rate. The personality make-up of many patients with this disease seems to be such that they accept the disease stoically but are unable always to conform to the regimen that is prescribed; for example, it may be impossible for the patient to eat the foods that he knows are best for him.

The treatment for ulcerative colitis is essentially medical. Blood transfusions are given for the anemia. If the patient is vomiting and is severely undernourished and dehydrated, parenteral fluids may be given. A high-protein, high-calorie, high-vitamin diet is usually urged to help the patient regain nutritional losses and to aid in the healing of the bowel mucosa. Sedatives such as phenobarbital are prescribed to alleviate nervous tension, and antispasmodics such as atropine and propantheline bromide (Pro-Banthine) are given to slow down peristalsis. Camphorated tincture of opium (paregoric) is also given to slow down peristalsis, but a real danger of addiction exists when this drug is used for a chronic ailment such as ulcerative colitis. Drugs such as kaolin and bismuth preparations (bismuth subcarbonate) are used to help coat and protect the irritated mucosa and give better consistency to the stools. Antibiotics may be ordered to prevent or to treat secondary infection. About 20 per cent of patients with ulcerative colitis require surgery because of complications such as hemorrhage or perforation.[10] A resection of the bowel is sometimes done in an attempt to cure the condition when the disease is so incapacitating that it makes an invalid of the patient and no improvement has been obtained from medical treatment over a period of time. Choice of surgery depends on the individual patient and on the physician; it is recognized that surgery does not remove the basic condition which led to development of the disease.

Nursing care of the patient with ulcerative colitis

The patient with ulcerative colitis may be admitted to the hospital for immediate supportive treatment during an acute exacerbation of the disease or for preparation for surgery during a remission. In either instance, if the disease is of long duration, the patient is usually thin, nervous, and apprehensive and is inclined to be preoccupied with his physical condition. These qualities caused by the illness are superimposed on the basic personality pattern of many patients with this disease—sensitivity, insecurity, and dependence are common characteristics. These characteristics of behavior plus the basic personality make it hard for the nurse to get to know the patient and sometimes hard for her to understand him. Yet, in the nursing care of no other patient are understanding and acceptance more necessary. The nurse should not hesitate to seek guidance from the physician in her approach to the patient. Sometimes psychiatric nursing or medical consultation is available. All members of the nursing staff should have the same approach to the patient. Although the patient may accept treatment and nursing care, he may remain restrained and withdrawn for a time; often he is depressed even though he appears resigned to his problems. Acceptance of his behavior, together with gentle, intelligent nursing care, will help the nurse gradually gain the patient's confidence and will increase his ability to accept certain essentials of his treatment, such as food.

All procedures and treatments should be carefully explained to the patient. Explaining to the patient, for example, that medication is available to him for controlling bowel movements sometimes seems to reduce his need. The nurse should listen carefully to the patient's own report of things that seem to stimulate peristalsis and cause frequency of bowel movements. If he has found that certain foods or combinations of foods cause diarrhea, this should be noted on the nursing care plan and reported to the dietitian. Other information, such as best time for bathing, whether soon after a meal (to permit a long rest period afterward) or later (when food is partially digested) should be on the plan.

The acutely ill patient may need to be

placed on bed rest. If he is very thin, care must be taken that bony prominences are protected. An alternating air pressure mattress is best; if this is not available, a large piece of sponge rubber should be placed under the buttocks. Sponge rubber mattresses are also useful in the prevention of pressure sores. Areas of friction against linen should be watched for; if the patient braces himself on the bedpan by leaning on his elbows thereby causing pressure areas, these areas should be massaged frequently with a light cream. If the patient spends most of his time on the bedpan, it should be padded with sponge rubber. If he uses the commode, it can also be protected with a piece of sponge rubber or with a rubber ring.

A record must be kept of the number, amount, and character of the stools, and specimens of stool should be sent to the laboratory as requested. Although each bowel movement may be very small, the commode or bedpan should be emptied as often as it is used. The patient wants the bedpan accessible at all times. He may even insist on keeping it in bed with him, and usually this is permitted. Air-Wick or electric deodorizers are sometimes used to dispel unpleasant odors in the room. Linen should be kept fresh, and the patient's perineum, buttocks, and anal region should be thoroughly washed several times a day. Nupercaine or other prescribed ointment may be applied to the anus to relieve discomfort. Tub baths are beneficial to the skin and circulation and are often permitted once a day provided the patient is carefully protected from chilling.

The patient should be kept warm, and drafts and chilling must be avoided. Extra covers should be provided so that the patient may use them as he wishes. Heat in the room and covers should provide enough warmth and protection to permit regular airing of the room to help remove odors and to supply fresh air.

Seeing that the patient follows the prescribed diet, in adequate amounts, and takes supplementary nourishment are essential parts of nursing care. Protein foods are very important. The ingenuity of the nurse will often be taxed in getting the patient to eat enough since sometimes a real distaste for food is a symptom of this disease. Any concession or consideration that promises to increase food intake should be made. The family should be permitted to prepare favorite foods at home and to bring them to the patient provided the foods are bland and otherwise conform to what the patient needs.

If infusions and transfusions are necessary, these procedures must be carefully explained to the patient since they often cause apprehension. Because the patient's blood pressure is often low and his veins "poor," and because he tolerates the annoyance of these procedures poorly, care is taken to anchor the needle securely and to use an arm board so that the needle does not become dislodged.

As the nurse cares for the patient during convalescence from an acute exacerbation of ulcerative colitis, she should be alert for any suggested problems. Since the physical causes of this condition are unknown and since the condition itself cannot be cured but only alleviated by the variety of treatments available, effort is made to learn of and to control the emotional components of the disease. The doctor may ask the social worker to talk to the patient and attempt to learn of social, economic, or other problems that are bothering him. The public health nurse may make a home visit before the patient leaves the hospital to determine whether or not he can be cared for properly at home and to report any other pertinent information. The family should be guided in ways to help the patient when he is at home, for example, preparation of food, maintenance of nutrition, and understanding and acceptance of the disease and the patient's behavior.

Surgical treatment and nursing care

An ileostomy is usually an operation that the patient elects so that he may again be an active member of society without the constant annoyance of the symptoms of ulcerative colitis. An *ileostomy* is a permanent opening of the small intestine (ileum) through the abdominal wall to the outside. Fecal material no longer passes through the large bowel to the rectum but is discharged through the opening in the abdominal wall. Special bags have been developed to collect this drainage since the contents of the ileum are semiliquid. Preoperative visits and talks with patients who have made successful adjustments to ileostomies are helpful and tend to make the patient less fearful of the operation and its consequences.

Three to five days before the operation, the patient is given a low-residue diet, and twenty-four hours before surgery he is limited to fluids. This decreases intestinal residue. Intestinal antibiotics such as Sulfathalidine or neomycin are given to lower the bacterial count of the intestine, which helps to prevent postoperative infection of the suture line. Immediately preoperatively, a gastric or intestinal tube is passed to keep the bowel decompressed.

An ileostomy and a *total* or *subtotal colectomy* (removal of all or part of the colon) are usually performed at the same operation. After a subtotal colectomy, the patient returns from the operating room with two openings, sometimes called buds or stomas, on the abdominal wall. The proximal opening which is usually on the right, is the ileostomy from which liquid stool will flow. The distal opening, usually on the left side, leads to the remnant of lower bowel that has not yet been removed. If a total colectomy was performed, the patient will have only an ileostomy since the large bowel and rectum are removed.

Ileostomy bag. A *temporary ileostomy bag* is placed over the opening to keep fecal drainage from running over the abdomen and into the incision while the wound is healing. The first few days after surgery the amount of drainage from the stoma may be very small; however, as soon as peristalsis returns and the patient begins to eat, fecal drainage begins. Enzymes in the contents of the small intestine can digest skin. The bag prevents these enteric enzymes from draining onto the skin and causing ulcerations that are difficult to heal and make later use of a permanent collection appliance less successful. The opening of the bag can be cut so that only the stoma (covered with normal bowel mucosa) is exposed to the drainage. The opening in the bag should be large enough so that it does not constrict the ileostomy but small enough so that fluid cannot escape onto the skin. The temporary ileostomy bag may be the disposable type or it may be made of a heavy, durable material. (See Figure 86.) Both types are adhered to the skin with skin adhesive; if the skin is intact and the bag properly applied, it will remain in place until pulled off or removed with ether or benzene. It usually needs to be changed every three or four days. Because the skin must be clean and dry for the application of the skin adhesive and the bag, the bag should be applied before the patient eats or several hours after eating when there is likely to be little or no drainage from the ileostomy. If a temporary bag is not available, a protective dressing of oiled silk and a gauze dressing similar to that used for urinary drainage can be applied around the ileostomy opening (see Figure 44).

It takes about six weeks for postoperative edema about the ileostomy stoma to disappear and for the stoma to shrink to its permanent size. At this time a *permanent ileostomy bag* may be fitted and applied. It is usually made of plastic material or rubber and lasts for from one to two years. The patient should be taught how to change the bag and how to care for the skin and bag. Many patients leave the bag in place for several days; they usually wear a belt to hold it securely. It can be emptied without being removed from the body; the elastic band at the bottom of the bag is removed and the feces allowed to flow into the toilet bowl. Then, with the use of a small glass or an Asepto syringe, the inside of the bag may be washed with lukewarm water and soap

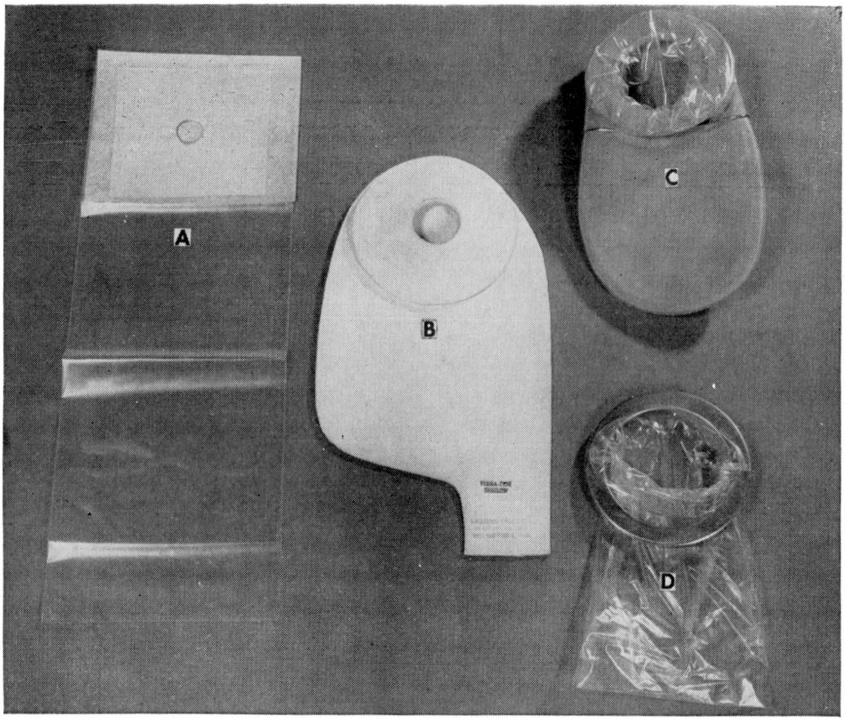

Figure 86

Various types of drainage bags are available for patients with an ileostomy or a colostomy. *A,* Temporary disposable drainage bag; the opening may be enlarged to fit any orifice. *B,* Permanent ileostomy bag. *C,* Permanent colostomy bag. *D,* Colostomy bag with metal frame and disposable bag.

and rinsed. When the bag is changed, the skin under it should be washed well. Most patients keep at least two bags so that the one most recently worn can be washed and soaked in a weak solution of vinegar or Clorox (1 teaspoon to 1 quart of water) and then aired thoroughly. This care will prevent odors and increase the life of the bag.

Many patients are concerned lest the bag show under their clothing. If loose, full clothing is worn, the bag is not noticeable at all. In fact, many women patients wear a girdle over the bag and are able to wear fitted clothes. As the patient gains weight and his strength returns, he may engage in any activities he wishes. Many engage in active sports, and even swimming is possible. If a woman wears a bathing suit with a full skirt and a man wears loose trunks, no one will notice the bag. Some women have become pregnant and had normal antenatal courses and normal deliveries after having an ileostomy.

Preparation for discharge and for secondary procedure. Some patients have difficulty in adjusting to the care of the ileostomy and need a great deal of encouragement and instruction. The patient should be able to care for his ileostomy before he leaves the hospital; however, if he seems reluctant to learn self-care, it may be advisable to teach a member of his family. Later, when the patient feels better physically, he usually takes over his own care. Groups of patients who have ileostomies have banded together to form "ileostomy clubs" in various parts of the country. They hold regular meetings to discuss mutual problems. If the patient seems interested and if there is a club in his area of the country, he may be referred to it. While most patients learn to handle their ileostomies very well, an occasional patient, unfortunately, will center most of his time and attention upon it.

Diet. There are few dietary restrictions for those who have an ileostomy; however, the patient needs to know that some foods, such as corn, will come through the ileostomy undigested and that foods such as cabbage will cause flatus. Certain foods, such as fresh fruits, usually make the stool more liquid and profuse and, therefore, should be taken in small amounts or avoided. Each patient learns what foods cause him difficulty and avoids them. Any food that has caused diarrhea or flatus before the operation probably should be avoided. Before the patient leaves the hospital his food intake should be carefully reviewed with him. He should know how to plan his meals so that the essential foods are included. Much good illustrative material is available and can be secured from local health departments and voluntary agencies such as the National Dairy Council.

Complications. Gastrointestinal upsets are much more serious for patients with ileostomies than for normal people. Fluid and electrolyte balance is easily upset, and the patient may go into acidosis or alkalosis (see Chapter 6). If nausea, vomiting, and diarrhea continue, medical attention should be sought.

Medical and nursing supervision. The patient who has an ileostomy must remain under medical supervision for some time. He may be readmitted to the hospital several months later to have the remainder of the large bowel and the rectum removed. This is done as an abdominoperineal resection, and in some instances this operation alters the ability of male patients to function sexually. The operation and the nursing care of the patient undergoing an abdominoperineal resection is described later in this chapter. After the second operation the patient's general condition and appearance are usually improved. His mental outlook is also better, and he may participate in a normal social life.

Before the patient who has had an ileostomy leaves the hospital after either the first or the second operation, he should be advised to have a public health nurse visit him in his home. She can assist in his adjustment and can supervise his health needs. The patient often does better if he knows that there is someone in the community to whom he may turn for advice and help in the simple details of daily care. He may have trouble with skin irritation, in obtaining new equipment, and in deciding on use of a new paste for the skin. He may have questions related to marriage, work, or recreation. The nurse can help him decide which of his questions and problems he should take to his doctor. It must be remembered that the basic personality of the patient is not changed by the operation, although the activities that the operation may make possible often produce remarkable changes in his attitudes and reactions toward himself and toward his problems.

AMEBIC DYSENTERY

Amebic dysentery is caused by the protozoan parasite, *Entamoeba histolytica,* which primarily invades the large intestine and secondarily invades the liver. The active motile form of the protozoa, the trophozoite, is not infectious and, if ingested, is easily destroyed by digestive enzymes. The inactive form or cyst, however, is highly resistant to extremes in temperature, most chemicals, and the digestive juices. When the cyst is swallowed in food or water, it easily passes into the intestines, where the active trophozoite is released and enters the intestinal wall. Here, it feeds on the mucosal cells, causing ulceration of the intestinal mucosa. While the disease varies in severity, the onset is usually acute, with symptoms developing within two to four days of exposure. Weakness, prostration, nausea, vomiting, and a griping pain in the right lower quadrant of the abdomen usually occur. The patient has numerous semifluid, foul-smelling stools a day. These may contain mucus and pus.

Prevention

It is estimated that from 10 to 20 per cent of the population of the United States have amebiasis.[10] While the disease exists chiefly in the tropical countries, it also prevails wherever sanitation is poor. The cyst, which is the infectious agent, can survive for long periods outside the body, and it is transmitted by direct contact from man to man, by insects, and by contaminated water, milk, and other foods. For this reason, people traveling in tropical countries should drink only boiled water and eat only cooked foods. The most infectious agent is the "carrier," who, although having few or no symptoms of the disease, passes the cysts in his stools. If his hygienic habits are poor and if he is a food handler, he can easily transmit the cysts to the food he prepares for consumption by others.

Treatment and nursing care

If either the trophozoite or the cyst can be found in the stool, a positive diagnosis of amebiasis can be made and definitive treatment started. It is easier to find the parasite in the stool during the acute stage of the disease than later. Immediately after defecation, a warm stool should be sent to the laboratory for examination. Several stool specimens from successive bowel movements may be requested. If the laboratory is at a distance, the specimen container should be transported on a hot-water bottle or in a pan of warm water.

The patient with a mild form of amebiasis is treated on an outpatient basis; 90 per cent of all patients usually respond to a course of amebicidal therapy.[10] The nurse should be familiar with drugs that are given for this disease and know their effects upon the patient. If the iodine-quinoline compounds such as Diodoquin, Vioform, and Chiniofon are given, the patient may have some diarrhea caused by them. Oral antimicrobials such as chlortetracycline (Aureomycin) and oxytetracycline (Terramycin) irritate the gastric mucosa and often produce gastrointestinal symptoms such as nausea, vomiting, and diarrhea; these drugs should be given after meals or with milk and crackers. Emetine hydrochloride may be used in the treatment of the disease, especially when liver involvement is suspected. The patient receiving emetine hydrochloride is placed on strict bed rest, and pulse rate and blood pressure are carefully watched since the drug is very toxic. Some of the many signs of toxicity to this drug include nausea, vomiting, diarrhea, generalized weakness, cardiac irregularity, fall in blood pressure, neuritis, desquamation of the skin, loss of the sense of taste, and mental depression. The drug is usually given only for a few days and then is followed by a course of antibiotic or Diodoquin treatment. The patient must remain on restricted activity for some time after the administration of emetine hydrochloride since, although it is given only for a short time, it is slowly excreted and cardiovascular symptoms may be late in appearing.

Some drugs such as Chiniofon may be given in a retention enema. The patient is first given a cleansing enema with a solution of sodium bicarbonate. He then receives by slow instillation approximately 300 ml. of solution (1 to 4 per cent concentration of the drug). The patient lies on his back with the hips elevated while the enema is given; then he lies for half an hour on each side and the rest of the time lies mainly on his back. The enema should be retained for at least six hours. Glucose solution may be given intravenously during this time so that food taken by mouth cannot stimulate peristalsis.

Amebiasis is a disease with remissions and exacerbations, and it may persist for years. During acute exacerbations, the patient may become dehydrated, exhausted, or anemic and require hospitalization. During these times the nurse gives any care required because of the patient's condition and assists with special treatments such as infusions and blood transfusions. She should review the patient's diet with him. He should eat a bland, low-residue diet, and alcohol and tobacco should be avoided since these tend to stimulate peristalsis.

A careful record of the patient's intake and output should be kept, and he should be encouraged to take generous amounts of fluid by mouth. The number and character of the stools should be described, and the bedpan should be emptied after each use. In handling the bedpan, precautions should be taken since some cysts are usually passed. Cleanliness should be stressed, and the patient should know why it is so important to wash his hands after bowel movements. Particular emphasis should be placed upon careful handwashing before meals to avoid reinfection.

DIVERTICULOSIS

A diverticulum is an outpouching caused by weakness of the muscular layers of the bowel wall or other structures of the body, such as the esophagus. The terms *diverticulosis* and *diverticulitis,* however, usually refer to the large bowel. The presence of many diverticula in the sigmoid and the descending colon is called diverticulosis. The cause of diverticula is unknown. About 5 per cent of the total population has this condition, which is much more common in middle-aged and elderly persons than in the young. In itself, a diverticulum is a benign condition usually causing no symptoms. It may, however, become impacted with feces and become irritated, inflamed, and infected. This is known as diverticulitis. Diverticulitis may sometimes be prevented by care in selection of food and avoidance of constipation. A fairly bland, low-residue diet is usually recommended, and mineral oil may be prescribed.

The patient with diverticulitis complains of a "nagging" pain in the left lower quadrant. There may be local tenderness, leukocytosis, and fever. The patient is usually treated conservatively with a low-roughage diet and with mineral oil. Antibiotics are given when there are signs of infection.

A possible complication of diverticulitis is perforation, with resultant abscess formation or generalized peritonitis. The inflammatory process may also cause bowel obstruction. The patient may require surgery for treatment of these conditions, and occasionally surgery is also done to remove a portion of the badly involved bowel. A colostomy is sometimes necessary (see page 581).

CANCER OF THE COLON

Malignant tumors of the large bowel caused 23,000 deaths in 1951.[11] They are thought to be increasing in frequency because of the increase in the life span. More people are now living to the age when cancer is common, and consequently more diagnoses of cancer are being made than was true years ago. While the cause of cancer of the colon is unknown, isolated polyps are known to undergo malignant changes. *Familial polyposis,* therefore, may predispose to the development of cancer of the lower bowel. Because, in the early stages, symptoms of cancer of the colon are vague and may be absent, it is now recommended that the yearly physical examination of those over 50 years of age include examination for the presence of this disease. Since carcinoma of the lower bowel is more common in men than in women, it has also been recommended that all men over 40 years of age have this examination; in some cancer-detection clinics, proctoscopic examinations are made routinely on all men past 35 years of age.

Anyone in whom constipation, diarrhea, or alternating constipation and diarrhea develops should seek medical attention at once. Changes in the shape of the stool, the passing of blood by rectum, and any change in bowel habits also should be reported. Weakness and fatigue are sometimes the first signs of cancer of the colon since constant loss of blood in the stool may go unnoticed and a severe anemia may develop.

Early discovery of the growth and its immediate removal offer a fairly good chance for cure. Cancer of the colon usually grows slowly and remains localized for a relatively long time. Eventually, it spreads either directly through the abdominal wall into the peritoneum or into other abdominal organs or indirectly through the lymphatics into the surrounding lymph nodes and through the blood vessels to the liver and other structures.

Symptoms of cancer of the colon vary with the location of the growth. Carcinoma of the colon on the right side (ascending colon) usually is a large cauliflower-like growth. It causes severe anemia, nausea, vomiting, and alternating constipation and diarrhea. A mass is usually palpable on the right side of the abdomen. There are no symptoms of obstruction as a rule, because the fecal contents in this portion of the colon are still liquid and able to flow past the growth.

Carcinoma of the colon on the left side (descending colon) often produces symptoms of partial obstruction. Although tumors in this area are usually smaller than those found in the colon on the right side, they proliferate fibrous tissue which, as it contracts, causes narrowing of the lumen of the bowel. Because the stool in the bowel on the left side is formed, it has difficulty passing by the tumor and through the stenosed area. The patient becomes progressively constipated, the stool may be small or flattened, "pencil-shaped," or "ribbon-shaped." Blood, mucus, and pus may be passed with the bowel movement. The abdomen may become distended, and rumbling of flatus and fluid may be heard. Fifty per cent of the cancers of the lower bowel occur in the sigmoid part of the colon.[11]

Diagnosis of cancer of the colon is made by physical examination, sigmoidoscopy, and barium enema examination. The treatment is always surgical, and the tumor, surrounding colon, and lymph nodes are resected; if possible, the remaining segments of bowel are anastomosed. If cancer of the ascending colon is found, the colon on the right side is entirely removed *(right colectomy)*, and the ileum is anastomosed to the transverse colon (ileotransverse colostomy). Growths of the descending colon or upper sigmoid are removed by a *left colectomy*, and the remaining sigmoid is anastomsed to the transverse colon. If the cancerous growth is such that it is not resectable, or if the growth has caused an obstruction with accompanying inflammation, an opening may be made into the cecum *(cecostomy)* or into the transverse colon *(transverse colostomy)* as a palliative measure to permit the escape of fecal contents. When the edema and the inflammation around the tumor subside, the growth is resected, the bowel is anastomosed, and the cecostomy or colostomy usually is closed. The preoperative and postoperative nursing care of patients who have resection of the bowel, a cecostomy, or a colostomy is discussed later in this chapter.

Occasionally carcinoma of the colon causes a complete obstruction, and the acute symptoms of obstruction may be the first indication that anything is wrong. Occasionally, the tumor perforates into the peritoneal cavity and peritonitis occurs before any other signs of illness have been noticed by the patient.

THE PATIENT WITH A HERNIA

A hernia is a protrusion of an organ or structure from its normal cavity through a congenital or acquired defect. Depending on its location, the hernia may contain peritoneal fat, a loop of bowel, a knuckle of bladder, or a portion of the stomach. If the protruding structure or organ can be returned by manipulation to its own cavity, it is called a *reducible* hernia; if it cannot, it is called an *irreducible* or an *incarcerated* hernia. The size of the defect through which the structure or organ passes (the neck of the hernia) determines whether or not the hernia can be reduced. When the blood supply to the structure within the hernia becomes occluded, the hernia is said to be *strangulated*.

The patient with a hernia complains of a lump in the groin, around the umbilicus, or protruding from an old surgical incision. The swelling may have always been present, or it may have suddenly appeared after coughing, straining, lifting, or other vigorous exertion. Age, sex, and obesity are contributory causes in the development of a hernia.

A hernia may cause no symptoms except swelling which disappears when the patient lies down and reappears when he stands up or coughs. If pain is present, it may be due to local irritation of the parietal peritoneum or to traction on the omentum. An incarcerated or strangulated hernia causes severe pain, and there are symptoms of intestinal obstruction such as nausea, vomiting, and distention. These complications require emergency surgery, and a portion of bowel may have to be resected if it has become gangrenous from impairment of its circulation.

Unless there are contraindications due to age or physical condition, most hernias can be successfully treated by an operation. When the patient is in good physical condition and when the hernia is causing little or no discomfort, elective surgery may be done. This obviates the serious complications of untreated hernias such as strangulation and incarceration. In 1948 in the United States the complications of hernias caused 5,000 deaths.[35] Patients who have unusual abdominal protrusions or enlargements, therefore, should be advised to seek medical advice. If a hernia is found during a pre-employment physical examination, employment may be deferred until the hernia is repaired; this is particularly likely when the work involves physical labor. Since hernias that "appear" after employment begins are compensable, the time and money involved in their treatment become of economic concern to the employer. Unfortunately, the patient too often seeks medical attention only if the protrusion becomes troublesome, if he fears it is malignant, or if he must have it repaired before he can be accepted for employment.

An *indirect inguinal hernia* is one in which a loop of intestine passes through the abdominal inguinal ring and follows the course of the spermatic cord into the inguinal canal. The descent of the hernia may end in the inguinal canal, or it may proceed into the scrotum (and occasionally into the labia). It is caused by the intestines being forced by increased intra-abdominal pressure into a congenital defect resulting from failure of the processus vaginalis to close after the descent of the testes in the male and after fixation of the ovaries in the female. Indirect hernias comprise 60 per cent of all hernias[11] and are much more common in men than in women. This higher incidence in men may be explained in part by their participation in more vigorous exercise and by the size of the testes which must pass through the inguinal ring during fetal life.

A *direct inguinal hernia* is one that passes through the posterior inguinal wall medial to the inferior epigastric vessels in the area bounded by Hesselbach's triangle.[11] It is caused by increased intra-abdominal pressure against a congenitally weak posterior inguinal wall. These hernias are more common in men. They are the most difficult to repair and are likely to recur after operation.

A *femoral hernia* is one in which a loop of intestine passes through the femoral ring and down the femoral canal. It appears as a round bulge below the inguinal ligament and is thought to be due to a congenital weakness in the femoral ring. Increased intra-abdominal pressure due to pregnancy or obesity probably causes the herniation through weakened muscle. Femoral hernias are more common in women than in men; this is thought to be because of the inclination of the woman's pelvis.

An *umbilical hernia* is one in which a loop of intestine passes through the umbilical ring. It is caused either by the failure of the umbilicus to close at birth or by a congenital defect in the umbilical scar, which opens in adult life under conditions causing increased intra-abdominal pressure, such as pregnancy, intestinal obstruction, or a chronic cough. Infantile umbilical hernias occur frequently in Negro babies. Umbilical hernias that occur in adults are seen most often in elderly, obese women.

An *incisional hernia* is one which occurs through an old surgical incision. It is caused by the failure of the resected and approximated muscles and fascial tissues to heal properly because of wound infections, drains, or poor physical condition. As a result of increased intra-abdominal pressure a portion of the intestine or other organs and tissues may protrude through the weakened scar.

Treatment

The patient can very often reduce the hernia by lying down with his feet elevated or by lying in a tub of warm water and pushing the mass gently back toward the abdominal cavity. If his physical condition does not permit an operation, the doctor sometimes advocates the use of a *truss* to keep the hernia reduced. However, this is not a cure. The truss should be applied before the patient gets out of bed so that the hernia is more likely to be reduced. If the hernia cannot be reduced, the truss should not be applied and the patient should seek medical treatment. The truss should be applied next to the body, since underclothing worn under it causes it to slide and decreases its effectiveness. Irritation of the skin under the truss can be overcome by daily bathing and the use of talcum powder. Unless the patient has a chronic cough, the truss should be removed when he is in bed.

The only cure for a hernia is surgical treatment. The structure or organ is returned to its cavity and the defect in the fascia or muscle is closed with sutures *(herniorrhaphy)*. To prevent recurrence of the hernia and to facilitate closure of the defect, a *hernioplasty* may be done using fascia, filagree wire, tantalum mesh, or stainless steel mesh to strengthen the muscle wall.

Nursing care

The preoperative preparation for a hernia repair includes a detailed evaluation of the patient's physical status to determine the presence of any diseases of the respiratory system which postoperatively might cause increased intra-abdominal pressure. A chronic cough due to bronchitis or bronchiectasis or excessive sneezing due to an allergy might cause weakening of the repair before the incision has completely healed. The operation is postponed until the patient recovers from any respiratory disorder that is discovered. The nurse should report to the surgeon any signs of incipient upper respiratory infection since these may occur after he has examined the patient.

In addition to good general postoperative care, the nurse, in caring for the patient who has had an operation for a hernia, should prevent tension on the newly repaired tissues. Postoperatively the nurse should be alert for signs of respiratory infection. If a cough occurs, medications such as terpin hydrate and codeine elixir are usually prescribed to depress the cough reflex. They should be given as ordered to prevent paroxysms of coughing and subsequent strain on the repair. The patient should be instructed to hold his hand firmly over the operative area when coughing or sneezing.

Since urinary retention often occurs after a herniorrhaphy, appropriate nursing measures should be taken to prevent the bladder from becoming overdistended. Catheterization is sometimes necessary. The patient is usually permitted to get out of bed to void on the operative day, and after the first day he has full ambulatory privileges.

The patient who has elective surgery for a hernia usually is permitted a full diet as soon as this is tolerated. If a local anesthetic is used and the abdominal cavity is not entered, there is usually no loss of peristalsis, and the patient is able to eat normally at once. If a general anesthetic is used, fluid and food are restricted until peristalsis returns. When an umbilical or a large incisional hernia has been repaired, a gastric tube may be used to prevent postoperative vomiting and distention with subsequent strain on the suture line. Fluids are given parenterally, and food and fluids are restricted by mouth. Abdominal distention following a hernia repair should be reported to the doctor at once. He may pass a stomach tube, or he may order a rectal tube inserted.

Because of postoperative inflammation, edema, and hemorrhage, swelling of the scrotum often occurs after repair of an indirect inguinal hernia. This is an extremely painful complication, and any movement of the patient causes discomfort. It is difficult to turn, to get in or out of bed, and to walk. Ice bags help to relieve pain. The scrotum is usually supported with a suspensory or is elevated on a rolled towel. Narcotics may sometimes be necessary for pain, and antibiotics may be given to prevent the development of epididymitis. When a patient has this trouble the nurse must check his voiding carefully; he may delay voiding because moving about increases pain and discomfort.

Wound infections occur in about 2 per cent of all hernia repair operations.[35] Such an infection interferes with healing and, if it is not recognized early and treated adequately, the repair may be weak. Infections are treated with antibiotics and with warm saline dressings.

The patient who has had elective surgery for a hernia is usually only hospitalized for seven days, but he is restricted from strenuous activity for at least three weeks. He should be advised to consult the doctor about when he may return to work. If his work entails lifting, he should be certain that the doctor knows this, and he should be instructed in good body mechanics.

HIATAL HERNIA

A hiatal hernia is the protrusion of an abdominal structure (usually a portion of the stomach) through a weakened diaphragmatic wall. Usually this occurs around the point where the esophagus passes through the diaphragm. The weakening may be caused by trauma or may be due to a congenital weakness which has not been enough to cause trouble until old age, when all musculature loses some of its strength and effectiveness. Most patients who develop symptoms of hiatal hernia are 60 years of age or over.

Symptoms of hiatal hernia include a feeling of fullness and discomfort after eating, belching, and vomiting of sour stomach contents particularly when the stomach is almost emptied of food during the night and when the patient has been lying flat. Occasionally there are also respiratory embarrassment from pressure on the lungs and palpitation from interference with heart action.

Hiatal hernia can be corrected surgically by a repair which may involve entering both the abdominal and thoracic cavities to return the stomach to the abdominal cavity and to repair the diaphragm. Many patients, however, are not sufficiently good surgical risks to make surgery advisable. Conservative treatment consists of sleeping with the head of the bed elevated (usually 4 to 6 inch wooden blocks are used), eating small meals and avoiding undigestible food that may cause distention, and maintaining as erect a sitting posture as possible, particularly during and after meals.

In recent years, hiatal hernia has been treated by injecting air into the abdominal cavity (pneumoperitoneum). This procedure has been found to be beneficial for some patients who did not respond sufficiently to the conservative measures mentioned and who were not suitable candidates for surgery. The air enlarges the size of the peritoneal cavity, elevates the diaphragm and thus causes the stomach to return to the abdominal cavity.[29] The patient who receives this treatment must return at regular intervals for "refills" of air; fluoroscopic examination may be made to determine the amount and location of air injected. This treatment is usually carried out on an ambulatory basis in the clinic, and the regular clinic visits offer the nurse an excellent opportunity to check on the patient's diet and his other health practices.

PERITONITIS

Peritonitis is an inflammatory involvement of the peritoneum caused by trauma or by rupture of an organ containing bacteria which are then introduced into the abdominal cavity. Peritonitis also can be caused by chemical response to irritating substances such as might occur following rupture of the fallopian tube in an ectopic pregnancy, perforation of a gastric ulcer, or traumatic rupture of the spleen or liver. Inflammation due to chemical causes, however, is so closely followed by invasion of blood-borne bacteria that it is only a few hours before organisms may be isolated from most fluids which accumulate in peritonitis.

Local reactions of the peritoneum include redness, inflammation, edema, and the production of serous fluid which becomes purulent as the condition progresses and bacteria become more numerous. Peristalsis is halted by the severe peritoneal reaction, and all the symptoms of acute intestinal obstruction may occur. These include nausea, vomiting, pain in the abdomen, electrolyte imbalance, severe distention, rigidity of the abdominal wall, and failure to pass anything by rectum. The patient's white blood cell count is usually high. Peritonitis also causes serious systemic symptoms, including high temperature, tachycardia, weakness, diaphoresis, pallor, and all other signs of severe systemic reaction and of shock. Peritonitis is a very serious disease that had an extremely high mortality rate before antimicrobial and bacteriostatic drugs were available.

Medical treatment and nursing care

Treatment usually consists of emergency measures to combat infection, to restore intestinal motility, and to supply lost electrolytes and fluids. Massive doses of antibiotic drugs are given. Intestinal and gastric intubation is usually ordered at once, and a rectal tube is inserted. Fluids and electrolytes are given intravenously, and the patient is prepared for surgery. He is not given anything by mouth, and narcotics and sedatives are given for severe pain and apprehension as soon as the diagnosis is confirmed and there is no danger of masking symptoms.

Nursing care of the patient having gastric and intestinal intubation has been discussed earlier in this chapter. The patient who has acute peritonitis needs constant nursing care since he is extremely apprehensive. Pain and discomfort may also be so severe that he cannot be expected to use good judgment in leaving the nasal tube in place and in keeping his arm still on a board when an infusion is being given. The patient should be given mouth care, and protection is needed to prevent drying and cracking of the lips since dehydration is usually marked.

Usually the patient is placed in a semi-Fowler's position so that gravity may help localize pus in the abdominal cavity into the lower abdomen or the pelvis. Also, in this position the patient can take deeper breaths with less pain, and deep breathing helps to prevent chest complications. Heat may occasionally be applied to the abdomen, but some doctors feel that heat is not advisable.

Surgery is usually done as soon as the patient's condition permits since, as long as the perforated structure continues to pour irritating or infected material into the abdominal cavity, the reaction will continue and perhaps will increase in severity. However, if the patient is in shock, it may be six or more hours before surgery can be safely performed. This operation usually consists of closure of the abnormal opening into the abdominal cavity and removal of the fluid that has accumulated. In the case of a ruptured fallopian tube in an ectopic pregnancy or traumatic rupture of the spleen, the organ is removed.

Before and after surgery, natural barriers are used in the body's attempt to control the inflammation. Adhesions quickly form in an attempt to wall off the infection, and the omentum helps to enclose areas of inflammation. These processes may result in only part of the abdominal cavity being involved and may finally narrow the infected area to a small enclosed one (abscess). As healing occurs, fibrous adhesions may shrink and disappear entirely so that no trace of infection can be found upon exploration of the abdomen at a much later date, or else they may persist as constrictions which may permanently bind the involved structures together; sometimes they cause an intestinal obstruction by occluding the lumen of the bowel. If abscesses form, they are usually in the lower abdomen. They may, however, be walled off elsewhere; for example, abscess formation following a ruptured appendix may develop under the diaphragm and can even perforate that structure and cause an empyema.

INTESTINAL OBSTRUCTION

Intestinal obstruction develops when intestinal contents cannot pass through the lumen of the bowel. It may be due to mechanical causes, neurogenic causes (paralytic ileus), or to vascular abnormalities. *Mechanical obstruction* is most often caused by strangulated hernias and adhesions, although cancer of the large bowel accounts for 70 per cent of the cases of mechanical obstruction in the colon.[11] Other mechanical causes are *volvulus* (a twisting of the bowel) and *intussusception* (telescoping of a segment of the bowel within itself; most common in emaciated infants and small children). Volvulus occurs most often in elderly persons, and the sigmoid loop of the large bowel is usually involved. Bands, strictures, and adhesions may be congenital but usually result from previous abdominal operations or from peritonitis. In *neurogenic obstruction* there is interference with the innervation of the bowel which causes peristalsis to cease or be markedly retarded. Paralytic ileus may be a complication of peritonitis, acute medical illness such as pneumonia, or changes in circulatory supply to the bowel. Other causes of paralytic ileus include handling of the bowel during surgery, spinal anesthesia, spinal cord lesions, electrolyte imbalance, or toxic conditions such as uremia.

Obstruction due to vascular disease is relatively rare and usually occurs in those who have evidence of other vascular disease. Occlusion usually occurs in the superior mesenteric vessels, cutting off the blood supply to a large segment of the bowel. When the affected portion of the bowel is unable to perform its muscular function, peristalsis ceases, the bowel gradually becomes distended with fluid, gas, and fecal contents and finally becomes gangrenous.

The symptoms of intestinal obstruction vary and depend on the degree and site of obstruction. In general, sudden acute mechanical occlusions located high in the intestinal tract produce more intense and earlier symptoms than those occurring lower in the system.[10]

When the lumen of the bowel first becomes obstructed, there is an increase in peristalsis above the occlusion in an attempt to move intestinal contents past the obstruction. As the peristaltic waves becomes more forceful, they cause sharp intermittent or cramping abdominal pain. The increased peristaltic activity also injures the intestinal wall, causing edema around the obstructed area. The intestine proximal to the obstruction becomes distended with intestinal secretions, food residue, and gas. Normally most of the fluid in the intestinal tract is absorbed through the intestinal wall, and this helps to maintain fluid and electrolyte balance. When the intestine is obstructed, however, the normal absorptive power of the intestinal mucosa is lacking because of irritation from hyperactivity, and fluid accumulates and distends the bowel. Most of the gas consists of swallowed air which, since it is composed of 70 per cent nitrogen, is slowly absorbed from the intestinal tract. The combined presence of fluid and nonabsorbable gas in the bowel causes increased tension and may occlude the blood supply, causing gangrene to develop. The bowel distal to the obstruction remains empty and constricted so that there is no passage of gas or stool by rectum.

Vomiting that occurs with intestinal obstruction may be frequent, copious, often projectile, and foul in odor (often fecal). Such vomiting is caused by *retrostalsis* or reverse peristalsis, as the intestinal contents are regurgitated into the stomach from which they are ejected. In general, the higher the obstruction, the earlier and more severe is the vomiting.[10] If the obstruction is in the large bowel, vomiting may not occur as the usually patent ileocecal valve permits fluid to enter the colon but prevents its passage back to the ileum.

Intestinal obstruction is an extremely serious condition which, if not treated promptly, can cause death within a few hours. Failure of the normal absorptive powers of the intestinal wall to continue and the loss of fluid through vomiting cause severe fluid and electrolyte imbalance. Bacteria and toxins escaping through the bowel may cause toxemia and peritonitis. The patient develops all of the signs of shock and requires immediate treatment.

Medical treatment and nursing care

The treatment for intestinal obstruction is intestinal intubation, the administration of fluids and electrolytes by infusion, and the relief of mechanical and vascular obstruction by surgery. Paralytic ileus is not treated surgically unless gangrene of a portion of the bowel has occurred. The operative procedure varies with the cause and the location of the obstruction and the general condition of the patient. If constricting bands or adhesions are found, they are cut, and it may be necessary to resect the occluded bowel and to anastomose the remaining segments. The surgeon may have to do a temporary cecostomy or colostomy and, later, when the patient is in better physical condition, do a resection and anastomosis of the bowel.

Nursing care includes caring for the intestinal tube, maintaining intestinal decompression, and keeping an accurate record of all intake and output. It also includes good supportive care. Pain and vomiting often leave the patient physically and emotionally exhausted; he may need assistance in simple activities such as turning in bed, and he needs encouragement and assurance that the intubation and other treatment usually result in lessening of symptoms within a short time. Skin and mouth care are essential. All vomitus should be immediately removed from the bedside since its foul odor may increase nausea; ventilation should have the nurse's careful attention. Since intestinal distention may cause respiratory distress, the patient usually is more comfortable in a Fowler's position. He should be encouraged to breathe through the nose and not to swallow air since this increases the distention and discomfort. A hot-water bottle or an electric heating pad may be ordered, and a rectal tube may be used to provide relief from lower abdominal distention. Enemas or colonic irrigations may be ordered, and the nurse must carefully observe the results of these treatments. She should be alert for signs that peristalsis has returned, and she should report the passage of flatus and any abnormal substances such as blood or mucus. Urinary retention due to pressure on the bladder may occur, and the patient may need to be catheterized. A total twenty-four hour urinary output below 500 ml. should be reported to the physician.

Nursing care of the patient having surgery of the lower gastrointestinal tract (resection and anastomosis of the bowel)

Preoperative care. Preoperative preparation of the patient who is to have surgery of the bowel varies in some aspects from that of preparation for other abdominal surgery. During the preoperative period the patient is usually given a low-residue diet so that the bowel will be free from formed stool when surgery is done. Vitamins and supplementary meals of food high in protein are usually given. Twenty-four hours before operation, the diet is usually changed to liquids and sometimes even to clear liquids. The reason for the diet changes should be explained to the patient so that he does not eat food other than that served to him.

Antibiotics specific for organisms found in the bowel are given beginning three to five days before surgery in an attempt to decrease the bacterial count of bowel contents, which helps to decrease the incidence of postoperative wound infection. Oral antibiotics used to "sterilize" the bowel are succinylsulfathiazole (Sulfasuxidine), phthalylsulfathiazole (Sulfathalidine), neomycin, streptomycin, and chlortetracycline (Aureomycin). These drugs are poorly absorbed from the gastrointestinal tract and thus their concentration in the blood stream is low. A cathartic such as magnesium sulfate may be given before they are administered, and then the drugs are given in large doses every four hours until the operation is done. The patient may also receive a daily cathartic or enemas followed by instillation of phthalylsulfathiazole into the bowel.

Since the passage of this tube from the stomach into the intestines may take as long as twenty-four hours, intubation of the upper intestinal tract is usually started the day before operation. As the tube passes through the small intestine, the bowel becomes "threaded" on it and thus is compactly held together and shortened while the operation is performed. Before and after surgery, the intestinal tube is usually attached to a suction apparatus for the aspiration of intestinal contents; this prevents the accumulation of gas and intestinal fluid around the suture line. If an intestinal tube is not used, a gastric tube is usually inserted the morning the operation is scheduled. (See page 531 for care of the patient requiring intubation.)

Postoperative care. Until peristalsis returns and the anastomosis is partially healed so that the patient is able to eat normally, the stomach or intestinal tube is used, and special attention must be given to fluid and electrolyte balance. The doctor carefully checks the amount of solutions needed and reviews the daily output from voiding and from aspiration through the tube. The nurse must be very certain that recordings of these are accurate and that all fluids given as infusions the previous day are also carefully included in the patient's record.

Since the patient may have some difficulty in voiding after bowel surgery, nursing measures should be instituted to prevent urine retention. Pain in the incision may be severe and may interfere with full respiratory excursion. The patient should be given narcotics as necessary for pain and must then be encouraged to cough and to breathe deeply. He must also be encouraged to change his position every hour or two and often needs encouragement and assistance in doing this during the first day or two postoperatively.

A rectal tube occasionally is sutured in the anus to be certain that it will be in place to facilitate the passage of flatus. This tube is attached to a drainage bottle, and the nurse must be sure that drainage is possible by having an extra opening in the bottle for an air vent if a cork is used and that there is enough tubing to allow the patient to move about freely in bed without traction on the tube. Discomfort from suturing of this tube can be severe and may require the use of analgesic drugs; often the tubing is anchored firmly to the thigh with wide bands of adhesive tape. Since ambulation is of great assistance in starting peristalsis, the patient may be assisted out of bed a day or two after surgery, even while the rectal tube and the gastric or intestinal tubes are still in use. The passage of gas or stool by rectum should be reported to the surgeon at once, since this usually indicates the return of peristalsis and means that the patient may begin to take something by mouth.

Until the intestinal tube is removed, the patient is not given anything by mouth, and total fluid needs are met by the parenteral route. After the tube is removed, the patient gradually is given additional foods until he has a full diet, although occasionally bland foods may be given for some time after surgery. It is not unusual for patients who have had a resection of the bowel to have some diarrhea after peristalsis returns. This is only temporary and soon disappears. When the stool becomes normal, the patient is advised to avoid becoming constipated because a hard stool and straining to expel it may injure the anastomosis.

If he has a tendency to develop constipation postoperatively, he should try drinking fruit juice and water in the morning or taking a glass of prune juice daily; he should not take laxatives without asking his doctor; the doctor may advocate that he take mineral oil or some mild cathartic at regular intervals.

Nursing care of the patient having a cecostomy

The patient with a growth in the transverse or the descending colon that is obstructing the bowel may have a cecostomy performed. When the patient cannot tolerate the major surgery that a bowel resection entails or the general anesthetic that would be necessary, a cecostomy provides an outlet for fecal wastes. Under local anesthesia, an opening is made into the cecum through a small incision in the right lower quadrant of the abdomen, and a large catheter is inserted into the bowel. The catheter is sutured to the skin so that it cannot slip out, and it is then connected to a drainage bottle. The catheter is left in until the obstruction is relieved; this usually requires a later operation and the cecostomy is maintained until after the resection and anastomosis of the bowel has healed. When the patient passes gas and stool by rectum following the second operation, the cecostomy tube is removed, and the opening gradually closes, healing by second intention.

The patient with a cecostomy experiences little postoperative discomfort, although his movement is somewhat restricted by the irritation of the large tube.

The tubing connected to the drainage bottle should have a large enough bore to permit passage of the fecal contents; special tubing usually should be kept for this purpose. It should be attached to the bottle through a cork to decrease odors, but there should be an air vent in the cork so the tube can drain. The tubing should be long enough so that the patient can turn freely, and it should be attached to the bed in such a way that there is no pull on the cecostomy tube as the patient turns. After it is inserted, the cecostomy tube may begin to drain almost immediately. If there is a large accumulation of intestinal contents in the bowel, gas and stool may be expelled with some force.

Although the contents of the colon on the right side (ascending colon) are normally fluid, the cecostomy tube may become plugged with small pieces of stool. To keep the tube draining freely, it usually is irrigated every four hours with a specified amount of fluid; normal saline solution is usually ordered. The doctor may do the irrigation on the first postoperative day; after this, it becomes a nursing procedure. An Asepto syringe without a bulb or a funnel is connected to the cecostomy tube, and the irrigation fluid is allowed to run into the bowel by gravity; no pressure should be used since there is danger of further traumatizing the obstructed bowel. The funnel is inverted to let the fluid return, or, if an Asepto syringe is being used, the fluid may be aspirated. If there is difficulty in instilling the fluid, the doctor should be consulted because the tube may be obstructed and may need changing.

Since there may be some leakage of fecal contents around the tube onto the abdomen, the skin should be washed with soap and water and dried and some protective ointment or dressing should be applied. Since dressings around the tube become stained, they should be changed to prevent irritation to the skin and to prevent odors. After the tube is removed, skin care and changes of dressings should be continued until all drainage ceases. Sometimes a temporary ileostomy bag can be used (see Figure 86).

Although the patient's first reaction to a cecostomy is that of relief of the severe abdominal distress from which he has suffered, he often experiences revulsion at the thought (and the sight) of fecal material draining onto the skin of his abdomen. Emotional reaction during the first day or two may be severe. If drainage of feces through this abnormal route is really believed to be temporary (not to be replaced later by a colostomy), the patient should be told this by the doctor. The nurse should report to the doctor the patient's questions and fears that indicate the need for explanation and reassurance. The dressings should be changed immediately when they are soiled and the skin should be carefully washed. The use of scented soaps are usually pleasing to women patients. Forceps may be used for cleansing, and during the first few days sterile gauze may be used in order to avoid introduction of any new organisms into the wound. Rubber gloves are never necessary and only serve to make the patient feel rejected.

Nursing care of the patient having a colostomy

A colostomy is an operation in which an artificial opening is made into the colon. It is done to permit escape of feces when there is an obstruction of the large bowel or a known lesion, such as cancer, which will eventually cause an obstruction. It also may be done to permit healing of the bowel distal to it after an infection, perforation, or traumatic injury since it diverts the fecal stream from the affected area. It may be done as a palliative measure in the treatment of an obstruction caused by an inoperable growth of the colon, or, if the rectum must be removed to cure cancer, it may be done to provide a permanent opening for bowel evacuation.

When the doctor first tells the patient of the probable need for a colostomy, the patient's immediate response is likely to be one of shock and disbelief. Whether the colostomy is to be temporary or permanent, he finds it very difficult to accept. Knowledge that it is a lifesaving measure, confidence in the surgeon, and sometimes explanation and acceptance of the proposed operation by members of his family may convince him to consent to the operation. It is not unusual for the patient to be sad, withdrawn, and depressed. So great is the emotional reaction that some women patients cry throughout most of their hospital stay. Occasionally a patient commits suicide in the hospital or abruptly signs himself out of the hospital when he knows that a colostomy is necessary. The nurse should anticipate and prepare for possible events and should help auxiliary nursing personnel to understand the emotional turmoil the patient is experiencing. The patient's reaction to a proposed colostomy will be based on the way he sees it affecting his life, his physical stature, his place in his family, his economic welfare and that of his loved ones, his social life, and many other situations that have meaning for him. His response will depend upon his social and cultural background and upon his emotional make-up, as well as on a number of other circumstances.

The nurse should be prepared to supplement any information given to the patient by the doctor, and she should try to determine how much information to give the patient during the preoperative period on care of the colostomy. Some patients definitely benefit from discussing the care, reading prepared materials, seeing equipment, and talking to persons who are living normal lives following a colostomy. Others find this too upsetting. The patient should, however, have at least superficial knowledge of the changes a colostomy may cause in his daily living pattern.

Some hospitals have prepared printed materials for patients who have had a colostomy.[26] If such material is used, it should be carefully discussed with the patient before it is left with him. After he has perused it, the nurse should plan to spend additional time answering any questions he may have. One of the advantages of this type of material is that the patient has a reference available after his discharge from the hospital; this adds to his security in caring for himself.

Members of the patient's family should be encouraged to visit him often since it is essential that the patient who has had a colostomy feel loved and accepted despite his misfortune. During the preoperative period, effort should also be made to augment the patient's confidence in the members of the medical and nursing staff, since the patient who has complete confidence in those who will treat and care for him is more likely to accept his situation postoperatively and be more willing to start to learn self-care. The patient watches every facial expression or gesture of the nurses and is extremely sensitive to evidence of distaste in care of problems such as he anticipates he will have. If others accept the colostomy as not unusual, it helps the patient to feel that it is not a calamity that has happened to him alone.

Occasionally a patient may reject the colostomy completely postoperatively and will make no attempt to learn to care for it. With help however, most patients will learn to care for themselves. Beginning in the immediate postoperative period, the nurse should take every opportunity to have the patient look at the colostomy and to assist her in small ways as she gives him care; in this way, fear and distaste for the task can usually be gradually overcome. Every effort should be made to keep the patient as clean and dry as possible; he may become emotionally upset and depressed at the sight of fecal drainage and particularly when the drainage is liquid and soils the bed and his gown in addition to dressings. Soiled dressings and materials should be disposed of neatly and quickly. Soiled dressings may make the patient socially unacceptable, interfere with his activity and his desire to eat, and delay his acceptance of the colostomy. Soiling of the bedclothes and the patient's clothing should be prevented if at all possible, but the patient should understand that, until defecation through the colostomy has been regulated, occasional soiling of bedclothes may occur. He should be reassured that this is not of major importance and that he should not let fear that the drainage "will run" keep him from moving about freely in bed. This is very seldom a problem in colostomy care. If it is, however, a disposable colostomy bag should be tried.

Although it is useless and even detrimental to "push" the patient to participate in his own care before he is able to accept this, the nurse should quietly, calmly, but persistently encourage increasing self-participation. A major psychologic hurdle for the patient is usually seeing the colostomy for the first time and observing while it is cared for. The nurse should carefully evaluate the patient's physical, emotional, and mental status in deciding how much participation she should expect from him. It is sometimes necessary to work with a member of the family and to teach him to care for the patient. If this is not possible or if there are no relatives, plans may need to be made for care in a nursing home or for a public health nurse to visit the home to give part of the regular care.

Transverse colostomy

When a colostomy is done for the temporary diversion of the fecal stream to relieve an obstruction or as a palliative measure, a loop of the bowel is usually brought out onto the abdominal wall, and the skin and underlying tissues are sutured around it. (See Figure 87.) A glass rod, the ends of which are connected to a piece of rubber tubing, usually is placed between the loop of the bowel and the skin to prevent the bowel from slipping back into the abdominal cavity. The rod is left in place until the wound is well healed and the loop of bowel has become adherent to the abdominal wall. This takes about ten days. The bowel usually is not opened to permit the escape of intestinal contents for from three to five days after the operation; this allows the skin incision to heal and prevents contamination of the abdominal cavity. A stomach tube is used until the loop of bowel is opened and the passage of gas and stool indicate the return of peristalsis. The bowel is usually opened by an incision made with a scalpel; the lumen is exposed but is not divided completely. It may also be opened with an electric cautery to minimize bleeding. The colostomy is usually opened in the treatment room since it does not cause pain and no anesthetic is necessary. Since the bowel has no sensory nerve endings, the patient may be assured that he will have no pain. If cauterization is done, however, the odor of burning flesh

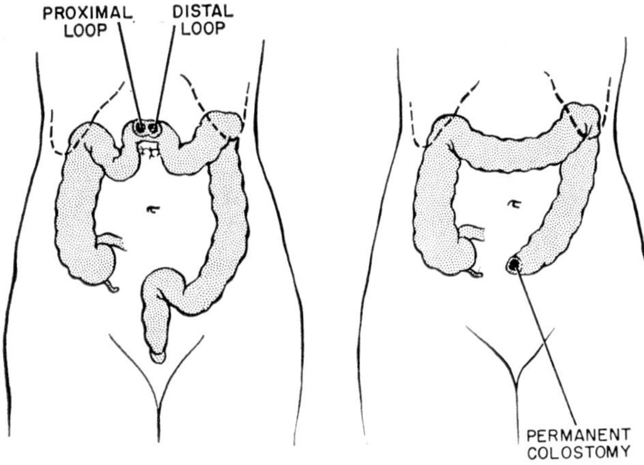

Figure 87

The diagram on the left illustrates a transverse colostomy which may or may not be permanent. The diagram on the right illustrates a permanent colostomy following an abdominoperineal resection.

may cause the patient to become nauseated.

The divided bowel now has a proximal opening leading to the functioning gastrointestinal tract from which stool and flatus will flow and a distal opening leading to the colon and rectum. This type of colostomy is often referred to as a *loop colostomy.* Since it may be difficult to establish which is the proximal and which is the distal opening, the nurse who assists the doctor in opening the bowel should obtain this information and make a drawing on the nursing care plan, indicating the proximal and distal openings. However, if such information has not been recorded, inspection will reveal the opening from which fecal material is coming; this is the proximal opening.

Care of a transverse colostomy. Because this type of colostomy is usually done on the transverse colon where the intestinal contents are still semiliquid, drainage from the opening may be fairly constant. The skin should be washed with soap and water, and the dressings should be changed as often as necessary to prevent skin irritation. A piece of oiled silk or other waterproof material, cut large enough to envelop the dressings and with an opening in the center cut to fit snugly around the colostomy bud yet not compress it, may be used to prevent fecal contents from getting onto the skin and staining the patient's gown or bed linen. This dressing is similar to that used for patients who have had ureteral surgery (see Chapter 21 and Figure 44). Montgomery straps may be used to hold the dressing in place and obviate the need for frequent removal and application of adhesive tape. Petroleum jelly gauze or a protective ointment such as aluminum paste is sometimes placed around the opening to keep the skin from becoming irritated; however, the paste must be removed at frequent intervals to ascertain that the skin under the protective coating remains in good condition. The use of pastes may make the appearance of the colostomy more objectionable to the patient.

The patient's bedside unit should be equipped with supplies needed for changing the dressings. It is best to keep the equipment on a tray that is easily available to both the patient and the nurse. The tray should be stocked with paper bags or newspapers for disposal of waste, gauze for dressings, cotton for cleansing the skin, abdominal pads for extra protection over the dressings, petroleum jelly gauze or protective ointments and tongue blades for their application, tincture of benzoin, and extra Montgomery straps.

As soon as the patient is physically able, he should be encouraged to assist in changing the dressings. Since this is not a sterile procedure, washed, used gauze or unsterile pieces of gauze may be used. The gauze should be rolled and placed about the opening in doughnut fashion since this prevents drainage from easily seeping out the bottom and sides of the dressing. If the gauze is opened and fluffed, it will be more absorbent than a flat piece.

The glass rod is removed eight to ten days postoperatively. After its removal the patient may wear a disposable or a "permanent" colostomy bag over the opening to collect fecal drainage (see Figure 86). In a loop colostomy irrigation is done regularly through the proximal opening; however, elimination through the opening rarely can be completely regulated so that there is no drainage between irrigations. The irrigation procedure is described in the discussion on care of the patient who has had a permanent colostomy. A colostomy bag is necessary for the patient who has a loop colostomy; without it, he may have difficulty in engaging in daily activities. Often, it is when the bag is to be worn that the patient first takes an interest in his own care. The bag tends to give him a feeling of security. The colostomy bag must be cleansed daily and immediately following its removal. It should be washed thoroughly with soap and water, dried, powdered to prevent the two surfaces from sticking together, and allowed to air for at least twelve hours. If this does not remove odors, the patient may be advised to soak the bag for half an hour in a weak solution of Clorox or vinegar.

Materials needed to care for the opening should be obtained during the early postoperative period so that they will be available for use before the patient leaves the hospital. He should not be discharged from the hospital until he or a member of his family is competent in caring for the colostomy or until other arrangements for his care have been made. This is extremely important since it may color the patient's ultimate adjustment to his situation. It is advisable to ask a public health nurse to visit the patient in his home (if he agrees to this) to evaluate the adjustment he has really made and to give him and his family additional help if necessary. The public health nurse should report her findings to the doctor or the nurse in the hospital or clinic. Most patients welcome the suggestion that a nurse may be available to visit them at home. The patient should remain under medical care and should feel that there is a nurse in the doctor's office, the hospital clinic, or the public health agency to whom he can turn for help in overcoming problems related to normal living following the colostomy.

Closure of transverse colostomy. If the colostomy was done to relieve obstruction or to divert the fecal stream to permit healing of a portion of the bowel, the patient will be readmitted to the hospital at a later date for further examination and for possible resection of the diseased portion of the bowel. The opening will subsequently be closed.

In preparation for a resection of the bowel and closure of the colostomy the doctor may order irrigations of the distal loop. Fluid, usually normal saline solution, is instilled into the distal loop through a catheter attached to a funnel or Asepto syringe. For this irrigation the patient should sit on the bedpan or on the toilet since, unless there is complete obstruction, the solution will be expelled through the rectum. Mucus and threads of necrotic tissue may be passed; the returns should be inspected before they are discarded. A nonabsorbable sulfonamide derivative, such as Sulfathalidine, dissolved in a small amount of water may be slowly instilled into the distal loop and rectum after the irrigation. The patient should be asked to retain this as long as possible since the antibiotic lowers the bacterial count of the bowel contents and lessens the risks of postoperative infection.

Permanent colostomy

The permanent colostomy that has been done in conjunction with the removal of the rectum consists of a single, small intestinal opening on the abdominal wall (see Figure 87); usually this is the end of the sigmoid colon. The colostomy bud may appear rather large and reddened at first due to local edema. However, it gradually shrinks and eventually appears as a small, pink bud of mucosa on the abdominal wall. Although there is no sphincter control, bowel movements from a sigmoid colostomy can be controlled by the administration of enemas at regular intervals. The stool in the sigmoid is formed and solid.

The patient usually returns from the operating room with the opening clamped off so that the incision can heal without fecal contamination. During the healing period, a gastric tube is used to drain stomach secretions and to help prevent distention. The clamp is usually removed from the colostomy stump in about three days. After its removal, protective dressings should be placed about the colostomy, and the incision wound should be sealed with collodion or wide strips of adhesive tape. As soon as stool or gas is passed through the colostomy, the stomach tube is removed and the patient is given nourishment by mouth. If there is no gastrointestinal distress, he may progress from a liquid to a regular diet quite rapidly.

Colostomy irrigation. About the fifth postoperative day the doctor usually does the first irrigation through the artifical opening; if the returns are satisfactory and the opening is patent, the nurse then assumes responsibility for subsequent irrigations. It is a nursing function to teach the patient how to establish regularity of evacuation through the colostomy and how to irrigate it.

Equipment needed for the irrigations should be assembled on a tray, and the patient should be encouraged to keep it in a convenient place when he returns home. While commercial irrigation sets are used by most patients, it is possible to improvise equipment, for example, a soft plastic container from the delicatessen may be used as an irrigating cup. Practical suggestions are contained in recent nursing periodicals.[36] Various types of commercial irrigation sets are available, but the principles of all are the same. The cup that fits over the bud has a small hole in the center through which to insert the catheter. It is usually plastic so that returns can be easily seen and is held snugly in place against the abdominal wall with elasticized straps. Outlet tubing attached to the cup allows drainage of the fecal material into the toilet or into a bucket if the patient does the irrigation in bed. The irrigator prevents uncontrolled drainage of the fluid and feces and helps to prevent the procedure from being "messy." The nurse should know that special cups are available for the patient who has an unusually large or high bud. Representatives of the various manufacturers are glad to give advice and assistance in such matters. Besides the irrigator, the patient needs a 2 quart enema can or bag, tubing 2 feet long, a glass connecting tip, a No. 16 or No. 18 Fr. catheter (usually a whistle-tip catheter is used), a tubing clamp, a pitcher for extra water, toilet tissue, petroleum jelly to lubricate the catheter, a paper bag or newspaper, dressings, and an irrigating pole or a hook on which to hang the bag. The patient may install a hook in his bathroom at home or he may use a clotheshorse. The hook should be so placed that there are no more than eighteen to twenty-four inches between the irrigating fluid and the colostomy opening. A small table or shelf on which to place equipment within easy reach should also be provided.

As soon as the patient is ambulatory, the irrigation should be done on a commode or on the toilet. Bathrooms which have poor ventilation and which do not afford privacy should be avoided since the procedure is a long one, taking at least one hour and often longer at first, and the patient is extremely self-conscious. At first it may be necessary to pad the toilet seat with sponge rubber and to provide some support for the patient's back; several bath blankets in a pillowcase can be used. When the equipment has been assembled, water obtained for the irrigation, privacy assured, and the patient comfortably settled on the toilet, the dressing is removed and the area around the colostomy opening cleaned with tissue that is disposed of in the toilet. Warm tap water, about 40.5° C. (105° F.), is used for the irrigation. After the air has been expelled from the tubing, the lubricated catheter is inserted through the opening in the cup and through the colostomy opening into the bowel. The cup is fastened snugly against the skin and the outlet tubing is allowed to hang between the patient's legs into the toilet bowl. When the catheter is inserted 4 to 8 inches, the clamp on the tubing is released and the solution is allowed to flow into the bowel. After about one third or one half of the solution has run into the bowel, the inlet tubing should be clamped until some of the fluid and fecal contents drain back. If, during the insertion of the fluid, the patient has abdominal cramps, the inflow should be clamped for several minutes. Excessive cramping usually means that the irrigating can is too high and the fluid is running in too rapidly. This should be avoided in order to lessen discomfort and because markedly increased peristalsis may hamper passage of material through the intestine. The procedure is continued until the returns are clear. For some patients this may require only 500 ml. of fluid, while others may need as much as 6,000 ml. of fluid.

The patient usually benefits psychologically from sitting on the toilet during the irrigation. Discarding tissues into the toilet and draining the bag directly makes him feel that his situation is not so far from normal as he had feared. If possible, the same nurse should assist the patient with this procedure for several successive days. (See Figure 88.) This saves the patient embarrassment and enables the nurse to give appropriate encouragement, reassurance, and assistance without the patient having to repeat his particular difficulties and problems.

When the irrigation is completed, the patient should be encouraged to massage the abdomen, to bend forward and from side to side, and to stand up once or twice before the cup is removed. Considerable variation in the time necessary for an irrigation exists among patients. Since it may take from fifteen to twenty minutes for the bowel to completely empty, some patients read during that time. Most patients leave the cup on and clamp off the bottom of its outlet while they take a shower, do household chores, or shave since there may be a small amount of drainage after they start to move about. If elimination has been regulated, only a small dressing such as a piece of cleansing tissue needs to be worn over the colostomy; this prevents the clothing from being stained with the small amount of mucus that may drain from the opening. When elimination is well regulated, it is preferable that the patient not wear a colostomy bag since this obviates any possibility of odors. Some patients, however, worry lest they have drainage and can only become regulated when one is worn. Since emotional upsets and worry hinder regulation, it is not always advisable to insist that the patient with a permanent colostomy go without a bag.

As the nurse helps the patient with the irrigations, she should explain what she is doing. Gradually the patient should take over one step of the procedure after another until, before discharge from the hospital, he is assembling his own equipment, doing the irrigation, and cleaning the equipment. The nurse should continue to do some part of the procedure occasionally so that the patient will not feel rejected.

A permanent colostomy should be dilated every day to prevent narrowing of the lumen due to shrinkage during and after healing. It is usually more convenient to do this dilatation just before the irrigation is begun. The procedure is usually initiated by the physician after the in-

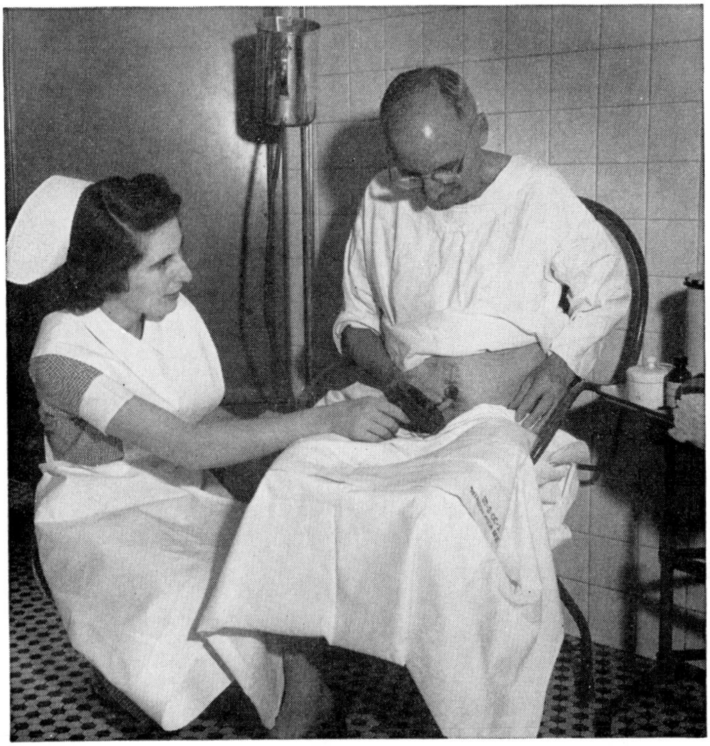

Figure 88

The nurse assists the patient in learning to irrigate his colostomy. (From Newton, Kathleen. Geriatric Nursing, St. Louis, 1960, The C. V. Mosby Co.)

testine becomes adhered to the abdominal wall; this is usually within ten days postoperatively. The nurse then assumes the responsibility for dilating the colostomy until the patient can be taught to do it. The patient is taught to insert his forefinger, covered with a lubricated finger cot, gently into the opening. The little finger may be used if the hands are especially large. The finger should remain in the opening for a few minutes and be carefully rotated to fully dilate it. If dilatation is neglected, the opening may become so narrow that a catheter cannot be inserted or the fecal contents expelled; such a complication requires corrective surgery.

Regularity through the colostomy depends upon setting up and maintaining a regular routine in its care. Before irrigations are started in the hospital, the nurse and the patient should try to determine the time of day it will be most convenient for him to do the irrigations when he returns home. He should remember that it will prevent use of the bathroom by others for at least an hour, and he must plan for his family's needs as well as his own. If possible, the irrigation should be done in the hospital at the time that will be best to do it at home so that a pattern of regularity will not have to be re-established when the patient goes home. Since the amount of solution needed to completely empty the bowel and to prevent any leakage until the next irrigation varies among individuals, it must be tested for each patient. After the irrigation, the nurse should note any incontinence. If incontinence has occurred, the amount of fluid should be increased. Some patients need to irrigate the colostomy every day, while others may need to do this only every two or three days. The latter is likely to be true if the patient normally has not had a bowel movement every day. An occasional patient may not have to irrigate at all; he may find that at the regular time for evacuation the colostomy empties spontaneously.

The patient may eat the food that he enjoys and that he was accustomed to before his operation. However, he should avoid foods that have caused diarrhea in the past. Most patients who have had a colostomy avoid gas-forming foods such as beans and cabbage, since the gas is not retained by the artificial opening which has no real sphincter.

When the skin incision is healed and the patient is physically able, he may bathe, swim, work, and engage in any physical or social activities he choses. The convalescent period usually lasts from two to four months. However, the care of the colostomy should be mastered and regularity should be established within two to four weeks. The patient should be encouraged to have a public health nurse visit him in his home since he often finds that some unanticipated adjustments need to be made after he is home. Many patients, if they have no one to turn to for assistance and advice in caring for the opening, have a feeling of insecurity that causes them to have diarrhea for several days after their discharge from the hospital.

Perineal colostomy. Sometimes the loop of sigmoid can be pulled out onto the perineum so that the colostomy opening is located in more nearly the normal position of the anus. The care of this type of colostomy is the same as for any permanent one except that it is more difficult to handle during the immediate postoperative period. The problems are similar to those of patients with uncontrolled incontinence. (See Chapter 8.) Once the patient learns to care for his colostomy, he may find the perineal opening more acceptable and its care not too awkward.

The patient with disease of the rectum and anal canal

Patients having surgery involving the rectum and anal canal may present special nursing problems. After these operations, the patient may have very sensitive external areas, particularly the area around the anus. Careful attention to these areas is needed to provide maximum comfort for the patient while healing takes place.

CANCER OF THE RECTUM

Cancer of the rectum and lower sigmoid comprises 7 per cent of all malignant tumors.[38] It occurs most frequently in men between 50 and 60 years of age. Cancer of the rectum metastasizes slowly, since the tumor extends by direct spread through the rectal wall to surrounding tissues before metastasis through the lymphatic and venous systems occurs.

The most common symptoms of cancer of the rectum and sigmoid are the passage of small amounts of bright red blood in the stool and alteration in bowel habits; either constipation or diarrhea may occur, or these two conditions may alternate. Early diagnosis and treatment are possible only if the patient reports early symptoms to a doctor; the importance of reporting these seemingly unimportant, but most significant, symptoms cannot be overemphasized to the public, since pain does not occur until the disease is far advanced. Cancer of the rectum can be accurately diagnosed by pathologic examination of a biopsy of the lesion taken during a proctoscopic examination.

Abdominoperineal resection of the bowel

Malignant growths in the rectum are removed by an operation known as an abdominoperineal resection of the bowel. The operation is performed through two incisions: a low midline incision of the abdomen and a wide circular incision about the anus. Through the abdominal incision, the sigmoid colon is divided and the lower portion is freed from its attachments and temporarily left beneath the peritoneum of the pelvic floor. The proximal end of the sigmoid is then brought out through a small stab wound on the abdominal wall and becomes the permanent colostomy. After the abdominal incision is closed, the patient is placed in lithotomy position and the perineal incision is made. Through this incision the anus and rectum are freed from the perineal muscles, and the anus, the rectum containing the growth, and the distal segment of sigmoid are removed. The perineal wound may be closed around Penrose drains, or it may be left wide open and packed with gauze and a rubber dam to cause it to heal slowly from the inside outward.

Preoperative care. Preoperative nursing care of the patient who is to have an abdominoperineal resection of the bowel is similar to that given the patient having other intestinal surgery. Such care is described earlier in this chapter. Some surgeons pass ureteral catheters preoperatively so that the ureters are not inadvertently tied off during surgery. A Foley catheter is inserted into the bladder and is attached to a straight drainage system to keep the bladder empty during surgery and thus prevent operative injury.

Postoperative care. Postoperatively the patient has a permanent sigmoid colostomy; the care of this is discussed earlier in this chapter. Because a large amount of tissue is removed at this operation, the patient is frequently in shock immediately postoperatively; blood pressure, pulse rate, and respirations should be noted frequently. Rectal dressings should be watched carefully for signs of excessive bleeding; the usual drainage is serosanguineous and profuse. The mattress, therefore, should be adequately protected and pads that can be changed without unduly disturbing the patient should be used. The dressing may need to be reinforced during the first few hours postoperatively. After the doctor has changed the first dressing (usually twenty-four hours postoperatively), the nurse may be requested to change the dressings as necessary. Since the dressing requires frequent changing, a T-binder gives the best support without causing skin irritation.

Because of the extensive surgery and because the patient must be in bed for several days to permit the pelvic floor to heal, postoperative complications may develop. Since the patient usually has severe pain while lying on his back, and since he finds it very difficult to turn, he usually prefers to find a relatively comfortable position on his side and remain there. He must, however, be encouraged to change his position frequently, to breathe deeply, and to cough productively. During the first few days the nurse should assist him in turning as necessary and should help him to do exercises in bed. For example, he must be encouraged to straighten out his knees, to dorsiflex the feet, and to tense the muscles of the legs. In her efforts to make the patient comfortable, the nurse must see that positions, such as flexion of the knees, that may predispose to development of postoperative thrombophlebitis, are avoided. Pillows should be used to add to the patient's comfort, but the nurse *must* assist him to change position at regular and frequent intervals. Some patients are comfortable in a prone position lying on a rubber air ring; others find that this causes a pull on the incision. The patient is most comfortable on a firm bed with pieces of sponge rubber placed to relieve pressure on weight-bearing areas and to support the perineal dressing when he is lying on his back.

The patient usually needs a narcotic for pain at regular intervals for the first two or three days postoperatively. If he is in the older age group, however, the narcotic should be given judiciously so that respirations and physical activity are not decreased too much. Smaller doses may be sufficient for older patients. If the nurse finds that the dose appears to depress the patient too much, she should discuss this with the surgeon.

The Foley catheter usually is left in the bladder postoperatively to prevent the bladder from becoming distended and from pressing against the repaired pelvic floor until it heals. Its use also eliminates the need for women patients to use the bedpan to void (a very painful procedure after this operation) and prevents contamination of the wound and dressings with urine. The catheter, however, fairly frequently causes irritation and infection of the bladder; after it is removed the patient may be unable to void or may void inadequately. It may then have to be reinserted for several more days, or the patient may be catheterized at specified intervals as necessary until he is able to void normally. It is not unusual, following this operation, for the male patient to require a prostatectomy for benign prostatic hypertrophy. Antibiotics and large amounts of fluid are given when a catheter is used. Special care should be taken that the catheter drains constantly so that residual urine does not remain in the bladder. (See Chapter 21 for discussion of care of patients using catheters.)

If the perineal wound has been packed, the packing is removed gradually. When this is completed, the wound is irrigated once or twice a day to remove secretions and tissue debris from the wound, to prevent abscesses from forming in the dead space which may be left, and to help ensure healing of the wound from the inside outward. The nurse should ascertain from the doctor how deep the catheter can be inserted and in what direction to insert it to accomplish this. Perineal wounds are often partially healed over yet contain sinus tracts. If fluid is not inserted into the cavity and completely returned from it, an abscess may form. Precise directions as to how to do the irrigation should be recorded on the nursing care plan of the Kardex (or equivalent record).

Normal saline solution or diluted hydrogen peroxide is frequently used as the irrigating solution. When the patient is permitted out of bed, sitz baths may be substituted for the irrigations, and as drainage from the wound decreases, a perineal pad may be substituted for the dressings. A rubber ring should be used when the patient takes a sitz bath so that water can flow freely around the incision; the response in healing is often quite remarkable when this is done. Since the patient is usually ready to leave the hospital before the perineal wound has completely closed, arrangements must be made for him to continue to take sitz baths at home. If he does not have a bathtub available, a large washtub may be used. A public health nurse should always be called upon to assist the patient and his family in procedures of this kind to avoid accidents and to give the patient the assurance of professional help as he cares for himself. He also usually needs her help with care of the colostomy.

The pelvic floor must be partially healed before the patient stands up or walks about so that danger of a perineal hernia is minimized. Because a longer time on bed rest is necessary than following most operations, the patient is usually weaker than most patients when ambulation is attempted. He should be very carefully assisted and closely observed until he is sufficiently strong to get about alone with safety. If a plastic-covered pillow, a piece of sponge rubber, or a rubber air ring, is placed on the chair, the patient is usually more comfortable and is able to sit up for a longer time.

Convalescence after an abdominoperineal operation is prolonged, and the patient may require months to regain his strength. During this time he should remain under close medical supervision. A well-prepared and detailed interagency referral from the nurse in the hospital to the nurse in the public health agency helps a great deal in assuring continuity of care for the patient. By this means the nurse in the home may contact one of the nurses who gave the patient care in the hospital or the doctor to discuss problems she encounters as she gives guidance and assistance to the patient and to his family.

This helps to prevent minor differences in procedures or in other instructions which may be upsetting to the patient.

DISEASE CONDITIONS OF AND ABOUT THE ANUS

While most conditions of the anus usually do not endanger the life of the patient, they are often a source of chronic discomfort and concern. They may cause a great deal of pain because the anus is well supplied with nerves. These diseases may prevent the patient from walking or sitting comfortably, may increase or initiate constipation, and may even cause so much local discomfort that the patient is unable to work. Even after treatment local discomfort may continue for some time, and although the treatment is minor, the patient may have difficulty in readily resuming normal activity. The nurse should be aware of the problems that patients with disease of the anal canal encounter, and she should try to anticipate nursing care that will prevent and relieve symptoms.

Hemorrhoids

Hemorrhoids are dilated veins located directly beneath the rectal mucosa or the skin of the anus. Infection invades the thin walls of the hemorrhoidal veins, causing a phlebitis which results in dilatation of the vein wall. Heredity, occupations requiring long periods of standing or sitting, the erect posture assumed by man, structural absence of valves in hemorrhoidal veins, and pressure caused by constipation, straining at defecation, and pregnancy are all factors predisposing to development of hemorrhoids.

External hemorrhoids are those which appear outside the anal sphincter; *internal* hemorrhoids appear above the internal sphincter. External hemorrhoids often cause pain especially when they become thrombosed, but they bleed relatively rarely. Internal hemorrhoids often bleed on defecation, and although the amount of blood lost may be small, continuous oozing over a long period of time may cause anemia. Internal hemorrhoids sometimes prolapse through the anus and become edematous and painful. Many patients have both internal and external hemorrhoids. Constipation often predisposes to the development of hemorhoids and usually becomes worse after they occur because the patient tries to restrain bowel movements which produce pain or bleeding. Other people resort to laxatives without competent medical supervision. Because constipation and bleeding may be symptoms of cancer of the rectum, by proctoscopic examination the doctor inspects the anal, rectal, and sigmoidal mucosa of all patients with these symptoms.

The local application of ice, warm magnesium sulfate compresses, and analgesic ointments such as Nupercaine give temporary relief from pain and reduce the edema around external hemorrhoids or prolapsed internal ones. Sitz baths are also extremely helpful in relieving pain. The doctor may prescribe mineral oil to lubricate the anal canal and to soften the stool. The treatment for hemorrhoids is digital dilatation of the rectal sphincter and removal of the hemorrhoids by ligation and then excision.

Postoperative care. Postoperatively a small rubber drain or wick of gauze usually is inserted through the sphincter to permit drainage of blood. Since there is usually very little drainage, only a small piece of gauze may be used over the anus or no dressing at all. The operative area, the dressing, and the bedding, however, should be inspected frequently for two or three hours postoperatively for signs of bleeding. While hemorrhage is not a common complication, it can occur. The drain is usually removed within twenty-four hours. The incidence of wound infection is slight due to local tissue resistance to the bacteria normally present in the rectum.

To prevent pressure on the anal area following a hemorrhoidectomy, the patient may be placed on his abdomen, although many patients prefer to lie on the back with a support such as a rubber air ring under the buttocks. Since the patient may have severe pain postoperatively, ice packs, warm wet compresses, analgesic ointments, and narcotics may be given. Since the operation is usually considered minor and dressings may not be used, the tendency may be to minimize this operative procedure. In reality it can cause the patient more discomfort than some much more serious operations. Sitz baths are usually started within twenty-four hours and often give relief from pain and discomfort; they should be supervised by nursing personnel until the patient can manage safely alone.

The patient often has difficulty voiding after a hemorrhoidectomy. This can usually be overcome by getting the patient out of bed to urinate. Sitz baths are also very helpful in stimulating voiding.

If the patient is not nauseated, a full diet is permitted immediately after surgery. Mineral oil usually is given once or twice a day beginning on the first postoperative day, and at any time the patient has a desire to pass gas or have a bowel movement he should be encouraged to do so. Care should be taken, however, as the bowel movement may be so painful that it may cause dizziness and even fainting. If a spontaneous bowel movement does not occur within three or four days postoperatively, an oil-retention enema followed by a cleansing enema is administered through a small rectal tube. The patient is advised to take a sitz bath after each bowel movement to keep the operative area clean and to relieve local irritation. This practice should be continued until he returns to the doctor (usually one to two weeks).

Following a hemorrhoidectomy, the patient is advised to avoid constipation by eating a diet containing adequate fruit and roughage, exercising moderately, drinking plenty of fluids, and establishing a regular time for daily bowel movements. The doctor may prescribe mineral oil or another mild laxative to be taken daily or every other day for a time.

Anal fissure

An anal fissure is an ulcer involving the entire thickness of the skin of the posterior anal wall. Upon inspection it appears to be a crack in the skin. It is the result of an anal infection, and the ulcer does not heal readily. Defecation initiates spasm of the anal sphincter and the patient has severe pain; this lasts for some time. Slight bleeding may occur, and constipation is usually caused by the patient restraining bowel movements to avoid pain.

Anal examination causes muscle spasm of the sphincter. Since this results in pain, the fissure must be examined under anesthesia. Treatment usually consists of digital dilatation of the sphincter under anesthesia, or the anal ulcer may be surgically excised.

Local pain and spasm sometimes can be relieved by warm compresses, sitz baths, and use of analgesic ointments. Mineral oil is usually ordered to lubricate the canal and to soften the stool. Postoperatively the care is similar to that given the patient who has had a hemorrhoidectomy.

Anal abscess

An anal abscess is located in tissues around the anus. It is caused by infection from the anal canal and may follow an anal fissure. If the abscess involves the anal, para-anal, or perineal tissues, there is throbbing local pain caused by pressure on the somatic sensory nerves in the perineum and local signs of inflammation. The patient finds it difficult to sit or lie on the area; in fact, any position is uncomfortable since he suffers from reflected pain.

If the abscess is located deep in the ischiorectal or submucosal tissues, however, the patient is aware only of vague discomfort until the disease spreads into an area where there are nerve fibers. The patient with an *ischiorectal abscess* is usually very ill; he has fever, chills, and malaise. The abscess must be incised and drained.

Postoperative care. Postoperatively the patient usually prefers to lie on his side or abdomen. Since most patients have some difficulty voiding, nursing measures should be initiated to prevent bladder distention. To void, the female patient needs to lie on her abdomen; this prevents pain and contamination of the wound. A small child's bedpan or an emesis basin is more comfortable for the patient to use in this position.

There is usually a large amount of seropurulent drainage from the wound, and the physician may order that the dressings be changed as necessary. The wound is usually packed with gauze, and the nurse may be asked to wet the pack with warm normal saline solution or to repack the wound with warm normal saline dressings at specified intervals. The packs should be inserted into the bottom of the wound since it is important that it heal from the inside outward. The skin around the wound should be protected with petroleum jelly to prevent irritation from drainage. The wet dressing should be covered with oiled silk or plastic material to prevent wick contamination and to prevent wetting the bed. The dressing can be held in place by Montgomery straps or a T-binder.

As healing progresses, sitz baths are usually ordered. If the wound is located near the anus, the patient is advised to cleanse the area carefully after defecation and to take a sitz bath after each defecation. Until healing is complete and all drainage disappears, a small dressing should be worn over the wound. Mineral oil may be given to prevent or to treat constipation. Antibiotics usually are given.

The patient is often discharged from the hospital before the wound has completely healed. He should continue to take sitz baths at home and if any difficulties are encountered should report to the doctor.

Anal fistula

An anal fistula is an inflammatory sinus or tract with a primary opening in an anal crypt and with a secondary opening on the anal, para-anal, or perineal skin or in the rectal mucous membrane. It results from the rupture or drainage of an anal abscess. The patient has a periodic drainage that stains his clothing. An anal fistula is usually a chronic condition, and unfortunately many patients attempt to treat themselves with patent remedies before they seek competent medical care.

The treatment of an anal fistula is a *fistulotomy.* The entire fistulous tract is opened under general anesthesia. The anesthesia relaxes the anal sphincter, making it easier to do the surgery. Following removal of the fistula the wound is packed.

Nursing care of the patient who has a fistulotomy is similar to that given the patient who has had an anal abscess incised and drained. The patient with a fistulotomy, however, is usually kept in bed until healing is progressing well. Bowel movements may be delayed by giving the patient lead and opium pills, and the patient may be given a liquid or a low-residue diet. After healing is well established, the constipating regimen is discontinued, and the patient may be given mineral oil and oil-retention enemas until a routine for regular elimination is established.

Pilonidal disease

Pilonidal cysts occur in the sacrococcygeal area and are thought to be congenital in origin. The cyst is lined with epithelium and hair. Pilonidal means "nest of hair." The cavity of the cyst communicates with the overlying skin by means of one or more short channels, each opening onto the skin in the midline. The lining of the channel or sinus is the same as the cyst, and tufts of hair are often seen protruding from the opening on the skin. These cysts or sinuses cause no symptoms unless they become infected. The patient then complains of pain and swelling at the base of the spine. An abscess forms, and it may rupture spontaneously or may require surgical incision and drainage. If the infection becomes chronic and the sinuses continue to drain, surgery becomes necessary.

Several types of operation may be done. The cyst may be excised and the wound closed. The patient remains in bed for several days after this procedure. To prevent contaminating the wound, the woman patient should void while lying on her abdomen. It is best if she practices this before the operation. The patient should be observed for complications of bed rest such as urinary retention and should be encouraged to cough, breathe deeply, and move his arms and legs often. Ambulation is gradual. The patient should not take large steps, and he should not sit for long periods since these activities cause tension on the incision. A low-residue diet is usually given, and foods such as orange juice or prune juice which may stimulate peristalsis are avoided for the first few days. Defecation usually is delayed several days if possible, and a small oil retention enema is sometimes ordered before the first defecation takes place. When the patient does have his first bowel movement, the surgeon usually wishes to be notified so that the dressing can be changed. Antibiotics are usually given prophylactically, and narcotics may be needed for pain.

If the cyst is excised and the wound widely exposed, the packing usually is removed within twenty-four hours after operation and the patient is then allowed to be out of bed. Sitz baths are usually ordered, and the wound is dressed daily and lightly packed with gauze. The nursing care is similar to that needed by patients who have surgery for anal abscesses. All patients with surgery about the rectum may be more comfortable when sitting on a protected pillow instead of a rubber ring.

REFERENCES AND SELECTED READINGS*

Common diagnostic tests and procedures

1 *Carmel, A. Gerson: Proctologic Nursing, Am. J. Nursing **48**:626-629, Oct. 1948.

2 Fuerst, Elinor V., and Wolff, LuVerne: Fundamentals of Nursing, ed. 2, Philadelphia, 1959, J. B. Lippincott Co.

3 Harmer, Bertha, and Henderson, Virginia (revised by): Textbook of the Principles and Practice of Nursing, ed. 5, New York, 1955, The Macmillan Co.

4 *Jay, Arthur: Is It Indigestion? Am. J. Nursing **58**:1552-1554, Nov. 1958.

5 *Loveland, Dorothy: Endoscopy, Am. J. Nursing **47**:732-734, Nov. 1947.

6 Smith, Tom E.: Proctoscopy and the Nurse, Am. J. Nursing **48**:232-233, April 1948.

7 Todd, James Campbell, and Stanford, Arthur Handley: Clinical Diagnosis by Laboratory Methods, ed. 12, Philadelphia, 1953, W. B. Saunders Co.

The patient with disease of the upper gastrointestinal system

8 Brown, Charles H.: New Blocking Agents, Am. J. Nursing **57**:877-879, July 1957.

9 Cassel, Chester: The Medical Management of Peptic Ulcer, Am. J. Nursing **52**:851-855, July 1952.

10 Cecil, Russell L., and Loeb, Robert F. (editors): Textbook of Medicine, ed. 10, Philadelphia, 1959, W. B. Saunders Co.

11 Davis, Loyal (editor): Christopher's Textbook of Surgery, ed. 6, Philadelphia, 1956, W. B. Saunders Co.

12 Diehl, Harold S.: The Textbook of Healthful Living, New York, 1955, McGraw-Hill Book Co., Inc.

13 Diller, Doris: Nursing Care in Esophageal Operations, Am. J. Nursing **47**:811-813, Dec. 1947.

14 Dragstedt, Lester R.: Gastric Vagotomy, Am. J. Nursing **48**:278-281, May 1948.

15 *Fisher, Jack A.: The Dumping Syndrome, Am. J. Nursing **58**:1126-1127, Aug. 1958.

16 Gordon, Betty Bason: Medical Nursing Care of Patients With Peptic Ulcer, Am. J. Nursing **52**:855-856, July 1952.

17 Hager, Catherine: Surgical Nursing Care of Patients With Duodenal Ulcer, Am. J. Nursing **52**:861-862, July 1952.

18 *Jay, Arthur N.: Colitis, Am. J. Nursing **59**:1133-1135, Aug. 1959.

19 Longmire, William P.: Esophageal Conditions and Their Treatment, Am. J. Nursing **47**:807-810, Dec. 1947.

20 Merrill, Isabel, and O'Neal, Louise: Nursing Care of the Patient With Peptic Ulcer, Am. J. Nursing **46**:520-523, Aug. 1946.

21 *Miller, Theodore: Gastric Cancer, Am. J. Nursing **56**:1420-1423, July 1956.

22 *Palumbo, Louis T.: Surgical Treatment of Duodenal Ulcer, Am. J. Nursing **52**:857-860, July 1952.

23 *Smith, Ann Valentine: Nasogastric Tube Feedings, Am. J. Nursing **57**:1451, Nov. 1957.

*References preceded by an asterisk indicate material particularly well suited for student reading.

24 Terracol, J., and Sweet, Richard H.: Diseases of the Esophagus, Philadelphia, 1958, W. B. Saunders Co.

25 *Woldman, Edward E.: Peptic Ulcer: Current Medical Treatment, Am. J. Nursing **59**:222-223, Feb. 1959.

The patient with disease of the lower gastrointestinal system

26 Booklet of Instructions for Persons With a Colostomy, ed. 2, New York, 1952, The New York Hospital.

27 Christian, Theresa: Nursing Care in Abdominal Surgery, Am. J. Nursing **50**:797-800, Dec. 1950.

28 Dericks, Virginia C., and Robeson, Kathryn A.: Problems of Colostomy Patients, Pub. Health Nursing **41**:16-18, Jan. 2, 1949.

29 Evans, Alberta, and Maisel, Bernard: Pneumoperitoneum in the Management of Hiatus Hernias, Am. J. Nursing **57**:1290-1293, Oct. 1957.

30 *Faust, Ernest Carroll: Amebiasis, Am. J. Nursing **54**:1507-1510, Dec. 1954.

31 Gale, Joseph W.: Intestinal Obstruction, Am. J. Nursing **48**:486-491, Aug. 1948.

32 *Hansen, Donald E.: Acute Appendicitis, Am. J. Nursing **55**:47-48, Jan. 1955.

33 Ingles, Thelma, and Campbell, Emily: The Patient with a Colostomy, Am. J. Nursing **58**:1544-1546, Nov. 1958.

34 Jaffee, Lila: The Patient and His Ileostomy, Am. J. Nursing **54**:68-70, Jan. 1954.

35 Lemner, K. E., and Watson, S. R.: Inguinal Hernia, Am. J. Nursing **53**:1471-1475, Dec. 1953.

36 *Linder, Janet: Inexpensive Colostomy Irrigation Equipment, Am. J. Nursing **58**:844, June 1958.

37 McDermott, William V.: Diverticulitis, Am. J. Nursing **54**:1231-1232, Oct. 1954.

38 Moseley, H. F.: Textbook of Surgery, ed. 2, St. Louis, 1955, The C. V. Mosby Co.

39 No One Knows I Have a Colostomy, Am. J. Nursing **51**:703-704, Dec. 1951.

40 Palumbo, Louis T.: Ulcerative Colitis: Medical and Surgical Care, Am. J. Nursing **55**:311-315, March 1955.

41 Secor, Sophie M.: New Hope for Colostomy Patients, Nursing Outlook **2**:642-643, Dec. 1954.

The patient with disease of the rectum and anal canal

42 Agnew, James W.: Abdominal-Perineal Resection, Am. J. Nursing **51**:225-228, April 1951.

43 Ferguson, Charles: Pilonidal Cysts, Am. J. Nursing **47**:68-69, Feb. 1947.

44 Frohman, I. Phillips: Constipation, Am. J. Nursing **55**:65-69, Jan. 1955.

The patient with disease of the liver and adjacent structures

Chapter 27

Study questions for review

1 Review the main functions of the liver.
2 What are the important constituents of bile? What is its function in digestion? Review the anatomy of the biliary system.
3 What are the practices in your hospital regarding use and sterilization of needles and syringes? Are sterile syringes used to draw blood? How are needles sterilized?
4 List some drugs you have learned about that are toxic to the liver.
5 Review from your notes on fundamentals of nursing the procedure and the nursing care given when a paracentesis is done.

The liver and the biliary system are affected by a variety of diseases. In this chapter general nursing care given when tests are ordered to determine liver and biliary function will be considered. Nursing procedures related to symptoms commonly seen in patients with liver and biliary diseases will be discussed before specific nursing care in some of the more common diseases is considered.

GENERAL NURSING CARE
Diagnostic examinations and tests

Several tests are used to determine whether or not liver disease is present and to distinguish the various causes of symptoms if some derangement of the liver or of the biliary system is evident. They include tests of liver function, procedures which demonstrate the amount and distribution of bile pigment, and roentgenograms which may show biliary malfunction.

Since the public is becoming better informed about diseases such as viral hepatitis, fear is usually present when liver disease is suspected. Many people have friends or acquaintances who have died of a liver disease or who have been handicapped for long periods of time. Therefore, the patient should be told the purpose of each test, what preparation is necessary, and what to expect during the test or examination.

Stools and urine. Stools and urine may be collected for study in liver and biliary disease. If the patient is ambulatory, but in the hospital, he should be told why he is asked to use the bedpan or urinal. Occasionally following an acute attack of biliary colic, the stools are saved to determine whether or not a stone has passed into the intestines. They may be sent to the laboratory or they may be crushed and strained for examination in the patient unit.

Stools may be examined for content of *bilirubin* and *urobilin*. In normal function, bilirubin is broken down in the intestine and absorbed for re-use by the liver, while urobilin is one of the end products which is normally excreted and gives the characteristic brown color to the stools. Since bile pigment is excreted in the urine in liver disease, urine specimens may be taken to test for the presence of abnormal bile pigments such as bilirubin. Total urine output for twenty-four hours may be requested to determine the amount of bile pigment being eliminated in the urine. Tests of the urine to determine the amount of bile pigment present may be done following an operation on the bile ducts in which an attempt has been made to establish passage of bile to the duodenum following obstruction.

X-ray examination. Several years ago is was discovered that a radiopaque substance could be administered which would be removed from the blood stream by a normal liver and stored and concentrated in the gallbladder. This test, sometimes called the *Graham* test or the *Graham-Cole* test after the physicians who first used it or more commonly a gallbladder series, shows the outline of a normal gallbladder and also reveals abnormalities in the biliary system in a roentgenogram. Stones, which are not radiopaque, show up as dark patches on the film. Visualization of the gallbladder depends upon absorption of the dye through the intestinal tract, isolation of it by the liver, and a free passageway from the liver to the gallbladder.

A synthetic drug, iodoalphionic acid (Priodax), in tablet form is now widely used. A newer preparation, Telepaque, is also used. The patient is given a low-fat evening meal, followed by six tablets of iodoalphionic acid (Priodax), 0.5 Gm. (7½ grains), to be taken by mouth, which is the average adult dose. Occasionally slight nausea may follow ingestion of the drug; if the pills are vomited, the doctor should be notified. He may ask that administration of the tablets be repeated in an hour or two when nausea subsides, or he may delay the test for a day or so. If vomiting persists, a radiopaque dye may be given intravenously; however, the preparation for the test is similar. The dye also may cause diarrhea. This should be reported to the doctor since the dye may have been eliminated through the gastrointestinal tract before enough was absorbed into the blood stream to reach the gallbladder.

On the morning of the examination the patient may have only black coffee, tea, or water. One or more enemas may be given to help remove gas from the intestinal tract which could interfere with a clear roentgenogram. The patient is taken to the x-ray department where two roentgenograms are taken during the morning. He is then given a high-fat noon meal, or more often a fatty substance, after which another roentgenogram is taken; ingestion of fat should stimulate flow of bile and emptying of the gallbladder.

The importance of following instructions regarding food restriction the morning of the test, as well as the need for the high-fat meal, even though he may not have sufficient appetite to enjoy this, should be explained to the patient. Severe hunger throughout the morning can be somewhat relieved by giving the patient small amounts of coffee, tea, or water. The dye is finally excreted in the urine, and some patients report slight temporary pain on urination following the test. If the results show a nonfunctioning gallbladder, sometimes the test is repeated to be sure that failure to visualize the gallbladder by x-ray examination was not due to insufficient dye.

Liver function tests. Liver function tests are used to determine the presence and the extent of liver damage and to check the progress of liver disease. They are of great importance in determining whether or not signs and symptoms are due to conditions that can be relieved by an operation or to medical conditions that will not benefit from surgery. It is estimated, for example, that about one half of all cases of jaundice can be cured by surgery while the other half, which are caused by disease within the liver or by excessive destruction of blood cells, are not amenable to surgical treatment.

Since the liver has many functions which are closely interrelated, single tests of liver function usually give information about the efficiency of several of the organ's activities. This is particularly true when metabolic functions are considered. Since most liver function tests involve taking samples of the patient's blood and many require that he fast preceding the test, causing inconvenience and discomfort for the patient, the nurse must do all she can to help so that tests need not be repeated. For example, if the nurse makes sure that blood samples are correctly labeled, urine specimens collected on time, and food withheld as necessary, she can help prevent the need for repetition of the tests. Since the rules of laboratories vary as to whether or not fasting should precede the taking of blood for some tests, the nurse should learn the practice in her hospital. If in doubt, it is usually best to have the patient fast, although the importance of regular meals for persons with liver disease must be kept in mind.

If the test to determine the *ratio of serum proteins* (A/G ratio) demonstrates alteration in the normal ratio, this may indicate degenerative liver disease. The serum albumin tends to drop below 4 Gm. per milliliter of blood while the serum globulin tends to rise above 2.4 Gm. per milliliter of blood in patients with liver disease. No fasting is necessary for this test of the patient's blood.

The *alkaline phosphatase test* is significant in that the result is only slightly elevated in liver diseases such as hepatitis and cirrhosis but is markedly elevated in biliary obstruction. Fasting is usually requested for this test.

A *quantitative determination of plasma cholesterol* may be done to determine liver function. It is known that patients with liver disease have a decrease in cholesterol esters in relation to total cholesterol. The normal blood serum cholesterol is between 140 and 220 mg. per cent, approximately 50 to 60 per cent of which is the cholesterol ester. In suspected or known liver disease a figure of 40 per cent or lower in cholesterol esters and a steady decrease in cholesterol esters are indicative of progressive liver disease and poor prognosis, while an increase in the cholesterol esters indicates improvement in the condition. Fasting usually is required for this test.

The *cephalin-cholesterol flocculation test* is performed to distinguish jaundice due to disease of the liver from obstructive jaundice. A colloidal suspension of a cephalin-cholesterol mixture becomes cloudy when normal blood serum is added but shows distinct flocculation and sedimentation when serum from the blood of a patient with liver damage is used; the latter is caused by failure of the diseased liver to make certain changes in the protein constituents of the plasma. The *thymol turbidity test* essentially is similar. Blood serum is added to a barbital buffer solution saturated with thymol, and the degree of turbidity indicates the amount of beta globulin present.[5] Fasting is usually requested for these tests.

Glucose tolerance and *galactose tolerance tests* determine disturbance in liver function in relation to carbohydrate metabolism. The galactose tolerance test is done as follows: The patient is not given anything by mouth on the morning of the test. The first morning specimen of urine is discarded, and the patient drinks 50 mg. of galactose dissolved in 500 ml. of water and flavored with lemon juice. After ingestion of this solution, urine specimens are collected hourly for five hours, numbered, and sent to the laboratory; the urine is examined for the total amount of sugar excreted. An excretion exceeding 3 mg. of sugar is considered indicative of disease. This test may also be performed by giving the galactose intravenously; 1 ml. of 50 per cent solution of galactose per kilogram of body weight is given after a sample of blood has been drawn. Another blood sample is taken one and one-fourth hours after injection of the galactose. A test on normal blood should reveal under 5 mg. of sugar per 100 ml. of blood in this blood sample. The glucose tolerance test is described in relation to care of the patient with diabetes (see Chapter 28).

Since one of the functions of the liver is excretion, tests which measure the rate with which dye is removed from the blood stream are useful, for example, the *Bromsulphalein test.* Fasting is necessary for this test. The patient is weighed and the dosage of the dye is calculated on the basis of 2 to 5 mg. per kilogram of body weight. The dye is injected into the vein, and blood samples are taken exactly five minutes and thirty minutes afterward. In some cases the nurse weighs the patient, injects the dye, and collects the blood samples, although usually the dye is injected by the doctor. The nurse participates in the scheduling of tests and should know that phenolsulfonphthalein tests for kidney function should not be scheduled for at least twenty-four hours after dye for a liver function test has been given.

Rose bengal instead of Bromsulphalein may be used as a dye for a similar test of liver function.

Tests also may reveal the amount of bile pigment in the blood serum which shows the functional capacity of the liver in breaking down, re-using, and excreting bile pigments. The *quantitative van den Bergh test* for serum bilirubin is one that is often ordered. Fasting is not necessary for this test. Normal serum should contain less than 1.5 mg. of bilirubin per 100 milliliters of blood. The *icterus index* is a test to determine the amount of bile pigment in blood plasma in which blood serum color is compared to a standard potassium dichromate solution. The normal reading is 4 to 6 units, although the reading may reach 15 units before jaundice is evident. Fasting usually is required for this test. Carrots eaten the day before the test will interfere with results because they color the blood serum.

The detoxifying capacity of the liver may be tested by means of the *hippuric acid test.* Hippuric acid results from the synthesis of benzoic acid and amino-acetic acid by the liver and is normally excreted at a regular rate in the urine. The test is done as follows: The patient is given a light breakfast of toast and coffee. One hour later, 6 Gm. of sodium benzoate, dissolved in 30 ml. of water and flavored with oil of peppermint, cherry syrup, or lemon juice is given by mouth. This may be followed by 100 ml. of water. The patient is then asked to void immediately, and this specimen is discarded; then he does not take anything by mouth and voids each hour for four hours. The specimens are labeled, numbered, and sent to the laboratory. Normal excretion should be approximately 3 Gm. of hippuric acid in the four specimens. Abnormal findings may show poor liver function such as occurs in hepatitis, cirrhosis, and malignant disease of the liver. In conditions in which jaundice is the result of obstruction in the biliary passages and in which the liver has not yet been damaged, the test is normal. Occasionally the test is done by giving sodium benzoate intravenously after the patient has voided and taken a glass of water. One urine specimen is collected an hour after the sodium benzoate solution has been administered.

Since prothrombin (and fibrinogen) is manufactured by the liver and functions in the clotting of blood, a *low prothrombin level* may indicate liver disease and may warn of danger of hemorrhage. A low prothrombin level that fails to respond to bile salts given by mouth and to parenteral administration of synthetic vitamin K indicates that jaundice may be due to liver damage and not to biliary obstruction. The prothrombin level is often lowered in cirrhosis of the liver and in metastatic carcinoma of the liver. Fasting is not necessary for this test.

Duodenal drainage. This test, also known as the biliary drainage test, consists of examination of bile obtained from the duodenum and may be done when the patient is ambulatory or while he is hospitalized. The preparation is similar to that for a gastric analysis (see Chapter 26). The patient is not permitted anything by mouth except small sips of water for twelve hours. A slender tube made of rubber is weighted at its tip with metal and marked with a series of rings to indicate the distance it travels as it is passed through the patient's mouth to his stomach cardia, pylorus, and the duodenum, respectively. After the tube has been passed into the stomach, the patient is placed on his right side with hips elevated about 6 inches so that the stomach movement, aided by gravity, will carry the tube into the duodenum. It may take a while for this to occur; when the tube finally reaches the duodenum, several specimens must be taken. The patient should be prepared for a somewhat lengthy procedure. He should know, however, that once the tube has been passed he will have little or no discomfort. The first specimen which drains from the duodenum is usually light in color and consists of bile coming from the common duct. Fifty milliliters of magnesium sulfate (25 per cent solution) are then introduced into the duodenum through the tube, and a second specimen is collected in from ten to fifteen minutes. This specimen is usually darker and more viscid, containing bile from the gallbladder which has flowed in response to the cholagogue action of magnesium sulfate. A third specimen containing bile coming from the hepatic duct and freshly secreted by the liver is sometimes collected.

Liver biopsy. A liver biopsy may be taken in an attempt to establish a diagnosis. In this procedure a double needle is inserted into the liver and a small piece of tissue is removed for study. Because of the danger of hemorrhage, many doctors consider this procedure unsafe if the patient is jaundiced. Vitamin K may be given parenterally for several days before the biopsy is taken. The doctor should explain the procedure to the patient; for example, the patient should know that he must hold his breath and remain absolutely still when the needle is introduced, since breathing may cause a tear in the liver covering. Most hospitals require that the patient sign his permission for the procedure to be done. A sedative usually is given about half an hour before the biopsy is to be done. The patient lies on his back. After the skin has been cleansed, it is anesthetized with procaine hydrochloride; the area selected may be between or below the ribs. A nick is made in the skin with a sharp scalpel blade. Then the patient is instructed to take several deep breaths and to hold his breath while the outer needle is introduced through the intercostal or subcostal tissues into the liver. A finer needle with a longitudinal slit is then passed through and beyond the outer needle, and the outer needle is advanced to separate the specimen, a tiny cylinder of liver tissue. Both needles are withdrawn together. For this procedure the doctor needs sterile gloves and a sterile tray containing drapes, syringe and needles for injection of the procaine hydrochloride, a No. 11 scalpel blade with handle, solutions to cleanse the skin, dressings to cover the wound, and a slide with 10 per cent formaldehyde or a sponge moistened with saline solution for the specimen. The procedure may be done with the patient sitting on a treatment table or in bed with his feet over the side and firmly supported on a chair or a stool. One nurse should give the patient encouragement, observe him closely, and support him if dizziness occurs, while a second nurse assists the doctor.

For several hours after a liver biopsy has been taken the patient should lie on his right side with a small pillow or folded bath blanket placed under the costal margin. He usually remains on bed rest for twelve hours. The dangers in this procedure, which is done relatively "blind," are accidental penetration of a small blood vessel, causing hemorrhage, and accidental penetration of a biliary vessel, causing a chemical peritonitis from leakage of bile into the abdominal cavity. The patient's pulse rate and blood pressure should be taken every half hour for the first few hours and then hourly for at least twenty-four hours. The nurse should check the equipment used and the specimen very carefully for any signs of discoloration from bile and report her findings to the doctor. Occasionally, a laparotomy must be done to treat complications of a liver biopsy procedure.

Jaundice

The liver, sometimes termed the chemical laboratory of the body, is one of the most complicated and versatile organs of the body. For descriptions of some of the many fascinating activities of this remarkable organ, the student is referred to specialized texts. One of the important functions of the liver is the production of bile and the re-use of some of the products of bile that are absorbed through the intestinal wall and returned by means of the blood stream.

Jaundice is a symptom complex characterized by a disturbance of the physiology of bile pigment. An excess of bile pigment in the blood is eventually distributed to the skin, mucous membranes, and other body fluids and body tissues. Jaundice is often described as catarrhal, infectious, or toxic, indicating that the cause is faulty liver action; mechanical or obstructive, due to intrahepatic or extrahepatic obstruction; and hemolytic, presumably caused by excessive destruction of blood cells.

Pruritus. Deposit of bile pigment in the skin often causes itching, although some patients have severe jaundice without pruritus. Bathing or sponging the skin with tepid water, followed by the application of calamine lotion with 1 per cent phenol, often helps relieve itching. Starch and sodium bicarbonate in the water often produce relief, but they are drying to the skin and their use should be followed by a gentle massage with a cream lotion. The antihistamine drugs are sometimes useful in controlling pruritus. Profuse diaphoresis sometimes occurs in liver and biliary disease, and bile-stained perspiration may color the bed linen. The linen should be changed at once for psychologic reasons as well as for physical comfort. Only soft old linen should be used for the patient with pruritus.

The patient's fingernails should be cut short and his hands kept clean, since itching may be so severe that the patient may excoriate the skin by scratching and may cause skin lesions which heal very slowly when jaundice is pronounced.

Emotional factors. The patient with marked jaundice is usually sensitive about his appearance. If he is ambulatory, dark glasses can be worn to conceal the yellow color of the sclera. The hospital room should be kept softly lighted; white or yellowish light bulbs make jaundice much less obvious than does fluorescent lighting. If possible, mirrors should be inconspicuously removed. The patient who is particularly concerned with his appearance may rest better in a room by himself and may wish to have visitors restricted.

Hemorrhage. The jaundiced patient has a low blood prothrombin level and bleeds easily; therefore, he is a poor risk for surgery and may bleed profusely from minor medical procedures. Normal production of prothrombin is dependent upon four things: (1) ingestion of foods which can undergo synthesis in the intestine, (2) presence of bile in the intestine, thus enabling the intestine to produce vitamin K from food constituents, (3) absorption through the intestinal wall of the vitamin K produced, and (4) use of the vitamin K by the liver in the formation of prothrombin. Since vitamin K depends upon the presence of bile salts for its manufacture and absorption in the intestine, bile salts are often given by mouth to patients who are jaundiced. Vitamin K may be given both orally and parenterally in the hope that this will enable the liver to form more prothrombin. If the liver is severely affected and unable to make use of the vitamin K provided, the prothrombin level will remain low despite the administration of bile salts and vitamin K. However, if the jaundice is due to obstruction in the biliary tract and not to liver damage it can be satisfactorily treated. The patient is given bile salts by mouth in dosages of 0.2 to 0.4 Gm. (3½ to 7 grains), three times a day; this improves production and absorption of vitamin K in the intestine. Menadione is a synthetic vitamin K preparation which can be given by mouth in dosages of 1 to 2 mg. daily (1/60 to 1/30 grain) in tablet or capsule form or by intramuscular injection. Bile salts should be administered when menadione is given by mouth. Menadione sodium bisulfite (Hykinone) is a preparation of vitamin K which does not need to be accompanied by bile salts when taken orally. The usual dose is 4 mg. (1/15 grain), given daily intramuscularly, hypodermically, intravenously, or by mouth.

The jaundiced patient may bleed more than usual from such minor procedures as drawing blood from a vein. To avoid repeated venous punctures, plans can be made for samples of blood to be taken for several desired tests and an infusion started at the same time. When giving intramuscular and hypodermic injections, the nurse should select the smallest needle that she can use safely and be particularly careful that the needle is sharp and that, following an injection, firm pressure is exerted for longer than is normally necessary. The patient's urine and stools should be checked for either old or fresh blood and specimens saved if bleeding is suspected. Steady oozing of blood from hemorrhoids is not unusual in severe jaundice.

Nutrition and elimination

Nutrition. Seeing that patients with liver and biliary diseases eat enough of the necessary foods is one of the most important nursing responsibilities in their care. The patient with a liver or biliary disease usually has difficulties with food. Disturbance of liver function and interference with normal flow of bile into the intestine upsets the entire digestive system and causes indigestion, poor appetite, flatulence, and constipation. The patient does not tolerate fatty foods well, and he may have learned over a period of months or years to avoid high-fat foods that tend to produce gas in the stomach and intestinal tract.

In recent years a great deal of attention has been given to diet and its relation to chronic degenerative disease of the liver. It is suspected that the liver's ability to excrete toxins and carry on its many other functions is seriously hampered by inadequate intake of protein and of vitamin B. If liver damage has occurred, the organ's ability to store glycogen and vitamins A, B complex, C, and D may also be lessened and the patient may be in much greater need of regular intake of complete foods than before his illness. Diet, therefore, becomes one of the most important parts of medical therapy.

A diet high in protein and vitamins, fairly high in carbohydrate (unless weight reduction is desired), and low in fat is often ordered. The nurse should learn what the patient likes to eat, what particular foods cause him most distress, and what foods he tolerates well. She should learn what meal schedule for the day seems to suit him best. For example, does he tolerate and enjoy frequent small meals? Does he like snacks between meals? Does he like the heaviest meal at noon or at the end of the day? She should convey this information to the dietitian so that meals for the hospitalized patient may not be too different from those at home.

Many doctors believe that the patient who has liver damage should have 100 to 300 Gm. of protein per day, but it is exceedingly difficult to have the patient eat this amount. Lean beef (broiled steak if it can be afforded), broiled chicken, and fish are some of the best high-protein foods. Egg white, gelatin, and cottage cheese provide large amounts of protein and can be prepared in a variety of ways; yeast is particularly high in protein and in vitamin B. Dried skimmed milk is very useful for fortifying drinks taken between meals and can be added to muffins, sauces, and many other foods. If the patient is hospitalized, members of his family should be permitted to bring in foods that he likes and will eat provided these foods conform to the diet prescribed. Almost any exceptions in dietary regulations should be made to get what the patient needs and will eat. Some hospitals have hot plates in the diet pantries where steaks, for example, may be cooked individually and thus made much more acceptable than regular hospital fare. Alcohol, however, to stimulate appetite or for any other purpose is practically never ordered for patients with liver disease since it may be taxing to an injured liver.

Mouthwashes before meals help to relieve the unpleasant sensation and taste in the mouth which interfere with appetite and which are so common in patients with liver disease. Meals should be attractively served, with hot foods hot and cold foods cold. Diversion during meals helps to improve appetite, often the patient eats best when not too much comment is made about appetite. Some patients find that drinking effervescent fluids instead of water during the meal helps to relieve nausea and the feeling of flatulance after meals. The patient should rest for half an hour immediately after concluding a meal.

Elimination. Clay-colored stools are caused by the absence of the bile pigment urobilinogen in the feces and by the presence of undigested fat. Constipation is common but is usually relieved by mild laxatives such as mineral oil or milk of magnesia. Bile salts taken orally also help to make intestinal evacuations more normal. If urobilinogen is not being excreted in the stools, the urine may be a dark brownish color. Dark urine should indicate to the nurse the need to examine the stool since changes in the color of urine or stools may be early specific signs of liver or biliary disease.

Protection from other diseases

The patient with severe liver or biliary disease is a ready candidate for *infection.* His resistance is low so that respiratory infections are easily acquired and shed with difficulty. Since infections produce toxins that must be dealt with by the liver, it is important that the patient be protected from exposure to infections of any kind. If he is seriously ill, he should be in a single room, and attendants who have upper respiratory infections should not be admitted. Visitors who have colds or other infections should be warned of the danger to the patient.

A large number of *drugs* are toxic to the injured liver. Furthermore, drugs may not be disposed of at the usual rate if liver function is impaired. Since drugs such as the barbiturates may have a delayed action, physical symptoms such as restlessness should be combated by nursing means so that medications can be avoided. For example, the usual nursing measures such as a back rub, attention to ventilation, and a warm drink should be tried before resorting to sedatives for sleep, and an ice cap should be tried before codeine is given for a headache. Even if the patient has little or no jaundice, the liver should be protected from possible additional injury by drugs.

INFECTIONS OF THE LIVER AND PANCREAS

Viral hepatitis

Viral hepatitis is by far the most important infection attacking the liver. Although the disease is not new, it assumed serious proportions during World War II and since that time has become a major public health problem. Viral hepatitis had existed in epidemic form during previous wars, but it was not until World War II that it was given extensive study, the nature of its spread fully recognized, and two strains of the virus identified. At the present time viral hepatitis is a common disease which presents a real threat to the health of the general population.

Causative agents—conduct and mode of transmission. Viral hepatitis is believed to be caused by filtrable viruses. Since these are not transmissible from man to experimental animals, study of the disease is difficult. The viruses of hepatitis appear to be extremely resistant to usual methods of destruction of pathogenic agents. They are known to survive freezing for long periods of time and heating to 56° C. (133° F.) for one hour. They have survived for several months in serum containing Merthiolate, 1:2000, and in a mixture of equal parts of phenol and ether in a 0.5 per cent solution.[18] There is evidence that the virus is more resistant to chlorination than are bacterial pathogens, and there is no proof that boiling for less than thirty minutes is effective in their destruction. Autoclaving is the best way to destroy the virus.

Viral hepatitis is caused by two distinct but similar viruses which produce almost identical symptoms but which vary in their incubation period and mode of transmision. These are known as the "A" or IH virus (short-incubation virus), causing infectious hepatitis, and the "B" or SH virus (long-incubating virus), causing homologous serum hepatitis. The incubation period for the IH virus is ten to forty days, for the SH virus, probably two to six months.[1]

Infectious hepatitis can be transmitted through natural channels or through any break in the skin, such as by parenteral injection. It is believed that infection usually occurs through personal contact, food, milk, water, or possibly insect vectors. The virus has been found in the gastrointestinal tract and in the blood, and the virus may remain for long periods of time in the feces of persons who have had the disease and in carriers. It is not known whether carriers are natural carriers or whether they have had the disease in mild and unnoticed form. It is known that mild subclinical disease which is not severe enough to cause jaundice can occur. Infectious hepatitis occurs throughout the world and seems to be more prevalent in low-income areas where there is crowding and limited sanitation. The incidence is highest in the fall and early winter, and susceptibility appears to decrease with age, being greatest between the ages of 6 and 25 years.

Homologous serum hepatitis is transmitted only parenterally through blood serum from persons who are infected or who are carriers of the virus. Pooled blood plasma, which is widely used during wartime, is a common source of infection. During the Korean War it was found that one out of five persons who received pooled plasma acquired the disease.[18] The increased use of blood transfusions in recent years has led to higher incidence of homologous serum hepatitis, although the chance of acquiring it by this means is much less than when pooled plasma is given. In the use of pooled plasma the chances are increased proportionately by the number of donors whose plasma is used. Any immunizing or therapeutic agent made from human plasma can be a means of transmitting the disease to those who receive the product by injection. There is no acquired immunity to homologous serum hepatitis, and anyone who is exposed may develop the disease despite age. Homologous serum jaundice can be transmitted from infected patients to medical, nursing, and other hospital personnel by accidentally pricking the skin with needles contaminated by a patient's blood.

Viral hepatitis is a serious disease. The large number of patients with mild clinical symptoms but no jaundice makes accurate reporting difficult. Fatality rate has been reported as less than 0.5 per cent.[2] Studies vary as to the mortality rate, but one series showed a death rate of 1.8 per 1,000 patients, while other smaller studies reported a death rate of 35 per cent in patients hospitalized because of the disease.[18] It is estimated that at least 10 per cent of all patients suffer some residual damage for as long as a year and that at least 2 per cent have liver damage persisting much longer. The disease has not been under study long enough to determine whether or not cirrhosis or other severe degeneration of the liver occurs many years after the acute onset of the disease. Homologous serum hepatitis has a somewhat higher mortality rate than infectious hepatitis, but it is thought this may be because many patients who are given plasma or blood transfusions are already quite ill and that lowered host resistance, rather than a higher virulence of the SH virus, may be the cause of death.[16] Recent studies show that pregnant women are highly susceptible to viral hepatitis during the second and third trimesters of pregnancy and that the mortality rate is extremely high in the last trimester.

One attack of viral hepatitis confers immunity for that strain of virus infection but does not protect against attack by the other virus. However, the disease can become chronic, with acute exacerbations occurring months after the first acute symptoms have subsided. Liver damage following attack by one virus naturally lessens the body's defenses if attack by the second virus should occur.

Prevention. It is in the area of prevention that the nurse can make her greatest contribution to control of viral hepatitis. Since there is no specific treatment for the disease and no available immunization, it is only by making use of what is known about the viruses that control can be accomplished.

Methods of destroying the viruses of hepatitis are limited; therefore, particular emphasis should be placed on *thorough handwashing* with soap and running water after possible exposure. Thorough washing of all equipment that might be contaminated lessens the danger to persons who must handle it and may help protect the next patient for whom the equipment is used. Since infectious hepatitis can be transmitted by infected foods and water, food handlers should be encouraged to pay careful attention to handwashing regulations.

At the present time dry heat and steam heat under pressure (autoclaving) are the only safe ways to sterilize needles and other equipment used to penetrate the skin. The adequate boiling time is still undetermined, and for this reason many hospitals are converting to autoclave sterilization almost entirely. While the nurse cannot set the policy in such matters for the hospital or the public health agency where she is employed, by careful planning she can often see that almost all equipment is autoclaved and that boiling is resorted to only in emergencies.

There are still situations in which boiling is the only way to sterilize needles and other equipment. If the nurse finds herself in such a situation, she should see that everything placed in the sterilizer is *covered completely* and *boiled* for at *least half an hour*.[6] The only way to be certain that equipment has been boiled the proper length of time is to mark the sterilizer and to time it accurately. Since the nurse is responsible for the work of auxiliary nursing personnel, it is her responsibility to see that they understand the importance of sterilization and that they do not drop pieces of equipment into the sterilizer during the boiling period or take other unsafe shortcuts. The danger of improper sterilization can be lessened by permitting only one person in the patient unit to use the sterilizer.

Both infectious hepatitis and homologous serum hepatitis can be transmitted from one patient to another when the "multiple dose–single syringe" method is used in which several doses are put into one syringe and only the needle is changed between patients. This is a dangerous procedure under any circumstances and should never be used. Regardless of the extra expense involved and the extra time and work entailed in preparation of materials for each injection, separate needles and syringes that have been autoclaved should be used. School immunization programs and practices in large outpatient clinics such as allergy clinics have been affected by recent recommendations in this regard. The nurse who is in charge often must help explain the need for the extra cost to administrative personnel. The nurse actually giving the injections and caring for equipment has a responsibility to handle it safely and carefully. Disposable syringes and needles are now available and, though not in general use at the present time, may save much breakage expense when many syringes must be handled.

If the nurse is in a position in which she is responsible for obtaininig blood specimens for laboratory tests, she should insist that only autoclaved lancets or needles be used to prick the skin and that only autoclaved needles and syringes be used in taking blood. All syringes should be autoclaved since a vacuum may be created that can draw contamination from the syringe into the patient's vein. Soaking equipment in alcohol or any of the commonly used antiseptics is useless; in fact, no chemical sterilization is safe against the virus of homologous serum hepatitis.[6]

Since there are carriers of the IH and SH viruses, all needles and other equipment that have penetrated the skin of any patient should be handled with the greatest care. Homologous serum hepatitis occurs quite frequently among hospital personnel. This is not surprising considering how often the nurse, the laboratory worker, or other member of the nursing staff may unwittingly prick himself with needles that have been used for a wide variety of parenteral treatments. The safest way to handle any needle is to rinse it carefully in plain water after use and to place it in a rack which can be immersed in a solvent or soap solution. This practice is now in use in some institutions and agencies where all needles are cared for by a central sterile supply department or by a special staff. Also, special washers that provide efficient cleansing of both needles and syringes with a minimum of handling are now available. Needles from infusion sets should be removed immediately from the tubing when an infusion is discontinued so that persons cleaning the equipment at a later time will not accidentally prick themselves.

It is recommended that patients with infectious hepatitis be isolated for seven days,[1] although there is no record of the disease being directly transmitted to those caring for a patient in the hospital. The greatest caution should be taken in handling the patient's fecal waste and in performing treatments that involve contamination of the hands. Bedpans should be isolated and should be boiled for an hour following the patient's discharge from the hospital. Rubber gloves are often advised when enemas are given. For the protection of the nursing personnel, the patient's temperature should be taken by mouth whenever possible. When small children must have the temperature taken rectally, the greatest care should be given to careful handwashing. At the present time there is no really safe and satisfactory method of sterilizing thermometers. Poor technique in carrying out temperature-taking procedures has been suspected as a cause of widespread infection from the IH virus in foundling homes and similar sheltered care facilities for children. All patients should have individual thermometers, and the thermometer used for a patient with infectious hepatitis should be discarded upon his discharge from the hospital.

Because the virus of infectious hepatitis has never been found in urine, no special protection is needed in the handling of urinary excretions. However, care should be taken in handling nose and mouth secretions. The patient should be instructed to use tissues which are placed in a paper bag and burned.

No isolation is necessary for homologous serum hepatitis since it is transmitted only by contamination from the patient's blood and blood plasma. If any doubt exists as to which of the virus diseases a patient has, it is safest to isolate him for seven days and take the precautions necessary in the care of patients with infectious hepatitis.

If a woman in the second or third trimester of pregnancy has been exposed to viral hepatitis, she should be urged to report this to her doctor. Gamma globulin offers some protection against infectious hepatitis, but it does not protect against the SH virus of homologous serum hepatitis. However, since often it cannot be determined which of the two diseases is involved, gamma globulin usually is given in the hope that exposure was to the IH virus of infectious hepatitis. Although gamma globulin and serum albumin are obtained from the blood, they do not transmit the virus of homologous serum hepatitis; therefore, their administration cannot expose the patient to this disease.

Symptoms and pathology. Symptoms and pathology in infectious hepatitis and homologous serum jaundice are almost identical, except that acute symptoms may be more severe in infectious hepatitis. Symptoms usually appear from four to seven days before jaundice is apparent and may consist of headache, anorexia, nausea and vomiting, chills, elevation of temperature, aches and pains, malaise, and tenderness over the liver. Often the patient who smokes has a sudden distaste for tobacco. Examination of blood cells reveals a leukopenia. The temperature usually returns to normal when jaundice appears, but the anorexia and nausea persist. The clinical symptoms often occur without being followed by jaundice making diagnosis difficult.

Viral hepatitis causes a diffuse degeneration of liver cells throughout the organ, with necrosis of cells either ultimately regenerated or replaced with fibrosis. Because the pathologic process is usually distributed evenly throughout the liver, biopsy has been particularly useful in studying and diagnosing the disease.

The disease may take several courses, and different terms describe each of these. Outcome of viral hepatitis may be affected by such factors as the virulence of the virus, the amount of liver damage sustained during the patient's life before exposure to the virus, his natural barriers to liver damage and disease, and the supportive care he receives when symptoms appear.

Fulminating *viral hepatitis* or acute yellow atrophy designates a sudden and severe degeneration and atrophy of the liver. This condition may follow acute poisoning, but it is most often associated with an overwhelming infection with the hepatitis virus. *Acute fatal hepatic necrosis* and *acute massive necrosis* are other terms used to designate this condition which begins as an infection and progresses rapidly to cause death. The liver may shrink in size to as little as 600 Gm. in contrast to a weight of 1,500 Gm. in a normal adult.[16]

Subacute fatal viral hepatitis causes acute massive necrosis which, even though it is not evenly distributed throughout the organ, finally destroys enough of the liver to cause death. This form of the disease may vary in duration from several weeks to several months, with apparent short remissions followed by exacerbations. In its late stages subacute fatal viral hepatitis is almost impossible to distinguish from cirrhosis of the liver in clinical manifestations and in liver function tests; however, history of exposure to viral hepatitis and symptoms of acute infection aid in diagnosis.

Viral hepatitis can become chronic. Although liver biopsy has been a substantial aid in studying the course of hepatitis in the liver and the regeneration that occurs, chronic forms of the disease are still not well understood. Signs of chronicity may persist in biopsied liver tissue when liver function tests show no abnormality and when no clinical signs are evident. However, the opposite may be true. It is suspected that the liver may not use all its cells at one time since jaundice occurs in patients when a relatively small part of the liver is destroyed, whereas in experimental animals it does not occur until 90 to 95 per cent has been removed, indicating that there are considerable reserves in the normal functioning organ.[10] Acute exacerbations of chronic viral hepatitis can progress to acute fatal hepatic necrosis.

Cholangiolitis is a condition in which stasis occurs in the bile canaliculi, while bile ducts within and outside the liver remain normal. It is thought to be due to viral hepatitis, although the same or very similar pathologic changes occur in the liver after ingestion of some poisonous drugs. Cholangiolitis is presumed to be caused by increased permeability of the cholangioles (ductules which carry the bile to the intrahepatic ducts) which causes bile to be regurgitated into the blood. Obstruction of the cholangioles follows since not all constituents of the bile are absorbed.

Medical treatment and nursing care. There is no specific medical treatment for viral hepatitis. The patient is kept in bed, and general care, including attention to good oral hygiene, skin care, and elimination, is necessary. Special attention should be paid to protecting the patient from infection. The nurse who cares for the patient in his own home should observe carefully for changes in the color of urine and stool and for jaundice and should report these at once to the physician.

If the patient's temperature is high and nausea and vomiting are severe, infusions containing glucose and salt are given, and occasionally solutions containing other electrolytes and protein hydrolysates are ordered. Fluid intake and output are recorded. During the acute stage of the disease, fluids are encouraged by mouth if nausea is not a problem; the desirable fluid intake usually is considered to be at least 3,000 ml. per day. Occasionally a daily weight is requested to determine whether there is water retention in acute stages of the disease, and when chronic disease has developed it is taken if ascites or edema is suspected.

During the first few days the patient feels ill, and keeping him contented in bed is not difficult; later, however, this becomes a nursing problem. Usually the patient must remain in bed several weeks although acute symptoms usually subside within two weeks. Wheeling the patient in his bed to the recreation area where he may view television or converse with others often helps him pass the day without boredom. Occupational therapy activities that can be brought to the bedside are useful in keeping the patient relatively content during the tiresome convalescent period. If the patient is isolated he should be told how long this is necessary.

Although foods with high protein and high carbohydrate contents have not been proved helpful in viral hepatitis,[2] a diet high in protein and high in carbohydrate is usually ordered. Vitamins may be given in an attempt to improve appetite. After the first few weeks the patient may feel well and begin to worry about his confinement. He becomes anxious to resume normal living and irritated by the circumstances requiring enforced inactivity. His irritation may be expressed by tiring of the hospital menu no matter how good the food may be. The family should realize that in the home he may also be critical of food for the same reason.

Liver abscess

A liver abscess may be caused by a variety of pyogenic organisms carried by the blood stream or traveling from the portal vein. Occasionally an infection in abdominal organs or other structures such as the appendix may lead to an abscess. The most common cause of liver abscess is infection with *Entamoeba histolytica*, the causative organism in amebic dysentery. Signs of liver involvement can occur several months after an attack of amebic dysentery.

Chloroquine and emetine are the drugs most widely used to combat amebic infections, but they are never given together because of the toxic effects, such as tremors, dermatitis, and nausea, they produce. An amebic abscess may be aspirated by needle, and emetine or another antiamebic drug introduced into the abscess cavity. Amebic abscesses do not respond well to surgical drainage.

Pancreatic disease

Pancreatitis. Pancreatitis may be caused by infection carried in the blood stream or traveling from the biliary system or the duodenum. It may follow obstruction of the pancreatic duct and subsequent congestion of the gland. Obstruction may be caused by a stone from the gallbladder or from regurgitation of bile into the pancreatic duct.

The most common type of *acute pancreatitis* is known as the *edematous* type and often is associated with chronic biliary tract disease. The patient has constant pain radiating to the back which may be so severe that he refuses to lie on his side. Nausea and vomiting, elevation of temperature, and elevation of white blood cell count often are present. The treatment is conservative, and most patients will recover without surgery. An elevated serum amylase level as shown by examination of the blood often helps the doctor to distinguish acute pancreatitis from other acute conditions of the abdomen which may require immediate surgery. Antibiotics are usually given, and fluids and food are provided intravenously. Food by mouth is withheld because of nausea and because it would stimulate the pancreas and aggravate symptoms. Nitroglycerin is sometimes helpful in relieving severe pain, but morphine or meperidine hydrochloride (Demerol) often is needed.

A much less common but more severe form of acute pancreatitis is known as *acute hemorrhagic pancreatitis.* This fulminating process may cause severe necrosis of pancreatic tissue with destruction by its own enzymes and hemorrhage into the gland with release of blood exudate into the abdominal cavity. The patient goes quickly into shock, and immediate treatment for shock is required. Operation may be done to drain blood or other fluid from the abdominal cavity. Despite intensive medical treatment and the best of nursing care, the mortality from this condition is high.

Pancreatitis can become *chronic* with calcification and fibrous replacement of normal duct tissue. Nausea, persistent pain, loss of weight, and occasionally jaundice occur. The danger of addiction to narcotics becomes a problem with these patients. Operation is sometimes done in an attempt to divert or increase bile flow at the sphincter of Oddi (entrance to the duodenum) and thereby reduce regurgitation of bile into the pancreatic duct.

Tumors. Tumors of the pancreas are usually malignant and occur most often in the head of the pancreas causing jaundice and obstruction. Men are affected much more often than women; usually the patient is past middle life and obvious signs may have been preceded by vague anorexia, nausea, and weight loss over a period of months. Surgery is usually done in an attempt to remove the tumor. If this is not possible, an operation is done to help restore temporarily a normal flow of bile and some pancreatic enzyme to the intestinal tract. The type of procedure performed depends on the involvement found at operation. For example, the gallbladder may be anastamosed to the jejunum, the remaining portion of the pancreas to the jejunum at its free end, and the stomach to the jejunum at a lower site. In this operation (Whipple operation) the head of the pancreas, the bile ducts, the duodenum, and the pyloric end of the stomach are removed. Postoperatively the patient must be carefully watched for signs of hyperinsulinism since the operative procedure may temporarily stimulate release of more insulin than is normal. In addition to routine postoperative care following abdominal surgery he must be watched for signs of peritonitis, gastrointestinal obstruction and jaundice until sufficient time for healing has elapsed and it is determined that all the anastamoses are successful. Stools should be observed, and frothy light-colored stools containing conspicuously undigested fat should be reported. If most of the pancreas was removed, the patient may have to take pancreatic enzymes in tablet form by mouth to aid the digestion of fat. If the pancreas has been completely removed, signs and symptoms of hypoinsulinism will occur and treatment with insulin will be necessary for the remainder of the patient's life. (See Chapter 28 for treatment and care of patients with too little or too much insulin.)

LIVER TRAUMA

Trauma to the liver is fairly commonly associated with automobile accidents or other injuries. There may be rupture of the liver with severe internal hemorrhage and death. Attempts are sometimes made to operate and suture the ruptured organ or to apply local pressure to stop the bleeding. Occasionally blood is aspirated from the abdominal cavity into a sterile receptacle containing sodium citrate to prevent coagulation and is then returned to the body through the usual transfusion route. The patient who has sustained rupture of the liver is almost always in severe shock, and all the medical and nursing measures used for shock may be employed (see Chapter 14).

Trauma to the liver can cause severe contusion, with subsequent degeneration of injured liver cells. Prognosis depends upon the amount of liver tissue damaged and other factors, and the final outcome for the patient may not be known for many years after the injury has been sustained.

CARCINOMA OF THE LIVER

Primary carcinoma of the liver is exceedingly rare. Secondary carcinoma, however, is very common and occurs in about one third of all patients in whom carcinoma has not been controlled by surgery before metastasis occurs. Metastasis to the liver should always be suspected when a patient with a history of carcinoma develops anorexia, weakness, loss of weight, secondary anemia, and general ill health. Jaundice and ascites are signs that the process is quite far advanced; the patient may then live only a few weeks. There is no treatment for carcinoma of the liver beyond symptomatic medical and nursing care. Radioactive gold (Au^{198}) may be injected into the peritoneal cavity. For further details of this and of care of the terminally ill cancer patient see Chapter 16.

DEGENERATIVE DISEASE OF THE LIVER

Degenerative disease of the liver can follow injury, infection, and damage by toxic agents such as incompatible blood. It can be caused by obstruction of biliary passages with subsequent pressure and damage to liver cells. It can also be due to the ingestion of substances toxic to the liver, to faulty nutrition, and possibly to other factors not yet understood.

Prevention

The nurse can help in the prevention of degenerative liver disease by teaching the danger of injudicious use of materials that are known to be injurious to the liver and by emphasizing the need for diet that is protective to the liver.

Since cleaning agents, solvents, and related substances sometimes contain products that are harmful to the liver, the public should read instructions on labels and should follow them implicitly. Dry-cleaning fluids used on clothing, upholstery, and rugs, may contain carbon tetrachloride that can cause injury if warnings to avoid inhalation of the fumes and to keep windows open are not heeded. If people must use these agents, a good practice is to open the windows wide, clean the materials as quickly as possible, and then vacate the room, the apartment, or the house for several hours, leaving the windows open.

The "do-it-yourself" movement has increased the danger of liver damage from poisons. Many solvents used to remove paint and plastic material and to stain and finish woodwork contain injurious substances and should be used outdoors and not even in the basement since dangerous fumes may spread throughout the house. Cleaning agents and finishes for cars should be applied with the garage door open or out-of-doors. Nurses in industry have a responsibility to teach the importance of observing regulations to avoid industrial hazards. Nitrobenzene, tetrachlorethane, carbon disulfide, and dinitrotoluol are examples of injurious compounds used in industry.

Some drugs that are known to cause mild liver damage must be used therapeutically. However, the nurse should warn the public regarding the use of preparations that are available without prescription that may be injurious. Many drugs reach the market before dangers of their extended use have been conclusively ruled out; for example, chlorpromazine which is being widely used to control "nerves" is now suspected of causing stasis in the canaliculi of the liver, and this may lead to serious liver damage. A safe rule to follow is to avoid taking any medication except that specifically prescribed by a physician for a specific ailment.

Evidence seems to be accumulating to show that liver damage can follow or be caused by poor nutrition to the liver cells. Protein and vitamin B complex appear to be essential in continuous amounts to ensure healthy liver function. For many years alcohol has been incriminated as the cause of cirrhosis, but recently it has been shown that the probable cause is not the alcohol but inadequate protein intake as a result of the haphazard fashion in which the alcoholic eats. There is no question but that cirrhosis of the liver and alcoholism often appear together. The National Institute of Statistics reports that France, a country which has been plagued with the problem of alcoholism during recent years, had 14,176 deaths from cirrhosis in a population of 43,000,000, or 32.5 fatalities per 100,000 in 1956. Of all alcoholics who died in France during that year, 80 per cent had a diagnosis of cirrhosis of the liver.[14] It is estimated that 70 million persons in the United States use alcohol and 5 million develop alcoholism.[12] Since she does not represent authority as a physician does, the nurse who does not have a judgmental attitude may make a real contribution in control of alcoholism. She should encourage persons who take large amounts of alcohol or who are increasing their consumption rate to seek the help of others, for example, their personal physician, a psychiatrist, or a lay group such as Alcoholics Anonymous.[12]

Toxic hepatitis

The treatment for toxic hepatitis is to remove or stop the cause if this is known. Rest in bed and general supportive care are usually all that can be done beyond the general measures used for patients with any liver disease. Some patients who have severe toxic hepatitis recover with apparently little, if any, residual liver damage; others have severe permanent damage and may develop all the signs and symptoms of cirrhosis of the liver. The patient who recovers from an attack of toxic hepatitis should be instructed to avoid additional injury for the rest of his life (see discussion on prevention of degenerative disease of the liver).

Cirrhosis of the liver

Cirrhosis of the liver usually refers to portal cirrhosis and is also called *Laennec's cirrhosis,* atrophic cirrhosis, and liver fibrosis. It is believed that malnutrition is the primary cause of cirrhosis, although other factors such as previous damage from toxins or infections may contribute. Alcohol has always been considered a major factor, but almost half of those who develop cirrhosis have never consumed alcohol. Cirrhosis sometimes follows rigid dieting by women intent upon retaining a slim figure but who do not choose proper foods. Although cirrhosis is considered a disease of late middle life, it may occur in younger persons.

The symptoms of cirrhosis are caused by degeneration of liver cells. There is proliferation of interstitial tissue with fibrosis, causing portal obstruction which the body attempts to circumvent by establishing collateral circulation. *Ascites* or fluid in the abdomen usually follows portal obstruction and occasionally is one of the first signs of the disease, although it usually does not occur until the disease is quite far advanced and jaundice has become marked. As the disease progresses, more and more liver cells are destroyed and many typical signs and symptoms of liver disease appear.

The patient with cirrhosis may have a long history of failing health, with vague complaints of gastrointestinal distress, fatigue, and low resistance to mild infections, and there may be weight loss, depression, headache, and slight elevation of temperature. As the disease advances, typical signs of severe anemia, including malaise and memory loss, may occur. Venules on the head and upper body become markedly distended, and spider angiomas (tiny bright red pulsating arterioles that disappear on pressure) frequently appear. Veins may be prominent in the lower extremities as the patient loses weight, the skin becomes thin and dry, and edema appears in the lower trunk and lower extremities. Sometimes jaundice, first apparent in the scleras, is the first sign that something is wrong. Because increased pressure in the portal vein increases the pressure in the esophageal veins which drain into this system, varicosities may develop in these veins. Occasionally, gastric hemorrhage following rupture of a varicosed esophageal vein and drainage of blood into the stomach are the first indications that the patient has advanced cirrhosis of the liver.

Medical treatment and nursing care. There is no specific treatment for cirrhosis of the liver. Once the disease is established, it usually advances slowly to cause death. Many patients, however, can be helped to live for years if they follow instructions to protect the liver from further damage. The liver has remarkable powers of regeneration. Sometimes sufficient collateral circulation can be established and sufficient repair of liver can be accomplished so that symptoms subside for long periods of time. At other times the patient appears to be doing

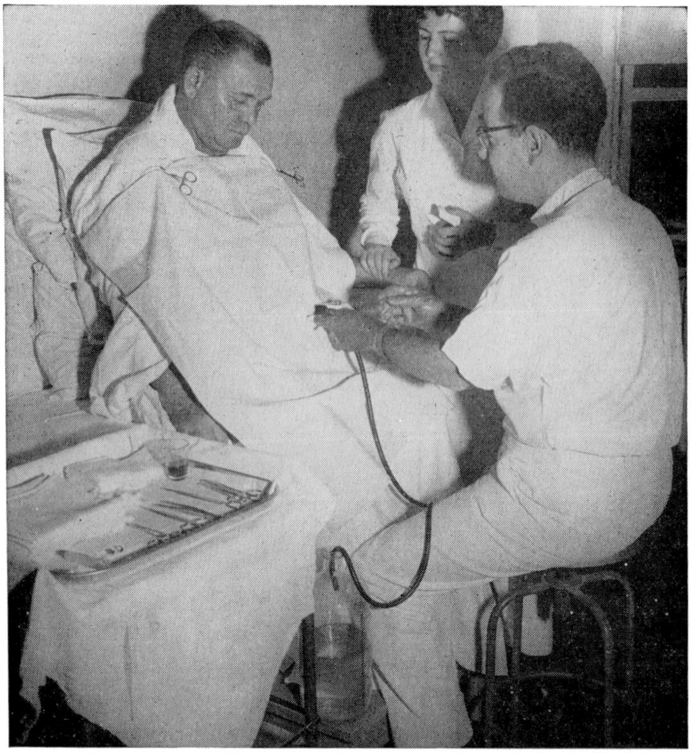

Figure 89

Careful observation is necessary during a paracentesis. Note the pillows supporting the back and arms of the patient. The patient's feet are resting on a stool.

fairly well when the liver suddenly gives up its battle and the patient dies in coma within a few days.

Rest, moderate exercise, avoidance of exposure to infections, and protection from toxic agents of any kind are emphasized in treatment, and alcohol is usually forbidden. As the disease progresses more and more effort must be made to compensate for the failure of the several functions of the liver. Vitamins may be given to compensate for the organ's lost ability to store vitamins A, B complex, D, and K. Because absorption of fat-soluble vitamin A and synthesis of vitamin K is poor due to insufficient bile salts in the intestine, bile salts are usually given if the patient is jaundiced. Transfusions may be given to combat marked anemia. Diet is the most important part of treatment and is the most difficult with which to cope. The patient needs constant encouragement to eat enough protein and carbohydrate.

Complications

Ascites. Ascites, or the accumulation of fluid in the abdominal cavity, is a fairly common complication of advanced liver disease. This condition may cause discomfort and difficulty in breathing and may require treatment by paracentesis. (For details of this procedure and the nursing care involved, see texts on fundamentals of nursing.) A paracentesis is not without danger to the patient with advanced liver disease. (See Figure 89.) Besides the usual complications that might occur, such as damage to the bladder, there is the danger of hemorrhage from the wound because of the patient's low prothrombin level. In far-advanced cases, fluid may form so fast that it exerts pressure on the small wound and prevents its healing, and fluid may drain continuously. This is uncomfortable for the patient and predisposes to infection in the wound.

Many physicians try to control edema and fluid accumulation in the abdomen by giving diuretics, while others believe that diuretic drugs such as mercurials may be too damaging to the liver to risk their use. Removal of fluid through the kidneys has the advantage of usually not removing essential body protein which is contained in fluid removed from the abdominal cavity. If paracenteses must be done at intervals, it is necessary to supply additional protein. One liter of ascitic fluid contains almost as much protein as 200 ml. of whole blood.[2] Restriction of sodium aids greatly in limiting the formation of ascitic fluid in liver disease. It is believed that limiting sodium restricts the antidiuretic hormone although the exact action is not understood.

Esophageal varices. Esophageal varices are varicosities occurring in the cardiac end of the esophagus and are caused by pressure within the portal venous system with subsequent backing up of venous blood. Esophageal varices occur in approximately 30 per cent of all patients with cirrhosis of the liver.[4] They may be caused too, by less common diseases such as Banti's disease and by thrombosis of the portal vein. The varices may rupture, with flow of blood into the stomach. Severe hematemesis may then follow with subsequent shock. This condition requires emergency treatment. The patient is kept absolutely quiet and is treated for shock. He must be attended constantly and given reassurance since vomiting blood is an extremely frightening experience. Blood transfusions are usually given. The patient is not given anything by mouth and is fed entirely by the parenteral route. During this time mouth care is very important.

There are several means by which attempts are made to stop the bleeding. Sometimes an esophagoscope is passed and effort is made either to inject the vessels with sclerosing solution or to seal them off by means of cauterization. A thoracotomy incision may be made and the vessels ligated; this is a somewhat strenuous procedure, however, for the patient who has a chronic disease and who has just sustained a serious hemorrhage.

The device most widely used to control hemorrhage from esophageal varices is the balloon (Blakemore-Sengstaken tube). This is a triple lumen tube which has two balloons attached to it (see Figure 90); one near the tip of the tube and another longer one directly above it. The tube is passed through the nose into the stomach with the balloons deflated. The tip of the tube has several openings so that stomach contents can be removed by suctioning through its connecting lumen. When the tube is in the stomach, the distal balloon is distended by injecting approximately 200 ml. of air through its corresponding lumen. The tube is then pulled back so that it is held tightly against the cardia. The upper or esophageal ballon is distended next through its connecting lumen with 40 to 60 ml. of air and to a pressure of 20 to 25 mm. of mercury. The pressure of this balloon against the mucosa of the lower third of the esophagus usually stops the bleeding. Tension is placed on the tube, and then it is secured against the patient's nostril. It may even be attached to traction to help maintain the pressure of the balloon against the varices. The opening of the lumen leading to the esophageal balloon is attached to a sphygmomanometer, and the pressure within the balloon is checked at intervals. If it drops below 20 to 25 mm. of mercury, additional air is pumped into the balloon. In most instances the tube is left in place until bleeding ceases. The doctor must decide between the possibility of tissue necrosis from pressure of the balloon and resumption of hemor-

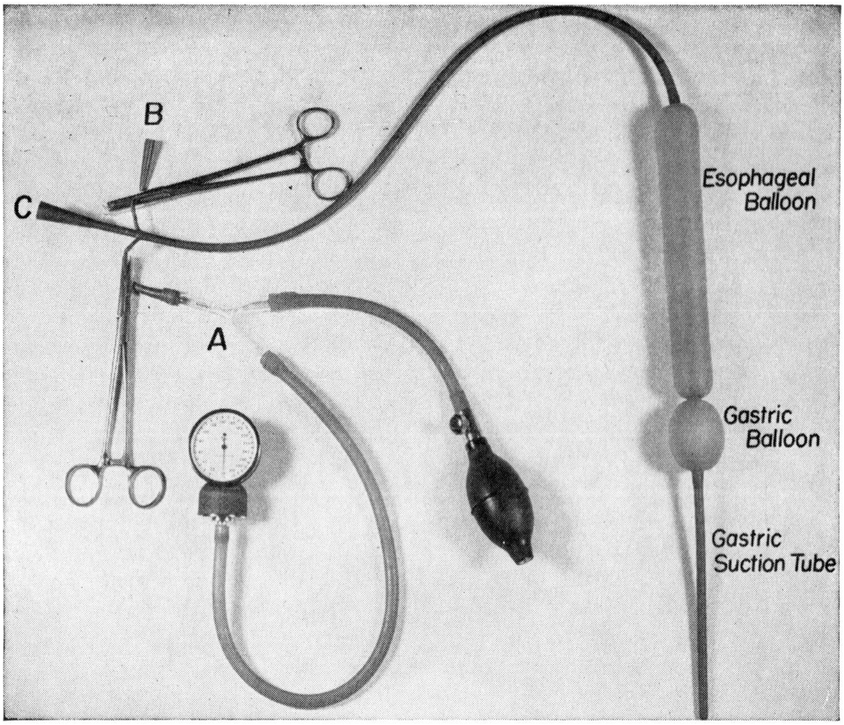

Figure 90

The esophageal balloon (Blakemore-Sengstaken tube).
A, Lumen leading to the esophageal balloon. *B,* Lumen leading to the gastric balloon.
C, Lumen for gastric suction. (See text.)

rhage if the balloon is removed too early. Before being removed the balloons are both deflated. A second balloon should be on the unit ready for immediate use in case of damage to the one being used. These balloons have the date of manufacture stamped on them; those over a year old should not be used because of deterioration of the rubber. Balloons are not reused.

Because the distended esophageal balloon occludes the esophagus, the patient may not take anything by mouth or even swallow his saliva. He should be provided with cleansing tissues and an emesis basin. The patient needs frequent mouth care. The nostrils should be kept clean, lubricated, and padded so that the tissues do not slough because of pressure from the tube. Cotton is used for this and should surround the tube as it leaves the nostril; a tiny piece of sponge rubber sometimes helps prevent pressure if the patient's position must be such that pressure is exerted against one side of the nostril. Care must be taken not to disturb the tube, and the nurse should consult with the doctor as to how much movement the patient is permitted. Passive moving of extremities is usually necessary.

Operative treatment. A *portacaval anastomosis* (portacaval shunt) is sometimes done to control bleeding from esophageal varices. By anastomosing the portal vein to the inferior vena cava the blood volume passing through the diseased liver is decreased and pressure on the esophageal veins is lessened (see Figure 91). Another operation less often used is the *splenorenal anastomosis* in which the spleen is removed and the splenic vein anastomosed to the left renal vein; this procedure relieves pressure on the portal vein since approximately 30 per cent of the portal vein blood volume comes from the splenic vein.[4]

Careful preoperative preparation is necessary since it must be remembered that the patient with liver damage severe enough to cause bleeding varices is not a good operative risk. If he also has marked ascites, the operation is not attempted. The patient is usually apprehensive about the recommended operation yet in selected cases it is known that the operative risk is much less than the risk from recurring hemorrhage. Vitamin K, antibiotics, and transfusions are usually given preoperatively.

Following surgery the patient needs close observation and often constant nursing attention. Narcotics should be given for severe pain but sedative drugs are usually kept at a minimum because of the liver disease. The patient must be encouraged to breathe deeply and to cough hourly. Fluid intake and output must be accurately recorded and lessening of output reported since renal function sometimes decreases for a time following this operation.

Some surgeons do not pass a gastric tube preoperatively because of danger of injury to the varices. Others pass a soft rubber tube and attach it to suction postoperatively since it is believed that postoperative distention may predispose to thrombosis of the portal vein. The patient is observed closely for pain, distention, fever, and nausea which may be signs of thrombosis at the site of anastomosis. *Regional heparization* may be employed to prevent thrombosis formation. A fine polyethylene catheter is inserted into the right gastroepiploic vein and the catheter then is brought out through the wound and attached to a bottle containing heparin and saline solution. The surgeon determines the rate of flow which is usually a slow continuous drip. This catheter may be left for five to seven days, and during this time the nurse must see that it is not obstructed or subjected to tension in any way. The patient remains

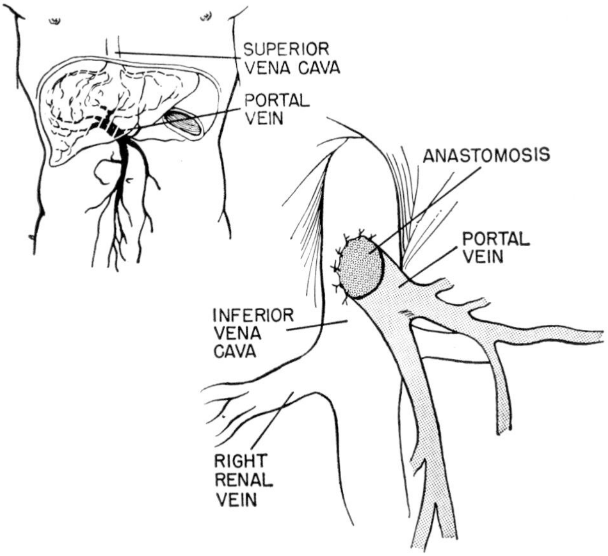

Figure 91

Schematic drawing of a portacaval shunt. Upper diagram shows the normal relationship of the portal vein to the superior vena cava. The lower illustration shows the anastomosis of the portal vein to the inferior vena cava.

in bed or can sit only by the bedside and does not walk about, therefore, particular attention must be paid to bed exercises so that thrombosis does not occur in the lower extremities.

Some surgeons prefer to keep the patient flat in bed for several days until the anastomosis is healed; others have their patients get out of bed on the day after the operation. Leg and arm exercises are begun on the day after surgery. The lower extremities must be carefully observed for signs of edema which may follow the sudden increase of blood flow into the inferior vena cava. Elevation of the lower extremities may be ordered, and the length of time the patient spends standing and walking should be medically prescribed.

Hepatic coma. Hepatic coma or liver coma is a relatively rare but serious complication following portacaval anastomosis. Signs and symptoms are the same as in the coma which may terminate the course of any degenerative liver disease. They include peculiar behavior, confusion, twitching and a characteristic flapping of the extremities, dizziness, stupor, and coma. The patient's temperature may rise markedly. Treatment includes eliminating protein from the diet or the tube feedings, giving high carbohydrate fluids in large amounts, and giving sodium glutamate intravenously in normal saline solution.

DISEASE OF THE BILIARY SYSTEM

Prevention

There are no specific means to prevent disease of the biliary system. However, since disease of this system occurs much more often in obese persons, it is reasonable to suppose that control of obesity may contribute to its prevention. Women are more often affected than men and the description, "fair, fat, and forty," is a fairly accurate one. In all health education, the nurse should stress the importance of avoiding excess weight. Since emotional need for gratification through food is often quite strong in obese persons, advice on food consumption may not be heeded.

If surgery has not been performed following an attack of acute cholecystitis or cholelithiasis, a reducing diet and careful avoidance of too much fat are usually recommended by the doctor. Patients who have had acute attacks are more strongly motivated to follow dietary instructions, and the nurse may be of real help to them in planning attractive dishes that are low in calories and fat. Married women who spend most of their time at home may add more calories than they realize by "eating up leftovers."

The patient who has had an operation for biliary disease with stones is usually cured. However, if stones have formed in the common bile duct stone formation may recur. Patients with biliary tract disease are usually advised to keep fat intake to a fairly low level for the remainder of their lives, although no rigid dietary regulations are needed. Patients who tend to form stones in the ducts are usually advised to be particularly careful of their fat intake and to take generous amounts of fluids. The nurse should emphasize the doctor's instructions in this regard.

Disease conditions

Cholecystitis. Inflammation of the gallbladder is called cholecystitis. This condition may be acute or chronic; the chronic form is usually associated with gallstones or other obstructions of bile passage. Cholecystitis is more common in women than in men, the ratio being 2.5:1. Sedentary obese persons are affected most often, and the incidence is highest in the fifth and sixth decades of life.

A large variety of organisms may contribute to acute disease of the gallbladder; colon bacilli, staphylococci, streptococci, salmonellae, typhoid bacilli, and many other organisms have been found. Infection may reach the gallbladder through the blood stream, the lymph system, or the bile ducts. Inflammation may be confined to the mucous membrane lining, or the entire wall of the gallbladder may be involved. Sometimes damage to the wall of the gallbladder results from increased pressure caused by obstruction of bile flow and from contractions of the smooth muscle as attempt is made to dislodge a stone occluding the lumen of one of the bile ducts.

Acute cholecystitis may be abrupt in onset, although the patient often has a history of intolerance to fatty foods and some general indigestion. Nausea and vomiting usually occur, and there is severe pain in the right upper quadrant of the abdomen. The patient's pulse rate and respiratory rate are increased, and temperature and white blood count are elevated. The chronic form of the disease is usually preceded by several mild acute attacks, and the patient gives a history of having learned to avoid fried foods and certain other food such as nuts that are high in fat.

The treatment for cholecystitis is surgical. There is not complete agreement as to when the gallbladder should be drained or removed if symptoms are acute. Some surgeons favor conservative treatment until the acute infection has subsided, whereas others believe that the danger of rupture and subsequent peritonitis is so great that immediate surgery for drainage is advisable. They recommend removing the gallbladder at a later time when the acute condition has subsided. Complications besides rupture and peritonitis that can occur are the spread of infection to the hepatic duct and the liver and inflammation of the ducts with subsequent strictures which may cause obstruction of bile flow and which are exceedingly difficult to correct surgically. The decision as to when to operate depends largely on the age and condition of the patient and the way he responds to immediate treatment. Immediate treatment includes antibiotics and infusions of 5 per cent glucose in physiologic solution of sodium chloride. Food is usually withheld until acute symptoms subside. Narcotics usually are necessary for pain.

Cholelithiasis. Cholelithiasis means the presence of stones in the biliary tract. The stones are composed largely of cholesterin crystals, although some contain calcium. Cholelithiasis may occur in either sex at any age, but it is more common in middle-aged women. It is not known why stones form in the gallbladder and in the hepatic duct. They may be present for years and cause no inflammation; sometimes they appear to be preceded or followed by chronic cholecystitis. Chronic cholelithiasis is aggravated by pregnancy, perhaps because of the increased pressure in the abdomen.

Gallstones vary in size and number. The small stones are most likely to cause attacks of acute biliary colic, since they pass more easily into the ducts. Stones may lodge anywhere along the biliary tract, where they may cause an obstruction which, if unrelieved, leads to jaundice, or they may cause pressure and subsequent necrosis and infection of the duct walls. Occasionally a stone, because of its location, blocks the entrance of pancreatic fluid and bile into the duodenum at the ampulla of Vater; this condition is difficult to differentiate from obstruction caused by malignancy.

There may be no signs of cholelithiasis until a stone becomes lodged in a biliary duct, although the patient often gives a history of indigestion after consuming rich fatty foods, occasional discomfort in the right upper quadrant of the abdomen, and more trouble than the normal person with gaseous eructations after eating. Gaseous eructations in cholelithiasis characteristically occur almost immediately following meals in contrast to those associated with gastric ulcer, which occur when the stomach is empty (usually several hours after a meal).

Gallstone colic, or *biliary colic,* can cause what is probably the most severe pain that can be experienced. It is caused by obstruction of a duct by a stone. The pain may come on suddenly and is probably caused by spasm of the ducts as they attempt to dislodge the stone. There is severe pain in the right upper quadrant of the abdomen and it radiates through to the back under the scapula and to the right shoulder. Pain may be so severe that the patient writhes in agony despite large doses of analgesic drugs. Morphine is avoided if possible because it increases spasm of the biliary sphincters and increases pressure which can cause further trauma to the walls of the biliary passages. The patient usually has nausea and vomiting, profuse diaphoresis, tachycardia, and occasionally complete prostration. Nitroglycerin or inhalations of amyl nitrite are sometimes helpful, and papaverine hydrochloride, atropine, and calcium gluconate are often given to help produce relaxation. A gastric tube passed through the nose into the stomach and attached to a suction apparatus often helps to relieve distention in the upper gastrointestinal tract and thereby lessen pain. If the attack is not too severe, barbiturates, hot compresses to the upper abdomen, and enemas may control the pain sufficiently. The treatment for cholelithiasis is surgical removal of the gallbladder and its contents as soon as the acute attack subsides and the patient can withstand an operation safely.

Carcinoma. Carcinoma can occur anywhere in the biliary system, and unfortunately, at present there is no way of diagnosing early carcinoma in the abdominal viscera. Jaundice may be the first sign and indicates that the lesion has developed sufficiently to obstruct bile passage at some point. The treatment for carcinoma of the biliary system is surgical, and an operation is performed as soon as the patient's condition warrants it in the hope that complete surgical removal of the lesion is possible. Patients often benefit from surgery when cure of the carcinoma is impossible, since various operations which help to restore the flow of bile into the gastrointestinal tract produce remarkable relief of symptoms, and the patient may feel relatively well for a time.

Surgical treatment and nursing care

Terminology. The terminology used to indicate specific biliary tract surgery sounds somewhat complicated but actually is self-explanatory. *Cholecystectomy* is the removal of the gallbladder, while *cholecystostomy* refers to the creation of a new opening into the gallbladder. *Choledochotomy* is a surgical incision of the common bile duct usually for removal of a stone *(choledocholithotomy).* Choledochoduodenostomy and choledochojejunostomy refer to anastomoses between the bile duct and the duodenum and between the bile duct and the jejunum, respectively. Cholecystogastrostomy is the surgical formation of an anastomosis between the gallbladder and the stomach. These operations are usually performed when carcinoma has been found or when strictures in the ducts make other methods of treatment unsatisfactory.

Preoperative care. A general medical examination preoperatively includes a roentgenogram of the chest, x-ray study of the gallbladder, and examination of the urine and stools. Usually an electrocardiogram is ordered to detect heart damage. Various tests of liver function may be made if liver disease is suspected, and if the patient is jaundiced, tests are done to determine the cause.

Prothrombin level is carefully checked preoperatively. It is usually low if there is jaundice. Vitamin K preparations may be given by various routes. Occasionally when the prothrombin level is quite low, yet surgery is imperative, transfusions of whole blood may be given immediately preoperatively. If the patient is taking food by mouth poorly, infusions containing glucose and protein hydrolysates may be given in an effort to protect the liver from potential damage and to ensure wound healing. Signs of upper respiratory disease should be reported at once since upper respiratory infections can lead to serious complications following surgery of the biliary tract.

Postoperative care. The patient is usually placed in a low Fowler's position upon his return from the operating room or the recovery room. Coughing and deep breathing should be encouraged. Because the wound is fairly high in the abdomen, breathing is painful, and the patient may hold his breath and take shallow breaths in order to splint the chest and lessen pain. Analgesic medications for pain should be given fairly liberally during the first few days, and the patient should then be urged to do deep breathing at regular intervals. He must also be helped and encouraged to change his position and to move about in bed the evening of the operative day and thereafter.

To control nausea and remove gas from the stomach, a stomach tube may be inserted through the nose into the stomach before or while the patient is under anesthesia. Upon his return to his room, this may be attached to suction equipment. Because essential electrolytes, as well as gas, are removed by this procedure, it is discontinued as soon as possible—usually within twenty-four hours. The patient is then given clear fluids by mouth and within a few days usually is able to tolerate a soft low-fat diet. Sweet effervescent drinks are usually best tolerated at first. Infusions of 5 per cent glucose in distilled water are almost always given; sometimes solutions containing electrolytes and protein hydrolysates are ordered. Appetite will probably remain poor if bile is not flowing into the duodenum.

The nurse should know exactly what surgical procedure has been done so that she may care for drains and check dressings intelligently. If the cystic duct has been ligated, a drain usually is inserted near its stump and brought out through a stab wound. This drains bile and small amounts of blood and other serous fluid onto the dressings and usually is removed in five to six days when drainage of bile has largely subsided. If drainage of an acutely infected gallbladder has been done, a drain is also inserted and drains bile, blood, and exudates from the infection. The amount of drainage and the length of time the drain is left in place depends on the nature and extent of the infection.

The nurse should check the dressings as often as every fifteen minutes for the first few hours postoperatively because though hemorrhage from the wound is rare it can occur. Internal hemorrhage also occasionally follows surgery of the gallbladder and bile ducts, particularly when the inflamed gallbladder was adherent to the liver and was removed with difficulty. Lowering of blood pressure, increase in pulse rate, and other signs of hemorrhage should be reported to the surgeon at once.

As soon as the patient responds from anesthesia, he should be told about any drainage tubes that have been used. He should know if much bile is expected on the dressings so he will not become alarmed by sudden soiling of dressings, his gown, or bedclothes. Outer dressings usually are changed frequently when there is much drainage, since the drainage is irritating to the skin and wet dressings interfere with the patient's comfort and rest. Montgomery straps make the changing of dressings much easier.

Any patient who has had surgery of the biliary tract must be observed carefully for signs that bile is being retained in the system. Postoperatively the bile should pass out of the body either through the surgical opening or through the intestine. If there are evidences that this is not occurring it can be assumed that bile is being reabsorbed by the system. The nurse must observe, report, and record early signs of this. The patient should be observed closely for signs of jaundice particularly in the scleras (see page 592). Urine should be examined grossly at each voiding for the dark yellowish color indicative of bile pigment and saved for the doctor's inspection if this is suspected. The nurse may observe the patient's progress by noting the stools: a light color is usual if all the bile is flowing out through the surgical wound (unless bile salts are being given by mouth) but the normal brown color should gradually reappear as drainage diminishes and finally disappears.

If exploration of the common duct has been done, a T tube with the short ends placed into the common duct will prob-

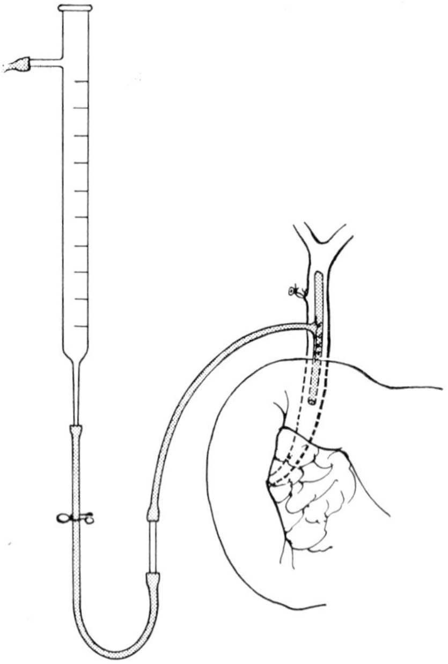

Figure 92

Schematic drawing to show a T tube placed in the common bile duct and attached to a manometer. The common bile duct has been brought from its normal position for better visualization of the T tube.

ably be used (see Figure 92). The long end of this soft rubber tube is brought through the wound and sutured to the skin. The tube is inserted to preserve patency of the common duct and to ensure drainage of bile out of the body until edema in the common duct has subsided enough for bile to drain into the duodenum normally. If the T tube was clamped while the patient was being transported from the operating room, it must be released *immediately* upon arrival in his room. The nurse should check the operative sheet carefully and make queries if directions on the chart are not clear. The tube may drain some blood and blood-stained fluid during the first few hours, but drainage of more than a small amount of blood should be reported to the doctor. Frequently, the tube is attached to a delicate manometer which determines the pressure of bile within the system (see Figure 92). The T tube usually drains bile to the outside for some time, although within ten days most of the bile should be flowing into the duodenum. At first, the entire output of bile (normally 500 to 1,000 ml. daily) may flow through the tube; the drainage bottle should be emptied and cleansed daily and the amount of drainage noted and recorded accurately. Occasionally the bile collected in the drainage bottle is administered to the patient through a stomach tube. If this is done, the funnel or Asepto syringe should be covered and the bile should be in a receptacle so that the patient does not witness the procedure. Digestion often improves greatly when this is done.

Observation for signs of jaundice, bile pigment in the urine, and lack of pigment in the stool is particularly important when a T tube is being used. Occasionally a radiopaque dye is injected through the tube in an effort to determine the location and kind of difficulty if drainage to the duodenum does not proceed as expected.

Usually the T tube is removed in ten days to two weeks. Before this is done, a radiopaque substance may be injected into the tube and a roentgenogram taken *(cholangiogram)* to verify the patency of the system. Following removal of the tube the patient should be observed closely; occasionally there is a violent local reaction with chills, fever, and prostration.[15] Abdominal pain must also be reported at once; occasionally flow of bile into the abdominal cavity causes peritonitis.

The patient is usually permitted out of bed the day after the operation (the T tube may be attached to a carrier). He may need help and encouragement since dressings are uncomfortable and he fears "spilling" the drainage when he moves about. He may still be receiving infusions, and transporting the infusion bottle is necessary (see Chapter 14). To prevent accidents, the elderly patient needs careful attention when he gets up. He often benefits from a regular schedule of getting up and sitting in a chair or walking with assistance.

Usually from ten days to two weeks of hospitalization are required following biliary surgery when no complications occur. The nurse should use this time constructively to teach the patient good general hygiene including the constituents of a good normal diet which has a minimum of fat. Special diets are seldom prescribed by the doctor following biliary surgery, but the patient is advised to avoid excess fats in his meals. The period of convalescence depends on the individual patient, but usually at least a month is needed before normal activities can be resumed safely.

Many patients who have gallstones also have stones in the common or the hepatic ducts. Effort may be made several days postoperatively to cause the body to expel fragments and small stones by stimulating secretion of bile. This procedure, sometimes known as "biliary flush," may be done at intervals (e.g., monthly) for an indefinite time postoperatively. In the hospital the nurse is responsible for seeing that the medications are given as ordered and that the high fat meal it taken. The procedure varies; one method is described in recent nursing literature.[15] She must also emphasize to the patient the importance of keeping medical appointments as requested for this when the doctor believes it is necessary.

REFERENCES AND SELECTED READINGS*

1 American Public Health Association: Control of Communicable Disease in Man, New York, 1955, The American Public Health Association.

2 Cecil, Russell L., and Loeb, Robert F. (editors): A Textbook of Medicine, ed. 10, Philadelphia, 1959, W. B. Saunders Co.

3 *Christensen, S. P., and Takayoshi, Masaki: Portal Hypertension and Nursing Care of Portal Hypertension, Am. J. Nursing **53**:1206-1209, Oct. 1953.

4 Davis, Loyal (editor): Christopher's Textbook of Surgery, ed. 6, Philadelphia, 1956, W. B. Saunders Co.

5 Eichenwald, Heinz F.: Viral Hepatitis, Pub. Health Service Publication No. 435, 1955, U. S. Government Printing Office, Washington, D. C.

6 Fuerst, Elinor V., and Wolff, LuVerne: Fundamentals of Nursing, ed. 2, Philadelphia, 1959, J. B. Lippincott Co.

7 *Heap, Beth: Sodium Restricted Diets, Am. J. Nursing **60**:206-209, Feb. 1960.

8 *Infectious Hepatitis—1954 Report of Outbreaks, Pub. Health Rep. **70**:543, June 1955.

9 Liebowitz, Hirsch Albert: Bleeding Esophageal Varices: Portal Hypertension, Springfield, 1959, Charles C Thomas, Publisher.

10 MacBryde Cyril Mitchell (editor): Signs and Symptoms, ed. 2, Philadelphia, 1952, J. B. Lippincott Co.

11 Mann, Marty: A New Primer on Alcoholism, New York, 1958, National Council on Alcoholism, Inc.

12 *McCarthy, Raymond: Alcoholism, Am. J. Nursing **59**:203-205, Feb. 1959.

13 Merck Manual of Diagnosis and Therapy, ed. 9, Rahway, N. J., 1956, Merck & Co., Inc.

14 New York Times, Aug. 4, 1957.

15 *Palumbo, Louis T., and Fisk, Jean E.: Present-Day Treatment of Diseases of the Biliary Tract and Nursing Care of the Patient With Surgery of the Biliary Tract, Am. J. Nursing **60**:50-55, Jan. 1960.

16 Popper, Hans: Hepatitis and Hepatic Tests, Ciba Clinical Symposia **8**:81-112, May-June 1956.

17 *Portis, Sidney A., and Williams, Elizabeth C.: The Treatment of Liver Disease and Nursing Care of the Patient With Cirrhosis of the Liver, Am. J. Nursing **54**:596-600, May 1954.

18 *Sborov, Victor M.: The Current Status of Viral Hepatitis, Nursing Outlook **2**:476-478, Sept. 1954.

19 Terracol, J., and Sweet, Richard H.: Diseases of the Esophagus, Philadelphia, 1958, W. B. Saunders Co.

20 Todd, James Campbell, Sanford, Arthur Hawley, and Wells, Benjamin B.: Clinical Diagnosis by Laboratory Methods, ed. 12, Philadelphia, 1953, W. B. Saunders Co.

21 *Weber, Robert W., and Elliott, Jane: Needle Biopsy of the Liver, Am. J. Nursing **56**:190-191, Feb. 1956.

*References preceded by an asterisk indicate material particularly well suited for student reading.

The patient with endocrine disease

Chapter 28

Study questions for review

1 Review the endocrine glands and the hormones secreted by each.
2 List the signs and symptoms of respiratory obstruction that might be caused by pressure on the trachea.
3 How would you explain to a patient who has a high basal metabolic rate that he needs increased amounts of foods? Name some foods which are high in carbohydrates.
4 Review the procedure for giving a medication by hypodermic injection, and outline a plan for teaching this procedure to a patient.
5 What is the price of a bottle of protamine zinc insulin? If the patient is to take a daily dose of 30 units, how long would one bottle of insulin last? What would be the monthly cost?

The endocrine glands are special glands or groups of cells within the body which secrete and release highly specific substances into the blood stream. These substances, known as hormones, are chemical compounds which affect the activities of body cells, and thereby influence growth, metabolism, function of end organs, and the activity of every system of the body. The actions of the endocrine glands are interrelated, one gland affects another in a chainlike reaction. For example, the thyroid-stimulating hormone (thyrotropine or TSH) secreted by the basophilic cells of the pituitary gland stimulates secretion of thyroid hormones. The anterior pituitary seems to be the "regulator" of the whole hormone environment, and it in turn appears to be controlled, at least in part, by hormonal influences from centers in the hypothalamus of the brain.[3]

Diseases of the endocrine glands usually are associated with their hyperactivity or their hypoactivity. These changes from normal activity usually are brought about by other hormonal interference of unknown cause, although occasionally they are stimulated by infection or by benign or malignant tumors in the immediate or the controlling gland. In some instances, hormones are secreted, but the organ or body system normally affected may fail to respond and symptoms similar to those caused by absence of the hormone appear. This is perhaps caused by some counteracting activity of other hormones in a total complex involvement not yet completely understood.[3] It is believed that both the production of hormones and the effect of hormones upon body cells can be affected by age, race, sex, season and climate, and disease.

Only a few of the more common endocrinologic diseases will be discussed in this chapter. Those occurring less often should be reviewed in appropriate specialized texts.

THE PATIENT WITH DISEASE OF THE THYROID GLAND

The thyroid gland secretes two hormones, *thyroxin* and *tri-iodothyronine,* that are similar but differ greatly in their rate of action. Both are closely associated with iodine metabolism; the thyroid gland alone contains approximately 80 per cent of all iodine in the body. An over-simplified description of the function of the thyroid gland is that it is the regulator of metabolism including use of oxygen and expenditure of energy. Symptoms of disease, therefore, consist primarily of changes brought about by derangement of this function. Diseases of the thyroid gland include functional *hyperplasia, hypertrophy* (with or without hyperplasia), functional *hypoplasia,* neoplasms, infections (thyroiditis), and anomalies. Certain diagnostic tests are useful in diagnosing any suspected disease of the thyroid gland. These will be discussed before some of the more common diseases and the related nursing care is given.

Diagnostic tests

Common tests for suspected thyroid disease with which the nurse will assist are basal metabolism, protein-bound iodine, blood cholesterol, and tests employing radioactive iodine.

Basal metabolism test. The basal metabolism test determines the amount of oxygen used by a person at rest during a given period of time. Results for each patient are compared with those of others of the same age, sex, and size (body surface). The results are expressed in percentage of deviation from the mean values obtained from a group of normal people. Thus, if the patient needs 15 per cent more oxygen than the control group, he has a basal metabolic rate (BMR) of plus 15 per cent. Normal basal metabolic rate ranges from minus 20 to plus 20.

Metabolic rates of patients who are at home and patients who are hospitalized may be determined. If the patient is in the hospital, he should be given time to become adjusted to the hospital routine before the test is scheduled. The mere fact that he is in a hospital may increase metabolism. In order for the test to be successful, the patient must have a good night's sleep before the examination, and he must be very quiet both physically and emotionally on the day it is done.

The patient needs detailed explanations of what to expect during the test and of the necessary preparations. Good results depend on how carefully the patient follows instructions. The nurse should explain that during the actual test the patient will lie on a comfortable bed, his nostrils will be closed with a clamp, and he will breathe through his mouth from a tube which supplies oxygen. A drumlike apparatus beside the bed will measure the amount of air he uses for several minutes. The test is simple, and the most unpleasant part is omitting breakfast.

The patient should rest and sleep as well as possible the night before the test, but without the aid of medications. His room should be quiet; if he is in a ward, the curtains should be drawn about his bed. Frequently a sign placed on the door or on the curtains helps to remind hospital personnel of the scheduled test and emphasizes the need for rest. If the patient is ambulatory, he usually is permitted to walk to the bathroom in the morning, but he is instructed not to bathe or carry out any other activity.

If the patient is at home, he should plan to have at least eight to ten hours of sleep or rest in bed the night before the test. He should take no food or fluid after the evening meal. In the morning he should omit most of the personal care he usually carries out and should dress slowly, avoid hurry in any way, and be driven to where the test is to be done. Basal metabolism tests usually are scheduled for after 9 A.M. so that rushing can be avoided.

Protein-bound iodine test. The protein-bound iodine test determines the thyroid function by measuring iodine that can be precipitated with plasma proteins in the blood. The blood for this test can be taken without regard to food intake, emotional state, or activity. It is important that the patient receive no medications containing iodine during the week before the test. Some cough syrups, for example, contain iodine. Tests in which iodine preparations are used, such as x-ray studies of the gallbladder or intravenous pyelograms, will interfere with accurate results by making the readings abnormally high if they have been done within several weeks. Because mercury interferes with the test, recent administration (twenty-four to forty-eight hours) of mercurial diuretics will cause readings to be abnormally low. The normal range of protein-bound iodine is from 3.5 to 8 micrograms per 100 ml. of plasma.

Blood cholesterol test. In hyperthyroidism the blood serum cholesterol usually tends to be subnormal, whereas in hypothyroidism it is increased in most instances. However, there is variation in opinion on the reliability of this test in diagnosing thyroid disease. No food is given on the morning of the test until 5 ml. of venous blood have been taken. The normal cholesterol reading is from 150 to 250 mg. per 100 ml. of blood.

Tests employing radioactive iodine. The most common test is called the *radioactive iodine uptake test* and tests the function of the thyroid gland by determining its ability to accumulate iodine that is ingested. Radioactive iodine (I^{131}), the location of which can be detected by using a scintillation detector or Geiger counter is used in the smallest amount (tracer dose) that will give a significant result. Radioactive iodine diluted in distilled water is colorless and tasteless. It is given by mouth. It is absorbed from the gastrointestinal tract, accumulated in the thyroid gland, and excreted by the kidneys. Since food delays absorption, the patient should fast or have only fruit juice and toast before taking the drug. Preceding the test no antithyroid compound should be given for at least three days and no medications containing iodine or foods with particularly high iodine contents should be given for a week preceding the test. No thyroid extract should be given for more than three weeks prior to the test and no test using dyes containing iodine should be done for several weeks before the test is scheduled. Apprehension at the thought of taking a radioactive substance usually is allayed by explanation to the patient by the doctor. The nurse should report to the doctor any fears the patient expresses so that further reassurance can be given if necessary. No isolation for radioactivity is necessary when tracer doses are taken.

Approximately twenty-four hours following the administration of I^{131}, a shielded Geiger counter or a scintillation detector is placed over the gland and the amount of accumulated radioactive iodine is calculated. The normal thyroid usually will accumulate 15 to 50 per cent of the drug within twenty-four hours while, if the patient has thyrotoxicosis, an uptake of 55 to 60 per cent may be shown. All iodine that is not concentrated in the thyroid is excreted by the kidneys. Most patients with thyrotoxicosis excrete from 5 to 40 per cent of the drug within twenty-four hours. Nursing care may include exacting attention to collection of all urine voided during the test since determinations of how much radioactive iodine is excreted usually are desired. This test is not done if the patient has poor kidney function, since the results are unreliable.

Simple goiter

Any enlargement of the thyroid gland is spoken of as a *goiter.* Simple goiter is most common in girls. Enlargement of the gland appears at puberty and may diminish or disappear between the age of 25 and 30 years. In temperate climates there is a seasonal variation; the greatest incidence is in late winter and in spring. This disorder may occur endemically or sporadically. In certain regions in the United States the disease is more common than in other regions because of the limited amount of iodine in the water and in the food grown and obtained locally. Most sea food contains iodine, and small amounts are found in green leafy vegetables. The regions in the United States where the incidence of simple goiter is greatest are the Great Lakes Basin, Minnesota, the Dakotas, The Pacific Northwest, and the Upper Mississippi Valley.

A simple goiter may grow unnoticed, or the patient may ignore it until it becomes nodular; toxicity may then occur, and occasionally malignancy develops. Pressure on the trachea and pressure on the esophagus may be the only symptoms. The nurse's greatest contribution to the prevention and control of simple goiter is in teaching the importance of eating foods that contain iodine and in encouraging those with signs of thyroid abnormality to seek medical counsel. When reviewing any person's diet, the nurse should ask about the amount of leafy vegetables and sea food eaten and the kind of table salt used. Particularly in parts of the country where there is a known defiicency of iodine in the natural water, she should question the kind of salt used. Using iodized table salt is an easy and inexpensive way of being certain that sufficient iodine is consumed. The average adult eats 6.2 Gm. of salt daily. This amount of iodized salt contains 0.01 per cent of potassium iodine, which provides more than twice the amount needed.

The nurse should notice the contour of the neck whenever giving care to any patient. If there seems to be enlargement, the patient should be questioned as to his awareness of it and whether he has consulted a physician about this. In the early stages of simple goiter, 1 drop of saturated solution of potassium iodide per week usually causes the goiter to disappear. If the goiter is moderately enlarged, it may be necessary for the patient to take thyroid extract as well as iodine. If the goiter is of considerable size and is causing pressure symptoms, it may be removed for this reason as well as for cosmetic improvement.

Hyperthyroidism

This disease, caused by hyperactivity of the thyroid gland has been called by many names including *thyrotoxicosis, toxic goiter, Graves's disease,* and *Basedow's disease.* In this condition the gland usually enlarges and it secretes excessive quantities of thyroid hormones. This increases internal combustion and production of energy. The process may be likened to opening widely the damper on a stove. More oxygen is used, fuel is burned, and heat output rises markedly. All metabolic processes are speeded up. The patient becomes nervous and jittery, tense, overly alert, and irritable. His reactions to situations may be exaggerated; he may weep or laugh out of proportion to what is expected normally. There is a fine tremor of the hands, and the patient may drop articles easily and may appear awkward or clumsy in his movements. He usually complains of weakness and fatigue. There often is loss of weight despite a normal or an enormously increased appetite. There is heat intolerance and increase in perspiration; the palms of the hands are warm and moist. Palpitations and breathlessness sometimes occur. Gastrointestinal motility is increased and diarrhea may occur. Hyperthyroidism is a serious disease which, if not checked, can lead to death from heart failure.

Exophthalmos or protrusion of the eyeballs is a characteristic although not uniformly present sign of hyperthyroidism. This condition may become so severe that the eyes cannot close. In this event the eyes should be protected to prevent irritation and possible corneal ulceration. The patient should sleep with an eye covering until a more permanent measure, such as a plastic operation on the lid, can be done. Control of the thyroid hyperactivity stops the progress of exophthalmos but does not cause the condition to regress.

Hyperthyroidism can occur at any age, but it is most likely to occur at puberty, following pregnancy, or at the menopause. Emotional trauma, such as loss of a parent, divorce, or financial crisis, sometimes precedes thyroid hyperplasia, but it has not been demonstrated that all patients with thyroid hyperplasia experience a serious emotional event preceding onset. The disease is more common in women than in men, the ratio being 4:1. Toxic thyroid disease often occurs in those who have other endocrine disturbance such as diabetes mellitus.

Every nurse should be alert to early signs and symptoms of hyperthyroidism. The public health nurse, particularly, encounters many persons who have beginning signs or early symptoms. This information may be revealed in ordinary discussion about home responsibilities or care of children. Physical signs may be obvious, but the patient's expressed complaints about his or her changes in behavior and management of usual activities may give many additional clues. Since the disease may become serious and often leads to heart damage, if unchecked, it is important that patients with the condition seek medical attention early when treatment is more effective and less difficult.

Medical treatment and nursing care. Medical treatment for the patient with hyperthyroidism endeavors to reduce the metabolic rate by rest, administration of antithyroid drugs, and a high-caloric and high-vitamin diet.

Environment. Severity of the condition, the home situation, and the patient's and his family's wishes will determine whether care is given in the hospital or at home. If the patient is to be at home, it is doubly important that his family understand him and the reasons for his behavior. The hospitalized patient should be in a single room if at all possible. The environment should be kept cool and quiet. Many patients are extremely restless, and having to remain in bed aggravates this. Rubber draw sheets are usually not used, and the bed is made with more than the usual amount of sheet tucked in at the head. The bottom part of the bed can be made more secure by using two full-sized sheets folded in half and placing one at the lower part of the bed and the other at the upper part. Bed linen should be straightened and tightened when necessary. Linen may need to be changed frequently because the patient with thyrotoxicosis usually perspires profusely. The patient may be embarrassed by the condition of the bed and the numerous "straightenings" of bed linen. To avoid this, the upper covers can be fanfolded to the foot of the bed during the day. Women patients will be more comfortable in pajamas so that covers can be completely removed if a sudden feeling of warmth occurs.

Rest. The greatest nursing problem in the care of patients with acute thyrotoxicosis is providing enough rest. These patients are often exceedingly sensitive and may be irritated by trivial incidents which are not easily forgotten and thus interfere with rest. It may be necessary to do small things for them, such as pouring water for medications and helping them into pajamas, even though they seem capable. They may drop articles or not be able to handle objects securely because of nervousness. This, too, causes embarrassment; if they drop things repeatedly, it becomes a source of real frustration.

Quiet activity in bed, such as handicrafts or reading, may be useful in helping a patient get rest. If unoccupied, the patient who is allowed to be out of bed may wander about the ward, and as a result of contacts with other patients who may misunderstand him may become more upset or disturb other patients. Some limited and guided activity may actually help him more than enforced absolute quiet and rest. Modifying routines also may be necessary; for example, permitting the patient to walk to the bathroom instead of insisting that he use a bedpan may be best.

Behavior. It is extremely important that the patient's family and auxiliary hospital personnel, as well as members of the professional staff, understand his symptoms. They should understand that sensitivity and irritability are a part of the disease. Much can be contributed to his recovery if there is thoughtful care in this regard. Surprise visits from the patient's family and too many visitors may tend to increase apprehension and overactivity. Disturbing news or discussion of controversial subjects should be avoided by both the family and the professional personnel. All personnel should remain calm in giving care, and the nurse should carefully explain the patient's mood and usual reactions to members of the nonprofessional nursing staff. If a staff member who has established good rapport with the patient is assigned consistently to care for him, this will help him to secure rest. If the patient has real difficulty resting, a sedative such as phenobarbital is given regularly.

Diet. Since appetite usually is increased and the diet should be high in caloric and vitamin contents, the nurse should see that the patient is getting sufficient food. If weight loss has occurred, extra protein may be needed to help rebuild lost tissues in addition to extra carbohydrate to meet the increased "fuel" requirements brought on by the disease. Self-consciousness and sensitivity about his enormous appetite sometimes keep the patient from eating as much as he really needs.

Occasionally the patient's appetite is not good, and yet he needs extra food. Finding out what he likes to eat and reporting this to the dietitian often helps. The patient should have repeated helpings of foods he likes and should have food between meals. Stimulating drinks such as tea and coffee should not be given unless withholding them really upsets the patient. Postum is a suitable substitute in many instances for those who are accustomed to a hot liquid with meals.

Drugs. Patients with hyperthyroidism are treated with several drugs. Preparations of *iodine,* such as Lugol's solution (potassium iodine), are still widely used in the treatment of hyperthyroidism since they temporarily inhibit release of thyroid hormones. Iodine preparations act quickly on the gland and are used to lessen its vascularity in preparation for surgery. Lugol's solution is given in small doses such as 0.3 ml. three times a day and should be diluted in milk or fruit juice. It should also be taken through a straw because it can cause staining of the teeth. Toxicity is rare, but a brassy taste in the mouth and sore teeth and gums are signs of chronic toxicity.

Thiourea and its derivatives such as *propylthiouracil* are used in the treatment of hyperthyroidism. They, too, block the release of thyroid hormones although their action is much slower than that of iodine; usually two weeks elapse before improvement is noticeable, and for this reason they may be given in combination with Lugol's solution in severe thyrotoxicosis. The usual initial treatment is with 225 to 300 mg. (38 to 50 grains) of propylthiouracil in divided doses. The usual daily maintenance dose is 25 mg. (2/5 grain) daily. The patient should be observed or should be instructed to look for toxic signs of the drug such as fever and skin eruptions. If toxic reaction occurs, blood counts may show leukopenia. Some patients may have good results from continued treatment with drugs, but others may need other treatment such as surgery. Continued use of thiourea derivatives may not be tolerated by some patients.

Radioactive iodine is now widely used in the treatment of hyperthyroidism. I^{131} with a half-life of eight days (half of its activity is expended in that time) is the preparation most often used. Usually a single dose of the drug is given and dosage is calculated on a basis of 0.16 millicurie per gram of estimated thyroid weight. As in the iodine uptake test, the drug is given by mouth. The patient who receives a treatment dose of radioactive iodine must be isolated for radioactivity. (See Chapter 16.) Occasionally remission is not achieved with one dose and the treatment is repeated after an interval of several months. This treatment is not generally used for persons under 40 years of age because of the undemonstrated but suspected possible effects on the germ plasm and the tendency of radioactive substances to stimulate carcinogenic activity.

A complication of treatment of thyroid disease with radioactive iodine is hypoplasia of the gland. Occasionally the hypoplasia is temporary and the thyroid resumes adequate function after a few weeks. The patient must be urged to keep appointments with his doctor or with the hospital clinic since it is important that he be followed medically for months to be certain that a normal rate of function remains and myxedema is not developing. This complication occurs in 10 to 20 per cent of all patients treated with radioactive iodine.[3]

Following administration of radioactive iodine the patient must be watched for thyroid storm. The treatment for this condition is discussed on page 623.

Hypothyroidism

The patient with hypothyroidism has signs and symptoms almost directly opposite those of the patient with a hyperactive gland. There is a general slowing up of the body's activities. This condition may occur at any age and may be due to a physiologic atrophy, overtreatment for thyrotoxicosis, thyroiditis, or a neoplasm. Congenital absence or atrophy of the gland leads to the condition in infancy known as cretinism. In adults the disease may follow a classic picture (myxedema) or there may be hypofunction of the gland without the classic signs of myxedema.

Hypothyroidism with myxedema. The patient with myxedema notices that he is more sensitive to cold than in the past, that he perspires little, and that his skin and hair are dry. If the condition has come on slowly, the hair may have become thin. The patient may also become forgetful and slow to grasp new situations. He may have noticed changes such as slowing up at work, falling asleep in the evening, and perhaps having an increase in minor accidents. Very often family members misjudge the patient and feel that he has grown lazy, or a new acquaintance may consider him slow mentally. Speech is slowed and the patient may have to plan sentences before speaking. All changes may occur so gradually that family members scarcely notice them.

Tests for hypothyroidism are similar to those for hyperthyroidism; the results of tests usually show opposite findings. The basal metabolic rate will be below normal, the amount of protein-bound iodine is lowered, the blood cholesterol is higher than normal, and very little iodine is accumulated from a tracer dose of radioactive iodine.

Since the gastrointestinal tract becomes sluggish, as do all other body functions, constipation with fecal impactions can occur. Even though appetite may be decreased, the patient tends to gain weight. Some added weight may be due to accumulation of water, but increased weight is due also to the lowered metabolic rate.

Treatment for myxedema is the administration of desiccated thyroid. The usual daily maintenance dose is from 0.09 to 0.12 Gm. (1½ to 2 grains). It is important that dosages be increased gradually because a sudden increase in the metabolic rate can cause death from heart failure. Since patients with hypothyroidism respond quickly to the administration of thyroid hormones, changes in appearance and in physical symptoms occur within two or three days. If hypothyroidism is discovered early, treatment is usually successful. Sometimes, however, there is derangement of the cortical and pituitary hormones, and this makes treatment more complicated and difficult.

General nursing care for the patient with myxedema is determined by his symptoms. Provision should be made for extra warmth. If the patient complains of drafts, his bed should be moved. In the home, the family will need to understand this need for warmth. It is important to give the patient time to carry out any activity. A minimum of soap should be used for bathing, and creams and lotions should be used to keep the skin in reasonably good condition. If constipation is a problem, the diet should consist largely of foods that are high in roughage. The doctor usually orders a diet fairly high in protein and low in total calories.

Hypothyroidism without myxedema. Medical authorities are not in full agreement as to whether or not this clinical entity really exists.[3,18] It is characterized by a low metabolism, fatigue, and general symptoms of neurasthenia. Weight is often normal. Some speculation has occurred as to the cause of this condition being the inability of the body to convert the hormone thyroxin into tri-iodothyronine in the tissues. Many patients appear to improve for a period of time with small doses of thyroid extract, but it is entirely possible that symptoms are not due to the thyroid gland at all. The conviction of some authorities that the long list of vague symptoms including constipation, some cases of obesity, anorexia, leanness, neurasthenia, dry skin, alopecia, anovulation, infertility, and habitual abortion may signify hypothyroidism without myxedema indicates the need for all persons to have regular physical examinations by competent physicians. Nurses should emphasize this need for regular physical examinations.

Operative treatment of thyroid disease

Part or all of the thyroid gland may be removed surgically depending upon the purpose for which the operation is done. In the case of a malignancy, the gland may be removed completely (total thyroidectomy) and the patient must then take thyroid hormones regularly. Hyperthyroidism is often treated surgically with removal of approximately five sixths of the gland and in most cases this permanently alleviates symptoms while the remaining thyroid tissue provides enough hormones for normal function. This operation is known as a *subtotal thyroidectomy.* Local anesthesia may be used if heart damage has occurred or if cardiac or other chronic disease makes the use of general anesthesia contraindicated.

The patient should know that he may be a little hoarse and have some difficulty swallowing after the operation. This is temporary and will subside after local irritation and edema disappear.

Postoperatively the patient usually is placed on his back in a low Fowler's or semi-Fowler's position, with the head, neck, and shoulders well supported. He should be reminded not to raise his head forward and, when he is moved, to support the back of his neck to prevent hyperextension. The patient should be assisted in coughing and in expectorating mucus. By the evening of the day of surgery he usually is permitted to lie partially on his side so that expectoration is easier. If secretions are thick and the patient is unable to raise them, suction may be necessary to ensure free passage of air.

To determine the possibility of laryngeal nerve injury the patient should be asked to speak as soon as he has reacted, and he should be encouraged to speak at intervals of from thirty to sixty minutes so his condition can be checked. Benzoin inhalations may be used in the room to soothe respiratory passage discomfort, which may be severe. Postoperative medications for rest and for relief of discomfort should be given as necessary. This will help the patient to breathe deeply and raise secretions.

The patient's pulse rate, respirations, and blood pressure are usually checked every fifteen minutes for several hours postoperatively and then, if they continue within normal limits, at longer intervals. The dressings should be watched for signs of hemorrhage; since blood may drain back under the patient's neck and shoulders, the nurse should slip her hand gently under the neck and shoulders to be certain this will be detected early. Any swelling around the dressing, any tightening of it, or increasing hoarseness or respiratory distress should be reported to the doctor at once since bleeding into the tissues may be the cause. If the patient is in acute distress, the dressing should be loosened even before the doctor arrives since thyroid dressings usually encircle the neck.

Intravenous solutions containing glucose are given, and as soon as postoperative nausea subsides the patient should take high-carbohydrate fluids by mouth and a soft diet if tolerated. Since the throat usually is sore for several days following surgery, the patient may have some difficulty taking nourishment. Giving an analgesic about a half hour before meals makes swallowing easier.

The patient who has had thyroid surgery usually is permitted out of bed on the first postoperative day. While supporting the back of his neck, the nurse should assist the patient from a side-lying position to a sitting position on the edge of the bed. He should "dangle" before being assisted to a standing position and then should walk about. On subsequent days, he has less discomfort. The nurse should teach the patient to place both hands at the back of his neck to support it as he rises to a sitting position (see Figure 93). A careful explanation of how to avoid hyperextension and flexion until the wound has healed should be given. When the doctor feels that sufficient healing has occurred, the patient can gradually prac-

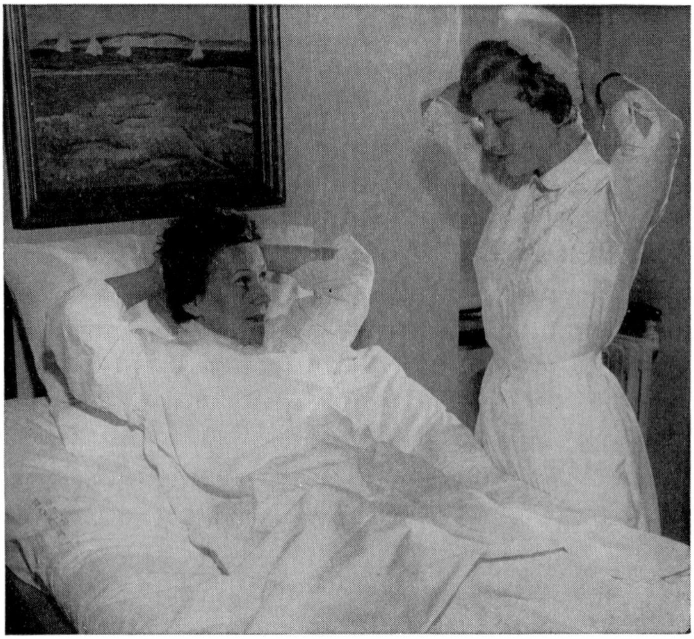

Figure 93

The nurse is teaching the patient who has had a thyroidectomy how to support the weight of her head as she attempts to sit up in bed.

tice full-range neck motion (see Chapter 4).

Generally, two to four days after the operation the dressings are changed by the doctor, and at that time if a small rubber drain has been used it usually is removed. Most surgeons use skin clips instead of ligatures, and the patient can be reasonably assured that the scar will hardly be noticeable within a short time. When the wound is well healed, the doctor often suggests that the patient lubricate it daily with cold cream.

Postoperative complications. Complications that the nurse should be alert for are laryngeal nerve injury, hemorrhage, tetany, and respiratory obstruction. Since the thyroid gland is so close to vital airways, there is danger or respiratory difficulty from a variety of causes. A tracheotomy set should be kept in the patient's room since this permits immediate surgical relief of respiratory difficulty without time spent in getting the patient to the operating room. Respiratory difficulty and difficult coughing and swallowing may indicate hemorrhage. Hemorrhage from an artery or a vein may not be obvious on dressings but will cause pressure on the trachea and epiglottis. If an emergency tracheotomy is necessary, the patient must then be taken to the operating room for resuturing of the wound or retying of blood vessels.

If the laryngeal nerve has been injured during an operation on the thyroid gland, the patient may have vocal cord spasm. If so, he will show signs of respiratory obstruction. As he attempts to pull air in through tightened vocal cords, a crowing sound is made and the tissues around the neck are retracted. A tracheotomy usually is necessary when this occurs. If there is paralysis of one vocal cord only, a hoarseness may develop. Within a few weeks the patient's speaking voice becomes normal, but the singing voice is permanently affected. A very rare complication is severence of the nerves supplying the vocal cords. This results in permanent loss of speech. The most common condition to suspect when the patient has difficulty speaking or breathing is edema causing pressure on the nerves.

A rare complication following thyroid surgery is the accidental removal of one or more of the parathyroid glands. This will cause symptoms of tetany which may appear from one to seven days postoperatively. The patient may complain of numbness or tingling of his hands and feet, or spasm (carpopedal spasm) may be the first sign (see Chapter 6). If not treated in time, this can cause respiratory obstruction, due to contraction of the glottis, and death. Calcium gluconate is given intravenously as immediate treatment. Daily oral doses are continued. If some, but not all, of the glands are removed, the remaining ones will hypertrophy so that the condition is only temporary. If all are removed, the patient must have continuous medical treatment.

Special care in surgical treatment of hyperthyroidism. The patient with hyperthyroidism usually undergoes a fairly lengthy program of preoperative preparation before surgery is scheduled. This may be at home or in the hospital. The acutely toxic patient usually has a short period of hospitalization under heavy sedation and then returns home for a time on a careful regimen of rest, high-caloric diet, thiouracil, and phenobarbital. Lugol's solution is also given preoperatively to help shrink the gland and make it less vascular. To detect evidence of heart damage an electrocardiogram is made before surgery. The usual criteria used to determine whether or not the patient is a suitable candidate for surgery include the return of thyroid function to normal (euthyroid) from its hyperactive state, a consistent weight gain, and a marked diminution of signs of thyrotoxicosis such as tachycardia.

A rectal anesthetic such as Avertin is sometimes used for patients who are extremely apprehensive at the prospect of surgery. The anesthetic is given in the patient's room. It is given as an enema, and the patient does not know that he is going to the operating room on that particular day. This is known as "stealing" the thyroid and seldom is practiced now.

Postoperatively the patient may be placed in an oxygen tent for the first twenty-four hours. Oxygen is used not only for supplying extra oxygen, but also for its cooling effect in hot weather. The intravenous fluids given postoperatively may contain Lugol's solution to help control any thyroid hormones that may have been spilled into the blood stream during the operation. Morphine sulfate is given at regular intervals to ensure rest and to slow metabolism. However, it must be given judiciously; respirations should not go below 12 per minute.

Thyroid storm, or *thyroid crisis,* is a rare complication which may occur following surgery in patients who have severe thyrotoxicosis or who have undergone too short a period of preoperative treatment with drugs, rest, and diet. Increased amounts of hormones are released into the blood stream as a result of emotional and physical stress caused by the operation. The cutting and compression of the gland during operation adds to this. The patient's temperature may rise to 41° C. (106° F.) in the body's attempt to release the heat formed from increased metabolism. The pulse may be very rapid, and there is marked apprehension, restlessness, irritability, and prostration. The patient may become delirious and finally comatose with death resulting from heart failure. Treatment includes oxygen, alcohol sponges, and ice bags to lower temperature, antithyroid drugs by mouth or intravenously, glucose, normal saline solution and sometimes blood intravenously, narcotic and sedative drugs and cardiac drugs such as digitalis preparations or quinidine as indicated by the heart action. Cortisone and prednisone may be given since it appears that cortical hormone action may play some part in thyroid crisis.

Thyroid storm or thyroid crisis may

also occur after radioactive-iodine treatment of patients who have severe thyroid toxicosis.

DISEASE OF THE PARATHYROID GLANDS

The parathyroid glands can become hyperactive or hypoactive. These glands maintain normal calcium and phosphorus contents of the blood. Any upset in this function causes symptoms of electrolyte imbalance. (See Chapter 6.)

Hypoparathyroidism

When there is insufficient hormone production or hypofunction of the parathyroid glands, blood calcium decreases and neuromuscular symptoms appear. These include numbness and tingling in the extremities, and carpopedal spasm as in tetany following thyroidectomy or in severe electrolyte imbalance due to other causes. The patient may have convulsions and muscular twitchings; laryngeal spasm may cause hoarseness of the voice. Other manifestations are prematurely gray hair with alopecia (loss of hair) and enamel defects of the teeth. If hypocalcemia continues, cataracts develop in the lens of the eyes. The main change is increased neuromuscular excitability.

Treatment of tetany is the intravenous administration of calcium gluconate. Calcium carbonate and calcium lactate solution is given by mouth to supply the body with sufficient calcium. Vitamin D may also be given in conjunction with this.

Nursing care of patients with tetany includes careful observation for beginning symptoms of neuromuscular disorder so that prompt treatment can be given and severe reaction, such as convulsions, can be prevented. If the patient does have a convulsive seizure, he should be protected against physical injury, and his tongue should be prevented from slipping backward in the throat and shutting off passage of air.

Hyperparathyroidism

Hyperactivity of the parathyroid glands is caused by tumor or by hyperplasia. The serum calcium is high and the phosphorus low. There is increased urinary excretion of calcium, and renal calculi are frequent. Other symptoms are anorexia, nausea, vomiting, and constipation. If the calcium intake is not increased, calcium is removed from the bones, and pathologic fractures can occur. Treatment is the surgical removal of the glands or tumor.

Nursing care should include precautions to prevent injury, particularly if there is evidence of demineralization of the bone. The patient should be moved carefully if he is confined to bed or to a wheel chair. He should be taught to avoid sudden moves or jolts.

DIABETES MELLITUS

Diabetes mellitus is a chronic metabolic disease involving a disorder of carbohydrate metabolism and subsequent derangement of protein and fat metabolism. Disturbance in production, action, or metabolic fate of insulin, a hormone secreted by the islands of Langerhans in the pancreas, is involved in the disease. The most common and characteristic symptoms of the disease are increased appetite (polyphagia), increased thirst (polydipsia), and increased urine (polyuria). These symptoms led to the name "diabetes" which comes from Greek and means "to pass through" or "to siphon." The word mellitus is the Latin word for honey. The disease has been recognized for centuries; it was noted that bees were attracted to the urine of persons who had the symptoms and its sugar content was suspected long before actual analyses for sugar were done.

The predisposition to develop diabetes is known to be hereditary and transmitted as a mendelian recessive characteristic. If both parents have diabetes, all their children, if they live long enough, will eventually develop the disease. If a person with diabetes marries one with no inherited tendency to the disease, none of the children will have diabetes although they will carry the recessive trait and in turn pass it on to their own children.

Signs and symptoms of diabetes are directly related to the faulty oxidation of carbohydrate and the chain of events which follows. Normally, glucose is oxidized by the body to form carbon dioxide and water, with production of energy to meet body needs. Any excess is changed to glycogen in the liver and is stored in the liver and in the muscles, or it is converted to fat and stored. However, insulin is needed for the formation of glycogen. Since in diabetes glucose remains in the blood stream and cannot be converted to glycogen because of insufficient insulin, the amount of sugar in the blood increases (hyperglycemia) and some of it is eliminated in the urine (glycosuria), after being diluted by the kidneys to cause the polyuria. Pruritus vulvae caused by the irritating effect of the urine with its high sugar content may occur. Despite a large appetite the patient often loses weight, weakness and fatigue are common, and normal resistance to infection is lowered.

Diabetes mellitus is found most frequently in persons over 40 years of age who are obese and who have a family history of diabetes, although the disease is now fairly common in children and in young adults. The incidence increases steadily until the seventh decade of life. Elderly persons usually have a much less severe form of the disease than younger ones, although complications may be severe. The elderly person's blood sugar level remains more stable and less rigorous treatment is required. It has been estimated that over 2 million persons in the United States have diabetes and that approximately one half of these cases have not yet been diagnosed.[8] There is a higher frequency among Jewish than among non-Jewish people.

From 70 to 90 per cent of persons with diabetes have a history of obesity. One theory is that since obesity presents an increased demand for insulin, the special cells within the pancreas which secrete insulin become exhausted, and diabetes develops. Diabetes is more common in women than in men and it is thought that this may be due to the higher incidence of obesity among women. It is also more common among married than single women. This may be linked to frequent occurrence of obesity in those who have borne children or to hormonal influences related to pregnancy.

In general, the increased incidence of diabetes can be attributed to the longer life span with more people in the older age group, to the lower mortality rate among younger people with diabetes since the discovery of insulin, to the increase in the number of persons with diabetes who now marry and have children, to the public's more acute awareness of the disease, and to the greater availability of detection facilities. In 1954, diabetes was the eighth cause of death in the United States; the rate that year was 15.5 per 100,000 population.[8] According to the Division of Special Health Services of the United States Department of Health, Education, and Welfare, "premature death from diabetes is estimated to cause a loss of 370,000 life-years every 12 months in the United States."[8]

The fact that this disease occurs in 13 out of 1,000 persons presents a sizeable public health problem of particular economic and social significance. The establishment of community diabetes programs is being urged by the United States Public Health Service. These programs should be directed toward (1) detection of diabetes and follow up of suspected cases to confirm the diagnosis and to give treatment, (2) prevention or correction of obesity, (3) keeping patients with diabetes under medical supervision and their condition under control, (4) promotion of understanding of diabetes through education of professional groups, the patient, family, and community as a whole, and (5) mobilization of community resources such as medical, nursing, social, and nutrition groups to aid those with diabetes.

The American Diabetes Association Inc., composed of physicians, furthers patient education, professional education, diabetes detection, public education, and research. It publishes a professional journal* that helps to keep physicians informed and a bimonthly magazine† for persons with diabetes. Each year there is a National Diabetes Week. This week is sponsored by the Association to stimulate early case finding in persons who do not know that they have diabetes and to educate the public about the disease. The Association has thirty-one local groups who work in their own areas; they sponsor camps for diabetic children and cooperate on nation-wide projects. The National Institute of Arthritis and Metabolic Diseases at Bethesda, Maryland, as part of the program of the United States Public Health Service, contributes much to research in diabetes.

Prevention

Since the cause of diabetes mellitus is unknown, specific measures for primary prevention are limited. However, much can be done by every nurse if she is aware of the hereditary nature of the disease and its probable association with obesity. If diabetes is part of a family history, the nurse can explain to relatives of the patient the significance of periodic testing for detecting the disease early and can encourage all members of the family to maintain normal weight.

It has also been suggested that closer study of women who have glycosuria during pregnancy and the possible administration of insulin therapy during this time might help to produce a more successful outcome of pregnancy and might delay or prevent development of diabetes in these women and in their children. Studies of women with diabetes have shown that there is a high fetal and neonatal death rate, an increased frequency of large babies with a high mortality rate, and a greater tendency toward other abnormalities in pregnancy. Thus, early prenatal care should be emphasized.

There is much the nurse can do to prevent complications in the person with known diabetes. These measures will be discussed as part of nursing care.

Local health departments have established multiple screening programs to detect diabetes. A test of the blood for sugar level and a test of the urine for sugar or either of these tests is used to detect diabetes. Case-finding programs can be carried out in health department clinics, hospital outpatient clinics, doctor's offices, industry, or in the community (at health fairs or by mobile testing units). Selected groups or whole communities can avail themselves of these services. Follow-up of any positive findings is essential for a successful program. Public health nurses can help by making home visits if diabetes is definitely established, if retesting needs to be done, if individuals have indicated they have no physician or are under no medical supervision, or if persons being tested request home visits by a nurse at the time of the first testing. Through her visits, misunderstandings about retesting can be cleared and family reactions to the possibility of diabetes can be determined.

Diagnostic tests

Urine tests. Urine testing is probably the most familiar test to the public. Most patients have been asked to give urine specimens when admitted to the hospital or when going to the physician's office for physical check-up. Four ounces of urine collected in a clean glass container are sufficient for complete analysis. Urine of patients suspected of having diabetes is tested for sugar and acetone. Three of the following tests, Benedict's, Clinitest, and Dreypak, are copper reduction methods.

Benedict's test. The Benedict test is very commonly used to test for sugar; 5 ml., or approximately 1 teaspoon, of Benedict's solution is placed in a test tube and 8 drops of urine are added. The urine and Benedict's solution are mixed and then either placed over a direct flame or in a water bath and allowed to boil for five minutes. A color chart is used to compare color results which are graded according

*Diabetes.

†American Diabetes Association Forecast.

to the following scale: if the solution remains blue, there is no sugar; green is considered 1 plus; yellow, 2 plus; orange, 3 plus; and red, 4 plus.

Clinitest. Clinitest is another method of testing the urine for sugar. Clinitest usually comes in a compact kit and is convenient for use because it is small and easy to carry and store. The kit contains a test tube, a medicine dropper, caustic tablets, a small pinch forceps, and a color chart. Ten drops of water and 5 of urine are placed in the test tube and a tablet is added. The tablet generates heat, and the color of the solution is graded just as for Benedict's solution.

Dreypak. Dreypak is a method in which a urine-impregnated strip of filter paper is dipped into boiling Benedict's solution. Color changes are the same as for Benedict's test.

Galatest. Galatest is a bismuth reduction method and comes in powder form. A drop of urine is placed on the powder, and the color changes are shades of gray to black. Since shades of gray are difficult to distinguish, this test is not widely used.

Tes-Tape and Clinistix. Tes-Tape and Clinistix are both enzymatic tests for sugar. The glucose is converted to gluconic acid. In the Tes-Tape test, strips of paper impregnated with the testing ingredients are dipped into the urine specimens. Clinistix is similar to a book match and is also dipped into the urine. Positive colors for sugar in both tests are green and blue.

Fractional urine collection. Although single specimens of urine may show the presence of sugar, the physician may wish to find out what time of day the excretion is heavy and may prescribe insulin accordingly. Fractional or group urines may be collected in four parts according to the time of day. The first collection extends from before breakfast to just before lunch; the second, from before lunch to just before dinner; the third, from dinner to before bedtime; and the fourth, from bedtime until the next morning.

Twenty-four hour urine collection. Twenty-four hour specimens may also be collected to determine the quantity of sugar excreted. In this collection the first specimen of the morning is discarded. All urine excreted thereafter until 7 A.M. on the next day is collected in a gallon bottle and is sent to the laboratory.

Blood sugar tests. Blood sugar levels are determined when diabetes is suspected. Ordinarily the normal blood sugar ranges from 80 to 120 mg. per 100 milliliters of blood. Blood specimens are taken before the patient has had his breakfast—when he is in a fasting state.

Glucose tolerance tests are done to reach a more conclusive diagnosis of diabetes. Most patients having a glucose tolerance test will be hospitalized. No food is allowed after midnight the night before the test. Samples of blood and urine are obtained, and the patient is asked to drink a mixture containing glucose, water, and lemon juice flavoring. The amount of glucose administered is proportional to body weight. Samples of blood and urine are taken at intervals of one-half hour, one hour, and two hours following the ingestion of the glucose mixture. Within two hours the normal person's blood sugar will drop to a normal level, whereas the diabetic person's will remain high.

Medical treatment and nursing care

Control. Although diabetes cannot be cured it can be controlled, to a large extent at least, by regulating the diet and giving insulin. There are two schools of thought on the control of diabetes. One medical group believes that the patient's urine must be kept sugar free and the blood sugar at a normal level. The other theory is that the disease can be *controlled* in the presence of an above-normal blood sugar and of sugar in the urine *provided* enough insulin is taken and enough food is eaten to meet metabolic needs and this is demonstrated by disappearance of signs and symptoms such as loss of weight and fatigue.

There is debated evidence that degenerative changes, such as retinal damage, occur more often in the presence of glycosuria *provided* enough insulin is given to enable the liver to convert sufficient glucose to glycogen and contribute to other metabolic function.[9] Exponents of the second school of thought maintain that until such evidence is forthcoming, the psychologic damage caused by insistence upon weighing food and testing urine more than outweighs the possible advantages. There is evidence, however, that complications such as retinal damage occur more often in persons who are not under medical supervision and treatment than in those whose disease is diagnosed and who remain under medical care.[1]

Emotional factors. The emotional response to a diagnosis of diabetes is often severe and is not easily dealt with. Part of this may result from fear of disability and eventual death. Since diabetes is so widespread, many people know of relatives and friends who have had the disease and who have eventually had amputations or have become blind. Perhaps an even greater cause of emotional reaction is that diabetes affects the patient's life pattern in regard to food. Food and eating have meaning beyond the actual meeting of nutritional needs (see Chapter 5), and changes in eating habits are extremely hard for patients to accept. Adolescents perhaps more than any other age group find restriction in eating almost intolerable and need the greatest of understanding in their early adjustment to the disease.

The patient's response to those who work with him, at the time of and soon after diagnosis is made, is tremendously important in determining his attitude toward his disease and in turn his ability to accept the treatment and restrictions that are necessary. Most medical authorities believe that the patient must know the potential seriousness of untreated diabetes. On the other hand, they believe that the simpler and easier the necessary changes can be made, the better for all concerned. If the patient with diabetes mellitus continues with the prescribed dietary regimen, takes insulin if it is ordered, follows other instructions and has periodic medical check-ups, his life can be very much like that of anyone else.

Only occasionally do adjustments in the patient's work need to be made. The patient who takes insulin regularly and who may possibly have hypoglycemic reactions (insulin shock) should not work where there is danger of injury to himself or to others. It is preferable that patients with diabetes work regular hours, but, if they must rotate shifts, plans should be made to avoid the 12 midnight to 8 A.M. rotation because the temporary change in eating pattern tends to upset control of diabetes.

Getting started on a suitable plan will often make a great difference in how the patient continues with it at home and can help him and his family avoid undue stress and concern. Most patients with diabetes are now treated in a doctor's office or a hospital clinic. Occasionally, when control is particularly difficult, when complications such as infection are also present, or when the patient is unusually apprehensive, a period of hospitalization affords the security that is needed.

General nursing care. Whether care and teaching are done in the hospital, in the clinic, or in the patient's home by the public health nurse, it is important that the nurse get to know the patient. In the clinic, for example, provision should be made for every newly diagnosed patient to have a conference with a nurse. This should be in a private conference room. The patient should be given an opportunity to express himself on what he thinks having diabetes will mean to him. At this time the nurse should attempt to learn what the patient knows about the disease and should make concrete plans with him for future teaching conferences.

Since the usual patient with diabetes has a chronic disease and must take daily medication and must adhere to a diet, he is taught early to take care of these particular needs himself or to have a member of his family assist him. The nurse works out a plan for the patient for self-injection of insulin, self-testing of urine (if this is necessary), preparation and measurement of food, and recognition of unusual symptoms. She also has the responsibility to review with him the general rules of good hygiene and of healthful living. If the patient is elderly, special care of the feet is taught since circulatory difficulties of the lower extremities often occur. The family should always be included in this plan even though they may not take an active part in the procedures involved. This helps them to understand what is necessary and to encourage the patient to carry out instructions and enables them to "take over" if this should become necessary.

The teaching plan should be arranged so that the patient is not rushed and has enough time for sufficient practice in self-care. If a member of the patient's family is to learn to inject insulin, prepare food, test urine, and detect untoward symptoms, it may require arrangements for this person to come to the hospital or the clinic at other than regular hours if work or home responsibilities make attendance at the usual times impossible.

As she works with each patient, the nurse gives him encouragement and notes how he appears to be accepting his disease. The necessity of having to take injections and perhaps to limit his diet for the rest of life is more than some patients can face. The patient may feel that he is "different" and must live a life different from that of other people. He may tend to dissociate himself from friends because he can no longer engage in much activity without fear of having insulin shock. He may be self-conscious about eating with others because he must avoid certain foods.

Each patient will need individual understanding and help to live as normal a life as possible. He can be assisted in planning a schedule for injections which will keep his diabetes under control yet will allow him as much freedom as possible. Help in learning diet substitution will aid him in overcoming unnecessary embarrassment when eating meals away from home. Safe methods of self-care can be learned, and satisfactory arrangements can usually be made in his social life. Throughout this adjustment period the patient needs emotional support and interest from his family and medical personnel who are familiar with his particular needs.

If the nurse is assigned to care for a patient with diabetes in the hospital, she should know whether the diagnosis is recent or whether the patient has had diabetes for some time. Patients who have diabetes often enter the hospital for treatment of another condition. If so, the nurse should find out early what the patient's usual diabetic regimen is and should help provide opportunities for him to follow it if his general condition permits. For example, he can continue to give himself insulin and to make his own food selection. If not allowed to continue his routine, he may have additional difficulty readjusting to it upon discharge from the hospital. Some patients become more dependent when a new illness occurs and are more than willing to have medical personnel assume complete responsibility for their care. Other patients may be seriously ill and actually physicially unable to continue self-care. The nurse should help to determine the best plan for each patient.

Diet. Depending upon the physician's experience and belief, the patient is placed on a weighed or measured diet or on an unweighed, unmeasured diet with elimination of concentrated sweets.

The nurse can do much to help the patient with diabetes to understand food values and to follow his prescribed diet. In each instance the patient's age, activity, medical condition, and general nutritional state should be considered when planning his meals. His social and economic background, as well as his eating habits and emotional needs, should be considered. For example, a patient who requires or normally has eaten a rather low-calorie diet should not have a 2,500 calorie diet planned. Working people may find they need to increase their caloric intake since they use more of their food for energy causing the blood sugar level to drop and leaving an excess of insulin which may cause signs of insulin shock. Extra food is also often necessary after unexpected exercise or emotional stress. It must be repeatedly stressed to all patients who have diabetes that insulin or tolbutamide (Orinase), if ordered, *must* be taken and meals *must* be eaten. Many patients assume that insulin and food can be safely omitted if they have a cold or other minor ailment and do not feel like eating. Full-liquid or clear-liquid diets can be prepared to provide the essential food for a short time, and the patient and his family should know how to do this. Any patient who cannot eat and who has insulin prescribed should consult his physician at once.

In planning the patient's diet, the six-food-exchange lists prepared jointly by the American Diabetes Association, The American Dietetic Association, and the Public Health Service are useful and should be available to the nurse. These lists have been published in a booklet* and are available for patients. They are set up according to calories and show how each food listed is equal in nutritional value to any other food on the list and give suggested menus. The exchange lists allow for substitution of one food for another, depending upon the patient's likes or dislikes or the general menus for the day. Exchanges are set up in seven categories; foods not needing measurement, vegetables, fruits, cereals, meats, fats, and milk. The patient may take as much as desired of foods not needing measurement such as coffee, tea, bouillon, sour pickles, asparagus, cabbage, celery, cucumber, greens, lettuce, and tomatoes. He must be cautioned not to use sugar, cream, or dressings on these, however, without planning for it in the total intake. A combination of glycine and saccharin is now available. It is reported to be less bitter than saccharin and comes in granulated form. However, each packet (2 teaspoonfuls) does contain 0.5 mg. of sodium, so it may be contraindicated if a low-sodium diet is necessary.

*Meal Planning and Exchange Lists, 620 North Michigan Avenue, Chicago, Ill., The American Dietetic Association, Inc.

If the nurse can help with menu planning on a weekly basis she can demonstrate how the patient can have variety and foods that he likes even though restrictions are necessary. Most patients find it helpful to see food portions especially such "unmeasurable" things as a small potato, an ounce of meat, or a slice of cheese. When possible, foods are measured using standard household measures such as an 8 ounce measuring cup, a teaspoon, or a tablespoon. All measurements are level and cooked foods are measured after cooking. The patient with diabetes usually does not need to buy special foods but can select his diet from the same foods purchased by the rest of the family. Canned fruits that are packed in water rather than in syrup should be suggested since sugar can be added by others as necessary. Vegetables can be prepared with those for the rest of the family except that the patient's portion should be removed before such things as extra butter, milk, flour, or cheese are added. Meats should be baked, broiled, or boiled. Any fat used must be accounted for in the measurements for the meal. Special diabetic foods are expensive, and the patient should also be reminded that they usually are not calorie-free and need to be reckoned in the daily dietary allowance.

In any situation in which a clinical dietitian is available, she usually participates in the diet teaching program. However, the nurse often must do this, and she always should work closely with the dietitian to assure adequate follow-up supervision. A good time for teaching the patient is during his meal.

The patient on a weighed diet actually weighs out specific amounts of food on a small scale. Food can be weighed for a day at a time; however, if the patient eats away from home, practice in estimating usual weighed amounts will be necessary. Specific amounts of carbohydrates, protein, and fat are prescribed. A usual diet consists of from 150 to 200 Gm. of carbohydrate, from 75 to 100 Gm. of protein, and fat in an amount which will make up the needed number of calories.

A measured diet is one in which the amounts are calculated according to household measurements or usual-sized portions. It is important to use reasonable-sized portions to avoid confusion and to simplify preparation for the patient and his family.

If the patient has a self-chosen, unmeasured diet, he should eat a well-balanced selection of food in moderate quantity and avoid overindulgence in sweets. On this regimen the patient usually must take insulin every day. He should eat regularly and eat at the accustomed time without skipping or delaying meals.

Insulin. Insulin is obtained from the pancreas of sheep, hogs, or cattle. From 50 to 70 per cent of the patients with diabetes in the United States require it in their treatment. There are now five types of insulin in general use, and each is effective in lowering blood sugar by aiding in the metabolism of carbohydrates. Insulins are either rapid acting or slow acting. Rapid-acting insulins include *regular insulin* and *crystalline insulin.* Regular insulin is a clear liquid which acts soon after injection, but its effects do not last. Its action begins approximately forty-five minutes to an hour after injection, reaches the peak from the third to the fifth hours, and loses effectiveness in six hours. Crystalline insulin looks the same as regular insulin but is a more refined product. It remains effective one hour longer than regular insulin and is less likely to cause local reaction at the site of injection.

Three types of insulin are slow acting. *Protamine zinc insulin* is a milky-appearing solution and is a combination of regular insulin and a chemical (protamine) and a small amount of zinc. If allowed to stand, the liquid separates into layers. In order to obtain an accurate dose of the active ingredient, the solution should be mixed by gently rotating the bottle between the palms of the hands; it should not be shaken or allowed to become frothy. Protamine zinc insulin begins to act from four to six hours after injection, reaches the height of activity between eighteen to twenty hours, and is effective for twenty-four hours. *Globin zinc insulin* is a clear, but slightly amber, solution which has a more rapid beginning action than protamine zinc insulin. It becomes effective in two hours, reaches its peak action at eight hours, and is effective for twenty-four hours. *Neutral protamine Hagedorn insulin* (NPH) is another type of protamine zinc insulin. It reaches maximum action from six to ten hours after injection and lasts from twenty-four to thirty hours. Since crystalline insulin has a rapid but short effect and protamine insulin has a slow but prolonged action NPH insulin is often used when an intermediate action is desired. Most patients receiving NPH insulin need an afternoon snack to prevent hypoglycemia.

Each individual patient has his own particular insulin need and suitable amounts as well as types are carefully selected by the doctor. It is important that the nurse understand the type and the rate of action of each kind of insulin prescribed for her patient. For example, it is imperative that the patient take food after the administration of rapid-acting insulin, and some patients may need more than one injection a day to enable them to use the carbohydrates eaten. Many patients are given the slower-acting insulins since this eliminates the need for several doses during the day. Other patients may need a combination of regular insulin and a protamine insulin. A supplementary meal at bedtime is usually necessary for the patient taking slow-acting insulin.

It is also important for the patient to take extra food after unusual exercise or during increased emotional stress. During these periods when insulin has been taken and available food has been used for producing energy, the blood sugar level drops and there is too much insulin in the blood. Colds and minor infections increase the need for insulin even if the patient remains at rest and neither the insulin nor the diet can ever be safely omitted. Any patient who feels that he cannot take the insulin prescribed and cannot eat should contact his doctor at once.

Insulin shock. All persons with diabetes should know about the signs and symptoms of insulin shock or too much insulin. Members of the patient's family should know about this and should be able to give treatment. If the patient follows his usual schedule of insulin injection, urine testing (if required), and prescribed diet, he may still have slight reactions at times, but marked reactions are usually caused by too large a dose of insulin or too little food. If the patient does not eat all of his food or if he skips between-meal and bedtime supplements of food that have been prescribed, he may have a reaction. Some patients alter the dose of insulin to cover excesses in eating. Vomiting, diarrhea, or added exercise may also be the cause of insulin shock. Every person who has diabetes should carry a card giving his address, the name and address of his doctor, the fact that he has diabetes, and his daily insulin dosage.

If for any reason the patient feels "different," is slightly nervous, perspires, is irritable or feels dizzy, he should take or be given additional food. These are the beginning signs of too much insulin. He may also feel weak or hungry, may have a headache, palpitation, tremor, blurring of vision, or numbness of the lips or tongue. Many persons with diabetes carry lump sugar or hard candies to be eaten in such emergencies. If the patient is at home he should drink a glass of orange juice or other fruit juice which he should keep available at all times. Sometimes the reaction comes on suddenly and the patient may not sense early signs; in such an instance a family member may have to give the orange juice or some other sweet fluid. If impending insulin shock is not treated immediately, the patient becomes stuporous and unconscious. Occasionally the tremor is very severe and convulsions may occur. When this happens and when the patient is unconscious, glucose usually is given intravenously. A stomach tube may also be passed through the nose and into the stomach when the patient is unconscious and cannot swallow safely.

Tolbutamide. Tolbutamide, commonly referred to by the trade name Orinase, is a sulfonamide derivative which appears to be helpful in the treatment of some elderly patients who have a mild form of diabetes. It is not effective in severe juvenile diabetes nor in middle-aged and older persons whose blood sugar fluctuates widely, nor is it of any use in the treatment of diabetic coma.

The action of tolbutamide is unknown, but it appears to influence the effectiveness of the insulin available. It does not take the place of insulin in experimental animals when the pancreas has been removed.

Tolbutamide, which is taken by mouth, is particularly helpful for elderly patients who have failing vision and shaky hands, thus making the administration of insulin difficult. It is a boon, too, for the patient whose emotional reactions make the taking of injections almost impossible. The usual dose is 1 to 2 Gm. (60 to 120 grains) taken daily after an initial dose of 3 Gm. daily for two to eight days.[3]

Toxic reactions to tolbutamide may occur and include skin reactions, depression, and urticaria. The drug does not appear to increase the utilization of glucose—acidosis may develop in the patient who increases his own dosage and eats more than his diet permits. The need to take only the amount of drug ordered and to adhere to the prescribed diet must be emphasized. The patient may feel that, since he is being treated with tablets and does not have to have "needles," his disease is minor and he may become careless about diet and general health care. This is particularly true of the elderly patient who accepts changes in his diet reluctantly. Exercise, routine care of the feet, and course of action in event of infection should be exactly the same as for the patient who takes insulin daily.

Teaching the patient to administer insulin. Typical trays for the injection of insulin and the testing of urine can be set up for use in demonstrations and for the patient to use in practice. The materials can be gathered in a cardboard box or on a tray. The nurse can discuss boxes or trays that the patient might have at home or suggest suitable purchases from the dime store. When the equipment is not in use, a piece of clear plastic can be used to cover it and the set should be placed on a shelf or in a closet out of the reach of children. The timesaving value of having all necessary equipment in one place and accessible is obvious.

Equipment needed for the *injection of insulin* includes an insulin syringe, several No. 25 hypodermic needles, a small jar for cotton or a box roll of cotton, a bottle of alcohol, and a small saucepan of sufficient depth to boil the syringe and needle. Many public health nursing agencies include a strainer which can be set into the saucepan. This makes it easier for the patient to drain and handle the equipment without breakage or contamination.

The patient can learn to prepare the needle and syringe for injection and can practice injecting water into an orange; then, on a gradual daily plan, he can proceed to inject himself, using the thighs as sites. When repeated injections are necessary, the site of injection must be rotated to assure proper absorption of medication. Irritation from repeated injections at the same site can cause induration so that the insulin is absorbed too slowly or not at all. The best method is to use a diagram of the thighs, numbering the sites to be used and rotating the sites as numbered. Injections should never be given in any one spot oftener than every two weeks and a safe rule to follow is not to use the same site oftener than once every thirty days.

Thorough cleansing of equipment and the use of only sharp sturdy needles, as well as adequate boiling time and sterile technique, should be emphasized. Careful attention to such matters will help to avoid local reaction or infection and pain. The patient should be shown how to sharpen needles on a small piece of soapstone. Sharpness can be maintained by careful handling of the needles and by storing them in cotton. The patient should learn to test needles for burrs before boiling them by drawing the shaft through a piece of cotton. Needles which bend or which are too pliable should be discarded.

Modifications in methods of administration. At times modifications in methods of administration of insulin may be necessary because of particular problems; for example, the patient may be elderly, may have unsteady hands, or may have failing vision. In these instances, measurement of insulin, as well as proper injection technique, will require closer attention and adaptation. The usual 40 to 80 unit insulin syringe may be too slender to grasp, and numbers may be too small for the patient to read easily. The Tru-Set syringe is one which often can be used. It has a capacity of 1 ml. and an adjustable metal marker that can be placed in the correct-amount position which prevents the plunger from drawing farther back. The patient draws up insulin until the plunger of the syringe will not go any farther. Even with very limited vision he can tell by feeling that he has the correct amount. Another kind of special syringe is the Cornwall syringe. This is a larger syringe which has a more elaborate stop regulator and can also be permanently set at the required dosage.

Patients who have failing vision also may use a small magnifying adaptor (C-Better Magnifier) which can be clipped to a syringe. The numbers on the syringe are magnified, and the patient can see that he has the correct amount of insulin in the syringe. Some of these special syringes and other aids are available from surgical supply houses. Some very practical suggestions as well as information as to sources of equipment are available in a publication, *Aids for the Blind.** Patients with poor vision have the danger of drawing air instead of insulin into the syringe. They must be cautioned to invert the bottle completely and to insert the needle only a short distance. Often they are ad-

---

*Prepared by the American Foundation for the Blind, Inc., 15 West Sixteenth Street, New York, N. Y.

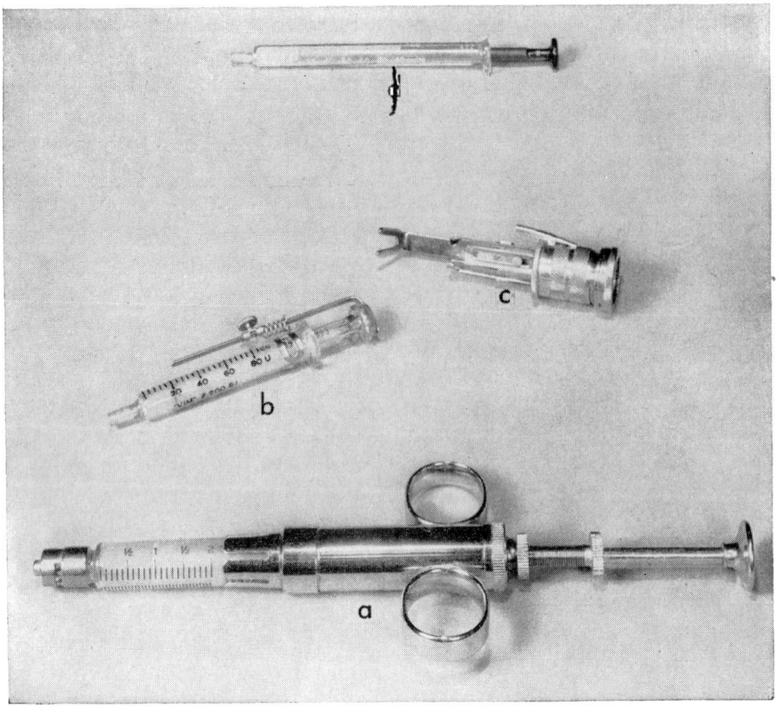

Figure 94

Special syringes are available for the diabetic patient who has visual difficulty. *a,* Cornwall syringe. *b,* Tru-Set syringe. *c,* Automatic injector. *d,* Regular insulin syringe.

vised to use only about two thirds of the bottle of insulin and to have on hand another full bottle. Some patients go to a clinic or have a public health nurse or a friend withdraw the last doses in a bottle of insulin for them.

Some patients are reluctant to put the needle through their own skin. This is difficult even for the calm matter-of-fact person and may be impossible for the tense nervous person. An automatic injector, however, can be used and is a great help to some patients. It can be attached to a regular 2 ml. syringe. When the medication is drawn up into the syringe, the automatic spring is set and the patient can wipe the site of injection with alcohol, pinch the skin, and press the spring release. The needle automatically and quickly enters the skin and the injection can be given slowly. (See Figure 94.)

Many elderly patients have a tremor of the hands which makes handling the equipment and giving themselves insulin quite difficult. Usually the patient has less tremor at certain times of the day and plans can be made by the physician and the patient so that insulin can be taken at the time of day that is best for the patient. A member of the patient's family may have to give the insulin. A family member should always know how to do this in case impending coma or other illness makes it impossible for the patient to give the insulin to himself.

Mixing two types of insulin. Since it may be necessary for a patient to take two types of insulin, the nurse must teach him to mix the two in the same syringe so that they may be given in one injection. A simple way of mixing insulin in the same syringe is first to insert a hypodermic needle in each of the bottles to be used. This equalizes the pressure within the bottle and will prevent the plunger of the syringe from being drawn in when the needle is inserted in the bottle, or, if the plunger of the syringe is loose, pressure within the bottle from blowing out toward the plunger and perhaps causing breakage. It also eliminates the necessity of having to inject air into the syringe equivalent to the amount of insulin to be removed. There is danger of accidentally mixing one type of insulin with the other in the bottle if the pressure is not equalized before beginning. Regular insulin and one of the zinc insulins is the usual mixture. After placing the needles in the bottles, the syringe should be attached to the needle in the regular insulin bottle without any air in the syringe. The correct amount of regular insulin is withdrawn, and the needle and syringe are withdrawn. Then the needle is taken from the zinc insulin bottle. The needle attached to the syringe containing regular insulin is inserted into the zinc insulin bottle, and the correct amount of insulin is withdrawn. The mixture should be shaken gently to obtain a well-distributed solution and then injected in the usual manner.

Teaching the patient to test urine for sugar. Urine testing equipment will depend upon the patient's wishes and finances. He may use a compact set such as Clinitest, or Benedict's solution which is cheaper. If the latter is used, he needs a clean empty can in which to place the tube for boiling, two to three test tubes, a teaspoon, a medicine dropper, and a bottle of Benedict's solution. A piece of wire can be bent to fasten over the sides of the pan and looped in the center to hold the tube in an upright position. The patient must be cautioned to avoid vigorous boiling which may cause the fluid to sputter and cause burning; the open end of the test tube must be directed *away* from the patient. A clock can be used for timing. Each patient who must test his urine should be provided with a color chart. Many times, these are available from pharmaceutical firms or are enclosed in the kits for testing urine. A helpful color guide can be made easily by any resourceful nurse using a piece of cardboard or paper and crayons and referring to a good laboratory textbook for accuracy of color.

What the patient *does* if his test is abnormal depends entirely upon the particular patient and the instructions from his doctor. These should be in writing. The doctor may, for example, instruct the patient to do nothing except repeat the test again during the same day and keep a careful record of urine reactions, increase or decrease his insulin dosage, increase or decrease his food intake, or get in touch with him at once. Some doctors may want certain patients to show a trace or even a plus one in their urine once daily as evidence that the blood sugar is not going too low while for other patients this would not be considered good control. The age of the patient and the stability of his disease affects the doctor's decision in advising a course of action. The nurse must emphasize to the patient that he must follow the doctor's instructions *exactly* and that he should have these in writing. Some patients, particularly young adults, take it upon themselves to alter dosage of insulin and diet for themselves and get into serious trouble by so doing.

Skin care. Since patients with diabetes are more susceptible to infection and since healing is generally slow, attention should be given to skin care. Oral hygiene and care of the nails, as well as over-all cleanliness, should be stressed. The legs and feet of the patient with diabetes are particularly vulnerable to infection. Bumps or bruises on the lower extremities should be avoided; if they do occur they should be observed carefully. (See Figure 95.) Maintenance of good circulation is extremely important for all adult persons who have diabetes. (For complete discussion of measures to improve and maintain circulation and to give good general care to the feet see Chapter 19.)

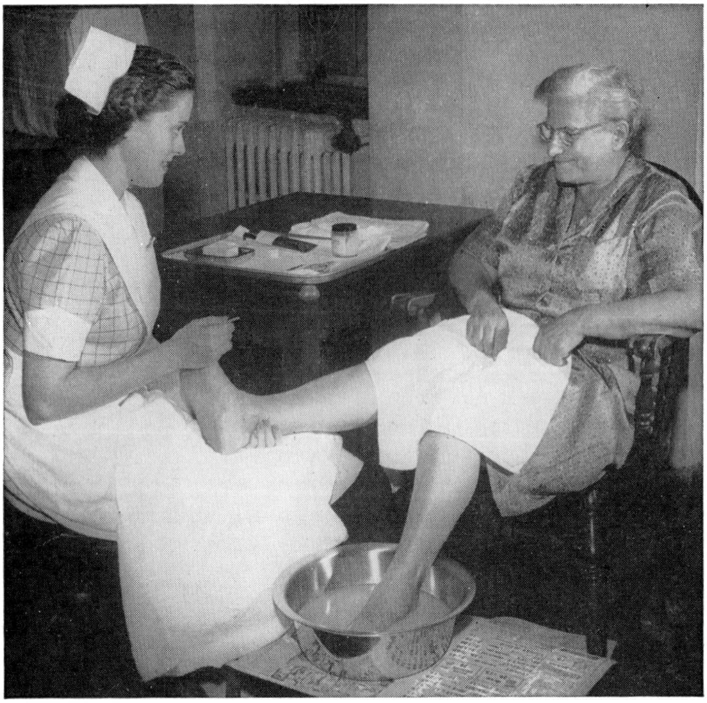

Figure 95

During visits to the clinic, the elderly patient with diabetes may learn to care for herself. Here the nurse is teaching the patient the proper care of her feet.

If the patient has pruritus vulvae, cleanliness should be stressed. The area should be sponged after each voiding, then thoroughly dried by blotting with a soft towel. Cornstarch can be used as a powder. Sitz baths may be ordered to be taken two or three times a day. Calamine lotion is sometimes helpful, and medicated ointment may be prescribed. When the diabetes is under treatment and the excretion of sugar and abnormal amounts of urine are decreased, the pruritus usually subsides.

Diabetic coma

Diabetic coma is a complication of undiagnosed or neglected diabetes, and is the result of prolonged and increasing acidosis. The series of events leading to the development of acidosis are difficult to describe and many questions regarding the metabolic processes involved have not yet been answered. As has been previously stated, the defect in carbohydrate metabolism is followed by derangement in protein and fat metabolism. For example, nitrogen is excreted in the urine of the poorly controlled diabetic patient; this is presumably because of the altered ability to store protein normally in the absence of insulin. Also, there then follows an abnormally rapid breakdown of fats into acetoacetic acid and beta-hydroxybutyric acid. These cannot be used by the body at the rate in which they are produced; their accumulation in the blood stream leads to ketosis and all the signs and symptoms of acidosis appear. (See Chapter 6 for further discussion of metabolic acidosis.)

Before the discovery of insulin, diabetic coma often caused death. *Immediate* care and treatment is still necessary, but with this care the outcome is usually good. The patient or his family should contact their physician at once if any signs or symptoms of acidosis occur. Carrying a card which states that he has diabetes helps to ensure prompt treatment in the event that coma develops while the patient is away from home. Such a card also helps prevent this condition from being mistaken for head injury, cerebrovascular accident, or drunkenness.

The patient in diabetic coma is given emergency treatment in the hospital emergency room or clinic, although he may be admitted to a ward. Hourly urine specimens may be obtained by catheterization and examined for sugar and acetone. Blood tests for sugar are done while the patient is given fluids, glucose, and insulin intraveneously. The amount of glucose and insulin is carefully prescribed by the doctor and changes are based on the blood sugar and urinalysis findings. The patient should be kept warm. Epinephrine may be given to raise the blood pressure. As soon as the patient can take fluids by mouth, he is given salty broth to help maintain electrolyte balance, then orange juice or other sweet fluids; insulin is given subcutaneously.

Continued care

Since, in many instances, the diagnosis of diabetes is made in a doctor's office rather than in the hospital, insulin regulation and diet will be prescribed and taught by the physician, or he may ask a public health nurse to work with the patient and his family. Those patients admitted to hospitals may need additional instruction or continued instruction at home. In this instance the hospital physician and nurse will discuss with the patient the possibility of continued care at home by the public health nurse. For one reason or another he may not be capable of learning the care he needs to give himself. If the patient lives alone and has no relative or neighbor who can be taught to give daily injections of insulin and to check on other aspects of care, it may be necessary for a nurse to visit the home to carry out these procedures.

The nurse in the hospital or in the home should always pass information along to other medical personnel as to what care has been given, what teaching has been accomplished, and probable future needs. This information enables the nurse and patient to continue his care without delays and repetition.

Complications of diabetes mellitus

Most medical authorities believe that persons in whom diabetes is under treatment and control may have complications later than those less controlled. Atherosclerosis, often affecting the coronary arteries, and arterial changes involving particularly the lower extremities, pyelonephritis, retinopathy, neuropathy, and intercapillary glomerulosclerosis (Kimmelstiel-Wilson syndrome) are the common complications. The alert nurse can help prevent the occurrence of complications in the lower limbs by teaching the patient to protect and make the best use of his limited vascular resources. Ulcerations heal very slowly in these patients, and amputation may be necessary if gangrene occurs. All patients with peripheral circulatory damage also have lessened nerve acuity; they need to be cautioned about possible traumatic injury from lack of sensitivity. (See Chapter 19.)

Kimmelstiel-Wilson syndrome, a nephrotic syndrome with albuminuria, edema, and hypercholesterolemia, has an unfavorable prognosis. Treatment is the same as for nephrosis from other causes. Pyelonephritis is treated with antibiotics. (See Chapter 21.)

Patients with retinopathy may have serious handicaps because of their needs for daily injections of insulin, urine testing, preparation of their own food, and general care. They present a great challenge to the nurse in helping them to accommodate to visual changes. (See Chapter 33.)

Patients with diabetes mellitus are particularly susceptible to tuberculous infection. They are treated for both diseases with as few modifications in treatment of each disease as possible.

DISEASE OF THE PITUITARY GLAND

The exact number of hormones secreted by the anterior lobe of the pituitary gland is unknown. Known hormones secreted by this gland stimulate other endocrine glands in the body, such as the adrenocorticotrophic hormone (ACTH; corticotrophin) which stimulates the adrenal cortex.

Hypofunction

Hypofunction of this gland may result from a tumor within the gland itself or tumors associated with contiguous structures. Metastatic carcinoma or inflammatory diseases such as syphilis and tuberculosis can cause glandular damage. One result of hypofunction is the effect upon body growth. In the adolescent, sexual growth and development may be arrested. If a tumor is present, the patient may have pressure symptoms such as visual disturbance and severe headache. Other symptoms due to pituitary failure will be exhibited elsewhere, depending upon which hormone insufficiency is manifested.

Treatment of pituitary failure depends upon the cause. Tumors are removed surgically, and substitution therapy with pituitary extracts is given during the preoperative and immediate postoperative periods. If failure continues postoperatively, hormone therapy is continued.

Diabetes insipidus. Diabetes insipidus is a disease caused by failure of activity of the posterior lobe of the pituitary gland. One of the actions of the pituitary hormones is the ability to increase reabsorption of water from the renal tubules. Patients with diabetes insipidus excrete a very large amount of urine; as many as 15 liters may be excreted daily. This causes fluid and electrolyte imbalance. They also have insatiable thirst (polydipsia), anorexia, weight loss, and weakness. Specific treatment usually consists of giving extracts of the posterior lobe of the pituitary gland. This is given as a powder which can be inhaled. Pitressin tannate in oil, 5 units, given intramuscularly will give relief up to forty-eight hours. A low-salt diet may also help.

Diabetes insipidus is a rare disease but its symptoms are being seen more often in recent years because it follows surgical removal of the hypophyseal gland in attempts to control metastasis of breast cancer (see Chapter 31).

Hyperfunction

Hyperfunction of the pituitary gland in an adult results in *acromegaly*. This is caused by a tumor of the eosinophil cells. The main symptoms or signs are those of excessive body growth. Bones enlarge transversely. The features become coarse and heavy. The lower jaw becomes particularly large; frontal sinuses are pronounced. Hands and feet become conspicuously wider, necessitating larger-sized gloves and shoes. Lips are heavier and the tongue is enlarged. Because the location of the gland makes surgery difficult, radiation is often used to destroy the tumor.

Striking changes in the patient's appearance may be noticed in comparing pictures of the patient taken some time before with his present appearance. Patients may be asked to bring pictures of themselves to the hospital to help in diagnosis. During diagnosis and treatment, the patient needs understanding care. Changes in appearance may have produced emotional reactions. Since physical changes are irreversible even if the disease is arrested, they may be doubly difficult to accept.

THE ADRENAL GLANDS

In recent years the adrenal cortex has been found to produce a large number of steroid compounds and thereby to affect a wide variety of body functions. Among these steroids are cortisone, corticosterone, hydrocortisone, desoxycorticosterone, dehydrocorticosterone, and aldosterone. The following are some of the vital functions affected by secretions of the adrenal cortex: regulation of sodium, potassium, and chloride metabolism, of water balance, of the metabolism of carbohydrate, fat, and protein, and of the development of secondary sexual characteristics, and control of skin and mucous membrane pigmentation, activities pertaining to hematopoiesis and tissue reactivity, and of gastrointestinal functions by control of stomach and pancreatic enzymes.

Nursing care in adrenal cortical steroid therapy

Because of the extremely wide range of body activities affected by adrenal cortical steroid secretions, these products are now used extensively in the treatment of an almost infinite number of diseases involving almost every system of the body. For this reason, the nurse should know about the activities of the gland, the secretions produced, the therapeutic effect, and the untoward effects that may occur. For more detailed information about the adrenal glands and the use of its secretions, the student should consult specialized texts. Current pamphlets and articles in recent periodicals[10] are particularly helpful since knowledge in this field is increasing rapidly. The nurse should know that cortical steroids are used in treating many conditions that do not appear to be related to endocrine dysfunction; their exact therapeutic effect is not understood too well but appears to rest primarily with their ability to control inflammatory reactions and the tissue repair that follows this.

There are many side effects and untoward reactions that can follow prolonged treatment with adrenal cortical steroids. The nurse should be aware of these and should report their early signs at once. They include disturbance in fluid and electrolyte balance partly contributing to the typical "moon face" so often described, disturbance of protein metabolism, alteration in secondary sexual characteristics, a predisposition to develop peptic ulcer, and a masking of signs of a developing infection.[10] A characteristic feeling of well being (euphoria) is characteristic so that the patient may feel much better than he really is. Another difficulty is that prolonged administration of the cortical steroids can suppress the secretions of ACTH by the pituitary gland and sudden withdrawal of the drug or marked decreases in dosage may precipitate adrenal cortical crisis (addisonian crisis), which is described later in this chapter. Errors in giving the medication and cancelation of orders when patients are transferred or when operations are scheduled can lead to serious consequences. Since one of the signs of adrenal cortical deficiency is low blood pressure, it is apparent that this situation may affect enormously the postoperative course of a patient whose blood pressure has already been lowered by an operation.

Since sodium tends to be retained and to increase the retention of water in the body, when adrenal cortical steroids are being taken, salt is almost always restricted. The nurse should question the diet of any patient who does not have an order for a low-sodium diet. She should also routinely record intake and output on any hospitalized medical patient and any patient having an operation who is being given adrenal cortical steroids.

Disease of the adrenal glands

Diseases of the adrenal glands are usually related to their *hyperfunction* or their *hypofunction* from a variety of causes. Study of these conditions is complicated by the fact that the adrenal cortex is affected by the pituitary gland and stimulation for increased or reduced activity may lie outside the adrenal gland itself. Only two of the most common, yet rare, diseases of the adrenal glands will be discussed here.

Addison's disease. Addison's disease is due to *hypofunction* of the adrenal cortex. Causes include tuberculous invasion of the cortex, inflammation of unknown origin which causes atrophy, and tumors of the cortex. It occurs in only one person in 100,000 of the population. Usually it is slow in onset and becomes chronic. Occasionally, however, an acute addisonian crisis may be the first sign of adrenal insufficiency and may accompany or follow other acute illness which increases the body's need for cortisone. Many early symptoms and signs are too nonspecific to be noticed and include lassitude, ease of fatigue, weight loss, amnesia, nausea, diarrhea, gastrointestinal discomfort, tension, irritability, and depression. Brown pigmentation of the skin, particularly over the knuckles and other joints is often the first sign observed. The skin may first appear tanned or bronzed and then become muddy, brown, and "unwashed" in appearance.

Medical treatment and nursing care. The disease is now usually diagnosed by means of a test which measures the adrenal cortical response to injection of pituitary corticotropin (ACTH), and the test is fully described in medical texts.[3] Techniques in conducting this test vary somewhat in different institutions. Urinary excretions of 17-ketosteroids and 17-hydroxycorticoids and eosinophile count in the blood stream are measured by the test. This test has almost completely replaced the several "nonspecific" tests which attempted to determine water excretion, response to salt deprivation, and other tests of adrenal cortical effectiveness. Obviously, important nursing responsibilities are to see that fluids are withheld as specified, that urine specimens are collected on time and preserved for study, and that equipment is available for injection of drugs and taking of blood samples.

Addison's disease is now effectively treated by giving cortisone in doses of 25 to 37.5 mg. daily and hydrocortisone in doses of 20 to 30 mg. (1⅓ to 2 grains) daily. Both drugs are given by mouth in divided doses at 8 A.M. and 3 P.M. Taking the second dose after 4 P.M. may lead to excitability and sleeplessness. Occasionally the drugs cause gastric irritation which can be avoided by taking the morning dose during breakfast and some food such as a glass of milk with the 3 P.M. dose.

Since cortisone and hydrocortisone control food metabolism but do not control salt depletion and water balance, the patient must have additional treatment to avoid hypertension and dehydration. Taking 10 to 15 Gm. of extra salt per day sometimes suffices, but usually small doses of desoxycorticosterone must be taken. Usually 2.5 to 5 mg. (1/6 to 1/3 grain) of desoxycorticosterone by mouth or 25 to 75 mg. (1 2/3 to 7 grains) of the long-acting form of the drug intramuscularly are taken monthly.

The patient with Addison's disease should carry a card stating his disease, the name and address of his physician, and what should be done in the event of sudden injury and unconsciousness. (Usually 25 mg. of cortisone is given by mouth every six hours or, if the patient is unconscious, 200 mg. is given hypodermically.) The patient should be taught to take particular care in the event of infection and to report to his physician if anything but the most minor indisposition occurs, since infection increases the need for adrenal hormones. Excessive mental or physical strain should be avoided.

Addisonian crisis or adrenal crisis. Addisonian crisis is really a severe exacerbation of Addison's disease. It may be precipitated by excessive activity, infection, or failure to take prescribed steroids. The signs of impending crisis are those of the disease in exaggerated form. Adrenal crisis is a very serious condition which quickly leads to death from severe hypotension, shock, coma, and vasomotor collapse. The treatment is immediate hospitalization and treatment with continuous infusions of normal saline solution and glucose and hydrocortisone given intravenously. The patient must do *absolutely nothing* for himself. He should be attended constantly and the temperature recording may be requested hourly since hyperthermia is common; the patient often complains of a severe headache. Blood pressure recording may be requested every fifteen minutes, and if hypotension is extreme the nurse should anticipate that Neo-Synephrine may be prescribed and should have shock blocks available for immediate use. If the patient is conscious, the nurse should caution him not to attempt to turn or otherwise help himself. He must be protected from members of his family and from hospital personnel who have colds or other infections. Sometimes penicillin or other antibiotics are given prophylactically because of the patient's extremely low resistance to infection.

Adrenalectomy, which is done for adrenal tumors, and bilateral adrenalectomy, which is done in an attempt to control some forms of malignant cancer cause symptoms similar to Addison's disease (see Chapters 21 and 31). The treatment and expected postoperative complications are similar.

Cushing's syndrome. Cushing's syndrome results from *excessive secretion* (hyperfunction) of 11,17-oxygenated corticoids, hydrocortisone, and cortisone by the adrenal cortex.[3] The most common cause is hyperplasia of the adrenal cortex although less often a tumor is found. If the cause is stimulation of the adrenal cortex by a tumor in the pituitary gland, the term "Cushing's disease" is used. Cushing's syndrome is a rare disease which is more common in women than in men and sometimes follows pregnancy.

Signs and symptoms of Cushing's syndrome include muscle wasting with resultant weakness, susceptibility to hemorrhage, peculiar fat distribution with deposition of fat in the face (moon face), neck, and trunk. Osteoporosis is also common and fracture of vertebrae may occur. The patient usually has hypertension and is irritable and changeable in mood. There may be disturbance of carbohydrate metabolism and accompanying diabetes mellitus. Women patients show signs of masculinization, often with cessation of menses, whereas adolescent or preadolescent boys may have precocious sexual development. Resistance to infection is often lowered and may lead to death.

Medical treatment and nursing care. Treatment depends on the cause. Tests are done to determine urinary secretion of steroids, and response to ACTH is also measured. X-ray examination of the adrenals and of the sella tursica surrounding the pituitary gland helps in diagnosis. Treatment may include administration of potassium chloride by mouth, adrenalectomy, and irradiation of the pituitary gland if no cause for symptoms is found within the adrenal cortex.

Nursing care of the patient with Cushing's syndrome requires careful recording of fluid and food intakes and of urinary output. The diet ordered by the doctor should be checked by the nurse to be certain that the patient receives the right food. Low-sodium and high-potassium foods are often given, and every effort must be made to have the patient eat the food that is ordered. Enteric-coated potassium tablets are often given with meals. Testing the urine for sugar and acetone and insulin treatment will be necessary if the patient also has diabetes mellitus.

The patient with Cushing's syndrome needs help in maintaining emotional stability. The nurse should notice and record on the nursing care plan those situations which seem to upset the patient and add to depression. Depression and emotional lability are pronounced and study of one series of cases showed that 5 to 10 per cent of deaths in this group occurred from suicide.[15] The nurse should be alert to the possibility of self destruction and should discuss early with the doctor any changes in the patient's mood and behavior.

When *adrenalectomy* is to be done, treatment with cortisone is begun preoperatively and continued postoperatively; it is continued indefinitely after a daily maintenance dose is established. Postoperatively the nurse should observe carefully for signs of hypotension, which may be severe if both adrenal glands have been removed. The patient must be turned at least every two hours, and intake and output measurements and recordings are extremely important since hypofunction of the posterior pituitary gland may occur and greatly alter urinary excretion. Measurements of steroids in the urine may indicate the level of activity of remaining adrenal tissues. If diabetes mellitus was a preoperative problem, urine is also tested for sugar and acetone until the blood sugar returns to normal. Indwelling ureteral catheters are usually used during this time.

Postoperatively the nurse should watch for signs of complications such as pneumothorax, atelectasis, and hemorrhage. The area of operation is close to the diaphragm and the inferior vena cava, and either could be damaged during surgery.

Patients with Cushing's syndrome often need long-term steroid therapy whether or not an operation is performed. They must be encouraged to visit their physician as requested and to take prescribed medications. If both adrenal glands have been removed, the patient will be treated medically in a manner very similar to the patient with Addison's disease.

REFERENCES AND SELECTED READINGS*

1 Adler, Francis Heed: Gifford's Textbook of Ophthalmology, ed. 6, Philadelphia, 1957, W. B. Saunders Co.

2 *Bortz, Edward L., and Burroughs, Deaconess Louise: The Control of Infections in Diabetic Patients, Am. J. Nursing **54**:1348-1350, Nov. 1954.

3 Cecil, Russell L., and Loeb, Robert F. (editors): A Textbook of Medicine, ed. 10, Philadelphia, 1959, W. B. Saunders Co.

4 *Conklin, Groff, and Conklin, Lucy: Good News About Diabetes, New York, June, 1954, New York Public Affairs Committee.

5 Cooper, Lenna F., Barber, Edith M., Mitchell, Helen S., and Rynbergen, Henderika, J.: Nutrition in Health and Disease, ed. 13, Philadelphia, 1958, J. B. Lippincott Co.

6 *Crile, George, Jr.: Radioactive Iodine in Treating Thyroid Disease, Am. J. Nursing **54**:828, July 1954.

7 *DeLawter, DeWitt E., and Moss, James M.: Tolbutamide, Am. J. Nursing **58**:1106-1108, Aug. 1958.

8 Diabetes Program Guide: Public Health Service Publication No. 506, Washington, D. C., 1956, U. S. Government Printing Office.

9 Duke-Elder, Sir Stewart: Parson's Diseases of the Eye, ed. 13, New York, 1959, The Macmillan Co.

10 *Frohman, I. Phillips: The Steroids, Am. J. Nursing **59**:518-521, April 1959.

11 Greenblatt, Robert B., Metts, James C. Jr., Reich, Barbara Hoffman, and Ault, Leilee Powell: Addison's Disease and Nursing Care of the Patient With Addison's Disease, Am. J. Nursing **60**:1249-1255, Sept. 1960.

12 *Hubay, Charles A., and Evans, Ruth D.: Hyperthyroidism, Am. J. Nursing **55**:1206-1210, Oct. 1955.

13 Martin, Marguerite M.: The Diabetic at Home, Am. J. Nursing **56**:1294-1298, Oct. 1956.

14 Martin, Marguerite: A Teaching Center for Diabetics, Am. J. Nursing **58**:390-391, March 1958.

15 Meakins, Jonathan Campbell (editor): The Practice of Medicine, ed. 6, St. Louis, 1956, The C. V. Mosby Co.

16 *Moss, James M., and DeLawter, Dewitt E.: Oral Agents in the Management of Diabetes Mellitus, Am. J. Nursing **60**:1610-1613, Nov. 1960.

17 Rouse, George P.: Pregnancy and Diabetes, Am. J. Nursing **58**:100-101, Jan. 1958.

18 Starr, Paul: Diagnosis and Treatment of Hypothyroidism, Postgrad. Med. **17**:73-80, Jan. 1955.

19 Tolstoi, Edward: Living With Diabetes, New York, 1952, Crown Publishers, Inc.

20 Unger, Robert H., and Davidson, Joseph W., Jr.: Current Status of Aryl Sulfonylureas in Treatment of Diabetes Mellitus, J.A.M.A. **162**:447-453, Sep. 29, 1956.

21 Williams, Robert H., and others: Textbook of Endocrinology, ed. 2, Philadelphia, 1955, W. B. Saunders Co.

---

*References preceded by an asterisk indicate material particularly well suited for student reading.

The patient with skin disease

Chapter 29

Study questions for review

1 Review the anatomy and physiology of the skin. What are its main functions?
2 What have you learned in fundamentals of nursing about skin care for the elderly patient, the malnourished patient, the dehydrated patient, the emaciated patient, and the obese patient?
3 Review techniques for bandaging various parts of the body.
4 What drugs fairly often cause skin eruptions?
5 How would you prepare 2,000 ml. of a 1:10,000 solution of potassium permanganate from a 1:1000 stock solution?

GENERAL SKIN CARE AND PREVENTION OF DISEASE

The nurse can contribute to the prevention of skin disease by teaching good care of the normal skin and by encouraging early referral of abnormal skin conditions to competent physicians. This can be done as she encounters people at work, in their homes, in school, in the hospital, and elsewhere in the community.

People vary in their resistance to skin disease. Some are born with tough skins which can resist irritation and infection quite well, while others have delicate skins which have little resistance to trauma, irritation, and infection. Usually the person with blond coloring has a more delicate skin than the person with a dark complexion.

General condition of the skin, color, and texture provide an excellent barometer of the state of a person's general health. Many conditions existing within and outside the body affect the development and progress of skin disease. Nutritional and vitamin deficiencies predispose to skin disease and slow the rate of healing. Hormonal influences are presumed to have a part in the progress of some skin diseases. Nervous make-up is known to affect skin lesions; for example, nervousness may lead to itching and to subsequent scratching; infection may then be introduced, and constant aggravation of the skin following the infection can seriously hamper healing. Occupational exposure to irritating substances and the removal of natural skin secretions also predispose to disease. For example, a person who handles fabrics or who washes dishes steadily may develop chapped hands and susceptibility to infection unless natural skin oils are replaced by creams and lotions; he may also develop a sensitivity to substances such as dyes and soaps.

The skin is affected by age. As age increases, the skin undergoes atrophy of underlying tissues and hardening of superficial arterioles which nourished the skin during youth. Sebaceous glands are less active, and the skin is thin, dry, and easily traumatized. Infections occur easily and often heal more slowly.

Cleansing

The old saying that cleanliness is next to godliness is probably not entirely true. People of cultures who do not have high standards of cleanliness do not necessarily have more skin disease. The outer layer of skin cells and the perspiration are acid in reaction, and their presence inhibits the life and growth of bacteria. Strong soaps that are alkaline in reaction may neutralize this protective acid condition of the skin and may also remove the oily secretion of the sebaceous glands which lubricate the outer skin layers and contribute to their health. However, mechanical removal of dead skin and excess oil appears justified because they can coat bacteria and prevent the antibacterial action of perspiration. Also, since these substances have an unpleasant odor after undergoing bacterial decomposition, bathing is necessary for esthetic reasons.

The skin should be washed often enough to remove skin excretions and prevent odors but not often enough to cause drying and irritation. Detergent cleansers that are neutral in reaction are often better than soaps. There is a great deal of individual variation in the bathing necessary to ensure cleanliness without causing skin irritation. The person who has an oily skin and who perspires freely may need to bathe twice daily in warm weather and wash his face several times, while the person who has a dry skin may have to use creams and lotions to protect the skin even when he bathes but once a day. Most people who have bathed daily from childhood are able to continue to do so without difficulty as they grow older. Skin secretions are decreased during cold weather so that protective creams and lotions may be needed to prevent skin irritation at this time. Hard, thickened skin areas should be rubbed daily with an oily substance such as cold cream, lanolin, or vanishing cream which may contain a small amount of salicylic acid to soften dry, thickened skin. The feet of elderly persons usually need this kind of care.

Observation of abnormalities

Care of the normal skin should include regular observation of pigmented skin areas, moles, or other apparently minor skin lesions, and any change in size, color, or general appearance should be reported to a physican at once. Pigmentation (lentigo) occurs on the face, neck, and backs of hands and arms of elderly people; these freckles, which are a source of annoyance to many elderly women, are harmless. They can be removed by abrasion but so-called "freckle creams" are useless. (For more complete details of care of the normal skin and hair, see texts on fundamentals of nursing.)

Skin diseases rarely cause death. They do, however, account for much human discomfort and for serious interruption of work and other activities. People should be urged to seek competent medical help when skin conditions develop. Many persons are inclined to rely upon the advice of friends or of the local druggist or upon medications they may have on hand. Each individual's skin reacts differently to treatment, and the skin that is already irritated or diseased may respond violently to inexpert treatment. Since the skin changes, medications prescribed even for a similar skin ailment in the same patient some time previously may not produce a favorable response. Also, drugs may deteriorate, and for this reason old medications are not safe. The patient may be spared much discomfort and expense if he turns to a specialist when symptoms first develop and before a mild skin condition becomes really troublesome. He should be advised to present himself to the doctor without changing dressings or otherwise "cleaning up" the lesion.

GENERAL NURSING CARE

Certain general principles of nursing care apply to most skin conditions and will be discussed before a few of the more common diseases are mentioned. Most nursing is directed toward making the patient more comfortable, controlling pain and itching, and encouraging healing.

Pruritus

Pruritus, or itching, was defined centuries ago as a disagreeable sensation that stimulates the urge to scratch. No better definition has yet been found. Pruritus is a serious problem in many skin conditions, because scratching leads to more itching, and a vicious cycle is formed. The sensation arises in the nerve endings in the skin; it is unknown in lesions in which skin layers have been destroyed. Pruritus is known to be aggravated by several circumstances within the body, such as dilation of capillaries, tissue anoxia such as occurs in venous stasis, and presence of abnormal constituents in the skin such as bile pigment. Some skin diseases, such as tumors and tuberculous and syphilitic lesions, are not accompanied by pruritus.

Pruritus can be exhausting and demoralizing to the patient. It is useless, however, to tell him not to scratch, for he may be unable to comply with this advice, and admonishing the patient may only increase his frustration and guilt and may make the pruritus worse. It is safe to assume that the normal person who has pruritus will stop scratching when the condition has been sufficiently controlled. Trauma from scratching can be partially prevented by cutting the fingernails short and by urging the patient to try such measures as pressing the itching lesion with the finger or with the back of the fingernail instead of using the ends of the nails. Hands should be kept scrupulously clean so that danger of introducing infection is reduced. Substitutions for scratching must be sought. These may include diversions which attempt to take the person's mind off the urge to scratch and sedatives to lessen the irritability which increases the urge to scratch and decreases will power. By counting to one hundred before scratching, some patients are able to control the urge until the strongest impulse is dissipated.

Cool, light clothing or bedclothes may help to allay itching. It is well known that wool is particularly likely to cause itching even in persons who have no skin disease but who have somewhat dry skins. Any clothing that constricts, rubs, or retains body moisture and heat in local areas should be avoided. Antihistaminic drugs often are prescribed for treatment of pruritus.

The patient with pruritus should be kept quiet. Activities of all kinds, both physical and mental, that increase metabolism also increase body heat and lead to pruritus. Attention must be given to room temperature and to humidity. Usually a room temperature of 20° to 21° C. (68° to 70° F.) and a humidity of 30 to 40 per cent are best. Pain in skin lesions is increased by warming or cooling the area beyond normal limits, and pruritus usually increases when the temperature goes up. The patient should not perspire because this moistens the skin and increases pruritus, particularly under dressings and on parts of the body where skin surfaces touch each other. Excessive drying of the skin from too high a temperature and too low a humidity can also increase pruritus; this occurs easily in the elderly patient who already has a dry skin.

Gentleness in handling

Gentleness in treatment and handling of all skin lesions is important. If the body is allowed to use its own resources, the skin has surprising recuperative powers. Usually, the more acute the skin disease, the gentler the treatment should be. Skin lesions should be patted, never rubbed, and irritation of the area surrounding the lesion should be avoided, because this stimulates circulation and leads to increased warmth and pruritus. Touching, rubbing, scratching, removing dressings, and inspecting the lesion are activities that interfere with healing and yet are a temptation to the patient both in the hospital and at home. Skin lesions may be overtreated easily. The conscientious ambitious nurse and the patient and his family should know that too much cleansing and treating can be more harmful than beneficial. The nurse must be certain that she understands exactly how much treatment the physician wishes.

Warmth in special situations

The patient who has a generalized flush, or erythema and the one who has an extensive exfoliative dermatitis may be losing body heat at an abnormally increased rate and may need a room temperature of 32.2° C. (90° F.) or more to maintain normal body temperature. Care must be taken to avoid chilling, particularly after baths and when compresses are used or when parts of the body are exposed. It is surprising how much body heat can be lost when cool moist compresses are applied to even a relatively small portion of the total body surface; for example, the patient who has cool compresses on a hand and arm or who has an uncovered weeping skin condition of one limb may suffer from generalized chilling if adequate covers are not provided for the rest of his body and if the room is not kept sufficiently warm.

Rest

All dermatologic patients need sleep and rest, yet skin conditions often interfere with these requirements. The patient in the hospital may be happier in a ward since this gives him opportunity to talk to others and thus to divert his attention from himself. Skin ailments and accompanying pruritus tend to become worse at night when surroundings are quiet and there are fewer distractions. The patient needs the benefit of nursing measures to induce sleep such as a warm drink, a back massage, elimination of light and noise, and attention to ventilation. If he awakens, he should be urged to call the nurse. A sedative such as chloral hydrate which seldom causes skin reaction may be given. Or he may be advised to turn on the light and read or otherwise occupy himself while resisting the temptation to scratch the skin lesions. This may make it necessary for the patient to have a private room in the hospital. However, if he does occupy a single room, he should be wheeled in his bed or in a chair to the sun porch or recreation room during part of the day so he will have contact with others. If he sleeps during the day, he should not be disturbed. Every effort should be made to help him get enough sleep without the aid of drugs since these may cause further pruritus or may even cause increased restlessness which is harmful.

Emotional support

Encouragement and emotional support are necessary for the dermatologic patient. Because many skin lesions are unsightly and slow in healing, the patient may become discouraged and upset. He fears that he is not accepted, not wanted, and not liked by others, particularly if there are unsightly lesions on exposed parts of the body. This response may be due in part to the idea that unsightly complexions are linked with unwholesome living and communicable disease. Such a response also may be because no one likes to be conspicuous. Members of the patient's family may need interpretation of the patient's reactions to them in the hospital or of his behavior at home. The nursing staff must make the patient feel that he is socially acceptable to those about him, and care must be taken not to show any distaste or rejection no matter how difficult care of the skin lesions may be. When the lesion, despite its appearance, is not communicable, the use of equipment such as gowns and rubber gloves is bad for the patient's morale and should never be employed. The nurse must know each patient and plan individual care accordingly. For example, one patient may be happier if he is permitted to change his own compresses and otherwise care for himself, whereas another patient, because he needs the attention and reassurance of having things done for him, may feel discriminated against if this is suggested. However, in almost all instances the nurse should give some care to the skin lesion, even though the patient may attend to his other needs, because it affords her an opportunity to observe the lesion carefully and because it helps the patient to feel accepted.

Occupational and diversional therapy is helpful in the care of most dermatologic patients either in the hospital or in the home. Any activity that keeps the patient busy and thus distracts his attention from the skin ailment or its feared consequences is justified. A program including occupational therapy during the day will often help the patient sleep during the night. Occupational therapy must be carefully prescribed because in some instances the patient may be sensitive to materials used in the activities.

Bathing and cleansing

The patient with skin disease should not be bathed either in the hospital or in the home until he has been examined by a physician. Clothing, dressings, and the lesions themselves with crusts or exudates should be left undisturbed unless a definite order has been given for their care. After the initial inspection by the physician, oil may be ordered for cleansing the skin. Mineral or cottonseed oil may be used and should be warmed slightly and applied with a soft pledget, with care taken not to rub or irritate the lesions or the surrounding skin. Gauze should not be used because of the danger of trauma. The nurse should anticipate a doctor's order for soaking hard crusts or thickened exudates with physiologic solution of sodium chloride, peroxide, pHisoHex in water, or a mild solution of tincture of green soap in warm water. Whether or not a sterile technique is used depends upon the lesions, but in any event the cleanest of techniques is necessary to avoid reinfection from soiled outer dressings.

Regular bathing is seldom permitted for dermatologic patients. Tepid sponge baths without the use of soap are often ordered. The water may be softened with a handful of bran or oatmeal or a tablespoonful of uncooked laundry starch to a basin of water. Borax and sodium bicarbonate are sometimes used to soften water and allay itching, but they are drying and, therefore, are seldom ordered if the patient is elderly or has a dry skin. Many patients simply do not feel clean and are greatly distressed when not permitted a shower or tub bath for several days. Local sponging of the genital areas is usually permitted. Cold creams and other perfumed cleansing preparations are usually prohibited, but some of the detergents, pharmaceutically approved rose ointment, and cold cream may be used to make the patient feel more comfortable and acceptable to himself and others.

Special collodial baths are often ordered. An oatmeal, soybean, or bran bath may be prepared as follows: (1) add 2 cupfuls of cereal to 2 quarts of boiling water and stir while boiling for five minutes; (2) pour into a mesh or gauze bag over the tub which is three-quarters filled with tepid water, 35° C. (95° F.); (3) stir the bag about in the bath for a few minutes. The bag may also be used as a mop to gently pat the skin and remove crusts and debris. A boiled-starch bath is prepared by pouring 2 quarts of boiling water over a cupful of cornstarch or laundry starch moistened with cold water and stirring as it thickens. This may be added directly to the bath without straining through a mesh bag. Cold uncooked starch also may be used in the same quantity. Sodium bicarbonate, ¼ to ½ cup, may be added to any colloidal bath if ordered by the doctor for its drying action on the skin.

Usually the patient should stay in a bath only from thirty to sixty minutes. Occasionally when itching is particularly severe, he may remain for over an hour. In this event, small amounts of hot water should be added to the bath at intervals to prevent its becoming too cool. The patient must be watched closely for signs of fatigue and must not be left unattended. After a bath, the skin should be patted dry with a soft towel. Skin medication should be conveniently placed so that it may be applied immediately, since pruritus may otherwise recur with intensity. Following a bath, the patient should remain in bed for at least one-half hour to avoid chilling. Soft old sheets should be used on the bed, and sometimes "neutral" linen is necessary. This is prepared by counteracting the excess alkaline of ordinary laundry soap by rinsing the linen in a mild acid solution. A tablespoonful of vinegar to a quart of water may be used in the home.

Compresses and dressings

When applying compresses and dressings, every effort must be made to prevent new infection of skin lesions. Hands must be thoroughly washed before any procedure is begun.

Compresses. Hot compresses are used to increase circulation and to hasten healing. The basin of solution is usually kept hot by placing it on an electric plate at the patient's bedside.

Cold compresses are used to reduce inflammation and to lessen itching. A solution of 3 per cent aluminum acetate (Burow's solution) or 5 per cent magnesium sulfate is often used for cold compresses in the treatment of conditions such as poison ivy dermatitis. Ice may be placed into the bowl of solution; in applying sterile compresses the basin containing solution must be placed in a bowl of crushed ice. If a piece of ice is used, the solution must be changed frequently since it will become diluted.

Equipment for compresses may be placed at the patient's bedside so that he may help with the treatment if he is able and wishes to do this. Compresses may be either sterile or unsterile, depending upon the skin condition. If sterile compresses are used, the patient needs special instruction before participating in his care. Two pairs of forceps are needed with which to wring out the compresses. Compresses are usually discarded after each use.

Dressings. Wet dressings are used to soften crusts, to promote and remove drainage, to combat infection, to allay itching, and to provide constant protection to healing tissue. A few of the many solutions used for wet dressings are potassium permanganate, 1:10,000, hydrogen peroxide and mineral oil in equal parts, acetic acid or vinegar, and physiologic solution of sodium chloride.

Pieces of worn-out linen are best for wet dressings, since they do not stick or hold in heat. If linen is not available, gauze is the best substitute. Cotton becomes soggy and uncomfortable and tends to hold heat and cause itching. Linen or gauze should be used generously, and the compress may be covered with waxed paper or oiled silk. Pliofilm and rubberized fabrics tends to hold in heat and increase itching but are sometimes used, depending upon the nature of the lesion being treated. An outer wrapping may be used, depending upon the purpose of the dressing. Old Ace bandages that have lost their elasticity are satisfactory as outer wrappings.

Wet dressings do not need always to be changed each time they are moistened but they may be moistened with an Asepto syringe carefully directed so that contamination is avoided. Care must be taken to moisten all parts of the inner dressing and yet to prevent fluid from running through outer dressings to other parts of the patient's body or onto the bed. The frequency with which complete change of dressings is necessary depends upon the type of lesion and the amount of drainage. Any skin maceration should be reported to the doctor. Wet dressings may be alternated with either powder dressings or exposure to a heat lamp. Certain solutions necessitate change of the entire dressing since moistening the dressing would increase the concentration of the drug used.

Either dry or moist dressings may be covered with rather bulky dressings made of gauze dipped in heavy boiled starch to provide a firm protection for the healing lesion. Such an outer dressing may be ordered when the physician suspects that the skin lesion may be self-inflicted or that the patient has an active part in preventing its normal healing. This circumstance is most likely to occur in patients with industrially associated skin lesions or in patients with strong attention-seeking motives. The patient needs close observation to be certain that he is not disturbing the skin lesion, and he should be given special consideration since his need for attention is greater than that of the usual patient.

Paste dressings. An *Unna paste boot* may be used in the treatment of stubborn eczematous lesions, stasis dermatitis, and ulcerations of the legs. The paste consists of water, gelatin, glycerin, and zinc oxide. It comes already prepared except for warming and melting. A dry, sterile dressing is placed over open lesions, and the paste is painted on with a 4-inch paint brush; layers of paste are alternated with layers of 3-inch gauze. Newer preparations are available with the gauze bandage already soaked in the paste material; these make the application of the boot much simpler. Since the patient who has a "boot" applied usually has poor circulation, he is kept at rest with the limb elevated for from twenty to thirty minutes before the bandage is applied. Care is taken to have the foot in good alignment. The bandage usually dries in from ten to fifteen minutes, and the patient may put on his stockings and walk about at that time. The "boot" is usually removed and the lesion examined in from two to three weeks, at which time another boot may be applied.

External medications and their application

The list of local applications for skin disease is endless. For detailed descriptions, the student is referred to texts on pharmacology. *Powders* are widely used for their cooling and drying effect and as vehicles for antibacterial or disinfectant drugs; DDT powder is an example. When large areas must be covered, *lotions* or powders suspended in liquids are often used for their cooling, refreshing, and antipruritic effects. One such preparation, calamine lotion, is widely used in the treatment of eczema, hives, and insect bites; it may be used with phenol, 1 per cent, which has an anesthetic effect and allays itching. *Liniments* are prepared with a medication and an oily substance emulsified in water. They facilitate the application of medication to large areas when dressings are not desired. Liniments are widely used by the laity following vigorous exercise for massage and for their counterirritant effect. *Ointments* usually are made with medications added to a base of petrolatum, lanolin, white wax, tallow, or cold cream. Ointments may be protective or antiseptic or have a variety of other uses. They may contain a *keratolytic* agent (salicylic acid) to soften the outer skin layers and enable other drugs to be effective. Some, such as tar ointments, are *antipuritic.* *Pastes* have 50 per cent or more of powder in the ointment base. *Cold cream,* in which water is emulsified into the ointment base, gives a more cooling reaction when in contact with the skin.

Before new medication is applied, any old medication that is on the skin often must be removed. Cleanliness and gentleness are important when this is done. The nurse must know exactly how much medication is necessary for therapeutic effect so that waste is avoided and so that excessive amounts may not be left on the skin to cause caking, stickiness, and discomfort. Lotions and liniments must be shaken well, and those that do not appear to mix thoroughly with shaking should be questioned. Lotions should be applied with gauze, not cotton, because cotton holds the powder solute. A paintbrush may be used with a firm gentle pressure so that "tickling" is avoided. Excessive use of powders on moist surfaces leads to caking and hardening which may cause trauma upon removal. Powders should be carefully handled, since sensitivity to inhaled powders is common. Ointments should be carefully applied in small amounts and removed at prescribed intervals with the solvent ordered. Trauma may be avoided in applying ointment by spreading the ointment or paste on a linen, muslin, or gauze dressing and then applying this to the lesion, with care taken to estimate correctly the size of dressing needed. Many healing ointments, such as scarlet red, and some liniments contain dyes that stain linen, so the oldest bed linen available should be selected for pa-

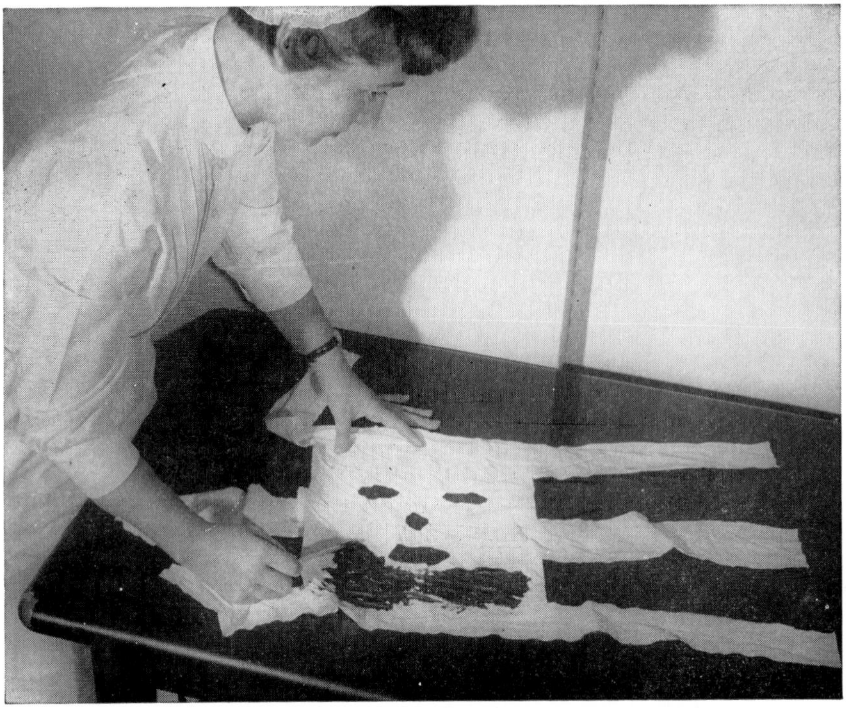

Figure 96

Ointment may be spread on a piece of discarded sheet that is to be used as a mask to cover the face. Note that the ointment is applied to the dressing rather than onto the patient's skin. In actual practice, the table would be protected from soiling.

tients receiving this treatment. (See Figure 96.)

Drugs and other preparations used for skin ailments are often costly. The nurse should know the cost of the preparation used, and if the patient is caring for himself at home, she should direct him to use only enough for therapeutic benefit. In the hospital it is well to have individual jars of ointment for each patient to prevent contamination between patients and to avoid waste of medication kept in large jars. Sometimes it is best to use clean fingers to apply costly ointments.

A large variety of dressings are needed in caring for dermatologic patients. The effectiveness of medications and dressings may depend largely upon the imagination and resourcefulness of the nurse. The nurse in a dermatologic unit often becomes a collector. She collects old linen, table napkins, muslin, binders, stockings, gloves, and the like. These may be cut up to prepare suitable dressings for every conceivable location on the body. The cheaper and older the dressings, the better for everyone concerned since they may become lost in the laundry or so soiled or stained that it seems best to destroy them. A white stocking makes an excellent head dressing when shortened and tied with attached chin straps. Old white cotton gloves or mittens are often better than dressings for lesions on the hands, and stockings with the foot cut off make excellent circular dressings for arms or legs. The stockinette used in the plaster room may be useful for arm and leg dressings.

Pieces of worn-out sheet may be cut into 4- or 6-tailed bandages which are useful to secure dressings under the jaw, on the chin, or on the scalp. (See Figure 97.) Old pillowcases can be used to make a mask to cover the face. The knitted finger dressings used in treating minor surgical wounds are useful in securing dressings on fingers and toes.

Many patients with skin diseases are not hospitalized. In the home and in the clinic the nurse must be specific in her instruction to the patient. It is often well to sit down with him and write out exactly what he must do. A common mistake that patients make when at home is to believe that if some is good, more is better; for example, while a skin ailment may respond to an ointment rubbed on very gently and lightly, trauma from vigorous rubbing may counteract all benefit and may even make the condition worse. The patient, in his eagerness to cure the condition, may not realize how vigorous his own administrations are. The nurse can help the patient to improvise equipment that he needs; she may need to teach him how to apply ointment and how to sterilize linen at home by scorching it with an iron and then folding it inward to avoid contamination.

DISEASE OF THE SKIN

There are many causes of skin disease. Some skin diseases are increasing in frequency as man spends his working day in

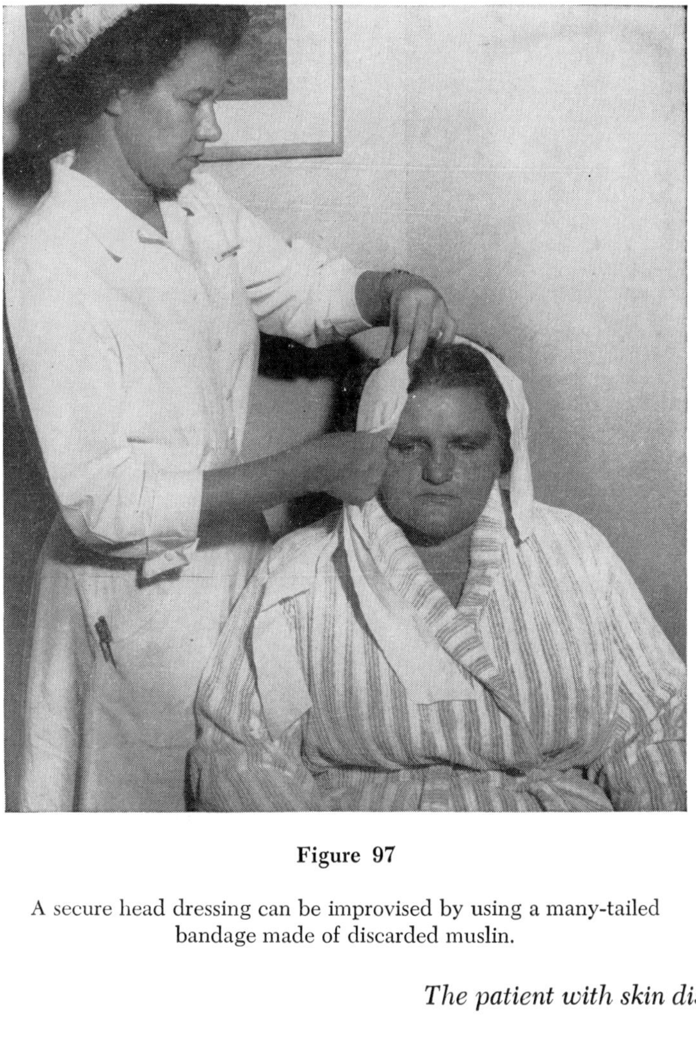

Figure 97

A secure head dressing can be improvised by using a many-tailed bandage made of discarded muslin.

a more complicated environment and surrounds himself with chemical substances unknown to his ancestors. Skin disease may be caused in some individuals by such substances as plastics, solvents, and petroleum products of various kinds both during their production and during their use in the home or in industry. Some of the many causes of skin disease are fungus and parasitic infections, response to bacterial organisms and viruses, reactions to ingestion of toxic substances, sensitivity to substances taken internally or encountered externally, and new growths. Some skin diseases are of unknown cause; others are part of a systemic disease which may or may not be communicable. Only a brief description of a few of the more common skin diseases can be given here, and grouping must be somewhat arbitrary in a book of this kind.

Dermatology is a complex subject with a vocabulary all its own. *Dermatoses* is the term used to designate conditions of the skin which are largely noninflammatory, while *dermatitis* is the term used to designate inflammation of the skin whether due to infection, irritation, or any other cause. Considerable time and effort must be spent in terminology drill if the specialty of dermatology is to have meaning for nurses. The following are some of the more common skin lesions that should be familiar.

macule a circumscribed discolored area, usually small, and not causing skin elevation.

papule a circumscribed area which is elevated, although usually not over 0.5 cm. in diameter.

vesicle a papule that is filled with clear fluid held beneath superficial skin layers.

pustule a circumscribed area containing pus and not usually over 0.5 cm. in diameter.

bulla a large elevation of outer skin layers containing either serous or purulent fluid.

nodule a large elevation of the skin usually involving the deeper skin layers and subcutaneous tissue.

excoriation a break or abrasion in the skin surface.

crust a dry exudate over a lesion.

scar a fibrous tissue covering of a lesion after healing and repair.

ulcer the erosion of skin substance.

scale the outer layer of epithelium as it loosens from the skin surface.

lichenification a leathery thickening of the outer skin layers.

Pruritus is a symptom, not a disease, and the best treatment is to remove its cause. Causes may include systemic disease, such as liver disease with jaundice and diabetes when sugar is not fully metabolized. Pruritus of the vulva, for example, may herald the onset of diabetes since sugar in the urine causes irritation and itching. Emotional stress is a real factor in the cause and control of pruritus, and even persons who have an average amount of emotional reserve will develop localized areas that itch excessively during periods of emotional strain. Pruritus is present in a very large proportion of all dermatoses and in almost all cases of dermatitis.

Insect pests

Several kinds of pediculi attack human beings: *Pediculus humanus* (capitis or head louse and corporis or body louse) and *Phthiris pubis* (pubic louse). Other lice from animals may bite human beings, but they have a short life unless the animal host is nearby. Head and pubic lice attach themselves to the skin and live on the host's blood; their eggs are laid along the shafts of the hair, along with a substance that encircles the hair shaft; the substance is dissolved fairly readily by an alkaline solution or an acid solution such as vinegar. *Pediculus humanus* var. *capitis* is grayish in appearance, 0.15 cm. (1/16 inch) long, and often can be found on the nape of the neck where it is most likely to lay its eggs. Pubic lice are small, 0.15 cm. (1/16 inch) or less in length, brownish, and crab-shaped. They may occasionally be found in the axilla and on the eyebrows, as well as in the pubic region. Body lice, about 0.31 cm. (1/8 inch) in length and dark in color, attach themselves to the underwear of the host, usually along the seams. The eggs, or nits, are yellowish and are laid in clumps along the seams of clothing. They are easily removed after they have been killed.

Pediculi are most often found among individuals who have poor personal hygiene habits. They may however, be easily acquired in city living. Many children get head lice from their classmates or in crowded buses. Pubic lice may be acquired from toilet seats. Pediculi produce much more consternation on the part of the patient or his family than is warranted. They are easily killed. One or more applications of 1 per cent benzene hexachloride in vanishing cream, when massaged thoroughly into the skin usually destroys the pediculi and their eggs. Satisfactory new preparations are appearing; some of these contain DDT. A powder containing 10 per cent DDT dusted on bedclothes and on inner surfaces of underwear is usually sufficient to destroy all body lice and nits. Underwear and bedclothes should be changed and boiled or autoclaved. Outer clothing which cannot be autoclaved or washed should be dry cleaned; pressing the inner lining with a hot iron sometimes suffices for clothing that cannot be washed or cleaned. Sometimes shaking clothing in a pillowcase or laundry bag containing DDT powder is adequate.

Bedbugs are dark brown, oval-shaped insects, about 0.45 cm. (3/16 inch) in length, which have an unpleasant odor. They hide in bed frames and mattresses, usually in poor housing units—but they may also be acquired on crowded city buses. They are destroyed by the same drugs that are effective in destroying pediculi. Mattresses should be autoclaved. If this is not possible, spraying with DDT solution or benzene hexachloride and extended airing in sunlight are usually sufficient.

Scabies caused by the itch mite, *Sarcoptes scabiei,* usually is found in persons who live in unhygienic surroundings and who bathe infrequently. The female burrows under the skin, leaving a dark trail behind her, and it is by this that a diagnosis is often made. The mite prefers the delicate skin areas such as the inner surfaces of the forearm and thighs, under the breasts, and between the fingers. Scabies responds readily to benzyl benzoate and DDT preparations. These drugs have largely replaced the sulfur treatment, which is complicated and time consuming. One application of benzene hexachloride ointment (1 per cent) thoroughly applied from head to foot also usually is effective. The patient may be sensitive to the medications used or may have irritation and infection from damage done by the insect pests. Usually mild antiseptic ointments or lotions such as calamine lotion are prescribed for the irritation. Antibiotics may be given for infection.

An important problem in treating patients with insect infestations is reinfestation. In large crowded families where there may be inadequate facilities for segregation of clothing, every member of the family may be affected and must be treated.

Fungus infections

Fungus infections can be either deep or superficial. The deep fungus infections, *actinomycosis* and *blastomycosis,* are extremely serious conditions and often lead to death. Fortunately they are quite rare. Potassium iodide, arsphenamine, and x-ray therapy are used to treat the infections, and some encouraging results have been obtained with corticosteroids.

Barber's itch (tinea barbae) is an extremely unpleasant superficial fungus infection causing lymph gland enlargement and swollen boggy skin tissue with softening of the hairs of the beard. It is treated with copper undecylenate or ammoniated mercury preparations, and x-ray therapy is used to remove the hairs. Barber's itch is entirely preventable by rigorous attention to cleanliness in barber shops.

Tinea of the scalp (tinea capitis), often incorrectly referred to as ringworm, is a disease of children. The condition often starts as a small reddish papule, although it may begin as a localized area of apparent dandruff with thinning of the hair. Sometimes scaling and pustule formation with matting of the hair and crusting are the first signs. As the roots of the hair become involved, the hairs drop out, leaving bald patches. Since tinea capitis is a disease of children, it is advisable to keep small boys away from barber shops as long as possible, because it is in these establishments that the disease is often spread. The condition is highly infectious among school children so that children with tinea capitis are often kept away from school. It is important to diagnose the condition and begin treatment at once. An important aid to diagnosis and determination of the extent of involvement is the Wood's light, obtained by a special filter from an ultraviolet lamp. The infected hairs fluoresce or appear luminous under the light. The doctor or technician usually works under the light and removes all infected hairs, which are loose and may be removed easily. X-ray therapy may also be used to help remove infected hairs. The area is then treated with a variety of drugs; often a preparation of copper undecylenate is used with success. Clothing should be boiled or destroyed and the scalp protected with a stocking cap during treatment. If the treatment has been adequate, hair will eventually return in the affected area.

Recently, the antifungal drug griseofulvin has been found to be effective in treating tinea capitis when comparatively large amounts are taken orally.[15]

Epidermophytosis. Epidermophytosis (athlete's foot; dermatophytosis) is caused by the *Trichophyton gypseum.* This is a superficial fungus infection which is widely spread through the use of showers, swimming pools, and common bath mats and by direct contact with those who have the infection. It thrives in moist skin areas. Often the first lesion appears as a crack between the fourth and fifth digits of the foot. The disease may spread to the entire foot and cause peeling, cracking, and itching of the skin. The groin, hands, and other parts of the body may become involved. Extensive involvement occurs easily in elderly patients, possibly because of poor circulation in the feet and legs.

The keynote to management of epidermophytosis is prevention. It has been said that the fungus cannot thrive on a dry skin. Therefore, after the daily bath, dusting between the toes with ordinary talcum powder after careful drying helps in prevention. Medicated powders such as those containing zinc undecylenate (Desenex) are considered even more effective. Persons who exercise vigorously, who stand for long periods at work, and whose feet perspire excessively should alternate from day to day with two pairs of shoes, leaving one pair to air and dry for a day between uses. During hot weather, shoes with straw or nylon mesh insets which permit ventilation to the feet are desirable. It is inadvisable ever to walk in public showers with bare feet; even the foot bath placed before the public shower at swimming pools is not sufficient protection. Paper slippers or one's own shoes should be used. Adolescents need instruction in the prevention of epidermophytosis; the habit of sharing bath towels even among the closest of friends should be discouraged.

Many agents have been used in the treatment of epidermophytosis. At the present time propionate-propionic acid and undecylenate-undecylenic acid ointments are widely used and are applied generously at night and removed in the morning. Powder is used during the day. Application of ointment may be preceded by soaks in potassium permanganate, 1:10,000 solution, which is an old and effective method of treatment. Cotton socks or stockings should be worn during treatment and should be changed and washed daily. Every effort is made to keep the feet dry. If it can be arranged, direct exposure to the sun is effective in treatment. Clothing should be boiled and shoes destroyed or treated with formaldehyde fumes; drying and sunning of shoes is not sufficient to kill the fungus. Bath mats and bedclothes should be boiled, and tubs and showers should be scrubbed with 0.1 per cent bichloride of mercury or 0.2 per cent creosol.

Diseases associated with infection

Acne vulgaris. Acne vulgaris is one of the most troublesome and most common skin conditions of adolescence. It is a condition about which the nurse must be informed, since she is often called upon in the home, the school, and the community to advise in the total management of young persons with this difficulty. Acne vulgaris is definitely known to have a relationship to hormonal activity. It usually makes its appearance at puberty, and in girls its activity can be clearly related to gonadal activity during different parts of the menstrual cycle. Hormonal activity produces hyperkeratosis of follicular orifices which leads to blocking of the secretions (sebum) and the formation of discolored fatty plugs or blackheads (comedones). Lack of cleanliness is often blamed for the development of the condition by the patient or his family when in reality cleanliness plays no part in the initial development of the condition. After the blackhead forms, there is hypertrophy of the sebaceous glands, and secondary infection occurs. A microorganism called the acne bacillus may contribute to this, and it is known that staphylococci are present in large numbers in the pustules that form. Sometimes cysts and nodules then form and unsightly scars result despite the best of treatment.

Unfortunately there is no specific treatment for acne vulgaris, although a wide variety of treatments is tried with varying success in individual patients. The face should be washed from three to five times a day with a mild soap, but the vigorous scrubbing so often undertaken by the patient in his effort to cure the condition often only makes it worse. Blackheads may be safely removed by applying hot compresses for fifteen minutes to half an hour and then using an instrument with a hole in a rounded metal tip that is especially made for this purpose. Pustules should never be squeezed or broken by the patient. The patient must be taught to avoid touching his face with his hands, since this may introduce more infection and may grind dirt or infection into open pores; it is often difficult for the patient to carry out this instruction, since he may try to hide his face with his hands and may develop the habit of resting his chin in his hands. Hormones are sometimes given but may cause undesirable systemic effects. The antibiotics are widely used and often produce marked improvement in the secondary infection, but they must be continued over too long a period to be satisfactory. Staphylococcal toxoid also is sometimes used. Often a quartz lamp is ordered for use in the home, and direct exposure to sunshine is thought to be helpful in destroying infection on the skin and improving its general resistance to organisms.

A variety of diets and other hygienic measures are usually advocated with varying success. Most authorities are in agreement that a diet low in carbohydrates, condiments, and fat is advisable and that certain foods, particularly chocolate and nuts, should be avoided. Rest appears to foster improvement in the condition. Regular elimination is stressed, although there is no evidence that autointoxication from faulty elimination has anything to do with the condition.

Probably most important is emotional support to the patient in the acute stages of the condition and assistance in his adjustment to any scarring that may occur. Unfortunately this condition appears at a time in life when the patient is adjusting to becoming an adult, and the disfiguring blemishes sometime precipitate serious emotional reactions. The greatest understanding on the part of all members of the family is necessary. The pancake make-up used by many adolescent girls in an attempt to hide the affliction often makes it worse. Among adolescent boys there is the mistaken belief that masturbation leads to acne. Some people believe that acne is aggravated by sexual abstinence and that it will be cured by marriage. This is not so, although acne is largely a self-limiting disease which tends to disappear at the marriageable age. Persons who have residual scars should known that a procedure known as *derm-*

abrasion or planing often helps tremendously in removing scars. (See Chapter 33.)

Acne rosacea. Acne rosacea, or rosacea, is a condition that usually affects people over 25 years of age. The actual cause is unknown. It begins with redness over the cheeks and nose, and this is followed by papules, pustules, and enlargement of superficial blood vessels. Many persons who have acne rosacea are of unstable emotional make-up. Achlorhydria has been found in many patients with this condition, and some favorable response has been obtained by giving hydrochloric acid. The treatment for acne rosacea is nonspecific and often not too satisfactory. Some patients respond to ultraviolet light treatment, and preparations containing naphthol and sulfur produce striking results in some patients. The condition is often accompanied by some pruritus, and the patient must be cautioned against touching the face since this may introduce infection and aggravate the condition.

Impetigo contagiosa. Impetigo contagiosa is a superficial skin disease produced by a form of streptococci. It is largely a disease of children and may be endemic in nurseries unless special precautions are taken. The disease begins as a blister or vesicle which becomes pustular and dries to form a honey-colored crust. Scarring does not result unless superficial infection or trauma occurs. Greatest care must be taken to isolate the patient and prevent reinfection with fingers and clothing. There is no common agreement as to treatment, but penicillin is now usually ordered either locally as ointment or systemically, or both locally and systemically. Other antibiotics may also be given. Ammoniated mercury ointment and gentian violet are old reliable methods of treatment.

Erysipelas. Erysipelas is caused by the hemolytic streptococcus. Elderly people with poor resistance are most often affected. The disease usually affects the face, and a bright, sharp line separates the diseased skin from the normal skin. Erysipelas was a serious disease before the advent of antibiotic and sulfonamide drugs but responds quickly to penicillin and to the sulfonamides.

Viral diseases

Verrucae. Verrucae (warts) are caused by a filtrable virus which may be transmitted from one person to another. Warts should be removed to prevent crops of them from developing. Electrodesiccation is one of the better methods of treatment and is safer than the use of acids, such as nitric acid, which may injure normal tissue. Warts sometimes disappear spontaneously, and this unexplained characteristic leads to the many tales of their being charmed by a variety of means. Warts may grow inward on the soles of the feet and cause severe pain and incapacity; these are treated by x-ray therapy or are removed surgically.

Herpes simplex. Herpes simplex, or the common cold sore, is caused by a virus thought to be related to the virus of encephalitis. It is probable that canker sores in the mouth and similar lesions about the genitals are of the same origin. The treatment of herpes simplex is not specific or too satisfactory. Strong caustics such as silver nitrate are not usually recommended, but some patients have excellent results from the application of copper sulfate to canker sores in the mouth. Hot compresses sometimes relieve the discomfort from lesions on the lips and on the genitals. Lip lesions sometimes respond to application of spirits of camphor. Sometimes smallpox vaccination is tried when the lesions recur frequently and are very troublesome to the patient.

Herpes zoster. Herpes zoster, or *shingles*, is thought to be due to a virus related in some way to that causing chickenpox. One attack of this aggravating condition usually confers immunity. The involvement is usually on the middle trunk, following the surface branches of the sensory nerves and, therefore, coming from the back forward. Small blisters form, and itching and pain may be severe. Herpes zoster can be a serious condition in any adult and may even lead to death from exhaustion in elderly debilitated individuals. It is one of the most drawn-out and exasperating conditions found in elderly patients and leads to discouragement and demoralization. Treatment consists of keeping the blisters dry and using local applications to allay itching. Calamine lotion with phenol is often prescribed. Alcohol injection of the offending nerves may be tried in an attempt to allay pain and itching, and general systemic medications, including sedatives and analgesics, are often necessary. Even after the blisters have crusted and disappeared, there may be severe pain and itching in the surrounding tissue. In extreme cases death and sloughing of involved tissue occur. Contrary to popular notions, the lesions, following the nerve pathways, never cross the midline of the trunk; whether or not they almost encircle the trunk has nothing to do with whether or not the outcome will be fatal.

Dermatitis due to sensitivity to internal and external toxic agents

Dermatitis is inflammation of the skin that usually goes through the stages of redness or erythema, vesicle or blister formation with oozing, and crusting, scaling, and thickening of the skin. *Eczema* is really the name for a symptom complex designating skin reaction to an irritating factor of endogenous origin and not acquired from the external environment. In the strictest sense of the word eczema most accurately describes the skin lesions of sensitive persons who often have asthma or hay fever. Infantile eczema, for example, often occurs soon after birth and may be outgrown only to be replaced by asthma or hay fever. The tendency to develop these conditions is inherited.

Contact dermatitis identifies the acute skin inflammations and reactions due to contact with irritating factors in the environment. Skin conditions caused by industrial products fall into this group. Primary irritants such as acids affect persons who must have their hands and arms in solutions during the larger part of their working hours, and sensitivity to chemical products such as nylon and plastics plague many workers in the dye and solvent industries. People whose work demands constant wetting of the skin often develop dermatitis. Use of detergents, petroleum products, tars, and resins may cause either direct irritation or sensitivity which may lead to contact dermatitis. Biologic products cause contact dermatitis in some persons, and nurses and doctors have been known to become so sensitive to penicillin and streptomycin that they must wear rubber gloves when handling the drugs; some people have had to abandon working where the drugs are used.

In the home, there are many materials that may lead to the development of contact dermatitis. Nail enamel and various cosmetics and related products such as deodorants and depilatories are examples. Some women develop contact dermatitis from contact with metal such as nickel which may be used in the clips of earrings or in other jewelry. The treatment for contact dermatitis consists of finding and removing the cause. In the home a large number of household cleaning agents, plastic products, and related materials must be considered. Occasionally the person who develops a sensitivity to materials encountered in his daily work must change his mode of employment permanently.

Neurodermatitis (atopic eczema) is due to neurogenic forces in susceptible people. Often allergens of various sorts are present. Pruritus is often severe in atopic eczema, and thickening and hardening (lichenification) of the skin occurs. Tar ointments are often used in an attempt to allay itching. Changes in the emotional life of the patient and in his general environment often are of most help in correcting this troublesome and stubborn condition.

A common form of contact dermatitis is due to contact with the oil of certain plants. *Poison ivy, poison oak,* and *sumac* are the most common offenders. This condition, *dermatitis venenata,* is largely preventable. Everyone should be taught to recognize the shiny leaves of the poisonous plants which are commonly found in his part of the country. Sensitivity to poisonous resins varies with individuals, but almost all people are sensitive to some extent. Some persons are so sensitive that minute particles of the irritating oil carried in smoke or borne in the air after someone has crushed the plant are sufficient to cause a severe skin reaction. Pets may carry the irritating resin to their masters, and it must be remembered that the resin can remain on clothing for several days. Dermatitis venenata can be a serious condition, incapacitating the person for long periods of time. The greatest care must be taken not to irritate new areas by contact with the exudate from active lesions. Symptoms vary from redness, with itching and burning, to blister formation and severe edema followed by secondary infection. Although the condition usually does not last over a week, it may persist in some sensitive individuals for many weeks and even months.

The best treatment for poison ivy dermatitis is prevention by wearing appropriate clothing when in areas where poisonous plants are found. If there has been known contact with the oleoresin, the skin should be thoroughly washed with alkaline laundry soap and then sponged with alcohol; preferably this should be done within ten minutes of exposure. Burow's solution (aluminum acetate) in a 1:20 dilution is often applied as cool compresses for from ten to twenty minutes every few hours, and a lotion such as calamine may be alternated with the compresses. The public should be taught the dangers of self-treatment in cases of extensive exposure to poison ivy, since secondary infections may occur.

Dermatits medicamentosa is the name used to designate reactions of the skin to drugs taken internally. Bromides are frequent offenders, and in recent years a large number of patients have suffered severe, prolonged drug reactions as a result of treatment with penicillin. Iodides, barbiturates, and sulfonamide drugs frequently cause skin eruptions. The skin lesions vary in dermatitis medicamentosa. In some instances they are highly colored and sharply defined, while in others they may resemble urticaria, with large flat wheals almost covering the entire body. The treatment for drug sensitivity consists of finding and discontinuing the offending medication. Pruritus must be relieved and infection prevented. It is important to reassure the patient since he may become panicky when a generalized eruption is superimposed on the illness for which the drug was given. The skin lesions sometimes disappear as suddenly as they appeared.

Exfoliative dermatitis is usually caused by drugs containing heavy metals such as mercury, bismuth, or arsenic. The condition is seldom seen since the antibiotics and the bacteriostatic drugs have largely replaced drugs containing the heavy metals. There are general redness, edema, and massive desquamation during which the patient may, for instance, lose the entire outer layer of skin from the soles of his feet and the palms of his hands. Colloidal baths are often used to allay the itching. Lotions may be used to reduce itching and to make the erythema and desquamation less conspicuous. Patients with exfoliative dermatitis also need constant reassurance.

Urticaria, or *hives,* is a disease of the skin characterized by wheals which may vary in size and appearance. The condition can be acute or chronic; when the lesions are very large and are accompanied by generalized edema, the term *angioneurotic edema* is used. Urticaria is generally conceded to be caused by the body's reaction to some foreign substance to which it is sensitive. In some instances the cause is easily determined; many people, for example, develop hives immediately after the ingestion of certain foods such as eggs, strawberries, and shellfish. In other cases the cause of hives is obscure. Urticaria may disappear spontaneously after a few minutes or may persist for hours. Usually there are severe itching, redness, and local heat. Calamine lotion is used for local relief of the pruritus, and the antihistaminic drugs are often given. Occasionally Adrenalin is used. The only real danger from this condition is the possible occurrence of giant hives in a vital area, such as on the mucous membrane of the larynx or glottis. Patients who have repeated attacks of hives are advised to take (and are taught to give themselves) an injection of Adrenalin when the hives appear or at the first sign of respiratory difficulty.

Other toxic skin reactions

Erythema multiforme may be of unknown cause or may be one of the body's responses to disease elsewhere in the body. Round, reddened, and slightly raised lesions appear along the shins and sometimes on the arms and thighs. The skin condition, which is painful, may be accompanied by headache, elevation of temperature, and joint pains. The treatment is primarily detection and treatment of the original pathology. Local treatment includes baths, soaks, and dressings. Fluids are forced, and the patient is encouraged to take a high-calorie diet. Lesions may appear in the mouth; if so, special care is needed, including frequent mouth irrigations with hot salt solution or alkaline solutions such as Dobell's solution.

The skin may respond to the toxicity produced by common communicable diseases. Examples are measles, chickenpox, and smallpox (the virus diseases); scarlet fever due to streptococci; the rose spots accompanying typhoid fever; and the several skin lesions (nodes and hemorrhagic spots) accompanying severe acute rheumatic fever.

Dermatoses of unknown cause

Psoriasis. Psoriasis is a very common benign skin disease of unknown origin. It causes a dry, scaly eruption on any part of the body but occurs most often on the elbows, back, shins, scalp, and chest. For some unknown reason psoriasis is often found in persons suffering from atrophic arthritis. The lesions have a shiny metallic (fish scale) appearance. A variety of medications is used in local treatment, but tar ointment is perhaps the most satisfactory in the majority of cases. Lesions may fade with local treatment, only to recur eventually in the same area or elsewhere. The patient should know that the condition is not transmitted to friends and relatives, that it is benign, and that while it probably will not get worse, it probably will never be cured. If the patient does not know these things, he may lose confidence in his physician and may seek a quick cure. Because psoriasis is so common (it comprises about 5 per cent of all skin disease) and so stubborn in response to treatment, manufacturers of patent remedies find a lucrative field for their products among those who have the disease. Anyone who reads the daily papers regularly has seen numerous promises of cure. The patient should be warned lest he take these advertisements seriously and waste his money.

Pemphigus. Pemphigus is a skin condition characterized by enormous pustules called *bullae* which appear all over the body and on the mucous membranes. The lesions break and are followed by crusts which heal and leave scars. The cause of pemphigus is unknown. The condition may appear to clear up, and there may be remissions lasting for months and even years, but invariably it returns and is finally fatal. Cortisone and ACTH (adrenocorticotrophic hormone) cause marked improvement in symptoms and prolong remissions. Lesions eventually appear in such large numbers that a large part of the skin surface is raw and oozing and becomes infected. The condition may appear similar to that following extensive burns, and the nursing care is equally difficult. Special mouth care, including frequent gargles with normal saline solution or alkaline mouthwashes, may be necessary if the lesions appear in the mouth. Sterile gown and mask may be worn in an attempt to prevent secondary infection. Bradford frames or Stryker frames may be used in an effort to move the patient as painlessly as possible and prevent weight-bearing on raw surfaces. Dakin's solution compresses may be used since these help to control odors. Fortunately pemphigus is a relatively rare disease, for it taxes the resources of the patient's family and medical personnel to the utmost. Emotional support and encouragement are extremely important. Members of the family should be prepared for their visits to the patient and should be encouraged to visit often and to behave as normally as they possibly can. The patient may fear that he is so repulsive that no one will take care of him. He needs constant reassurance that the nursing staff is interested in him as long as he is conscious and able to benefit from this reassurance.

Mycosis fungoides. Mycosis fungoides is one of the most dreaded of all skin diseases. It begins as an itching, thickened lesion in the skin. This progresses to a tumor stage, which finally breaks down and destroys the skin. A large, soft, mushy vegetative lesion develops which destroys all the normal adjacent structures. Lesions may break out in several parts of the body. While the patient lives, all resemblance to his normal self is lost, and the disease is invariably fatal. X-ray therapy is sometimes used to allay itching in the early stages, and nitrogen mustard is sometimes given intravenously. Cortisone delays the process somewhat but does not affect the final outcome. In the late stages, the nursing care for mycosis fungoides is similar to that required for pemphigus.

Collagen diseases

The collagen or connective tissue diseases are a group of not too well known and not too well understood clinical entities in which there is derangement of collagen substance. Collagen and elastic substances are the fibrous constituents of connective tissue and connective tissue makes up the extracellular framework around which cells develop and organs and other essential structures are formed and carry out their function. The collagen substance may respond to unknown causative factors with inflammation and degeneration. Its extremely wide distribution in the body makes it obvious that disease involvement is widespread also. There are several collagen diseases including polyarteritis, scleredema, and dermatomyositis. Only two, systemic lupus erythematosus and progressive systemic sclerosis (scleroderma), which have quite definite skin manifestations will be discussed here.

Systemic lupus erythematosus. Systemic lupus erythematosus is a serious disease involving the collagen substance of connective tissue in the skin, blood vessels, and serous and synovial membranes. It is now known to be fairly common and young women are most often affected. Since the use of a new test—the L.E. cell phenomenon[3]—it has been learned that less than half of all patients with this disease have skin lesions. *Discoid* and *acute* and *subacute disseminated lupus erythematosus* are terms referring to the skin lesions.

The cause of systemic lupus erythematosus is unknown. It may be acute or chronic and usually runs a long course with exacerbations and remissions. There may be cardiac, lymphatic, neurologic, pulmonary, hematologic, hepatic, and gastrointestinal involvement. No specific treatment is available. Adrenocortical steroid therapy is used to control active manifestations. With this treatment and supportive treatment of systems involved, many patients live for years. Bed rest and salicylates are used and antimalarial treatment with chloroquine is sometimes surprisingly helpful.

A common skin manifestation of systemic lupus erythematosus is an erythema usually in a butterfly pattern over the cheeks and bridge of the nose. The margins of the lesions are usually bright red and the lesions may extend beyond the hair line with partial alopecia (loss of hair) above the ears. Lesions also occur on the exposed part of the neck. Rest in a darkened room during the acute stages and permanent avoidance of sunshine are usually prescribed. Chronic discoid lesions are also fairly common and these may undergo vascularization, degeneration, and subsequent atrophy.

Progressive systemic sclerosis (scleroderma). Skin manifestations of scleroderma are only part of a generalized systemic disease involving the collagen substance throughout the body. The cause of this relatively rare condition is unknown. Middle aged persons are most often affected, and women are affected more frequently than men. Essential organs such as the heart, kidneys, and liver may be affected and may suffer fatal impairment. Chest expansion may be impaired by firming of the skin so that respiratory failure threatens.

The name *scleroderma* means "hard skin" and describes the skin manifestations accurately. Usually local areas such as the face and fingers are first affected and sometimes the condition is confused with rheumatoid arthritis and with Raynaud's disease in the early stages. Usually there is pain on joint motion but no joint involvement. The skin may first appear slightly edematous, then turns pale and becomes steadily more firm and finally fixed to underlying tissues and mildly pigmented. The face becomes masklike and chewing may be impossible; finally all body motion becomes so restricted that the patient has the appearance of a living mummy.

There is no cure and no specific treatment for scleroderma and the outcome is fatal within a period of months or years. Death usually is caused by failure of involved organs or systems such as the liver or the circulatory system. Intensive treatment with cortisone in the early stages has proved helpful in some cases. Salicylates and mild analgesics are used for joint pain and physical therapy is ordered to slow the development of contractures and deformity. In advanced stages of the disease, meticulous nursing care is imperative; this includes mouth care, care in eating, skin care and prevention of decubiti, and attention to the emotional problems of the patient who is becoming more helpless daily.

Degenerative skin diseases

Corns. Corns are thickened skin lesions that have a center core that thickens inwardly and causes acute pain upon pressure. They are often caused by the pressure of ill-fitting shoes. They are best treated by correction of shoes and by the use of small felt pads with a hole in the center placed over the corn to relieve pressure on the center. Popular corn remedies seldom produce a cure, since their active ingredient is usually salicylic acid, which is keratolytic and only dissolves the outer layer of skin. As soon as the medicated pad is removed, a new layer of skin will form unless pressure is relieved. Soft corns occur between the toes where the skin is moist and are extremely painful and difficult to treat; sometimes x-ray treatment is required to effect a cure.

Calluses. Calluses often appear on the plantar surface of the foot when the metatarsal arch has fallen and there is constant pressure against the sole of the shoe. They are often successfully treated by relief of the pressure and by regular massage with softening lotions and creams. They must be distinguished from *plantar warts*, caused by a virus, that have a central core growing inward and that may require irradiation or electrosurgery under anesthesia for satisfactory removal.

Stasis dermatitis. Stasis dermatitis is a common condition in older persons who have poor circulation. It is usually preceded by varicosities and poor circulation. Irritation in the tissues is produced by substances normally carried away by the circulation. The skin is often reddened over some generalized edema, and pruritus may be quite severe. Breaks in the skin are often caused by scratching, and infection is introduced by the hands, clothing, and other sources. The most important treatment for stasis dermatitis is prevention by careful attention to circulation during middle life and special measures at the first sign of limitation of normal circulation. Unna paste boots are often ordered for this condition. Other nursing procedures are discussed with vascular disorders in Chapter 19.

Seborrheic keratoses. Seborrheic keratoses occur most often in persons past middle age. The lesions resemble large, darkened, greasy warts and are often found around the trunk, on the back, and under the breasts. They seldom become malignant but should be observed at intervals for any change. They often can be easily removed with dichloracetic acid or carbon dioxide snow.

Angiomas. Angiomas are tufts of blood vessels that may occur spontaneously either as tiny bright red lesions or as deeper purplish vascular lesions. The lesions should be closely watched, for although they do not usually become malignant, they may suddenly develop extensive vascular channels which may be difficult or impossible to remove surgically.

Malignant and premalignant lesions

Malignancies of the skin are more accessible to treatment than are those in any other part of the body. Education of the patient in reporting suspicious lesions and prompt action by nurses and doctors when such lesions are reported should make malignancies of the skin an entirely controllable disease.

Leukoplakia occurs as raised, flat, shiny areas of various sizes on the mucous membrane of the mouth and also of the genitals in women. About 25 per cent of the lesions become cancerous if not removed. Surgical removal is the treatment of choice; however, if the lesions are too extensive to be removed by surgery, radiotherapy or electrodesiccation may be used. In the early stages leukoplakia of oral mucosa may be controlled by careful mouth hygiene. The patient who smokes should stop smoking at once and should never smoke again, because smoking is definitely known to aggravate the condition. Any loose or jagged teeth are removed, periodontal treatment is given if necessary, and frequent mouth irrigations with an alkaline solution are advised.

Senile keratoses usually begin as scaly excrescences in exposed parts of the body. The lesion is firm to pressure, and there is usually an elevated surface or border that bleeds easily. Senile keratoses require prompt surgical treatment, because they undergo malignant degeneration and metastasize quickly in many instances.

Pigmented moles are often precancerous. These skin lesions may be present at birth or may appear at any time of life. The darker the lesion, the more dangerous it seems to be; the blue or greenish-black type (melanotic nevus) is the most dangerous of all. Yellow and brownish moles are less likely to become malignant. Blue or black moles should be removed even if they are not raised above the normal skin surface. Any mole that shows signs of growth or that is in a part of the body where it is traumatized by clothing should be removed at once.

Squamous cell carcinomas occur in areas of irritation, such as on the bridge of the nose in those who wear glasses or on the lip of those who smoke pipes. If they are not diagnosed and treated early, squamous cell carcinomas metastasize very rapidly.

Sarcoma and *fibrosarcoma* are lesions that may develop quite suddenly from seemingly innocuous nodules somewhere in the skin. Unfortunately metastasis often occurs before the original node shows much change. For this reason any nodule in the skin should be reported to a competent physician at once.

REFERENCES AND SELECTED READINGS*

1 *Bozian, Marguerite Wilkinson: Nursing Care of Patients Having Dermatologic Conditions, Am. J. Nursing **52**:873-875, July 1952.

2 Cecil, Russell L. (editor): The Specialties in General Practice, Philadelphia, 1951, W. B. Saunders Co.

3 Cecil, Russell L., and Loeb, Robert F. (editors): A Textbook of Medicine, ed. 10, Philadelphia, 1959, W. B. Saunders Co.

4 *Cormia, Frank E.: Acne Vulgaris, Am. J. Nursing **57**:198-201, Feb. 1957.

5 *Goldman, Leon: Itching—Causes and Relief, Am. J. Nursing **53**:1203-1204, Oct. 1953.

---

*References preceded by an asterisk indicate material particularly well suited for student reading.

6 Harmer, Bertha, and Henderson, Virginia (revised by): Textbook of the Principles and Practice of Nursing, ed. 5, New York, 1955, The Macmillan Co.
7 Hollander, Lester: Care of the Skin in Older People, Am. J. Nursing **47**:219-222, April 1947.
8 Iverson, Preston C., and Staneruck, Isabella D.: Dermal Abrasion, Surgical Care and Nursing Care After Dermal Abrasion, Am. J. Nursing **57**:860-864, July 1957.
9 Jeghers, Harold: Herpes Zoster, Am. J. Nursing **54**:1217-1219, Oct. 1954.
10 Klauder, Joseph V.: Some Aspects of Occupational Dermatoses, J.A.M.A. **160**:442-448, Feb. 11, 1956.
11 Lea, Walker A., and Hackett, Angela M.: Rouges and Rashes, Am. J. Nursing **58**:84-86, Jan. 1958.
12 Morris, George E.: Prevention and Treatment of Dermatitis in Industry, Nursing Outlook **2**:582-584, Nov. 1954.
13 Noojin, Ray O.: Common Scalp Conditions, Am. J. Nursing **56**:870-872, July 1956.
14 Ormsby, Oliver S., and Montgomery, Hamilton: Diseases of the Skin, ed. 8, Philadelphia, 1954, Lea & Febiger.
15 Osment, Lamar S.: Tinea Capitis, Am. J. Nursing **60**:1264-1266, Sept. 1960.
16 Piper, William N.: Poison Ivy, Poison Oak and Poison Sumac, Am. J. Nursing **54**:814-816, July 1954.
17 *Torrey, Frances: Care of the Normal Skin, Am. J. Nursing **53**:460-463, April 1953.

The patient with burns

Chapter 30

Study questions for review

1 What are some of the precautionary measures you have already learned that must be observed when applying heat to the skin?
2 From your knowledge of anatomy and physiology, list the harmful effects of loss of a large area of skin.
3 From your notes in fundamentals of nursing review the principles and techniques of surgical asepsis.
4 Name some ways of helping a patient increase fluid intake. What kinds of food are high in protein? What are some ways in which high-protein foods may be given to the critically ill patient?

Burns are wounds caused by excessive exposure of the body to heat, radiation, x-rays, electricity, and certain chemicals such as strong acids. Heat in various forms such as flame, air, water, and steam is the most common cause, and this chapter is devoted mainly to the nursing care of patients who have been burned by these agents. Burns are classified as first second, and third degree, depending upon their depth. A *first-degree burn* is one in which the outer layer of skin is injured and reddened without blister formation; mild sunburn is a good example. A *second-degree burn* is one in which a blister, or bleb, forms beneath the upper layer of skin in which deeper layers are not destroyed; thus regeneration of epithelium can occur. First-degree and second-degree burns are likely to be painful because nerve endings have been injured and exposed. A third-degree burn is one in which all layers of skin are destroyed, thus making regeneration impossible. Such burned areas eventually must be covered either by scar tissue or by skin taken from elsewhere on the body. Nerves, muscles, and bone may also be injured and are sometimes destroyed in third-degree burns.

Approximately 6,700 persons died of burns in the United States in 1958.[1] Many of these deaths could have been prevented. Nurses have a positive part to play in the prevention of accidental burns, particularly by participating in general health education and by promoting legislation to control some of man's thoughtless practices and to make his working and living environments as safe as possible. Public health nurses are in an unusually advantageous position to recognize unsafe practices in the home and to help families develop safer habits of living.

Excessive sunburn should be cautioned against, as even a relatively mild first-degree burn of a large part of the body can cause change of fluid distribution and kidney damage. Camp nurses should keep this in mind in their educational programs for children and camp counselors. (For further discussion of sunburn see Chapter 15.)

The occurrence of accidental burns in and about the home is common. Kerosene, used to light stoves indoors and wood fires outdoors, causes many burns by igniting clothing. Explosions resulting from defective gas stoves and heaters also lead to many deaths each year. Serious burns to children often result from permitting pot handles to project beyond the stove top and from allowing children to have access to matches. Smoking in bed and falling asleep in an upholstered chair with a lighted cigarette are two of the most easily preventable, yet most common causes, of fatal burns in the home.

A large number of children have been burned to death or maimed for life by firecrackers. Legislation in many states now prohibits the sale of firecrackers, but violations of the law and accidents still occur. Because aged persons are frequently housed in old and poorly equipped structures, many of them have been burned to death. Each year brings increased demand for careful inspection and regulation of places in which the ill and infirm are housed. Attention is being focused on places in which large numbers of people congregate; laws now require that doors in public buildings be hinged to swing outward, that draperies and decorations in night clubs be fireproof, and that stairways with special fire doors be used in new apartment buildings and hotels. These laws have been the outcome of serious fires in which many persons lost their lives. Rigid enforcement of laws requiring that industrial products be labeled when known to be flammable and that new products be carefully tested for their flammable qualities before being placed on the market is further evidence of governmental effort to protect the public from accident by fire.

EMERGENCY CARE

The nurse may be called upon to assist with injuries at the scene of a fire. If flame is involved and the victim's clothing is on fire, his first panic reaction is to run, which only fans the flame. Rolling the burning person in a blanket on the ground to exclude oxygen, thereby putting out the fire, is one of the best things to do.

As soon as the fire is out, several things should be done at once. The patient should be kept quiet and lying down, and, if the burn is at all severe or extensive, immediate plans must be made to send him to a hospital. Loss of natural body heat may be prevented in part by covering the victim with blankets, coats, or whatever is available; external heat should not be applied, since this may cause dilation of blood vessels and further loss of body heat. If clothing adheres to the burned surface, it should not be removed. Exposed burned surfaces should be covered with sterile dressings or with the cleanest material available. If the burn has occurred in the home, pieces of sheeting can be ironed and used as sterile dressings for large areas; these can be dipped in boiled water and sodium bicarbonate (baking soda), using 1 tablespoonful of sodium bicarbonate for each quart of water. Outer covering must then be applied lest this dressing cause chilling, particularly if large burned areas are so treated. Oils and salves relieve pain and are harmless in a first-degree burn; however, since it is difficult to determine the depth of the burn, it is better not to use them; they make initial cleansing and débridement much more difficult in second-degree and third-degree burns. Burns occurring about the eyes should be lavaged with copious amounts of cold, clean water, and if the burn was caused by acids, the procedure should be repeated in from ten to fifteen minutes. A few drops of any mild oil such as mineral oil, castor oil, or olive oil should then be put into the eyes and the help of a doctor sought at once.

No layman and no nurse should attempt to estimate the degree and severity of a burn; all patients with burns other than the most trivial should be seen by a doctor. As a general rule it is safe to assume that the burn is more severe than it first appears. Occasionally, deep third-degree burns are almost painless, since nerve endings have been destroyed, and for the first few minutes the patient may appear not too badly affected. Usually, however, some part of the body has sustained first-degree and second-degree burns which cause immediate pain. If the burn appears fairly extensive, it is best to get the patient to a hospital immediately; if possible, the hospital should be notified that he is on the way so that preparations can be made for his arrival. During this period, warm fluids can be given by mouth if the patient can tolerate them. Pain is best controlled by gentle and minimal handling and by the exclusion of air from the burned skin surfaces.

MEDICAL TREATMENT AND NURSING CARE

Early supportive care

The severely burned patient presents one of the most taxing assignments that doctors and nurses can encounter. However, the lives of many persons who are badly burned are now being saved, since in recent years more has been understood about what takes place within the body when a severe burn is sustained.

Fluid and electrolyte balance. Most of the emergency treatment of patients with severe burns in the first twenty-four to forty-eight hours centers about the fluid and electrolyte balance, since sudden and very serious changes occur in the fluid distribution in the body. When the capillary beds are traumatized by a burn, interstitial fluid and blood plasma rush to the injured area. This causes the local edema and weeping of the burned area. The fluid outside the cells (extracellular) constitutes about 20 per cent of the entire body weight. Three fourths of this surrounds the tissues and one fourth is in the plasma of the blood stream. (See Chapter 6.) As much as one half of this 20 per cent can suddenly shift from its normal distribution to the site of severe burns. For a person weighing 67.2 kilograms (150 pounds), this means that from 10 to 15 pounds, or from 5,000 to 7,500 ml., of fluid are removed from the interstitial spaces and the blood stream. The result is a tremendous drop in blood pressure, shock, inadequate blood flow through the kidneys, which in turn leads to further shock and anuria, and death within a short time if treatment is inadequate.

The doctor estimates the amount of burned body surface and determines the quantity of plasma and other fluids which will be needed. The "rule of nine" is usually used in making such estimates. Each arm is considered as 9 per cent of the total skin surface; each leg and thigh, 18 per cent; the front and back of the trunk, each 18 per cent; the head, 9 per cent; and the throat, 1 per cent. (See Figure 98.) For a patient with a burn of over one fourth of the body surface, the necessary fluid replacement may be as much as 6,000 ml. of plasma, 3,000 ml. of 5 per cent glucose in distilled water, 3,000 ml. of 5 per cent glucose in saline solution and 500 ml. of whole blood in the first forty-eight hours.[11] Authorities differ somewhat concerning the total amount of fluids needed, but all agree that the largest portion (approximately one half) of the forty-eight hour requirement should be given during the first twelve hours. If vomiting occurs, as it often does following severe burns, fluids containing other electrolytes in addition to sodium and chloride are given intravenously in an attempt to replace those lost in the vomitus. Ringer's solution, Hartmann's solution, and Tyrode's solution are examples of fluids that may be requested.

Approximately one half of the estimated fluids are usually given during the first twelve hours, one fourth during the second twelve hours, and one fourth during the second twenty-four hours. Ideally, intravenous treatment should be started within an hour following a severe burn, which explains why it is necessary that the hospital be notified that the patient is to be admitted and that the nurse have equipment and solutions ready for immediate use.

Because no estimate of the severity of a burn can be really accurate, it is important that the nurse observe the general condition of the patient and report any changes promptly. Persistent vomiting must be noted and the amount recorded, since this loss must be considered in estimating the total amount of fluid needed. If a sphygmomanometer can be applied, blood pressure should be taken as often as every fifteen minutes. Rate and volume of the pulse should be carefully noted. Skin color and level of consciousness are often important in determining whether or not progress is favorable. The patient who has been burned by hot air or steam must be closely watched for signs of respiratory complications; difficulty in breathing, coughing, and cyanosis are signs that the trachea and the lungs may have been burned. These signs must be

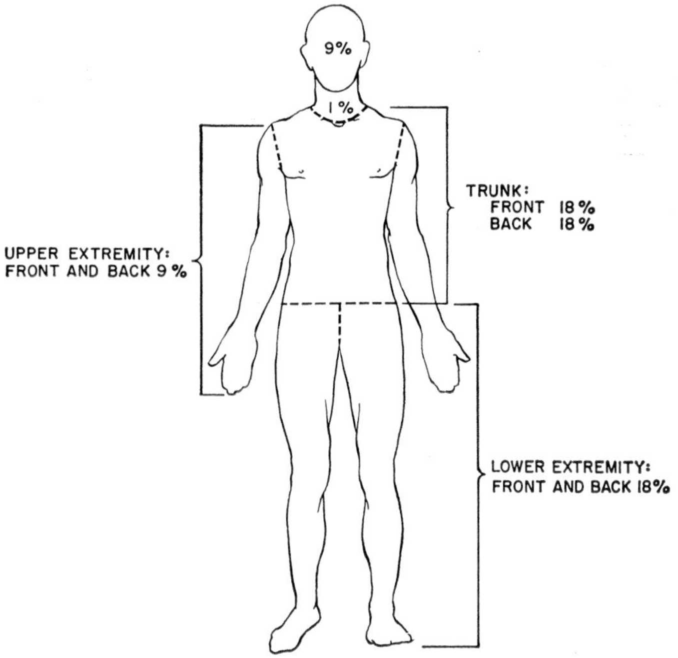

Figure 98

The "rule of nine" is used to estimate the amount of skin surface burned.

reported immediately. Depending upon the severity of the symptoms, emergency treatment may include oxygen, suctioning, and postural drainage. Tracheostomy may be necessary if severe edema of the throat develops.

Prevention of infection. While the nurse must give primary attention to assisting the doctor to re-establish a safe fluid balance for the patient, she also has other responsibilities. Many times the patient's clothing must be cut off in order to estimate the amount of burned body surface and to prepare for local treatment. Every effort is made to prevent introduction of infection to the burned area. All who attend the patient wear masks, and no one who has an upper respiratory infection is permitted near him. Good aseptic surgical technique is used in the emergency room; sometimes the patient is transferred to the operating room where even better surgical technique can be carried out and where a general anesthetic may be more easily given if this is necessary. The extent of local cleansing depends upon the severity of the burn and the judgment of the doctor; sometimes soap and detergents are used, and a rather extensive débridement may be carried out at the initial cleansing. The wounds are then treated by either the open or the closed method which will be described later in this chapter. Room temperature is carefully checked and should be kept at about 24° C. (76° F.) when the patient is exposed; patients lose more heat from burned surfaces than from the normal skin surface, since there is no vascular bed to contract and retain heat in the body.

Pain. Morphine may be ordered for pain. Subcutaneous injections are often poorly absorbed in severely burned patients because of the alterations in fluid distribution in the tissues and the low blood pressure; the intravenous route of administration must sometimes be used. Usually one of the antibiotics is given at once; if possible, the oral route is used in preference to subcutaneous injection. Large doses of analgesics and sedatives are avoided because of the danger of respiratory depression and because they may mask other symptoms.

Kidney function. Kidney function is one of the surest gauges of the patient's progress, and hourly checking and measuring of urinary output for several days is one of the most important responsibilities of the nurse. Usually a retention catheter (Foley catheter) is inserted and drained into a calibrated bottle. The nurse must be sure that the tubing is not kinked or otherwise hampered in providing constant drainage. The record of output is kept either by noting the amount in a calibrated bottle or by emptying the bottle and accurately measuring the amount. If the output drops below 20 ml. per hour, the doctor should be notified; an output of 15 ml. or less per hour for three or more consecutive hours indicates that insufficient fluid is being given or that kidney function has failed.[8] A urine flow of 30 to 50 ml. per hour is considered optimal.[8] Hematuria may also occur, indicating severe kidney damage. Usually by the fourth to sixth day sudden marked diuresis occurs; the exact cause of this is undetermined. Body fluid that has rushed to the burned area is as quickly redistributed, and if intravenous fluid is not drastically reduced, overloading of the circulatory system and pulmonary edema may occur. Therefore, the doctor must be notified at once if the output rises to 75 ml. or more per hour.[8]

Local treatment and general care

Pressure dressings. The closed method of pressure dressings came into wide use during World War II. Theoretically, by initial cleansing and the application of petroleum jelly gauze and massive pressure dressings, which are often held in place with elastic bandages, some fluid is held in the tissues and infection is reduced. The patient is able to move about more freely, and some patients with quite severe burns, particularly of the extremities, are mobilized within a few days and may be able to feed and partially care for themselves. Mobilization improves circulation and speeds healing, helps to prevent deformity, and contributes to the patient's morale. Treatment by use of pressure dressings seems to lend itself better to burns of the extremities and to small areas than to extensive burns of the trunk. Dressings are changed every four to ten days. This treatment is continued up to the time when skin grafting is done, which may sometimes be as early as one week after the initial burn. When large areas are involved, the patient may be taken to the operating room and a general anesthetic given while a change of dressings is carried out. Treatment of burns with pressure dressings is very time consuming and the materials are expensive. It has been pointed out that, in the event of major disaster such as atomic attack, it would be impossible to procure sufficient dressings despite stockpiling of equipment for initial dressings.

When assisting with the application of pressure dressings, the nurse should help to see that the affected part is placed in such a position that a deformity, such as foot drop, will not occur. If dressings are changed frequently, position is somewhat altered from time to time. If the nurse is responsible for the dressings, she must be sure that no two skin surfaces are left in contact; petroleum jelly gauze can be placed between toes and fingers, between the ears and scalp, and between genital folds. After the dressing is applied, the nurse watches for signs of impaired circulation such as numbness, pain, and tingling. Signs of infection, such as odor on the dressings and increased pulse rate and temperature, are reported to the doctor. Odors may be caused from sloughing tissue even when no active infection is present. Deodorizers in the room often are helpful for this.

Open method of treatment. The open method of treatment of burns seems to be

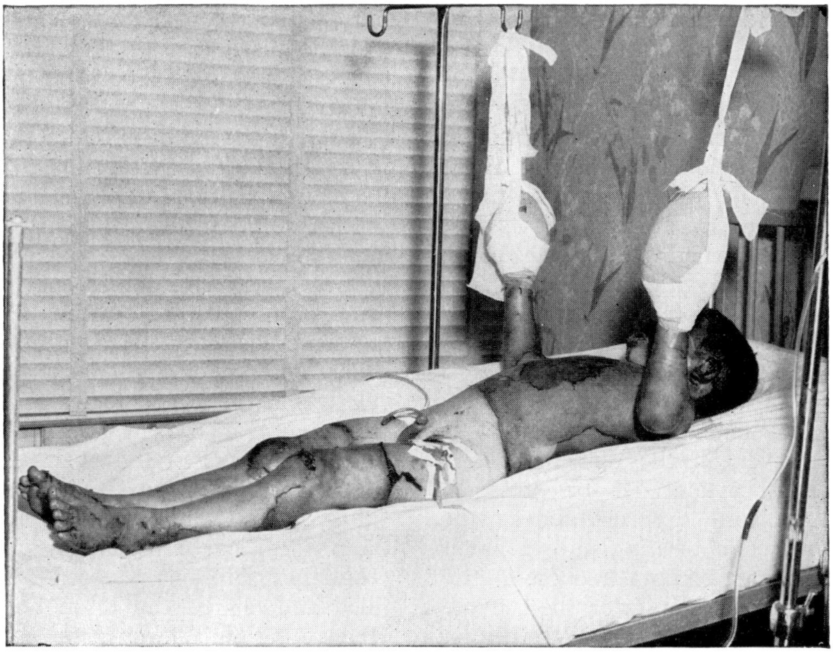

Figure 99

The open method of treating burns is now widely used.
(From Baker, T. J., and Peterson, J. E.: An Apparently Proteolytic Fungus Isolated From a Burn Patient, Plast. & Reconstruct. Surg. **24**:209-213, Aug. 1959.)

gaining in popularity at the present time. This is a modification of the method of treatment used about twenty years ago when local applications of drugs were used to produce a crust or eschar. Eschar treatment has been discarded, since it is believed that infection may develop beneath the eschar and that this may contribute to toxicity. In the present method, no drugs are applied locally; the area is cleansed and left exposed to the air. The serous exudate dries to form a crust which appears to be conducive to good healing and to the control of infection. (See Figure 99.) The open method of treatment was accidentally discovered to be effective in 1888 when, during a serious steamboat fire on the Mississippi, those in attendance ran out of bandages and later observed that the neglected persons fared better than those who received more intensive local treatment.[5]

Since the patient's resistance is usually lowered and cracks occur in the crusts, effort is made to protect him from exposure to infection. He should be placed in a ward or room where only "clean" surgical cases are cared for. He is usually placed on sterile linen. Sterile cornstarch can be sprinkled on the bed to help prevent sticking caused by drainage from cracks in the crust as he moves about. In summer months, screen doors should be used to keep out flies which may introduce direct infection or lay eggs in the open wounds. A cradle with lights or a gooseneck lamp may be used for warmth, since no clothing or top bedclothes are allowed directly over a burned area. If the burn is extensive, it is often satisfactory to place the patient on a "burn bed," which is prepared by draping a Balkan frame with sheets to make a tent. This may then be equipped with a chain of small electric bulbs to provide warmth. A thermometer should be hung within the canopy, and a small section of the canopy should be left open to prevent humidity from rising and softening the crust; the temperature in the tent should be maintained at about 24.4° C. (76° F.). If there are no burns about the face, sometimes patients rest and sleep better when wearing sunglasses, while others find that cloth eyeshades are helpful in keeping light from their eyes.

There are many advantages in using a "burn bed." Adequate covering of the patient is often difficult if a gown cannot be worn. However, in the tent the extensively burned patient can be protected from embarrassing exposure and can be kept warm while wearing only a halter and loin cloth. Maximum freedom is provided for him to get on or off the bedpan, move about, and perform exercises for the prevention of contracture and the improvement of circulation. Many patients prefer to turn themselves, and, if dressings are used to cover small areas, they may wish to help remove the dressings; they should be permitted to help themselves since this is often less painful and more acceptable to them. The nurse caring for the patient should wear a sterile gown and mask. In most hospitals it is fairly simple to make up a "burn pack" to be autoclaved. This pack can include sheets for the canopy and bed, loin cloth and halter, bath blankets, pillowcases, towels, washcloths, and bedpan covers, as well as gowns and masks for those in attendance.

Stryker frames and Foster beds are used in the care of some severely burned patients, since they facilitate the use of the bedpan and permit larger skin surfaces to remain free from body pressure than is possible when the patient lies in bed. These are particularly useful when both back and front of the trunk, thighs, and legs have been burned. They allow turning of the patient with a minimum of handling and thus help to decrease pain. A regular schedule for turning the patient must be set up to prevent thrombophlebitis, emboli, contractures, and decubiti. (For details of use of these frames, see Chapter 34 and textbooks on orthopedic nursing.)

Diet. If they can be tolerated without nausea, food and fluids should be given by mouth. Salty solutions such as meat broths are often given to replace sodium chloride lost in the oozing from the burned surfaces. Effervescent beverages are also an acceptable means of supplying some necessary electrolytes as well as sugar. Sodium citrate (packaged in envelopes) to be added to water has been stockpiled for use in treating severely burned patients in the event of atomic disaster. A solution containing 1 teaspoonful of table salt and 3 teaspoonsful of sodium bicarbonate in 1 quart of water (Haldanes' solution) flavored with lemon juice and chilled can often be retained when other fluids would be vomited; it supplies electrolytes as well as fluid.

The patient may have nausea and vomiting to such an extent that nutrition must be provided entirely by the intravenous route. For the first few days, while the patient is dehydrated, the hematocrit reading is high, but when the patient is hydrated, severe anemia is shown to have occurred. Because of the marked anemia and because the damaged or destroyed tissue must be replaced, a diet of about 3,500 calories per day, with 250 Gm. of protein, is often recommended.[11] This is several times the average daily protein requirement. Because of the patient's poor appetite, every bit of imagination and ingenuity on the part of the dietitian and the nurse is called upon to persuade him to eat what he needs. Sometimes relatives are helpful in suggesting favorite foods, and the patient's knowledge that special preparations are being made in the hospital will motivate him to take more food. If self-feeding is possible, even though slow, it may help to improve the patient's appetite. It is important that painful and disagreeable changes of dressings and other treatments be timed so they do not immediately precede meals.

The high-protein powdered milk preparations are valuable in masking the amount of protein taken and often seem to leave the patient with less of a feeling of oversatiation than may result from large servings of meats such as chops, which are often high in fat. They are also valuable because the very ill patient can take fluids more easily than he can chew and swallow solid foods.

Bulk foods must also be stressed in the diet of one who is rendered as inactive as the severely burned patient. A before-breakfast glass of prune juice seems to be unusually effective in helping ensure regular elimination.

Contractures. Contractures are among the most serious long-term complications of burns. A large responsibility for their prevention rests with the nurse, because she is with the patient more than anyone else, and it is the nurse who should note whether or not he is assuming the same position for the major part of each day or night. The newer practice of early skin grafting now prevents many contractures by mobilizing the patient sometimes months earlier than would otherwise have been possible. Despite this, it is still necessary to guard against contractures. Many patients are now undergoing painful reconstructive surgery as a part of rehabilitation which would not have been necessary if those attending them had been alert to the prevention of contractures.

Burned patients often have severe pain as healing progresses; they are anemic, debilitated, and depressed. The nurse's temptation may be to leave them in what appears to them the most comfortable position, promising herself that change will be made tomorrow. The nurse must never let her sympathy for the patient lead her to overlook her concern for his ultimate good. She must make gentle, but determined, efforts to have the patient maintain range-of-joint motion and thus prevent scars from healing in positions that will result in deformity. The problem is even worse in children, since normal skin and normal tissues grow while scar tissue does not grow or stretch—it shrinks instead. Thus what begins as a minor deformity in childhood may become a major one with increased growth. For a definite interval of time each day, patients with burns should lie prone and also flat on their backs with no pillow or elevation of the head of the bed. Prolonged rest in a semi-Fowler's position and with the pillow pushing the head forward must be avoided; many patients like this position because it enables them to see about the room better. The resourceful nurse can often turn the bed so that the same objective can be reached without jeopardizing complete recovery. It is often advisable to change the bedside table from one side of the bed to the other at intervals. Mirrors help these patients keep in better touch with their environment, provided that viewing disfiguring burns on the face can be avoided.

If burns have been sustained about the neck, chin, and face, the patient should lie in a position of hyperextension of the neck for a period of time each day; a pillow may be placed under his shoulders and the bed lowered to a completely level position. Facial exercises are encouraged to prevent scars from tightening as they form. Chewing gum and blowing balloons provide exercise for this purpose.

Burns on the hands can easily result in contractures unless the part is kept in a position of hyperextension at least part of each day. If the patient has only one hand burned, he can be taught to exercise his own affected hand. Tight scarring in the axilla may be prevented by bandaging the arm loosely to the head of the bed in a position of external rotation for a period of time each day. Splints and shell casts may be used to prevent contractures of knees and plantar flexion deformity of the foot; these deformities can result from poor position during sleeping hours.

Exercises for prevention and correction of contractures may be more easily done in an occupational therapy or physical therapy department where the patient may also benefit from a change in environment. If the burned areas have healed sufficiently, the patient may be sent to the department of physical medicine where exercises are often done under water and are supervised by a physical therapist. The occupational therapist also helps the patient improve his range of motion in a satisfying and efficient fashion by teaching him to type, to weave, and to engage in a host of other activities. The nurse must know what the patient is being taught by the physical therapist and the occupational therapist so that progress can be continued when he returns to his room.

Skin grafting. After the fluid in the local edema has been redistributed, the patient continues to lose fluid and protein through oozing of the burned area. The best treatment for this has been found to be early skin grafting. Early skin grafting of burns is probably the most significant change that has taken place in the care of burned patients in several decades. It is now known that it is unnecessary and even undesirable to wait for granulation tissue to form before grafting. Skin grafting is often done between the seventh and fourteenth days after the initial injury, with the result that patients who otherwise might have been hospitalized indefinitely may leave the hospital in about a month.

Split-thickness grafts are usually used. These include the upper layer of the skin and part of the under layer but are not taken so deep as to prevent regeneration of skin at the part of the body where they are removed (donor site). They grow as normal skin on the burned areas (recipient sites), and thus the skin at the donor site has actually been doubled. These grafts are removed with a dermatome from almost any unburned part of the body. They are sutured into place, and gentle pressure dressings are applied. The donor site, which presents an oozing, painful surface, is covered with sterile gauze and a pressure dressing. In most instances, it heals within two weeks. Many patients complain of quite severe pain in the donor site, and the nurse should not hesitate to give medications that are ordered for pain, since the pain should subside within a day or two. Sometimes an odor develops from dead tissue at either the donor or recipient site, and this is distressing to the patient. Odor should be reported to the doctor; occasionally it may be due to infection, although usually infection is controlled by giving antibiotics before and after grafting. In occasional emergencies, the skin of other persons is taken to cover burned surfaces and prevent fluid loss; however, this is a temporary measure since, with the exception of the case of identical twins, the skin of another person is incompatible and dies and sloughs within one to three months.

Dressings and soaks. Local application may be ordered to stimulate healing of burned areas. Some of these include nitrofurazone (Furacin), cod-liver oil ointment, scarlet red ointment, and balsam of Peru. When any of these is used, old or discarded linen should be obtained for bandages since most of them stain linen badly.

Infection is prevented or controlled by giving penicillin or other antibiotics, maintaining as clean and nearly sterile an environment as possible, and using soaks or dressings on infected areas. Saline dressings are used to treat small infected areas. It is important to keep these moist, because drying causes the dressing and the exudate to shrink; this causes pain and may cause hemorrhage from newly developed superficial blood vessels.

Tub baths at 37.7° C. (100° F.) may be used to soak off extensive dressings over infected areas. The patient should never be left unattended during this procedure, because fainting and injury might occur. Those in attendance should wear gowns and gloves and the patient must receive careful personal care so that fecal contamination is minimal. The water in the tub cannot be kept sterile. In spite of this, many patients benefit a great deal from the cleansing effects of the water and from the fact that dressings are removed so much more easily and less painfully.

Emotional aspects of care. The emotional impact of severe burns is enormous. During the first few days the patient is too ill to fully comprehend what has happened, but then comes the long healing period and the realization of endless implications. The patient's reaction is determined by his own personality make-up, by his degree of total adjustment to life, and by the extent and location of the burns. Burns on the face make adjustment particularly difficult. All sorts of fears arise to harrass the patient. Will my husband (or wife) still care for me? Can I ever let my children see me? To the adolescent, the thought of being diferent or conspicuous may be unbearable. Fears about not being taken back on the job often haunt the wage earner who is badly burned. If possible, the patient should not see facial burns until a good deal of healing has taken place, and sometimes he should not see his face until skin grafting has been done. One way to reassure patients is to show them pictures of patients with burns in the early stage and several years after treatment; the recovery is almost unbelievable in some instances. He should be told that the redness that accompanies burns in the early stage and newly healed skin will often fade a great deal within a few months. He must have an opportunity to talk about his problems and his fears. He may discuss these with the nurse when he cannot express them to relatives, and she must take time to listen. Almost every burned patient needs the help of the social case worker for himself and for his family; the nurse should recognize this need and initiate the referral. The patient's relatives may give the nurse many leads to further understanding of the patient and of his particular needs; visiting hours can be used to learn from relatives how to give better care to the patient who is severely burned.

Long-term problems and rehabilitation. Complete recovery and rehabilitation of the badly burned patient may be a long and costly process. Many industries have compensation insurance to cover part of the cost, and the patient should be encouraged to discuss his financial problem with his doctor and with the social case worker if one is available. If the patient is under 21 years of age, he will be eligible for care financed in part by the Children's Bureau through its aid to states for their programs for crippled children. This care will cover surgical procedures and care, special rehabilitative services, and social service.

Patients who have been burned should have medical checkups at regular intervals indefinitely and should be advised to report any unusual change in the burn scar to their doctor at once. There is a fairly high frequency of malignant degeneration of scar tissue following burns; this is particularly true when the burn is caused by electricity or by x-rays.

REFERENCES AND SELECTED READINGS*

1 Accident Facts, Chicago, 1959, National Safety Council.

2 *Armistead, Nancy B.: Preventing Deformities Following Severe Burns, Am. J. Nursing **50**:162-163, March 1950.

3 *Baker, Thomas J., and others: Open Techniques in the Management of Burns and Nursing Care of the Burn Patient, Am. J. Nursing **59**:1262-1268, Sept. 1959.

4 *Blocker, Truman G., and others: The Care of Patients With Burns, Nursing Outlook **6**:382-387, July 1958.

5 Cockshott, W. P.: The History of the Treatment of Burns, Surg. Gynec. & Obst. **102**:116-124, Jan. 1956.

6 *Cornell Conference on Therapy, vol. 6, New York, 1953, The Macmillan Co.

7 Davis, Loyal (editor): Christopher's Textbook of Surgery, ed. 6, Philadelphia, 1956, W. B. Saunders Co.

8 *Division of Medical Sciences of the National Research Council, Am. J. Nursing **53**:179-182, Feb. 1953.

9 MacGregor, Frances Cooke, and others: Facial Deformities and Plastic Surgery, A

*References preceded by an asterisk indicate material particularly well suited for student reading.

Psychological Study, Springfield, Ill., 1953, Charles C Thomas, Publisher.
10 *Milner, Constance W.: Nursing Care of Severely Burned Patients, Am. J. Nursing **54**:456-459, April 1954.
11 *Moore, Francis D.: Treatment of Severe Burns, Am. J. Nursing **54**:454-456, April 1954.
12 Statland, Harry: Fluid and Electrolytes in Practice, Philadelphia, 1954, J. B. Lippincott Co.
13 Whitney, John M.: National Medical Civil Defense Planning and Requirements, J.A.M.A. **160**:1195-1201, April 7, 1956.

The patient with disease of the breast

Chapter 31

Study questions for review

1 Review the anatomy of the breast and adjacent structures.
2 What are some of the psychologic reactions to be expected when a patient faces disfiguring surgery?
3 Review the normal range of motion of the shoulder joint. What daily activities involve the full use of this joint?
4 Describe how you would teach a person to apply a sling.

The most common diseases of the breast are dysplasia, or "cystic disease," carcinoma, and fibroadenoma in that order. These conditions occur almost entirely in women and are known to surgeons as the "big three" of breast disease. Because carcinoma is by far the most important, the nursing care for this will be discussed in some detail before other breast diseases are mentioned.

CARCINOMA OF THE BREAST

The nurse has three main responsibilities in regard to carcinoma of the breast: educating women so that breast cancer may be discovered and treated early; caring for the patient in the hospital when a breast has been removed because of carcinoma and assisting with physical and emotional rehabilitation; helping the patient and her family in the home and in the hospital when the lesion is inoperable or when metastasis has occurred.

Development, mortality, and prognosis

Carcinoma of the breast is the most common malignancy in white women and exceeds even carcinoma of the uterus as cause of death from cancer.[6] Over 20,000 women die from this disease each year. In 1920 there were 6,665 deaths reported in a population of 105,710,000; in 1958, there were 22,261 deaths reported in an estimated population of 168,368,000.[15] This increase is due partly to changes in the age distribution of the population with proportionately more older women. Although many cases are found in young women, carcinoma of the breast often immediately precedes or follows the menopause and continues to develop in those past the climacteric. Most tumors of the breast in women past the menopause are malignant since fibroadenomas occur largely in younger women and dysplasia in those between the age of 30 years and the menopause. The older the woman becomes, the more likely she is to develop carcinoma of the breast. With present life expectancy, figures show that in New York State one woman in every twenty-five will develop this disease.[9]

There is some evidence that carcinoma of the breast is increasing in incidence as well as in prevalence.[12] The incidence is highest between 40 and 49 years of age when involutional changes occur in all organs associated with reproduction. It is conspicuously more frequent in women whose breasts have never functioned normally.[6,9] It occurs more often in single women and in married women who have not borne children than in women who have had children. Carcinoma of the breast is somewhat more common in the economically well favored.[6] The incidence of carcinoma of the breast also rises when there is a familial history of breast cancer.

Causes of carcinoma of the breast are not known, although it is fairly definitely established that hormones have some relationship to its development and, certainly, to its rate of growth. There is a considerable difference in the rate of growth and in the likelihood of metastasis among individuals, and this "genetic determination" is suspected by some authorities to be an extremely important factor in controlling the outcome for the patient.[6] It is believed that injury does not lead to breast cancer, although a lump in the breast is often discovered after a minor injury has been sustained, perhaps because the one injured feels her breast at this time and notes a mass which was already present. There is little evidence that dysplasia or cystic disease predisposes to the development of carcinoma, although these conditions make it much more difficult to diagnose an early carcinoma.[9]

Carcinoma may develop anywhere in the breast or on the nipple; however, the upper outer quadrant is the most commonly affected. The early lesion may be discovered only by careful palpation of the entire breast. Signs that the lesion is well established and has invaded surrounding tissues are dimpling of the skin (orange rind appearance) over a hard lump, puckering of skin and changes in skin color over the lesion, alteration of contour of the breast, raising of the nipple if the lesion is in the upper quadrant of the breast, serous or bloody discharge from the nipple, and unusual scaling or inversion of the nipple.

Paget's disease is a condition in which there is a shiny-appearing scaling of the nipple which progresses to bleeding and ulceration of the nipple and areolar structures. This is a precancerous lesion in its early stages, but it always becomes malignant if untreated; the treatment is total mastectomy as soon as a diagnosis is made.

Pain is seldom a symptom of early cancer. In the advanced phases of neglected cases there may be ulceration of the skin, with subsequent infection in necrotic tissue. Because of the distribution of the lymph vessels and because there are no lymph nodes between the two breasts which might delay spread of malignant cells, metastasis may spread rapidly through the lymph vessels to the opposite breast and to the mediastinum. Spread to the axillary lymph nodes also occurs early. Sometimes discovery of enlarged lymph nodes is the first indication to the patient that anything is wrong, particularly when the lesion is deep in the breast tissue and routine palpation of the breast has not been carried out.

Prognosis in carcinoma of the breast depends greatly upon early diagnosis and complete surgical removal of all tissue containing malignant cells before metastasis occurs. Since the disease arises in such a relatively accessible part of the body, it is tragic that diagnosis is not made earlier in more patients so that their lives can be saved. Approximately 80 per cent of patients having radical mastectomies survive for five years when the disease appears confined to the breast, and 40 per cent survive when axillary nodes are involved.[12] The American Cancer Society, Inc. reports that the five-year survival rate is only approximately 25 to 40 per cent when axillary lymph nodes are involved despite radiation and hormone therapy. At the present time the only hope for cure lies in complete early removal of the entire breast and its surrounding tissue, yet it is estimated that only approximately 60 per cent of all patients who seek medical attention for cancer of the breast are suitable candidates for radical mastectomy; the disease is too far advanced in the others for satisfactory surgical treatment.[14]

Self-examination of the breasts

For years, surgeons have been urging women to examine their own breasts routinely. This practice ensures much more frequent examination than is practicable or possible by a physician, and many women can learn to detect lesions early. Authorities[6,9] believe that all women should be taught to examine their own breasts each month and that those over 30 years of age who have a familial history of carcinoma of the breast should have a medical examination twice a year. All women should have an annual medical examination that includes palpation of the breasts.

The nurse working in industry, in the clinic, in the doctor's office, or in the community nursing agency has the responsibility of teaching women how to examine their breasts and of explaining why it is necessary to do this. A movie prepared by the American Cancer Society, Inc. that describes a good method of self-examination is available for loan from local chapters of the Society. In most large cities the local committee of the American Cancer Society, Inc. will arrange for showing the film for an audience of fifty or more. In smaller communities the film may sometimes be obtained through the local health department.

Self-examination of the breasts should be done regularly each month. The best time is at the conclusion of, or a few days following, the menstrual period. Some women have engorgement of the breasts premenstrually, and the breasts may have a lumpy consistency at that time; this condition usually disappears a few days after the onset of menstruation although occasionally lumpiness and tenderness may extend throughout the menstrual cycle. Because of this possible change it is important that the breasts be examined at the same time each month in relation to the menstrual cycle. Women who have passed the menopause should check their calendars and examine their breasts on the same day each month.

Self-examination of the breasts as outlined by the American Cancer Society, Inc.* should include the following steps:

Step 1. Sit straight before a mirror, arms relaxed at sides. Study the contour of the breasts. Has there been a change since the last examination?

Step 2. Next, raise the arms high above the head and observe whether there is any deviation from normal in size or shape of the breasts or abnormal puckering or dimpling of the skin.

Step 3. Lie down, place folded towel under shoulder, and raise arm above head on the side being examined. With flat of the fingers, feel gently the inner half of the breast.

Step 4. Then, bring the arm down to side and feel gently the outer half of the breast, giving special attention to the upper outer section. Examine the other breast in the same way.

Some women need help in learning to examine themselves; they may, for example, feel a rib when examining the lower half of the breast and become alarmed. However, most women learn quite readily. If a lump of any kind is discovered, it should not be rubbed or touched excessively; it should be left alone, and the advice of the family physician should be sought at once. The woman who finds a lump in her breast should not become panicky and decide that she has cancer. She should know that there are other causes for a mass in the breast besides cancer. The lump may be caused by a benign tumor or by a cyst; only the doctor can determine this. All women should know that a tumor in the breast need not be painful to be of significance. Actually, pain in a mass in the breast is a heartening sign in that few cancers of the breast cause pain.

Women need to be taught that the prognosis for cancer of the breast could be much better if the cancer is discovered early and treatment instituted immediately. National statistics on deaths from this cause are widely publicized, however, and women fear the disease so much that many have a negative attitude which leads

*Leaflets on self-examination of the breasts are available free of charge from local chapters of the American Cancer Society, Inc. for distribution to all women.

them to delay seeking medical help. Almost every woman knows of a relative or a friend who has died from the disease, yet the average woman tells only her very closest friends when a breast has been successfully removed for cancer. As a result, deaths from the disease are much better known than are cures by surgery with no recurrence. Some women wish to avoid the expense of examination, do not wish to face the embarrassment of an examination, or rationalize that their trouble would appear trivial to the busy doctor. Sometimes they seek the advice of nurses, and it then becomes the nurse's responsibility to stress the urgency of getting medical advice at once. A safe rule to follow is to suspect that any lump in the breast is cancer until proved otherwise.

Medical treatment and nursing care

Although doctors can develop remarkable skill in distinguishing benign from malignant tumors by inspection and palpation, the only way to determine this conclusively is by microscopic examination of a portion of the tumor. Most surgeons believe that it is safer to remove the entire mass if there is the slightest possibility of cancer rather than to risk permitting a malignant tumor to remain. Small pieces of a tumor are seldom removed surgically because there is danger of releasing malignant cells into the blood and lymphatic systems at the time of operation. Sometimes, as when axillary nodes can be felt, the diagnosis of malignancy can be made with relative certainty before operation, and an axillary node may be excised for microscopic study.

Preoperative care. Before surgery is scheduled, the patient is given a thorough medical examination to determine her general physical condition and to discover any metastasis. Evidence of metastasis means that radical breast surgery will not control the cancer and such surgery is therefore contraindicated. The finding of metastasis in the spine, for example, means that radiation and hormone therapy are the usual treatments that will be used to control the disease for a time and that there is no hope of cure. A roentgenogram of the chest is always made and may reveal metastasis to the lungs, the pleura, the mediastinum, or the bones of the upper trunk.

An electrocardiogram is usually ordered preoperatively for the patient who is 40 years of age or over to help rule out heart disease. Blood-typing and crossmatching are also done preoperatively so that immediate extensive surgery may be done if an excision and frozen section examination of the tumor prove it to be carcinoma. If the diagnosis is carcinoma, the first incision is then closed; drapes, instruments, and gloves are changed to help prevent possible spread of cancer cells, and the more extensive operation is performed. This prevents the patient's having to endure preparatory procedures a second time.

Emotional preparation. The surgeon usually discusses the entire situation with the patient and sometimes with her family. This may be done in the doctor's office prior to the patient's coming to the hospital or in the hospital a day or two before surgery is scheduled. He explains the operation, why it is necessary, and what he hopes can be accomplished. The patient who comes to the hospital for removal of a breast tumor is always worried and upset although she may try to hide her fear from hospital personnel. Fear of mutilation and fear of death are the two main reasons why some women delay seeking treatment and hesitate to risk the confirmation of their fears when a tumor is found. These fears lead others to the doctor's office in a state of near panic when a mass is discovered in the breast. The patient needs the greatest understanding from all who care for her in the preoperative period. Visits from her husband and other close members of her family should be permitted at any time. Some women benefit from a short visit by a patient who has had a mastectomy and has made a satisfactory adjustment. The nurse must observe the patient closely and be guided by what she learns. For example, some patients are helped by a concise discussion of breast prostheses, while others are much too upset by the thought of the loss of a breast or the threat to life to even consider the use of an artificial breast. The nurse should report to the physician if she finds that the patient has not understood his explanation clearly and has misunderstandings that are adding to her worry.

In our culture the breasts have become a primary source of women's identification with femininity. So much emphasis is placed on the female breast as a symbol of attractiveness that the thought of loss of a breast becomes almost intolerable to many women. This is particularly true of those who depend largely on physical attractiveness to hold the esteem of others and to secure gratification of their personality needs. Psychologists have pointed out that there is a symbolic connection between the breasts and motherhood which is severely threatened when a breast must be removed.[12] All women, including single women and those past the menopause, are seriously threatened emotionally by the loss of a body part which is so closely bound up with sexual attractiveness and motherliness. The single woman or the married woman who has no children may feel even greater privation than the married woman with children who can be assured that her breasts have served their essential functions. Carcinoma of the breast often occurs at the menopause and soon afterward when women already feel that they have lost much of their sexual attractiveness; it occurs when normal women take stock of their relative degrees of satisfaction with their own femininity. The patient may feel that the operation, although it may save her life, ends her life as a woman. Surgeons often discuss the implications of the loss of a breast with the patient's husband since his attitude and behavior can help in the patient's acceptance of the decision regarding surgery and in her future rehabilitation.

Most patients are helped by a kindly, yet matter-of-fact, attitude toward loss of the breast and by the assumption that there need be no change in appearance or mode of living. Mention of ways by which clothing can be adjusted to preserve normal contours often helps. The patient may be told that bathing suits and evening dresses can be worn following surgery if there is evidence that this information will be comforting.

If it is likely that a total mastectomy will be done, the patient should be prepared for what she will experience postoperatively. She should be told that it may be necessary for her arm to be held against the body for a few days to prevent strain on the wound and that she will probably be able to get out of bed the day after the operation. She should know that, if the breast is removed, there will be a tendency for her shoulder to droop on the unoperated side because of the inequality of weight and that she can prevent this by close attention to posture. Poor posture may give more evidence that a breast has been removed than will a slight inequality in breast contours. While padding and prosthetic devices can be used to take the place of the breast and give normal contours to the upper body, stooped, awkward posture cannot be hidden. Telling the patient about this helps to give her the feeling that there is something in the situation that she can control and contribute to, and thus aids in a positive attitude toward rehabilitation.

Operation. If there are no gross signs of extension of the carcinoma, the entire breast, the pectoral muscles, the axillary lymph nodes, and all fat, fascia, and adjacent tissues are removed in one piece. This is a *radical mastectomy*. The judgment of the surgeon regarding the amount of overlying skin that can safely be left to cover the defect determines whether or not a skin graft is to be done. The surgeon may order preparation of the anterior surface of a thigh in addition to the routine preoperative preparation discussed in Chapter 14.

A mastectomy may take several hours, and since 600 to 800 ml. of blood may be lost a transfusion is usually started in the operating room. Some surgeons insert a drain in one side of the wound next to the axilla to help remove serous fluid which may collect under a graft delaying its attachment and thus predisposing to infection. Pressure dressings are then applied. These may be made of gauze, marine sponge, rubber sponge, or cotton reinforced with mechanic's waste, depending on the preference of the surgeon; they are held in place with wide bands of adhesive tape.

Postoperative care. When the patient returns from the operating room or the recovery room, she is usually placed on her back; the head of the bed may be slightly raised to facilitate breathing. The upper arm is usually held against the side with adhesive tape, the elbow bent at a right angle, and the lower arm supported in a sling. The hand and elbow are free. The dressings are usually quite snug in order to help control serous oozing from the wound and to provide even pressure on the graft. If a graft has been taken from the thigh, this area will be covered with a firm pressure dressing and the patient may complain of severe discomfort in this wound as soon as she responds from anesthesia.

Immediate postoperative nursing care includes checking dressings as often as every fifteen minutes for the first few hours to detect hemorrhage or excessive serous oozing; evidence of hemorrhage or excessive serous oozing should be reported to the surgeon. The bedclothes under the patient must be examined since blood may flow from the axillary region backward and go unnoticed unless special care is taken. Dressings must also be checked to be certain that they do not hamper circulation. Swelling and numbness of the lower arm or inability to move the fingers must be reported at once. The nurse, however, should never loosen dressings without specific instruction from the surgeon.

The patient must be encouraged to take deep breaths and to cough deeply at frequent intervals since this helps to prevent congestion in the lungs. She may complain of a feeling of constriction over the chest which causes discomfort and interferes with deep breathing; medications for pain often help this. Because the patient may be drowsy from sedation and may not remember a spoken reminder, it is best to remain with her and see that deep breathing is done. By supporting the dressings over the wound while the patient coughs, pain may be lessened. Pain may be quite severe, and narcotic drugs should not be withheld for the first few days following a total mastectomy provided deep breathing and coughing are done routinely every few hours.

A firm mattress helps to splint the chest wall and lessen pain and discomfort when the patient moves. The elbow should be protected from pressure by pillows. Pillows can also be used to support the arm when position is changed and thus lessen general discomfort. The patient may be more comfortable sitting up straight while getting back care since turning toward the affected side may be exceedingly painful. A pull rope attached to the foot of the bed will help her to raise herself to a sitting position. The patient should be encouraged to take fluids by mouth as soon as she has completely reacted from anesthesia. Her time of voiding postoperatively should be noted.

Ambulation. The patient usually is allowed out of bed the day after a mastectomy. She needs help when she gets out of bed to use the commode, to sit in a chair, or to walk about for the first time, since her ability to maintain normal balance is hindered by the tight awkward dressings and by the loss of weight of the breast and the inability to swing the arm on the affected side for balance. She must be cautioned not to get out of bed without assistance until she learns to handle herself safely and until narcotic drugs are given less frequently. Nursing assistance should be given when she walks even when she can walk safely since the nurse should at this time encourage her in her progress and urge her to begin to check her posture regularly. The patient should try to relax the affected side yet use trunk and shoulder muscles to prevent inequality in height of her shoulders.

Dressings. Dressings usually are not

changed for several days after the operation. The skin sutures are often removed on the sixth to the eighth postoperative day. If a drain has been used, it is removed on the second to fourth postoperative day depending upon the amount of drainage. If a skin graft has been used, a catheter attached to suction set at low pressure may be used instead of the usual drain. By this means fluid is not permitted to accumulate and prevent the graft from growing.

Exercises. The surgeon decides when specific postoperative exercises should be begun. This may depend upon the extent of the operation and whether or not grafting has been necessary. The nurse should ask for specific orders if she is not certain of the doctor's wishes. Usually the patient is encouraged to flex and extend her fingers immediately upon return to her room even when the lower arm is held partly immobile in a sling. She should also be encouraged to pronate and supinate her forearm; simply turning the palm up and down will do this.

Exercises are essential to prevent shortening of muscles and contracture of joints and to preserve muscle tone so that the affected arm can be used without limitations. The nurse should explain to the patient why exercises are necessary and should encourage her in carrying them out; she should make the patient understand that by exercising and giving attention to dress she need have no handicap in use of her arm on the operated side or in her general appearance. Everyone finds it easier to follow routines that are well established and that are scheduled for specific times. An exercise routine also helps to keep the patient occupied and thus lessens postoperative depression which usually occurs a few days after surgery. It is best for the nurse and the patient to work out a schedule of specific exercises. Exercises are tiresome at best. As soon as possible, normal household activities should take the place of exercises, provided the patient knows what particular exercises can be accomplished by specific household tasks.

A small handbook entitled *Help Yourself to Recovery** is available for use by nurses in teaching patients and for distribution to patients, provided the surgeon agrees that the booklet will be useful to them. Smith[13] has outlined exercises for the patient who has had a mastectomy which should be helpful to nurses in working out appropriate exercises for patients. The following list is only suggestive and is adapted primarily from the two sources just mentioned. Again, it should be emphasized that it is not enough simply to ask the patient to comb her own hair or to wash her own back. She must know what motion is intended in each exercise. For example, the patient may brush her hair with the arm on the affected side but she may lower her head and hunch her shoulders in such a way that she does not get normal use of the shoulder joint and attached muscles. The whole intent of the exercise may, therefore, be lost. All exercises should be done with good normal standing or sitting posture. The patient should relax as much as possible and try to develop smooth rhythmic function. It helps to do as many exercises as possible in front of a mirror. The following are a few examples of recommended exercises.

Care of the hair. This may be done first by resting the elbow on books on a small table and brushing only the front part of the hair on the affected side. The exercise should eventually include brushing the hair on the top of the head and doing upward sweeps on the back of the neck. It can include pinning curls in the nape of the neck if this was the patient's practice before surgery.

Climbing the wall. (See Figure 100.) This exercise is usually started while the patient is in the hospital. At home it helps if the patient places a mark on the wall so that each successive day's progress can be noted. (1) Stand with toes as close to the wall as possible and face the wall; (2) bend the elbows and place the palms of both hands against the wall at shoulder level; (3) work both hands up the wall parallel to each other

---

*Published by The American Cancer Society, Inc., 1957; available from local chapters of the Society.

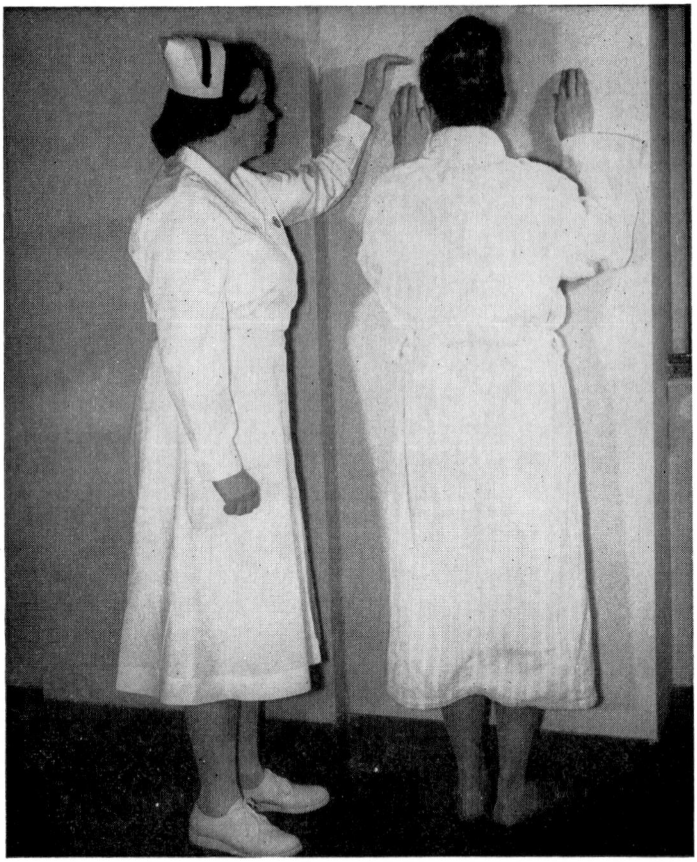

Figure 100

The patient needs help and encouragement in doing postmastectomy exercises.

as far as possible (eventually the arms should be completely extended with the elbows straight); (4) work the hands down to the starting position. Housework such as reaching into high cupboards or closet shelves, hanging out clothes, washing windows, and dusting upper walls gives this exercise.

Arm swinging. (See Figure 101.) This exercise should be started from the standing position with the feet well separated and the body straight. (1) Bend forward from the waist, permitting both arms to relax and fall naturally; (2) swing both arms together sideways, describing an arc as when sweeping (keep elbows straight and arms parallel). Another arm swinging exercise is as follows: (1) Bend forward from the waist, permitting both arms to relax and fall naturally; (2) swing the right arm forward and the left arm backward; (3) swing the left arm forward and the right arm backward.

Attaching a rope (a skipping rope is good) to a door knob and twirling it with a rotary motion alternately in one direction and then in the other, using first the affected arm and then the unaffected arm, gives good exercise to the shoulder. The wrist and elbow must be kept straight. Putting the rope over the shower rod and, grasping each end, alternately lowering and raising the rope until the affected arm is almost directly overhead is another beneficial exercise. It is good because it gives exercise to both arms at once. Some experts believe that the best exercises are bilateral ones in which the patient uses both arms simultaneously.[16]

Back buttoning. Stand straight with the feet well apart. Bend the elbow of the arm on the

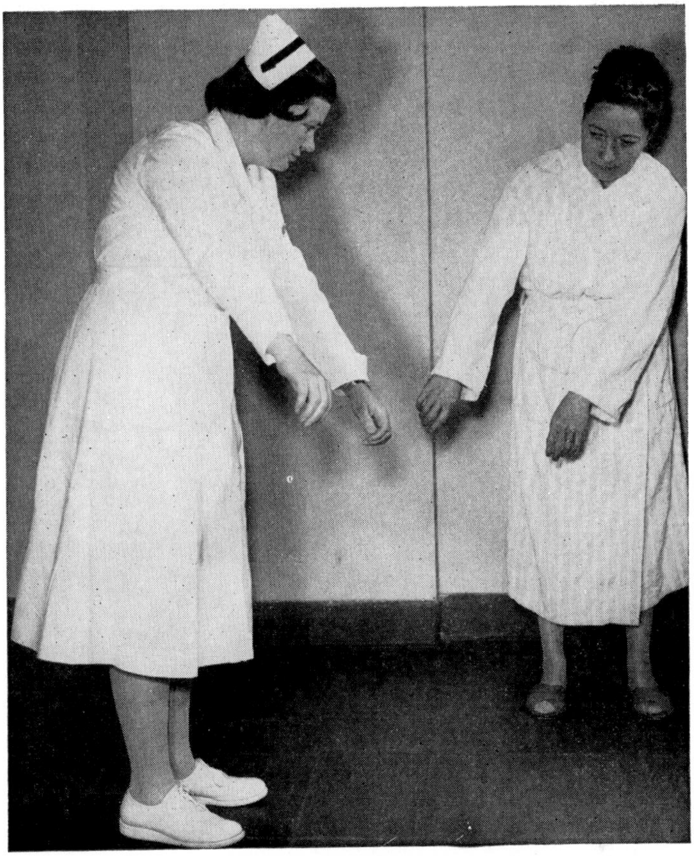

Figure 101

The nurse demonstrates the swinging exercise to a patient who has had a radical mastectomy.

unoperated side and reach back until the fingertips reach the opposite shoulder blade. Repeat using the operated side. This exercise can be accomplished by fastening a brassière, washing the back, or massaging or scratching the opposite shoulder blade.

Elbow pull-in. Stand straight with the feet well apart. (1) Clasp the hands at the back of the neck; (2) raise the elbows and bring them forward until they touch; (3) with the hands still clasped behind the neck, bring the upper arms out at right angles to the body.

Elbow elevation. Stand straight with the feet well apart. (1) Place the hand of the affected side on the opposite shoulder; (2) raise the elbow to chin level. Equivalent exercise is obtained in adjusting shoulder straps or pulling a garment over the shoulder and upper arm.

Care of the scar and breast prostheses. Rate of healing determines when dressings can be completely removed and a prosthesis worn. If a small open area remains to heal by formation of skin around the wound edges it may take several weeks. The patient should be encouraged to look at the scar before she leaves the hospital. She should be told that the skin will look a little irregular and that sensation may be lessened and may never fully return to the scar tissue. Any signs of redness, infection, or swelling within or outside the scar must be reported at once to the physician. The patient should be told that the scar will remain but that it will

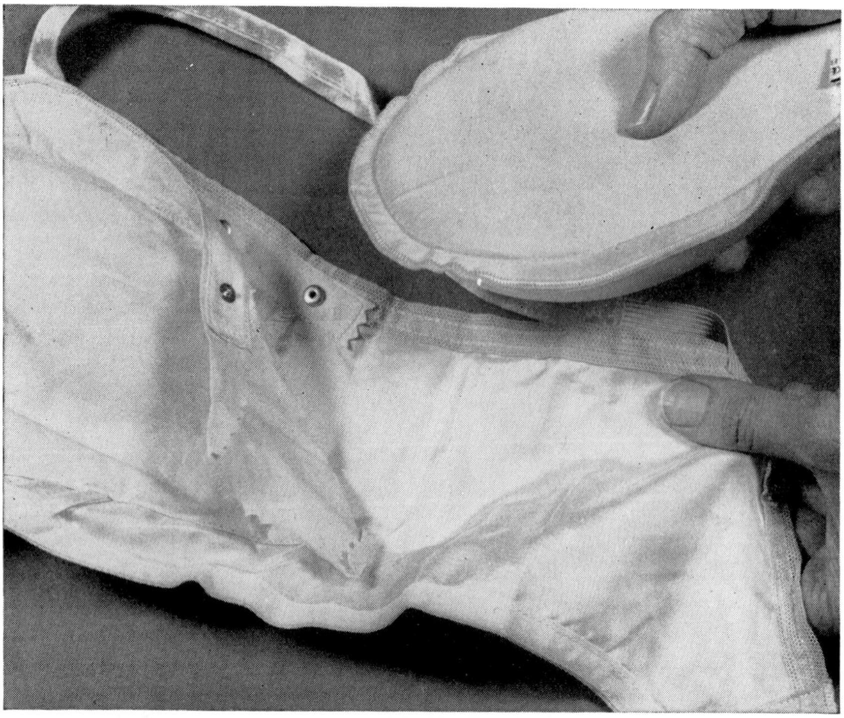

Figure 102

An inner pocket which will hold the padding or prosthesis securely can be made in the patient's own brassière. Note the snaps which simplify removal of the padding.

become softer, smaller, and more normal in color in time. She should bathe the area with a soft washcloth as soon as the wound heals and should pat the skin dry. The scar can be gently massaged with cocoa butter or cold cream. Itching of the scar is a fairly common complaint, especially during warm weather; talcum powder often helps to relieve this. If a heavy prosthesis is worn regularly, such as one filled with fluid, it is wise to wear a brassière padded with lamb's wool for several hours during the day so that there will be freer circulation of air over the scar.

It should be assumed that the scar is a usual one and that the patient's situation is no different from that of many other women. Night brassières can be worn and usually are comfortable and do not interfere with normal sleep. If the patient is married, however, she should be encouraged to let her husband see the scar and not try to hide it unduly. While the patient is in the hospital, her plan of living when she leaves should be discussed. The surgeon usually begins this by telling the patient how much rest she should have and what she should be able to do at once. The nurse should follow this explanation with encouragement to continue life normally. Many patients remain at home, avoid their friends, hesitate to engage in social activities with their husbands and families, and thus make life unhappy for themselves and their families when this is unnecessary. The reasons for withdrawal from social participation are usually more psychologic than physical. It should be pointed out to the patient that she will be able to do everything she could do before the operation although total muscle strength in the arm and shoulder may be slightly lessened. Actually, bathing suits can be fitted so that the loss of a breast is hidden, and swimming is excellent exercise for the patient who has had a mastectomy.

The nurse can help the patient with her immediate preparations to return home. A needle, thread, and scissors will be needed. The brassière worn to the hospital or one brought from the patient's home can be used to demonstrate to her how light padding can be used until the scar has completely healed and a prosthesis can be worn. (See Figure 102.) Plain cotton can be covered with gauze and lightly tacked with thread to the inside of the brassière. The family can bring the dress the patient will wear when she leaves the hospital and the nurse should help her to tack similar padding into the front of the dress if this seems better for the individual patient than padding the brassière. This can sometimes be anchored satisfactorily by using an attractive pin on the outer blouse or dress.

The patient should have help with the selection of an artificial breast before she leaves the hospital. The term "falsie" seems more acceptable to most women when speaking of an artificial breast, probably because the term is used to denote breast enhancement by those who have not had an operation. There are several kinds of artificial breasts, and some hospitals have manufacturers' literature and samples which can be demonstrated. Sponge rubber prostheses are preferred by many patients since they are light and are easily washed. Other patients prefer the prostheses filled with fluid since their weight more nearly approximates that of the normal breast. Still others prefer the artificial breasts that are filled with air. (See Figure 103.) In large communities the patient can usually be referred to a special corset shop where there are people prepared to fit her properly. The artificial breast should fit comfortably and should be covered with a correctly fitted brassière; the top of the brassière should

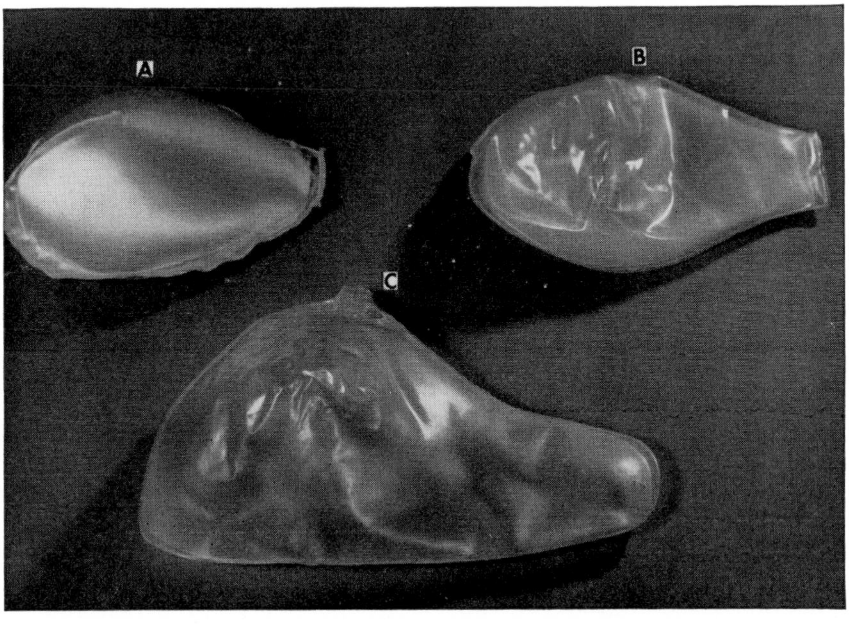

Figure 103

Several types of breast prostheses are available. *A*, Foam rubber prosthesis. *B*, Prosthesis containing fluid. *C*, Prosthesis containing air.

touch the skin lightly even when the patient bends forward. If the brassière tends to slip upward on the operated side, a V-shaped piece of elastic can be attached to the lower edge of the brassière and to a garter belt or girdle. Lengthening the brassière strap on the operated side helps to prevent discomfort from pressure of the strap. Erect sitting posture helps keep the prosthesis in the correct position when the patient is seated.

Lymphedema. Some patients have difficulty with swelling of the arm following a mastectomy. This follows interruption of lymph channels and infection. If there is a tendency for edema to occur, the patient is usually advised to sleep with the affected arm elevated on a pillow. For short periods several times each day, she should sit with the arm elevated on a table or on the arm of a sofa. Care must be taken when minor infections occur since they spread quickly. The patient is advised to take particular care in cutting her nails; she must remember to wash her hands thoroughly before doing this, and she must be careful not to cut the skin. Creams help to keep the skin in a healthy condition. Gloves should be worn during activities in which there is danger of trauma or gross contamination of the hand. Hangnails should be cared for by a doctor; any sign of infection should be reported to the doctor at once since even apparently minor infections can become really troublesome.

Treatment when metastasis occurs

X-ray treatment. X-ray therapy may be given if there is suspected or known metastasis. Treatment can be started as soon as the day after surgery and may be continued on an ambulatory basis after the patient leaves the hospital. (For details of care of patients receiving x-ray treatment, see Chapter 16.)

Hormone therapy. When surgical removal of the breast and x-ray therapy are unable to control cancer of the breast with metastasis, hormone treatment may be used. This is particularly effective in controlling the progress and also the pain when there has been metastasis to the bones. For example, bone cells may be regenerated in decalcified areas in the spine and pathologic fractures may heal as a result of hormone therapy. It is estimated that, with hormone treatment, approximately one half of patients with metastasis have relief of symptoms for one year or more. Testosterone is the hormone most often used. Testosterone (a synthetic male hormone) is usually given in doses of 50 mg. intramuscularly twice a week for an indefinite period. Treatment with testosterone will cause secondary changes which are distressing to the patient and which include deepening of the voice, coarsening of the skin, and appearance of hair on the face and the rest of the body. The patient usually gains weight. She should be warned that these changes may occur, and she may need to pay greater attention to details of personal grooming than formerly was her practice.

Surgical procedures. Estrogens are thought to be necessary for the growth and maintenance of the malignant cells of breast carcinoma. Several somewhat radical operative procedures are now occasionally being used to remove estrogen supply from the body in an attempt to prolong the life of the patient who has metastasis of breast cancer.

Bilateral oophorectomies are done to remove the major estrogen supply. See Chapter 22 for the nursing care of a patient having bilateral oophorectomies.

Since the adrenal glands secrete small amounts of estrogen, a *bilateral adrenalectomy* as well as oophorectomy may be done. See Chapter 28 for a discussion of the nursing needs of a patient who has insufficient adrenocortical hormone.

Removal of the pituitary gland (hypophysectomy) suppresses the function of both the ovaries and the adrenal glands. A hypophysectomy is performed through a right frontal craniotomy. The nursing care is the same as that required by any patient with a frontal craniotomy. However, since the "master gland" has been removed, many metabolic disturbances may occur. The patient must be watched carefully for polyuria; this is controlled by the administration of pitressin. Adrenal insufficiency may also develop. (See Chapter 28.) Symptoms of thyroid insufficiency occur and are counteracted by giving thyroid extract. If the patient is operated upon before the menopause, she will also have symptoms of the menopause and these may be quite troublesome because of their abrupt onset.

Psychologic considerations. The patient who has metastasis needs encouragement and help to continue to carry on her normal work either in the home or elsewhere for as long as possible. Some patients who have had to wear a brace because of metastasis to the spine have returned to their jobs for a year or more. Nothing contributes more to the patient's morale than continuing to work and participate in life around her. Appetite improves and probably the resultant general improvement in health delays complete invalidism for some time. Patients may even continue to work or to carry on normal social activities when they have severe pain that requires regular narcotic or other analgesic treatment.

NONMALIGNANT DISEASE OF THE BREAST

Dysplasia and fibroadenoma

Dysplasia. Dysplasia is characterized by thickened nodular areas in the breast which usually become painful during or prior to menstruation. A variety of changes take place in the breast tissue, among which is cystic formation in some cases. The condition is thought to be caused by hormonal imbalance and increases with changes preparatory to the menopause when hyperinvolution takes place. The nodules may be singular or multiple; they may increase in size or remain the same. Usually they are fairly soft and tender on palpation and are freely movable, sliding under the examining fingers. The woman who discovers such a mass (or masses) in her breast should seek the advice of her family doctor, who will decide whether or not the lesion should be measured and checked at frequent intervals or whether surgery should be considered. There is little, if any, evidence that dysplasia predisposes to the development of malignancy, but the presence of nodules in the breast make the early detection of malignant lesions much more difficult.

Fibroadenoma. Fibroadenomas are usually firm, round, freely movable, nontender, and encapsulated. They occur most often in young women under 25 years of age and are caused by an overgrowth of fibrous connective tissue. The woman who discovers such a mass should not delay in seeking medical consultation. Usually the tumor will be removed under local anesthesia and will be examined microscopically. The hospital stay is short, and sutures are removed after the patient leaves. Patients who are admitted for removal of a tumor which is thought to be benign, however, need thoughtful nursing care since they are usually extremely fearful of cancer.

Infections

Infection of the nipple. Infection usually follows cracks in the nipple during lactation. This condition is less common than previously since women are taught to "toughen" the nipple during pregnancy so that cracking is less likely to occur.

Infections of the breast. Infections can occur in the breast by direct spread from cracked or infected nipples and following congestion or "caking" during lactation when a portion of the breast becomes engorged from blockage of gland ducts. Manual expression of excess milk and hormone treatment for women who are not going to nurse their infants have reduced the incidence of infections of the breast. Infections in the breast can also occur with no specific cause and perhaps follow infections elsewhere in the body; these infections can occur at times other than during pregnancy or lactation.

Infections of the breast cause pain, redness, swelling, and elevation of temperature. The treatment is usually conservative. Penicillin or other antibiotics are usually given systemically. Sometimes local heat is used, and at other times ice packs may be prescribed. If the condition does not subside with conservative treatment and becomes localized to form an abscess, surgical drainage is necessary.

An increase of epidemic breast infections in nursing mothers, caused by the antibiotic resistant staphylococcus, is being reported in the literature.[5] The staphylococcus is transmitted to the mother's breast from the nasopharynx of the newborn who has been exposed to infected infants and hospital personnel. This infection occurs three or four weeks after childbirth and usually locates in the deeper tissues of the breast; it is difficult to treat in the absence of effective antibiotic drugs. The increase in this infection in recent years points out the need for strict aseptic technique in nurseries for newborn infants and the prevention of all infected persons (carriers) from contact with patients.

REFERENCES AND SELECTED READINGS*

1 *Alexander, Sarah E.: Nursing Care of a Patient After Breast Surgery, Am. J. Nursing **57**:1571-1572, Dec. 1957.

2 American Cancer Society, Inc: A Cancer Source Book for Nurses, New York, 1950, The American Cancer Society, Inc.

3 *American Cancer Society, Inc.: Help Yourself to Recovery, New York, 1957, The American Cancer Society, Inc.

4 Ca: A Bulletin of Cancer Progress **6**:48-60, New York, March 1956, The American Cancer Society, Inc.

5 *Carrington, Elsie R.: Epidemic Puerpural Breast Abscess, Am. J. Nursing **58**:1683-1685, Dec. 1958.

6 Davis, Loyal (editor): Christopher's Textbook of Surgery, ed. 7, Philadelphia, 1960, W. B. Saunders Co.

7 Davis, J. B.: Ovariectomy and Adrenalectomy for Treatment of Metastatic Cancer of the Breast, Am. J. Surg. **96**:492-495, Oct. 1958.

8 Galente, Maurice, and others: Adrenalectomy for Metastatic Carcinoma, J.A.M.A. **163**:1011-1016, March 23, 1957.

9 Haagensen, C. D.: Diseases of the Breast, Philadelphia, 1956, W. B. Saunders Co.

10 Higginbottom, Sarah: Arm Exercises after Mastectomy, Am. J. Nursing **57**:1573-1574, Dec. 1957.

11 Pearson, Olof, and others: Hypophysectomy in Treatment of Advanced Cancer, J.A.M.A. **161**:17-21, May 5, 1956.

12 *Renneker, Richard, and Cutler, Max: Psychological Problems of Adjustment to Cancer of the Breast, J.A.M.A. **148**:833-838, March 8, 1952.

13 *Smith, Genevieve Waples: When a Breast Must Be Removed, Am. J. Nursing **50**:335-338, June 1950.

14 *Sugarbaker, Everett D., and Wilfley, Lucy E.: Cancer of the Breast, Am. J. Nursing **50**:332-335, June 1950.

15 Summary of Vital Statistics, Public Health Service, Publication No. 600, U. S. Department of Health, Education, and Welfare, National Office of Vital Statistics, Washington 25, D.C.

16 Wolf, Edith S.: Personal communication.

*References preceded by an asterisk indicate material particularly well suited for student reading.

Study questions for review

1 What reaction does the average person have when he encounters someone with a facial abnormality? What types of work would probably not be available to the person with such a deformity? List as many recreational activities as you can that would be difficult or impossible for a person who has a marked deformity of the right hand.
2 Review the anatomy of the skin. How does skin differ from granulation tissue? Describe how new skin forms at the edges of a wound.

The patient needing plastic surgery

Chapter 32

Plastic and reconstructive surgery has been attempted for centuries. Surgery of this kind was done during the era of the Roman Empire and even earlier. Hindu records describe some very good results from efforts to alter deformities caused by disease or other misfortune. In the sixteenth century, Italian surgeons did remarkable work in plastic surgery, and there was interest in the emotional aspects of facial deformities. The discovery of anesthetics and of the cause of infection enabled surgeons to make strides in this field. Disfigurements resulting from World Wars I and II challenged the imagination of surgeons so that new techniques were developed, and the extensive surgery that is now undertaken in treatment of cancer of the mouth and face has led to much more interest in maxillofacial reconstructive surgery.

There is every reason to believe that plastic and reconstructive surgery will become a more important part of medical care as time goes on. The main purposes of such surgery are to restore function, prevent further loss of function, and cosmetically improve the defects left by congenital deformities, disease, or trauma. Occasionally, plastic surgery may be done purely for cosmetic improvement. Congenital anomalies such as cleft palate and cleft lip require plastic and reconstructive surgery. Medical science has made some progress in learning the cause of some congenital anomalies; for example, a woman who has German measles during the first trimester of pregnancy may deliver a child who has a congenital anomaly. It is not possible, however, to control the development of many congenital anomalies, and it is reasonable to suppose that many more children will be born who will need treatment for this condition. The cause of cancer is still unknown, and extensive surgery will continue to be used until a better method of treatment is discovered. Trauma such as that sustained in automobile accidents often necessitates plastic and reconstructive surgery, and it seems likely that the number of people requiring such treatment will increase. Plastic and reconstructive surgery is often needed following loss of skin and scarring from burns. *Keloid tissue,* the thick weltlike masses of overgrowth of scar tissue which occur particularly in Negroes, often requires plastic surgery. Posttraumatic scars in which subcutaneous tissues are separated from or are adherent to underlying structures such as bone may be corrected by plastic surgery.

GENERAL NURSING CARE

The nurse has two important functions relating to patients needing plastic and reconstructive surgery. She should direct persons who may benefit from plastic procedures to appropriate medical care, and she is an important member of the team which cares for the patient undergoing plastic and reconstructive procedures.

Many people do not know that it is possible to correct a congenital defect. Some parents may delay seeking medical care for a child with a defect due to a congenital anomaly because of their own guilt feelings. They may hope that somehow, miraculously, the child will "outgrow" the condition. Often they do not realize that the normal development of the child depends upon early treatment of some conditions. Defects may interfere with the use of a part of the body so that normal growth does not take place. This follows the principle that form follows function; for instance, a child's deformed and therefore unused hand does not grow at the same rate as the hand that is used normally. Contractures of joints and atrophy of muscles occur with disuse, thus increasing the defect and handicap; for example, facial asymmetry can result from contractures in the neck which prevent uniform action of the muscles of both sides of the face even though the muscles themselves are not affected.

Parents need to know that healthy emotional development in the child is dependent upon normal physical appearance. When a defect is allowed to persist, there may be emotional maladjustment which will affect the patient's whole life. For example, conspicuous patches of brightly discolored skin present at birth and known as birthmarks or port-wine stains are quite common. These stains, particularly if they are on the face or neck, cause the patient great emotional distress and sometimes lead to serious personality maladjustment. Yet many people do not know that they may sometimes be effectively treated by tattooing.

The patient's emotional reaction to a deformity or defect must not be underestimated. One's pride in himself, his ability to think well of himself, and to regard himself favorably in comparison with others are essential to the development and maintenance of a well-integrated personality. Every person who has a defect or a handicap, particularly if it is conspicuous to others, suffers from some threat to his emotional security. The extent of the emotional reaction and the amount of maladjustment that follow depend upon the individual's make-up and upon his ability to ward off emotional insults. Disfigurements almost invariably lead to disturbing experiences. The child who has webbed fingers may be ridiculed at school; the adolescent girl who has acne scars may be a wallflower at school parties; and the young man with a post-traumatic scar on his face may be refused a salesman's job. Under any of these circumstances it is not unusual for the individual to withdraw from a society that is unkind. The defect may be used to justify failure to assume responsibility or to justify striking out against an unkind society by such reactions as becoming a "problem child" or, in some extreme cases, a criminal.

Many parents do not know that financial resources are available to cover costs of plastic and reconstructive surgery for children. Every state in the country has a plan for medical care of crippled children. This program is partially supported by matching funds from the federal government, administered by the Crippled Children's Division of the United States Children's Bureau, which was formed soon after the first White House Conference on Child Care held in Washington, D.C. in 1912. Children and adolescents up to 21 years of age with defects requiring plastic and reconstructive surgery are eligible for care under this plan. If the nurse encounters a child who might benefit from medical treatment, she should first ask the family if they have a family doctor with whom she can discuss the matter. If the family has no personal physician, the local hospital may conduct a clinic or may recommend a physician designated to care for eligible children in the area or the state. Small community hospitals may not have clinics of their own but may refer patients to larger hospitals or special clinics in near-by cities.

In larger communities, the school nurse is usually well informed about available resources.

Plastic and reconstructive operations may require repeated and long hospitalizations. These may place serious financial strain upon the patient and his family if they must assume responsibility for the major part of the expense. Clinic nurses, public health nurses in the community, social workers, and welfare agency personnel can help in preparing the patient for this problem and in helping him to meet it. If the patient is an adult, leaves from employment, financial support while undergoing treatment, and plans for convalescent care and rehabilitation are examples of problems that must be faced in many instances. The patient should be encouraged to discuss his problems freely since their solution does affect his medical treatment.

Preparation for surgery. It is believed that any plastic and reconstructive surgery for an obvious defect is justified if it helps the patient to feel he has a better chance for recognition among his fellowmen. The nurse cannot possibly know what the disfigurement means to the individual patient and should avoid judging whether or not surgery is necessary. It has been learned, however, that some people blame an apparently trivial physical defect for a long series of failures in their lives when the major defect lies within their own personalities. Because of this, the patient is usually carefully evaluated before surgery is planned; it is necessary to know what the patient expects the operation to accomplish before the doctor can decide whether or not such expectations are realistic. The plastic surgeon may reshape a nose or repair a deformed hand so that an emotionally stable person will have more assurance among others; however, it is foolish to assume that reconstructive surgery alone will correct a basic personality problem. It is necessary to learn about the social standards and cultural mores in the community in which the patient lives and his adjustment to them. His economic contribution as a citizen and as a member of a family, his characteristic pattern in interpersonal relationships, and whether or not he has previously sought medical treatment for the particular problem should be known. The social worker is often called upon to assist the surgeon in his efforts to learn as much as possible about the patient. By observing and reporting the patient's behavior at home, in school, in the clinic, upon arrival in the hospital, and during preparation for the operation, the nurse can help the surgeon in his study of the patient. Sometimes the help of specialists in psychology and psychiatry is sought. Before surgery, the doctor will tell the patient what probably can be done and what changes are possible. It is important that the nurse know what the patient has been told so that she can increase the patient's confidence in his surgical treatment and can avoid contributing to misunderstandings and misinterpretations.

The patient who is admitted to the hospital for plastic and reconstructive surgery may have extensive scarring and deformity and may be exceedingly sensitive to scrutiny by the people he encounters. On the other hand, the patient may have little apparent deformity, and it may be difficult to understand what brought the seemingly well person to the hospital for surgery. The nurse may be inclined to concentrate her efforts on the more physically ill patients, yet it is important for her to learn about each patient who is to have plastic surgery and to assure him of her interest.

The patient should be in the best possible physical condition before plastic and reconstructive surgery is begun. When the plans are made for elective surgery, the patient may be advised to eat a diet high in protein and vitamins for a short time prior to coming to the hospital because it is thought that this may help in the "take" or healing of the graft. Hemoglobin and clotting times are usually determined, and many surgeons request that the blood protein level be assayed.

The wound which is to receive the graft must be free from infections which

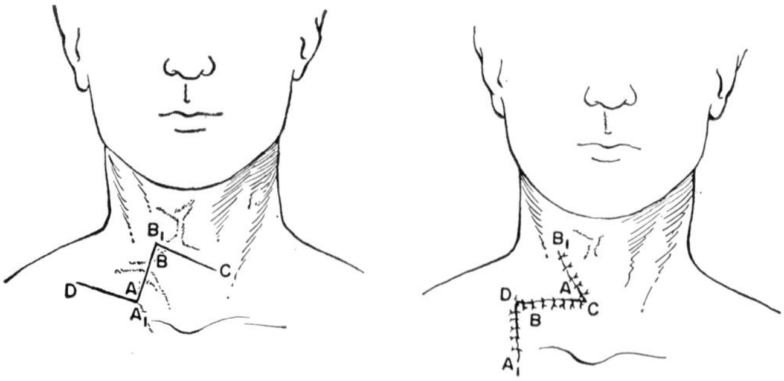

Figure 104

By means of Z-plasty operations, scar tissue can be removed and defects can be covered without the need to transplant skin.

would delay healing, lead to more scar tissue formation, and cause death of the graft. Infection is treated by the administration of antibiotics and by the use of warm soaks and compresses; a sterile physiologic solution of sodium chloride is the solution most often used. Before skin grafting is attempted, any dead tissue that is adherent to the wound is removed by débridement; otherwise this will interfere with the graft's healing.

The donor site (area from which skin is to be taken) is shaved and scrubbed with soap and water or with a detergent solution the evening before surgery, and this cleansing may be repeated the morning of operation. Strong antiseptics are avoided because they may irritate the skin. If the recipient site (site to receive the graft) is not an open wound, it is cleansed in the same way.

It is important to explain to the patient the measures used to prepare him for surgery, and he should be prepared for the postoperative experience. It must be repeatedly explained to him that the immediate results may not meet his expectations. Postoperative tissue reaction may distort normal contours, suture lines may be reddened, and the color of the newly transplanted skin may differ somewhat from that of surrounding skin. The patient may become alarmed and discouraged if he has not been prepared for the normal appearance of skin grafts and reconstructed tissue immediately after surgery. Preferably he should not see the operative site until it is well healed. If it is not possible to remove all mirrors to prevent the patient from inspecting the results, after facial surgery, dressings may be left on longer than necessary to cover wounds. Members of the patient's family should also know what to expect so that they will not be unduly worried and so that they can give support to the patient if apprehension occurs.

SPECIAL PROCEDURES FOR CONTRACTURES

Plastic surgeons make excellent use of the natural elastic quality of the normal skin. Operations knows as a *Z-plasty* and a *Y-plasty* are often done. Scar tissue can often be removed and the Z- or Y-shaped incision enables the surgeon to undermine adjacent skin, draw the edges together, and cover the defect without using skin from another part of the body. (See Figure 104.) These procedures are naturally limited by the size of the scar and its location since elasticity of skin varies in different parts of the body. Z-plasty and Y-plasty procedures are suitable for such locations as the axilla, the inner aspect of the elbow, and the neck and throat; they are not so useful in treating defects on the back or the palmar surfaces of the hand because the skin in these areas cannot be undermined and stretched.

TYPES OF GRAFTS AND RELATED NURSING CARE

Nearly all plastic and reconstructive surgery requires moving tissue from one part of the body to another. The moved tissue, or graft, is known as an *autograft,* and skin, bone, cartilage, fat, fascia, muscle, or nerves may be taken. Tissue transplanted from another person is called a *homograft.* The latter may be necessary when the patient's condition is poor and autografting is impossible, for example, when the patient is in shock but must have large burned areas covered by grafted skin. Homografts survive only about one to three months and will then die and slough; they can be used only as temporary grafts in extreme emergencies. When bone, cartilage, or blood vessels are obtained from sources other than the patient, it has been noted that they do not become part of the patient's body but act as a framework around which the body usually lays down cells of its own. The homograft is then gradually absorbed over a period of time.

Plastic surgery may be done by means of free grafting, cutting tissue from one part of the body and moving it directly to another part. It may also be done by leaving one end of the graft attached to the body to provide a blood supply for the graft until blood vessels form at the new place of attachment. The surgeon selects skin for grafting which is similar in texture and thickness to that which has been lost; he studies the normal lines of the skin and its elasticity to avoid noticeable scars. Scar tissue contracts with time, and in normal circumstances this is good because it produces a complete closure of the line of injury. However, in some cases it may contract in such a way that surrounding tissues are pulled out of normal contour and distortion may result. The plastic surgeon is an artist as well as a surgeon and he studies cosmetic and many other aspects of the patient's problem before he decides upon the type of graft or plastic procedure that will be most effective.

Free Grafts

Free grafts are those that are lifted completely from one part of the body to another. There are several kinds of free grafts, and each has its advantages and its limitations. *Reverdin* or *pinch grafts* are widely used because they grow easily and can sometimes be used to cover wounds that have been recently infected such as those that result from varicose ulcers. In such a graft, the skin at the donor site is picked up with a needle, and tiny pieces, about 0.5 cm. in diameter, are removed by means of a razor or sharp knife and placed on the recipient site about 1.5 cm. apart. Because the full thickness of skin is taken, the grafts regenerate epithelium around their edges until finally they coalesce on the recipient surface. The donor site, on the other hand, regenerates new skin around the edges of the small wounds left when the grafts are taken. Pinch grafts are easy to obtain and, if a few of them die and slough, no serious damage has been done. The disadvantages are that the resultant skin has a bumpy unattractive appearance and there are permanent small scars at the donor site.

Ollier-Thiersch, or razor, *grafts* are thin layers of the outer skin which are removed from the donor site (usually the front of the thigh) by a long razorlike knife or by a dermatome. The use of these grafts is limited because they contract easily, often become shiny and discolored, and have poor wearing qualities. Their advantages are that they will often grow on bony and tendinous areas where blood supply is poor, they can be taken in large pieces to cover large defects, and new skin regenerates quickly and without scarring at the donor site. Razor grafts are often used to replace mucous membrane in reconstructive surgery of the mouth and vagina.

A modification of the Thiersch graft is the *split-thickness graft* which is very widely used. This graft consists of the outer layer and part of the middle layer of skin. It does not wrinkle, contract, and become discolored as easily as the razor graft, yet the donor site is able to regenerate completely since the deeper layers of skin are not removed. Split-thickness grafts can be used to cover almost any part of the body. They can be cut in large pieces with a dermatome which is set to ensure a uniform thickness of the graft.

Wolfe's grafts, or *full-thickness grafts,* include all three skin layers and are used mainly to cover small areas where matching skin color and texture are important, as on the face. One disadvantage of the Wolfe graft is that only a moderate-sized piece of full-thickness skin can survive as a free graft under the best of circumstances because blood supply cannot become established quickly enough to provide essential nutrition. For nourishment these grafts depend entirely upon existing lymph until their own blood supply can be established. If the graft dies, the skin is irretrievably lost to the body since regeneration of skin at the donor site is not possible. Surrounding skin at the donor site is usually undermined so that the skin edges can be brought together, and grafting of the donor site is not necessary. This means that full advantage has been taken of the elastic quality of the skin and another graft probably cannot be taken from the same place at least for some time. It takes at least two weeks for blood supply to become established, although it is usually possible to tell within a week whether the graft is going to survive.

Skin flaps and sliding grafts

When a large and deep defect is to be covered, a skin flap may be used. Sliding, rotating, and pedicle grafts are examples of these grafts, which are never removed from a source of blood supply. Flap grafts may include skin, subcutaneous tissue, and sometimes fat and cartilage or bone; when the edges of the graft are sutured together to form a tube, it is known as a pedicle, or suitcase-handle, graft. This modification is often made when the skin is to travel a good distance because the danger of infection is much less than if it were open. Tissues such as fat and cartilage can also be easily transferred within the tube. This type of graft might be used to cover a defect on the back of the neck with skin from the abdomen. For example, the piece of skin taken from the abdomen may be grafted to the wrist, then, when circulation is safely established there, the attachment on the abdomen may be released and attached to its final location in the neck. The attachment on the wrist is maintained until circulation is established in the neck, at which time the graft is freed from the wrist and the tube opened and sutured into place to cover the defect. Circulation from the new attachment is often tested by putting a rubber-covered clamp or tourniquet about the pedicle close to its oldest attachment and noting the color and warmth of the pedicle at intervals of from ten to fifteen minutes. Usually it takes from three to six weeks for new blood vessels to become established. These grafts are less likely to die than are free grafts, but strangulation can occur from pressure, and tissue can be lost from infection. Pedicle grafts are often taken from the abdomen, where fat and subcutaneous tissue are available, to support skin in areas of the body that are subject to pressure, such as the heel, the sole of the foot, and the palm of the hand. The piece of skin taken is fairly narrow, and adjacent skin is undermined so that edges can be sutured together. When this wound has healed, a small gauze dressing is usually placed between the pedicle and the suture line to keep the area dry and free from the accumulation of dead skin.

Nursing care

Maintaining pressure dressings as ordered and preventing infection of grafted areas are important responsibilities of the nurse in caring for patients who have had plastic surgery. The life of the patient is not usually at stake in plastic surgery, but time, discomfort, and economic and emotional factors are involved. Sometimes a procedure that is not successful cannot be repeated because necessary skin is lost and too much scar tissue may have formed. Moreover, the patient undergoing extensive reconstructive surgery has usually suffered a great deal both physically and emotionally. His ability to cope with the disappointment of unsatisfactory results may be limited.

A graft must be in constant contact with the underlying tissue to attach itself and to grow. Some grafts, such as pinch and razor grafts, are left free, but usually grafts are carefully sutured into place with horsehair or silk sutures. If anything comes between the undersurface of the graft and the recipient area, such as a discharge caused by infection, excess serous fluid, or blood, it will float the graft away from close contact and may cause it to die. To prevent this from happening, some surgeons insert tiny drains at strategic spots along the edges of the graft. A wide variety of materials are used as dressings, depending upon the kind of graft and the surgeon's preference. Petrolatum gauze is perhaps most widely used at the present time, but some surgeons use Xeroform gauze and silver foil. Occasionally no dressings are used. Pinch grafts, for example, may be protected with a fine wire mesh cage and left uncovered in the belief that better healing is promoted with less danger of infection. Often the graft is covered with a piece of coarse-mesh gauze anchored to the adjacent skin edges to give firm, gentle pressure. The first dressing may be covered with a sterile normal saline compress and then protected with cellophane or some other waterproof material. When flap grafts are used, slings and casts may help to keep parts of the body in the correct relationship for healing. (See Figure 105.) A continuous pressure is necessary to keep the graft adherent to the recipient bed, but it should not be so firm as to cause death of the graft from pressure. Marine sponges, rubber sponges, cotton pads, and mechanic's waste may be applied as outer dressings by the doctor to provide the amount of pressure he desires. The patient may be placed on an oscillating bed to improve circulation to the graft and to help prevent circulatory complications such as thrombophlebitis.

The nurse should observe the dressings closely for drainage and bleeding; she should make sure that they are secure and that they have not become too tight because of local edema, thus interfering with circulation. She must also be certain that the patient does not lie on the dressing and thereby exert too much pressure on the graft. Dressings are almost always changed by the surgeon from one to twelve days after the operation, and it is usually possible to know then whether or not the result of the operation is satisfactory. Sutures that may be hampering circulation may be removed at this time.

Some surgeons believe that grafts are stimulated in their effort to establish blood supply by the use of warm moist compresses, and sterile normal saline solution is usually ordered for this purpose. The greatest care must be taken that infection is not introduced when compresses are being changed and moistened. The nurse must remember to wash her hands before handling dressings or changing compresses and must follow the most meticulous technique so that infection does not occur. She must be careful, too, not to traumatize the newly grafted skin; the temperature of the compress solution should not be over 40.5° C. (105° F.), and compresses should be applied with sterile forceps. Compresses may sometimes be covered with a sterile petroleum jelly dressing and moistened by gently directing fluid from a sterile Asepto syringe under the edge of the dressings. Sterile tubes with tiny openings (Dakin's tubes) may also be placed through the outer compresses to provide a means of moistening the inner dressings without disturbing them and without introducing infection.

The patient who must be in a cast for one or more stages of plastic and reconstructive surgery requires special care. Sometimes it is helpful preoperatively for the patient to assume the position that will be necessary for the next stage of the procedure so that he may become accustomed to a posture that may cause tedious strain on joints and muscles. Immediately after application and frequently there-

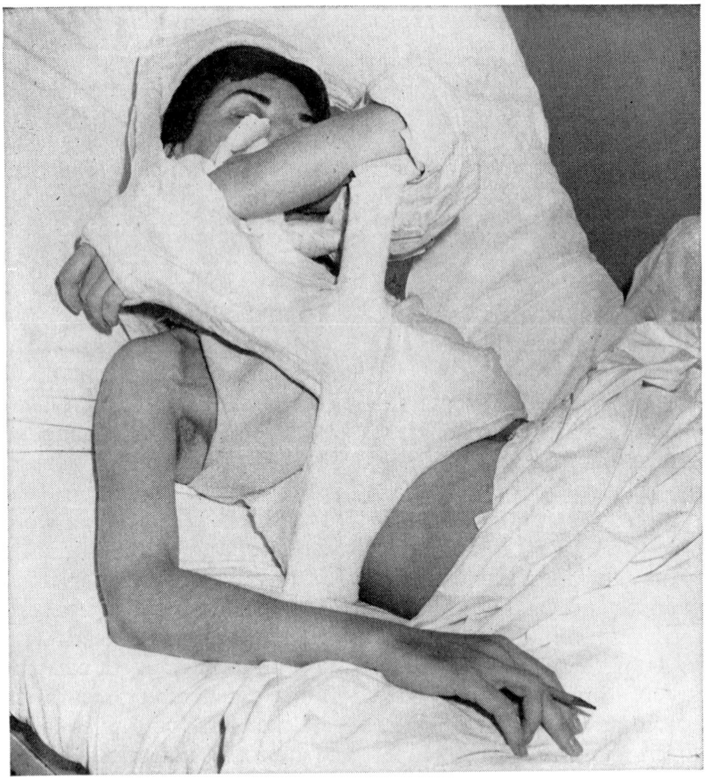

Figure 105

Plastic operations sometimes require the patient to be in extremely awkward positions. Eating, mouth hygiene, and communicating with others are problems in caring for this patient. Note the pencil used for communicating.

after, the cast must be checked for cracks or breaks which will interfere with support for the graft, and it must be carefully checked to make certain that no excessive pressure is being exerted. Pillows can be used to give support and to lessen strain on body parts; sometimes overbed bars and side rails help the patient to shift his position if he has one free arm and is otherwise able to do so. The patient who is in an extensive cast for several weeks must be reminded to do muscle-setting exercises for limbs in the cast and to exercise actively the limbs that are not confined.

Arrangements should be made for the patient to see what goes on around him. Sometimes this is made possible by changing his position in bed or the position of the bed in the room. In some instances putting the patient "head to foot" in the bed is helpful. A mirror may be attached to the bed and arranged at such an angle that it enables the patient to see at least a part of the room if his head, neck, and shoulder movements are restricted by a cast.

Occupations must be planned to keep the patient busy and to keep his mind off his discomfort. If he cannot engage in handwork, then passive activities such as listening to radio, reading, and watching television should be arranged. Even the patient who appears to be in a very complicated cast and in an awkward position can be placed on a stretcher or wheeled in his bed to a solarium or to other locations where he may have a change of scene and engage in some activity with others. Members of his family should be encouraged to visit the patient as much as possible and try in every way to assist him to maintain his community relationships that have been temporarily interrupted by his hospitalization.

The nurse may also help the patient to think along constructive lines in regard to what he will do when surgery is completed. Since a long period of rehabilitation is sometimes necessary, it is important to keep the patient in the best possible physical condition so that he will be ready to undertake specific rehabilitation activities and not require corrective therapy for disabilities acquired during hospitalization. For example, the patient who is having extensive skin grafting for a large traumatic wound on one leg should not be found to have foot drop on the unaffected limb when reconstructive procedures are completed.

The patient may tire of the hospital menu and may need to be encouraged to eat a well-balanced diet to promote healing of the graft, to reduce the chance of infection, and to maintain muscle strength during hospitalization. If he is on bed rest for a long time, it is important that bulk foods be eaten in sufficient quantities to help in elimination and that plenty of fluids be taken so that bladder complications do not develop.

TATTOOING

Tattooing has been found useful in plastic surgery for changing the color of grafted skin so that it more closely resembles the surrounding skin. This treatment is usually given on an ambulatory basis. Pigment is carefully selected and blended with the normal skin coloring by a skilled technician who then impregnates the grafted skin, using a tattooing needle. The procedure is painful, since no anesthetic is used. Sometimes the patient is given a sedative such as phenobarbital or is instructed to take such medication approximately one hour before coming to the clinic or the doctor's office. Prior to the tattooing, the skin is cleansed with a gauze sponge moistened with alcohol or normal saline solution. There may be a slight serous oozing from the skin, and this should be left to dry and crust. Sometimes a piece of sterile gauze can be placed over the tattooed area, and an ice bag may be applied if severe discomfort follows the treatment.

Tattooing is usually done in several stages; the amount done at one time depends upon individual circumstances, such as the location of the part treated and the emotional reactions of the patient. For example, treatment of the skin close to the eye is often quite painful and is extremely trying for the patient; therefore, usually only a small amount of tattooing is done at one time. Children may be given a general anesthetic for treatment around the eyes. Grafted skin may change in color with time, so tattooing done for the purpose of changing the color of grafted skin may have to be repeated.

Port-wine stains that are too large to treat by excision and grafting have also responded to this method of treatment with excellent results. The whole area may be treated at one time and the treatments repeated so that the color changes slowly. This is a tedious procedure if the stain is large and dark but, finally, in some cases the stain is barely apparent to the casual observer.

DERMAL ABRASION

Pockmarks, scars from acne, and certain other disfiguring marks may be removed from the skin by abrasive action. While the results vary depending upon the type and extent of the condition, there is usually noticeable improvement in the patient's appearance. Preoperatively the patient is prepared by the doctor for the degree of improvement to be expected so that his expectations are realistic. He is also informed about the face bandage he may wear, postoperative swelling, discomfort, crusting, and the erythema which may persist for several weeks. The procedure is done under local or general anesthesia, depending on the size of the area to be treated, the individual patient, and the preference of the doctor. It may be done in the clinic, the doctor's office or the hospital, again depending on the extent of the procedure and the preference of the physician; hospitalization is necessary if a general anesthetic is used.

The skin is first cleansed with soap and water or a detergent and then with alcohol or an antiseptic such as benzalkonium chloride. Ethyl chloride or other less flammable spray anesthetics, such as Frigiderm, are used most often for local anesthesia. After the skin preparation has been completed, the skin is stretched and its superficial layers are removed either by sandpapering or by using an abrasive machine (Dermabrader). If the procedure has not been extensive and oozing is slight, the area may be left uncovered. Usually it is covered either with an ointment or by moist compresses moistened with an antiseptic solution such as benzalkonium chloride and then by a pressure dressing which covers the entire face except for the eyes, nose, and mouth. Prepared dressings that adhere less readily to the skin surface, such as Telfa dressings, are also used.

If the patient has had a general anesthetic he must be turned to his side to prevent the dressings from becoming wet or contaminated in the event of vomiting or excessive salivation. The dressings should be checked for signs of bleeding, and the patient must be observed for signs of respiratory embarrassment which may be caused by pressure from the dressings. Pressure dressings usually are removed after forty-eight hours and the patient is discharged to return to the doctor's office or the clinic. Washing the face and shaving are seldom permitted until all the crusts have fallen away but some physicians permit the patient to wash his face gently with a mild soap as soon as the dressing has been removed. If the patient's face feels dry after healing has occurred, gentle lubrication with substances such as cold cream usually is advised. Dermal abrasion may be done in stages; at least two weeks and often longer may intervene between treatments.

MAMMAPLASTY

Some women develop conspicuously large and pendulous breasts which they wish to have reduced in size. Large breasts are embarrassing to some women and make it difficult for them to participate in sports, maintain good posture, and buy clothes that fit. Such women often respond to reconstructive surgery remarkably well.

Reconstructive surgery of the breast is usually major surgery and requires the use of general anesthetics and a hospital stay of about two weeks. Pressure dressings are kept in place for about a week postoperatively. The patient is advised to wear a firm, supporting brassière both night and day for several months after surgery. If the patient cannot make necessary adjustments in clothing she already owns, brassières are sometimes especially made. It is important that the fit be such that firm constant support is provided when the patient is in the prone position.

MAXILLOFACIAL SURGERY

Maxillofacial surgery is a specialty requiring a surgeon with unusual preparation and nurses with special knowledge and experience. Maxillofacial surgery received impetus as a result of the injuries sustained in World War II and the increase in radical surgery now being done for malignancies of the face. The surgeon works closely with the dental surgeon and with the specialist in problems of the nose and throat. Preventing infection, ensuring an airway, and providing nourishment for the patient are some of the greatest nursing problems. (For details of nursing care see Chapter 24.)

The emotional reactions of patients who undergo extensive maxillofacial surgery are severe, and one of the biggest nursing problems is attempting to keep up the patient's morale. The patient may be helped by seeing someone else who has undergone a similar operation with a good result and who has made good adjustment. When damage has been so great that reconstruction with living tissue is impossible, it is sometimes possible to construct prosthetic parts of the face that are so true to natural color and contour that they are not easily detectable. For example, a side of the nose may be replaced by a prosthetic part which is colored to match the patient's skin and disguised with marking to resemble skin. Rubber and a variety of plastic materials are used.

COSMETIC SURGERY

The most common operation for purely cosmetic effect is removal of some of the cartilage from the ears in order to flatten them against the head. This procedure is relatively simple for the plastic surgeon and requires only a short hospitalization.

Rhinoplasty, or reconstructive surgery of the nose, is another common cosmetic operation. Bone and cartilage may be removed from the nose if it is irregular or they may be inserted if defects such as saddle nose are being corrected. A local anesthetic is often used for these procedures unless it will interfere with a study of contours during the operation; if this is so, intravenous or rectal anesthetics may be used. The incision is usually made at the end of the nose inside the nostril so that it is not conspicuous. A nasal splint made of plaster, tongue blades, or crinoline may be used for protection. Immediately after the operation there will be ecchymosis and swelling around the eyes and nose; ice compresses and an ice bag may be used to help prevent these reactions. The patient must anticipate waiting several weeks before evaluating the final result of the operation.

Meloplasty is commonly called "face lifting." An incision is made at the hairline and excess skin is separated from its underlying tissue and removed. The remaining skin is pulled up and sutured at the hairline, thus removing wrinkles and giving firmness and smoothness to the face. A gentle pressure dressing is then applied and left in place for approximately a week. This procedure is sometimes repeated at intervals of five years or more.

REFERENCES AND SELECTED READINGS*

1 Barsky, Arthur J.: Principles and Practice of Plastic Surgery, Baltimore, 1950, Williams & Wilkins Co.
2 Conway, Herbert, and Stark, Richard B.: Plastic Surgery at the New York Hospital One Hundred Years Ago, New York, 1953, Paul B. Hoeber, Inc.
3 Davis, Loyal (editor): Christopher's Textbook of Surgery, ed. 6, Philadelphia, 1956, W. B. Saunders Co.
4 Iverson, Preston C., and Staneruck, Isabella D.: Dermal Abrasion—Surgical Care and Nursing Care After Dermal Abrasion, Am. J. Nursing **57**:860-864, July, 1957.
5 Kessler, Henry H.: Rehabilitation of the Physically Handicapped, New York, 1953, Columbia University Press.
6 *MacGregor, Frances Cooke: Some Psychological Hazards of Plastic Surgery of the Face, Plast. & Reconstruct. Surg. **12**:123-130, Aug. 1953.
7 MacGregor, Frances Cooke, and others: Facial Deformities and Plastic Surgery, Springfield, Ill., 1953, Charles C Thomas, Publisher.
8 National Research Council and Representatives of the Medical Department, U. S. Army: Plastic and Maxillofacial Surgery, Philadelphia, 1943, W. B. Saunders Co.
9 *Pearlman, Louis M.: Plastic Surgery, Am. J. Nursing **51**:618-620, Oct. 1951.
10 Stafford, Edward S., and Diller, Doris: Textbook of Surgery for Nurses, ed. 2, Philadelphia, 1954, W. B. Saunders Co.

*References preceded by an asterisk indicate material particularly well suited for student reading.

The patient with disease of the eye

Chapter 33

Study questions for review

1 Review the anatomy of the eye.
2 Is there an organization in your community which is concerned primarily with aid to the blind? If so, how is it financed?
3 From what you have learned in health hygiene classes or elsewhere in school, list some measures that everyone should take to preserve eye health.
4 Review the technique for application of sterile eye compresses.

Vision is one of man's most priceless possessions. It is essential to most employment and is necessary in countless experiences that make life enjoyable and meaningful. Yet each year in the United States many people are totally or partially blinded. Many of these suffer needlessly. For example, during each year 100,000 school children sustain serious accidental eye injuries. Glaucoma causes about 20,000 persons to become blind each year and industry loses an estimated 10 million dollars from unemployment due to this disease alone.[7] It is estimated that an additional 500,000 persons do not know that they have glaucoma and are currently sustaining eye damage which may lead to blindness.

Public education in the prevention of eye disease and help in assuring early medical care when disease symptoms appear have been traditional responsibilities of public health nurses. More recently, these activities have been recognized as appropriate functions for all nurses—those who work in hospitals, schools, and industry, and also those who marry and leave the profession.

This chapter deals with health education, as well as general nursing, in eye disease. At the conclusion of the discussion on general nursing, specific nursing procedures for a few of the more common eye conditions are discussed.

HEALTH EDUCATION IN CARE OF THE EYES AND IN PREVENTION OF DISEASE

By knowing a few simple facts, all nurses can teach the measures for maintenance of eye health and conservation of sight.

Normal eyes. Normal healthy eyes do not need special local treatment. The normal secretions of the conjunctiva are protective and should not be removed by frequent bathing with unprescribed solutions. Boric acid solution and numerous trade preparations recommended to cleanse the eyes are usually unnecessary. While these preparations are generally harmless, some proprietary solutions contain substances which may cause allergic reactions in sensitive persons.

If an individual complains of itching or burning of the eyelids after reading, or of the sensation of needing to "wash out his eyes," he should be advised to consult an ophthalmologist. Care should be taken not to irritate the eyes or introduce bacteria into the eyes by rubbing them. Children sometimes develop the habit of rubbing their eyes and this may persist into adulthood. Rubbing the eyes is a natural response of many persons under nervous strain. It may, however, be due to eczematous scaling, infection of the lids, or occasionally, to louse attachment on the lashes.

Nurses should be able to explain the complex structure of the eye and to clarify unfamiliar and misused terms. The term eyestrain is widely used and many people believe that this condition causes permanent eye damage. Eyestrain actually refers to strain of the ciliary muscles when there is difficulty in accommodation; it causes a sense of fatigue but does not produce serious damage to the eyes.

A good light should be used when reading and doing work that requires careful visual focus. Extremely fine work should not be done for long periods of time without giving the eye muscles periodic rest. Looking at distant objects for a few minutes helps to rest the eyes after close work. The eyes should be protected by goggles or special dark glasses from prolonged exposure to very bright light, such as sunlight over snow. They also need special protection from sudden flashes of light and heat that occur in some industrial occupations.

In the school and in the home, as well as in health agencies, the close relationship between diet and good eye health should be taught. One extensive 10-year study gave the amazing information that fully two thirds of a large group of boys and girls had eye difficulties related to dietary deficiencies.[17] Sometimes habit is the reason for poor nutrition. Older persons and those of teen age are perhaps the worst offenders in this respect. Elderly people may not have the energy or the incentive to prepare and eat proper meals. Teen-age boys and girls may eat poorly because of poor habits established in early childhood and because of adolescent notions and group preferences; an example is the so-called jitterbug diet, consisting mainly of soft drinks, frankfurters, potato chips, and ice cream. A lack of vitamin A in the diet can cause changes in the conjunctiva and corneal epithelium. Secretion of tears is reduced and the lid margins become reddened and inflamed. Sensitivity to light is often present, and some loss of visual acuity is noticed at night, although this must not be confused with true night blindness. This condition responds rapidly to a diet high in vitamin A. Lack of vitamin B in the diet can cause damage to the retina, and the public should know that damage due to poor nutrition may be irreversible if it continues too long. Emphasis in all teaching should be upon the daily essentials of good nutrition (see Chapter 5). A good practice is to have patients keep food-intake charts for a week. Many persons who believe that they are eating a well-balanced diet discover, on close scrutiny, that their eating practices are really poor. Sometimes there are financial reasons, and help may be needed in the selection of inexpensive but nutritious foods, such as dried milk and cheaper cuts of meat, to supply protein.

Terminology. There is widespread confusion and misunderstanding on the part of the public as to the proper specialist to consult about visual problems. This is particularly true of the aged and the foreign born who have trouble with our terminology. People who demand the best care when other medical and surgical problems arise may fail to seek help from an ophthalmologist when they have eye difficulties. Many persons do not understand the difference between the *orthoptist* who directs eye exercises, the *optician* who grinds and fits lenses, the *optometrist* who adjusts lenses to changes in accommodation of the eye, and the *ophthalmologist* or *oculist* who has had intensive medical training and experience in the diagnosis and treatment of eye diseases. In their search for help, a surprisingly large number of people respond to radio advertising and may even purchase glasses from store counters or use glasses originally prescribed for friends or relatives. These people need to understand that eye conditions cannot always be remedied simply by the purchase of a pair of glasses or a change of lenses.

Special teaching. Eye specialists now realize that examination of the eyes without examination of the rest of the body may lead to serious consequences. The eyes cannot be considered alone since they are often profoundly affected by conditions within the rest of the body. In fact, nearly all diseases of man cause some eye change that is diagnostically important.[6] The nurse who is teaching eye health must be aware of total health. When apparently minor disease or abnormality of the eyes occurs, she must be particularly alert for other signs of illness. Many serious medical conditions, such as diabetes, renal disease, and generalized arteriosclerosis, may be diagnosed through early recognition of eye symptoms and examination of the eyes by a medical specialist.

A dangerous but common belief is that eye drops and other medications which the patient or others have used at some time in the past can be useful in treating a new eye ailment. Most persons fail to realize that there is a variety of disorders that can effect the eyes and that many different drugs are used, each of which has a specific purpose. For example, two drugs may have completely opposite effects. Since liquids may evaporate and drugs may deteriorate, use of preparations that the patient or his friends may have on hand can contribute to actual damage. Real danger lies in self-treatment with proprietary remedies. Much valuable time for treatment can be lost by such dangerous practices.

Another detriment to good eye care is the natural human tendency to put things off, to reject any obvious fact that is unpleasant or disturbing, and to assume that an eye condition will "clear up" within a few days. Despite the fact that the average person thinks of loss of vision as a major catastrophe, he is careless in giving early attention to eye difficulties which, if neglected, may become serious. The danger of procrastination must be stressed since some eye diseases progress rapidly and irreparable damage may occur quickly. Neither the patient nor the nurse can know, for example, whether an irritation of the eyes is a simple conjunctivitis or an incipient acute glaucoma. The patient must never be permitted to postpone treatment and thus risk further infection or progress of disease.

A nurse should recognize danger signs. Without making the persons whom she encounters unduly apprehensive, the nurse should guide them in seeking appropriate treatment if signs of eye disease appear. Frequent headaches associated with reading indicate the need for medical care. Constant dull pain in the eyes, blurring of vision, spots before the eyes, rings around lights, and noticeable changes in visual acuity are signs that eye function is affected and should be investigated. Frequent changes of lenses and history of repeated visits to optometrists for lens changes indicate the need for complete medical examination. Every person 45 years of age or over should have this examination at least every two years and preferably each year.

Nurse-teachers and teachers should be alert to changes in the vision of children during the school year. Sometimes the more acute symptoms of a brain tumor in a child may be preceded by difficulties in seeing material on the chalkboard that is read easily by others, and seriously progressing nephritis in children may be heralded by visual difficulty before any other signs become apparent. Behavior problems in children are sometimes caused by eye difficulties. Irritability, restlessness, inability to concentrate, rubbing the eyes, and frowning may be signs of need for medical attention to the eyes.

One of the most tragic areas of neglect is that of *strabismus* in young children. Parents are naturally reluctant to face the fact that something about their child may not be quite normal. They are likely to believe and hope that the child will outgrow the condition, and they often believe that no accurate medical examination can be done until the child is able to read. Infants should have acquired binocular vision at about 6 to 9 months of age. If they do not, the mother should be advised to mention it to her doctor. Strabismus can be treated with glasses, exercises, or surgery, or a combination of these. The decision as to what is the best treatment should always rest with the ophthalmologist. It is most important, however, that treatment be started in the first year of the child's life, because prolonged strabismus can cause serious permanent damage to vision. Strabismus sometimes can be treated with glasses, and, if the glasses are worn before the end of the child's second year, no other treatment may be needed. Questions of parents as to whether or not glasses will have to be worn for the child's entire life should be referred to the specialist, because there is no safe answer for all cases. Glasses may or may not be discarded in later life, depending entirely upon the child's particular problem, his age when treatment is begun, and his progress. Wearing glasses, however, is not a serious handicap to normal play nor is it the threat to normal life that many parents fear. The vogue for attractive frames makes the wearing of glasses more acceptable to teen-age boys and girls.

Accidents. Prevention of accidental injury to the eyes should be stressed in child and parent education. Sling shots, BB guns, and even the seemingly harmless rubber bands and paper wads can be dangerous.

First-aid measures necessary in the event of eye injury should be known by everyone; these may be taught in schools. The nurse can help physical education teachers and others to be alert to hazards in gymnasiums and on playgrounds. The sight of many persons could be saved each year if everyone understood the need for immediate copious flushing of the eye with water when an acid or other irritating substance has been accidentally introduced. Much damage is done by the layman's well-intentioned efforts to remove foreign bodies from the eye, and the important rule of always washing the hands before attempting to examine the eye or to remove a foreign body is not always obeyed. Everyone should know that a person who has a foreign object lodged on the cornea must be referred to a physician; the layman should never attempt to remove it. The eye should be closed to prevent further irritation, the lids held shut and loosely covered with a dressing or patch anchored with a piece of cellophane or adhesive tape, and the patient should be taken to a doctor at once.

Special glasses and lenses. Nurses are often questioned about sunglasses, plastic lenses, and contact lenses. *Sunglasses* should be carefully ground and should be large enough to exclude bright light around their edges and dark enough to exclude about 30 per cent of the light. Tinted glass such as rose or green is of no particular value. The person who wears glasses regularly should have dark ones made from his prescription. Eyestrain can occur if correctly prescribed glasses are not worn by those who need them even though they wear dark glasses when in bright sunlight.

Light *plastic lenses* are useful for some persons who must wear thick lenses which are heavy when made of glass. Plastic lenses are useful for individuals engaged in vigorous activities since they do not break and splinter, and they do not fog easily in cold weather; they are often prescribed for active children. Plastic lenses must be carefully cleansed with soap and water; abrasive materials such as those contained in cleansing papers should not be used since they may scratch the plastic material. Experiments are being conducted on plastic lenses to be inserted in the eye when an opaque, crystalline lens (cataract) is removed. At the present time the procedure is still in the experimental stage, and persons who inquire about it should be referred to a medical specialist.

Contact lenses are expensive (average cost is $125) and are not suitable for persons who may not be able, physiologically or psychologically, to tolerate the constant presence of a foreign object. However, contact lenses have been perfected so that they can be worn continuously by some people. No artificial lubrication is needed because the normal conjunctival secretions accumulate behind the lenses in sufficient amounts. Contact lenses sometimes are prescribed for persons who have a cone-shaped deformity of the cornea (keratoconus) which may prevent satisfactory fitting with the usual glasses. They also may be prescribed for cosmetic reasons, particularly for those in public life such as the theater. Because they do not fog and are not easily broken, contact lenses are useful for persons engaged in active outdoor sports. The person who wishes contact lenses should be encouraged to discuss his particular need with an ophthalmologist.

GENERAL OPHTHALMOLOGIC NURSING

Examination of the eyes

Refraction is one of the most common eye examinations. This procedure reveals the degree to which the various light transmitting portions of the eye bring light rays into correct focus on the retina. Refractive errors account for the largest number of impairments to good vision. The refractive error is tested by means of trial lenses and the Snellen chart. Suitable glasses are then prescribed.

Some specific terminology must be understood before refractive studies can be meaningful. *Emmetropia* refers to a normal eye, while *ametropia* indicates that a refractive error is present. *Accommodation* is the ability to adjust vision from near to far objects; this is normally accomplished by the ciliary muscles which flatten or thicken the lens as need arises. *Myopia*, or nearsightedness, is caused by an unusually long anteroposterior dimension of the eyeball which causes light rays to focus in front of the retina. *Hyperopia*, or farsightedness, is caused when the anteroposterior dimension is too short so that light rays focus behind the retina. *Astigmatism* is a condition caused by asymmetry or irregular curvature of the cornea so that rays in the horizontal and perpendicular planes do not focus at the same point. *Presbyopia* occurs in persons past 40 years of age when the lens becomes more firm and responds less to the need for accommodation in viewing near and far objects. Blurring of near objects results, and those who require different lenses for distant and for close vision must get bifocal lenses.

Before refraction is performed the nurse may be asked to instill eye drops containing a medication which paralyzes the muscles of accommodation (cycloplegia) and dilates the pupil (mydriasis). A relatively new drug, Cyclogyl, has largely replaced atropine, which was previously used for children, and homatropine, which was used for young adults. Cyclogyl is effective in half an hour and the effect is worn off completely by the end of six hours. Homatropine usually requires one hour to take effect and causes some dilation to persist for at least twenty-four hours, while atropine must be instilled at intervals for three days prior to examination of children and persists in its action for about ten days. Therefore, Cyclogyl is much more convenient for the patient and for the doctor since the examination can be made at the first visit. Cyclogyl also lessens danger of accidents occurring as a result of poor vision following use of other cycloplegics. Persons over 40 years of age are usually given eye examinations without the use of cycloplegic drugs, because the power of accommodation has become sufficiently weak to permit satisfactory examination without their use.

The nurse who works in a clinic, in an ophthalmologist's office, or in schools must know how to do *vision screening* and how to teach others to do this. Distance vision is usually determined by use of a Snellen chart. Examination is done with the patient standing 20 feet from the chart. The chart consists of rows of letters or numbers or other characters arranged with the large ones at the top and the small ones at the bottom. The uppermost letter on the chart is scaled so that it can be read at 200 feet and the successive rows so that they can be read by the normal eye at 100, 70, 50, 40, 30, 20, 15, and 10 feet, respectively. Visual acuity is expressed as a fraction, with a reading of 20/20 considered normal. The upper figure refers to the distance of the patient from the chart, and the lower figure indicates the distance at which the smallest letters can be read by the person being tested. For example, the person who is only able to read at 20 feet the line which should be readable at 70 feet has 20/70 vision in that eye.

The distance from the chart to where the patient stands must be carefully measured. The person doing the testing usually stands beside the chart and points to the line to be read so that no mistake occurs; each eye is tested separately and its performance is carefully recorded. When testing vision, it is best to have the person being examined hold a piece of cardboard over his unused eye rather than have him attempt to read the line with first one and then the other eye closed. The Snellen chart examination is only a basic screening test. Additional detailed procedures must be done to test for nearsightedness, color blindness, and many other abnormalities.

Meticulous care must be taken to ensure cleanliness of all equipment used in eye examinations. The most common instrument used by the ophthalmologist is the *ophthalmoscope,* which comes close to the patient but not in direct contact with him. This instrument cannot be sterilized by boiling or autoclaving, but it should be wiped with a damp cloth after each use; alcohol is sometimes used. Special care should be taken if the patient has any evidence of an acute eye condition which might prove to be infectious.

Accurate determination of the intraocular pressure by use of a tonometer is becoming common in medical care. The general medical practitioner, as well as the eye specialist, now does this test quite often, because it is such a useful means for detecting early glaucoma. The Schiøtz tonometer is a delicate instrument that is placed directly on to the cornea and measures the pressure within the eyeball; 15 to 30 mm. Hg is considered normal. Before the test, the cornea is anesthetized with a drug such as Pontocaine, 0.5 per cent, in three doses. Cocaine is avoided, because it increases intraocular pressure and may soften the cornea and predispose it to damage. Some ophthalmologists use an antiseptic ointment or solution to protect the eye following this examination, and others have the patient wear a patch over the eye until the sensation of a foreign body in the eye disappears. Because the tonometer comes into direct contact with the eye, it must be carefully cleaned. Although it cannot be boiled, cleansing with soap and water followed by an antiseptic solution such as benzalkonium chloride is satisfactory. If alcohol is used, it must be thoroughly removed because it is irritating to the cornea.

Areas of opacity within the eye may be detected by means of a fine beam of light projected through the eye from a *slit lamp.* The limitation of visual field is determined by means of a *perimeter.* Pins are placed on a dark field to outline the patient's field of vision when he is seated a specific distance from the field. This tracing can then be transferred to the patient's chart for reference. Neither of these two eye examinations requires specific nursing assistance.

Local treatments

Accuracy in the administration of medications and treatments is essential. Irreparable damage can follow instillation of unprescribed or deteriorated preparations into the eyes. In the hospital all medication bottles must be checked frequently for smearing or obliteration of labels; solutions that have changed in color, that are cloudy, or that contain sediment should not be used. The nurse must know the usual dosage and strength of medications she uses. The following is a safe rule: Question any dosage that is over 1 per cent in strength unless one is completely familiar with the drug, with the patient, and with ophthalmologic nursing. The nurse who is assigned to care for patients with eye disease should immediately familiarize herself with the drugs most commonly used, the therapeutic dosages of these drugs, and their toxic signs. The nurse caring for the patient with an eye condition at home or teaching members of the patient's family to give care must be equally careful. The basic rule of checking labels three times should be adhered to. Checking must be done in a quiet environment and with careful thought so that it does not become a meaningless routine. Medicine cards must be carefully verified and the identity of the patient conclusively determined before eye medications are administered. In the home the patient should be protected from the use of incorrect drugs from the family medicine cupboard. Medications for the eyes should be placed carefully in a separate part of the cupboard and dangerous drugs removed if the patient is to select and administer his own medications.

Drugs. A large variety of drugs is used for treatment of eye diseases, and most of them are applied locally as drops, irrigations, or ointments. *Mydriatics* are drugs which dilate the pupil; *cycloplegics* paralyze the muscles of accommodation. Atropine, 0.5 to 1 per cent, homatropine, 2 per cent, and Cyclogyl, 1 per cent, are cycloplegics, whereas Neo-Synephrine is only mydriatic in its action. *Miotics* or drugs which contrict the pupil include physostigmine hydrobromide (eserine), 0.25 to 1 per cent, and pilocarpine, 1 to 2 per cent. *Local anesthetics* such as tetracaine (Pontocaine), 0.25 to 1 per cent, and cocaine, 1 per cent, are widely prescribed and often used with Adrenalin chloride, 1:10,000. Physiologic solution of sodium chloride or mild silver protein (Argyrol) are used as cleansing agents. Antibiotics such as penicillin are widely used in treating eye infections and may be given both locally and systemically. *Astringents* such as zinc sulfate preparations are often useful in chronic conjunctivitis, and fluorescein is employed to stain and thereby outline injury to the cornea.

Techniques. Nursing techniques for doing irrigations, applying compresses, and instilling eye drops are fully described in texts on fundamentals of nursing, therefore techniques will not be given in detail here. Gentleness is extremely important in performing all treatments. The natural sensitivity of the eye and the reluctance of the normal person to have anything done to his eyes is increased by pain, discomfort, and fear. Nature's powers of repair may be retarded by trauma resulting from pressure on the irritated or inflamed tissues. Hands must be thoroughly scrubbed before doing any eye treatment, and all materials placed in the eyes should be sterile. If the patient is being treated for an active infection, individual medicine bottles, droppers, tubes of ointment, and other equipment should be used. This would be necessary if an infected eye were being treated with an antibacterial drug such as penicillin and the same medication had been ordered prophylactically for the other eye. Many eye medications to be instilled as drops now come in bottles with droppers attached to the stopper. These can be used safely to dilate the eyes for examination and to treat noninfectious conditions such as glaucoma since the dropper does not touch the patient when proper technique is used.

A good light is necessary when giving treatments, but care must be taken to protect the patient's eyes from direct light. If one eye is affected with an inflammatory disease, the other eye may be covered to prevent the infection from spreading to it. A shield may be made from a watch glass or an eye patch covered with waterproof materials; the cover should be anchored to the skin with cellephone or adhesive tape. The covered eye should be inspected daily and any discomfort reported to the doctor immediately. Occasionally the good eye is covered to ensure more rest for the affected one, while at other times it is left uncovered. If severe emotional reaction to total, though temporary, blindness is anticipated, the unaffected eye usually is left uncovered.

Compresses. *Hot compresses* are used to relieve pain and improve circulation. They should be large enough to cover the entire orbit. Compresses are prepared in a variety of ways; they may be sterile or unsterile, depending upon the eye condition. If both eyes are involved and the condition is infectious, separate trays must be prepared and the hands carefully washed between treatment of each eye.

Compresses may be heated in a basin placed on an electric plate at the patient's bedside, or they may be heated in a strainer placed in steam and then applied with sterile forceps. A good unsterile compress is made by filling a large wooden kitchen spoon with gauze or cotton secured with gauze bandage. This is then dipped into the warm solution, pressed fairly dry with the rounded side of another spoon, and applied to the eye until it cools. An alternate spoon provides continuous treatment for the prescribed time. The spoon is easy for the patient to hold. The temperature of the solution used for compresses should not be over 49° C. (120° F.), and the treatment usually lasts for ten to twenty minutes and is repeated hourly or several times a day. Great care must be taken not to exert pressure on the eyeball when applying compresses. If there is evidence of irritation of the skin about the eyes, a small amount of sterile petrolatum can be used, but it should not be allowed to enter the eyes.

Cold compresses are often ordered to help control bleeding immediately following eye injury, to prevent or control edema in allergic conditions, and to attempt to prevent spread of infection in the early stages of such conditions as conjunctivitis. A small basin of sterile solution may be placed in a bowel of chipped ice at the bedside; sterile forceps are used to wring out and apply the compress. If the compress does not need to be sterile, pieces of gauze or cotton may be placed on a piece of ice at the patient's bedside. A rubber glove packed with finely chipped ice may be adjusted to the eye and necessitates fewer changes of compresses.

Irrigations. Eye irrigations are done to remove secretions, to cleanse the eye preoperatively, and to supply warmth. Pillows should be protected with waterproof material, and irrigations should always be done with the patient lying comfortably toward one side so that fluid cannot flow into the other eye. A rubber bulb syringe is usually used unless very large amounts of fluid are needed. Physiologic solution of sodium chloride is most often prescribed since it is considered more soothing and less likely to cause pain than plain sterile water. Irrigating fluid is directed along the conjunctiva and over the eyeball from the inner to the outer canthus, and care is taken to avoid directing a forceful stream onto the eyeball or to touch any eye structures with the irrigating equipment. If there is drainage from the eye, the nurse should wrap a piece of gauze about her index finger to raise the lid and ensure thorough cleansing.

Instillation of medications. Eye drops should be sterile. Each patient should have his own bottle of medication; however, if stock solutions are used, only enough should be drawn out for use at one time. If the bottle is small, it may be warmed slightly by holding it in the hands for a few moments. Eye droppers must be sterile. The dropper is held downward so that medication does not flow into the rubber bulb since foreign material from the bulb can contaminate the solution. When instilling eye drops, the lower lid should be gently turned outward, and the dropper should approach the patient's eye from the side and not directly. Drops are placed on the conjunctiva; care should be taken not to touch the eyelids, the conjunctiva, or the eyeball with the dropper. The eyelids should then be closed and, unless eye motion is contraindicated for some reason, the patient instructed to roll his eyes a few times to ensure even distribution of the medication.

A small, sterile, glass spatula may be used to apply ointments to the eyes. The most common and satisfactory method, however, is to express the ointment directly on to the conjunctiva from a small individual tube. Care is taken not to touch tissues with the tube.

The patient's environment

Most patients with acute eye conditions are more comfortable in a darkened room, provided it is not dreary and depressing. Screens or curtains should be arranged so that bright light does not enter the room. Bright artificial lighting should be shaded. Persons with chronic eye diseases also are more comfortable in a room that is not too well lighted. The patient in the hospital is usually happiest in a room with others, especially if both eyes are covered or if he is unable to see. The sound of voices and normal activity around him tends to relieve the feeling of isolation that the blinded person experiences; he benefits from having others around him who may, for example, share newspaper headlines with him. Radios also help the patient to keep up with everyday events.

Accidents present a real hazard when eye disease occurs. If the onset of visual loss is slow, the patient and his family may have sufficient time to eliminate common household hazards such as stairs without banisters. The partially blinded person who receives care on an ambulatory basis is taught to have someone accompany him to the doctor's office or clinic because he may need additional help for a short time after certain treatments. In the hospital, special measures to prevent accidents are necessary. Side rails are usually needed on beds, and low beds are safer, particularly for older patients who may forget that they are in a hospital bed. Particular effort should be made to have the space around the patient's bed and chair uncluttered; for example, gooseneck lamps and electric plates used for compresses must have short cords that do not fall to the floor. If the patient has serious visual difficulty, hot plates for compresses are not kept at the bedside because the patient may burn himself. Furniture should be firmly anchored with casters locked; rails along hallways and in bathrooms are also helpful.

Emotional factors in loss of sight

Emotional reactions to temporary or threatened loss of sight is often severe. Even if the individual has been careless with his eyes, he is much disturbed at the thought of losing his vision. Fear of learning that what he suspects is true may lead the patient to reject danger signs and delay medical attention. Worries over finances and family support and of being conspicuous among others may be added to concern over losing vision. Often the medical social worker can help the patient by talking through his many problems.

Picture the young man who has a traumatic injury to his eye; one day he sustains what appears to be a relatively minor eye injury, the next day he learns that the injury was deeper than was first believed, and the next day he is told that his eye must be removed. Emotional reaction to news of this sort is so great that it cannot be expected that the patient will behave rationally. The patient may be demanding and impatient when he fears that his vision is threatened. Treatments must be done on time, because delay in treatments is of vital significance to the patient even when adherence to a rigid schedule may be irrelevant from a therapeutic point of view.

Sudden or jerky movements must be avoided in caring for any patient with eye disease since the natural reaction, blinking, may be painful or impossible. Jerky movements and haste tend to make the patient "on edge" and hamper release of tension and rest.

The person with visual loss depends upon immediate sound and tactile sensation to maintain his feeling of security and kinship with those around him. He must be spoken to frequently in a quiet and reassuring voice. This is particularly important when he is in a strange hospital environment awaiting diagnostic procedures and perhaps surgery.

It is upsetting to the patient who cannot see to be touched without first being spoken to; this can be irritating and humiliating as well as actually dangerous. The nurse must teach all who attend the patient and who are under her supervision the importance of making their nearness known to the patient before touching him. The elderly patient who is also deaf presents a real problem, for then there is no alternative but to touch him gently to make one's presence known. Elderly persons who use hearing aids are urged to bring them to the hospital when surgery such as a cataract extraction is anticipated. Frequent physical contact must be made with the patient who is both deaf and blind if he is to remain in contact with his environment. The nurses should speak and let the patient know when they are leaving the room so he is spared the embarrassment of talking to someone who is not there. A small bell is often used instead of a call signal; this gives the patient who can hear the assurance that his request has been made since he is not able to see the light flick on in response to pulling a signal cord.

Life for the patient who has both eyes covered should be made as normal as possible. If he is used to smoking, he should be permitted to smoke although someone must be in attendance to prevent a fire. Visitors should be allowed, though sometimes they need assistance in learning how to conduct themselves when they are with the patient who cannot see. They should be as natural as possible; for example, they should not make a conspicuous attempt to avoid such common phrases in speech as "see what I mean." Common sense makes it obvious that gifts should appeal to other senses than vision; scented colognes and soaps or a small bouquet of highly scented favorite flowers should be brought, for instance, instead of a large display bouquet of flowers.

Restraints are sometimes necessary to prevent the patient from disturbing his dressings during sleep. These can be psychologically traumatizing unless carefully explained to the patient. Restraints should be very light in weight and loosely attached to the wrists; usually a 2-inch gauze bandage is used. A boxing glove type of hand restraint is also used. It must be clearly explained to the patient that the restraints are used only to cause him to awaken and recall where he is and what has happened so that he will not touch his dressings. If this is not sufficient to prevent disturbance of dressings, the patient should be constantly attended rather than restrained. The use of side rails should be explained in the same fashion. They are primarily to assist the patient in carefully shifting his position without turning, if this is permitted, and to remind him not to get out of bed; they are not used to keep him in bed forcibly.

Preoperative care

Routines for preoperative treatment and care vary with the part of the country, the institution, and the eye surgeon. If a complete medical examination has not been given before hospitalization, the patient usually spends a few days in the hospital preoperatively. The patient's general condition and his reaction to the anticipated surgery must be closely observed and reported. He should meet the staff in the unit and get to know other patients; this is especially important if he is to have both eyes covered following surgery. The patient often benefits from meeting and talking to another patient who has successfully recovered from a surgical treatment such as he is to receive. He should be prepared for the routines necessary for his care following his return from the operating room.

Sedatives may be given the night before and on the morning of surgery. Unusual reactions to sedation must be carefully observed and reported. Enemas may be given if a general anesthetic is to be used and if the patient is to remain in bed for some time following surgery. The patient may be taken to the operating room in his bed, and sometimes the operation is performed without removing him from his bed. When this is to be done, the patient is placed head to foot in the bed for the convenience of the surgeon.

Local preparation of the eye may be started in the unit, although some surgeons prefer that part or all of this preparation be done in the operating room. The eyelids may be gently washed with a very mild soap, the lashes cut, and the eyes irrigated with physiologic solution of sodium chloride at body temperature. A topical anesthetic such as tetracaine, 1 per cent, Butyn, 2 per cent, Holocaine,

1 per cent, or cocaine, 2 per cent, may be instilled into the eyes at specified times before the patient goes to the operating room. Antibiotics may be instilled in the eyes as many as twenty-four hours preoperatively. Some surgeons wish for the eye to be covered with a pad following local preparation; others may prefer to have the eye left uncovered, in which case it can be identified more easily by marking the eye or cheek with a colored solution.

Procaine hydrochloride (Novocain), 2 per cent, with Adrenalin may be injected into the conjunctiva, and cocaine, 4 per cent, may be used to anesthetize the site of operation. Occasionally a general anesthetic must be used when the patient has generalized pain and for certain operations such as removal of an eye. General anesthesia is avoided when possible, because restlessness may occur as the patient reacts, and this may be damaging to the surgical wound. If a general anesthetic is needed, thiopental sodium (Pentothal sodium) given intravenously or Avertin given rectally is most often used.

Postoperative care

It is impossible to outline routines for postoperative care following eye surgery since they have changed so much in recent years and are still changing. In the past, most eye surgery was associated with long periods of immobilization, and the patient did not even move for several days following some surgery. Now much more freedom of movement is permitted. The nurse should expect routines to vary with different hospitals, and she should learn the routines of the institution in which she is employed. Only a few principles of general postoperative care will be included here.

It is reasonable to assume that the patient should be quiet no matter what the current regimen for rest or freedom of activity may be. Immediately after the operation the patient probably should keep his head fairly still; he should not jerk suddenly, cough, strain, or vomit. If a general anesthetic has been given, care must be taken that dressings are not loosened or removed as the patient awakens. Dressings should be adjusted by the doctor if they are tight or uncomfortable. Bleeding and drainage of serous fluid may occur when an eye has been removed or other extensive surgery performed; this should be reported to the eye surgeon at once.

The patient who has had eye surgery may develop the same postoperative complications as other surgical patients, and the same attention should be given to deep breathing, moving the limbs, muscle setting, and other permitted activity that prevents complications such as thrombosis, emboli, and lung congestion. Backache is a problem if the patient cannot turn, be raised in bed, or be out of bed. This may be relieved by placing a very small pillow under the curve of the back, by slipping one hand under the patient and lightly massaging the back at frequent intervals, and by having the patient alternately raise his knees and consciously extend his legs, thereby changing tension on the back muscles. Backache can cause greater discomfort to the patient than the eye operation.

General care, including mouth hygiene and giving enough fluids, may be difficult if the patient's activity is curtailed. Urinary and bowel elimination must be carefully noted and recorded. Mineral oil is often given to lessen difficulty in having bowel movements.

A soft diet may be ordered for a few days postoperatively, although some doctors feel that a diet which permits moderate chewing will decrease distention and discomfort. If both eyes are covered, the patient may be fed as long as dressings are in place. Otherwise, whether or not he needs assistance depends on the amount of vision he has and his general condition. When feeding the patient who cannot see, it is important to identify the kind of food he is to receive. The nurse must not allow the feeding of her patient to become a routine procedure and she must not appear hurried. If he is to have visual limitation for some time, he must be helped to learn to feed himself.

Postoperative confusion is a problem, particularly in elderly persons and in those who have both eyes covered. Since the eyes move together, it is considered best to cover both when rest is necessary for healing. This should be fully explained to the patient preoperatively and the explanation repeated postoperatively. If confusion does occur, the surgeon may decide that the danger of this activity is worse than activity resulting from having one eye uncovered. For this reason, many surgeons no longer attempt to cover the unoperated eye.

The nurse must help the patient and his family develop patience and learn not to expect an immediate cure from the operation. This demands understanding by both the patient and his family. Even though the problem has been explained by his doctor, the patient often expects that the moment the dressings are removed he will be cured. He may never be cured but only have his eye condition improved, and he should know this. It may take weeks and even months for him to become accustomed to the type of glasses he must wear.

After surgery the patient should follow his doctor's instructions carefully and keep appointments as specified. Many patients must return to the doctor's office or the clinic periodically for a long time, some indefinitely. The nurse caring for the patient in the hospital has a responsibility to teach him this when he is most receptive to teaching. The nurse working in the community can be invaluable in arranging for clinic care and in helping the patient and his family to avoid discouragement, to administer medications as prescribed, and to report to the doctor regularly.

A big problem in the patient's adjustment is that he or his family often know or know of someone who had the same diagnosis. That person perhaps did better or improved faster than the patient, and the patient becomes dissatisfied unless he realizes that there is a great deal of difference in each patient, even though the diagnosis may be the same.

Removal of the eye

An eye, with or without its supportive structures, may be removed for four reasons: (1) in an attempt to save life when a malignant tumor has developed, (2) to save sight in the other eye when sympathetic ophthalmia is feared or threatens, (3) to control pain in an eye blinded by disease such as chronic glaucoma or chronic infection, or (4) for cosmetic reasons following blindness from trauma or disease. *Enucleation* is removal of the eyeball, and *evisceration* is the removal of the contents of the eyeball, leaving only the sclera. Occasionally, the entire eye with the surrounding structures must be removed (exenteration) because of a disease such as cancer. If feasible, the eyeball alone is removed, leaving the surrounding membrane (Tenon's capsule) and the muscle attachments. A gold ball or a piece of body fat may be inserted and the capsule sutured over this. This provides a stump for support and motion to the artificial eye and therefore a more normal appearance. The gold ball is left in place permanently.

Hemorrhage, thrombosis of blood vessels, and infection are possible complications following enucleation, exenteration, or evisceration of an eye. Moist sterile dressings are usually applied at the conclusion of the operation, and these are not changed for one or two days unless unusual bleeding or drainage is observed. Pressure dressings may be used for one to two days to help control possible hemorrhage. Headache or pain in the operated side of the head should be reported at once since meningitis occasionally occurs as a complication following thrombosis of adjacent veins. The patient is usually allowed out of bed the day following surgery.

An *artificial eye* can be used as soon as healing is complete and edema has disappeared. This is usually from six to eight weeks after operation, although many patients begin to wear an artificial eye after

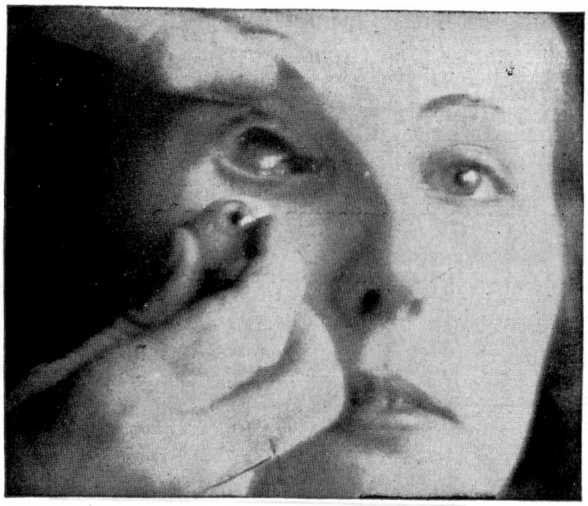

A

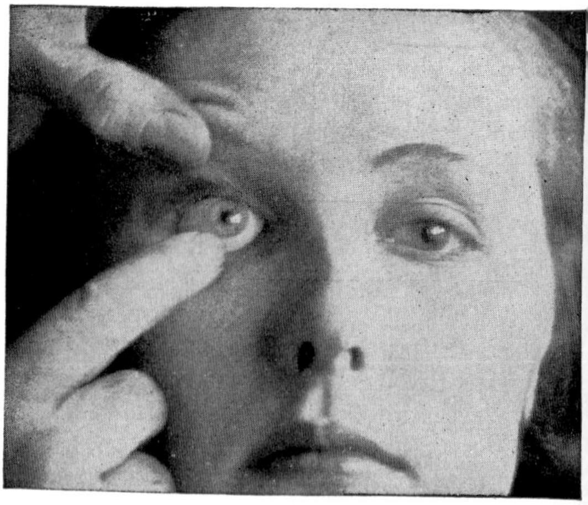

B

Figure 106

A to *D*. Steps in inserting an artificial eye. (From Parkinson, Roy H.: Eye, Ear, Nose, and Throat Manual for Nurses, St. Louis, 1959, The C. V. Mosby Co.)

only three weeks. Artificial eyes are made of glass or plastic materials. Glass eyes last longer if not broken, but they are heavier; plastic ones must usually be replaced every year or two because they become roughened around the edges, and this may be irritating to the conjunctiva. There are two kinds of artificial eyes: the shell-shaped and the hollow artificial eye. The choice for the individual patient depends on what operation has been done. Artificial eyes may be bought in shades which closely match the normal eye or they may be especially made. Stock eyes of plastic cost approximately $50 and glass ones $15; the prices for custom-made eyes are about $110 for the plastic and $35 for the glass. Artificial eyes that almost exactly match the natural eye can be made, but the pupil must, of course, remain fixed.

Even young children can be taught to care for their own artificial eyes. Usually the eye is removed before retiring and kept either in a clean dry place after cleansing or in a glass of normal saline solution. The eye should be cleansed immediately after its removal and care taken not to scratch the surface. The eye is removed by gently pressing upward on the lower lid, being certain that the cupped hand is held against the cheek so the eye does not fall to the floor and break or become lost. It is inserted by gently everting the lower lid, being certain that the narrower end of the eye is placed next to the inner angle of the orifice. Then by grasping the upper lashes and gently raising the upper lid, the eye is easily slipped into place. (See Figure 106.) Most people who wear prosthetic eyes keep an extra one in case the eye in use should be lost or broken.

More important than care of the artificial eye is care of the remaining eye. The person who has only one eye is advised to wear protective nonbreakable glasses. He is also instructed to avoid excessive strain on the eye, for example, strain which might be caused by extended television viewing. The patient must be prepared for the adjustment necessary in learning to carry on normal activities with only one eye and of the accident hazards entailed. Driving a car, for example, is dangerous for the person who suddenly must use only one eye. With patience, however, almost all normal activities are possible—

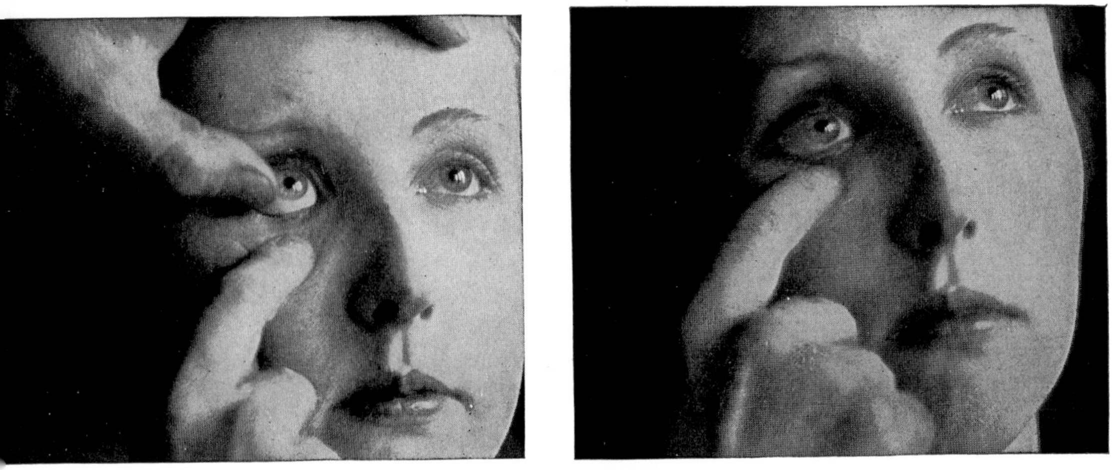

C D

Figure 106 (**Cont'd**)

For legend, see opposite page.

even surgeons who have had an eye removed have been able to learn to operate successfully using only one eye.

Blindness

Despite the best efforts of all concerned, some patients will become blind. It then becomes the responsibility of the nurse, working with other members of the health team and with the patient, to help him adjust to his blindness.

There are now approximately 350,000 blind persons in this country.[16] It is likely that the number of blinded persons will increase in the future since glaucoma, cataracts, and degenerative disease associated with arteriosclerosis occur in older people, and this part of our population is increasing faster than the population as a whole.

Two thirds of those who are blind lose their vision after the age of 20 years, so it is necessary for a majority of the blinded to learn a completely new way of life. It is estimated that between 20 and 30 per cent of those who become blind are employable, and many state and voluntary services have been established to assist them in rehabilitation.

The decision as to whether or not the patient should be told of approaching blindness or of certain blindness must rest with the doctor. Usually it is considered best for the doctor to be completely honest and frank with the patient, provided he is certain that blindness will occur or is irreversible. The patient who has a little time before becoming blind may then use it to good advantage by beginning certain rehabilitative activities (for example, learning braille), and he is spared the period of wishful hoping during which no rehabilitative activities are begun.

When the patient has been told that he will become blind, it is to be expected that he will be depressed for a while. This is a normal reaction and is described by psychiatrists as a period of mourning for his dead eyes which the patient must undergo before he can begin to think and plan for his new life.[8]

The nurse can help the patient during his period of adjustment to partial or complete blindness. She can merely listen to him talk of what blindness means to him, she can report any exaggerated reactions

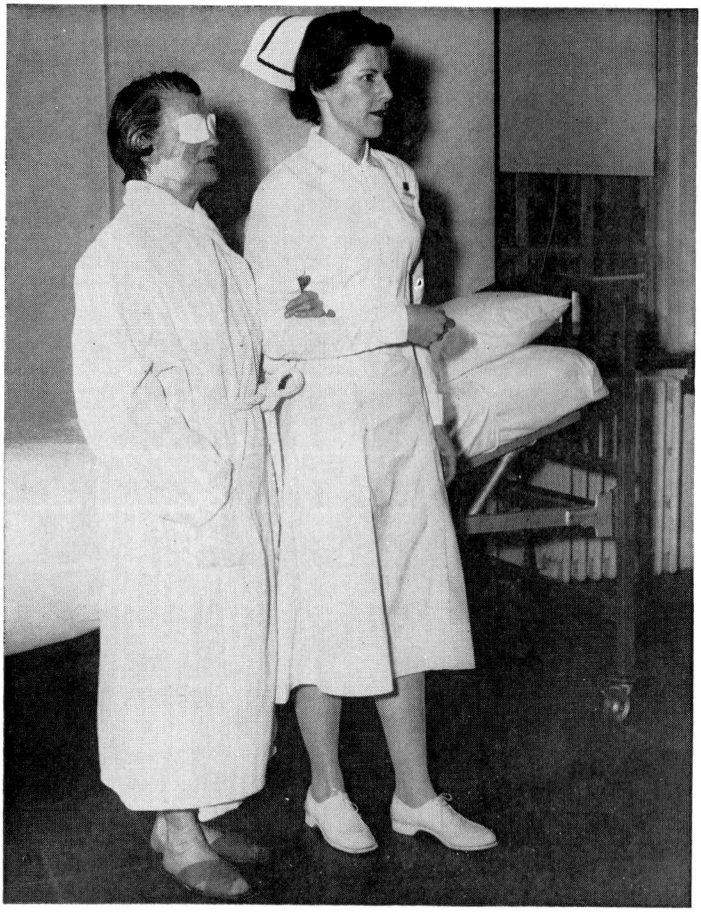

Figure 107

Ambulation of a patient who cannot see.
Note that the patient holds onto the nurse's arm and is thus lead
to her destination without being held.

which might indicate thoughts of self-destruction, she can direct the patient's thinking gradually along positive constructive lines, and she can help to make available to him the resources that he will need.

Rehabilitation. Important contributions that the nurse can make to rehabilitation are to begin to teach the patient as soon as he becomes blind and to encourage him to carry out the activities of daily living. (See Figure 107.) She can also help members of his family see the importance of letting the patient experience the satisfaction of his own independence. It is imperative that the patient be given an opportunity to preserve his self-respect and esteem by caring for his personal needs. He should be urged to feed, clothe, bathe, and otherwise care for himself. The family needs expert counseling and guidance since the natural tendency is to overprotect the patient and thus render him completely helpless. The nurse can suggest ways in which the home may be arranged to prevent accidents and to permit the blinded person to get about without embarrassment.

The patient will have many questions and many needs. He may, for example, want to go to the occupational therapy department of the hospital to learn to type, or he may want to know how he may arrange to learn braille and what cost is involved. The patient may be impatient to know his chances of learning a new occupation. The nurse's actual participation in giving direct help will depend on whether she works in a hospital which has a social service department and other good rehabilitation resources or whether she works in a rural public health nursing agency where she may have to seek specific answers for the patient rather than refer his questions to others. The nurse who works with patients with eye disease and blindness should familiarize herself with the local resources in her own community. Religious groups such as Catholic Charities, the Salvation Army, and others often have programs in local areas. Almost every state has a voluntary organization devoted to this need, and the nurse can learn about it by writing to the state health department. Some state health departments also have their own special programs. If the patient qualifies, help may also be available through the Veterans Administration.

National voluntary organizations. Two national voluntary organizations concerned with blindness and the prevention of blindness are the American Foundation for the Blind* and the National Society for the Prevention of Blindness.† Both of these have literature which is available to nurses and patients upon request. The American Foundation for the Blind distributes a booklet entitled *Tools and Aids for the Blind* which contains a list of aids for the blind and the partially blind; for example, magnifying glasses that can be carried in the pocket and used to see street signs are described and a variety of special syringes and aids for giving injections are described for the partially blinded person who has to give himself injections of insulin or other medication. The primary functions of the National Society for the Prevention of Blindness include research, education, and preventive services. Pamphlets and films are available for both lay and professional use. The quarterly publication of this voluntary organization, *The Sight Saving Review,* is available to nurses and covers many aspects of sight conservation and eye health.

Legal blindness. A person is considered legally blind when his vision in the better eye is reduced to 20/200 or less even with the use of corrective lenses. This means that he is able to see at 20 feet what the normal person can see at 200 feet. Legal blindness entitles a person to certain federal assistance. The Social Security Act in 1952 made provision for assistance to the blind and now all fifty states and all territories have approved plans for such aid. Assistance through this program is based on need. In April 1959, 109,500 persons received aid to the blind, with a national average payment of $68.56.[16] The Internal Revenue Act of 1948 permits blinded persons an extra deduction ($600) in reporting income. In 1943 the federal government established a counseling and placement service for the blind in the Office of Vocational Rehabilitation; it shares cost of rehabilitation with the states. The Veterans Administration provides a substantial pension for the single veteran who has enucleation of both eyes even when he has no other physical defects.

Schools. Progress has been made in improving school opportunities for the blind. In 1953, thirty-eight cities and fourteen states had provisions and facilities for blind children to attend the public schools, and 1,500 pupils were enrolled. Eighteen states have legislated funds to provide higher education for the blind and to provide readers for them.[15]

*The American Foundation for the Blind, 15 West Sixteenth Street, New York 11, N.Y.

†The National Society for the Prevention of Blindness, 1790 Broadway, New York 17, N. Y.

DISEASE CONDITIONS AND RELATED NURSING CARE

Trauma

Trauma may damage the eyelids and adjacent structures, the outer surface of the eyeball, and the deep structures of the eye. (For details of first aid in event of eye injury, see Chapter 15.) Lacerations of the eyelids should be treated by an eye specialist, because there is danger of scar formation as healing occurs. Any injury to the eyeball should be referred immediately to the specialist; no attempt should ever be made to remove a splinter or foreign object that has penetrated the cornea. Sometimes very small sharp objects may penetrate the eyeball without the patient knowing that more than the outer surface of the eye has been injured.

Hospital treatment of eye injuries may include cold compresses to attempt to stop bleeding within the eyeball, followed by warm compresses and other forms of heat in an attempt to increase absorption of blood and serous fluid. Infection is a serious complication and occurs easily since some of the eye structures such as the cornea are sparsely supplied with blood vessels. Antibiotics are usually given systemically and topically, and antitetanus serum is usually given to all patients who sustain eye injury.

The most dreaded sequel to eye injury is *sympathetic ophthalmia;* it occurs in about 2 per cent of all penetrating injuries which involve the uveal tract (ciliary body, iris, and choroid). Sympathetic ophthalmia causes inflammation and destruction of the good eye, and, once established, it is not arrested by removal of the injured eye. Sometimes the onset of sympathetic ophthalmia is delayed for several months. The cause of this condition is unknown, although it is speculated that an allergic reaction to the pigment of the injured iris may be a cause, since sympathetic opthalmia never appears earlier than twelve days after the injury and never develops if the injured eye is removed within a week of the injury. Before the use of cortisone it usually resulted in total or almost complete loss of vision of both eyes. When cortisone has been given immediately following the injury or at the first sign of involvement of the good eye, it has saved the vision of many patients. The decision as to whether or not the involved eye should be removed rests with the surgeon and often depends on the amount of damage to the uveal tract. Fever therapy is used, and large doses of salicylates are sometimes given in an attempt to prevent progress of sympathetic ophthalmia, but their usefulness is unproved.

Infections and inflammation

Infections and inflammation can occur in any of the eye structures and may be due to the presence of organisms, to mechanical irritation, or to sensitivity reactions.

Styes. Styes (hordeola) are relatively mild but extremely common infections of the small lubricating glands of the lid margins. Staphylococci are often the infecting organisms. If warm moist compresses are used, styes usually open and drain without surgery. These infections come in a series (recur at intervals), affecting those who use their eyes a great deal and those who need glasses but do not use them. Poor nutrition and lowered resistance to infection may also be contributing causes.

Chalazion. A chalazion is a cyst of the meibomian glands in the tarsal plate of the lids. Cysts present a hard, shiny, lumpy appearance as viewed from the inner side of the lid, and they may cause pressure on the cornea. If they become infected they are red and painful and usually require surgical excision after warm moist compresses have been used. Chalazions are usually removed in the doctor's office or the clinic under local anesthesia; an antibacterial ointment such as penicillin is then instilled into the eye, and a pad is worn for a day or two.

Conjunctivitis and blepharitis. Conjunctivitis, or inflammation of the conjunctiva, and blepharitis, or inflammation of the eyelids, are common infections and have a variety of causes. They may result from mechanical trauma such as that caused by sunburn, or infection with organisms such as staphylococci, streptococci, gonococci, or viruses may be the cause. Inflammation is often due to allergic reactions within the body or to outside irritants such as poison ivy. "Pink eye" (conjunctivitis caused by the Koch-Weeks bacillus) is common in school children and is highly infectious; however, it responds to treatment with penicillin.

Treatment for conjunctivitis depends upon the cause. Specific antibacterial drugs may be used systemically and locally. Compresses, irrigations, eye drops, and ointments are often prescribed. The patient must be cautioned not to touch his eyes since the inflamed tissues are susceptible to new infection, and trauma delays healing. If only one eye is involved, he must be cautioned to leave his good eye strictly alone; frequently the good eye is covered for its protection. Patients with blepharitis or conjunctivitis rest better in a darkened room than in a well-lighted one. They must be carefully observed for progress of the eye condition; infections of the conjunctiva can be stubborn and can even lead to involvement of the cornea with serious consequences to vision, and blepharitis can extend to the conjunctiva. Before the Credé method of protecting the eyes of newborn infants by instilling silver nitrate solution and before the discovery of penicillin to treat gonorrhea, the most common cause of blindness in children was destruction of the cornea. This followed an overwhelming infection of the conjunctiva caused by gonococci from the birth canal.

Corneal ulcer. A corneal ulcer indicates either an abrasion or infected lesion on the surface of the cornea. They may be caused by trauma or by infections of the conjunctiva which have spread to the cornea. Persons with a low resistance to infection may develop ulcers from little apparent cause (for example, the individual who has diabetes). The extent of the ulcer can be outlined by using fluorescein, a green, harmless dye. Treatment for corneal ulcers includes rest for the eye and locally and systemically administered drugs to prevent and control infection. When a traumatic abrasion has occurred, a drop of sterile oil is placed in the eye and a pad is worn until the lesion heals. Infected corneal ulcers may be exceedingly stubborn and difficult to cure; occasionally they progress despite all medical effort and, depending on their location, may cause partial or total blindness.

Keratitis. Inflammation of the cornea is called keratitis. It causes severe pain in the eye, tearing and redness; it may be acute or chronic and superficial or deep (interstitial). The cause of keratitis is often difficult to determine; however systemic infection or allergic reaction may contribute to its development. A virus may be the cause. It is sometimes caused by disease such as tuberculosis and syphilis; chronic interstitial keratitis frequently is known to accompany congenital syphilis. There is no specific treatment unless the causative organism is known; for example, penicillin may be given if the patient has a positive serologic test for syphilis. Hot compresses decrease pain and perhaps alleviate the condition, and cortisone has been found useful for some patients. Keratitis can produce clouding of the cornea and loss of vision.

Corneal grafts (keratoplasty) taken from other human beings have been a boon to many patients with loss of vision resulting from corneal ulcers and interstitial keratitis. Such grafts have been surprisingly satisfactory when done by skilled ophthalmologists. Donors or their relatives usually make the arrangements before death, since the cornea must be removed within six hours of death and used within twenty-four hours (a longer period of time is sometimes considered safe). The present practice is to keep a waiting list of persons who need grafts, since eye banks are not able to keep up with the demand. Eye Bank for Sight Restoration, Inc. is a nonprofit organization founded in 1945 which collects and distributes donated eyes throughout the country.

Corneal transplantation cannot be done if there is any infection, and it is usually performed under local anesthesia. Only the operated eye is covered, and the patient is permitted out of bed the day after surgery. It takes approximately two weeks or more for the graft to heal and longer to be certain that the results of operation are satisfactory. There are several complications of corneal transplant operations; blood vessels may grow into the new cornea (compensatory neovascularization), and clarity may be lost or the new cornea may become cloudy for no apparent reason. The operation can usually be repeated, but this depends on the condition of the patient's eye.

Iritis. Iritis (inflammation of the iris) often occurs in combination with inflammation of the ciliary body and the choroid; then the term *uveitis* is used. Iritis and uveitis produce pain, redness, sensitivity to light (photophobia), and diminished vision, and they result from several causes. They may be associated with a systemic disease, such as syphilis or tuberculosis; in these circumstances hot compresses and atropine used with systemic treatment of the underlying cause produce a cure. Other infections also cause the disease, and, if discovered and removed, the inflammation usually disappears. At other times there seems to be no known cause for the inflammation, although a toxic reaction to some foreign substance may be the causative factor. Some patients respond favorably to corticosteroids, but others resist almost all forms of treatment. Complications of the two diseases are adhesions (synechiae) of the uveal tract and related structures with secondary glaucoma and loss of vision.

Atropine is instilled into the eyes of the patient with iritis in the hope of preventing the iris from becoming adherent to the lens capsule, thus interfering with the flow of aqueous fluid into the posterior chamber, since this would lead to increased intraocular pressure and secondary glaucoma. Salicylates are sometimes given, but their action is not specific.

Fever therapy is an old standard form of treatment for uveitis and is still used when other treatment is ineffective. Typhoid vaccine ordinarily is used for adults and boiled milk for children; both are given intramuscularly. Since the reaction to fever therapy is sometimes severe, this treatment is not given until the patient has had a careful medical evaluation, and the status of his heart has been determined. A temperature elevation of 40.5° C. (103° F.) is considered desirable; usually at least six bouts of fever are produced. The treatment is given every other day or several times a week.

When fever therapy is ordered, the nurse prepares the patient for the chills and discomfort that he will experience. The patient must be attended closely during the stage of fever; adequate covers should be available for the period of chilling and warm fluids should be forced. Temperature and pulse rate are taken every fifteen minutes when temperature begins to rise (usually one-half to one hour after administration of the foreign substance) and until it subsides, which is usually in three to four hours. Any rise of temperature above that desired by the doctor should be reported at once; patients have been known to sustain severe reactions to this treatment with response far beyond that which is generally anticipated. The patient should remain in bed during the course of fever treatment and usually an ice cap applied to the head adds to comfort. After the temperature has passed its peak and diaphoresis occurs, a sponge bath may be given and fluids again forced. A course of fever therapy may be debilitating to the patient. He must be encouraged to take extra amounts of high-calorie foods between treatments; care must be taken to prevent accidents when he gets out of bed following a bout of fever.

Strabismus

Strabismus, or squint, may be present at birth and be caused by birth injury; it may appear a year or later after birth and may be caused by eye differences, or it may follow severe trauma, such as skull fracture, at any age. Only strabismus occurring in early childhood will be considered here.

When the infant with normal eyes is born, his eyes do not focus together. At the age of 6 to 8 weeks, his eyes begin to work harmoniously, and by the age of 9 to 12 months he should have developed fusion (the ability to see a separate image with each eye and fuse them into one image). Occasionally an infant is born without this ability, and it can never be acquired. In most cases of strabismus, however, fusion is present but underdeveloped. In the normal person, when one eye fixes, the other eye also fixes and there is normal vision. Peter explains this complicated process as follows:

In the more common type of squint, a fusing power is present at birth but is weak, as are all other mental faculties. It grows and develops and begins to assert itself six to eight weeks after birth and increase in power up to the seventh year.

*If no other defects were present, the growth of fusion would continue uninterruptedly and the eyes would remain straight. Unfortunately, farsightedness of high degree is a second factor which interferes with normal progress. Vision is not sharp because of the far sight. In most instances vision is better in one eye than in the other and the eye with the better sight will habitually fix while the image of the weaker eye is ignored. If the fusion faculty is normally developed, the eyes will remain straight, but when fusion is not strong, the weak eye will tend to turn in. This act causes confusion because double images appear. If the eye turns to a considerable extent, the child can better ignore the image in the weak eye. Medically, this is known as suppression. Suppression means the image is ignored, and as a consequence, from nonuse, central vision becomes less and less acute. This adds another factor to the vicious circle. Vision falls rapidly in the eye which turns in and renders the squinting habit easier.**

Early medical attention is important in strabismus both to save vision and to prevent the emotional trauma which is always associated with cross-eyes. Treatment should begin by the end of the first year of life or sooner. Contrary to popular belief, glasses (with harness frames) can be safely worn by children only 5 to 6 months of age.[5] Treatment of very young children may consist of prescribing glasses and having the child wear a cover on alternate eyes. Fifty per cent of all children with strabismus would need no further treatment if glasses were worn before the end of the second year of life. One serious difficulty, however, is that it is almost impossible to have some small children wear glasses consistently. Exercises to strengthen weak muscles are used, but often they cannot be started until the child is about 4 years of age.

Treatment for strabismus includes testing vision, fitting glasses, preventing further loss of vision in the weak eye, awakening the faculty of fusion, or surgery. Surgery may be necessary and can be performed when the child is only 2 or 3 years of age. Up to the sixth year there is still hope that normal vision of both eyes can be restored, but, after that time, surgery can usually only achieve cosmetic improvement.

Surgery for strabismus can be and may have to be repeated, and the child's family should understand this. The operation is a simple one, consisting of shortening the weakened muscles. The child wears a dressing over both eyes for a few days and is permitted to move freely in bed and to be out of bed. Absorbable sutures may be used so that they need not be removed. Surgery is usually followed by the prescription of corrective glasses and exercises, depending on the individual patient. Parents must be cautioned to con-

*From Peter, Luther C.: Facts and Fallacies Concerning Squint (Cross-Eye), New York, 1932, The National Society for the Prevention of Blindness.

tinue with medical treatment for as long as is recommended, sometimes indefinitely. They may believe that the condition is completely cured and may neglect medical attention until a conspicuous squint again appears. By this time damage to vision may have occurred, and the condition may be exceedingly difficult to correct. This happens in some families who move and are tardy in establishing medical contacts in new places of residence. The nurse who works in schools should be particularly alert to notice children who show any signs of strabismus and should inquire to be certain that they are under competent medical care.

Glaucoma

Glaucoma is a disease that is increasing with the proportionate increase in older people in our population. It is seldom seen in persons under 35 years of age, but it is the greatest enemy to vision in older people. Treatment of glaucoma is often much more difficult than treatment of cataracts, which also occur in older people.

There are several types of glaucoma, but they all have one common characteristic: fluid is formed in the eye faster than it can be eliminated, so pressure within the eyeball rises. Pressure is often increased by some faulty mechanism of reabsorption of aqueous fluid in the anterior chamber of the eye. This, in turn, leads to destruction of the retina and blindness unless diagnosis is made early and treatment is effective and continued.

Primary glaucoma is of unknown origin. A predisposition to the disease may be inherited; primary glaucoma occurs most often in persons who have a family history of glaucoma and who are of somewhat unstable emotional make-up. Secondary glaucoma may follow another disease, such as uveitis or a tumor.

Glaucoma may be acute or chronic, the latter being much more common. *Acute glaucoma* may cause general symptoms of nausea and vomiting in addition to eye pain and dilation of the pupil. There is edema of the ciliary body and the cornea and an increase of tension within the eyeball. Marked increase in tension for twenty-four to thirty-six hours may lead to complete and permanent blindness, hence the necessity for immediate treatment. Treatment usually consists of miotics to constrict the pupil, narcotics for pain, and complete rest. If symptoms do not subside within a few hours, an emergency operation may be performed to provide a means of escape for superfluous fluid.

Chronic glaucoma may come on slowly, and, at first, symptoms may be absent. Chronic glaucoma gives one characteristic sign which is important: before central vision becomes affected, the peripheral visual fields are impaired so that objects to the side are ignored. This may lead to automobile accidents. Limitation of vision may not be so apparent as in other eye diseases, and much damage can occur before medical aid is sought. The patient may bump into others in the street or fail to see passing vehicles, yet not realize that the fault lies in his own vision. The community nurse who recognizes this may be most helpful in early case-finding and in promptly referring patients to the ophthalmologist.

Chronic glaucoma usually begins in one eye, although if left untreated, both eyes often become affected. Symptoms are most apparent in the morning when a persistent dull eye pain may develop. Frequent changes of glasses, difficulty in adjusting to darkness, and slight blurring of vision are fairly early signs of glaucoma. Then follows a steamy appearance to the cornea and further blurring of vision. Tearing, misty vision, blurred appearance to the iris which becomes fixed and dilated, headache, pain behind the eyeball, nausea, and vomiting can then occur. Halos, resembling street lamps seen through a steamy windshield, may be seen about lights. Symptoms may be increased by watching movies or television. Early symptoms have been confused with sinus trouble and treatment delayed for this reason. Symptoms of acute glaucoma may be precipitated by severe emotional disturbance, worry, or general poor health.

There is no known cure for glaucoma; all treatment is directed toward reducing intraocular tension and keeping it at a safe level. Miotics are widely used to try to ensure better drainage of aqueous fluid through the canal of Schlemm, but surgical measures are often necessary. Surgical procedures for glaucoma are used to produce a permanent filtration pathway for aqueous fluid. There are many operations for glaucoma, a few of which are *iridectomy, iridencleisis, cyclodialysis,* and *corneoscleral trephining.* If a piece of tissue, such as a portion of the iris, is brought through the newly made opening, healing and closure are not likely to occur, which ensures a passageway for the aqueous fluid. Following surgery the patient is usually allowed out of bed at once, although one or both eyes may be bandaged for several days.

The patient with glaucoma needs assistance in learning to accept his disease. Despite explanation from his physician, he frequently hopes that the operation will cure his condition and that no further treatment will be necessary, and perhaps that the sight he has lost will be restored. He must realize that the vision lost cannot be restored but that further loss can usually be prevented. The patient is often advised to avoid stimulants of any kind, including tea, coffee, and certain soft drinks. He should avoid anything that will increase his blood pressure and, in turn, his intraocular tension. A few of these are emotional situations such as arguments and quarrels, tight-fitting clothing such as constricting collars, constipation with straining at defecation, and heavy lifting. Watching movies and television, driving a vehicle, and work involving close watching of moving objects must often be limited.

The person with glaucoma must be under medical care for the rest of his life, receiving either drug or surgical therapy, or both. Following the operation he must return regularly to the doctor since one operation does not necessarily mean that drainage will be continued. Any obstruction or closing of the artificial pathway will result in reappearance of symptoms and further visual damage. The patient and his family must know specifically what to do if essential eye drops are accidentally spilled; for example, they should know what local drugstore is open at night and during holidays. They need constant encouragement about progress and reminders to continue administration of eye drops as ordered and to pay attention to general health.

Cataract

A cataract is a clouding or opacity of the lens which leads to blurring of vision and eventual loss of sight. Cataracts can be congenital, occurring most often in infants whose mothers had German measles during the first trimester of pregnancy. Congenital cataracts respond favorably to a simple operation known as a *discission* procedure. A very small opening is made in the capsule surrounding the lens and a small sharp needle knife is passed in pendulum-like manner through the lens. This procedure is also referred to as a "needling" operation. The operation permits aqueous fluid to pass into the cloudy lens and cause the cloudiness to disappear. Congenital cataracts are usually operated upon when the child is about 3 years of age. A general anesthetic is used, no immobilization in bed is necessary, and the child may be permitted to go home within a day or two of the operation. The results from discission of congenital cataracts in children are remarkably good, but unfortunately the operation is not effective for adults with cataracts.

Cataracts can occur at any time of life and may be associated with iritis, uveitis, and other conditions such as diabetes; they may follow the ingestion of injurious substances such as dinitrophenol, which was taken for weight reduction a decade or so ago. Operative treatment, including removal of the lens, is the only satisfactory treatment for these cataracts. Surgery, however, cannot be attempted if any signs of inflammation are present.

Cataracts occur so often in the aged that the term senile cataract is used. At 80 years of age, about 85 per cent of all people have some clouding of the lens. Senile cataracts are listed as the most common cause of blindness in older persons,[15] yet the response of the condition to surgery is often excellent. Patients who are in their nineties can often be operated upon with good results.

Nurses may be asked about when a cataract can be operated upon, because many people believe that they must wait until the cataract is "ripe" before surgery is satisfactory. The trend is toward early removal of cataracts by the intracapsular technique in which the capsule is removed with the lens. Most cataracts can be removed at any stage by this method. Decision as to when to remove the cataract depends largely on the individual patient and the use he makes of his eyes. It is the nurse's responsibility to refer the patient with a cataract to an ophthalmologist and to urge him to accept treatment as recommended.

Cataracts are usually removed under local anesthesia. They may be removed within their capsule (intracapsular technique), or an opening may be made in the capsule and the lens lifted out without disturbing the membrane (extracapsular technique). Usually only one eye is operated upon at a time lest some complication should arise or some unexpected behavior of the patient interfere with good results. If the patient has cataracts in both eyes, both may be removed during one hospitalization. This plan for treatment must be explained to the patient and his family or else he may feel that time is being spent in the hospital unnecessarily.

Following an operation for cataract, a dressing is applied to the eye that was operated on. The unoperated eye may also be covered, but usually it is left free. The patient is normally allowed out of bed the day following surgery. Dressings are changed by the surgeon in one to three days, and, at the end of a week or ten days, all dressings are removed and temporary glasses may be used.

The elderly patient sometimes finds it hard to adjust to removal of a cataract. He may be surprised to learn that he needs glasses before he can use his operated eye, that the color of objects seen with the eye from which the lens has been removed is slightly changed, that if he has the lens removed from only one eye he will use one of his eyes at a time, but not both together, and that he must wait at least three months before he can have permanent glasses prescribed. He needs to know that it will take time to learn to judge distance, climb stairs, and do other simple things. The little remaining ability to accommodate the eye is lost when the lens is removed, and the patient must wear glasses at all times. Bifocal lenses are often ordered, and the patient must have perseverance in becoming accustomed to their use.

Detachment of the retina

Detachment of the retina is a condition in which there is separation of the layers of the retina and elevation of the inner layer (the rods and cones) from a normal position where the retina lines the posterior three fifths of the eyeball. There are many causes of this condition, some of which are unknown or poorly understood. Normally the vitreous is gelatinous in consistency, and it helps to hold the retina in normal position. In retinal detachment, tears appear in the retina and some of the vitreous fluid which has become liquefied seeps through. The vitreous may develop fibers which become adherent to the retina and pull it forward, or it may shrink, thereby lessening its support to the retina. Tumors behind the retina, disease of the choroid, hemorrhage, or adhesions from a long-standing inflammation may cause detachment of the retina. Poor general health may contribute to detachment of the retina since separation will not occur, despite changes in the vitreous, if the retina is entirely normal and healthy.

Detachment of the retina may occur suddenly or develop slowly. It may follow sudden severe emotional shock, physical trauma, or physical exertion, especially in persons who are debilitated. The symptoms include floating spots or opacities before the eyes, wavy vision, flashes of light, and progressive constriction of vision in one area. The area of visual loss depends entirely on the location of the detachment. Visual loss is usually greater when the upper part of the retina detaches, because it may fall downward over portions of normal retina. When detachment is extensive and occurs quickly, the patient may have the sensation that a curtain has been drawn before his eye. In detachment associated with systemic or degenerative disease, it is common for both eyes to be affected or for involvement to occur eventually in both eyes, even though symptoms may begin in a single eye.

Immediate care for detachment of the retina includes keeping the patient quiet in bed and covering the eyes to prevent quick eye movements. Excitement, nervous tension, and physical exertion of any kind must be avoided. The patient may be placed on his back with the head of the bed lowered, in the hope that gravity may help the detached retina settle against the posterior surface of the eyeball and become adherent to it. This may or may not be successful, depending on circumstances surrounding the detachment. For example, liquefied vitreous may seep back through the tear to its normal location in front of the retina as the retina is aided by gravity in returning to a more normal position. On the other hand, retinal detachment, caused by adhesions to the vitreous, may not be affected by this measure.

Extended conservative treatment for detachment of the retina has not been successful,[6] and early surgery is now the approved method of treatment. The surgeon usually explains the procedure fully to the patient and his family. The nurse may refer the patient's misinformation and lack of understanding to the physician so that explanations may be clarified or repeated if necessary. The results of surgery are much less predictable than for eye conditions such as senile cataracts, and the family needs to know this. When tears in the retina are large and the area of detachment is three quarters or more of the retina, the chances of surgical benefit are poor. Old age and general debility also lessen the chances of good results, although age alone is never considered a contraindication for surgery.

Cyclogyl or Neo-Synephrine are used to keep the pupils widely dilated so that tears in the retina may be identified during the operation. The surgery may be done either under local or general anesthesia; inhalation anesthetics are avoided because of the fear of coughing and vomiting postoperatively. All operative procedures are designed to bring about reattachment of the retina. Many different procedures to reattach the retina are used and new methods are constantly being devised. An attempt may be made by electrocoagulation using diathermy to produce multiple points of inflammatory reaction in the sclera and choroid underlying the detached area which will cause adhesions to form and hold the retina. Air may be injected into the posterior chamber to help increase pressure of the vitreous in the posterior chamber or under the choroid, where its presence will cause bulging into the posterior chamber and lessening of its capacity. Air and normal saline solution may be introduced into the anterior chamber again to increase pressure within the eyeball and to help force the retina against its normal attachment. Draining of the vitreous fluid behind the retina is often attempted. An operation known as a "buckling" operation or *scleral resection* is now being used widely. An attempt is made to lessen the size of the eyeball when the condition appears to be the result of shrinking of the vitreous which causes a dead space that leads to lack of support of the retina; in this operation the choroid is raised against the defective portion of the retina.

Dressings are usually changed daily, but it is about a week before the eye can be fully examined and determination made as to whether or not the operation has been successful. It may be possible to reoperate upon eyes when surgery has not been successful, although this is usually delayed for at least one or two weeks. Hemorrhage is the worst complication of an operation for detachment of the retina; this may result from electrocautery destruction of blood vessels or from trauma at the time of operation.

The patient's postoperative position will depend on the extent and location of his retinal detachment. Because postoperative routines vary a great deal, the nurse must be certain that orders for bed position and for ambulation have been written by the surgeon, and that she understands exactly how much activity he wishes the patient to have. She must then explain the reason for this to the patient and be certain that orders are followed. Vomiting, coughing, laughing, and any sudden jerking motion may be dangerous. If the patient does vomit, great care must be taken that he does not choke and raise his head; emesis basins should be conveniently placed to receive the vomitus.

The patient may be allowed out of bed the day after operation or he may be kept flat in bed for a week to ten days, with only enough turning to facilitate back care. When dressings are removed, the patient is usually required to wear pinhole glasses which permit some vision, but which tend to limit eye movement. The length of time that these are necessary varies.

After operation for detachment of the retina, the patient is urged to avoid heavy lifting and straining of any kind for several months. Because of this he may have to be away from work for a long time, or he may even have to alter his mode of earning a living entirely.

Eye disease resulting from nutritional deficiency

There seems to be a direct relationship between good nutrition and eye health. A lack of vitamin A in the diet can cause an eye disease with changes in the conjunctiva and corneal epithelium. Tears are reduced, and eyes and lid margins become reddened and inflammed. Sensitivity to light is often present, and some loss of visual acuity is noticed at night, although this condition should not be confused with true night blindness. Signs of vitamin A deficiency often disappear rapidly when a diet high in vitamin A is eaten.

Pathologic changes can occur in the retina as a result of nutritional deficiency, particularly of vitamin B. This condition is found in persons who ingest large amounts of alcohol and who pay little attention to their diets. The disease has been thought to be due to alcohol, and the name tobacco-alcoholic amblyopia is used. Patients who suffer from optic atrophy as a result of nutritional deficiency will often respond miraculously to a diet high in vitamin B, even though they may continue to take alcohol. Occasionally when damage to the nerve tissue of the retina has been severe and prolonged, a diet high in vitamin B and all other essentials can accomplish only partial recovery.

Eye disease resulting from degenerative disease

Characteristic changes occur in the retina when nephritis with high blood pressure is present. It is often possible for the ophthalmologist to make a diagnosis of nephritis merely by looking into the patient's eyes. No local treatment to the eyes is of value, and sometimes the condition causes complete blindness. Treatment is directed toward control of the kidney ailment and reduction of the blood pressure before vision is entirely lost.

Certain pathologic changes occur in the eyes of persons with diabetes, but their true cause is obscure and debatable. Corneal ulcers and iritis occur most often in persons with diabetes, but the diseases are thought by some to result from the general state of malnutrition and debility that accompanies diabetes before diagnosis is made and insulin given.

Degeneration of the retina, often called diabetic retinopathy, is caused when the increased fragility of blood vessels results in many small hemorrhages in the retina, leading to its destruction. It is definitely known that this condition appears in conjunction with diabetes, but it has not been proved that a high blood sugar level is a factor in its development. Diabetic retinopathy, is more closely related to the length of time the person has had diabetes than to whether or not the blood and urine sugar levels are carefully controlled. Some physicians believe that the appearance of retinal damage is an indication to give strict attention to blood sugar levels; they feel that progress of the disease can be partially arrested in this manner.

There is no treatment for diabetic retinopathy other than possible the adherence to a strict insulin regimen. Most patients with diabetic retinopathy eventually become blind if death from other causes does not intervene. Realistic care consists of helping the patients to remain independent and self-sufficient as vision is gradually lost.

Senile degeneration of the retina is a rather common cause of blindness in the very elderly. There is gradual atrophy of the retina, possibly from impaired nutrition to the retina resulting from arteriosclerosis or artherosclerosis. It may or may not be associated with high blood pressure. There seems to be no real control of this condition at the present time, although attention to an adequate diet high in vitamins may assist in retarding the degenerative process.

Night blindness is due to pigmentary degeneration of the retina and affects the peripheral visual fields first. This condition is fairly common in the aged and became a problem in England during World War II when blackouts made it extremely difficult for elderly persons to get about safely.

Visual loss may follow vascular accidents to vessels anywhere in the eye or in the main blood vessels outside the eye. A cerebral vascular accident may cause hemianopsia or total blindness, depending upon its location. Thrombosis of the central vein or arteriosclerotic involvement of the central artery of the eye may cause blindness. Generalized arteriosclerosis involving the vessels of both eyes may cause partial or complete loss of vision in both eyes.

Retrolental fibroplasia

Retrolental fibroplasia is a condition in which there is derangement of the vascular structures in the retina with projection through the vitreous to the lens capsule and other adjacent structures. It occurs in premature infants, most often in those born in the sixth and seventh month of gestation. The incidence of retrolental fibroplasia increased in the past few decades since better medical care enabled many premature infants to live who formerly would have died. Retrolental fibroplasia is responsible for a fairly large amount of the blindness found in school children today. It is now known that there is a definite relationship between the administration of oxygen in high concentration to premature infants and the development of retrolental fibroplasia. The relationship of oxygen to the disease is not understood, but, by controlling the administration of oxygen to premature infants, it is now possible to control the disease. Supplementary oxygen is now given for very short intervals, and concentrations of more than 40 per cent are not used. It is hoped that new cases of of retrolental fibroplasia will become unknown within a few years.

REFERENCES AND SELECTED READINGS*

1 Adler, Francis Heed: Gifford's Textbook of Ophthalmology, ed. 6, Philadelphia, 1957, W. B. Saunders Co.

2 *Blake, Eugene M.: Glaucoma, Am. J. Nursing **52**:451-452, April 1952.

3 Blodi, Frederick C., and Honn, Ruth C.: Tumors of the Eye—Medical and Nursing Care, Am. J. Nursing **56**:1152-1156, Sept. 1956.

4 Brinkley, Dorothy: Focus on Vision, Am. J. Nursing **53**:1224-1226, Oct. 1953.

---

*References preceded by an asterisk indicate material particularly well suited for student reading.

5 *Burian, Hermann M.: Strabismus, Am. J. Nursing **60**:653-655, May 1960.
6 *Calhoun, F. Phinizy, Kilgo, Alice P., and Mills, Elizabeth: Detached Retina, Am. J. Nursing **53**:1316-1321, Nov. 1953.
7 Cecil, Russell L. (editor): The Specialties in General Practice, Philadelphia, 1951, W. B. Saunders Co.
8 Cholden, L.: Some Psychiatric Problems in Rehabilitation of the Blind, Bull. Menninger Clin. **18**:107-112, May 1954.
9 *Clark, Graham, and Shaw, Cora L.: The Patient With Retinal Detachment, Am. J. Nursing **57**:868-870, July 1957.
10 Duke-Elder, Sir Stewart: Parson's Diseases of the Eye, ed. 3, New York, 1959, The Macmillan Co.
11 Esposito, Albert: Contact Lenses, Am. J. Nursing **57**:462-463, April 1957.
12 *Gamble, Richard C.: The Medical Eye Examination, Am. J. Nursing **57**:1590-1592, Dec. 1957.
13 *Gibbons, Helen, and Cunningham, Florence: Finding and Helping the Partially Seeing Child, Nursing Outlook **7**:524-526, Sept. 1959.
14 Harmer, Bertha, and Henderson, Virginia (revised by): Textbook of the Principles and Practice of Nursing, ed. 5, New York, 1955, The Macmillan Co.
15 Kuhn, Hedwig S.: Eyes—Facts and Fallacies, Field of Vision **9**:3, June 15, 1954.
16 Kurtz, Russell H. (editor): Social Work Yearbook 1960, New York, 1960, National Assn. of Social Workers.
17 News Item, Field of Vision **9**:2, March 15, 1954.
18 Perera, Charles A. (revised and edited by): May's Manual of the Diseases of the Eye, ed. 19, Baltimore, 1947, Williams & Wilkins Co.
19 Peters, Luther C.: Facts and Fallacies Concerning Squint (Cross-Eye), New York, 1932, The National Society for the Prevention of Blindness.
20 *Rones, Benjamin: The Eyes and Vitamins, Am. J. Nursing **52**:728-729, July 1952.
21 Ruedemann, Albert D.: Headaches Caused by Eye Defects, Am. J. Nursing **52**:1093-1094, Sept. 1952.
22 *Weaver, Helen E.: Glaucoma: A Problem for the Public Health Nurse, Pub. Health Nursing **41**:92-95, Feb. 1949.
23 *Weaver, Helen E.: The Nurse in Sight Conservation, Am. J. Nursing **51**:553-555, Sept. 1951.
24 *Weiss, M. Olga: Psychological Aspects of Nursing Care for Eye Patients, Am. J. Nursing **50**:218-220, April 1950.
25 Yudkin, Arthur M.: The Ocular Manifestations of Vitamin Deficiencies, New York, 1947, Prevention of Blindness Service, Commission for the Blind, New York State Department of Social Welfare.

The patient with neurologic disease

Chapter 34

Study questions for review

1 Review the anatomy of the nervous system.
2 What vital centers are located in the brain? What bodily functions would be affected by pressures on these centers?
3 Outline a plan for moving and changing the position of a completely dependent patient. What nursing measures can be used to maintain normal body alignment and function?
4 Describe the procedure for giving tube feedings.
5 If a patient is unable to speak, what methods of communication could you devise?
6 From among patients on your ward or among members of your family or acquaintances, select a person who has a chronic neurologic disease. How has his disease affected family life? How has the community been affected?

The specialties of neurology and neurosurgery are complicated and demand special knowledge, skill, and experience. Before the nurse can give good nursing care to a patient with neurologic disease, she must have knowledge of the nervous system, of any pathology present, of the surgical procedure if one is performed, and the general nursing needs of neurologic patients. It is suggested that the student nurse review the anatomy, pathology, treatment, and nursing care needed for each neurologic patient encountered in her daily practice on any service.

Many neurologic patients have serious emotional and even psychiatric disturbances. Psychiatry, however, is concerned largely with functional disorders, whereas neurology is concerned largely with disorders that have a demonstrable organic or physical cause. There may be neurologic involvement in such general diseases as pernicious anemia, diabetes, and severe infections, but many diseases are caused by pathology which is primarily in the nervous system. Only a few of the commonly seen neurologic diseases and their nursing care will be considered in this chapter. General nursing care which is common to many neurologic diseases will be discussed before a few of the more common diseases and neurosurgical procedures are described.

GENERAL NURSING CARE

Loss of function and control. Neurologic disease may occur suddenly, as in cerebrovascular hemorrhage or traumatic spinal cord injury, or may be slow in onset, as in multiple sclerosis or Parkinson's disease. The loss of some motor or sensory function is common in most neurologic diseases. Because of this it may be difficult for the patient to carry out daily activities that require coordinated movement. The ability to move about at will and control one's actions is precious to every human being. Regardless of the speed of its occurrence, the loss of the ability to function independently or to predict one's movements is psychologically traumatizing. Irritability, defensiveness, fear, and other signs of threat to emotional security are likely to appear and must be met with calmness, patience, and kindness by all who work with the patient.

If the patient has a nonprogressive limitation of function due to neurologic damage, he needs reassurance that his condition will not become worse. Unfortunately, however, cure is not possible in many neurologic diseases. The nurse needs to know what the doctor has told both the patient and his family about the prognosis. If assurance of arrest or of improvement of the disease cannot be given, the patient must be helped to live a relatively full life as long as possible, and it is the nurse who often gives much of this help.

The nurse must protect the patient from close observation and comment by persons who have no part in his care. This is particularly true when he is in a general hospital or in his own home. The peculiarities of gait, mannerisms, or loss of control so common in neurologic disease seem to interest people who should have no concern with them. The unfortunate quality of morbid curiosity in human nature must be faced. The patient should be told how common his particular condition is and that he is not alone with his affliction. The nurse can help him by making him feel that she is interested in him as a person and not primarily in his physical ailment. She may find that he turns to her as someone with whom he can discuss his reactions to his disease when he cannot discuss these with his family. Listening attentively to the patient's problems is an essential part of neurologic nursing. Knowing when problems are too involved and beyond the nurse's sphere of knowledge is equally essential. A medical social worker can often be of great help to the patient in thinking through his feelings about his disease.

It is useless to argue with the patient or to try to talk him out of his fears. Giving a word of encouragement on small achievements, changing the conversation to other topics, and introducing some diversional activity sometimes help. Emotional tension seems to be released by working with one's hands. Making something useful in the occupational therapy department of a hospital or in his own home may be most satisfying to the patient. The patient may get more satisfaction from weaving a belt or making a wallet than from spending an equivalent amount of time watching television or in a similar passive time-killing activity. He must not, however, be urged into activities that do not interest him. For example, the patient at home may get more satisfaction from washing dishes and peeling vegetables than from making some decorative object.

The desire of the patient and his family to shop for a cure is understandable when the diagnosis of a chronic and incurable neurologic disease has been made. The nurse should help to prevent the loss of time and of financial and emotional resources which this practice usually entails. She must take particular care to build up the confidence of the patient and his family in the doctor and in the clinic or hospital where he is receiving care. She must have patience and understanding in answering questions about advertised remedies, news items that may be misleading, and reports from neighbors and friends. At times she may need to refer questions to the doctor. Many patients with incurable neurologic disease live out their years in the hope that a cure will be found during their lifetime. They need to feel sure that those responsible for their care are alert for new discoveries that may be helpful to them.

Provision for self-care. Physical facilities should be arranged so that the patient can do as much as possible for himself to maintain his self-esteem and to give him some satisfaction. Hand rails along hallways, firm locks on bed casters and bedside tables, low beds, and rails along the sides of the tub and toilet help the patient to handle himself even though his movements are uncertain. It is important to most people to be able to feed themselves; appetite is better and disposition improves when this is possible. Even a patient with poor coordination may be able to feed himself if food is cut into bite-sized pieces. A special spoon with a large handle may be helpful. If he is clumsy and untidy while eating, he will usually want to be protected from the scrutiny of others. The nurse should be calm about failures in attempts to master an activity or else she should ignore them. Emotional outbursts as a result of frustration should be treated in a matter-of-fact fashion. The nurse needs to know what the patient can do and must keep him aware of her faith in his ability to do these things for himself. Statements such as "You're not trying" or "You couldn't be tired yet" only add to the patient's discouragement and should be avoided. She must use good judgment in deciding what the patient may safely do without assistance; if any doubt exists, she should consult the doctor. She must know what activities are dangerous for the patient. Great frustration may result from attempting activities that are beyond his abilities because they accentuate his limitations. Activities that are steppingstones to greater accomplishments will result in satisfaction for the patient and will motivate him to further self-help.

It is fortunate that many neurologic diseases progress slowly so that the patient has time to adjust to necessary changes. As difficulty in walking progresses, the patient may benefit from special shoes. These may need to be built up in a variety of ways to provide a stable base of support. They should have low rubber heels, fit well, and give good support for the arches. As disease progresses, many patients must use a cane; this is a painful step for the patient in his acceptance of the disease, even though built-up shoes and a cane may be less conspicuous than the patient's gait would be without these aids. The nurse can help by suggesting the activities that are safe and possible with the use of a cane. Eventually, many patients must resort to a wheel chair. The light wheel chairs now available make it possible for the quite helpless patient to get about safely in his home and to be taken in a car for trips away from home. Collapsible wheel chairs should be used only for special occasions because most of them do not give enough support to foster good sitting posture.

The nurse should help the patient to plan the necessary adjustments needed in the home so that he can continue to be at least partially self-sufficient. Furniture can be arranged to allow the patient to get about more easily in his wheel chair, cupboards and shelves can be lowered, and special equipment such as lamps and the telephone can be placed on lower tables.

If the patient has difficulty using his fingers and hands for fine movements, the use of shoes with elasticized insteps or of elastic laces instead of the usual ones and use of metal grippers on clothing instead of buttons may help him to remain self-sufficient. (See Chapter 4 for additional suggestions.) When the patient is hospitalized, the activities he can perform should be noted on the Kardex sheet or other equivalent record form. If he is at home, the family should know what he can and cannot do so that he is not overprotected.

Aphasia. Aphasia is a disorder of language caused by damage to the speech-controlling area of the brain. Cerebral hemorrhage and cerebral thrombosis are the most common causes of such damage, but tumors, multiple sclerosis, and trauma may also lead to aphasia. Aphasia caused by cerebral edema following trauma is usually temporary. Occasionally a patient cannot speak following a cerebrovascular accident because the vocal cords are affected, not because of cerebral damage. This is not true aphasia.

A variety of abnormalities in speech can occur. The patient may be unable to comprehend the spoken or written word (sensory aphasia), or he may comprehend yet be unable to use the symbols of speech (motor aphasia). He may have both disorders at the same time. He may be able to write but not to speak; he may be able to speak but may use the wrong words or have a selective loss of words; he may be able to read but be unable to speak or to write. It is unusual for a patient to be unable to understand the spoken word or to know what he wishes to express. Sensory aphasia is much more difficult to deal with than motor involvement. Explanations are difficult, and it is hard to reassure the patient who may become completely confused and undirected in his efforts to speak.

Each patient reacts to language difficulty in a different way, depending on his pattern of adjustment to life's problems. Most patients with aphasia become tense and anxious. They may be irritable and emotionally upset because they are unable to evoke the words they need, and they become discouraged easily in their efforts to speak. Some may quickly refuse to attempt to communicate; others feel ashamed and withdraw from people, including even their family and close friends. Yet desire to communicate and persistence in efforts to do so are the essential ingredients in speech rehabilitation.

Nursing care is directed toward decreasing tension. This should be started as soon as aphasia occurs since this helps the patient to make a more satisfactory adjustment to his limitation and makes later rehabilitative efforts less difficult. The nurse should anticipate the patient's needs so that he will not need to make repeated attempts to ask for things. She should try to help him understand that he may relearn speech and should teach him ways in which he may communicate with others at this time. She must also help his family and friends and the auxiliary nursing staff to learn how to communicate with the patient and thus spare him humiliating experiences. She can help other patients to understand and help the patient by talking with him, avoiding any show of amusement or embarrassment, and making him feel that he is one of the group. Calmness and avoidance of hurry and impatience on the part of the nurse are essential to the patient's acceptance of his difficult program of practicing the use of relearned words and patterns of speech.

The patient's environment should be quiet. Those who care for him should guard against speaking loudly; the patient with aphasia is seldom deaf. Although he cannot respond, he should be talked to and have procedures explained in the same manner as done for any patient. Recreational activities should be quiet. Music is often relaxing and the patient may enjoy listening to radio. If patients are able to read and comprehend the written captions on television, watching television will sometimes be particularly gratifying. Other patients may be made irritable by radio music they do not enjoy or television programs that they do not like or cannot follow; watching the patient's facial expression may give the nurse a useful clue to the satisfaction derived from these activities.

Tests must be done to determine what language abilities have been lost. In some hospitals a trained therapist may be available to do an initial evaluation and to guide members of the nursing staff in making appropriate nursing care plans concerning the patient's speech problems. Sometimes, however, this assistance is not available, and the nurse must do simple tests which have been ordered by the doctor. These may be conducted as follows. Spread several familiar objects, such as keys, a pencil, a book of matches, a penny, and scissors, before the patient: (1) Ask him to name each object; (2) as you name each object, ask him to point to it; (3) ask him to write the name of each object as you point to it; (4) ask him to write the name of each object as you say the word; (5) show him a card containing the printed name of each object and ask him to read the word orally and point to the object. It may be too fatiguing for the patient to do all the tests at one sitting and some must be delayed. As a result of these tests one can determine the best way to communicate with the patient. If he can only read, one should give him cards with the words and phrases needed in asking for the most common daily necessities. Words needed by most ill persons include yes, no, bedpan, urinal, hot, cold, headache, pain, doctor, nurse, turn, sit up, lie down, bed, pillow, sheet, gown, water, thirst, hunger, comfortable, chair, light, telephone, wife, or husband. If the patient is unable to recognize the written word, he may be able to recognize pictures of objects. If he can write or draw a picture of his needs, he should be given a writing pad and pencil with which to do so.

As the nurse cares for the patient, she should name common objects and encourage the patient to handle them, to speak their names, and to write or copy their names. The patient should be helped to relearn the names of members of his family and friends; the family can supply these words and others that are particularly important for the patient. Speech retraining should be done for short periods of time because it is exceedingly trying, and fatigue tends to increase dysphasia. The slogan of the National Hospital for Speech Disorders is "slow and easy." Praising the patient for each small improvement and encouraging him to take his mistakes good naturedly help to make this difficult problem more bearable. The patient's progress in language retraining will depend on his level of intelligence, his age (older patients have more difficulty), the severity of the damage, and whether or not the brain lesion is a progressive one. Complete language rehabilitation may require months of painstaking work on the part of skilled therapists.*

Personality changes and prevention of accidents. Personality changes are common in neurologic disease, and occasionally their slow development is the first and only sign of a serious neurologic disorder. Changes should be watched for carefully and reported accurately. Physical changes caused by neurologic disease may affect the personality; reporting these changes may help the doctor in his diagnosis and treatment of the patient. Frustrations resulting from restrictions and attempts to get about, anxiety from increasing helplessness, and the fear of helplessness may also cause personality changes.

Changes in judgment and in intellect may become serious. The patient may make poor investments or other unwise decisions in business or family matters. Multiple sclerosis, Parkinson's disease, cerebrovascular arteriosclerosis, and brain tumors are examples of neurologic disorders that may seriously alter judgment. Handling such a situation is extremely difficult because strong emotional reaction may follow curtailment of the patient's freedom in managing his own affairs. The problem is usually dealt with by the doctor and the family with the assistance of the medical social worker. The nurse should not tell the patient that she knows of measures taken to prevent the consequences of errors in his judgment.

Judgment defects may lead to behavior that is dangerous both to the patient and to others. It is believed that many automobile accidents are caused by persons with neurologic disease; for example, patients with multiple sclerosis may have blind spots (scotomas), and those with epilepsy may lose consciousness for only a few seconds—long enough for an accident to occur. Unfortunately, these two diseases appear in young people, who feel very keenly the restriction of such activities as driving an automobile. The need to avoid certain other dangerous activities must be stressed; for example, swimming is dangerous for the patient who has convulsive seizures. Emphasis must be positive, however, and must be upon the many things that the patient can do. Members of the patient's family should be helped to plan so that the necessary restrictions are not obvious; for example, hiking and camping may be substituted for swimming or horseback riding if the patient has convulsive seizures.

The neurologic patient must be protected from accidents in his daily living. Measures to prevent accidents must be

*Some institutions that specialize in working with patients who have aphasia are The National Hospital for Speech Disorders, New York, N. Y.; The Institute for the Crippled and Disabled, New York, N. Y.; The Institute of Logopedics, Wichita, Kan.; and the Vanderbilt University Hospital Clinic, Nashville, Tenn.

carefully introduced because the patient may resent his limitations so much that he is inclined to reject precautions for his safety. Personality changes and judgment defects again may interfere with the patient's acceptance of measures which would help to ensure his personal safety. Elderly persons with arteriosclerotic brain damage are often great trials to their families; for example, they may decide to paint the outside of the house, when standing on a ladder is obviously dangerous.

The bathroom is a common location of accidents. To prevent falls in the bathtub, hand rails should be installed beside the tub and the tub should be made slipproof. This can be done by applying a rough paint to the floor of the tub; if this paint is not available, a less satisfactory method is to place a rubber mat in the tub. When limitations are severe, it may not be advisable for the patient to take a tub bath without assistance. Sitting on a stool or preferably in a small metal wheel chair in the shower and using a spray attached to the faucet is safest and is usually satisfactory for the patient.

Bathroom doors should not lock from the inside, since there is danger that the patient may lock himself in and, in the event of accident, prolong the time needed to reach him. Bath water should be drawn and tested before the patient steps into the tub. This is particularly important if the patient is elderly or if his sensory perception is impaired; patients have received severe and even fatal burns from stepping into a tub of water that was too hot or from fainting or suffering a stroke or heat attack as hot water was running into the tub.

Accidents in and about the home can be prevented by special attention to sources of accidents by the nurse and the patient's family. Scatter rugs should never be used, and any upturned, curled rug edges should be nailed down. Wall-to-wall carpeting is best. Floors should not be highly waxed. Toys, lamp cords, or other accident hazards on floors should be removed. The patient should wear firm slippers or shoes. Bathrobes should have buttons instead of long cords or sashes. Good lighting is essential. Night lights at the bedside, in hallways, and in bathrooms are desirable.

Railings and firm casements on steps and ramps often enable the patient to get about independently for a longer period. It is advisable to caution the family to lock basement doors and even front and back doors when persons who have neurologic disease with judgment defects are living in the house. They may open the wrong door and fall down basement steps or go into the street at odd hours and come to harm.

Contractures. Patients with neurologic disease are likely to develop contractures and deformities. Many changes come on so gradually that they are barely noted by the patient until they are relatively fixed. Warm baths often relax tightened muscles enough so that joints can be put through a range of motion. In this way limitation of joint motion may be prevented or delayed. Since muscle and joint stiffness come from prolonged sitting or lying in one position, the patient should be advised to change his position frequently.

Failure to keep the body in good alignment, both while up and while in bed, may lead to deformity. If the patient is rational and able to help himself, the nurse can teach him to help prevent deformity and preserve his best possible function. In the home, as well as in the hospital, much can be done to prevent the progress of deformities. A firm mattress and chairs that provide good support are essential. Pillows may be used to support paralyzed parts, and change of position, both in and out of bed, help to prevent deformities from developing. A comfortable arrangement can be made so that the patient may stand supported for short intervals during the day. In many communities a walker may be rented, but home-made substitutes fashioned of wood are sometimes quite satisfactory. Standing for even a few minutes each day will prevent the development of contractures at the hips caused by prolonged sitting. The nurse, the doctor, the physical therapist, and the occupational therapist may all give useful suggestions to members of the patient's family for improvising equipment for use in the home.

Body parts that are paralyzed must be put through the normal range of motion daily so that range will not be limited if and when the ability to move is restored. The nurse can determine the patient's range of motion as normal or limited by comparison with her own range of movement. She must allow for individual variations and for changes due to age and to any joint disease the patient may have. Since range of motion for some joints cannot be achieved with the patient in the supine (back-lying) position, it is necessary that he lie prone at least once each day. The nurse should know any special exercises prescribed for the patient so that she can assist with them at intervals during the day if this is desirable. They should be written or typed. Stick drawings help the patient to understand such details as the angle and arc of motion. (See chapter 4.)

Pressure areas and skin care. When the nerve supply to a body part is affected by disease, nutrition of that part is impaired because the arterial and venous blood flow which is dependent upon normal muscle action is often decreased as a result of disturbance of nerve impulses. It is well to consider how often the normal person changes his position during both waking and sleeping hours; some change is made in distribution of weight on weight-bearing parts of the body every few minutes. When the patient is paralyzed or unable to move, the pressure of body weight further curtails adequate circulation. The skin breaks down easily, and pressure sores may be difficult or impossible to cure. Therefore, the patient with a neurologic disorder who is confined to bed or chair must be reminded to change his position frequently if he is able to do this. If he cannot move himself, he must have assistance. If he is unconscious, he will sense no need to move or be moved. An important nursing responsibility is to change the patient's position at regular intervals or to remind others to do so. Light massage of the dependent areas should be given each time the patient is turned. If the patient is completely paralyzed, aged, or particularly devitalized, regular turning and massage may not be adequate to prevent decubiti and an alternating air pressure mattress, sponge rubber, or sheepskin under the bony prominences should be used. Attention should be given to a well-balanced diet since this helps to maintain healthy tissues.

Turning patients who are helpless or unconscious involves physical labor. The nurse and auxiliary workers who help her need to apply the principles of good body mechanics. This will make the difference between ending the day with a feeling of normal tiredness and satisfaction and ending it with the feeling of discouragement and undue fatigue. (For principles of good body mechanics, see texts on fundamentals of nursing.)

It is necessary to keep the skin clean and dry. Incontinence is sometimes a problem in care of the patient with neurologic disease. (See Chapter 8.)

The patient's family. Few illnesses tax the entire physical and emotional resources of the patient's family as do the chronic neurologic diseases. It is imperative that the family participate in long-term plans for the patient. Members of the family may have severe emotional reactions and difficulties in adjustment which may require the assistance of specially trained persons such as the psychiatrist. The medical social worker or the spiritual adviser can be invaluable in listening to close members of the family and in helping them to think through their own futures. From this the family may determine a constructive plan of action for caring for a loved one who has a serious neurologic disease. Both the patient and his family need time. Sometimes the enormity of the significance of the diagnosis cannot be grasped for weeks or even months by either the patient or his family. Severe paralytic poliomyelitis in a young husband and father and multiple sclerosis in a young mother are examples of problems of such magnitude that long-term plans cannot be made quickly.

The family may need help in accepting the concept of self-help and independence for the patient. Upon learning the diagnosis, their first reaction may be to do too much for the patient and thus to hasten his complete dependence upon them. Later, when the reality of the burden becomes clearer, they may tire of the restrictions imposed upon them and become impatient or needlessly exhausted. Care of the patient may fall too much on one relative who most readily assumes the burden. Sometimes this family member eagerly takes on the greatest responsibility yet resents it; she may complain that others do not contribute, yet avoids their assistance when it is offered. By reacting in this way she may be meeting some particular emotional needs of her own. Family crises may sometimes be prevented by careful initial family planning in which each member assumes some specific part of the total responsibility. The medical social worker is usually the key person who brings about joint planning by the family.

The relative who is to give nursing care to a chronically ill or terminally ill person should be taught how to do this with a minimum of strain to herself and a minimum of discomfort to the patient. Sometimes the relative may enroll in a home-nursing course given by the local chapter of the American National Red Cross and thus be prepared for the time when the patient will need more physical help. In the hospital, at the bedside of the patient, or in the clinic she may learn specific techniques and procedures that will be needed. She should know that public health nurses from local agencies are available to give assistance and instruction in the home. In many instances, before the patient leaves the hospital, it is well for the public health nurse to visit his home to review the plan of care with responsible relatives and to consult, if necessary, with the doctor or with nurses in the hospital. Members of the family should be prepared for anticipated changes.

THE NEUROLOGIC EXAMINATION

The patient with neurologic disease dreads examinations and tests more than many other patients. He may fear that certain procedures, such as a spinal puncture, will cause further disability, and he may be reluctant to have his limitations proved or exposed. He may sense a serious prognosis yet dread its confirmation. It is essential that all tests and procedures be thoroughly explained to the patient before they are begun. Even the neurologic examination itself is trying and exhausting. Usually the patient wears little clothing, and he may be examined by more than one person. It is upsetting to him to be examined for alteration in gait, equilibrium, hand grip, and other similar abilities even when this is done with the greatest kindness.

The neurologic examination includes a complete history, with detail not solicited in a general physical examination. The patient should be prepared for a long and tedious procedure which is sometimes done in stages, depending on the condition of the patient and the urgency for completing the study.

Equipment needed. In addition to the necessary materials for a routine examination, the neurologic examination tray should contain the following: a straight pin that is usually stuck through a tongue blade and a safety pin to be used for testing the sensation of pain, a wisp of cotton and a fine soft brush to test the sensation of touch, tuning forks to test vibratory sense and hearing, a dynamometer to measure hand grip, substances with distinctive odors such as peppermint, vanilla, coffee, and tobacco to test the sense of small, test tubes for hot and cold water to test heat and cold sensations, and sugar, salt, vinegar, and quinine or cascara to test the sense of taste. Areas of abnormal reaction are indicated on a diagram of the anterior and posterior surfaces of the body. This helps the doctor determine the nerves involved and may indicate the location of the primary lesion.

Vocabulary and definitions. Certain neurologic signs are of interest to the nurse. Also, she must learn a special vocabulary if the study of the patient's symptoms and the results of the examination are to be meaningful to her.

A positive *Kernig's sign* indicates irritation of the meninges. The sign is positive when there is pain upon extension of the lower leg while the thigh is maintained in a flexed position upon the abdomen. This sign is elicited with the patient in a back-lying or sitting position.

A positive *Brudzinski's sign* also indicates meningeal irritation. The sign is considered positive when attempts to flex the head on the chest result in involuntary flexion of the ankle, knee, or hip. This test is done with the patient lying on his back or sitting on the side of the bed.

A positive *Babinski's sign* (or reflex) indicates lesions in the pyramidal tract. The sign is positive if the great toe extends upward when the sole of the foot is stroked. Usually a broken tongue blade is used for this test.

A positive *Romberg's sign* indicates locomotor ataxia. The sign is positive if there is inability to maintain body balance when standing with the feet close together and the eyes closed.

An *area of anesthesia* is one in which sensation is absent. *Hyperesthesia* means that sensation is intensified, and *paralgesia* indicates a painful sensation. *Paresthesia* is an abnormal sensation such as burning, pricking, or itching.

Hemiplegia is paralysis of one half of the body (linear division), *paraplegia* refers to paralysis of the lower half of the body, and *quadriplegia* means that all four extremities and the trunk are paralyzed.

The terms used to describe spasms and convulsive movements are as follows: *tonic movements* are fixed contractions of the muscles which usually draw joints into a position of flexion and *clonic movements* are alternating contractions and relaxations of muscles. *Spastic* refers to a state of muscular rigidity or tenseness, while *flaccid* or flail-like means that the involved part is completely relaxed and limp; these terms usually describe the more common kinds of paralysis or partial paralysis. A *spasm* is an involuntary, sudden movement or convulsive muscular contraction that the patient cannot control; a *tic* is a spasmodic muscular contraction usually of the face, neck, or shoulder muscles that may be involuntary or the result of habit. *Ataxia* means lack of coordination in attempting to perform a planned purposeful motion.

Tests of special nerves and groups of nerves. The first cranial or olfactory nerve is tested by blindfolding the patient, covering each nostril in turn, and having him smell and identify certain odors such as coffee.

The second or optic nerve is tested grossly by having the patient count the number of fingers one holds up and more minutely by having the patient identify letters on a Snellen's chart (see Chapter 33 for details of examination of the eyes). Visual field examinations test not only the ability to see directly ahead but also over a broad normal field. The test, performed on each eye separately, may be done crudely by standing behind the patient and moving the fingers toward the eyes from various points above, below, and at either side of the field of vision; the patient indicates when he sees them. If the test is done in a dark room, the results may be specifically plotted on a diagram with the use of a flashlight and a special chart known as a perimetry chart. This method identifies patients who may have lesions which press on one side of the optic nerve, cutting off half the vision of each eye.

Examination of the eyes with an *ophthalmoscope* reveals the condition of the blood vessels in the retina. Congestion of the optic nerve head (choked disc) can be seen by an ophthalmoscopic examination and is particularly indicative of increased intracranial pressure.

The third, fourth, and sixth cranial nerves are examined by noting the size and reaction of the pupils and the movements of the eye. Double vision (diplopia), squint (strabismus), and involuntary rhythmic movements of the eyeballs (nystagmus) may indicate involvement of these nerves.

The fifth cranial or trigeminal nerve is tested by noting sensation caused by pricking or lightly brushing the face. The patient is asked to make chewing and biting movements and to open his mouth against resistance. If the fifth nerve is involved, severe pain radiates to the midline of the face and neck in the involved side.

The seventh, or facial, nerve is tested for its motor components by having the patient raise his eyebrows, close his eyes and resist attempts to open them, show his teeth, smile, frown, and whistle. The sense of taste on the anterior two thirds of the tongue is tested by applying liquid testing solutions along the outer part of each side of the tongue and having the patient identify the taste as sugar, salt, acid, or bitter.

The eighth, or acoustic, nerve is tested by having the patient listen to whispering, the tick of a watch, and a tuning fork at prescribed distances. Special hearing tests with an audiometer give more accurate information about the acoustic nerve. (See Chapter 24.)

The ninth and tenth cranial nerves are tested by noting the movements of the tongue, and the gag reflex and by having the patient speak and cough. If there is involvement of the vagus nerve, the voice is weak and hoarse, and coughing is not effective.

The eleventh or spinal accessory nerve is tested by checking the sternocleidomastoid and trapezius muscles for atrophy or weakness, by having the patient rotate his head and by having him shrug his shoulders against resistance.

The twelfth, or hypoglossal, nerve is tested by having the patient stick out his tongue; lateral deviation indicates paralysis of the nerve on the side to which the tongue turns.

Motor and sensory function of the trunk muscles are checked in detail. For example, asking the patient to close his eyes and place his index finger on his nose tests both his coordination and his sense of touch and of position. Reflexes throughout the body are tested; the patellar reflex (knee jerk) and Achilles tendon reflex (foot flexion) tests are familiar to all nurses. Sense of position may be tested by having the patient close his eyes and tell the examiner where his hand or foot has been placed. Sense of touch may be tested by having the patient feel and identify materials of various textures. The autonomic nervous system is examined by noting the general appearance of the skin, whether its temperature and color are normal, and whether perspiration is either excessive or less than normal.

SPECIAL EXAMINATIONS

Special examinations of the nervous system include study of the cerebrospinal fluid, x-ray study of the spinal cord and brain, and measurement of electric waves elicited from the brain.

Examination of cerebrospinal fluid. The cerebrospinal fluid normally is a water-clear fluid which is formed in the lateral ventricles of the brain. It passes through the third ventricle, the aqueduct of Sylvius, the fourth ventricle, and finally into the cisterna magna at the base of the brain. From this location between the arachnoid and the dura mater, the fluid bathes the entire brain surface and passes down to surround the spinal cord. The main purpose of the spinal fluid appears to be to provide mechanical protection for the brain and spinal cord. The exact manner of its production and absorption is not entirely clear nor is the rate of its production clearly determined. It is thought that approximately 150 to 200 ml. of spinal fluid circulate within the system.

Spinal fluid normally is under slight positive pressure; 80 to 180 mm. of water is considered normal. This is measured on a manometer when a spinal puncture is done. When a brain tumor or other space-occupying lesion is within the cranium, the spinal fluid pressure usually is greatly increased. For this reason a lumbar puncture is not done lest the quick reduction in pressure produced by removal of spinal fluid cause the brain structures to herniate into the foramen magnum; this would put pressure upon vital centers in the medulla and might cause sudden death. The experienced neurologist often writes "no spinal tap" on the patient's chart to be certain that no other medical staff member attempts this procedure.

Normally, each ml. of spinal fluid contains 0 to 10 leukocytes. An increase in the number of cells may indicate an infection. Tuberculosis and viral infections may cause an increase in lymphocytes, while pyogenic infections may cause increase in polymorphonuclear leukocytes which may be in large enough numbers to make the fluid cloudy. Bacterial infections such as tuberculous meningitis often lower the sugar level from the normal level of 40 to 60 mg. per hundred milliliters (approximately one-half the normal blood sugar). They may also reduce the chloride level from the normal of 720 to 750 mg. per hundred milliliters. In the presence of degenerative diseases and when a brain tumor is present, the spinal fluid protein is usually increased from the normal level of 30 to 50 mg. per hundred milliliters. Study of the spinal fluid may occasionally reveal the actual organism causing disease. The serologic test for syphilis may be positive in spinal fluid even when the blood serology is negative.

Blood in the spinal fluid indicates hemorrhage somewhere in the system. It may be caused by a fracture of the base of the skull which has torn blood vessels, or it may be due to the rupture of a blood vessel such as may occur with a congenital aneurysm. Occasionally, the first specimen of spinal fluid contains blood from slight bleeding at the point of the puncture; for this reason the specimens of fluid are numbered and the first one is not used to determine the cell count.

The strictest aseptic technique is mandatory in all procedures in which the cerebrospinal fluid system is entered. The nurse is responsible for seeing that all equipment is sterile and that good technique is used throughout the procedure. She explains the procedure to the patient and sees that a permit for treatment is signed if hospital policy requires this. If the patient is uncertain about any details of the procedure, the nurse should not hesitate to ask the physician to give him further explanation. The nurse tells the patient what to expect during the procedure and how he may help to make it as simple as possible.

Details of the *spinal puncture procedure,* the equipment needed, and the nursing required are covered in texts on fundamentals of nursing. It should be explained to the patient that the needle will be inserted below the level of the spinal

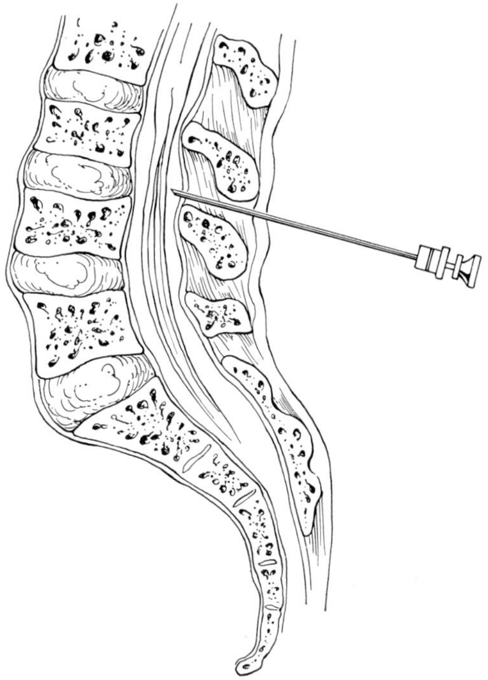

Figure 108

This diagram shows the position and angle of the needle when a lumbar puncture is done. Note that the needle is in the fourth lumbar interspace below the level of the spinal cord.

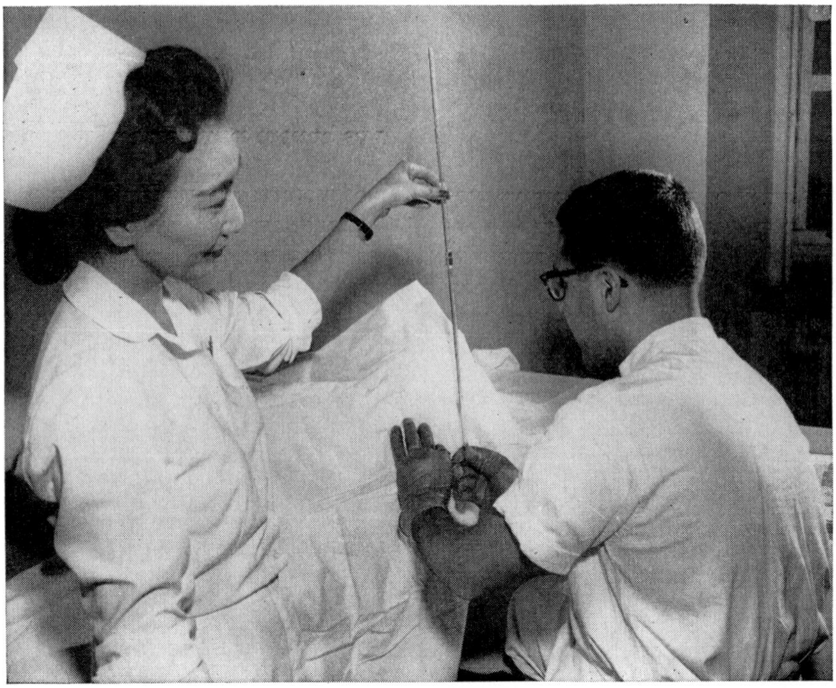

Figure 109

The nurse assisting the doctor with a lumbar puncture may support the manometer and record essential readings.

cord so there is little danger of injury. (See Figure 108.) He should know how to lie with both his knees and his head acutely flexed and should have constant nursing attention during the procedure. The patient should be reminded not to move suddenly. He should know that he may possibly experience a sharp shooting pain down one leg; this is caused by the needle coming close to a nerve and is similar to hitting one's "funny bone"; however, the nerve is actually floating in fluid and is safe from injury. Even when a local anesthetic is used (usually 1 per cent procaine), the patient should be prepared to feel slight pain and pressure as the dura is entered.

The nurse prepares the equipment, assists the doctor, watches the patient during and immediately following the procedure for signs of reaction such as pulse changes, arranges for suitable labeling and disposition of specimens, and replaces equipment. She may hold the manometer during the procedure. If so, she must hold it above the point where the doctor's hands need to come in contact with it since her hands are not sterile. (See Figure 109.) The nurse may be asked to compress the jugular vein first on one side, then on the other side, and finally both sides at the same time and to help the doctor to recall the spinal pressure under each of these circumstances. The pressure should be exerted with the fingers flat against the patient's neck, avoiding his trachea. This test, known as the *Queckenstedt test,* is simple but may alarm the patient who has not been informed that pressure may be exerted on his neck for a few seconds.

Headache is fairly common following a lumbar puncture. Although its exact cause is unknown, it is thought to be due to loss of spinal fluid through the dura. Sharpness and size of needle used, the skill of the doctor, and the emotional state of the patient are probably the determining factors in whether or not a headache will develop. If one does develop, it is treated with bed rest, an icecap to the head, and acetylsalicylic acid. Most headaches from this cause disappear within twenty-four hours.

Lumbar punctures are often performed on patients who are ambulatory and who go home immediately after the procedure is completed. It has been found that they suffer no more from headaches than do those who are treated more conservatively with bed rest and no elevation of the head.

In a *cisternal puncture*, the cerebrospinal fluid system is tapped by inserting a short-beveled needle immediately below the occipital bone into the cisterna magnum (see Figure 110). This procedure may be more frightening to the patient than a lumbar puncture since the approach is closer to the brain. The patient should have a detailed explanation by the doctor before any head preparation is done or before he is placed in the required position. A permit for operation is usually required. The back of the patient's neck may be shaved and he is placed on his side at the edge of the bed or on a treatment table with his head bent forward and held firmly by the nurse or another assistant. The patient is observed immediately following the procedure for dyspnea, apnea, and cyanosis, but these complications seldom occur. A cisternal puncture is often done on children. In some outpatient departments it is commonly done because it is considered less likely to be followed by headache than is a lumbar puncture.

Pneumoencephalography. Pneumoencephalography combines a spinal puncture with an x-ray examination. Air or oxygen is injected to replace spinal fluid that is withdrawn; the gas rises in the spinal canal to the ventricles, where its presence can be noted upon x-ray examination. Abnormal shape, size, or position of the ventricles or failure of the ventricles to fill with the gas is diagnostically significant. The procedure usually is done under local anesthesia, but a general inhalation, rectal, or intravenous anesthetic may be used for nervous or unstable patients. Headache is usually severe during and following pneumoencephalography; nausea and vomiting are not uncommon. A nurse must be in constant attendance to observe the patient while a second person assists the doctor.

Preparation for a pneumoencephalogram includes a bath, an enema, a sedative given the night before, and omission of food and fluid for six hours prior to the procedure. The patient must sign a permit. A sedative such as Nembutal is usually given one hour before the procedure is to be begun, and atropine and codeine or Demerol is given by injection one-half hour before. Hair pins, bobby pins, and false dentures are removed, and temperature, pulse rate, respiratory rate, and blood pressure are recorded on the chart.

The procedure may be started in the patient's room or in the treatment room. The patient is then taken to the x-ray

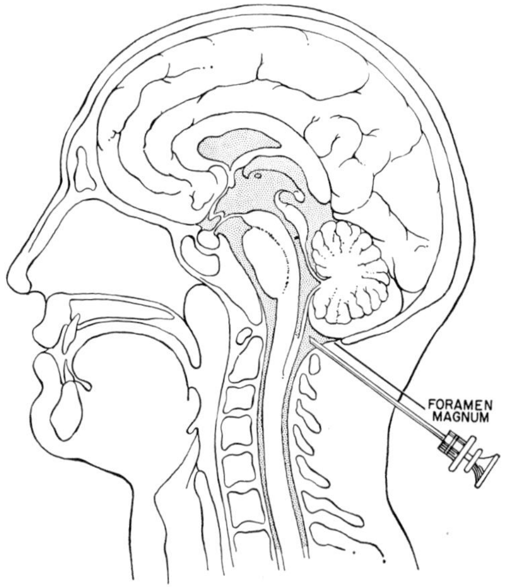

Figure 110

This diagram shows the position of the needle when a cisternal puncture is done. Note the needle length and the short bevel.

department where the pictures are taken. The equipment needed is the same as that for a spinal puncture with the addition of a three-way stopcock, a 20 ml. syringe with which to withdraw spinal fluid and inject air, a calibrated glass to measure the fluid that is removed, and an ampule of caffeine sodium benzoate and an ampule of Adrenalin for use in case of respiratory distress. Emergency oxygen equipment is also often requested.

The pressure of the spinal fluid is taken as soon as the needle is inserted into the lumbar spine. From 5 to 10 ml. of fluid are withdrawn at a time, and an equal amount of air or oxygen is injected. This is continued until the spinal fluid is drained; usually 75 to 100 ml. of fluid are removed. As the procedure is carried out, the patient is watched carefully for headache, nausea, and vomiting, and his pulse rate, respiratory rate, and blood pressure, and also his color are noted and recorded. The head of the bed or table is gradually raised and some physicians like to have the patient's head gently rotated after each 20 ml. of air have been injected in the belief that this gives better filling of the lateral ventricles.

Upon return from the x-ray department the patient is placed in bed with the head flat; usually he is more comfortable without a pillow. If a general anesthetic has been given, he is kept on his side and constantly attended until awake. Blood pressure, pulse rate, and respiratory rate are taken every fifteen minutes for the first hour, then every half hour and every hour for several hours or until they become stabilized. They are then taken every four hours. Any changes should be reported to the doctor at once. Fluids containing salt should be forced as soon as nausea subsides, since they may possibly increase the production of spinal fluid and the absorption of air. The patient who has a severe headache may benefit from an icecap to the head, and he should be given fluids through a straw so that his head is not raised. Acetylsalicylic acid, codeine, and Demerol are given for severe headache. If the patient complains of noises in his head, he should be assured that this is temporary since it is caused by gas in the ventricles and will disappear when the gas is absorbed. If the patient has any history of convulsions or unpredictable behavior, side rails should be placed on the bed and a mouth gag should be at the bedside. Often an emergency tracheotomy set is kept at the bedside for forty-eight hours after this procedure.

Reactions to pneumoencephalography can be severe, including continued vomiting, convulsions, shock, and signs of increased intracranial pressure with respiratory difficulty. Severe prolonged headache may also follow this diagnostic procedure, although headaches usually disappear after from twenty-four to thirty-six hours. For the first day or two the patient should be fed and encouraged to be as quiet as possible; he should have assistance even in turning from side to side. Usually after forty-eight hours he can be out of bed gradually. He may find that his headache and nausea increase when he is up, but these will be relieved by lying flat again.

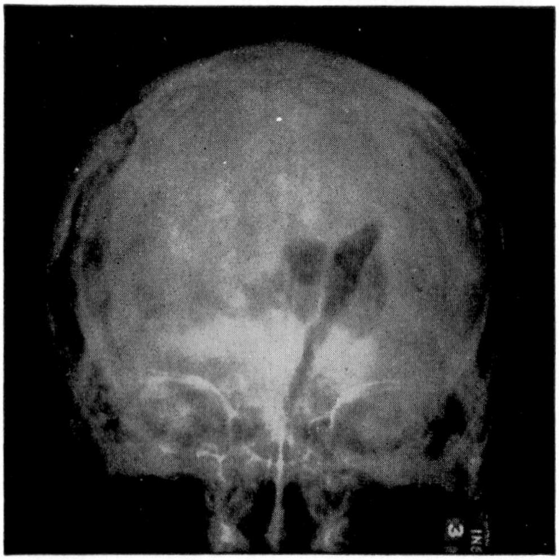

Figure 111

A ventriculogram showing marked ventricular shift. (From Moseley, H. F. [editor]: Textbook of Surgery, St. Louis, 1959, The C. V. Mosby Co.)

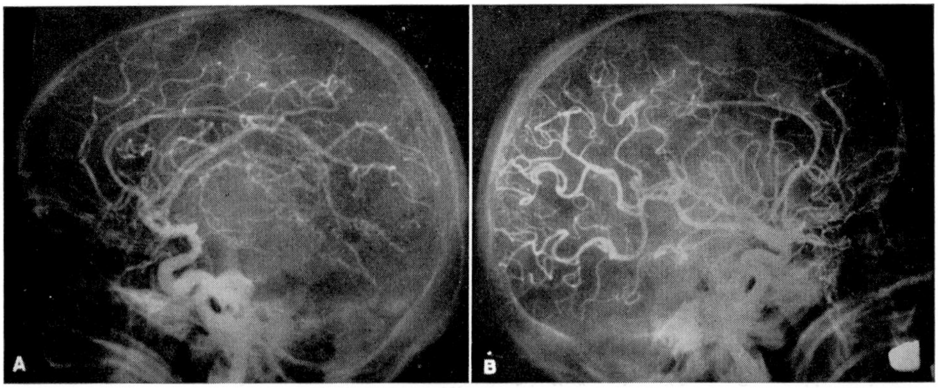

Figure 112

A, Arteriogram showing elevation of middle cerebral arteries by glioblastoma multiforme containing abnormal vascular network. *B*, Arteriogram showing the opposite normal side for comparison. (From Moseley, H. F. [editor]: Textbook of Surgery, St. Louis, 1959, The C. V. Mosby Co.)

Ventriculography. Ventriculography is similar to pneumoencephalography except that air is introduced directly into the lateral ventricles through trephine openings (burr holes) in the skull (see Figure 111). This procedure is always done in the operating room. It may be used when the suspected diagnosis is such that a spinal puncture is contraindicated because of extreme pressure within the skull or because the spinal canal is blocked. The preparation is similar to that for an encephalogram except that the top or the back of the head must be partially shaved depending on the doctor's orders. An intravenous or general anesthetic is usually used, and the patient may go directly from the x-ray department to the operating room for attempted removal of a tumor or for other necessary brain surgery. If the roentgenogram is normal, the patient is cared for in a manner similar to that following a pneumoencephalogram. The burr holes will be sutured and covered with a collodion dressing.

Arteriography. In this diagnostic procedure a radiopaque substance is injected into the carotid artery; roentgenograms taken immediately afterward may reveal an intracranial aneurysm, anomaly, or ruptured vessel. The large blood vessels of the circle of Willis at the base of the brain and the larger vessels penetrating the cerebrum can often be seen by this means. (See Figure 112.) Before the test is performed, a permit is signed by the patient or a responsible relative. A sedative is given the night before if necessary, and scopolamine or atropine sulfate and Demerol or morphine sulfate are given one-half hour before the procedure is done. A general anesthetic may be given; if this is necessary, the procedure is usually done in the operating room. If the dye can be injected directly into the carotid vessel without surgical exposure of the artery and if no general anesthesia is necessary, the procedure may be done in the x-ray department.

Following the test, the patient is watched for changes in the vital signs such as pulse, blood pressure, and respirations. Decreased hand grip, plantar pressure, or facial weakness on the side opposite the injection are significant. Convulsive seizures or aphasia may occur. Occasionally a delayed reaction to the dye occurs, and this may be serious. Ice collars applied to the neck help to prevent leaking from the vessel and local edema

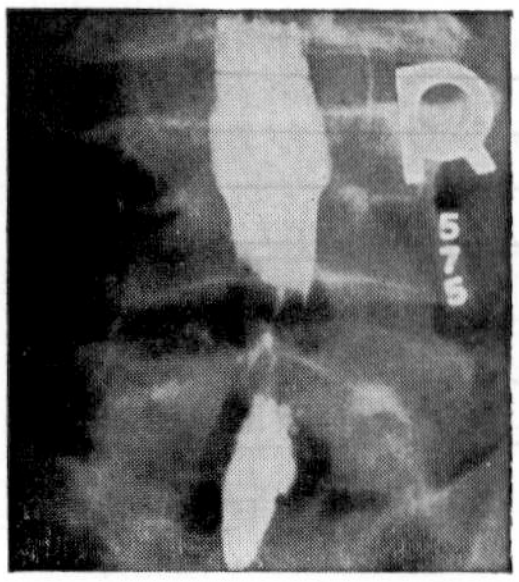

Figure 113

A myelogram showing an almost complete block of the interspace between the fourth and fifth lumbar vertebras. (From Moseley, H. F. [editor]: Textbook of Surgery, St. Louis, 1959, The C. V. Mosby Co.)

which might cause respiratory difficulty. A tracheotomy set is kept at the bedside. Usually, however, the patient experiences little, if any, discomfort and can resume his usual activities within a few hours.

Myelography. In this test either a gas or a radiopaque liquid is injected into the subarachnoid space, usually in the lumbar area, in an attempt to visualize a lesion of the spinal cord or in the spinal canal by means of the distortion it produces in the adjacent subarachnoid spaces. (See Figure 113.) This test is most often done as part of the diagnosis of cord tumor and occasionally when herniation of an intervertebral disc is suspected. The procedure is similar to that for a spinal puncture except that after the radiopaque substance is injected, the patient's head is elevated on two pillows and he is taken to the x-ray department. After fluoroscopic examination and roentgenograms are completed, the doctor removes the dye by doing another lumbar puncture. All the material must be removed, because it may cause serious irritation to the meninges. If some of it remains, care is taken to keep the patient's head elevated, and repeated attempts to remove the dye are made under fluoroscopy. One disadvantage of this test is the irritating quality of the available dyes; therefore, the test is not done when relatively certain diagnosis can be made by other means.

Electroencephalography. The electroencephalogram is an electric recording of the activity of the brain amplified many times and recorded in a manner similar to that of the electrocardiogram. Certain characteristic patterns in the record are normal, and by study of the recordings of brain action, areas of abnormal action can sometimes be detected. This is only an adjunct to other diagnostic tests, but it may be helpful in locating the site of the lesion. Before the examination the patient should be quiet, and the procedure should be explained to him so that no undue excitement occurs. The scalp should be clean, but no other local preparation is necessary. Approximately sixteen tiny electrodes are attached to the scalp with collodion, and the patient should be prepared for this; no hair need be cut, which is often reassuring to the patient. (See Figure 114.) Occasionally the electrodes used are tiny pins which are stuck into the scalp. The patient should know that this will not be really painful because there are very few nerve endings in the scalp. The examination is done in a special room where outside electrical activity is eliminated. The patient usually sits in a comfortable chair or lies on a stretcher or table with his eyes closed. The test may last for an hour or more.

Radioactive iodine-tagged albumin test. Albumin tagged with radioactive iodine has proved useful in locating tumors within the skull cavity; approximately 70 per cent can be localized by this means.[28] Solutions containing the radioactive substance are injected intravenously; location of a tumor can be determined by using a Geiger-Müller counter since tumor cells tend to hold the radioactive substance.

Caloric testing. Testing the equilibrium by dropping water into the auditory canal often is done to differentiate neurologic disorders (see Chapter 24).

DEGENERATIVE DISEASES

Multiple sclerosis

Multiple sclerosis is a common neurologic disease in northern climates, although it is practically unknown in trop-

, and meat, and cereal increase acidity. Eating polished rice only causes beriberi. Newbor are low in vitamin K because it is not synthesized for the first week of life.

Children diabetics are not usually obese. Eat polyunsaturated fats to prevent atherosclerosis ., and lower blood cholesterol, therefore avoid fried foods and fricassees, eggs and cheese, milk and lard. Oleic fatty acid is mono-unsaturated. Linoleic and linolenic are polyunsaturated. Skim milk is free from cholesterol. Corn oil is polyunsaturated. Guide a patient, do not force him. Dumping syndrome requires six small meals to provide gradual emptying of stomach and abosrption; no fluids at meals; B 12 medication because stomach secretions are lessened. Motives for reducing must come from the person reducing himself. The only reason for not losing weight is calories are not low enough. Exercise helps weight loss by using calories. Eating meat rather than cereal, fruit or vegetable will increase blood pressure. Soft drinks and sugar are not allowed on reducing diets because they supply calories but nothing eseential. Worst food pattern is no breakfast. Know signs of too much and not enough insulin. Multiply cho by 4, pro by 4, fat by 9. If diabetic does not eat bread, give her only 3 soda crackers. Egg is same as 1 ounce of meat or cheese. But bacon, cream cheese are fat substitutes. Cheese protects longest against insulin reaction.

Vitamin A in yellow vegetables and yellow fats. Orthodix Jews, no meat and milk products at the same meal. Americans eat little grains. Near East eats lamb and fruit. Far east eats pork and eggs. Gluten means grain, chiefly wheat foods. If diet is low in grain it is low in thiamin. If low in fat it is low in carotene (vitamin A). Vitamin A needs bile salts for absorption, especially if in the form of carotene. Celiac disease is treated by gluten-free diet (no wheat, oats, barley or rye). In ulcers eat fat to inhibit gastric secretion. Protein should be from animal and vegetable sources. Iron is added to enriched bread. Yellow fruits and molasses are high in iron. Citrus fruits are low in iron. Leagy vegetables are high iron. With talkative child, tell him a story while feeding him. Ask patients what they customarily eat. 1 quart of milk is 32 ounces and furnishes 32 grams protei Skim milk is the same as whole except in fat. In toxemia measure protein and salt. Inadequate diet does not diminish the quantity of breast milk. Lactose is in both human and cow's milk. Arginine is essential for growth but not for adults. Ask mothers about quantity of protein foods served daily, rather than variety. Candy is not important unless it spoils the food pattern for other foods. Quart of milk is not as essential as acceptance of solid food at proper age. Giving protein for tissue building is practical only if other calories are furnished for energy.

Nutrition in Medical and Surgical Nursing Curriculum Guide (By American Dietetic Association for the National League for Nursing and American Hospital Association).

In visiting nursing ,question mother on the diet of the weaned child. Deficiencies: kwashiorkor, endemic goiter(lack of iodine) pellagra(too much corn)myxedema(lack of thyroxin,causing rise in blood cholesterol. Hygiene:handwashing, refrigeration of all foods,especially meat.Fever requir increase in calories,protein and thiamin to aid appetite.Riboflavin deficiency : stomatitis and dermatitis.Thaimin deficiency : loss of appetite.Vitamin A deficiency : keratinization of the epi thelium. Vitamin D deficiency : beading of ribs. PKU causes mental retardation. Vitamin D defici cy : rickets. Toxicity from excessive vitamins A and D. Vitamin C deficiency, flexed muscles,crie when handled(needs orange juice). Salt deficiency : result of perspiration in cystic fibrosis of pancreas. Noted for calcium : milk and spinach .Sodium in hotbreads,crackers etc must be consider as well as table salt. Avoid salads on a bland diet. Increase calories and protein in hepatitis. Negative nitrogen balance is more out than in,may occur in weight reduction. Increase albumin if alb in in the urine; increase calcium if calcium in urine. Emphasize the four basic food groups in teac ing patients. Child copies tension of mother in feeding problems.In menu problems, avoid negative directions, question mother about other items the child eats. Apply dietary pattern and 4 food groups to all menus. There is no egg in French dressing or in gelatin dessert. [illegible]

Know World Health Organization for clinical aspects and Food Agricultural Organization for food problems. Rules for food additives: manufacturer must prove them harmless before marketing them. If glucose (or glycogen) accumulates and calories remain excessive, deposition of adipose tissue results. NRC allowances are minimum and for normal people. Excess vitamins are wasted. Vitamin C builds connective tissue. Intrinsic factor promotes the absorption of B 12. Pernicious anemia is characterized by defective gastric secretions. Deficiencies are often prevented by abundances of other food. Read labels on packaged cereals because they differ in potassium and salt content. Pellagra is due to lack of niacin and cured by foods high in niacin or foods as milk which contain tryptophan which is converted into niacin. Iron is most needed by children and women. Hepatic coma is caused by ammonia in blood producing neurologic symptoms, treated by restricted protein, and high cho to prevent catabolism of tissue proteins; since protein is low it should be high quality. Know foods high and low in potassium and sodium. Acid ash and alkali ash foods and exceptions. Diabetic exchanges and unusual listings (ex. ice cream for bread etc). Avoid glandular meat as liver on low purine diet. Liver damage is prevented by protein to rebuild liver cells and high calories. Low residue diet forbids nuts and skins. Milk is high in residue. Salt or water retention is not the cause of obesity. Do not treat obesity by low salt. Fish, cheese and peanut butter are high in salt. Garlic salt and ketchup are high in salt. Urea results from the catabolism (destruction)

Eck 312

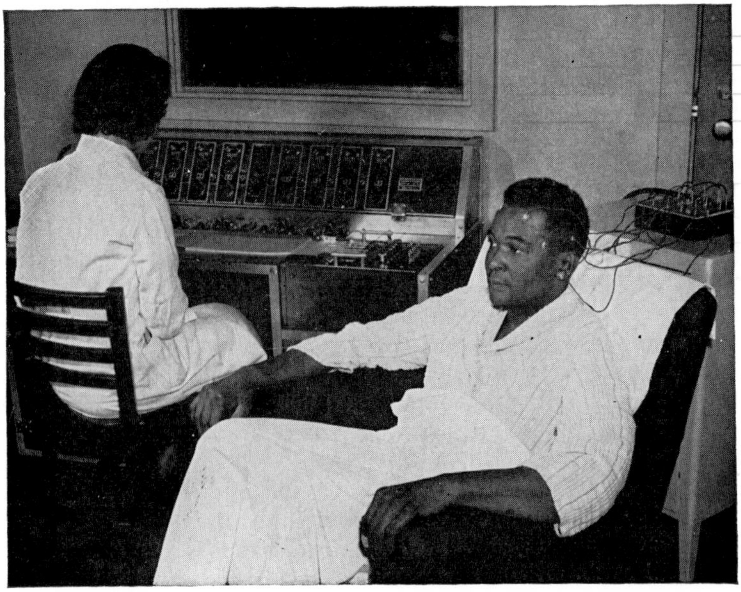

Figure 114

A patient ready to have an electrocencephalogram.
(From de Gutiérrez-Mahoney, C. G., and Carini, Esta: Neurological and Neurosurgical Nursing, St. Louis, 1960, The C. V. Mosby Co.)

ical countries. The exact prevalence of the disease is not known since in many instances a diagnosis is not made, but probably at least 300,000 persons in the United States are affected.[19] The onset of symptoms usually occurs between 20 and 40 years of age; symptoms rarely occur before 15 or after 50 years of age. Multiple sclerosis has serious implications for family life since it affects men and women in the active productive years when their responsibilities are the greatest. Men and women are affected about equally.

The cause of multiple sclerosis is unknown. Mineral deficiency, toxic substances, viruses, and disturbance of blood clotting mechanisms are a few suspected contributory causes, but there is no real evidence that any of them is involved. Patchy, irregular areas of degeneration appear in the white matter of the brain and in the outer part of the spinal cord. The outer myelin sheath of the spinal cord can be compared to the insulation on an electric wire, and its destruction causes interruption of nerve pathways. Because of the wide distribution of areas of degeneration, there is a larger variety of signs and symptoms in multiple sclerosis than in any other neurologic disease.

There is evidence of partial healing of the areas of degeneration, which accounts for the transitory nature of many early symptoms. The scarring that occurs at the site of the degenerative lesion gives the name sclerosis to the disease.

Multiple sclerosis may be acute or chronic. Usually there are acute exacerbations and remissions which may last for a year or more, although eventually exacerbations will recur. There is no record of any patient having recovered from the disease, although many have lived for twenty or more years and have died from other causes. Exacerbations may be aggravated or precipitated by fatigue, chilling, and emotional disturbances.

Early symptoms are usually transitory and may include double vision (diplopia), spots before the eyes (scotomas), blindness, tremor, weakness or numbness of a part of the body such as the hand, fatigue, susceptibility to upper respiratory infections, and emotional instability. Many patients with early multiple sclerosis are considered neurotic by their associates and sometimes by their physicians because of the wide variety and temporary nature of symptoms and because of their emotional instability. As the disease progresses, symptoms may include nystagmus, disorders of speech, urinary frequency and urgency, constipation, and changes in muscular coordination and gait. Late symptoms may include urinary incontinence, difficulty in swallowing, and severe muscle spasm and contractures. Pain is not a symptom of multiple sclerosis except when there is severe muscle spasm.

In the hospital, the nurse may care for the patient for short periods when he is admitted for diagnosis or for some other condition. She may also participate in terminal care of those with advanced disease. Because many patients with multiple sclerosis are not hospitalized, she is likely to encounter them when she works in patients' homes as a public health nurse.

Medical treatment and nursing care. There is no specific treatment for multiple sclerosis. Warm baths, physical therapy, psychotherapy, and specific drugs for acquired infections are helpful. Effort is made to keep the patient working for as long as possible, and many men have worked for from five to ten years and even longer after the onset of the first symptoms. Women can be helped to plan their shopping, housework, and other duties so that they may continue to function as wives and mothers even when the disease is advanced. The decision as to whether or not the patient is told his diagnosis rests with the doctor, and there is not full agreement among doctors as to the proper course of action. Usually the decision is made on an individual basis and depends on the patient's emotional make-up and upon his family's ability to cope with the economic, social, and emotional problems that a situation of this kind presents.

The patient with multiple sclerosis should have a daily routine for rest and activity, and he should adhere to it strictly. Rest must be balanced with adequate exercise. The patient is usually advised to exercise regularly but never to the point of extreme fatigue. Because he almost always feels tired, he must look for some special sign that tells him he has exercised enough. If he does more, he may suffer ill effects. For example, a tight feeling in the chest may indicate that the patient must rest or else have severe discomfort. After an exacerbation, it may be difficult for the patient to resume exercises, but it is usually best for him to return to an established schedule as soon as possible.

One side of the body is usually affected more than the other, and the patient may learn to stabilize his gait by leaning toward his good side. The annoyance of having the foot slap forward in taking a step may sometimes be overcome by the patient if he puts the heel down in a pronounced fashion and rolls the weight forward on the side of the foot.

The patient with multiple sclerosis needs a peaceful, relaxed environment. He should never be hurried and should not be expected to respond quickly either physically or mentally. He may have slowness in speech and slowness in ability to respond, and these should be ignored by those around him. Members of the family and friends need help in understanding this reaction and in meeting it calmly. The patient may have sudden explosive emotional outbursts of crying or laughing brought on by such simple acts as putting something hot into the mouth. Close members of the family must protect both the patient and visitors from the embarrassment of prolonged emotional outbursts. Reminding the patient of something sad may stop him from laughing and holding the mouth open will sometimes stop the crying.

A sense of optimism and well-being (euphoria) seems to be characteristic of persons with multiple sclerosis, especially during remissions. It is suspected that this is due largely to the patient's attempts to reassure himself that his condition is not so serious as is supposed. This response is helpful to the patient in many ways, but sometimes it may lead him to overdo and thus increase symptoms.

Good general hygiene is necessary for the patient with multiple sclerosis. This includes a well-balanced diet with plenty of high-vitamin foods and fluids. Obesity must be avoided, because it makes it more difficult for the patient to handle himself and detracts from his appearance. The patient should sleep eight hours each night and should have a rest period after lunch. Fresh air and sunshine are good, but chilling and overheating must be avoided because they may aggravate symptoms or bring on exacerbations.

Since association with others is good for physical and mental health, the patient with multiple sclerosis must be encouraged and helped to remain an active participating member of his family and his community for as long as possible. Personal cleanliness adds to a feeling of acceptance and well-being; consequently these patients should be encouraged to pay careful attention to personal appearance even though they may sometimes feel too tired to put forth the effort. The patient should be encouraged to develop interests and hobbies that will help make up for things he should not do, such as driving a vehicle, and which will help to fill the time when physical activity becomes more difficult. Music, writing, reading, and question games are good hobbies to develop. Interests in politics and in world affairs which may be followed on the radio if sight is lost may stand the patient in good stead. Study of philosophy and the development of a faith should be encouraged.

The National Multiple Sclerosis Society* is a national voluntary organization founded in 1946. Its functions are to encourage and finance research, to gather statistics, and to act as an information center for patients and for the public. Membership is open to doctors, nurses, and other health and welfare workers and to patients and their families. Local organizations are located in many of our larger cities.

Paralysis agitans (Parkinson's disease)

Parkinson's disease is a slowly progressive degenerative disease of unknown cause in which there is destruction of nerve cells in the basal ganglia of the brain. It may follow encephalitis and occasionally occurs following carbon monoxide poisoning. The disease usually affects older persons and is often associated with arteriosclerosis, although this is not thought to be a direct cause. Approximately 200,000 persons in the United States have the disease, and it appears to be increasing. Since the disease is more common in persons past their mid-fifties, the increase is probably the result of the increase in the number of persons in this age group.[12]

Parkinson's disease begins with a faint tremor and progresses so slowly that the patient is seldom able to recall its onset. There is no true paralysis and no loss of sensation. Tremor and muscle rigidity are the two outstanding signs of the disease. Muscle rigidity seems to prevent normal response in commonly performed acts and leads to characteristic changes which make the diagnosis almost unmistakable to those who have observed patients with the disease. There is a masklike appearance to the face and slowed monotonous speech; drooling may occur because of the difficulty of swallowing saliva. This may cause skin irritation which is best prevented or treated by frequent sponging followed by protecting the skin with an emollient such as cold cream. There is a characteristic shuffling gait in which the patient tends to walk on his toes; the trunk is bent forward and the arms fall rigidly at the sides and do not swing as in a normal rhythmic gait. Neuromuscu-

*Home office: Academy of Medicine Building, Fifth Avenue and 103rd Street, New York, N. Y.

lar control may be altered so that the patient is unable to stop his propulsive gait until he meets an obstruction; finally, he may become unable to walk at all. The patient usually has a moist oily skin. Judgment defect and emotional instability may occur, but intelligence is not impaired. The appetite may be increased, and there is heat intolerance probably because of the activity of the tremor. All signs and symptoms increase with fatigue, excitement, and frustration.

Medical treatment and nursing care. Treatment for Parkinson's disease is only palliative. Drugs which produce relaxation such as atropine sulfate and related drugs (hyoscine and stramonium) are widely used. These are more effective in lessening muscle rigidity than in controlling the tremor. One of the disadvantages in the use of these drugs is that in order to get the desired effect upon the muscles, the dosage must be such that unpleasant side effects, such as dryness of the mouth, occur. Also there is danger of atropine poisoning in elderly patients whose liver and kidney functions are limited. Many newer drugs are being tried in attempts to find some that are effective yet produce fewer side effects. One synthetic atropine-like preparation, *trihexyphenidyl* (Artane), appears promising. The dosage is usually 2 mg. in tablet form given by mouth three times a day. Phenobarbital and bromides are used to allay excitement and thereby decrease the tremor and treat the insomnia which is common in this disease.

In recent years a surgical procedure has been used with some success in treatment of selected patients with Parkinson's disease. Descriptions of successful operations in popular magazines have led some patients and their families to believe that a cure for all patients has been found. The nurse should refer those asking her about the operation to a qualified neurologist. Many patients cannot be treated surgically. Results seem to be best in younger patients with unilateral involvement following other disease and who have marked tremor and rigidity. Treatment consists of destroying portions of the globus pallidus (relieves rigidity) and/or the thalamus (relieves tremor) in the brain by means of cautery, removal, or by injection of a chemical (alcohol). Medical reports of success and of surgical risks vary. Nursing care includes seeing that medications are discontinued and attention to nutrition preoperatively. Postoperative care includes the most careful attention to the vital signs, use of side rails to prevent accidents in the event of convulsions, disorientation or temporary hemiplegia, and frequent turning and moving to prevent respiratory and circulatory complications. Excessive salivation and difficulty in blinking the eye on the operated side may be problems requiring special nursing care. If a needle has been left in the trephine opening in the skull for repeated injections of alcohol, the patient requires special care to assure its remaining in position. This care is fully described in current periodicals.[14]

The progress of Parkinson's disease, a condition which often lasts for years, may be slowed by good nutrition, sufficient rest, moderate exercise in fresh air, and other measures which improve general health. Special attention should be paid to posture. Lying on a firm bed without a pillow during rest periods may help to prevent the spine from bending forward, and lying in the prone position also helps in this. Holding the hands folded behind the back when walking may help to keep the spine erect and prevent the annoyance of the arms falling stiffly at the sides. The tremor often is less apparent when the patient is sitting in an arm chair since he can grip the arms of the chair and partially control the tremor in his hands and arms.

The patient with Parkinson's disease should continue to work as long as possible. Most physicians advise this unless the occupation is such that continued work is dangerous. The patient should reduce his regular work gradually while he builds up hobbies and interests in which he may engage when the disease becomes more advanced. Relatives must have a complete understanding of the circumstances so that they may intelligently assist in the adjustments that will eventually be necessary. Such problems as danger of accidents, personality changes, and progressive helplessness must be anticipated. While drooling and difficulty in swallowing often limit the important social outlet of eating at group gatherings, the patient should have his meals at home with the family as long as possible. Feeding the patient becomes a real problem when the disease is far advanced because of the danger of choking in attempts to swallow; eventually, aspiration pneumonia may terminate the patient's life.

Myasthenia gravis

Myasthenia gravis is a relatively rare disease of unknown cause. It usually occurs in young adults. The outstanding symptom is severe fatigue to the point of exhaustion which comes on quickly and, in the early stages of the disease, disappears quickly with rest. Weakness of arms and hands first may be noticed when shaving or combing the hair. Muscle fatigue becomes so severe that it may cause weakness or drooping of muscles; facial muscles innervated by the cranial nerves are often affected. There is a flattening of the facies, and it may not be possible for the patient to hold his eyelids open, to keep his mouth closed, or to chew and swallow. He may have double vision and a weak voice. Occasionally the fatigue becomes so great that the patient cannot breathe and a respirator must be used. The symptoms are due to failure of nerve impulses to pass to the muscles at the myoneural junction and not to central nervous system involvement.

There is no known cure for myasthenia gravis. There is, however, a very marked improvement in symptoms following the administration of neostigmine or Prostigmin. These drugs block the action of cholinesterase at the myoneural junction and allow action of acetylcholine, a chemical necessary for transmission of impulses to the muscles. Treatment is planned so that the patient may be maintained on the amount of drug which he can tolerate without side effects and yet carry out activities essential for normal living; usually the patient is permitted to adjust his own dosage. Patients with myasthenia gravis must often change their method of earning a living. The nurse can help the patient and his family plan so that a minimum of energy is used in activities that are essential to his remaining relatively self-sufficient.

The patient with myasthenia gravis should take particular care of his health. Upper respiratory infections may be serious, because he may not have the energy to cough effectively and may develop pneumonia or strangle. The patient who is living at home may feel more secure if he has a suction apparatus and a member of his family knows how to use it if an emergency arises.

During acute episodes of the disease a tracheotomy set is kept in the patient's room ready for immediate use. Often it is necessary to use suction before the patient eats. If swallowing is too dangerous, a gastric tube is used, and great care must be taken to be certain that the tube is in the stomach before fluid is introduced, since the patient cannot cough to indicate its presence in the trachea. When caring for the patient with severe symptoms of myasthenia gravis, the nurse must remember that he is too weak to do anything for himself. Therefore, the patient may not take a drink and may not turn over in bed unless the nurse thinks of helping him.

HEADACHE

Headache is the most common of all neurologic conditions. Probably over 98 per cent of all persons suffer from this condition at some time in their lives. Headache is not a disease but is a symptom of disease, of bodily reaction to harmful substances such as drugs or to excessive psychic pressure. The conditions that cause headache are almost infinite in number. Headaches may be caused by systemic disease or infection, by hypertension, and by pressure from a lesion such as a tumor. They may be caused by drugs, by foreign substances to which the person is sensitive, and by anoxia or inhalation of poisonous gases. They may be caused by eyestrain, by congestion in the sinuses, and by excessive contraction of neck and scalp muscles. Headaches often occur either before or during the menstrual period.

Headaches often vary, depending on their cause. For example, frontal headache may be caused by sinusitis and is characteristically relieved if the patient sits up and if local heat is applied to the sinus areas of the face. Brain tumors often cause dull constant headaches. Headaches caused by emotional tension are usually steady and bandlike and usually precede or follow periods of tension and become worse as the day wears on.

Headaches are probably treated by the laity more often than any other condition, including even the common cold. However, the public should know that persistent headaches are abnormal and need investigation by a physician. Patients have been known to "doctor" a headache for months in the belief that it was due to a sinus infection, only finally to learn that it was due to hypertension or to a brain tumor. Persistent headaches, even when physical cause has been ruled out, indicate that the patient should review his mode of living and make some adjustments. The nurse can sometimes help him see the wisdom of this course. She can also advise against the widespread use of the coal-tar analgesics in treatment of headaches. Occasional use of acetylsalicylic acid by the laity for minor indispositions is considered safe by most medical authorities. The use of phenacetin and other similar preparations is not advisable unless prescribed by a physician; prolonged and excessive use of these preparations has caused changes in blood cells and may be responsible for other serious signs and symptoms.

Migraine syndrome

The layman' s term for migraine headache is "sick headache." This condition is now believed to be much more common than was previously supposed. Before the acute onset there may be fatigue, chilliness, and irritability; these symptoms occasionally precede the acute attack by as much as a day or more. The acute symptoms vary in intensity but may be severe. Usually the headache is present upon awakening in the morning, and one side of the head is more affected than the other. Pain is usually keenest in the temporal area but may be anywhere in the head, and sometimes the face is also affected. There may be spots before the eyes, partial blindness, dizziness, nausea, and vomiting. The pain is often so intense that the patient is forced to seek isolation in a dark room; the acute attack usually lasts from a few hours to a day but occasionally may last for a week or even longer.

The precipitating cause of migraine headache is a constriction and then a dilation of cerebral arteries. The cause of this is unknown, but it has been repeatedly demonstrated that nervous tension contributes to attacks. The person who develops migraine headaches is usually one who works hard and strives for perfection; migraine headaches often follow a period of overwork and overstrain. After an attack, the patient feels better, probably because he has been forced to rest. Hope for a cure of the condition lies in changing the patient's attitudes toward the world and toward himself, and usually this is not easy.

Acetylsalicylic acid is seldom effective for the true migraine headache. The one drug that is quite effective is ergotamine tartrate. For best results ergotamine tartrate should be given early—before the condition is full-blown. The usual dosage is 3 mg. by mouth or 0.25 mg. (1/240 grain) hypodermically, but it can also be given intravenously for quicker action. The disadvantages of the drug are that it causes nausea and vomiting, tingling sensations, and muscle tightness. The weekly dosage should not exceed 0.5 mg. (1/120 grain) if given hypodermically or 10 mg. (1/6 grain) if given by mouth.[4]

CONVULSIVE SEIZURES

Convulsions may occur in many illnesses such as uremia, eclampsia, tetanus, and infections accompanied by extremely high temperature. Convulsions may be caused by poisons such as strychnine and may occur with increasing intracranial pressure such as that produced by a brain tumor. Children are more susceptible to convulsive seizures than are adults, presumably because their nervous systems are less stable; children may have generalized convulsions when temperature is elevated in many infectious diseases or with relatively minor conditions such as gastrointestinal upsets. Convulsions may be hysterical in origin rather than due to an organic disease; in such a case the patient seldom injures himself during the seizure. Actually, these are not true convulsions. By far the most common cause of convulsive seizures is epilepsy.

The nurse should observe the patient during a seizure and note the kind of convulsion that is occurring. In a *tonic convulsion* all muscles contract at once, while in a *clonic convulsion* opposing muscle groups alternately contract and relax, giving a jerking convulsive movement of the body. Convulsions may start in one muscle or group of muscles and may spread to parts or all of the body; this is known as a *jacksonian seizure.* A brain lesion may be the cause, and the part of the body in which the convulsive movements start may give a clue to its location.

If the nurse is present during a seizure, she should protect the patient from injury, and she must observe the seizure closely. If the patient is in a precarious location where he might fall or otherwise injure himself, he should be lowered to the floor gently and a pillow or soft object placed under his head. Any equipment that might be harmful, such as an electric fan, should be placed out of reach. If the patient has fallen to the floor at the onset of the seizure, no attempt should be made to move him to a bed or sofa during the attack. A rubber wedge or tongue blade should be placed between his back teeth to prevent the tongue from being bitten. In the hospital, a padded tongue blade is kept at the bedside when seizures are anticipated. Care must be taken not to pry open the front or side teeth in an attempt to insert the gag since this may loosen them and cause the patient more inconvenience than a bitten tongue. Tight clothing should be loosened, but no restraint should be used. The duration of the seizure should be noted. The nurse should observe whether the patient convulses equally in all parts of the body, whether his eyes turn to one side or to the other, and whether his pupils dilate or constrict. She should note how pulse and respirations are affected and whether there are changes in skin color; grinding or clenching of the teeth, unusual diaphoresis, and urinary or fecal incontinence should be reported. Following a seizure she should question the patient to determine his state of consciousness and to learn if he knows where he is and if he has headache or any other complaints. Convulsions should be described in detail in the nurse's notes or on the patient's chart and should be reported to the physician at once.

Genetic epilepsy

Epilepsy is one of the oldest diseases known to man; it was described in detail by Hippocrates. The term epilepsy means seizure or "state." The disease was at one time thought to be of divine origin and perhaps for this reason has been linked in the public mind with the occult, the strange, and the unmentionable. No disease has been more carefully concealed within families, and many attitudes toward the disease have persisted from early times to the present day. Attitudes may also be affected by the frightening experience of having seen a person during a severe seizure, by the belief that mental deterioration always occurs in epilepsy, and by the belief that epilepsy is inherited and runs in families.

Genetic or *idiopathic* epilepsy is a disease of unknown cause. The disease is not directly inherited, although abnormal brain waves, as shown in the electroencephalogram, are found in many relatives of persons having seizures, and it is likely that a predisposition to the disease is inherited. It is believed that some alteration of chemical balance touches off the seizure in susceptible persons. There are over 800,000 persons in the United States with some form of epilepsy, or approximately one out of every 200 of our population.[9] Epilepsy is largely a disease of younger people, approximately three fourths of sufferers having seizures before the age of 20 years.[9] The life expectancy of persons with epilepsy is less than for the population as a whole, primarily because the person often dies of an accident incurred during a seizure.

Types of seizures. There are several types of epileptic seizures: grand mal seizures, petit mal seizures, and psychic equivalents. Status epilepticus is the term used when the patient goes from one grand mal seizure to another without regaining consciousness. A common name for seizures is "fits." However, the term has an unpleasant connotation. "Attacks" is the best term to use in conversation with the laity.

Grand mal seizures (the big sickness) refers to major convulsions in which the patient may lose consciousness for minutes. These are preceded by an *aura* or warning sensation in about 50 per cent of all patients.[8] This aura may be dizziness, spots before the eyes, numbness, or a wide variety of other sensations which the patient may find difficult to describe but which give him conclusive warning of the impending seizure. It serves a useful purpose in that it enables the patient to seek safety and privacy before the onset of the seizure. Occasionally it occurs as much as a day before the seizure so that the patient who works can remain at home and his fellow workers need not know of his attacks.

The grand mal seizure is usually heralded by a sharp cry as air is rapidly inhaled. Expiration of air does not follow naturally, the muscles are held rigid in a tonic contraction, and the patient's skin becomes cyanotic. After what seems to the observer to be a long time (usually only a few seconds), a jerky (clonic) movement and quick irregular respirations begin and continue for as long as a minute or more. Often there is frothing at the mouth; this may be streaked with blood if the tongue or lips have been bitten during the convulsion. During the clonic phase there may be fecal or urinary incontinence. As the convulsion subsides, the patient usually falls asleep, awaking moments or hours later with a dull headache and depression. There is no actual pain from the seizure, and many patients who have seizures during sleep realize this only when, upon awakening, they find blood on the pillow or soiling of the bed. If convulsions occur often during sleep, it is necessary to protect the bed; however, this should be done as inconspicuously as possible. Side rails are sometimes necessary, and these are likely to disturb the patient. It is possible that depression following seizures is caused in part by the knowledge that they have occurred.

The *petit mal attack* (the little sickness) is a momentary loss of consciousness. It occurs frequently in children and in adolescents at the onset of puberty. It does not produce the frightening spectacle of the grand mal seizure, but it can be most disconcerting to the patient and is seldom preceded by an aura. Petit mal attacks may be more difficult to control with the drugs available than grand mal seizures. While talking, the patient may stop for a moment and stare into space or drop his head and then go on talking without realizing that his conversation was interrupted. The child may be considered awkward by his parents, since, as he loses consciousness, he may appear to stumble and starts to fall but then regains consciousness before he really falls. He may drop his fork or glass of milk during meals, and again the reason may not be discovered for a time. A serious problem is the momentary loss of consciousness during play, such as when riding a bicycle in traffic, walking on a high fence, or climbing a tree.

Psychic equivalents, or *psychomotor epilepsy,* is a condition in which consciousness is lost or amnesia occurs but in which no convulsion ensues, and activity which in some ways appears normal may be continued during the attack. When the attack is over, the patient has no recollection of what took place. During the attack, he may appear drowsy, intoxicated, or violent, behave normally, or engage in violent antisocial activity. Since serious crimes have been committed by persons with psychic equivalents, diagnosis in such persons is sometimes of great interest to lawyers and judges as well as to medical scientists.

Status epilepticus, or a *continuous major convulsion,* is relatively rare, but it can lead to death from exhaustion. Emergency medical and nursing measures are often needed, and padded side rails must always be used. Inhalation anesthesia or large doses of barbiturates may be given in an effort to halt seizures. Concentrated solutions of glucose may be given intravenously to cause dehydration, and magnesium sulfate (50 per cent) may be given intramuscularly to promote relaxation. Oxygen and cardiac stimulants should be readily available. A suction machine is often needed, and occasionally the head of the bed is lowered if there is danger of aspiration of mucus. The patient should be kept in a quiet room and noise and confusion reduced to a minimum.

Medical treatment and nursing care. Some authorities believe that the only prevention for epilepsy is applied eugenics since the predisposition to develop the disease appears to be inherited.[4] There is no known cure for idiopathic epilepsy, although seizures can sometimes be controlled by dehydration, quieting the emotional state, increasing the acidity of the body, and using certain drugs. Treatment consists of attempting to lower the threshold at which the nervous system can no longer control the seizure. Bromides have long been considered helpful in the treatment of epilepsy, and phenobarbital has been widely used for years. Phenobarbital is usually given in small doses four or more times each day. However, so much of the drug may have to be given in order to control seizures that its sedative effect may give others the impression that the patient is mentally sluggish. One of the most satisfactory drugs is *diphenylhydantoin sodium* (Dilantin sodium) which was first used in Boston in 1936. This drug has an antispasmodic effect with less of a sedative effect than the barbiturates. The dosage is often 0.1 Gm. (1.5 grains) three times a day by mouth for adults, but this depends on the reaction of the individual patient to the drug and the severity of his symptoms. Tremor, nystagmus, gastric disturbances, rash, and hypertrophy and bleeding of the gums are signs of toxicity from Dilantin sodium. Hypertrophy of the gums may be controlled in most instances by regular, vigorous massage.

Many newer drugs are being used in the treatment of epilepsy. *Trimethadione* (Tridione) is one that has been particularly useful for petit mal seizures, but it causes a peculiar photophobia (glare phenomenon) in which objects are perceived as if they were reflected from a bright snowy surface. This condition is relieved by wearing dark glasses. *Methylphenylethylhydantoin* (Mesantoin) is particularly helpful for grand mal seizures and for psychic equivalents. Most of the drugs which are helpful in epilepsy produce toxic effects, including severe kidney and liver damage, if given in too large doses and if patients are sensitive to them. The patient must remain under careful medical care, and an important nursing function is to emphasize to the patient that he must take the drug as ordered. He must not take more lest he have ill effects; neither must he decrease his dosage lest he have recurrence of convulsions. Patients with epilepsy tend to indulge in wishful thinking, to hope that they have "outgrown" the disease, and to believe that they can "get by" without taking the drug if they have gone for some time without a seizure.

Special diets in the treatment of epilepsy are prescribed less often than formerly. The *ketogenic diet,* planned to produce a mild ketosis or acidosis, is so high in fat that it is not acceptable to most patients, but it is still ordered occasionally for children. A general well-balanced diet is usually recommended, with avoidance of excess foods or fluids. Most patients seem to have fewer seizures when they are mildly dehydrated; presumably this is because there is less danger of cerebral edema. Alcoholic beverages, particularly beer, are likely to contribute to attacks. The patient should be advised to avoid excesses of any kind, both physical and emotional. This advice may be hard for the young person to follow since the need to participate with those in his age group often makes it difficult for him to avoid physical and emotional stresses.

Home care. Members of the family must learn to care for the person during and following a convulsion. They should have a mouth gag on hand at all times and should know how to insert it correctly, and they should be alert for accident hazards. One of the most important things for the family to learn is the need to be calm and accepting in regard to the patient's seizures. They should attempt to keep him from engaging in activity that may be dangerous and from exposure to the curious during convulsions, but they should not contribute to the patient's feeling that he is different from others.

Public attitudes. One of the most important aspects in epilepsy is changing the public's attitude toward the disease. The patient and the public must be made to look upon convulsive seizures not as bizarre catastrophes but as relatively normal events which should be dealt with rationally. Many persons with epilepsy lead normal productive lives. Indeed, many outstanding figures in world history had seizures, including Julius Caesar, Lord Byron, and Napoleon Bonaparte. Recent studies do not bear out the popular assumption that there usually is mental deterioration with epilepsy. Nor is there any evidence that personality changes are the result of pathologic progress; they are probably the result of society's attitude toward the person with epilepsy. For example, most people who are found to have epilepsy are automatically and immediately suspended from their work even when it is such that they are not dangerous to themselves or to others. It is almost impossible for a person with known epilepsy to get new employment, yet at least 80 per cent of all persons with epilepsy are employable. The patient is haunted by fear of being seen during a seizure, fear of being found to have seizures, fear of losing his job, and fear of losing the companionship of others. Children with epilepsy have been segregated in separate schools, and only recently have some major cities passed laws ensuring children with epilepsy the right to attend the public schools if they are under adequate medical care. Children in many schools are barred from the classroom depending on the inclination of the teacher. Limitation of environment and of educational opportunity often limits the patient's knowledge, but this does not mean that his learning capacity is poor.

Interest in the field of epilepsy and in the problems of the epileptic person has been increased by various organizations such as the National Association to Control Epilepsy, Inc.* and the National Epilepsy League, Inc.† Membership in these organizations is open to medical science personnel, to those with epilepsy, and to other interested citizens. The nurse should encourage public-spirited citizens to support these organizations.

VASCULAR DISEASE

Cerebral vascular accident is the most common disease of the nervous system and in 1959 was the third highest cause of death in the United States. The condition is often associated with vascular disease of the heart, the kidneys, other organs, and the peripheral blood vessels. Usually the vessel involved in a cerebral

---

*Headquarters: 22 East Sixty-seventh Street, New York 21, N. Y.

†Headquarters: 130 North Wells Street, Chicago 6, Ill.

accident is a relatively large one and affects one side of the brain, which leads to partial or complete paralysis of the opposite side of the body (hemiplegia). *Shock, hemiplegia,* and *stroke* are other terms used in referring to cerebral vascular accidents.

Vascular lesions of the brain are often categorized as due to embolus, hemorrhage, or thrombosis. Cerebral embolism is usually caused by an embolus breaking away from a thrombosed blood vessel elsewhere in the body. This condition has been less frequent since the treatment of bacterial endocarditis with antibiotic drugs. Anticoagulant drugs given in treatment of coronary artery disease and early ambulation now also prevent much thrombosis of peripheral blood vessels in hospitalized patients.

Cerebral hemorrhage is due either to the rupture of a congenital aneurysm or weakened area in a blood vessel or to the rupture of a sclerosed blood vessel in persons who have high blood pressure. Although the symptoms of rupture of an aneurysm and of hemorrhage due to arteriosclerosis and high blood pressure may be similar, the treatment is different; therefore, the nursing care will be considered separately. Cerebral thrombosis is due to the formation of a thrombus or clot in the blood vessel of the brain. Because the nursing care of patients with cerebral vascular hemorrhage due to arteriosclerosis does not differ too much from that for cerebral thrombosis, it will be considered in one discussion.

Cerebral thrombosis and cerebral hemorrhage

Cerebral thrombosis and cerebral hemorrhage may occur at any time, although thrombosis is more likely to occur when the patient is sleeping and the hemorrhage when physical and emotional stress is encountered. Both cerebral thrombosis and cerebral hemorrhage may be preceded by headache, vertigo, flushing of the face, momentary loss of consciousness, and foreboding that something is wrong. The patient may fall and lapse into total unconsciousness, and convulsions may occur immediately following the accident. Loss of consciousness may come on slowly or quickly and may last for a few minutes or continue until death, which usually does not occur for several days. The pulse is rapid and bounding, the respirations labored or stertorous, and the blood pressure elevated; vomiting may also occur. The pupils may not react normally to light, and one side of the body may appear limp. If the paralysis is on the right side of the body, the patient may not be able to speak even if consciousness returns, because the speech center in right-handed persons is located on the left side of the brain along with the sensory and motor areas for the right side of the body. If the patient is hospitalized, a spinal puncture is usually done which may reveal blood in the spinal fluid if hemorrhage has occurred in an artery that communicates with the spinal fluid system.

Emergency care. Cerebral vascular accidents may occur when the patient is at work or elsewhere outside his home and may be confused with convulsive seizures, diabetic coma, and drunkenness. Emergency care at the scene of the episode consists of turning the patient carefully on his affected side (determined by the puffiness of the cheek on this side) and elevating the head without tilting the neck forward, since tilting may cause congestion of blood within the skull. Turning the patient on his affected side permits saliva to drain out of the mouth and lessens the danger of aspiration into the lungs. Elevation of the head may help to prevent edema of the brain. Clothing should be loosened about the throat to further help prevent engorgement of blood vessels in the head, which may lead to cerebral edema. The patient should be kept quiet, moved as little as possible, and protected from chilling. Medical aid should be sought at once.

General nursing care. Nursing care for the patient with cerebral vascular accident does not differ whether he is in the hospital or in his own home, although oxygen is more likely to be given in the hospital. Dicumarol and heparin may be given to the patient when he is in the hospital if it is certain that the cause of the trouble is cerebral vascular thrombosis and not cerebral hemorrhage.

If the patient survives the first few days, he may begin to regain consciousness and some of the paralysis may disappear. It is then that the greatest understanding is needed by persons attending him. He may realize that he cannot talk, that he drools, that he cannot move a hand or a leg, or, if he can move the limbs, that the motions are shaky and uncertain. This is a terrible shock to the patient, and it is then that the nurse's active part in rehabilitation begins. By her quiet assurance she must make the patient feel that his progress toward recovery and self-sufficiency has begun and will continue. She can help by telling him what she is going to do even though he cannot answer her. If the patient is right-handed and cannot speak, he has the added difficulty of having to learn to write with his left hand in addition to being partially speechless. The nurse should try to anticipate the patient's needs and should make every effort to understand his indistinct speech, since repeated attempts to make himself understood only augment his misery and frustration. Usually, if partial speech is present at the time of return to consciousness, there is likelihood that speech will improve, and the patient is heartened by the knowledge of this fact. Speech may be affected because of involvement of the tongue, mouth, and throat, as well as because of damage to the speech center in the brain.

Rest and quiet are important even if the accident has not been serious enough to cause complete loss of consciousness. No attempt should be made to rouse the patient from coma, although respiratory and circulatory stimulants may be prescribed by the physician. The vital signs should be carefully checked, watching for such things as a rise in temperature within the first day or two, slowing of pulse and respirations, and deepening of the coma. All of these indicate pressure on the vital centers and a poor prognosis.

The patient's eye on the affected side should be protected if the lid remains open and there is no blink reflex; otherwise damage to the cornea can lead to corneal ulcers and blindness. Irrigations with boric acid solution or physiologic solution of sodium chloride, followed by drops of sterile mineral oil, sterile castor oil, or sterile petroleum jelly are sometimes used. After gently closing the lid, an eye pad may be taped over the affected eye. If a pad is used, it must be changed daily and the eye cleansed and carefully examined for signs of inflammation or drying of the cornea. Eye shields are preferable to pads because they lessen danger of lint getting into the eye.

Mouth care is difficult to give since the patient may be unable to retain fluid and is likely to choke if it is introduced into the mouth. (See Chapter 9 for details of giving mouth care to the unconscious patient.) Mouth care should be given every four hours during the day and night, and special attention must be given to the paralyzed side of the mouth and tongue.

Fluids may be restricted for the first few days after a cerebral vascular accident in an effort to prevent edema of the brain; then regular diet and fluid intake are desirable. Patience and persistence are necessary in giving food and fluids to these patients. The nurse must make the patient feel that the problem is not discouraging and that time taken to assist him to eat is well spent. He may encounter so much difficulty getting food and fluids beyond his partially paralyzed mouth and throat that the effort may not seem worth while. Therefore, each small step in improvement should be brought to the attention of the patient. Turning him to his back or to the unaffected side may spare the annoyance and embarrassment of having food spill from the affected side of the mouth. Foods that may cause choking, such as mashed potatoes, stringy meats, and semicooked vegetables, must be avoided. Since food may collect in the affected side of the mouth, it must be irrigated after eating to prevent accumulation of food with subsequent poor mouth hygiene. The patient should assist in feeding himself as soon as possible, since the helplessness of having to be fed by others is detrimental to emotional health. Foods such as meats must, of course, be cut up. A covered plastic cup is now available with a small center opening through which a straw can be introduced, or one can be improvised by using a straw and a covered plastic food container. This is useful for the patient who can draw through a straw but whose hands are unsteady. If the patient can swallow but cannot draw through a straw, an Asepto syringe with a piece of rubber tubing on the end or a pitcher must be used. Turning the patient to his unaffected side before introducing fluids into his mouth often helps him to control the mouthful of fluid and to swallow it successfully. The patient with dentures should have them placed in the mouth as soon as possible since this also improves his morale and will increase his interest in eating.

Urinary output should be noted carefully and recorded for several days after a cerebral vascular accident. Retention of urine may occur, but it is more likely that the patient will be incontinent. If urinary incontinence occurs, the patient must be reassured and told that his control of excretory function probably will improve day by day. A retention catheter may be used for the first few days for women patients, and offering them a bedpan immediately after meals and at other regular intervals helps them to overcome incontinence.

Fecal incontinence is fairly common following a cerebral vascular accident, and again the patient must be reassured that as general improvement occurs this condition will be overcome. Other patients develop constipation, and impactions develop readily. Elimination must be noted carefully since diarrhea may develop in the presence of an impaction, thus causing it to go unnoticed for several days. Small daily doses of cathartics may be ordered, and an enema may be given every other day. Massage to the abdomen may be helpful in starting peristalsis, but is done only when ordered by a physician. Warm oil-retention enemas are sometimes given regularly in an attempt to prevent impactions and when impactions occur. Mineral oil by mouth is often given, since straining in the act of defecation must be avoided. The patient must be cautioned not to strain and must be assured that the enema can easily be repeated if no results are obtained. He usually needs assistance in getting on and off the bedpan. Side rails which he can hold on to to turn himself or a trapeze which he can reach with his unaffected hand is useful if he is permitted this exertion.

The length of time the patient remains in bed depends entirely on the type of cerebral accident suffered and the judgment of the doctor in regard to early mobilization. Some physicians prescribe fairly long periods of rest following cerebral vascular accidents, while others believe that early mobilization is best. However, the trend is toward early mobilization of the patient with cerebral thrombosis, sometimes beginning a day or two after the accident has occurred.

While the patient is in bed, he must be moved frequently to avoid danger of circulatory stasis and hypostatic pneumonia. Care must be taken to see that body weight is not borne on the paralyzed side or on the back for long intervals, because decubitus ulcers occur very easily. Pillows should support the upper-most limbs when the patient lies on his unaffected side to prevent strain on shoulder and hip joints. The patient can suffer complete dislocation of the hip joint from lack of support to the limb when he is placed on his unaffected side and when the flaccid thigh is allowed to fall forward and downward, because the muscles take an active part in holding the head of the femur in its socket. The patient may be turned to a face-lying or partial face-lying position, with pillows again being used to maintain good body alignment. This position is good for the patient who is not fully conscious, since it lessens the danger of aspiration of mucus.

Specific rehabilitative nursing measures. If there is ability to use the arm when consciousness returns, there is reason to believe that the leg action will return sufficiently for the patient to walk. Return of motor impulses and subsequent return of function are evidenced by a tightening and spasticity of the affected part. This often appears from the second day to the second week after the cerebral vascular accident. It is significant for the future use of the affected part but presents new nursing difficulties. Muscles which draw the limbs toward the midline become very active, and the arm may be held tightly adducted against the body. The affected lower limb may be held inward and adducted to, or even beyond, the midline. Muscles which draw the limbs into flexion are also stimulated, with the result that the heel is lifted off the ground, the heel cord shortens, and the knee becomes bent. In the upper limb, flexor muscles draw the elbow into the bent position, and the wrist is flexed and fingers are curled in palmar flexion. This is often seen following a vascular accident.

Persistent nursing effort must be directed toward keeping any part of the body from remaining in a position of flexion long enough for muscle shortening and for joint changes to occur which might interfere with free joint action. If physical therapists are not available, the total responsibility for this may rest with the nurse. Every minute counts in this contingency, and the nurse must not miss one opportunity to take a moment from her busy day in the hospital to move the patient's adducted or flexed limbs back to the correct position. In the home she must teach members of the family who are caring for the patient to exert this same careful attention.

If the patient is lying on his back, a pillow can be placed between the upper arm and the body to hold the arm in abduction. A roll made of one or two washcloths serves as a good support to prevent flexion of the fingers, and a splint made from a padded tongue blade may be used to ensure straightening of the thumb or other fingers for periods during the day. A firm box at the foot of the bed holds the foot at right angles and prevents contractures in drop-foot position.

Range of joint motion should be preserved, and passive exercises are often begun early. The nurse needs no order to put the patient's limbs through complete range of joint motion passively once or twice each day. (See Chapter 4.) But passive exercise in which the limb is to be exercised more than this should be done only when so ordered by the doctor. If she does not have a written order, the nurse should consult the physician as to the amount of passive exercise he wishes the patient to have. Passive exercise stimulates circulation and may help to reestablish neuromuscular pathways. No difficulty is encountered with these procedures until tightening of the muscles begins to appear. Then other physical measures are needed, and the patient's treatment should be under the direction of a physical therapist.

Active exercise of the affected side also may be started early. This is ordered by the physician and, in the hospital, may be directed by the physical therapist. Under guidance of the physical therapist the nurse checks the exercises while the patient is in the hospital, and she or the physical therapist may teach the exercises to the family in preparation for the patient's return home.

Since the patient will depend a good deal on his unaffected arm and leg when he begins to move about, the unaffected part of the body needs attention to prevent contractures and preserve muscle strength. Even while he is in bed, the patient should exercise his good arm and use it in all normal positions. The unaffected leg should be in a position of slight *internal rotation* most of the time while the patient is in bed, and the knee should be bent several times each day. Exercise to strengthen the quadriceps muscle should be done because the quadriceps is the most important muscle giving stability to the knee joint in walking. Exercise against resistance is obtained by placing two small sand bags that are fastened together saddle fashion over the ankle and having the patient raise his leg. One of the best exercises for strengthening the quadriceps is to have the patient straighten the knee against resistance when he is sitting on the edge of the bed or in a chair; a bucket of sand may be used, but care should be taken to protect the skin of the ankle from pressure; an ordinary cooking pan with a bucket handle may be used in the home.

Before standing or walking, the patient may practice raising himself up in bed and may sit on the side of the bed while holding firmly to an overbed table or to a strap with his good hand and pressing his feet on a chair or stool. The patient benefits from wearing shoes, since this is good for his morale and keeps his paralyzed foot in good position.

If preparation for walking has been adequate, the patient usually needs only one crutch when he begins to walk, and from that he progresses to the use of a cane. When he first begins to walk, the nurse must remain close to him to allay his fear of falling. He may practice balancing himself by standing between parallel bars or by leaning on the backs of two chairs (provided the chairs are heavy enough to support weight safely). Good walking patterns must be established early, because incorrect patterns are difficult and sometimes impossible to change. A sideward shuffle should be watched for and avoided. The patient should begin by leaning rather heavily upon his crutch or cane and lifting his body sufficiently to bring the leg and foot forward so that the toes point straight ahead and not inward. The cane must *always* be held in the hand opposite the damaged side of the body.

The patient may be taught to help with his own improvement by using his unaffected hand to help straighten out the flexed fingers on the affected side; because he is unaccustomed to his clumsy and uncooperative limbs, he becomes easily discouraged. Careful and detailed instructions on how to hold and support himself will save him much embarrassment and confusion. The patient can move his affected arm to a position where, with the weight of gravity, the elbow will be straightened; usually he needs help in securing abduction of the shoulder.

Home care. The patient may receive care in his own home where most of his care is given by family members assisted and taught by the nurse. The pamphlet *Strike Back at Stroke** written for patients and their families should be familiar to all nurses. It is available to any patient who has his doctor's approval for its use.

Long-range plans. General care and the pattern of living that should be followed after a cerebral vascular accident vary for each patient and are determined by his own circumstances, the amount of recovery he has, and the guidance he received in the early stages of his illness. Despite all effort he may, for example, never be able to negotiate stairs. The medical social worker and the public health nurse are indispensable in helping to arrange the patient's home so he may live with a moderate amount of self-sufficiency and independence. Members of the family often need help in assisting the patient to accept his limitations, both physical and emotional. They must also make adjustments to actual circumstances. Almost all persons who have cerebral vascular accidents need health supervision for the rest of their lives.

While it is not uncommon for cerebral vascular accidents to recur, the patient may go for years with no further difficulty and eventually die of some other cause. The physician usually explains this to the patient and to his family. The nurse should know what explanation he has given and must sometimes help in interpreting it to the family. Some patients

*Prepared and published by U. S. Departments of Health, Education, and Welfare, P.H.S., Bureau of State Services, Division of Special Health Services, Chronic Disease Program.

must curtail activity to such a point that they have little enjoyment in living and still have recurrences, whereas others may be active and escape further accidents for many years.

The patient who has sustained a cerebral vascular accident and who has high blood pressure is usually advised by his physician to change his mode of life so that more rest is assured and strain and excitement are avoided. If his work is strenuous, he may be urged to take longer and more frequent vacations. He may be advised to lose weight if obesity is putting an extra strain on his circulatory system and to avoid the use of tobacco because of its effect on blood vessels. Activities of daily living may be modified; for example, the patient may be advised to sit while shaving. If the doctor feels that the danger of cerebral hemorrhage is imminent, he may advise against any activities which promote dilation of cerebral blood vessels, such as vigorous exercise, hot or cold baths, violent coughing or laughing, straining at defecation, and sexual activity. Occasionally, retirement at an early age is necessary. Relocation in a warmer climate or in a more rural area is helpful to some people provided they can afford it and it does not upset the living pattern of the patient and his family too much.

Cerebral arteriosclerosis and multiple small thrombi

Cerebral arteriosclerosis may lead to deterioration of brain tissue, even though vascular accidents do not occur. This condition, which usually is associated with high blood pressure, may occur in people in their fifties, though it is usually considered a disease of old age.

Multiple small thrombi may occur in persons whose blood pressure is normal or even below normal if atheromatous changes have occurred in the lining of arteries. This condition causes frequent, small, and barely perceptible strokes. Both cerebral arteriosclerosis and multiple small strokes from thrombi may produce personality changes. The person who has arteriosclerosis is likely to have a more consistent downward course, while the one suffering from multiple small thrombi may have periods of apparently normal physical and mental response between episodes of confusion.

Both cerebral arteriosclerosis and multiple small thrombi cause slowly progressing changes that are particularly distressing to members of the patient's family. Complete brain deterioration may occur. The patient may feel irritable and unhappy with apparently little cause, and no amount of reassurance can make him feel better. The family must be prepared for gradual deterioration in the patient's condition and should make provision for his safety and for the results of the poor judgment he may demonstrate; for example, he may forget to dress appropriately, may give away family possessions, and may enter into unwise business dealings. The family needs help in learning how to treat the patient as an adult yet deal with his limitations. The doctor, the social case worker, and the nurse can help the family care for the patient in such a way that their own lives are not completely disrupted and yet are not plagued by guilt feelings when the patient dies. Institutional care is sometimes necessary, and the family needs encouragement and help in arriving at joint decisions that serve the best interests of all its members.

Cerebral aneurysm

A cerebral aneurysm is a weakening and outpouching of the wall of a cerebral artery usually caused by a congenital weakness in the vessel wall. The most common site is at the circle of Willis. Hemorrhage occurs when the aneurysm ruptures and the blood seeps into the subarachnoid spaces. This condition accounts for the sudden death of young people from "strokes" during strenuous exercise or excitement that causes the blood pressure to rise. The aneurysm commonly ruptures between the ages of 20 and 40 years. Signs and symptoms include sudden explosive headache, nausea and vomiting, loss of consciousness, shock, convulsions, a full bounding pulse, and noisy labored respirations.

The immediate treatment for *subarachnoid hemorrhage* is to keep the patient absolutely quiet. He should be very gently moved to bed, and sometimes it is not advisable to move him to a hospital. He must be kept flat in bed in a darkened room and attended constantly to be sure that he does not raise his head. If he is conscious, he is given small amounts of water by mouth, but this must be given through a straw so that the head is not elevated. Intravenous fluids may be given by slow drip, and often an indwelling catheter is inserted to avoid exertion. Bowel elimination is usually ignored for several days, and then oil-retention enemas may be given. Under no circumstances should the patient be permitted to strain, cough, or otherwise exert himself. Visitors must be carefully prepared so that they will not upset the patient, and no mail should be given to him unless it is certain that no disturbing information is contained therein.

About 50 per cent of those with rupture of an aneurysm recover from the initial episode, but at least 50 per cent of these will have recurrences of hemorrhage if untreated.[22] Recurrence may occur within two weeks, and the danger of death increases with each recurrence. If the aneurysm is not obliterated by surgery, the patient may die eventually from a recurrent hemorrhage.

The only satisfactory treatment for congenital aneurysm is surgery. This consists of applying a metal clip around the artery on each side of the aneurysm or applying a metal clip across the neck of the aneurysm. The location of the lesion can often be demonstrated by angiographic study. If the lesion is in a portion of the brain where it is inaccessible to surgery or if it is in a vital vessel which cannot be ligated, an attempt is made to decrease the flow of blood through the vessel by ligating the carotid arteries, provided the patient can carry on normal brain function with the blood supply which will remain.

If the aneurysm is in the internal carotid artery and ligation of the external carotid is to be attempted, the surgery must be done in three stages to allow for gradual rechanneling of blood to the part of the brain supplied by these vessels. In the first stage, the common carotid artery is ligated; this still allows blood to flow through the external carotid artery and the anterior cerebral artery. About seven days later, the internal carotid artery is ligated leaving only the anterior cerebral artery to furnish the blood supply to this part of the brain. The first two stages are performed under local anesthesia through small incisions in the neck.

Although actual surgery is minor in the first two stages, the patient must be closely observed because there may not be adequate blood supply to a part of the brain. The nursing care and observation are identical with that following arteriogram. Any signs of muscle weakness in the face or in either extremity on the side opposite the incisions should be reported to the surgeon at once. Immediate removal of the ligatures, which are placed so that they may be quickly released, may prevent irreversible complications such as hemiplegia, aphasia, and loss of consciousness. If symptoms of inadequate blood supply appear, further surgical treatment cannot be done safely.

The third stage in surgical treatment is usually done within two days of the second stage if the patient's response to the second stage has been satisfactory. The carotid artery is ligated above the aneurysm after it has been exposed through a craniotomy. Thrombus formation with resultant cerebral embolism may complicate the patient's postoperative course following either the second or third stages.

Before surgery for aneurysm is attempted, the surgeon usually explains the hope for cure and the risks involved to the patient's family. The nurse must appreciate how distressing the situation is for the family and must realize that the time spent waiting to know whether or not the outcome will be favorable seems interminable to them. The reasons for details of nursing care should be explained to them if they are with the patient. For example, it is important that both the patient and his family know that blood pressure, pulse rate, and respiratory rate and other pertinent observations will be taken frequently, since these procedures can be most upsetting if not explained.

If the surgery is successful, the patient will be cured, although usually he will be advised to avoid strenuous exercise and emotional stress for the rest of his life. Occasionally, he may have a severe physical or mental handicap resulting from damage to brain tissue during surgery.

If the aneurysm cannot be successfully treated, however, the family should be aware that there is always the danger of sudden death. The patient must be protected from strenuous activity and excitement. He may have a severe physical or mental handicap resulting from damage to brain tissue.

Arteriovenous fistula

Since the internal carotid artery passes the cavernous sinus (a venous sinus), an aneurysm at this point may cause pressure on the first division of the fifth cranial nerve, as well as on the third, fourth, and sixth cranial nerves. The aneurysm may not necessarily rupture, but the patient may complain of frontal headaches, double vision, ptosis of the eyelid, dilated fixed pupil, and inability to move the eye laterally. These symptoms will all occur on the side of the aneurysm. If the aneurysm has ruptured into the sinus, the patient often complains of a noise (bruit) over the eye on the affected side, and the eye may become infected due to venous engorgement. The noise is caused by the rush of blood between the artery and the venous sinus. The condition is referred to as an arteriovenous fistula, and the treatment is similar to that for aneurysm of the carotid artery.

Arteriovenous anomaly

An arteriovenous anomaly is a congenital malformation of the cerebral vessels in which the capillary bed is congenitally absent. There is a resultant loss of nourishment to the brain tissue supplied by the vessels. Symptoms are rarely manifested before the patient is between 20 and 40 years of age. The patient may complain of the sudden onset of headache, stiff neck, and low-grade fever because of leakage of blood through the thin vessel walls into the subarachnoid spaces. Convulsive seizures that involve only one part of the body are common, and hemiparesis may occur because of loss of nutrients and oxygen to the brain tissue. It is not unusual for unconsciousness to occur.

Diagnosis is made by the detection of a yellowish spinal fluid which indicates bleeding into the subarachnoid space, a bruit, the visualization of a wormlike cluster of vessels on the arteriogram, and the visualization of intracranial calcification on roentgenograms of the skull.

Treatment for arteriovenous anomaly is usually conservative and is similar to that given the patient with cerebral aneurysm during episodes of acute hemorrhage. Surgical treatment is rarely attempted if the tangle of blood vessels is in the dominant hemisphere (the left side of the brain in right-handed persons) or in any vital area, because control of speech and the important acts of daily living may be seriously threatened. Hemorrhage from this lesion is seldom fatal, and the leakage of blood usually causes only moderate symptoms. The patient is usually urged to plan his entire mode of living so that physical and emotional stresses and strains are avoided. In this way, blood pressure may be kept at a safe level and severe symptoms avoided.

INFECTIONS

The nervous system may be attacked by a variety of organisms and viruses and may suffer from toxic reactions to bacterial and viral disease. Sometimes the infection becomes walled off and causes an abscess, sometimes the meninges or coverings of the brain and spinal cord primarily are involved, and sometimes the brain itself is affected most. Pyogenic and syphilitic infections are much less common now than before the advent of antibiotic drugs which have prevented their progress and spread. Chronic sinus and middle ear infections, if not adequately treated, can spread to the brain and its coverings and cause disease.

Meningococcal meningitis (epidemic), viral encephalitis, and poliomyelitis are reportable communicable diseases. Because they are becoming less common and because they are discussed in specialized texts on communicable disease nursing they will only be mentioned briefly here.

Meningitis

Meningitis is an acute infection of the meninges usually caused by pneumococci, meningococci, staphylococci, or streptococci. The incidence of meningitis is higher in fall and winter when upper respiratory infections are common. Children are more often affected than adults because of frequent colds and ear infections. The incubation period for epidemic meningitis is from two to ten days.

The onset of meningitis (except when due to tubercle bacilli) is usually sudden, with severe headache, stiffness of the neck, irritability, malaise, and restlessness. Nausea, vomiting, delirium, and complete disorientation may develop quickly. Temperature, pulse rate, and respirations are increased. The diagnosis is usually confirmed by doing a lumbar puncture; usually the offending organism can be isolated from the spinal fluid and, if a pyogenic organism is the cause, the fluid is cloudy. Treatment consists of large doses of the antibiotic most specific for the causative organism; this antibiotic may be given directly into the spinal canal as well as administered by other routes.

Nursing care. Isolation is required for the patient with epidemic meningitis until the acute illness is over. Particular care should be taken in handling discharges from the nose, mouth, and throat. Nursing care for the patient with meningitis includes the general care given a critically ill patient who may be irritable, confused, and unable to take fluids, yet dehydrated because of elevation of temperature. The room should be kept darkened, and noise should be curtailed as much as possible. The patient must be observed very carefully and must be constantly attended if he is disoriented. Side rails should be placed on the bed.

Residual damage from meningitis includes deafness, blindness, paralysis, and mental retardation. However, these complications are now rare, because the infection is effectively treated with antibiotics before permanent damage to the nervous system occurs.

Encephalitis

Encephalitis is inflammation of the brain and its coverings; occasionally the meninges of the spinal cord are also involved. Encephalitis can be due to a variety of causes. A generalized inflammation of the brain can be caused by syphilis, and encephalitis can follow exogenous poisoning, such as that following the ingestion of lead or arsenic or the inhalation of carbon monoxide. It can be caused by reaction to toxins produced by infections such as typhoid fever, measles and chickenpox, and occasionally it follows vaccination.

Encephalitis caused by a virus and occurring in epidemic form was first described by von Economo in Austria, and the name von Economo's disease is still used to identify the widespread epidemic in the United States which followed the influenza epidemic in 1918. This form of the disease has not recurred since 1926. Von Economo's disease was also called encephalitis lethargica and sleeping sickness, a term still used by the layman.

Encephalitis or encephalitis lethargica caused by poisoning can lead to a chronic form of the disease in which paralysis agitans (Parkinson's disease) develops. This is slowly progressive and is irreversible. The form of encephalitis which complicates diseases such as measles, as well as the current viral forms, seldom causes this sequela.

Viral encephalitis. Viral encephalitis appears to be caused by a number of viruses, some of which may be interrelated. Many names are used to identify the kind of virus; e.g., St. Louis, western equine, eastern equine, and Japanese B. All are believed to be transmitted by the bite of a mosquito, to have an incubation period of from five to fifteen days, not to be transmissible from man to man, and to leave no serious sequelae though the acute illness may be severe.

The onset of viral encephalitis may be sudden, with death occurring within twelve to twenty-four hours of the onset of symptoms, although usually the height of symptoms is reached in approximately forty-eight hours. Symptoms vary and include severe headache, malaise, dizziness, nausea and vomiting, restlessness, irritability, lethargy, sleeplessness, vague feelings of fear and misgiving that can be poorly described, difficulty in speech, and twitching and tremor in muscles of the face and hands. Temperature, pulse rate, and respirations may be moderately elevated and, upon neurologic examination, there may be some reflexes absent or otherwise abnormal. The patient's white blood cell count may be normal, and the spinal fluid is usually normal or shows only slight increase in protein and in lymphocytes. Upon postmortem examination, visible clouding of the meninges can be seen grossly, and small petechiae and degeneration of brain cells can be found upon microscopic examination.

Nursing care consists mainly of symptomatic care and careful observation. Any change in appearance or behavior must be reported at once since the progress in this disease sometimes is extremely rapid. The patient is kept in bed, and side rails are used if disorientation develops. The patient must be constantly attended to prevent injury. If the temperature is high, sponging may be ordered; frequent changes of linen may be necessary if perspiration is excessive. There is no specific medical treatment for this disease, and mortality ranges from 5 to 60 per cent. No isolation is necessary.

Poliomyelitis

Poliomyelitis is an acute febrile disease caused by three different strains of one of the smallest known viruses. With discovery of the Salk vaccine and its wide use since 1956, and with the recent availability of a safe "live virus" vaccine, this disease, which has been a serious crippler of children and young adults, promises to become quite rare. The vaccine contains three strains of the virus, one of each type, grown in monkey kidney tissue and inactivated by formalin. Salk vaccine is now available to everyone and is given in three injections: two injections one month apart and a third injection at least seven months later. Some authorities now recommend a fourth injection or "booster" a year after the third injection. An important responsibility of the nurse is to help prevent poliomyelitis by encouraging immunization. Since this dreaded disease is now largely preventable, it is deplorable if all children and young adults do not receive protection.

Poliomyelitis is probably transmitted by secretions from the nose and throat of infected persons and by means of the gastrointestinal tract. The virus has been found in milk, is known to remain active in sewage for many months, and has been found on insects such as flies. However, none of these has been proved to be a source of epidemic spread. The disease is not easily transmitted, and very few infections have occurred among medical and nursing personnel caring for acutely ill patients. Several members of one family, however, often have the disease in varying degrees of severity. It is believed that, for every person who develops paralysis, there are many who have a milder form of the disease without paralysis and who develop an immunity to subsequent exposure. The incidence of poliomyelitis is highest in the summer and early autumn, and it is higher among rural than urban dwellers. The general health of the person before exposure does not seem to affect his resistance to the disease, although immediate bed rest upon the onset of symptoms may lessen the severity of symptoms.

The incubation period for poliomyelitis is from seven to twenty-one days. The virus attacks the anterior horn cells of

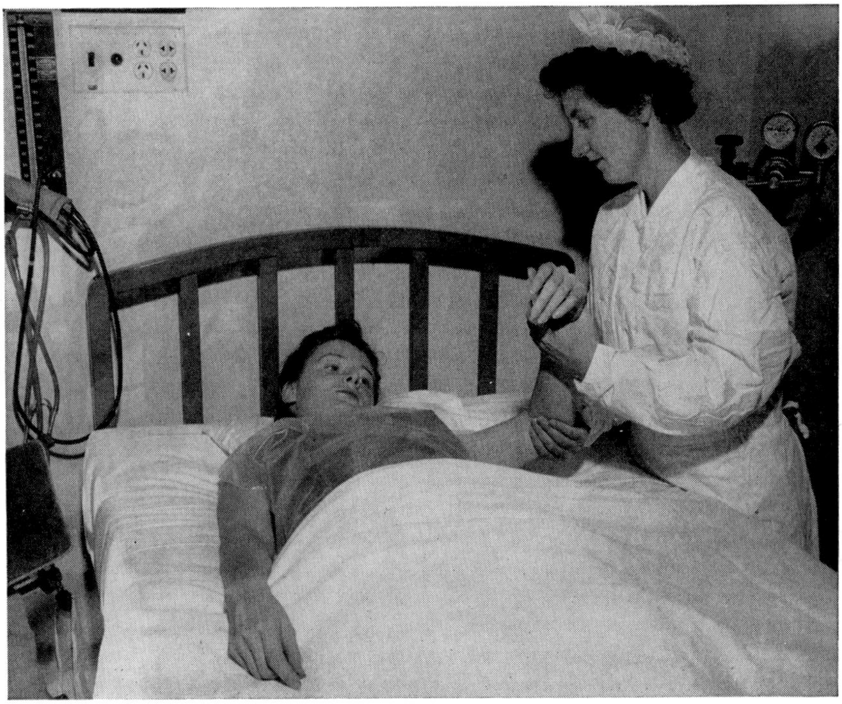

Figure 115

Nursing care of the patient acutely ill with poliomyelitis calls for a variety of skills. Note the isolation gown, the oxygen ready for immediate use if necessary, and the convenient wall equipment for frequent taking of blood pressure. This patient is receiving lay-on packs in an attempt to improve her breathing and avoid the use of a respirator. Note that the affected upper limb is handled at the joints, thus avoiding pressure on sensitive muscle bellies.

the spinal cord where the motor pathways are located and may cause motor paralysis. Sensory perception is not affected since posterior horn cells are not attacked. Poliomyelitis sometimes takes a somewhat different form and attacks primarily the medulla and basal structures of the brain, including the cranial nerves; the term bulbar poliomyelitis is used for this form. Many patients have both bulbar and spinal involvement, and when this occurs the spinal involvement is more likely to be in the upper trunk, involving the arm, shoulder, and respiratory muscles. Mortality rate varies with epidemics, but it is highest when there is bulbar and respiratory involvement. If the patient recovers from acute bulbar poliomyelitis, however, there is seldom any serious residual paralysis. Symptoms of bulbar paralysis include weakness or paralysis of muscles about the face and neck. There may be difficulty in swallowing, excessive salivation, nasal voice, and speech impairment. These often occur with involvement of muscles of breathing which causes protrusion of the abdomen from weakening of the diaphragm, unequal chest expansion, and use of the auxiliary muscles of respiration.

Medical treatment and nursing care. The treatment of acute poliomyelitis is largely symptomatic. There is no specific drug, and antibiotics are given only to prevent superimposed infection. The patient should be kept warm and quiet, and fluids should be given freely provided there are no signs of bulbar involvement. Narcotics and sedatives are not given because they may mask symptoms of oncoming bulbar involvement. The application of warm moist packs to tender muscles and warm tub baths often lessen pain and give comfort if they can be given without causing fatigue and pain from moving. (See Figure 115.) Urinary retention occurs quite often and may require use of an indwelling catheter. This is disturbing to the patient, and he must be assured that the condition is temporary; bladder function is always regained within a few weeks. A careful record of bowel elimination must be kept since constipation is common.

For the first few days when pain is severe and the patient is generally quite ill, he should assume any position that is comfortable. After that time attention must be given to good bed posture, keeping weakened muscles in a protected position and being certain that normal range of joint motion is maintained. Often the patient is admitted to a bed especially prepared with a fracture board to assure good alignment of the spine, bath blankets instead of sheets to help prevent chilling, and a board at the foot against which his feet may rest in good alignment. Responsibility for retraining and redeveloping weakened muscles is assumed by the physical therapist, but the nurse must see that postural deformities do not develop, that uninvolved muscles do not undergo unnecessary atrophy, and that range of joint motion is preserved.

Sudden loss of muscle function, with resultant helplessness, is a severe shock to any patient. The nurse should expect the patient to be irritable and depressed. She can make his adjustment to dependence upon others easier by doing things simply and calmly, by anticipating his needs so he will not have to ask for simple things such as having the bed covers pulled up, and by helping him as he devises methods to substitute for normal ways of caring for himself. For example, the patient whose right hand is severely involved may need help in cutting meat and buttering bread when he uses his left hand. Eventually, if paralysis continues in his right hand, he will learn to use his left hand more effectively or to use his involved hand in a different way. In the first few weeks of illness, however, even mention of this may be too depressing for the patient.

The nurse's ability to move the helpless patient easily adds tremendously to his physical and mental comfort. The patient in whom both lower limbs are paralyzed, for example, cannot possibly pass the night without discomfort and strain on back, joints, and muscles since normally he shifts frequently during sleep. If the nurse knows the correct method of moving him without strain on herself, he may not hesitate to ask for her help. However, if he must endure the nurse's helpless and ineffectual tugging at his paralyzed limbs, he may lie awake without asking to be turned and may feel that his situation is hopeless. (See fundamentals of nursing texts for correct methods of turning and lifting patients.)

Any patient with acute poliomyelitis should be watched closely for signs of sudden progress particularly to the muscles of respiration or for bulbar involvement. The approach to the patient should be calm and reassuring so as not to alarm him, but every patient with this diagnosis should be observed every half hour for at least twenty-four hours after admission. If there are any signs of respiratory or bulbar involvement, the patient should be attended constantly, since symptoms of bulbar involvement can progress with startling rapidity. Every effort should be made to have the patient remain calm and quiet since becoming upset only increases his breathing and swallowing difficulties.

Nursing care of the patient with bulbar and respiratory involvement is difficult but not beyond the capacity of any nurse who has a background in the basic principles of good nursing. Since all patients

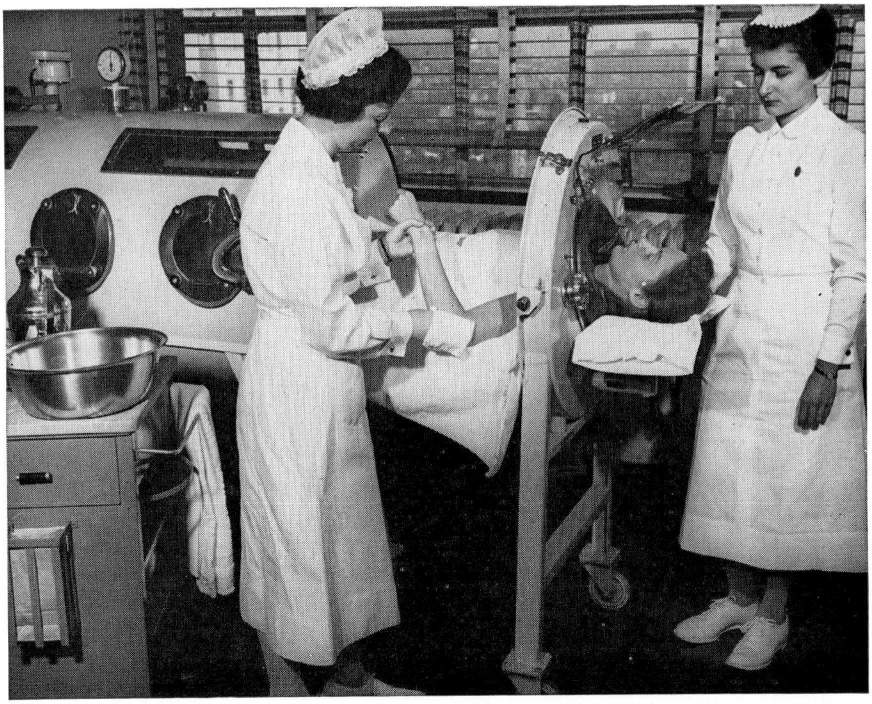

Figure 116

A patient being weaned from a respirator needs encouragement. Short periods out of the respirator are also used to give essential care.

with acute poliomyelitis are isolated for at least a week from the onset of symptoms, and longer if the temperature remains elevated, nursing care includes isolation technique as well as careful observation of an acutely ill patient, use of oxygen, use of suction, and sometimes care of the patient having a tracheostomy.

Nursing care of the patient in a respirator. Respirators are mechanical devices used to substitute for normal respiratory action by creating a negative pressure outside the chest wall. This causes air to enter the respiratory passages. A mechanical device is a poor substitute for normal respiration and, therefore, is usually used as a last resort. For example, the rate of inhalation and rate of exhalation are the same when a respirator is used, whereas in normal respiration the time for inhalation is less than that for exhalation.

Since respirators are used in emergencies, it is essential that they be checked often and kept in working order at all times. If they are housed on a ward or unit of the hospital, a regular day each week should be designated for their routine inspection. There are two main kinds of respirators and several makes of each. The tank respirator encases the entire body except the head and imposes handicaps on persons who attempt to give nursing care. The chest respirator may enclose the entire chest or may consist of a shell held firmly against the chest with straps and attached to a suction device. Chest respirators permit the patient much greater freedom and simplify nursing care. The shell type cannot, however, be used for long periods of time since it does not assure good aeration of the posterior portion of the lungs.

Respirators can be dangerous in inexperienced hands. Too much negative pressure can cause inspiration to be too deep and thus traumatize the alveoli of the lungs. The respirator must be tested before the patient is placed in it. This is done by closing all arm ports and other openings and turning the pressure gauge until approximately the desired pressure is reached. The head opening can be closed by holding a pillow firmly against it. Pressure must be carefully regulated when the patient is placed in the machine.

If the patient is conscious, it is imperative that the procedure of placing him into the respirator and the purpose of this treatment be explained to him. Usually he is told that the treatment has been ordered so that he can relax and breathe more easily and thus get necessary rest and sleep. Often the patient is so exhausted from having to remain awake and consciously use his accessory muscles of respiration in an effort to breathe that he welcomes use of the respirator. Occasionally he becomes panicky and "fights" the machine so that adjustment is extremely difficult. A nurse must always remain with the patient and help him to breathe with the machine until he becomes accustomed to it; respiratory rate is stipulated by the doctor and is usually a little slower than the patient's rate at the time he is placed in the machine.

Before the patient is placed in a respirator, provision must be made for his relative comfort and for care that will be necessary. The mattress should be covered with small sheets in sections that can be easily removed through the arm holes, and the following supplies should be in the patient's unit: a piece of plastic material to protect the sheet under the buttocks, bath towels, bath blankets, foot supports, and a thermometer. Soft material such as an old diaper or chamois skin should be used to protect the patient's throat and neck from the rubber collar.

The patient in a respirator must never, under any circumstances, be left alone. Patients have been known to die because an electric cord was inadvertently disconnected or because some other mechanical failure occurred. Auxiliary nursing personnel, relatives, and volunteers are often asked to help in emergencies.

An important concept to remember in care of the patient in a respirator is that the patient needs exactly the same care as he would if he were not in this awkward enclosure. He needs to be turned, to have skin care, to have joints flexed and extended, to void, and to defecate regularly. He needs to take fluids and food in normal amounts. Teamwork is essential, and planning should be done so that several essential activites can be carried on at once. For example, when turning the patient to relieve pressure on the sacrum, one can also sponge the back, flex the knees, and massage the ankles provided equipment for these procedures has been placed in the respirator before the patient has been turned. If the patient can be out of the respirator or can breathe on his own for a short time, this time is used by several nurses and attendants to give essential care (see Figure 116).

The greatest care must be taken in helping patients to swallow when in the respirator. It is extremely difficult for anyone to swallow comfortably when lying on his back or in mild hyperextension, much less when breathing cannot be controlled. Swallowing must be done on exhalation. The patient should first try small amounts of liquid or semisolid foods; foods that tend to cause choking, e.g., mashed potatoes, must be avoided. A suction machine should always be on hand when the patient first attempts to swallow when in a respirator. If the patient vomits, he must be removed from the respirator at once to prevent aspiration.

Preparation for leaving the respirator should begin as soon as the patient is placed in the machine. Although some patients are overly anxious to be out of the machine, others become overly dependent upon it. Effort is made to stop the machine for a few seconds or minutes at intervals. Oxygen may be given during this time and a nurse stands at the patient's head, encouraging him to breathe normally and timing his efforts while others give physical care. At first the patient

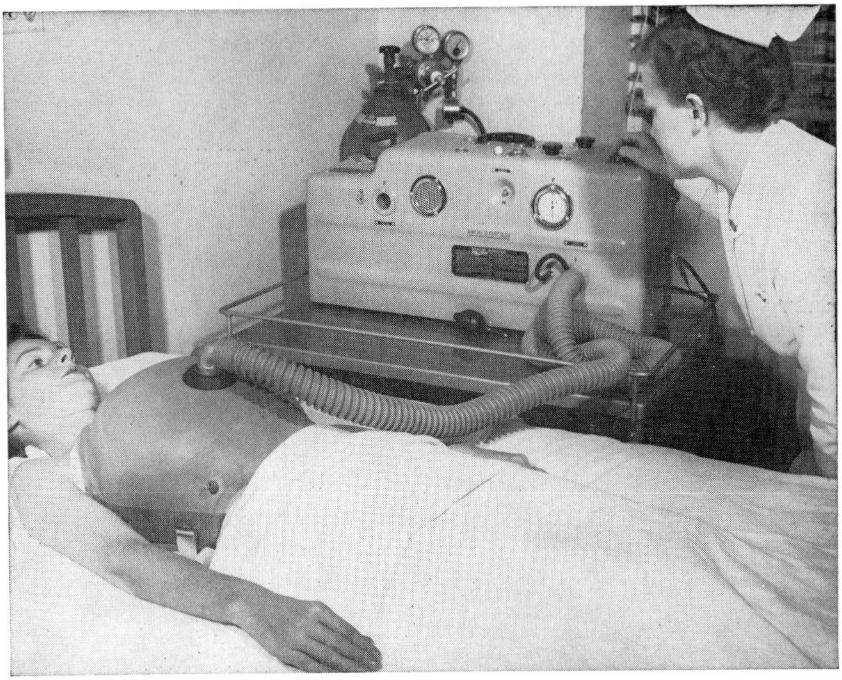

Figure 117

The patient for whom a chest respirator is needed requires constant nursing care. Here the nurse is checking to be certain that the pressure is maintained as prescribed. Some patients are more comfortable in a low Fowler's position.

is left on the carriage of the machine so that he knows that its use is immediately available. He may then be moved to bed where a chest respirator may be used (see Figure 117) or to a *rocking bed* which tilts at a specified rate and thus assists in breathing; as the head of the bed goes down, the viscera fall against the diaphragm and assist in exhalation, while, as the head goes up, the diaphragm falls toward the abdominal viscera and assists in inhalation. The convalescent and rehabilitative stages in poliomyelitis are long, and much special treatment and care is necessary. (For details of this, see texts on orthopedic nursing.)

Syphilis

In the late latent or chronic stages of syphilis, infection may involve the brain and spinal cord. The oculomotor nerves may be involved, causing inability of the pupil to react to light (Argyll Robertson pupil). *Tabes dorsalis* is the name given to the involvement of the posterior columns of the spinal cord and the posterior nerve roots. Since the sensory nerves are primarily involved, sensory symptoms predominate. The patient may have severe paroxysmal pain anywhere in the body, although perhaps the most common location is in the stomach. This condition known as *gastric crisis* may be confused with ruptured peptic ulcer or other acute conditions of the stomach or gallbladder. There may be areas of severe parathesia on the skin. A common finding in tabes dorsalis is loss of position sense in the feet and legs. The patient is unable to sense where he places his feet, and his resultant slapping gait is highly characteristic of the disease. He has real difficulty walking at night because he depends on sight in placing his feet normally; visual loss or even total blindness also occurs. Tabes dorsalis can cause trophic changes in the limbs and changes in the joint so that stability is lost (Charcot's joint).

General paresis is the term used to designate another late manifestation of syphilis in which there is degeneration of the brain with deterioration of mental function and varying evidences of other neurologic disease. Since patients with this condition occupy many beds in mental hospitals, the disease is discussed quite fully in texts dealing with nursing care of the mentally ill. (See also Chapter 17.)

BRAIN TUMORS

Brain tumors are relatively uncommon, but every nurse should recognize their early symptoms, since, unless the tumor is diagnosed and treated promptly, death from irreparable brain damage will occur. Fifty per cent of brain tumors are benign,[38] but even these may cause death; as the tumor grows within the cranial cavity, it eventually exerts lethal pressure on vital centers of the brain. Hemorrhage and abscess may cause symptoms similar to those caused by brain tumors.

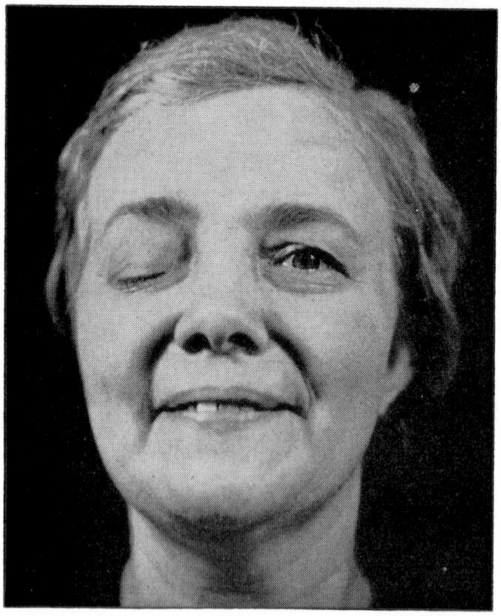

Figure 118

This patient has a marked ptosis of the right eyelid. (From Davis, Loyal: The Principles of Neurological Surgery, Philadelphia, 1942, Lea & Febiger.)

Brain tumors are named for the tissues from which they arise. The more common types are gliomas, arising from the connective tissue; meningiomas, arising from the meningeal coverings; and neuromas, arising from the cranial nerves. Glandular tumors such as pituitary tumors may occur, and tumors which have metastasized from elsewhere in the body are fairly common.

Brain tumors cause symptoms by direct irritative or destructive effects on the brain and by damage from increasing intracranial pressure. In many instances, especially if the tumor is infiltrating brain tissue, an alert observer may recognize subtle changes suggesting the need for neurologic examination before symptoms of increased pressure appear. The symptoms depend on the part of the brain affected. They usually are transitory at first but become more frequent as the tumor grows. The first noticeable symptom may be a change in personality or judgment. If motor areas are involved, there may be weakness of a leg, an arm, or any other part of the body (see Figures 118 and 119). Sometimes the patient complains of paresthesia or anesthesia of a part of the body. He may complain of unpleasant odors, a sensation which often accompanies tumors of the frontal lobe. If the speech center is involved, the patient may be unable to use words correctly or he may become unable to understand the written or spoken word. He may complain of loss of visual acuity or of double vision; these signs indicate pressure on the optic nerve or on one or both of the abducens nerves. The patient may have a change in his gait, perhaps staggering, veering to one side, or walking with an unusually wide base of support. These symptoms often occur with cerebellar tumors. Convulsions occurring for the first time after middle adulthood are suggestive of a brain tumor.

Pituitary tumors may cause a variety of symptoms, depending on their type. *Gigantism* and *acromegaly* (overgrowth

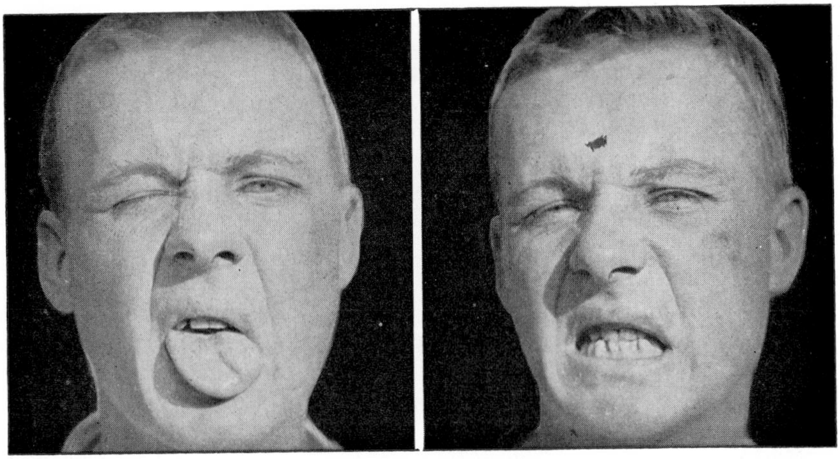

Figure 119

This patient has weakness of the left facial nerve and hypoglossal palsy. Note the deviation of the tongue and the drooping of the mouth on the left side when the patient clenches his teeth. (From Davis, Loyal: The Principles of Neurological Surgery, Philadelphia, 1942, Lea & Febiger.)

of bone) are caused by eosinophilic adenomas of the pituitary gland. *Cushing's syndrome,* characterized by hyperglycemia, a grotesquely obese trunk with thin extremities, and an abnormal amount and distribution of hair, is caused by a basophilic adenoma. Gigantism and Cushing's syndrome seldom cause signs of intracranial pressure; they both are treated by endocrine therapy (see Chapter 28). However, chromophobe tumors of the pituitary gland compress the surrounding brain structures and are treated surgically. The most common symptom is a decrease in vision caused by pressure on the optic chiasm. Signs and symptoms such as sallow skin, sparse thin hair, impotence, amenorrhea, and a low basal metabolic rate may follow pressure on or destruction of secreting portions of the pituitary gland.

Unfortunately, some tumors do not produce any symptoms until they become large enough to displace brain tissue or until they block the flow of cerebrospinal fluid, causing *increased intracranial pressure.* The patient then often complains of slight dimming of vision which is caused by papilledema or swelling of the optic nerve head (choked disc). He may have projectile vomiting that is not preceded by nausea. Persistent dull headache, most severe in the morning, often accompanies these signs. Blood pressure progressively rises, and pulse and respirations become slower because of pressure on regulatory centers in the medulla. One of the first signs of increased intracranial pressure may be change in level of consciousness. The patient may first be irritable and restless and then gradually become lethargic and stuporous.

Nursing care of patients having brain surgery

When a patient suspected of brain tumor is admitted to the hospital, both he and his family may be extremely apprehensive. If the patient has marked personality changes, aphasia, or convulsions, the family may even be afraid of him. Because they are unaware that he may fully understand, they may make tactless remarks in his presence. It is often desirable to have the patient escorted directly to his room and then to take the family aside to ascertain their insight into the situation. This gives the nurse valuable information for beginning a nursing care plan, and it gives her an opportunity to help interpret the patient's actions and responses so that his family may not inadvertently upset him.

When admitting the patient, the nurse should carefully observe his physical and mental status. Limitations of movement, muscle weakness, difficulty in following instructions, speech impairment, loss of vision or hearing, and any symptomatic complaints can easily be noted at this time. Blood pressure, temperature, pulse rate, respirations, and pupil reaction also should be carefully recorded, since the doctor often needs this information later as a basis for comparison. Even before the doctor examines the patient, necessary plans for nursing care related to his personal needs, such as help in eating, assistance in walking, placement of the bedside stand if he has limitations of movement in the upper extremities, the need for side rails on the bed, a mouth gag at the bedside, and appropriate means of communication, should be made.

The patient may be well oriented and most fearful about the probable diagnosis or the anticipated surgery. The nurse should encourage the patient to talk, listen to what he says, and reassure him as to the skill of his surgeon. The nurse who has a positive feeling about the surgery will be most convincing.

The nurse may be able to help the doctor localize a brain lesion by accurately reporting and recording her observations. For example, noting that the patient has less severe headache when his head is in a certain position may be important, because it suggests that this position relieves the pressure. If possible, the exact location of headache should be noted. Careful description of the course of convulsions may help locate a tumor. Any symptoms indicative of increasing intracranial pressure should be reported to the physician at once.

Occasionally a patient enters the hospital with signs of severe intracranial pressure, or signs of increased pressure may come on suddenly while he is undergoing a period of observation and diagnosis. If the latter happens, treatment for relief of pressure must be given at once. Hypertonic solutions such as 10 to 50 per cent glucose in physiologic solution of sodium chloride may be given intravenously. Magnesium sulfate, given intramuscularly, by mouth, or rectally by retention enema or proctoclysis, may also be given to cause dehydration. A lumbar puncture may be done to remove cerebrospinal fluid and thereby release pressure, provided it is assured that this will not result in more pressure on the vital centers in the medulla as pressure in the spinal canal lowers. Immediate operation, known as decompression of the skull, may be done to allow for expansion outside the cranial cavity, thus releasing pressure.

Preoperative care. If immediate surgery is not necessary, the patient is given a thorough physical examination and a complete neurologic examination. If a pituitary tumor is suspected, complete endocrine studies may be done. Roentgenograms of the skull are always taken, and an electroencephalogram is also ordered routinely when a brain tumor is suspected. The patient may need a pneumoencephalogram or a ventriculogram. Since a ventriculogram requires that the patient have general anesthesia, the operation is usually performed immediately after the test if the results show evidence of a tumor.

Written permission for operations on the brain must be given by the nearest relative unless the patient is able to do this himself. Even then, close relatives are usually consulted, and the doctor obtains their consent before doing surgery. Brain surgery is very threatening to the patient and to his family, so every effort should be made to inspire confidence in the surgeon, members of the nursing staff, and the hospital. It often gives members of the family reassurance to know that the patient will return after surgery to the same floor where the members of the nursing and medical resident staffs are known to them. As before any other major surgery,

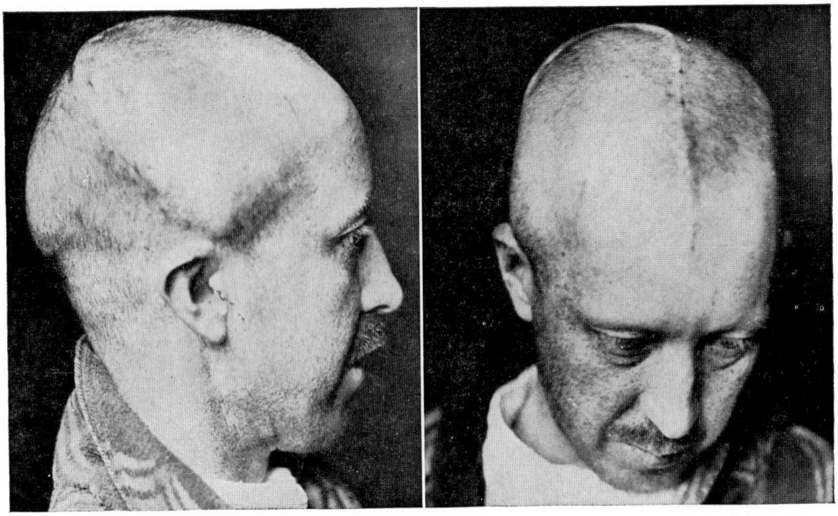

Figure 120

Subtemporal decompression combined with unilateral frontal flap. This photograph was taken one week after operation. The only place the scar might show is in the middle of the forehead. The scar is imperceptible if made accurately in the median line. Note the slight bulging of the right subtemporal decompression. (From Sachs, Ernest: Diagnosis and Treatment of Brain Tumors and Care of the Neurosurgical Patient, St. Louis, 1949, The C. V. Mosby Co.)

they should be encouraged to have their spiritual adviser visit them.

Treatments and procedures should be explained to the patient even though he may not seem to understand too clearly. Enemas may not be given because of the danger of increasing intracranial pressure by exertion and absorption of fluid. Narcotics, except codeine, are rarely ordered preoperatively since they may cause further depression of cerebral function; any order for their use should be carefully verified by the nurse. The hair is usually not shaved until the patient is in the operating room and under anesthesia. Long hair should not be discarded but should be returned to the unit because the patient may wish to have it made into a wig for use until her hair grows again. It is rarely necessary to shave the entire head. Hair along the front hairline can often be left so that after the operation it can be drawn backward to cover the scar.

Surgery. A surgical opening through the skull is known as a *craniotomy.* The meninges are opened, and the tumor is removed if possible. Brain surgery usually is done under hypothermia to lessen bleeding during the procedure. Hypotensive drugs also may be given (see Chapter 13). Fluorescein sodium may be given intravenously one hour preoperatively to help localize the tumor. Tumor tissue tends to retain the substance which can then be seen under ultraviolet light. This drug will cause the skin and the scleras to appear jaundiced for several days. The nursing staff, the patient, and the family should be aware of this.

When the brain lesion is in the *supratentorium* (the cerebrum), the incision is usually made behind the hairline (see Figure 120); when the incision is into the *infratentorium* (the cerebellum and brain stem), it is made slightly above the nape of the neck. Neither of these incisions is

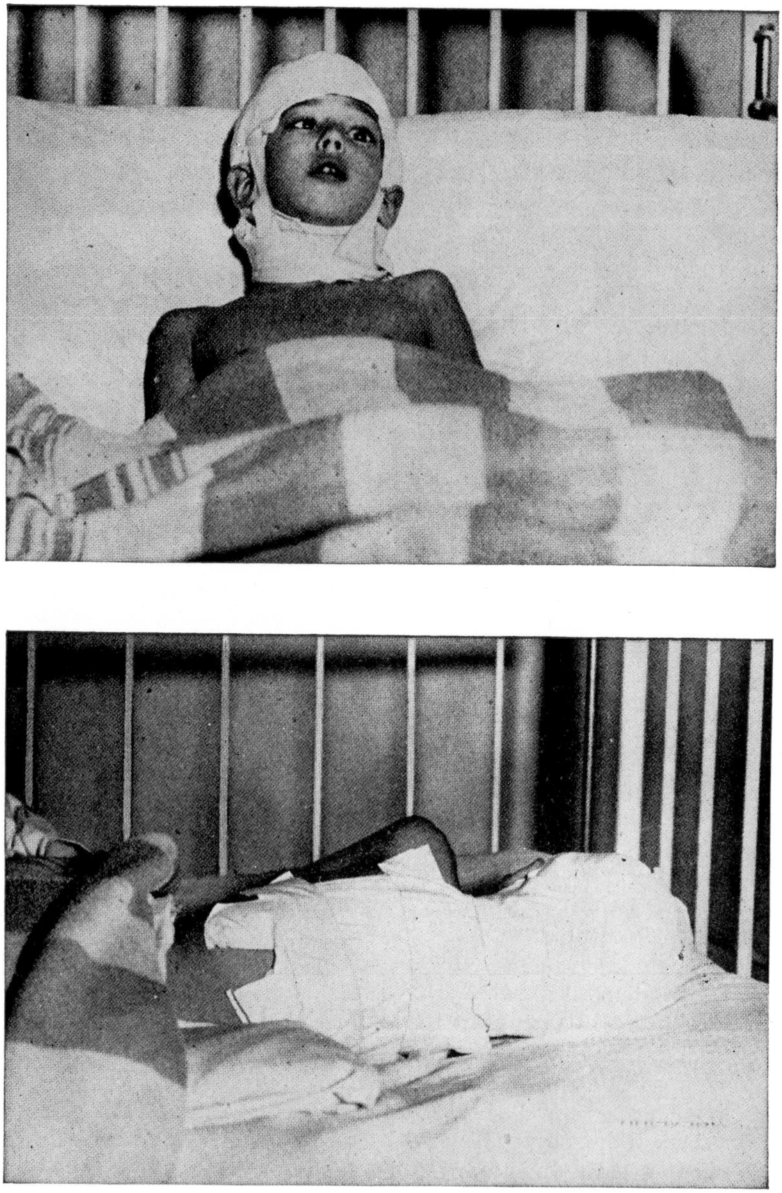

Figure 121

This patient has had an infratentorial craniotomy. Note that the adhesive straps extend down the back to prevent the patient from flexing his neck. (From Sachs Ernest: Diagnosis and Treatment of Brain Tumors and Care of the Neurosurgical Patient, St. Louis, 1949, The C. V. Mosby Co.)

apparent when the hair has grown. The scalp is incised, and a piece of the bone over the site of the suspected tumor is removed with a small electric saw. The bone flap is carefully saved, since it usually is replaced following the operation. The bone flap, however, may be left out to prevent pressure from edema postoperatively or to permit expansion of an inoperable tumor. It may be replaced weeks or months later, or a Vitallium plate may be used instead of the preserved bone.

Although a portion of the frontal lobe can be removed with little residual damage, limitation of some functions may necessarily follow complete removal of tumors elsewhere. The operative mortality of all types of brain tumors is between 10 and 20 per cent.[38] In about one half of the cases the tumors can be completely removed; if the patient survives the operation, he has about a 66 per cent chance of returning to useful life.[38] Patients with meningiomas, pituitary adenomas, acoustic neurinomas, and cysts of the cerebellum are likely to have the best prognosis.

Immediate postoperative care. Before the patient returns from the operating room, the nurse should assemble the following special equipment: a bed made up "head to foot" so that inspecting and changing the head dressing will be made easier, side rails on the bed, a suction machine with No. 14 Fr. and No. 16 Fr. Robinson catheters, a rubber airway, a mouth gag, a lumbar puncture set, and an emergency medication tray containing caffeine sodium benzoate, theobromine, sodium Amytal, syringes, intravenous and hypodermic needles, and a tourniquet. If there has been an infratentorial incision or if an acoustic neurinoma has been removed, a tracheotomy set should be in the room since sudden severe respiratory obstruction may develop.

Immediately after the patient returns from the operating room, he is placed on his side to allow for an adequate airway. If a large tumor has been removed, he must not be turned onto the affected side since this may cause displacement of brain structures by gravity. Otherwise, he may be turned to either side. If there has been supratentorial surgery, the head gatch on the bed is elevated 45 degrees and a large pillow is placed under the patient's head and shoulders. This should lessen the possibility of hemorrhage, provide for better circulation of the cerebrospinal fluid, and decrease cerebral and other tissue edema. If an infratentorial tumor has been removed, the head dressing will extend down to the shoulders, holding the head in slight hyperextension. The bed should be kept flat with only a small pillow under the nape of the neck. (See Figure 121.)

The protective head dressing (a helmet of crinoline and starch) should be inspected to make sure that it is thoroughly dry. (See Figure 122.) If it is not dry, a hair dryer turned to "cool" should be used. The dryer should never be turned to "hot," because this would burn the patient, and the face and neck should be covered with a towel since air blowing over them may be very annoying. Serosanguineous drainage on the dressings should be outlined in ink, as is done on other dressings, so that it can be accurately checked for an increase in amount. Yellowish drainage should be reported immediately to the doctor, because it probably indicates loss of spinal fluid. If the head dressing appears to be soaked with any kind of drainage, it should be covered with a sterile towel held in place with adhesive tape. Every half hour the towel should be removed and the dressings checked and reinforced with sterile towels if necessary. An unprotected wet dressing may cause the wound to become infected, and this might even cause meningitis.

The nurse should observe the patient carefully, recording his blood pressure, rectal temperature, pulse rate, respirations, state of consciousness, pupillary responses, muscle strength (hand grip), and ability to move. If he is unconscious or semiconscious, she should note his response to painful stimuli. Specific observations are usually made and results recorded every thirty minutes for six hours, every hour for at least a day, and every every three to four hours until the third or fourth postoperative day. Frequency of making and recording specific observations depends on the patient's condition. His temperature is usually taken every hour for four hours, and then at least every four hours for twenty-four hours.

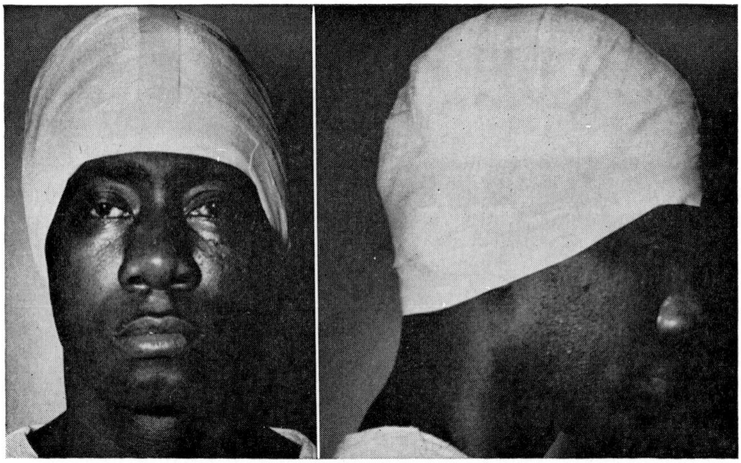

Figure 122

Typical head dressing for the patient who has had a supratentorial craniotomy. (From de Guitérrez-Mahoney, C. G., and Carini, Esta: Neurological and Neurosurgical Nursing, St. Louis, 1960, The C. V. Mosby Co.)

If the lesion was in the infratentorium, the temperature may be taken every two hours for two or three days, because edema of the brain stem might occur and upset the temperature control center in the medulla. (The treatment for hyperthermia is discussed in Chapter 9.) Any change in the patient's vital signs, state of consciousness, or ability to use muscles should be reported at once. If he appears to be restless, he should be watched closely for further signs, since restlessness may forewarn of hemorrhage or of irritation to the brain. Irregular or fixed pupils indicate pressure or disturbance that may be due to hemorrhage. A patient who has intracranial bleeding has elevation of blood pressure and a drop in pulse rate as the hemorrhage increases intracranial pressure.

The family during the postoperative period. The family should be prepared to see the patient. They should know that he will return from the operating room with a helmetlike headdressing and that edema may distort his features. If he is unconscious or has any noticeable limitations such as aphasia, they should be told of this before entering his room. If he is alert, members of the family should be advised to sit quietly at the bedside since talking will tire the patient. If a supratentorial incision has been made, the family should be warned that when they see him on the day following surgery he may be unable to open one or both eyes, may have generalized facial edema, and may have discoloration of the skin about the eyes (ecchymosis). (See Figure 123.) Periocular edema is caused by postoperative cerebral edema; it usually improves in three or four days. Iced compresses to the eyes may make the patient more comfortable.

Fluids and food. Fluid intake and output should be accurately recorded. If there is no special medical order to the contrary, 2,500 to 3,000 ml. of fluid should be given each day. If the patient shows signs of increased intracranial pressure, the fluid intake may be limited to 1,500 ml. in twenty-four hours.

Since the gag and swallowing reflexes may be depressed or absent after infratentorial brain surgery, fluids by mouth are usually withheld for at least a day and intravenous fluids are substituted. These should be run very slowly to prevent increased intracranial pressure. The doctor tests the patient's reflexes; if they are present, water is carefully given by mouth. A nurse should help the patient until she is sure that there is no danger of his choking or aspirating fluid; then a competent nurse's aid may be assigned this task. The patient should be placed on his side or in a semisitting position. Fluid is most easily given by placing the rubber-protected tip of an Asepto syringe into the patient's mouth and allowing him to suck through it. Fluid should not be injected into his mouth. If he coughs or cannot swallow, the fluid feeding should be discontinued.

A regular diet is usually given as soon as tolerated. After supratentorial surgery this may be on the second postoperative day. Any patient who has had a craniotomy, however, should be fed for at least forty-eight hours to prevent undue fatigue. This may need to be continued longer to ensure adequate food and fluid intake. If the patient is unable to take food and fluid by mouth, tube feedings are started forty-eight hours postoperatively. (See Chapter 9.)

Urinary output. Care must be taken to see that the patient voids. If a pituitary tumor has been removed, special attention must be paid to urinary output because surgery on the pituitary gland may alter the function of the adrenal glands which control water balance. There may be a marked increase in urinary output accompanied by excessive loss of electrolytes. Usually there is an order for vasopressin (Pitressin) to be given if the urinary output exceeds a given amount. If this is ineffective in decreasing output, the doctor should be notified. The doctor should also be told if the patient complains of feeling "jittery" or has abdominal cramps following administration of the drug. Patients who have had surgery of the pituitary gland usually are given prophylactic doses of adrenocorticotrophic

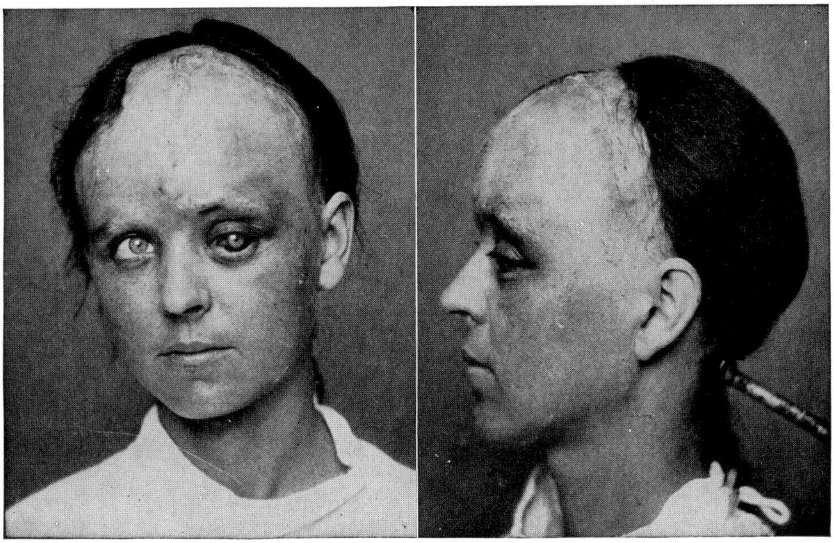

Figure 123

This patient had surgery for a left-sided brain tumor eight days prior to the taking of this photograph. The conjunctiva of the left eye still shows ecchymosis. Note the area of hair and eyebrow shaved. (From Sachs, Ernest: Diagnosis and Treatment of Brain Tumors and Care of the Neurosurgical Patient, St. Louis, 1949, The C. V. Mosby Co.)

hormones (ACTH) for from twenty-four to forty-eight hours and smaller doses of cortisone until adrenal function returns to normal.

Bowel function. Because straining increases intracranial pressure, the patient is urged not to try to have a bowel movement until three days postoperatively. On the second and third postoperative days he may be given a cathartic, and on the fourth postoperative day a small, low, enema. He should be instructed not to strain in an attempt to expel the enema. If an impaction develops, it must be removed manually by the doctor.

Headache. Patients who are conscious after intracranial surgery complain of severe headache for twenty-four to forty-eight hours. Codeine sulfate usually is given hypodermically every four hours for this, and acetylsalicylic acid may be given by rectum or by mouth if fluids can be swallowed. An icecap may be placed on the head, and sudden movement and jarring are avoided. Even if the patient is conscious, he should be turned with a turning sheet for the first forty-eight hours since the effort needed to move himself may cause further headache, increased intracranial pressure, or hemorrhage. The turning sheet should be placed well above the level of the patient's head. General hygienic care for the patient during the first forty-eight hours is the same whether he is conscious or unconscious.

Ambulation. The patient who has had surgery for a supratentorial lesion usually is allowed out of bed on the third to fifth postoperative day. Activity should be gradual, and he should be watched carefully for signs of increased intracranial pressure. First, the head of the bed should be elevated to a high Fowler's position and then the patient should sit on the edge of the bed, with his feet hanging over its side. If he tolerates this, four to six hours later, with the help of two persons he may be assisted to a chair and usually may sit up for half an hour. He then progresses to normal activity as quickly as he desires and is able. The patient who has had surgery for an infratentorial lesion is not permitted up until the tenth postoperative day. His initial progress needs to be slower, since patients who have been kept flat in bed for some time may be dizzy upon arising until the circulatory system readjusts to the positional change.

Head dressings. If a drain has been used, the head dressing is changed by the doctor in twenty-four to forty-eight hours. Otherwise it is not disturbed until the sutures can be removed. This is usually the third postoperative day following supratentorial incisions and the fifth postoperative day following infratentorial incisions. A head dressing is reapplied; if no complications follow, it is usually removed on the seventh and tenth postoperative days, respectively. Special equipment and techniques are needed to change head dressings of this kind. The wound is covered with gauze dressings. Two-inch crinoline bandage or a special head dressing (neurosurgical roll) is then applied in a recurrent fashion from the back to the front of the head. After this has been anchored, a coating of heavy laundry starch is applied; occasionally a thin plaster-of-Paris cast is used. This must be thoroughly dried with a hair dryer. The crinoline and starch dressing gives an even pressure to the dressings and affords some protection from injury. The dressing may be too tight when it dries; signs of this, such as edema, must be reported to the doctor, who may slit the dressing, taking care to avoid the operative site.

When final dressings are removed, the scalp needs care. It should be gently cleansed with hydrogen peroxide to remove dried blood. Crusts can be loosened with mineral oil. The head may then be shampooed, with care taken not to rub the operative area or put traction on the healed suture line. The patient is often given a head covering. This protects the healed wound from dirt and helps to remind the patient not to scratch. Some doctors prefer that a stockinette cap be worn at first because this readily reveals any bulging of the wound. A cap may be made by tying one end of a 10-inch piece

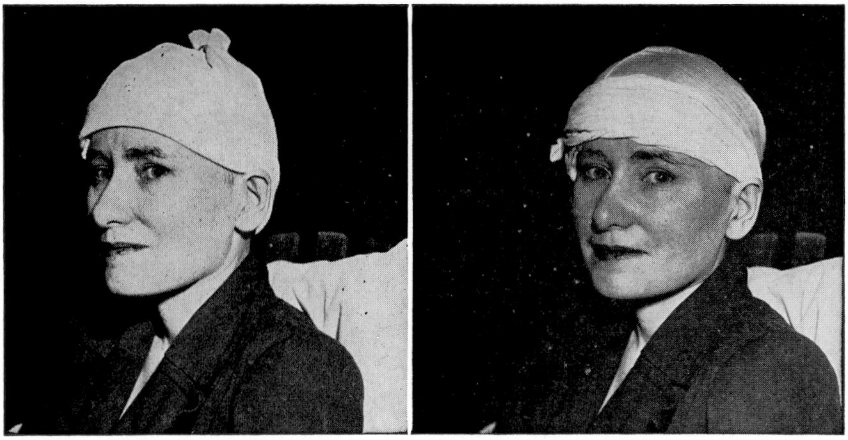

Figure 124

The patient convalescing after brain surgery. In one picture she wears a stockinette cap; in the other, a turban. Note that she wears make-up. (From Sachs, Ernest: Diagnosis and Treatment of Brain Tumors and Care of the Neurosurgical Patient, St. Louis, 1949, The C. V. Mosby Co.)

of tubular stockinette. For women patients, it is psychologically important to cover the operative scar; many doctors prefer that women patients wear attractive bandanas. (See Figure 124.) The nurse should inspect the wound at least twice a day. The patient who has had a piece of bone left out will eventually have a depression in the scalp, and he should be warned of the danger of bumping his head in this area. Women patients should be encouraged to have the remaining hair restyled. If the hospital has beautician service, restyling may be done, with the doctor's permission, before the patient leaves the hospital.

Protective measures. Sometimes the patient must be protected from self-injury after a brain operation. If he pulls at dressings or a catheter, scratches, or hits himself, he should have constant nursing care and occasionally some kind of hand restraint may have to be used. A large mitten made of combination pads, bandage, and stockinette and fastened at the wrist with adhesive tape may be used. Mittens usually upset the patient less than arm restraints since with mittens he can move his arm freely. The fingers should be separated with gauze to prevent skin irritation and should be curled around a large bandage roll in the palm to prevent hyperextension of the fingers. The hand is then well covered with combination pads held in place with bandage. A piece of stockinette is closed at one end and everted to avoid danger of the tied end causing injury to the eye; it is then slipped over the bandaged hand and fastened securely at the wrist with adhesive tape. The hair should be shaved from the wrist and the skin protected with tincture of benzoin before adhesive is used. At least every other day the mitten must be removed, the hand washed in warm water, and passive exercise given to the fingers before the mitten is reapplied.

Ventricular drainage. Occasionally a catheter is placed in a ventricle of the brain to drain excess spinal fluid and prevent increased intracranial pressure. This is usually attached to a drainage system on a level with the ventricle. The collection bottle is frequently attached to the head of the bed. The tubing and drainage receptacle should be sterile, and care must be taken to prevent kinking of the tubing.

If drainage seems to stop, the doctor should be notified. The catheter is usually left for only twenty-four to forty-eight hours and is then removed by the surgeon.

Complications. *Meningitis* is a relatively rare complication of brain surgery; it can follow infection during the operation or thereafter. Following supratentorial surgery, the nurse should watch for any clear watery drainage from the nose. This may be present if there has been a tear in the meninges, which causes subsequent loss of cerebrospinal fluid. The treatment consists of keeping the patient very quiet, avoiding any suctioning or blowing of the nose, and administering antibiotic drugs. The leakage usually subsides spontaneously. Because of the danger of causing damage which might be followed by the drainage of cerebrospinal fluid through the nose, many surgeons request that the nose never be suctioned when supratentorial surgery has been done; a sign with this caution may be placed at the head of the bed.

Respiratory collapse may follow infratentorial surgery. This is caused by edema of the brain stem or edema above the brain stem causing herniation into the foramen magnum and pressure on the respiratory center. Any irregularity of respirations, dyspnea, or cyanosis should be reported to the surgeon at once. Equipment should be ready to administer oxygen, to do a ventricular tap, and to do a tracheostomy. Some doctors routinely do a tracheostomy on any patient who has surgery for an acoustic neurinoma since respiratory difficulty most often follows removal of this tumor. (For details of nursing care of the patient with a tracheostomy see Chapter 24.) Occasionally a respirator is used.

Convulsions are not unusual after a craniotomy, and because of this a mouth gag should be at the bedside and side rails should be used even if the patient is unconscious and it is believed that he cannot move. Phenytoin sodium (Dilantin sodium) may be ordered prophylactically to prevent convulsions. The drug may be given by rectum until the patient is able to take it by mouth. If the patient has a history of seizures before the operation or if convulsions occurred in the postoperative period, he may be given this drug for several months postoperatively.

Loss of the corneal reflex may follow brain tumors or brain surgery. If the eye appears inflamed or the patient does not seem to blink when objects approach the open eye, the doctor should be notified. Special eye care, such as that given patients who have had cerebrovascular accidents or who have surgery for trigeminal neuralgia, may be necessary.

The patient may complain of *double vision* after brain surgery. This condition is often temporary, and the patient should know that it will probably improve. It can be relieved by placing an opaque eye shield over one eye. The eye covered should be altered each day to prevent disuse atony of eye muscles.

X-ray therapy is given to many patients following surgery for brain tumors. (See Chapter 16 for discussion of nursing the patient with radiation sickness.)

Long-term care. Some patients who have had cranial surgery will have physical and mental limitations. The patient may have hemiplegia, aphasia, and personality changes, including severe depression. The rehabilitative care and planning both for the patient and for his family are the same as for other patients with chronic and permanent neurologic disease. Specific rehabilitation for patients with hemiplegia and aphasia is similar to that following cerebrovascular accidents. Preventive exercises should be started at the first signs of muscle limitations. No matter what the eventual prognosis, each patient should be helped to be as independent as possible for as long as possible.

The patient who has had brain surgery may need the same protection from injury as do other patients with neurologic disease when judgment defect, disorientation, or locomotor difficulties make it unsafe for him to move about without assistance.

HEAD INJURIES

With the increase in automobile accidents, almost every nurse will be called upon to care for a patient who has an accidental head injury. These vary from minor scalp wounds to concussions and open fractures of the skull with severe damage to brain tissue. The amount of apparent injury is not necessarily indicative of the seriousness of the trouble. Scalp lacerations for example, bleed profusely and may be frightening to the patient and to others. Most of them are relatively minor, however, if bleeding is controlled before too much blood is lost.

The brain can be seriously injured, yet there may be no break in the skin and no evidence of skull fracture when a roentgenogram is taken. When the bony skull strikes a solid object, the soft tissues within the cavity continue to move. This action can be likened to what happens as one stops suddenly when moving quickly with an open dish of fluid—some of the fluid spills. The only difference is that, instead of spilling, the soft contents of the cranial cavity strike the bony covering forcibly and many sustain severe damage. This injury is known as *concussion* and is suspected whenever a patient loses consciousness for even a few moments at the time of or immediately after an accident.

If lethargy or unconsciousness develops after consciousness has been regained following an accident, an *extradural hemorrhage* should be suspected. This may occur even when consciousness is not lost at the time of injury. Usually one pupil becomes dilated, and the patient may vomit. Bleeding is usually caused by the tearing of the middle meningeal artery. This injury is fairly often sustained in baseball, football, and other vigorous sports.

If the patient has been conscious for several weeks or even months following a head injury and then shows neurologic signs suggestive of a lesion, he may have a *subdural hematoma* caused by slow venous oozing after the accident. This may occur following even seemingly inconsequential blows to the head. Careful observation and recognition of subtle changes may bring patients to medical attention before irreparable brain damage has occurred. Extradural or subdural hemorrhage may, of course, accompany other serious injury causing unconsciousness.

Fractures *of the base of the skull* usually result in serious damage and cause a high mortality, whereas *linear fractures* of the skull may be of little significance. When a basal fracture has been sustained, the brain tissue and vital nerve pathways may be permanently damaged. Trauma and edema often cause interruption in the flow of cerebrospinal fluid, with resultant increase in intracranial pressure. If the injury has caused a direct communication between the cranial cavity and the middle ear or the sinuses, meningitis or a brain abscess may develop. Bleeding from the nose and ears is highly suggestive of a basal fracture; occasionally there is serosanguineous drainage which may contain cerebrospinal fluid.

Medical treatment and nursing care

Although the period of unconsciousness usually varies directly with the extent of brain injury, even severely injured patients may regain consciousness, recover almost completely, and return to an active life. Medical and nursing care is directed to lifesaving measures immediately following the accident and maintaining normal body function until recovery is accomplished.

Care at the scene of the accident. The patient with an obvious head injury should be kept absolutely quiet. The wound should be covered with the cleanest material available, and pressure applied to the bleeding scalp *provided* there is no evidence of a depressed fracture. If it is apparent that a sharp instrument has penetrated the bone or if brain tissue is protruding through the wound, the wound must be left strictly alone and no attempt should be made to remove the instrument of injury. No matter how serious the injury seems to be, no patient should be regarded as hopeless; some truly remarkable recoveries have followed injuries in which contents of the cranial cavity were exposed. The patient should be kept warm, and a clear airway should be assured. If there is bleeding into the mouth, he should be turned carefully to one side, provided that several persons are available to help with this. The patient must be turned "in one piece," with the greatest care taken that the cervical spine is kept absolutely straight; a support must be placed under the head when the patient is on his side. No other moving of the patient should be permitted until an ambulance has arrived and experienced help is available.

Any person who has sustained a blow to the head must be watched closely following the accident. Even if consciousness has been regained almost immediately, the patient should sit quietly and not attempt to help others. Pulse and respiratory rate should be noted and cyanosis watched for. Vomiting may be a sign of increased intracranial pressure following injury, although sometimes it is an emotional response to shock.

Hospital care. The patient who has a skull fracture or other serious head injury must be attended constantly. Usually the doctor orders that the bed be kept flat, though some doctors believe that the danger of edema may be reduced by slight elevation of the head of the bed. The patient should be kept absolutely quiet. No vigorous effort should be made to "clean the patient up" during the first few hours after an accident. Rest is much more important. Sudden noises, flashes of light, and the clatter of equipment can increase the patient's restlessness and should be avoided. Portable units are usually used to take roentgenograms; the nurse must remain in the room with the patient to help move him and to protect him from exertion. Side rails should always be on the bed, since restlessness may come on suddenly and convulsions may occur.

Usually the blood pressure, pulse rate, and respiratory rate are taken and recorded every fifteen minutes until they return to within safe limits. Leaving the deflated blood pressure cuff on the arm helps to prevent disturbing the patient unduly when the pressure must be taken so often. Developing the habit of not forcing the mercury column much above the expected reading also sometimes enables the nurse to take the blood pressure and yet barely disturb the patient. The eyes should be observed for inequality of the pupils and the lips and fingernails for cyanosis. Slowing of the pulse, sudden rise in temperature and in blood pressure, and deepening of the unconsciousness or coma are important signs of increase in pressure which must be reported at once. Twitching or convulsive movement of a body part should be recorded and reported. Narcotics are avoided despite restlessness, because they depress the respiratory center.

Drainage from the ears and from the nose should be observed, but no attempt should be made to clean out these orifices. Loose sterile cotton may be placed in the outer openings only; this must be done with caution so that it does not in any way act as a plug to interfere with free flow of fluid. The cotton must be changed as soon as it becomes moistened. Usually the flow of fluid subsides spontaneously. Antibiotics are given routinely when a basal fracture has been sustained. Suctioning of the throat may be necessary but suction must never be used to remove nasal secretions.

Effort may be made to dehydrate the patient and thereby try to lessen intracranial pressure. Fifty milliliters of 50 per cent glucose in distilled water may be given intravenously, and magnesium sulfate may be given by stomach tube or by rectal instillation (proctoclysis). If the patient is unconscious, fluids by mouth are withheld, and the amounts of intravenous infusions are carefully calculated. Mouth care must be given often.

If possible the patient's urinary output should be accurately recorded. No attempt is made to have the patient have a bowel movement for several days following a head injury.

Lumbar punctures are rarely done following head injuries because of the danger of lowering spinal fluid pressure in the spinal canal, followed by herniation of the brain stem into the foramen magnum with resultant severe pressure on vital centers. If a spinal puncture is done, the patient must be watched exceedingly carefully during and following the procedure for signs of pressure in vital centers such as change in respiratory rate and pulse rate.

If hyperthermia develops, it is cared for as described in Chapter 9. General nursing care as described in Chapter 9 is necessary for the patient with a head injury who remains unconscious for some time. Some patients are unconscious for as long as a month or more and yet finally make a satisfactory recovery provided good supportive care has been given.

Because of the danger of *extradural hematoma,* many doctors believe that any patient who has sustained any injury to the head with loss of consciousness should be hospitalized for at least twenty-four hours. If he is asleep during this time, he should be awakened hourly to determine his state of consciousness. Some doctors believe that fluids should be restricted to from 1,000 to 1,500 ml. for the first day and that a dehydrating substance such as 50 ml. of 50 per cent glucose should be given intravenously. If the patient does remain at home, the family should be told to watch him closely for signs of increased intracranial pressure, to awaken him hourly during the night after injury, and to bring him to a hospital at once if drowsiness, stupor, paralysis, or convulsions occur. The treatment for extradural hematoma consists of making burr holes through the temporal bone to relieve the pressure caused by the bleeding and to attempt to control the bleeding. Occasionally the patient has so much damage to the soft tissue of the brain that he dies despite relief of pressure caused by the bleeding; usually such a patient is unconscious for an indefinite time after the accident and is taken to a hospital at once.

Often when a person has sustained a serious head injury, members of his family are in a state of shock and need special attention. Occasionally the doctor orders sedatives for them. If they are not permitted to see the patient because he is in the operating room or undergoing tests, they should be kept informed of his progress. A quiet, pleasant waiting room and a helpful word as to where such facilities as the telephone are located do a great deal to make them more comfortable.

Convalescence. The length of convalescence will depend entirely on how much damage has been done and how rapid recovery has been. Patients are usually urged to resume normal activity as soon as possible, since this seems to decrease the tendency to develop psychoneurotic responses to the injury. Patients may complain of headache and occasional dizziness for some time following a head injury. Occasionally convulsions develop due to the formation of scar tissue in injured brain substance or in its coverings. Such scar tissue may often be surgically removed to effect a complete cure. Loss of hearing and strabismus (cross-eyes) sometimes complicate basal skull fractures and require a long period of rehabilitation; sometimes corrective surgery can be done for the strabismus.

SPINAL CORD INJURIES

The spinal cord may be damaged by a primary lesion or by a tumor within the cord itself. The more common cause of injury, however, is compression by surrounding structures. Metastatic tumors growing in the vertebral bones may cause injury by direct extension and pressure or by destroying the bony support around the cord. Rupture of an intervertebral disc with protrusion of the nucleus pulposus into the spinal canal is a common cause of cord compression. Accidents involving the spine may cause fractures of the vertebras or laminas, with resultant tearing or compression of the cord and edema, which also causes compression. Since the spinal cord is located within a bony canal, slight edema of the cord, small tumor growths, and minimal protrustions of tissue into the canal may cause symptoms of cord compression. Paralysis may occur in body

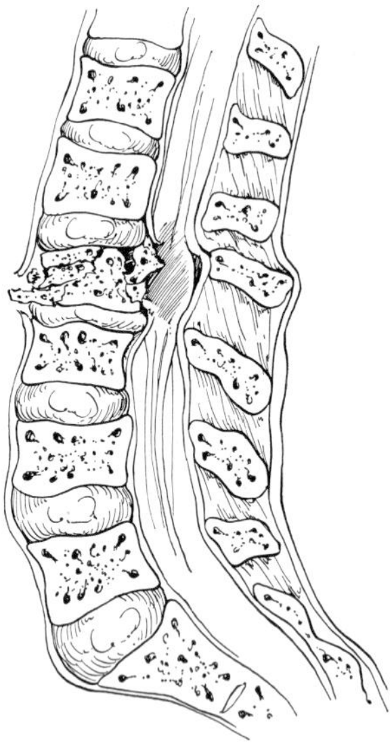

Figure 125

Schematic drawing showing damage to the spinal cord and distortion of adjacent structures that may occur in traumatic injuries to the spine.

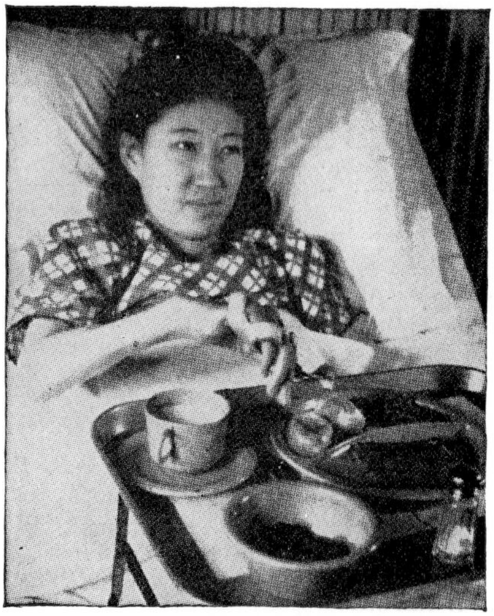

Figure 126

If the injury is high in the spinal cord, the patient may be quadriplegic. Here the patient practices using a hand device for self-feeding. (From Morrissey, Alice B.: Am. J. Nursing **49**:550, 1949.)

parts supplied by nerves leaving the cord below the level of injury. (See Figure 125.)

The symptoms of cord compression depend on the level at which the compression occurs. (See Figure 126.) Cervical injury may cause paralysis of all four extremities and the trunk. Perspiration may be absent in the paralyzed parts, the patient is unable to void and has fecal incontinence. Since the diaphragm and intercostal muscles are paralyzed, respiratory failure may result, and the patient may die unless he is placed immediately in a respirator. A pulmotor is sometimes used for short periods of transportation to a hospital where a respirator is available.

Compression of the spinal cord in the thoracic region causes paralysis of the lower extremities, bladder, and rectum; the paralysis is flaccid at first but becomes spastic. Compression of the cord in the lumbar region causes a flaccid paralysis of the lower extremities, bladder, and rectum; this paralysis remains flaccid.

Diagnosis of cord compression can usually be made by the history and the neurologic examination. Roentgenograms of the spine may be taken and lumbar punctures done; myelograms also may be made. Any inability to move an extremity or any loss of sensation should make one suspicious of cord compression, and the patient should be treated accordingly until it has been proved otherwise. This may prevent such disastrous results as permanent paralysis or death.

General principles of care

Position and movement. Before moving a patient with acute spinal or cord injury onto a bed from the stretcher on which he is admitted, the doctor should be consulted about the type of bed he wishes used. The selection will depend on the doctor's preference, the type of injury, the size of the patient, and the equipment available. If a regular bed is to be used, a full-length fracture board should be placed on top of the bedspring (if there is a separate mattress) or under the mattress. This prevents sagging of the bed and motion of the spine. If the bed is to be gatched, the board must be hinged, or two or more boards must be used with breaks correctly placed. Mattresses containing springs should not be used. Instead of springs and one mattress, some doctors prefer two hair mattresses placed on top of the fracture board. Some use the knee gatch to provide hyperextension to the spine; the bed must then be made up "head to foot." Sponge rubber mattresses are widely recommended and, when available, are usually used when there is the possibility that for some time the patient will be moved very little and with extreme difficulty. If available, an alternating air pressure mattress should be used unless a sponge rubber mattress is being used. Since it may be dangerous to move the patient for some time and since he may have loss of sensation and paralysis of part of the body, pressure areas develop easily. The air pressure mattress alternates the points of pressure at regular intervals and helps to stimulate circulation in the skin. The mattress and entire bed foundation must be well protected with rubber or plastic sheeting so that incontinence will not cause damage.

Before moving the patient, the bed foundation should be completely adjusted with gatches raised as ordered, bolsters placed in the desired positions, and a turning sheet available so that a minimum of motion will be necessary. Three or five people are needed to move the patient from the stretcher to the bed, depending upon his size and the location of injury. The doctor should supervise moving the patient. The body should be supported in proper alignment, and, if necessary, a doctor should apply manual hyperextension to the spine as the patient is moved. (See Chapter 15.)

Observations. The nurse must carefully observe the patient with spinal fractures, cord tumors, and ruptured intervertebral discs for signs of cord compression. The motion, strength, and sensation in the extremities should be tested at least four times a day and more frequently if specifically ordered. Any loss of motion or sensation should be reported at once, since immediate surgery may be needed to relieve pressure on the cord. Some of the laminas may be removed to prevent pressure from edema.

General hygiene. If cord damage has occurred, nursing care will depend on the level of the injury. Patients with cervical lesions, for instance, will be unable to do anything for themselves. Meticulous skin care, maintenance of correct body alignment, preservation of range-of-joint motion, and attempts to preserve muscle tone are imperative nursing measures in the care of any paralyzed patient. No external heat such as a hot-water bottle should be used if the patient has loss of sensation and will not feel a burn. Care should also be taken to be sure that bath water is not too hot, and paralyzed areas should be inspected daily for any signs of skin irritation. There will be no perspiration below the cord injury. At first this may cause the patient to have a fever, which may be treated as in the unconscious patient. (See Chapter 9.) Later there may be excessive perspiration of the unaffected areas, and these will need to be bathed frequently.

Diet. If the patient's arms are paralyzed or if he is not allowed to move them, he will need to be fed. The diet for any patient who is immobilized because of spinal injuries should be high in protein to increase the resistance to decubiti. Fruit juices and foods high in calcium may be limited since urinary calculi tend to form quite easily in patients who are completely immobilized and in those who have fractures. Unless otherwise ordered, at least 3,000 ml. of fluid should be given daily.

Urinary output. The patient may have urinary retention because of injury to spinal nerves. Since he may have no sensation of needing to void, the nurse should check carefully for voiding and for distention of the bladder. A Foley catheter may be inserted into the bladder, or a cystostomy may be done. Later, if the injury is not in the lumbar area, automatic bladder function may be established. (See Chapter 8.)

Gastrointestinal function. Following an acute injury to the spinal cord, the patient often has trouble with abdominal distention. A rectal tube may be used, and Prostigmin is often given hypodermically to stimulate peristalsis. A stomach tube or a Miller-Abbott or Cantor tube attached to suction equipment may be tried. Cathartics and enemas may be required to maintain normal bowel function. A permanent loss of bowel control may occur. (See Chapter 8 for care and rehabilitation measures for patients with fecal incontinence.) If the injury is in the lumbar area, no recovery of automatic control can be hoped for, since the bowel is permanently flaccid, unless partial recovery eventually occurs.

Pain. Patients with spinal injuries often have a great deal of pain at the level of the injury which radiates along the spinal nerves. A thoracic injury causes chest pain, while a lumbar injury causes pain in the legs. Analgesics such as acetylsalicylic acid are ordered, and narcotics usually must be given for some time. However, if the patient has a high cervical injury, no narcotics should be given because respirations may be further embarrassed. Sometimes the paravertebral nerves are injected with 95 per cent alcohol to relieve thoracic pain. This may give relief for several weeks or even months.

Prevention of respiratory complications. Respiratory complications are common following injury of the spinal cord. The patient should be encouraged to take frequent deep breaths, fully expanding the lungs. If he cannot be turned, deep-breathing routines should be supervised, and he should take ten to fifteen deep breaths at least every two hours. Patients who can be turned should have position changes at least every two hours and should be encouraged to take deep breaths. If coughing is not contraindicated, this also should be encouraged, but the doctor should be consulted before urging the patient to cough. Patients who have injuries of the thoracic spine tend to splint their chests and have shallow breathing. Narcotics may be given to control the pain which causes this.

Rehabilitation. As the patient recovers, every possible effort should be made to help him do as much as possible for himself. Supplies should be placed within his reach on special trays or on overbed tables, and he must be given time to give what daily personal care he can manage for himself. Diversional activity should be started to keep him constructively occupied. An occupational therapist can help the nurse in selecting practicable activities; however, if one is not available, any light handiwork that the patient enjoys and that is feasible can be used provided he can use his arms. A radio, television set, and reading material may help to pass the time. If the patient's neck is hyperextended, books that can be flashed on the ceiling are useful provided they do not cause eyestrain. Volunteers are exceedingly helpful in reading to patients. The patient's family and friends should be encouraged to visit often and to keep him up to date on activities in his home and community.

Possible rehabilitation depends on the extent of the cord injury, the emotional reactions of the patient, his age, and other factors. (See Figures 127 and 128.) Muscle exercises often can be started long before the patient is allowed up, and this practice lessens the period of rehabilitation necessary for returning to activity. The patient should be kept in proper body alignment at all times to prevent shortening of muscles and contracture of joints. The patient who must be kept on his back should have a small round bolster placed under the knees so that the proximal end of the tibia is supported without any popliteal pressure. A bath blanket or a small pillow can be used to fashion such a bolster. A firm, flat pillow should be placed under both calves, and the feet should be firmly dorsiflexed against a footboard. Foot drop and contractures at the hips and knees may take months to overcome, and they may prevent the paralyzed patient from being

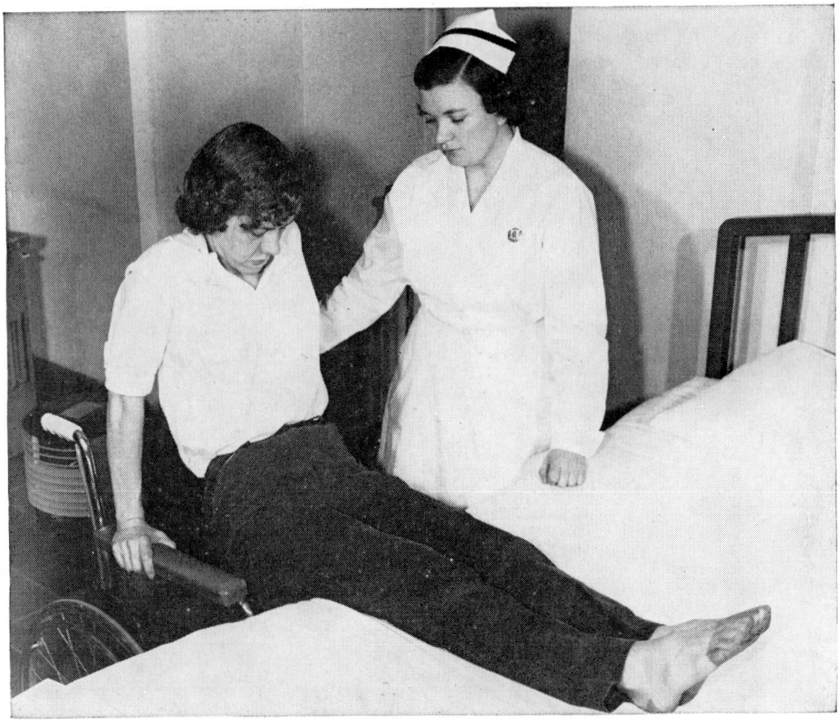

Figure 127

The paraplegic patient moving from bed to wheel chair. Note placement of the chair. The patient pushes up with her arms when moving the buttocks into the chair seat. The paralyzed legs rest on the bed and must be lifted down. Patients with spinal tumors or injuries are frequently paraplegic.

able to walk even with braces and crutches.

Before the patient is permitted to be up following a spinal injury, a brace may be prescribed. A *Taylor back brace,* made of padded and covered metal bars to support the back, is often used. It has leather straps which come forward to be fastened over a muslin "apron." Patients who have ruptured lumbar intervertebral discs may be fitted with a heavy muslin corset with firm stays. All braces and corsets must be custom made and are quite expensive; the cost usually is at least $75 for a brace and, of course, it cannot be reused by another patient. The brace or corset should be applied before the patient gets out of bed, and he will need help in getting into it. The patient should wear a thin knitted undershirt next to the skin to keep the brace clean. Correct placement so that the brace fits contours of the buttocks and chest as designed makes a great deal of difference in the patient's comfort. Care should be taken that the apron is smooth and that tapes are not twisted. The patient's emotional reaction to wearing a brace or a corset is important, since it vitally affects ultimate rehabilitation. Attention to small details that help in initial acceptance of this somewhat uncomfortable and unfamiliar piece of "clothing" is important. The patient should practice putting the brace on while he is in the hospital if he must wear it for some time. A close member of his family may visit the hospital and learn to assist him. Patients who live alone and who are unable to care for their braces themselves may need to have

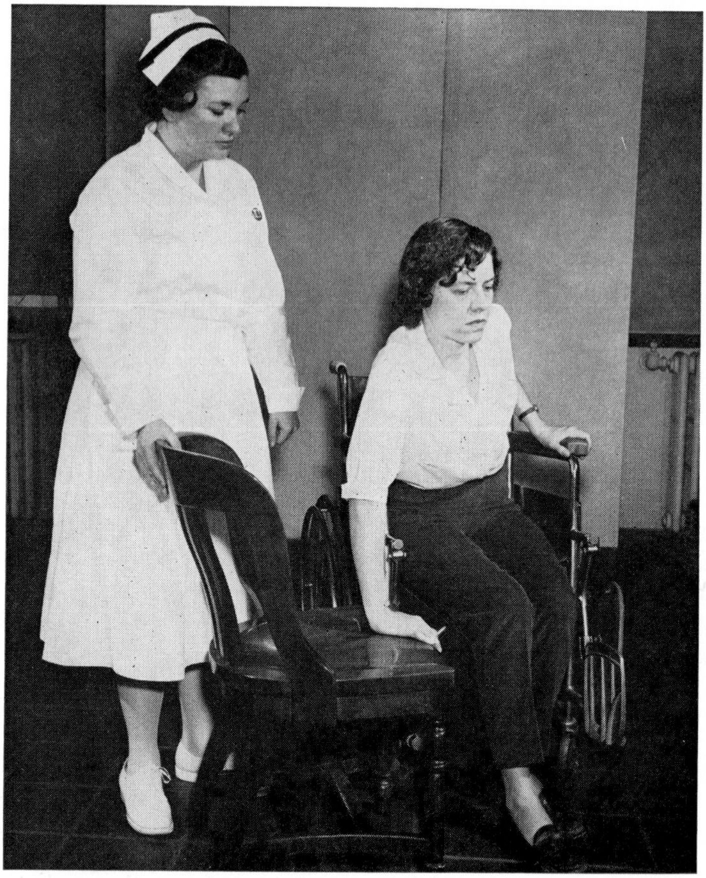

Figure 128

Teaching the paraplegic patient to move from wheel chair to a straight chair. The same motion is used in moving from a wheel chair to the toilet seat. The patient should push up, turn toward the straight chair, and then swing the buttocks around onto the chair seat.

a public health nurse help them in the home or teach someone else to assist. The patient wearing a brace should be especially careful in crossing streets and in engaging in activities such as walking down stairs, since he is limited in his ability to shift his balance quickly to prevent an accident.

Following fracture of a cervical vertebra, a neck brace may be ordered. This fits in such a manner that the chin rests on a cup, and the neck is kept in slight hyperextension. Patients who have a ruptured cervical disc may also be given a neck brace, and the *Thomas collar* is often used. A Thomas collar can be quite cheaply and easily made as follows: (1) cut a piece of firm cardboard the depth desired; (2) pad this with cotton or combination pads and secure with bandages; (3) cover the collar with stockinette and carefully stitch at the top and bottom, avoiding bumps or knots that may irritate the skin. The collar is usually anchored at the side with wide adhesive tape and must never be removed without specific orders from the surgeon. The collar extends well up under the chin and prevents flexion of the neck. The patient who wears any brace to hyperextend the neck has difficulty in seeing where he is going and must be cautioned about this, because accidents can occur easily during everyday functions—such as crossing streets and going down stairs.

All patients who have had spinal injuries should wear shoes with firm lasts and low heels. If the woman patient has always worn moderately high heels, she should continue to wear them rather than to wear flat-heeled shoes. Shoes that tie are preferable. The patient is usually asked to have his family bring his shoes to the hospital so that they may be examined by the doctor and can be worn when he first walks about in the hospital.

Nursing care of the patient with a fracture of the spine

Fractures of the spine may cause compression of the bodies of the vertebras or smashing of the laminas, with or without dislocation of parts, and compression of the spinal cord may result. The emergency care for patients suffering fracture of the spine is discussed in Chapter 15. Nurses should know and be able to teach others what symptoms indicate spinal fracture and how to care for a patient with a spinal fracture so that cord damage is not caused or increased. Spinal fractures should be suspected after automobile accidents, falls, and diving accidents.

Hyperextension. The patient with a spinal fracture may be placed in hyperextension since this position causes the least pressure on the spinal cord. This may be accomplished by various means. Skeletal traction may be used. Small burr holes are drilled in the outer portion of the skull over each parietal region. *Tongs* (usually Crutchfield) are then inserted into the holes, the skin around the tong is sutured, and a collodion dressing is applied. From ten to twenty pounds of weight are attached to a rope coming from the center of the tongs and extending over a pulley attached to the head of the bed. If Crutchfield tongs are to be used, the bed should be made up "head to foot." The nurse must be sure that the patient does not slip up in the bed enough for the weights to rest on a rung of the bed or on the floor. The rope should be free of the mattress or any other obstruction that might decrease the amount of pull needed and do the patient harm. (See Figure 129.) Sandbags are often placed above the patient's shoulders to help prevent his slipping to the head of the bed. It is sometimes desirable to make a trough in the mattress for the patient's head; this is done by fastening wide strips of adhesive tape to the mattress, starting at the level of the gatch, pulling the tapes taut, and securing them to the bottom of the frame. The trough should be about 10 inches wide. No pillow is used under the patient's head. Occasionally the head of the bed may be elevated by placing the bed on blocks to give counteraction and to prevent the patient from slipping to the head of the bed; since this increases

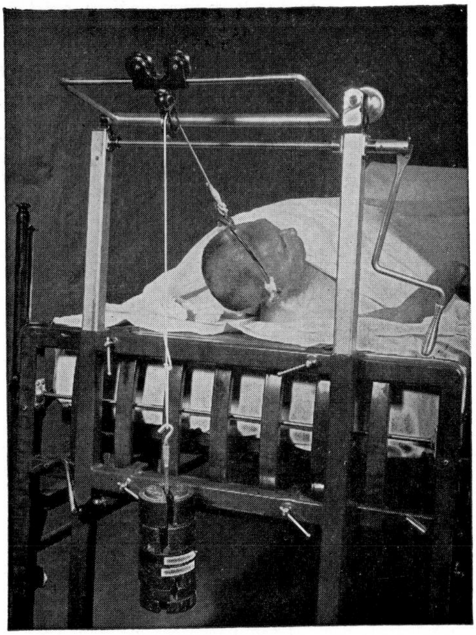

Figure 129

The patient has skull traction with Cone-Barton ice tongs. Note that the head and neck are free from support by a pillow or the mattress. (From Moseley, H. F. [editor]: Textbook of Surgery, St. Louis, 1959, The C. V. Mosby Co.)

the traction, it must not be done without a specific order from the doctor.

In order to obtain traction and hyperextension, a leather chin strap (Sayre strap) attached to a pulley and weights, as described for use with tongs, may be used. The strap fits snugly under the chin and against the occipital protuberances. Leather straps from front and back meet a metal spreader to which the pulley rope is centrally attached. Skin care of the patient's chin is extremely important when this kind of traction is used. The amount of pressure on the skin and soft tissues depends on the amount of weight used. Traction must not be released without the doctor's order, but the chin may need to be gently massaged as often as every hour. The nurse can exert gentle pressure on one side of the chin as she massages the other side with her other hand. Alcohol and powder should be used, and frequent sponging of the skin is necessary to protect the leather from perspiration and to make the patient more comfortable. A small piece of rubber sponge, sheep's wool, or chamois skin is helpful if signs of skin irritation and pressure occur. When feeding the patient care must be taken not to soil or moisten the leather chin strap.

Hyperextension may be accomplished by gatching the bed with the patient head to foot in the bed and placing him so that the high point is directly under the fracture. If the bed gatch is not at the desired position, a small firm round bolster, the width of the mattress, may be placed under the top mattress at the desired level. Several tightly rolled bath blankets may be used to make a bolster of the desired size. Obviously a fracture board must be used to give firm support, and this must be hinged to permit use of the gatches. This method of obtaining hyperextension is commonly used following fracture of a thoracic vertebra.

Members of the family should be prepared for seeing the patient in head or neck traction. Tongs are particularly frightening to them. Both the family and the patient should understand that the tongs do not go through the skull but only into the outer layer of bone. Actually, many patients get so much relief from pain from this type of traction that they accept it surprisingly well. An adjustable mirror attached to the head of the bed enables them to see about the room. Usually they are happier and more content when in a ward with others around them.

The patient who is placed in hyperextension cannot be moved about in bed; he must stay flat on his back for as long as six weeks. He must understand why this is necessary, since a sudden movement might cause irreparable cord damage. A drawsheet may be placed over the abdomen and tucked in at the sides of the mattress to remind the restless patient not to move. Occasionally, sandbags are placed on either side of the body; this is done most often during sleeping hours. If the patient is very restless or unable to cooperate, he must be constantly attended to prevent his moving about in bed.

Patients who are immobilized in head or neck traction or kept in hyperextension develop pneumonia easily. The patient must be instructed to take from ten to fifteen deep breaths regularly each hour when he is awake. The nurse must remind him to do this and should remain with him to see that it is done at least several times each day. Arms and legs usually may be exercised passively if the patient is paralyzed and unable to move himself, but a doctor should be consulted before this is done.

Care of the skin is a major responsibility of the nurse, and the patient must be given back care at least every two hours. The nurse's work is made much easier if the patient is on a sponge rubber mattress, since two nurses working together can give the patient back care without moving him. Each nurse depresses the mattress with one hand and massages the patient's skin with the palm of the other. No part of the back should be neglected, although not all the surface of the back must be done at once, since this might tire the patient too much. Using a bedpan presents a problem, but a child's bedpan may be placed under the patient without moving him if two nurses work together. The mattress under the buttocks should be depressed with one hand and the bedpan slipped into place with the other. To maintain correct spinal alignment, a small towel roll should be inserted at the small of the back directly above the bedpan.

Extreme care must be taken in feeding any patient who is in hyperextension and lying on his back, since it is difficult to swallow in this position. Obviously if the patient chokes he cannot turn or be raised forward. A suction machine should always be on hand for immediate use in case the patient should aspirate into the trachea. The patient should practice swallowing saliva before he attempts to take fluids or solid foods. Usually he does best when given fairly soft food, such as baked custard, at first, because liquids tend to flow into the nasopharynx quite easily. Feeding the patient, at least until he has become fully accustomed to the awkward position, is a nursing responsibility that should never be delegated to a nonprofessional worker. Since feeding the patient takes time, this must be planned for; he must not be allowed to feel that he is a nursing problem on this account. Adequate food intake is necessary to prevent pressure areas from developing and to preserve general tissue health. Also, since meals are psychologically important to all people, the patient needs the emotional support that attractive meals will give when carefully fed to him.

Stryker frame and Foster bed. If the patient with a spinal injury can be placed flat in bed but cannot be turned in bed, a Stryker frame or a Foster bed may be used. These beds make it possible to change the patient's position from abdomen to back without altering his alignment. Usually the patient on this bed is turned every two to four hours. The bed cannot be used for very obese patients because space between the frames is inadequate and cannot be adjusted sufficiently. The beds have two metal frames to which canvas covers are attached. The canvas used for the back-lying position has an opening under the buttocks to allow for use of a bedpan, and that used for the prone-lying position can be cut out so the male patient can void. When the patient is in the prone position, the canvas should extend from below the shoulders to the ankles and a narrow head strap used to support the forehead. In the prone position the patient can eat, read, and do light activities with his hands. The canvasses may be covered with thin sponge rubber mattresses cut the same size as the canvas and covered with bed linen. To turn the patient, the linen, mattress, and the opposite canvas and frame are placed in that order over the patient. The frame fastens to a metal attachment at head and foot. Straps are placed around both frames, and then two people release pivot pins at either end of the frame and slowly rotate the patient on the frame from his abdomen to his back or vice versa. The pins are reinserted, and the upper frame, canvas, and mattress are removed. The bed has armboard and footboard attachments to use, if desired, for permissable activity or for good alignment. The patient may be quite apprehensive about being placed on this bed, and, if possible, a demonstration of turning should be given to him before he is moved onto it. This type of bed is unsafe for a very restless or disoriented patient, although the straps may be used to give some security and protection. A real advantage of these beds is that they wheel easily, so that the patient may be taken to a sun porch or recreational area for a change of surroundings.

Plaster jacket. A plaster jacket which extends from the shoulders to below the hips is sometimes used to treat the patient with a fractured vertebra below the cervical area. A fracture board and a firm mattress should be used. As soon as the patient returns from the plaster room, the nurse should check the cast at the top and bottom for crumbs of plaster which can usually be removed at first but later are difficult to remove as they work downward or upward. The cast should be examined to be certain it is cut out enough to permit use of a bedpan. If it is not, the nurse must remind the doctor, since it must be done before the patient has a bowel movement. The patient can usually urinate safely without soiling the case. Plastic material may be used to cover the cast edges, and the head of the bed may be raised on blocks. The gatch must never be raised without the doctor's order, since this may cause the cast to crack. When the cast is dry, its edges should be bound with small pieces of adhesive tape to protect the skin from irritation. This is known as "petaling" the cast. The lower portion should be covered with plastic material fastened on the edge and pushed up under the cast so it will remain in place when a bedpan is used. This can easily be removed and changed if it becomes soiled.

If abdominal distention is troublesome, a "window," or opening, may be cut in the cast over the abdomen. The edges of this opening must also be bound. Such a window is useful in checking for distention of the bladder. Skin under the cast should be massaged with alcohol and powder. The nurse should slip her hand palm downward as far as she can reach to feel for crumbs or bits of plaster and any areas of skin tenderness which may be due to pressure or irritation. The cast is usually loose enough to permit threading a thin piece of terry cloth toweling from top to bottom under the cast to partially cleanse the patient's skin. This is done by having the patient lie down which permits the toweling to be pushed along the upper surface of the body that "falls away" from the cast while he is in this position. The patient then turns slowly and supports himself by holding the upper rungs of the bed. Pillows may be needed to support the cast at the hips. The toweling must not be too wet or the lining of the cast will become moist, but soap may be used and scented colognes are often gratifying to women patients.

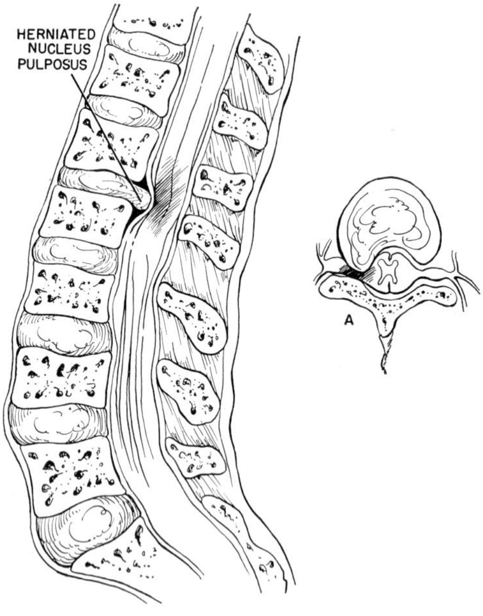

Figure 130

Note compression of the spinal cord caused by herniation of nucleus pulposus into the spinal canal and pressure on nerves as they leave the spinal cord.

Nursing care of a patient with a ruptured intervertebral disc

Rupture of an intervertebral disc with protrusion of the nucleus pulposus into the spinal canal is a common spinal injury among middle-aged persons engaged in manual labor. (See Figure 130.) With age, the annulus fibrosis or fibrous capsule within which the nucleus pulposus (a soft cartilaginous pad) is enclosed becomes less elastic. Although the disc may rupture at any level in the spine, the most common sites are the last two lumbar interspaces. Rupture of a disc at the fifth and sixth cervical interspaces is seen less frequently.[36]

Principles of body mechanics. Injury to an intervertebral disc usually is caused by stress on the back while it is in acute flexion. Much back injury of this type could be prevented if persons doing a good deal of lifting and pulling were taught to observe principles of good body mechanics. When lifting heavy objects, the knees should be flexed and the back

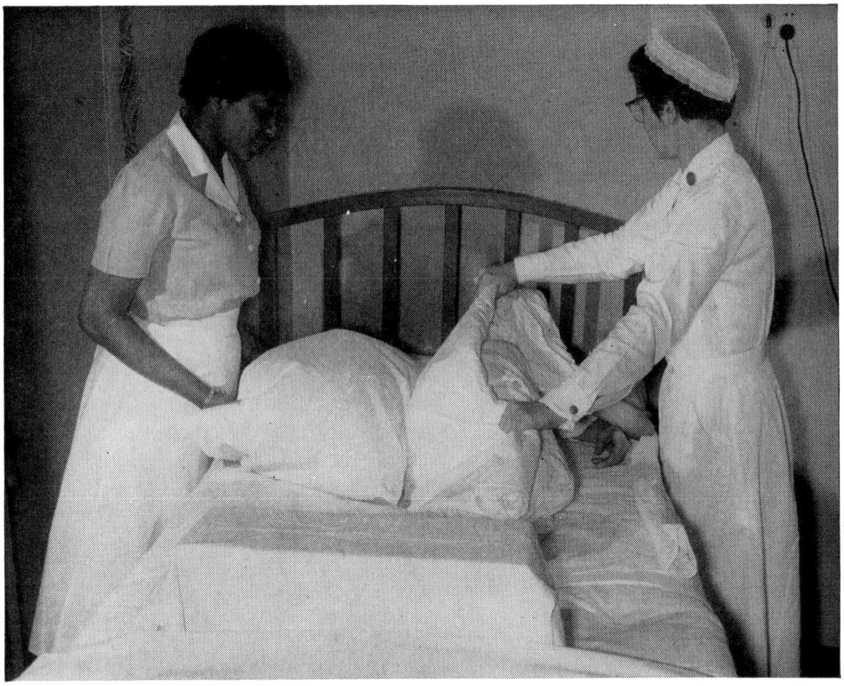

Figure 131

The nurse and the aide are turning the patient who has had surgery for the excision of a ruptured disc. Note that the nurse holds the turning sheet taut with one hand at the level of the patient's shoulder and the other below his buttocks.

kept straight. In this position, the large muscles of the thighs and the buttocks carry the weight—not the back muscles which give support to the spine. It is always better to pull than to push, and the body should be kept in correct alignment and not twisted to one side whenever one bends, lifts, or carries heavy objects. In lifting objects from a high shelf, both hands should be used; this will place the weight of the object on the arm muscles, not the cervical spine.

In bedside nursing the nurse must frequently move patients and heavy objects; therefore, she must learn and practice the principles of good body mechanics. The incidence of back strain and ruptured intervertebral discs is high among nursing personnel. The nurse should be responsible for teaching the principles of good body mechanics to persons who work with her. The industrial nurse may have many opportunities to help workers improve their body mechanics and avoid back injury. (For complete discussion of body mechanics in nursing, see texts on fundamentals of nursing.)

Diagnostic measures. The diagnosis of ruptured intervertebral disc usually is made from the history and neurologic examination. The patient with a ruptured lumbar disc typically has a sciatic pain when the leg on the affected side is raised straight up without bending the knee (Lasègue's sign). This is because the protruding nucleus pulposus presses against the sciatic nerve. Motor and sensory losses can be traced along the course of the impinged spinal nerves, and manual pressure on the juglar veins will cause increased pain since this causes a rise in intracranial pressure. A lumbar puncture is often done to differentiate this condition from an intervertebral tumor; the cerebrospinal protein is elevated in the presence of a tumor. Roentgenograms of the spine are taken, and a myelogram sometimes is done. The latter procedure is most useful in differentiating a herniated disc from an intervertebral tumor; some doctors do it routinely, whereas others believe that there is danger of meningeal irritation from the medium used.

The patient with a ruptured intervertebral lumbar disc. The patient with a ruptured intervertebral lumbar disc usually complains of acute pain in the lower back. This pain usually appears suddenly when stress is placed on the back, such as when opening a window or soon thereafter. Later the pain begins to radiate over one buttock and into the leg, often extending as far as the ankle. It is unilateral since the nucleus pulposus usually presses on nerves arising from one side of the spinal cord. Activities such as sneezing, coughing, bending, or straining to defecate cause increased pain since they temporarily increase intracranial pressure which puts additional pressure on the pinched spinal nerves. Since motor and sensory nerves to the leg and foot may be impinged upon, the patient may limp and have paresthesia or hyperesthesia in the leg and foot on the affected side. He typically walks on either his toes or his heels because of muscle spasm in the leg. The severity of neurologic damage is indicative of the amount of compression on the cord and may dictate the treatment, since immediate operation may be imperative to prevent permanent cord damage. The nurse should urge anyone who has injured his back to seek immediate medical attention.

Conservative treatment. If possible, patients with ruptured intervertebral lumbar discs are treated conservatively. The patient is placed on bed rest for several weeks. The bed should be kept flat, and a firm mattress should be used to maintain good body alignment and alleviate pain caused by stress on the affected disc. This may be accomplished by placing a bedboard under the mattress. If the patient is at home, table leaves or a door may be used. The patient should be taught to turn himself in a log-rolling fashion: to cross his arms over his chest, bend the uppermost knee to the side to which he wishes to turn, and then to roll over. (See Figure 132.) This position helps him to maintain good spinal alignment. If there is any motor nerve loss, a footboard should be used to prevent foot drop. The patient may complain of burning sensation in his feet because of paresthesia, and a footboard helps by keeping the bedclothes off the feet. If the patient has a sensory nerve loss, hot-water bottles or heating pads should not be used on the feet or legs, and other precautions should be taken to prevent further injury. A small bedpan should be used and a small towel roll should be placed directly behind it to support the arch of the lower back. (See Figure 133.) The patient should roll onto the bedpan instead of lifting his hips so that the bedpan can be slid into place. He should be advised not to strain to defecate since this will increase pain. Constipation is frequent. The patient is urged to increase the amount of roughage eaten, and fresh fruits are helpful. At least 3,000 ml. of fluid should be taken each day, and a regular time for defecation should be established. A mild laxative such as milk of magnesia may be needed.

Many patients with a ruptured lumbar intervertebral disc suffer from severe muscle spasm in the lower back. A heating pad may relieve this, although codeine and acetylsalicylic acid are often necessary. Physical therapy in the form of infrared heat, massage, and active and passive muscle exercises done in warm water may also be ordered to help relieve the muscle spasm. Exercises are more easily performed in water, and the heat helps to relax muscles. The patient should be transferred to the physical therapy department by stretcher, and extra covers, such as a towel to wrap around the head if the hair becomes wet, should be sent

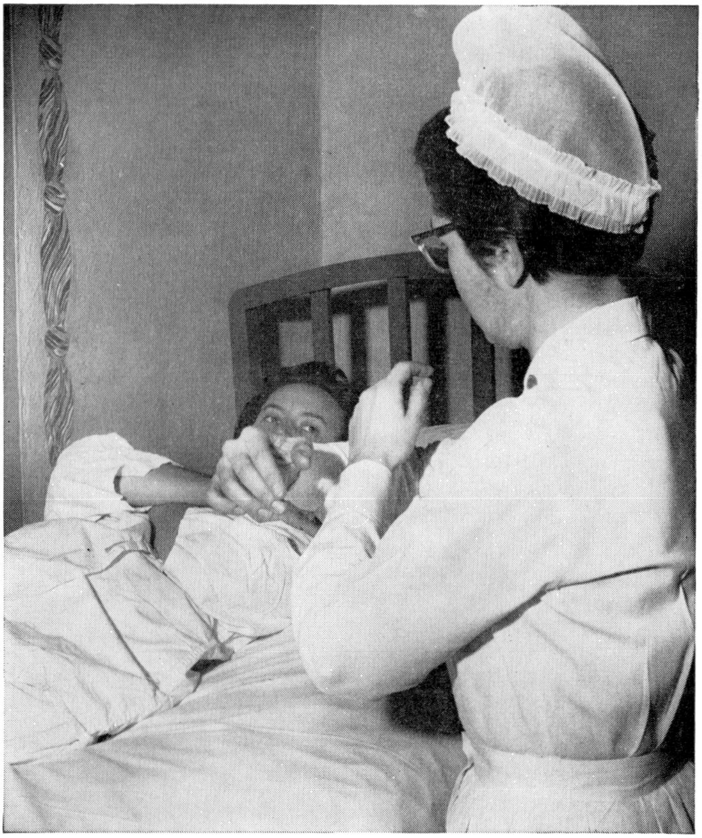

Figure 132

The nurse is teaching the patient with a ruptured disc how to fold her arms preparatory to "log-rolling."

with him to avoid chilling after the treatment.

The patient with a ruptured disc may be discouraged by the prospects of a long period of bed rest and possible surgery. If he has motor or sensory losses, he worries lest he become unable to walk. To some people the words spinal surgery are synonymous with paralysis. The patient may worry about his family, his finances, and his job and about collecting compensation if the injury was sustained at work. Doctors, nurses, other professional team members, and the patient's spiritual adviser may need to help alleviate his fears and anxieties. He may be more content if the head of the bed is elevated on 6-inch blocks, since this increases his range of vision and allows him to eat more easily. He may also find it easier to use the bedpan in this position. Diversions such as reading, visiting with others, and light handicrafts should be encouraged.

During this time of inactivity, the nurse should teach and demonstrate principles of body mechanics to the patient since he will need to be particularly careful in lifting. Some patients may be encouraged by the doctor to change their type of work.

While the patient is still in bed, he should be measured for a corset so that it will be available when he gets up. He should have walking shoes and socks brought to the hospital. The corset should be put on before arising. Since straight

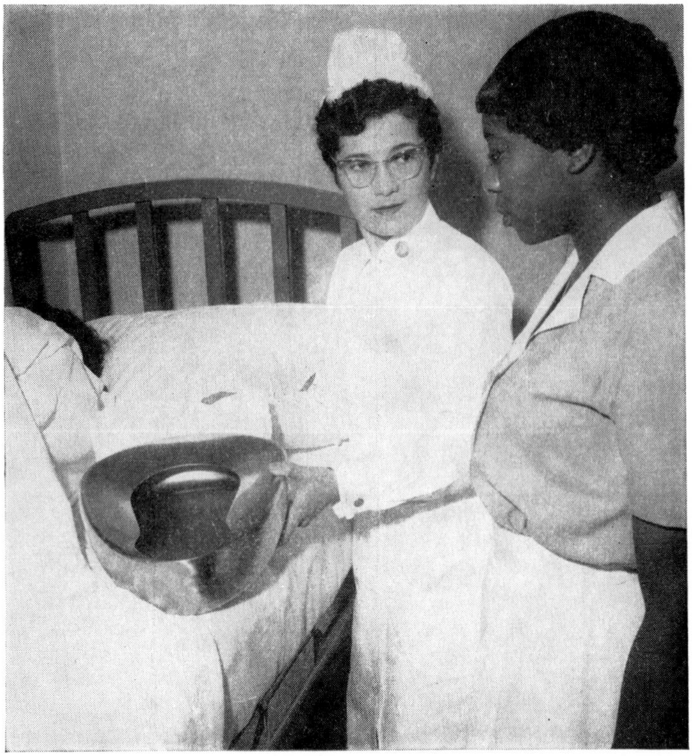

Figure 133

The nurse is demonstrating to the aide
how to place a rolled towel behind the bedpan for the patient who
has a ruptured disc. This prevents arching
of the back and makes the patient more comfortable.

leg raising and bending at the waist should be avoided, the patient may need assistance in getting into shoes and stockings. However, it is permissible to bend the knees to bring the foot up, and most patients learn to dress themselves.

Movement and positions that cause poor alignment of the spinal column and put strain on injured nerves should be avoided until approved by the doctor. This will usually be about six weeks after the patient is allowed out of bed. A firm straight chair should be used instead of an overstuffed one. The knees should not be crossed or the feet or legs elevated on a footstool. It is inadvisable for the patient to drive a car since this would necessitate stretching the legs. Stairs should be climbed as infrequently as possible, and great care should be taken in walking over rough ground or in stepping off curbs to avoid sudden twisting of the back. In taking a tub bath, the knees should be bent. The corset should be worn by the patient when he is out of bed except when bathing and taking a shower. In picking things off the floor, the knees should be bent and the back held straight. (See Figure 134.) Weights heavier than five pounds should not be carried.

If, on resuming activity, the symptoms recur, surgical excision of the ruptured portion of the nucleus pulposus will usually be necessary. This is done through an opening made by removing part of the bone surrounding the spinal cord. The procedure is called a *laminectomy.* If more than three intervertebral discs are ruptured, a *spinal fusion* usually is done. In a spinal fusion the spinal vertebras in the affected area are ankylosed; this permanently prevents movement of this portion of the spine. The bone used is often taken from the iliac crest. The skin incision for both a laminectomy and a spinal fusion is made directly over the spinous processes and is about 10 centimeters (4 inches) long.

The postoperative nursing care of patients having surgery for a ruptured lumbar intervertebral disc is similar to that given the patient being treated more conservatively, with a few additional considerations. The patient should be observed carefully for signs of hemorrhage or leakage of spinal fluid from the wound and for compression of the cord caused by edema at the site of operation. Evidence of hemorrhage or a loss of spinal fluid can usually be seen on the dressings. The doctor should be called at once; usually he changes the dressings, since moisture on the dressings may predispose to infection. The patient who is bleeding from the wound may be placed on his back and the head of the bed elevated on

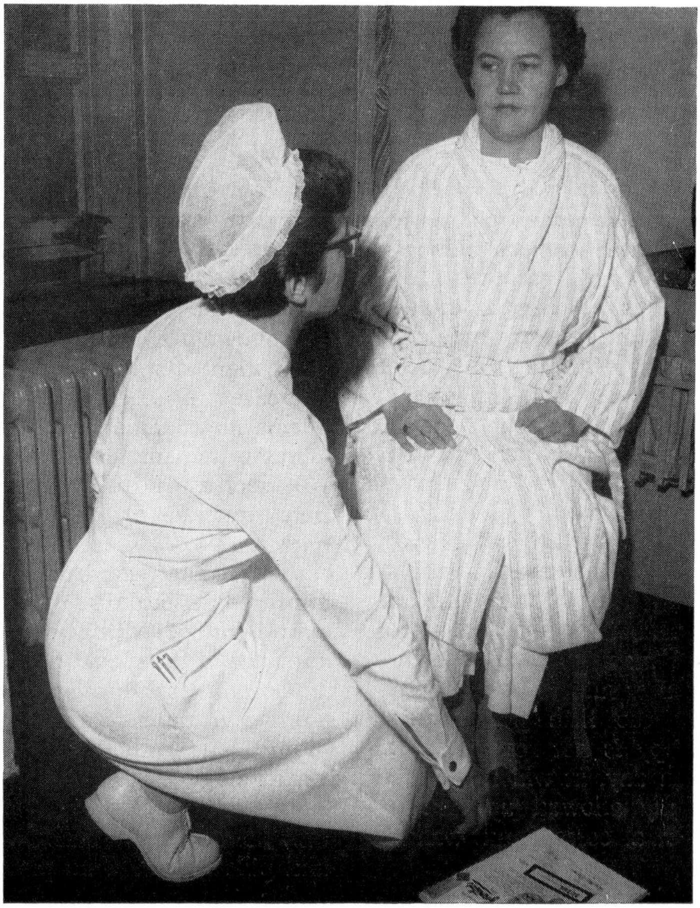

Figure 134

The nurse is demonstrating to a patient with a ruptured disc how to stoop to pick something from the floor. Note that her back is held straight and that her knees and hips are flexed sharply.

blocks, since this causes the spinal fluid to put pressure on blood vessels in the area.

Before the operation the patient should be warned that pain will persist for some time postoperatively because of local edema. Time is also needed for the nerve to recover from damage caused by the pressure on it preoperatively. The patient may complain of severe spasm in the back and thigh muscles. This is a result of the nerves being touched during surgery. The spasm may be relieved somewhat by moving the legs in bicycle fashion while the patient is lying on his side. This exercise can be started on the first postoperative day. The patient may have bladder and bowel dysfunction for several days; these complications are treated in the usual manner—with Foley catheters, rectal tubes, Prostigmin, and carminative enemas.

Some doctors order bed rest for about ten days after a laminectomy for excision of a protruded lumbar nucleus pulposus; others have the patient get up on the operative day. If the patient is on bed rest, he should be turned every two hours by two people using a turning sheet. (See Figure 131.) He should make no attempt to help himself for forty-eight hours to prevent strain on the operative site. It is better if the patient and the nurse practice turning preoperatively, since postoperatively the patient may have a great deal of pain and may be tense and frightened. He should be told not to try to reach toward his bedside table but to ask for help. Heat and massage treatments are started the day after sutures have been removed, usually the fifth postoperative day. Hydrotherapy is not resumed until around the tenth day, at which time the patient is usually allowed up and required to wear a corset and walking shoes.

If the patient is to get up on the operative day, he must be fitted with a corset preoperatively. He should be watched closely for weakness or fainting, and the dressings should be checked for signs of hemorrhage or leaking of cerebrospinal fluid. These patients may be given special exercises to do, such as the "goose-step," raising the knees high as they walk, and "wood chopping," which consists of raising both hands over the head and letting them fall to below the knees. The exercise should be done from five to ten times three times a day. Exercises help to relieve muscle spasm in the back and thighs. Patients may be discharged from the hospital by the fifth postoperative day. They should continue to sleep on a firm bed.

Patients who have had spinal fusions are kept in bed for varying lengths of time and resume activity slowly. A jacket cast sometimes is applied. When such a cast is used, ambulation is possible at an earlier time.

The patient with a ruptured cervical intervertebral disc. The patient with a ruptured cervical intervertebral disc usually complains of pain and muscle weakness in the arms. Immediate operation may be necessary to relieve cord compression, since the compression may cause respiratory failure.

Following surgery for a cervical disc, the patient should be closely watched for decrease in chest expansion because edema may temporarily paralyze the diaphragm and intercostal muscles. If there is a decrease in chest expansion, the patient must be placed in a respirator at once.

The patient who has had surgery for a ruptured cervical disc is placed flat in bed postoperatively with only a small pillow at the nape of the neck. The head should not be flexed, because pressure many then be exerted on the cord and cause respiratory failure. The patient may be turned, but the turning sheet should extend above the head. On the third postoperative day he may be placed in a semi-Fowler's position and pillows should be placed well down under the shoulders. Arm movements, even to eat, are prohibited until this time. The patient is allowed up on the fifth postoperative day, and a Thomas collar may be used to prevent forward flexion of the head for several weeks.

Nursing care of the patient with an intravertebral tumor

It is fortunate that intravertebral tumors are infrequent, since they are extremely difficult to remove surgically without causing serious damage to the spinal cord. Tumors of the spinal cord are both intramedullary, involving primarily the substance of the cord, and extramedullary, involving primarily the meninges. Metastatic tumors often involve the vertebras and may also invade the spinal cord and its coverings. Obviously, tumors involving the meninges are more likely to be successfully removed than the other types. Even when complete removal is not considered possible, surgery is often done to remove part of the tumor and to remove some of the bone surrounding the spinal column. This is called a *spinal decompression operation.*

The patient first complains of tenderness over a spinous process which is aggravated by movement and by bed rest. He may also have pain in the areas innervated by the cord at that level. A cervical lesion causes pain in the arms; a thoracic lesion, in the chest; and a lumbar lesion, in the legs. Foot and hand pain are rare, but there may be numbness and tingling. As the lesion grows and further compresses the cord, motor and sensory losses occur until eventually the patient loses all functions below the level of the tumor.

Nursing care for a patient with a tumor of the spinal cord is the same as that given other patients with spinal injury and its resultant neurologic symptoms. The care after a decompression operation is similar to that given the patient who has had excision of a ruptured nucleus pulposus, except that recovery is much slower. The patient often has severe pain and requires narcotics.

Convalescent care and rehabilitation depend entirely on the kind of tumor and whether or not it has been successfully removed. Even if it is not removable, the decompression operation may give relief from symptoms for months and sometimes years. X-ray treatment may be given while the patient is recovering in the hospital and continued after his dismissal. The family often needs help in caring for the patient and in meeting the problems that his condition entails. The patient often either knows or guesses if little can be done for him medically because he does not have mental dulling which often accompanies brain tumors and sometimes accompanies cerebrovascular accidents.

INTRACTABLE PAIN

When pain becomes unbearable and cannot be controlled by more conservative means, it is sometimes possible to alleviate it by surgery. Pain may involve the nerve endings in the skin, and scars such as those seen after an attack of herpes zoster may cause severe pain. Such pain usually can be relieved by resecting a piece of the nerve going to the skin and cutting off pathways to the damaged nerve endings.

Neurectomy

When pain is localized in one part of the body, it can be relieved by interruption of the peripheral or cranial nerves supplying the area. The nerve fibers to the affected area are severed from the cord (cell body) in an operation known as a neurectomy. (The nerve may also be effectively destroyed by injecting it with absolute alcohol, but the results are unpredictable.) Not only pain fibers are interrupted by these procedures, but also fibers controlling movement and position sense. Therefore, this type of treatment cannot be used to control pain in the extremities. A neurectomy probably is most often done to relieve the suffering of patients with trigeminal neuralgia, in which case it is referred to as a *fifth nerve resection.* It may also be done to control incapacitating dysmenorrhea. The latter procedure is called a *presacral neurectomy.* (See Chapter 22.)

Trigeminal neuralgia. Trigeminal neuralgia, or tic douloureux, is characterized by excruciating, burning pain which radiates along one or more of the three divi-

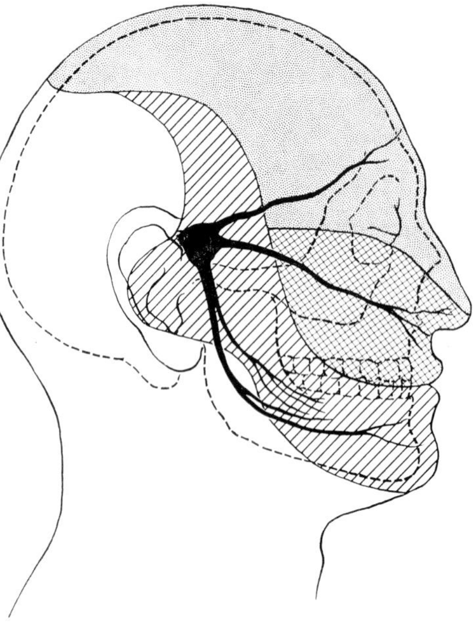

Figure 135

Diagram showing pathway of the trigeminal nerve and the facial area innervated by each of the three main branches.

sions of the fifth cranial nerve. (See Figure 135.) The pain typically extends only to the midline of the face and head since this is the extent of the tissue supplied by the offending nerve. There are areas along the course of the nerve known as "trigger points," and the slightest stimulation of these areas may cause pain. Patients with trigeminal neuralgia usually are very unhappy individuals who try desperately to avoid "triggering" the pain. It is not unusual to see them lying in bed with the covers over their heads in an effort to avoid drafts. They frequently have been unable to eat properly for some time, since chewing causes pain. They may, therefore, be undernourished and dehydrated. They may have slept poorly and not have washed, shaved, or combed their hair for some time. Oral hygiene must often be neglected because of pain.

In caring for the patient with trigeminal neuralgia preoperatively or in caring for the patient who is being treated medically, it is important that members of the nursing staff be sympathetic toward the patient's behavior. Every effort should be made to avoid placing the patient in a draft and to avoid walking swiftly to his bed, because the slight motion of air created may be enough to cause pain. The bed should not be jarred or the bedclothes fanned. It is unwise to urge the patient to wash or shave the affected area or to comb his hair, since he may either become upset in feeling that it is required or he may comply and set off another seige of pain. He will probably prefer to do things for himself if touching his face is involved. It is sometimes possible for him to give himself mouth care if applicators and a lukewarm mouthwash are provided. Often a purèed diet or lukewarm fluids taken through a straw are all that can be tolerated.

Fifth nerve resection is an elective operative procedure. Although surgery relieves pain, some patients find that the side effects due to the numbing are almost unbearable. The patient is usually treated conservatively with such drugs as nicotinic acid, thiamine chloride, potassium chloride, cobra venom, analgesics, and sedatives for a time and surgery is done only when the condition becomes unbearable. The recently discovered drugs, Banthine and Diparcol (diethazine) are now being used. Their action is similar to that of thorazine. The peripheral branches of the fifth cranial nerve may also be injected with 95 per cent alcohol; this may give relief for several months.

Postoperatively it is important to know what branches of the nerve have been cut in order to provide the necessary protection. If the upper branch is completely severed, the patient may lose the corneal reflex on that side. An attempt is made to save a few fibers of the nerve, since even a few seem to preserve this vital reflex. Until the doctor has tested the corneal reflex and verified its presence, an eye shield is used to prevent dust or lint from getting onto the cornea and causing injury.

The patient should be instructed not to touch or rub his eye but to blink it often, since this helps to lubricate the eye. Mineral oil or other medications should be used only as ordered by the doctor. If the reflex is completely missing, the eye must be washed out twice a day with normal saline solution or a weak boric acid solution. (See Chapter 33.) The lids should not be dried, since any material such as cotton, gauze, tissues, or towels may leave lint. The patient should be taught to care for his eye when he returns home and should do this twice daily using an eye cup. Any contact with the eye should be carefully avoided when washing the face. The eye should be inspected several times a day, and medical attention should be sought if it becomes inflamed. Patients are safer outdoors if they wear glasses, since this protects the eyes from dust and other flying particles.

When the lower branch of the fifth cranial nerve is interrupted, the patient needs to avoid hot foods, since he will not be aware if the mucous membrane is burned. He may have some difficulty chewing and swallowing at first and should be instructed to place the food in the unaffected side of the mouth. Since food may be retained in the mouth on the affected side, mouth care should be given immediately following meals. Dental caries on the affected side will not cause pain; therefore, the patient should visit the dentist routinely every six months. He should tell the dentist that he has had a fifth nerve resection so that trauma is avoided. Care must be taken in shaving to avoid nicking the insensitive skin.

Within twenty-four hours after a fifth nerve resection, most patients develop herpes simplex (cold sores) about the lips. It is believed that perhaps the virus causing this condition is harbored in the trigeminal nerve. Campho-Phenique, applied frequently, seems to give more relief than any other treatment. Usually the lesions clear in about a week.

Recently an operation has been devised by which the myelinated sheath of the fifth cranial nerve is partially removed, this permits the nerve to expand. Since the nerve is not resected, there is no sensory loss. However, the operation necessitates an infratentorial craniotomy.

Other cranial nerve surgery. Other cranial nerves may be interrupted if necessary. It is sometimes necessary to resect both the fifth and ninth nerves to relieve severe pain caused by carcinoma of the sinuses. The nursing problems in each instance are related to the areas that have been desensitized and the resulting handicaps. Often there is temporary and sometimes permanent loss or a change of facial expression. This may cause severe psychic problems. When any nerve is resected, whether it be peripheral or cranial, the patient must understand that all sensation in this area is lost so that he will need to avoid injury especially from heat, cold, and trauma.

Rhizotomy

Resection of a posterior nerve root just before it enters the spinal cord is known as a rhizotomy. This procedure frequently is useful in controlling severe pain in the upper trunk such as that caused by carcinoma of the lung. However, it cannot be used to relieve pain in the extremities since position sense is lost. The incision is made high in the thoracic or low in the cervical area and involves a laminectomy. The postoperative observation and care are similar to that necessary for any patient who has had a laminectomy, except that the patient who has had a rhizotomy is usually a poorer operative risk and may be suffering from a severe debilitating disease and therefore develops complications, such as decubiti, more easily. It is important for both the patient and the nurse to realize that this operation will not prevent pain at the level of incision because the resected nerves affect only the area below the incision.

Chordotomy

A chordotomy is an operation done to relieve intractable pain in the lower trunk and legs and is most often done for patients with extensive carcinoma of the pelvis. The incision is made high in the thoracic area, two laminas are removed, and the pain pathways in the spinothalamic tract (anterior and lateral aspect of the cord) on the side opposite the pain are severed. If the pain is in the midline, the interruption must be done bilaterally; however, the two operations must be done separately to avoid extensive damage to the cord from edema.

Following surgery, nursing care is similar to that given a patient who has had a cervical laminectomy for removal of a protruded nucleus pulposus. Frequently temporary paralysis, or at least leg weakness, and loss of bowel and bladder control follow a chordotomy due to edema of the cord and will gradually disappear in about two weeks. Back care, with special attention given to pressure points, should be given every two or three hours since position sense is lessened and the patient is often debilitated. It is advisable to use an alternating air pressure mattress until the patient is allowed out of bed. Sometimes Foster beds and Stryker frames enable the nurses to give the patient better care. Because of the decreased position sense, special attention needs to be given to placing the patient in proper body alignment by using foot blocks. If quadriceps setting exercises are begun in the early postoperative period, retraining in walking will be less difficult for the patient. It usually is easier for the patient to use a walker when he first begins to walk, but he should progress to a cane. Many patients will always feel more secure with a cane. Occupational therapy should be designed to strengthen the leg muscles. The use of a treadle sewing machine or a treadle sander will give exercise to the ankle. A bicycle jig saw provides for hip and knee flexion and extension. This can be started as soon as the patient can be out of bed comfortably for at least two hours at a time.

Temperature sensation is permanently lost, so the nurse must be cautious of burning or of inflicting other injury to the lower trunk and legs, and she must teach the patient and his family the danger of this. The lower portion of the body, especially the feet, should be inspected routinely for any breaks in the skin or unnoticed infection.

Many patients who need to have a chordotomy already have a colostomy which should be irrigated regularly. The patient will need to be taught to notice how much fluid he uses since he may not feel the usual cramping sensation. If the patient has a normal bowel, he will need daily enemas at first to prevent incontinence. He must guard against constipation and impactions since he will not be aware of the usual signs which stimulate evacuation of the bowel. He should try to defecate at a regular time each day.

It is usually necessary to leave a Foley catheter in the bladder for a week after a chordotomy has been done. Routine catheter care should be given. Some doctors order tidal drainage to restore or maintain the bladder tone. When the catheter is removed, the patient, because of diminished sensation, may need to be taught to void at regular intervals using the Credé method (see Chapter 8).

The patient is likely to have severe pain in the incision and to need narcotics frequently for the first three or four postoperative days. The pain should be described accurately, since occasionally not all the nerve fibers are cut, and a second operation may be necessary. Most doctors feel that the best results are obtained from a chordotomy if it is done before the patient becomes addicted to narcotics.

The patient may need much reassurance, because he has suffered intensively before surgery and may have a low pain threshold. The operative course is a long one, and recovery takes time. The patient frequently becomes worried and depressed. Emphasis should be placed on daily progress, and any new independence should be praised. Since the hospital stay is likely to be an extended one, some plan should be made to provide both occupational and recreational therapy. These activities not only help in the physical restoration, but also are an acceptable outlet to release the hostility, anger, and irritability that invariably are felt by the patient.

Because of the danger of temporarily paralyzing the diaphragm and the intercostal muscles, a bilateral high cervical chordotomy cannot be done safely. Occasionally a chordotomy is done unilaterally, however, to interrupt pain fibers to the upper part of the arm and the chest. This relieves chest pain that radiates into the arm.

Prefrontal lobotomy

A prefrontal lobotomy is rarely used because of the prolonged retraining in activities of daily living that is necessary. The patient also may have marked loss of inhibitions to the point that he is socially unacceptable. The surgery does, however, relieve pain in those patients with a low pain threshold, leaving them euphoric. (For further information on the nursing needs of patients having a prefrontal lobotomy, see textbooks which include psychosurgery.)

REFERENCES AND SELECTED READINGS*

1 American Public Health Association: Control of Communicable Disease in Man, New York, 1955, The American Public Health Association.

2 *Baker, Elmer, E., and Sokoloff, Martin: Teaching Aphasic Patients to Talk Again, Am. J. Nursing **52**:831-832, July 1952.

3 Boyce, Helen E.: Rehabilitation in Multiple Sclerosis, Nursing Outlook **3**:549-551, Oct. 1955.

4 Cecil, Russell L., and Loeb, Robert F. (editors): A Textbook of Medicine, ed. 10, Philadelphia, 1959, W. B. Saunders Co.

5 Danca, Eleanor Drexler: The Aphasic Patient, Am. J. Nursing **46**:234-236, April 1946.

6 de Gutiérrez-Mahoney, C. G., and Carini, Esta: Neurological and Neurosurgical Nursing, ed. 3, St. Louis, 1960, The C. V. Mosby Co.

7 *Fritz, Edna L., and Wolf, George A., Jr.: Multiple Sclerosis, Am. J. Nursing **47**:519-522, Aug. 1947.

8 *Lennox, William G.: The Epileptic Patient and the Nurse, Am. J. Nursing **46**:219-223, April 1946.

*References preceded by an asterisk indicate material particularly well suited for student reading.

9 *Lennox, W. G.: Epilepsy—A Problem in Public Health, Am. J. Pub. Health **41**:533-536, May 1951.

10 *McCluskey, Audrey: The Patient in a Chest Respirator, Am. J. Nursing **51**:260-262, April 1951.

11 *MacKenzie, Marguerite, and Baldwin, Maitland: Cerebral Seizures, Am. J. Nursing **57**:312-316, March 1957.

12 *Magee, Kenneth R., and Elliott, Alta: Parkinson's Disease—Neurologic Management and Nursing Care, Am. J. Nursing **55**:814-818, July 1955.

13 Meakins, Jonathan Campbell (editor): The Practice of Medicine, ed. 6, St. Louis, 1956, The C. V. Mosby Co.

14 *Olsen, C. Kent, and Tollefsrud, Valborg, E.: Chemosurgery for Parkinsonism and When the Patient Has Chemosurgery, Am. J. Nursing **59**:1411-1416, Oct. 1959.

15 *Pirnie, Florence A., and Baldwin, Maitland: Observing Cerebral Seizures, Am. J. Nursing **59**:366-369, March 1959.

16 *Posture Fundamentals Illustrated: The Nurse, Am. J. Nursing **46**:122-123, Feb. 1946.

17 *Ray, Bronson S.: New Methods in the Diagnosis of Intracranial Tumors, S. Clin. North America **32**:491-503, April 1952.

18 Roseman, Ephriam, and Taylor, Anne: Progress in Treatment of Epilepsy, Am. J. Nursing **52**:437-440, April 1952.

19 Schumacher, George A., and Palmer, Mary Ellen: Multiple Sclerosis and Nursing the Patient With Multiple Sclerosis, Am. J. Nursing **57**:751-755, June 1957.

20 Smith, Genevieve Waples: A Stroke Is Not the End of the World, Am. J. Nursing **57**:303-305, March 1957.

21 Turner, Gwendolyn E.: The Cerebral Vascular Accident Patient, Nursing Outlook **8**:326-330, June 1960.

22 Uihlein, A., and Dollfe, R.: Aneurysms of the Cerebral Carotid Arteries, Am. J. Nursing **51**:492-496, Aug. 1951.

23 *Walters, Mary Ellen: Surgical Procedures in the X-Ray Department, Am. J. Nursing **57**:623-625, May 1957.

References specially related to neurosurgery

24 *Evans, Joseph P.: Acute Head Injuries, J.A.M.A. **149**:322-324, May 24, 1952.

25 *Bailey, Jean: Care of the Patient With a Taylor Spine Brace, Am. J. Nursing **44**:665-668, July 1944.

26 Campbell, Eldridge, and Whitfield, Robert

D.: Surgical Treatment of Intractable Pain, S. Clin. North America **30**:349-362, April 2, 1952.
27 *Chandler, Fremont A., and Bruck, Helen: Laminectomy and Nursing a Laminectomy Patient, Am. J. Nursing **51**:156-161, March 1951.
28 Covalt, Donald A., Cooper, Irving S., Hoen, Thomas I., and Rusk, Howard A.: Early Management of Patients With Spinal Cord Injury, J.A.M.A. **151**:89-94, Jan. 10, 1953.
29 *Hodges, Lucien R., and Taufic, Marjorie: Tumors of the Brain and Rehabilitation After Craniotomy, Am. J. Nursing **58**:58-63, Jan. 1958.
30 *Howorth, M. Beckett: Posture in Adolescents and Adults, Am. J. Nursing **56**:34-36, Jan. 1956.
31 *Janes, Joseph M., and Stifter, Rosina: Spinal Fusion, Am. J. Nursing **55**:1062-1065, Sept. 1955.
32 Martin, John, and Craig, Iris: The Early Care of Patients With Injury of the Spinal Cord, Am. J. Nursing **55**:936-939, Aug. 1955.
33 *Mullan, John F., and Van Schoick, Mildred R.: Intractable Pain, Am. J. Nursing **58**:228-230, Feb. 1958.
34 Palumbo, Louis: Some Recent Advances in Surgery of the Autonomic Nervous System, Am. J. Nursing **52**:700-702, June 1952.
35 *Raney, Rupert B.: The Minor Concussion, Am. J. Nursing **57**:1444-1445, Nov. 1957.
36 Ray, Bronson, S.: Lesions Stimulating Disk Protrusion, American Academy of Orthopaedic Surgeons Instructional Course Lectures, vol. 7, Ann Arbor, Michigan, 1950, J. W. Edwards, Publishers, Inc.
37 Ray, Bronson S.: Management of Head Injuries, American Academy of Orthopaedic Surgeons Instructional Course Lectures, vol. 7, Ann Arbor, Michigan, 1950, J. W. Edwards, Publishers, Inc.
38 Ray, Bronson S.: Brain Tumors, The Mississippi Doctor, March 1954.
39 *Schlesinger, Edward B., and Haber, Martha E.: Trigeminal Neuralgia and Nursing Care of the Patient With Trigeminal Neuralgia, Am. J. Nursing **58**:853-858, June 1958.
40 *Seidel, Eleanora S.: Tidal Drainage–Its Present Status, Am. J. Nursing **50**:702-706, Nov. 1950.
41 *Skinner, Geraldine: Nursing Care of a Patient on a Stryker Frame, Am. J. Nursing **46**:288-293, May 1946.
42 *Stimson, Barbara B.: Backache, Am. J., Nursing **51**:672-674, Nov. 1951.

The patient with arthritis

Chapter 35

Study questions for review

1 What main types of joints are there in the body? Review the range of motion for the hip, shoulder, knee, elbow, ankle, wrist, and finger joints, and give examples of daily activities for which these joints are used.
2 What are the harmful effects of immobilization of a joint?
3 What is the therapeutic action of acetylsalicylic acid? What are the toxic effects?
4 What are the therapeutic effects of heat? What are some of the measures used to provide heat and the related nursing care?
5 Select a patient from your ward, a member of your family, or an acquaintance who has arthritis. How does this person earn his living? What financial problems has the disease presented? What major modifications in the patient's life have been necessary because of the disease? How has his need for recreation been affected?

The word arthritis means inflammation of the joint. This term is used to designate any disease of the joints although not all such diseases are accompanied by inflammation. Arthritis and the related rheumatic diseases are among the most common chronic illnesses of our times. It is estimated that approximately 10 million persons in the United States suffer from arthritis or related disorders; 4½ million have arthritis, and 190,000 of these are completely disabled, while 1,143,000 are partially disabled.[9] Rheumatic disease is estimated to be responsible for 92 million man-days per year lost from productive employment and untold millions of hours of human suffering.[8]

Arthritis is one of the oldest diseases known to man. Except for cases resulting from bacterial infections, such as those caused by the gonococcus and the tubercle bacillus, which respond to therapy, the condition has not yielded permanently to any of the new drugs of modern times. However, much progress in the diagnosis and treatment of arthritis has been made. Most persons with this disease can benefit substantially from modern physical medicine and rehabilitation provided they have good supportive care physically, socially, and emotionally from the time of the onset of their illness.

The nursing care required by patients with arthritis presents many problems. The patient may have been ill for some time; he may be worried, irritable, pessimistic, or resigned. He may be impatient and harm himself by overexercise, or he may be discouraged and not try to help himself at all. Progress is often very slow, and the nurse may tend to become discouraged. She must have a truly optimistic attitude based on her conviction that arthritis need not be a hopeless disease. She must help the patient set up realistic goals. Then, as each small, but definite, step toward these goals is achieved, she must help him to realize that progress is being made. The nurse shares several responsibilities with the physician and other members of the health team. She has a part in the prevention of the disease and in its detection and treatment in early stages when hope for arrest is most promising. It can be assumed that poor health habits do play some part in the predisposition to develop arthritis. By teaching the importance of a well-balanced diet, a careful schedule of rest and exercise, avoidance of exposure to infections, and avoidance of severe emotional strain, the nurse may be contributing to prevention. She may discover sufferers from arthritis who do not know that help is possible. On a home visit to someone else, she may find such a person; in the hospital, while talking to a patient, she may learn of such a member of his family and direct him to medical care.

The nurse gives supportive care during acute episodes of illness in order to control pain, prevent deformity, and assist the patient and his family to adjust to the social, economic, and emotional consequences of a long-term illness. She also helps to correct the deformities of those with long-term illness, including those who have been neglected and those whose disease has progressed despite all medical effort.

To carry out her responsibilities, the nurse must have some understanding of the disease process involved and of what the doctor, the physical therapist, and others are trying to accomplish. Since atrophic arthritis is most likely to cause crippling, it is toward this condition that the most intensive medical and nursing care in the prevention of crippling must be directed. While much of the following discussion of nursing care refers primarily to atrophic arthritis, it also applies to certain phases of other types of arthritis and other rheumatic disease.

DISEASE ENTITIES AND THEIR PREVENTION

Rheumatic fever

Rheumatic fever is a systemic disease causing an elevation of temperature and acute inflammation of the joints with pain and swelling. It occurs most often in children but can occur at any age, and it is particularly important because it is often a precursor of acute rheumatic heart disease. The inflammation tends to move from joint to joint, and, although the pain and swelling may be severe, no permanent joint damage or deformities occur. The incidence of rheumatic fever is higher in the lower economic groups, and conditions such as poor housing, dampness, lack of sunshine, poor nutrition, and repeated exposure to upper respiratory infections seem to be predisposing factors. Some association seems to exist between rheumatic fever and streptococcal infections. Prevention of the disease appears to lie in the improvement of environmental conditions, the early treatment of respiratory infections, and immediate medical care if streptococcal infections occur in those who have had previous attacks of rheumatic fever.

Atrophic arthritis (rheumatoid arthritis, arthritis deformans)

Atrophic arthritis attacks young adults most often and attacks women more often than men. Again the incidence is higher in those who are less favored economically. The cause of atrophic arthritis is unknown, though it sometimes appears to be associated in some way with streptococcal infections. General debility, overfatigue, endocrine imbalance, emotional instability, and psychic trauma all apparently play a part in its development. Thin, asthenic persons seem more susceptible to the disease than others. Atrophic arthritis, a systemic disease, is characterized by fatigue, poor appetite, low-grade fever, anemia, mild leukocytosis, and increased blood sedimentation rate.

Atrophic arthritis begins in the synovial membrane of a joint. The membrane is inflamed, the cells proliferate, the joint becomes swollen, and the process gradually extends to the outer structure of the joint. Often the hands are affected with early involvement of proximal interphalangeal joints, which gives a characteristic tapering appearance to the fingers. Several joints may be involved at the same time, and the disease may progress steadily to other joints if it is not arrested. Eventually the entire joint may be destroyed and is replaced by a solid mass of spongy bones, thus causing complete loss of function (ankylosis). Spasm occurs in muscles which are attached to involved joints, and the wasting of these muscles is disproportionate to their lessened activity. Because the collagen substance of the connective tissue is involved, atrophic arthritis is now considered a collagen disease (see Chapter 29).

Atrophic arthritis appears most often during the productive years of life when family responsibilities are at their height. The patient may overlook the first signs, hoping that they are of no significance. The dangers of delay in reporting early signs and symptoms should be stressed in all health teaching, since precious time may be wasted while the patient hopes that nothing is really wrong. The public should be taught that the outlook for atrophic arthritis is not necessarily hopeless but that the disease has a tendency to relapse and to recur in more severe form if not treated early. If intensively treated, some patients recover from the first attack and, with careful attention to their general health, never suffer any recurrences. Approximately 10 to 15 per cent progress to crippling despite any kind of treatment.

Prevention of atrophic arthritis consists mainly of preventing relapses and disease progression by continuous medical supervision and care. The nurse may be helpful in stimulating the patient to seek and continue competent medical care. There is a tendency on the part of patients with discouraging, long-term illness of this kind to shop about in search of a quick cure. The patient with arthritis may find himself the victim of quacks and quick-cure advertisements and may spend his money futilely.

Because most patients with arthritis remain ambulatory, a large part of the nurse's work will be in the home and in the clinic. Warm human interest from others does a great deal to help the patient meet the pain, worry, and expense. He needs constant encouragement, and possible plans must be explained to him so that he can understand why they are necessary. The nurse must, of course, know what the doctor has told the patient and must build on this information. There is an increasing tendency on the part of physicians and other health workers to take the patient into full confidence in the planning of a program of care. It is only when the patient understands and accepts his condition and participates actively in determining his long-term goals that he can contribute effectively toward his own recovery.

Atypical forms of atrophic arthritis

Nurses should be familiar with two atypical types of arthritis. *Marie-Strümpell disease*, or *ankylosing spondylitis*, primarily affects the spine in young men and is thought to be a form of atrophic arthritis. The sacroiliac joint is most often first involved. The disease progresses upward in the spine and, unless arrested, causes a severe forward-bending deformity. Marie-Strümpell disease sometimes responds to x-ray treatment, and sometimes fusion of the spine is done to prevent further progressive deformity.

Atrophic arthritis which affects children is called *Still's disease*. The clinical findings and the progress of the disease are almost identical as in adults; the percentage of patients who develop severe deformities is fairly high.

Hypertrophic arthritis (osteoarthritis, degenerative arthritis)

Hypertrophic arthritis is primarily a disease of older people. Almost everyone past 40 years of age has hypertrophic changes in the joints. These may become symptomatic, depending on their severity and on such mechanical factors as poor posture, obesity, and occupational strain. Weight-bearing joints such as the knees, hips, and spine are most often affected.

Changes within the joint consist of thinning of the articular cartilages and deposition of calcium on the bone surfaces and in the joint spaces. Some enlargement of the joint occurs, but there is no swelling. There are some discomfort and limitation of motion, but there is no severe crippling deformity. The patient needs reassurance that pronounced deformity will not occur. Pain is often intermittent, tending to follow chilling, and is possibly due to muscle tension from the cold. Small fragments of bone or cartilage known as joint mice occasionally break off, causing severe pain on movement and must be removed surgically.

Although hypertrophic changes in the joints cannot be prevented, their attendant discomforts can be controlled to some extent. This is true particularly if prevention is considered early in life. Obesity should be controlled because it places considerable strain on all weight-bearing joints. Trauma and excessive use of certain joints could lead to hypertrophic arthritis fairly early in life. Examples of professions or occupations which seem to be associated with hypertrophic involvement of the upper spine and shoulder joints are dentistry, barbering, and dishwashing. It seems likely that the position assumed during working hours contributes to this. Public education and industrial practices that consider the dangers of prolonged work in a position of strain may help to prevent some people from developing symptoms. The orthopedic principle of alternate rest and activity to prevent strain on particular joints and muscles has real application in the prevention of hypertrophic arthritis. Poor posture throughout life contributes to hypertrophic arthritis. The child should be taught to stand correctly so that strain due to prolonged hyperextension does not occur in joints such as the knee joints. Holding the pelvis correctly with a forward tilt will prevent increased curvature of the lower back with its resultant strain on muscles and joints. Correct mechanical use of the body, such as stooping rather than bending, prevents strain on muscles which may pull the joint out of alignment just enough for osteoarthritic changes to develop or to cause symptoms. Holding the head up and back takes a great deal of strain from the joints of the upper spine. It is surprising how many older patients can benefit from posture improvement even though the damage which may date from childhood cannot be completely corrected.

Gout

Gout, or gouty arthritis, is arthritis caused by the deposit of sodium urate crystals in the joints. Eighty-five per cent of all patients with gout show a familial tendency to develop the disease, and 95 per cent of all patients with gout are men. Probably too much emphasis in fiction and elsewhere has been placed upon overindulgence in food as a cause of gout. Actually the disease occurs most often in the economically less favored, provided the familial predisposition is present. Although the distal joints of the great toes are often first affected, any joint of the body may become involved. Subcutaneous deposits of urates in such locations as the ear and known as *tophi* occur in about a third of all patients who have gouty arthritis. Gout is truly a chronic disease, although acute exacerbations occur, causing high temperature, malaise, and headache. Treatment is directed toward control of acute attacks, since permanent joint damage and deformity can follow repeated attacks. Kidney stones and resultant kidney damage also occur when acute attacks are repeated over an extended period of time. Prevention of recurrences depends mainly on taking specific prescribed medications to increase the output of urates, on increasing the intake of fluids (particularly those which are alkaline-ash in reaction), and on weight reduction if obesity is present. Foods high in purine elements, such as brains and glandular meats, are often restricted, but there is no evidence that other protein foods contribute to the formation of urate crystals.

Other types of arthritis

Almost any organism can affect the joints. The typhoid bacillus, tubercle bacillus, gonococcus, and staphylococcus

Table 10 Summary of characteristics of various types of arthritis

Characteristics	*Rheumatic fever*	*Atrophic arthritis*	*Hypertrophic arthritis*	*Gout*
Synonyms	—	Rheumatoid arthritis Arthritis deformans	Osteoarthritis Degenerative arthritis	—
Average age of onset	5-11 yr.	30-50 yr.	50-70 yr.	20-40 yr.
Sex (ratio)	—	Women 3:1	Women 5:1	Men 19:1
Build and weight	—	Asthenic—underweight	Stocky—overweight	Overweight
Joints involved	Any; moves from joint to joint	Any; often fingers, other joints; progressive	Weight-bearing joints—knees, hips, spine, fingers; localized	Terminal great toe of feet—spreading to any joint
Subcutaneous lesion	Rheumatic nodules over tendon surfaces; indicate poor prognosis	Nodules over bony prominences; painful on injury; no prognostic significance	Heberden's nodes on fingers; painful at times; no prognostic significance	Tophi; prognostic of difficulty in control of blood urates
X-ray findings	None	Clouding of fluid space, fraying of inner joint margins, lessening of joint space	Lipping of bony margins, lessening of joint space	Clouding of joint spaces
Outward appearance of joints	Swollen, tender, reddened, painful	Swollen, painful, reddened, shiny	Enlarged; no swelling	Swollen, painful, reddened, shiny
Termination	No joint damage or limitation of motion	Ankylosis and deformity	Some limitation of motion, little deformity, no ankylosis	Limitation of motion, deformity; possible kidney stones

were common causes of arthritis before the discovery of the specific antibiotic drugs and the control of communicable diseases. Arthritis can also result from trauma to the joint, or it may be associated with new growths within or about the joint or with neurogenic changes.

Nonarticular rheumatic disease

Bursitis may be acute or chronic. It is caused by trauma, strain, and overuse of the bursa, and sometimes by toxins and infection. The shoulder bursa is the one most often affected and may be exceedingly troublesome. The main treatment consists of application of local heat, control of pain with medications, and immobilization of the part with a sling. X-ray treatment is sometimes given and may give excellent results. Sometimes the joint may be aspirated and the irritating calcium deposit causing the pain washed out; sometimes the calcium forms larger particles and surgery is necessary for their removal. Chronic bursitis follows very slow absorption of calcium and slow body response to irritation. In addition to control of pain, the main problem in chronic bursitis of the shoulder is preservation of range of joint motion in the shoulder. Pendulum exercises are almost always ordered; in some cases recurrence of bursitis may be prevented by avoiding excessive use of the joint. The patient with

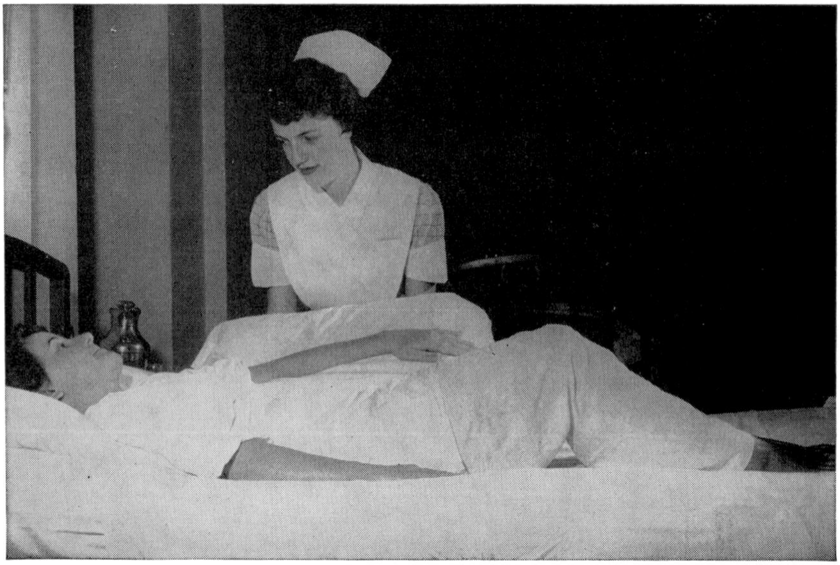

Figure 136

Supporting the painful part on a pillow lessens discomfort when the patient must be moved.

chronic bursitis should continue physical therapy and exercises as prescribed by the physiatrist. He also needs reassurance and needs to know that many people who avoid overuse of the involved joint never have recurrences.

There are many other forms of non-articular rheumatism. Lumbago, stiff neck, tendinitis, and tenosynovitis are examples. These conditions can be very painful and may cause distress out of all proportion to their seriousness as far as the lesion is concerned. So far, unfortunately, there seems to be no specific cure for any of them, and the greatest comfort comes from the use of local heat and mild analgesic drugs such as acetylsalicylic acid. Constant pain is demoralizing to the patient, and one of the things he needs most is a sympathetic person to listen to his problems and to give encouragement.

MEDICAL TREATMENT AND NURSING CARE

General nursing care

Pain may be exquisite in acute stages of rheumatic fever, atrophic arthritis, and gout. The patient requires the greatest care and gentleness when he must be moved. Fear of pain often makes the patient irritable and can lead to muscular resistance which makes the pain worse. Care must be taken not to jar the bed. Heavy bedclothes may cause added pain; if cradles are used, the greatest caution must be taken not to accidentally bump an involved part of the body when adjusting or removing the cradle. Footboards help to relieve the pressure of covers, provided the patient can be kept warm during their use. Patients with atrophic arthritis must be encouraged to change position often since their general nutrition is often poor and pressure sores and contractures develop easily. Sometimes a very painful joint such as a wrist, elbow, or ankle can be placed on a pillow, and the pillow and the limb can be moved together when the patient must turn over or otherwise adjust his position. (See Figure 136.)

Despite acute pain, personal hygiene must not be neglected. The patient with acute rheumatic fever often has profuse, sour-smelling perspiration and needs refreshing warm sponges at least daily, as does the patient with an acute attack of gout. The patient with atrophic arthritis is often too tired and discouraged to keep himself as well groomed as he should be, yet few things contribute so much to general morale as attention to personal hygiene. The nurse should give time to cutting fingernails and should assist women patients to set and arrange their hair. The man with atrophic arthritis should be encouraged to shave regularly, and those in nursing attendance can help by having equipment conveniently placed and by providing time for this activity. If the patient is having much pain, the nurse should see that drugs for pain are given about one-half hour before a procedure is started. While care is being given, the nurse should get to know her patient. Nothing is more important in the care of the patient with arthritis, whether in the home, the clinic, or the hospital, than a friendly interest in him and in his particular problems. His relationship to his family should be considered. The family may be overprotecting the patient and thus contributing to his becoming a permanent invalid. On the other hand, they may be tired of the problems the patient is causing, and he, in turn, may be greatly disturbed over the burden he is, or may become, to his family. It is at such times that a well-placed word from the thoughtful nurse may help to direct the patient's thinking along positive lines and may suggest new opportunities that are within his physical limitations and that may contribute immeasurably to his rehabilitation. In almost all instances, the assistance of a social case worker is needed by the patient in thinking through and talking through his family problems. If the patient is not hospitalized and lives at home, the nurse may refer him to a family service agency for help with his problems.

Rest, furniture, and exercise

Rest. Bed rest is usually ordered for the patient who has an elevation of temperature; when the temperature becomes normal, a careful balance of rest and activity is planned. Every patient with arthritis should have his whole schedule of rest and activity carefully examined by the physician. For the ambulatory patient, this involves consideration of work, recreation patterns, family and community life, and responsibilities. The importance of regular vacations and routine exposure to sunshine is usually stressed. In most instances, a change of climate is not advised, since the personal disadvantages for the patient often outweigh the advantages.

The nurse may help the woman patient with atrophic arthritis to cut down on her work load at home. Sitting down with a piece of paper and plotting the activity for each hour of the day is a good way to help the patient see what changes may be made. It is possible that home arrangements can be altered to save energy. Such simple things as using lightweight aluminum pans, sitting while preparing vegetables and ironing, and using a lightweight iron may be all that are necessary to enable a woman to remain at home and care for her family. Properly fitted shoes that give support to the feet should replace soft bedroom slippers for wear about the house, and frequent changes of shoes also help. The patient is usually gratified at the difference these changes make in how she feels after several hours on her feet.

Furniture. Furniture should be such that good posture can be maintained during working and recreational hours with a minimum of drain on vital energy resources. There are five criteria of a good chair; the seat should be deep enough to support the thighs but not so deep that circulation in the popliteal spaces is hampered; the seat should be high enough so that feet rest firmly on the floor and do not dangle, thereby putting strain on knee joints; the seat should be level or tilted slightly forward so that flexion of the knees and hips is at a minimum and not at less than a right angle; the chair should have arms so that arm and shoulder muscles can provide leverage to help in moving from the chair; the rungs must be such that one foot can be placed partially under the seat in preparation for rising so that the patient is better able to stabilize his center of gravity when he assumes an erect position. Chairs with a seat a little higher than is usually considered comfortable provide better leverage when arising. If the patient has been sitting for some time and finds his knee stiff upon attempting to move, he should remember to flex and extend his knees several times before attempting to rise from the chair. By eliminating some of the stiffness before trying to bear weight, he will find that he is much steadier on his feet. Many patients who otherwise find an evening at the movies intolerable are able to enjoy such recreation by remembering this simple practice.

In the home or in the hospital, the bed should have a firm mattress, and often bedboards are needed. Boards should be long enough and wide enough to rest firmly upon the main side and end rails of the bed—not on the bed springs. A firm bed lessens pain by preventing motion and consequent pull on painful joints and helps to keep the spine in good alignment. The person with arthritis should either use no pillow or should use one small pillow that fits well down under the shoulders so that forward bending of the cervical spine is not encouraged. Knees should not be flexed on pillows, and all patients who must be confined to bed most of the day should lie flat on the abdomen for a part of each day. Splints may be used during sleeping or waking hours to help prevent the deformity caused by muscle spasm. Splints should be well padded and should be removed frequently, and the skin should be carefully checked for signs of pressure, particularly over bony prominences. In the home, night splints may be made from chicken wire carefully covered and padded. Often the patient finds that he must take aspirin on awakening to relieve pain and stiffness. Many patients set their alarms a little earlier than usual and take aspirin kept at the bedside. They then rest for about half an hour before beginning their preparations for the day. Each patient must work out his own schedule. The Arthritis and Rheumatism Foundation has prepared a pamphlet* which should give the nurse many helpful hints in working with her patients.

Exercise. Most patients with atrophic arthritis must do special exercises prescribed for them by the physiatrist and taught to them by the physical therapist. The nurse should know what these exercises are; she must not only encourage the patient to do his exercises regularly but also should occasionally watch him do them. She must know that, to be beneficial, all exercises involve steady, prolonged contraction before relaxation—not merely "wiggling" the part. Exercises are necessary to preserve range of joint motion, to strengthen muscles, and to prevent shortening of muscles. It should be remembered that muscles are very important in holding joints in good position and that without muscle action joints themselves could not produce motion. Exercises are often prescribed to be done two or three times a day. Pain experienced during the exercise and disappearing soon afterward is not significant, but pain persisting throughout the rest of the day or into the night probably is an indication that the exercise has been too strenuous and should be decreased. In this case, the physician or the physical therapist should be consulted. Some patients are so eager to get well that they are too vigorous in exercising and may cause aggravation of the disease and damage to the involved joints. Others who are tired and resigned to their fate may sit passively, not moving their limbs sufficiently because of slight pain, and thus negate the whole purpose of the exercises.

The patient needs to know why exercises are ordered, why it is so important for him to do them regularly, and what changes take place in muscles and joints when motion is not maintained. If he can

*Home Care of the Arthritis Patient; The Arthritis and Rheumatism Foundation, National Headquarters, 10 Columbus Circle, New York 19, N. Y.

understand this explanation, then he will know why his position in bed is important and what the correct positions are. He needs to understand the normal range of motion for every joint in his body and should be helped to appreciate why the daily efforts demanded to prevent limitation of any involved joints is so important in his long-term outlook. Drawings and pictures help in this explanation, which is usually given by the doctor and augmented by the nurse and the physical therapist. Members of the patient's family also should be taught the exercises so that they may help the patient if assistance is needed; however, they should encourage the patient to do without help those that he is capable of performing alone. Members of the family also need to thoroughly understand the importance of the exercise regimen as determined by the physician. Activities should be planned to keep joints limber.

It may be helpful for the patient to take aspirin about one-half hour before doing exercises and, if he is able, he may prefer to do routine exercises while lying in a tub of warm water. If bath oils and bath salts can be afforded, their use makes this routine more enjoyable. Use of heat before beginning the exercises is of great help in making them easier for the patient; the patient may prefer a heating pad, a heat lamp equipped with a 25-watt bulb and placed at least twelve inches from the skin, or warm moist packs applied for short periods. Bath towels wrung out in hot water and applied directly to the skin are often used, since moist heat seems more effective than dry heat in causing muscle relaxation and alleviating pain. Warm baths rather than moist packs may be preferred by the patient who is caring for himself and who may have difficulty in wringing out the towels.

Heat therapy

Many forms of heat are used in the treatment of arthritis to increase circulation to the affected joints and to lessen muscle spasm thereby decreasing pain. Hot wet packs applied locally and hot tub baths are often ordered. A cradle with electric light bulbs is sometimes used to supply dry heat and diathermy is also used for this purpose; however, in some cases diathermy increases joint pain.

Paraffin may be used to provide an excellent form of penetrating heat. Sometimes the patient is instructed by his physician to use paraffin at home, and usually he is advised to use this form of therapy before doing the prescribed exercises. The nurse may be called upon to help the patient or his family with this procedure in the home. Usually from eight to ten pounds of paraffin are slowly heated in the top of a large double boiler until it is melted and vaporizes slightly. It is then removed from the stove and cooled until a thin film appears on the surface. At this point it is at the right temperature for use. The skin should be shaved before application. From eight to ten coats may be applied with a brush, or the part may be immersed the same number of times. Wax paper or Pliofilm is then wrapped about the part, and the part is then covered with a bath towel while the patient rests for about half an hour. The paraffin is then peeled off and saved to be reused. During and following this treatment, the patient must be protected from drafts and chilling. If the paraffin appears too hot for comfort, soaking the part in hot water preceding the treatment sometimes helps. Another device is to use an ounce of mineral oil in the paraffin to lower its melting point and therefore its temperature.

Paraffin can be dangerous unless carefully used. Since it is inflammable, the greatest care must be taken if gas or other open flame is used for heating. Panhandles must be watched, since accidental spilling of hot paraffin can cause serious burns. It goes without saying that this procedure should never be carried out when children are playing nearby. Clothing should be protected from wax by using an old work apron, and floors can be protected with old newspapers. Care must be taken not to clog plumbing with wax.

Diet

There are no special diets that will cure or even materially alter the course of any type of arthritis. Yet thousands of patients follow special and expensive diets in the hope of cure. More patients with arthritis than with any other disease are the victims of advertising and diet fads. The essentials of good nutrition, which include fruits, vegetables, protein, and vitamins, are recommended for patients with atrophic arthritis. Since the patient with atrophic arthritis is often underweight, a high-calorie diet with vitamin supplements to stimulate appetite may be needed. Sunshine and fresh air also stimulate appetite. The patient with hypertrophic arthritis is often overweight, and general weight reduction may be advised. The patient with gout is instructed to avoid foods high in purine, such as brains, kidneys, and sweetbreads, to avoid too much fat, and to avoid alcohol. Meat, fish, and fowl do not form uric acid, and the patient with gout may be encouraged to have a fairly high-protein diet in an effort to lose weight. Fruit juices, mineral waters, and alkaline-ash fluids of all kinds are beneficial for the patient with gout, partly because they help supply extra fluid so that any uric acid crystals may be flushed from the kidneys more easily and partly because they inhibit uric acid precipitation. The daily urine output for the patient with gout should be about 2,000 to 3,000 ml. per day, or two to three times that of the average person.

The patient should be permitted to indulge his food likes and dislikes within the range of the essentials of good nutrition with the few exceptions mentioned. He should be urged to eat regular meals and should be given plenty of time for meals. Even the patient with marked limitation of movement should be urged to feed himself, even though food may sometimes have to be cut up or otherwise prepared beforehand. Built-up handles on eating equipment may enable the patient with severe limitations to handle the utensils independently.

Drugs

Drugs play a part in the arrest of arthritis and in the control of pain. Salicylates are ordered almost universally in the treatment of acute rheumatic fever and are often helpful in other forms of arthritis, particularly gout. Sodium bicarbonate is usually given with the salicylates, and fluids are forced. The signs of salicylate poisoning, such as ringing in the ears, nausea, vomiting, and tachycardia, should be watched for. Acetylsalicylic acid (aspirin) is widely used for patients with arthritis and has been found to be effective in almost all types of arthritis. It can be taken over a long period of time without toxicity occurring or tolerance being acquired. A newer drug, phenylbutazone (Butazolidin) has an analgesic and possibly anti-inflammatory effect in atrophic arthritis and in gout; the usual dosage is 100 mg. (3⅓ grains) four to five times per day for one to two days. The drug is a pyrazol derivative and may cause edema, nausea, gastritis, anemia, and agranulocytosis. Codeine and other habit-forming analgesics are avoided whenever possible because of the danger of addiction in diseases of such long duration as the arthritides.

Antimalarial drugs such as chloroquine (Aralen) and hydrochloroquine phosphate (Plaquenil) appear to have some ameliorating effect upon rheumatoid arthritis and are being used by some physicians in the treatment of this disease.

Gold salts. Although gold salts do not effect a cure, they seem to have a specific effect in controlling symptoms in many patients with atrophic arthritis. Solganal-B and Myochrysine are two forms of the drug used. The dosage is usually 10 mg. (1/6 grain) intramuscularly as a first test dose. If no ill effects are encountered, a second dose of 25 mg. (2/5 grain) is given and then 50 mg. (4/5 grain) are given at weekly or biweekly intervals until 750 mg. to 1,000 mg. (12½ to 16½ grains) have been given.[2] A rest period of at least four weeks is usually planned before another series of injections is given, although in some clinics a maintenance dose of 25 to 50 mg. is given every four weeks for months and sometimes years. The nurse must be alert for symptoms and signs of toxicity to gold and should instruct the patient to report any signs and symptoms promptly. The most common sign is skin reaction; any signs of dermatitis should be suspected when gold is being taken. Other toxic signs are stomatitis, salivation, nausea, vomiting, and diarrhea. Gold salts have been known to cause serious and even fatal kidney and liver damage; signs of jaundice must be watched for, and urine must be tested frequently for albumin.

Steroids. Hydrocortisone is often given directly into the joint in atrophic arthritis and appears to be helpful in controlling local joint inflammation. It is usually injected under sterile precautions after the joint has first been aspirated. ACTH (pituitary adrenocorticotrophic hormone), cortisone, and hydrocortisone are given by injection or by mouth for atrophic arthritis and produce very satisfactory, though temporary, results in many patients. When these drugs are given, salt should be restricted since fluids tend to be retained in the tissue; a typical moonface often follows the accumulation of fluid. These drugs cause a marked euphoria and decrease pain so that exercises can often be done, thus sometimes preventing deformity that might otherwise have occurred. Unfortunately the effects are only temporary, and extended use of the drugs causes voice changes, growth of hair on the face, and other disturbances of endocrine function and sometimes may mask symptoms of other latent disease such as tuberculosis. (See Chapter 28.) Each year, however, yields new knowledge of the effects of this group of drugs, and it is not beyond the realm of possibility that with them may rest the ultimate secret to the control and cure of atrophic arthritis.

Colchicine and other drugs. Colchicine, which has been used for at least six centuries, is the standard drug used in the treatment of gout. When an acute attack of gout is imminent, the usual treatment is 0.5 mg. (1/120 grain) of the drug each hour by mouth until nausea develops. Camphorated tincture of opium (paregoric) is then sometimes given as treatment for the gastrointestinal irritation. The usual maintenance of colchicine (0.5 mg.) is administered daily or two or three times per week. Some patients may require medication two or three times each day. There is no evidence of damage to the body from therapeutic doses of colchicine even when it is taken for years. Acetylsalicylic acid also helps to increase the uric acid output and may be regularly prescribed over long periods of time.

Since probenecid (Benemid) furthers the excretion of uric acid through the kidneys, it is another drug that has been ordered for the treatment of gout in the last few years. The usual dosage is 0.5 Gm. (7½ grains) daily by mouth for one week, followed by 1 Gm. daily for months. The drug may cause gastric distress and is best tolerated if taken with meals. Large amounts of fluid must be given to prevent formation of stones in the kidneys. Since the drug works best in an alkaline medium, sodium bicarbonate, 5 to 7.5 Gm. (7½ to 10 grains) daily, is often ordered; however, this may disturb the acid-base balance of the body if continued for too long. The nurse may be asked to check the patient's urine with litmus paper each time he voids or to teach him to do so and to record the results for the physician. One limitation in the use of Benemid is that salicylates cannot be given at the same time since this combination diminishes the benefit derived from both drugs.[3]

Operative care

The patient with advanced atrophic arthritis who has ankylosis and deformity may sometimes benefit from surgery. Surgery is done to correct deformity and to improve function. For example, severe alteration of alignment may prevent the wearing of normal shoes or may make the wearing of shoes unbearably painful; contractures at the hip may make it impossible to get the patient up on crutches or otherwise rehabilitated. An *arthrodesis,* surgical fixation of a joint by fusion, may be performed to stabilize an affected part, such as the knee, which has become distorted from normal alignment because of muscle spasm, muscle weakness, and joint disease. As a result of this operation pain is lessened and the stabilized joint can be used more in body function. Usually a cast is applied following operation, but sometimes bandaging, slings, and traction are used.

There are particular problems in caring for the arthritic patient following any type of surgery because of the danger of further stiffness and limitation of joint movement throughout the body. Bed posture and bed exercises are important. Muscle-setting exercises in which a muscle may be consciously contracted may be ordered if the patient cannot move freely. The patient should be urged to do things for himself to help prevent further stiffness and to improve his morale, but he must be given more time than the average patient.

Mobilization of the patient is difficult following surgery on his joints. Many joints may be involved, and the patient may have been tired and discouraged even before the operation took place. He is cautious and fearful of falling, and rightly so, since he does not have the quickness of action at his command that is necessary for the prevention of many accidents. A walker is usually used and is much safer than crutches for the patient beginning to walk. To prevent accidents the greatest care must be given to see that the floor is dry and not slippery, to provide good supporting shoes, and to see that no bathrobe cords are dangling for the patient to trip over. Morale usually improves visibly when the patient can be up to spend time on the sun porch with other patients.

Habit-forming drugs are used as little as possible following surgery for arthritis because of the chronic nature of the disease. The nurse can help to make sedatives less necessary by giving attention to simple details of patient comfort. A firm bed, a small, correctly placed pillow, a warm drink, and appropriate bed coverings all help to induce rest. The patient with arthritis feels drafts and changes of temperature more than most patients who move about more readily. If the affected limb is in traction, for instance, it is often a good idea to put a warm sock on the foot or to wrap the whole limb in a light, warm blanket provided this can be done without interfering with the traction. Sometimes wrapping an exposed limb in cotton batting and then in a light towel or blanket affords protection from drafts.

The patient with atrophic arthritis often anticipates too much from his operation. He may have been ill a long time and may have made many major adjustments, yet he hopes that an operation will produce a cure. This feeling is often true even in the patient in whom many joints are involved when it is obvious to everyone else that the particular operation is only one small step toward improving his ability to care for himself. He will often need an understanding person to talk with when he begins to accept this reality.

Attempts have been made to restore partial function to joints which have become ankylosed. By far the most successful of these operations is an *arthroplasty* in which a Vitallium cup is placed into the acetabulum after the head of the femur has been removed from the socket and spongy ankylosing bone has been scooped away. Following this operation, the patient is usually placed on a firm bed in traction. Motion of the hip joint must be started within three or four days if effective use of the joint is to be obtained. A favorite and very satisfactory method used to facilitate this exercise is to place the foot on a roller skate, which in turn is placed on a firm shellacked board. Then, using this setup, the patient is able, by an arrangement of pulleys, to exercise the hip joint in adduction and abduction. It is important to prevent external rotation of the hip joint, since this will result in an awkward flat-footed gait with the entire extremity turning outward. A full-sized bed sheet folded over to form what is usually referred to as a *trochanter roll* and tucked inward at the crest of the ilium will often suffice to keep the thigh and leg from rolling outward. If the patient's arms are in good condition, the time in bed is well spent in doing resistance exercises to strengthen the arms; for example, holding sandbags on the palms of the hands to strengthen the triceps in anticipation of ambulation first in a walker and then on crutches.

Rheumatic nodules may sometimes be removed surgically if they have become irritated by trauma or pressure or if they are particularly unsightly. Hospitalization for this treatment is usually of only one day's duration. In a similar fashion, the tophi of gout may be excised, particularly if they have opened and are draining or are causing pain.

Patients with hypertrophic arthritis may be operated upon when bony prominences, or exostoses, develop and cause pain, particularly on weight-bearing areas such as the heel. Calcium deposits within the joint that are causing pain are also removed surgically in some instances. Occasionally a joint is fused when pain is persistent and severe, but, generally speaking, surgery is not indicated in hypertrophic arthritis.

REFERENCES AND SELECTED READINGS*

1 *Barckley, Virginia, and others: Arthritis and a Narrow Perspective Do Not Mix, Nursing Outlook **6**:638-639, Nov. 1958.

2 Cecil, Russell L., and Loeb, Robert F. (editors): A Textbook of Medicine, ed. 10, Philadelphia, 1959, W. B. Saunders Co.

3 Goodman, Louis S., and Gilman, Alfred: The Pharmacological Basis of Therapeutics, ed. 2, New York, 1955, The Macmillan Co.

4 Holmquist, Emily W.: The Patient With Atrophic Arthritis, Am. J. Nursing **49**:302-306, May 1949.

5 *Jaschik, Eva, and Olsen, Catherine: Nursing Care of the Arthritic Patient at Home, Am. J. Nursing **55**:429-432, April 1955.

6 *Jesser, Ralph A., and Hollander, Joseph Lee: Types of Arthritis and Their Medical Treatment, Am. J. Nursing **55**:426-429, April 1955.

7 Larson, Carroll B., and Gould, Marjorie: Calderwood's Orthopedic Nursing, ed. 4, St. Louis, 1957, The C. V. Mosby Co.

8 Lowman, Edward W.: Rehabilitation of the Patient With Chronic Rheumatoid Arthritis, J. Chron. Dis. **1**:628-637, June 1955.

9 *McDermott, Ita K., and Wensley, Edith: We Can Help Arthritic Patients, Nursing Outlook **3**:582-585, Nov. 1955.

10 Margolis, H. M.: Rheumatoid Arthritis, Am. J. Nursing **47**:787-793, Dec. 1947.

11 Medical and Scientific Committee of Arthritis and Rheumatism Foundation: Manual for Nurses—Arthritis and Related Disorders, New York, 1954, Arthritis and Rheumatism Foundation.

12 Miale, Julie E., and Plotz, Charles M.: Nursing Care of Patients With Rheumatoid Arthritis During Therapy With Cortisone, Am. J. Nursing **53**:290-293, March 1953.

13 *Talbott, John H.: Gout and Gouty Arthritis, Nursing Outlook **2**:540-543, Oct. 1954.

*References preceded by an asterisk indicate material particularly well suited for student reading.

The patient with a fracture

Chapter 36

Study questions for review

1 Describe the anatomic structures of bone. What are the functions or purposes of the skeletal system?
2 What are some of the changes that might be observed in the skin if circulation is impaired?
3 Review the methods of assisting a patient in and out of bed and to and from bed to a wheel chair.
4 What are some of the exercises to preserve muscle tone in the legs and arms that you might teach the patient?

The nursing care of patients with fractures is discussed here because fractures are so often encountered by nurses on the medical and surgical wards of general hospitals and by nurses who visit patients in their homes. Application of the principles of body mechanics—often referred to as orthopedic principles—are part of all nursing and have been included in previous chapters. Nursing care of patients with many orthopedic ailments requires specific knowledge which is beyond the scope of this book. Since there are excellent orthopedic nursing textbooks available, the student nurse should turn to these when she encounters a patient with an orthopedic condition on the medical or surgical floors of the general hospital.

This chapter includes only a few of the more important general principles of care of all patients with fractures and nursing responsibilities when surgical treatment is used. Prevention of fractures and first-aid care are considered in Chapter 15, amputations and crutch-walking in Chapter 19, skull fractures and back injuries in Chapter 34, arthritis in Chapter 35, and fracture of the jaw in Chapter 25.

GENERAL STATEMENTS

Definitions and terminology. A bone is said to be fractured or broken when there is an interruption in its continuity. This is usually caused by a blow or injury sustained in a fall or other accident. A fracture may also occur during normal activity or following a minimal injury when the bone is weakened by disease such as *cancer* or *osteoporosis;* this is called a *pathologic fracture* and causes collapse of the bone. Osteoporosis involving usually the hip or the lumbar spine is becoming increasingly common with the increase in age of the population. The real cause of the condition is obscure, but it is thought to be definitely related to hormonal activity.[4] The nurse should bear in mind the possibility of this condition being present whenever she cares for an elderly patient, and she should urge the elderly patient with low back pain to report it to his doctor so that treatment can be begun before marked collapse of bone occurs.

There are several classifications of fractures. A fracture is *complete* when there is complete separation of the bone, producing two fragments; it is *incomplete* when only part of the bone is broken. The part of the bone next to the body is referred to as the *proximal* fragment, whereas the one away from the body is called the *distal* fragment. The proximal is also called the *uncontrollable* fragment since it can seldom be moved or manipulated in an attempt to bring the separate fragments into correct alignment. The distal is referred to as the *controllable* fragment since it can usually be moved and manipulated to bring it into the correct relationship to the proximal fragment. Fractures in long bones are designated as being in the proximal, middle, or distal third of the bone.

If the skin is intact, the fracture is classified as *simple* or *closed.* If there is a break in the skin, with or without protrusion of bone, the fracture is called *compound;* if a bone fragment, such as a rib, has penetrated an internal structure, such as a lung, the fracture is called *complicated.* When the two bone fragments are in good alignment with no change from their normal position despite the break in continuity of bone, the fracture is referred to as a fracture *without displacement.* If the bone fragments have separated at the point of fracture, it is referred to as a fracture *with displacement;* this may be slight, moderate, or marked.

The line of fracture as revealed by x-ray examination or fluoroscopy is usually classified as to type. It may be *greenstick* with splintering on one side of the bone (this occurs most often in young children with soft bones), *transverse* with a break straight across the bone, *oblique* with the line of fracture at an oblique angle to the bone shaft, or *spiral* with the fracture lines partially encircling the bone. The fracture may be referred to as *telescoped,* if a bone fragment is forcibly pushed against and into the adjacent fragment. If there are several fragments the fracture is referred to as a *comminuted* one.

Symptoms of fracture and related injury. The signs and symptoms of fracture vary according to the location and function of the involved bone, the strength of its muscle attachments, the type of fracture sustained, and the amount of related damage.

Pain is usually severe and immediate following a fracture. It may continue and is aggravated by attempted motion of any kind and by pressure at the site of injury. Loss of function is another characteristic sign; if the patient attempts to use the injured part, he may be unable to do so. If there has been marked displacement of fragments, there will be obvious gross deformity, and there may be motion where motion does not usually occur. Upon moving the fractured limb gently, there may be a characteristic grating sound (crepitus) as the bone fragments come in contact with each other. The nurse should never, under any circumstances, attempt to elicit this sign since it may cause further damage and increase pain. It is possible, though unusual, for a fracture to occur with no displacement of fragments, little or no swelling, and pain only when direct pressure is applied to the site of fracture or upon use of the limb or body part. Fractures of this kind might be missed if x-ray examinations were not routinely ordered when there is any reason to suspect that a fracture might have occurred.

Since the bones are firmer than their surrounding structures, any injury severe enough to cause bone fracture will also cause injury to muscles, nerves, connective tissue, and blood vessels which may be evident by hemorrhage externally or into surrounding tissues. Bleeding may not be fully apparent for several hours, and discoloration of the skin (ecchymosis) may not be apparent until several days after injury. Edema may follow extravasation of blood into the tissues and localization of serous fluid at the site of injury, and paralysis or other evidence of nerve injury may develop. Occasionally a large nerve becomes locked between two bone fragments and causes immediate paralysis. The patient who has a fracture usually has signs and symptoms of injury of both bone and surrounding tissues. He may go quickly into shock if the injury is severe and if he has intense pain.

IMMEDIATE CARE

Perhaps the most important basic principle in care of a patient with any fracture is to provide some kind of splint before moving him. This is constantly emphasized in the emergency care of patients at the scene of accidents; it is equally important for the nurse to remember when caring for patients who are in traction or other mechanical apparatus to preserve body alignment.

When a patient with a known or a suspected fracture is to be admitted to the hospital, his bed should be provided with a fracture board. This is a good routine to follow because the patient with a known fracture of the ankle, for example, may be found, upon further examination, also to have a fracture of the pelvis or of the spine.

Since it can be assumed that edema will occur following a fracture, the injured part usually is elevated routinely. One or more protected pillows should be used, and these can support the extremity if moving must be done. If a temporary splint has been applied, this should not be removed without orders from the doctor no matter how crude or soiled it may be. The limb encased in the splint can be elevated.

Careful observation is necessary for local changes in color, sensation, or temperature. Care should be taken that emergency splinting bandages do not cause constriction as edema develops. Tingling, numbness, or burning pain may indicate nerve injury; coldness, whiteness, or cyanosis may indicate interference with circulation; increased warmth and swelling may indicate infection. Gas bacillus infection is a dreaded complication in grossly contaminated compound fractures. Sudden increase in edema and pain associated with darkening of the tissues should be reported to the doctor at once. Tetanus immunization usually is given when a compound fracture has been sustained (see Chapter 11).

General observation is necessary to detect early signs of shock. If the injury has been severe or if there are signs of impending shock, the blood pressure is taken every fifteen minutes for several hours, and the pulse and respiratory rates are noted and recorded frequently.

The nurse should anticipate that the doctor may order cold local applications during the first twenty-four hours following a fracture, since these help to reduce hemorrhage and edema and contribute to the patient's comfort. Ice bags are often used and must be covered to prevent skin damage.

Pain is usually relieved in the first few hours by giving acetylsalicylic acid or narcotics. Adjustment to sudden immobilization is difficult for the patient, and the nurse must appreciate what it means to him to be unable to move about freely. Even a fracture of an arm bone may make the patient quite helpless at first. He may be unable to move or use the rest of his body without severe pain; sometimes treatment of the fractured bone makes it physically impossible for him to care for some of his most basic physical needs. The patient almost always needs sedation such as phenobarbital to help him sleep the first few nights after he has sustained a fracture.

Very occasionally an air or fat embolus may result from compound fractures or from severe comminuted fractures with extensive soft tissue injury. The signs of an embolism of this kind are similar to those of other emboli and consist of sudden severe pain in the chest, pallor, dyspnea, shock, prostration, and collapse. Treatment includes administering oxygen and stimulants and keeping the patient absolutely quiet. (See Chapter 23.)

Ischemic paralysis (contracture) is a somewhat rare complication of fracture and develops when an artery is injured by trauma or pressure so that arterial spasm occurs. This occurs most often in the arm when the radial artery is involved. The condition leads to an ischemic contracture (Volkmann's contracture) and a permanent flexion deformity of the hand if pressure upon the artery is not released surgically as soon as symptoms appear. Occasionally a nerve may also become caught between bone fragments during the process of manipulation to reduce the fracture.

COMMON METHODS OF TREATMENT AND RELATED CARE

Objectives in treatment

Objectives in the treatment and care of fractures include reduction of the fracture, maintenance of the fragments in the correct position while healing takes place, prevention of complications, and maintenance of good general health so that, with return of the fractured bone to usefulness, the patient can continue as before his accident or injury.

Reduction of fractures

Reduction is the term used for the return of bone fragments to their normal position; this may be accomplished by closed manipulation, traction, or operation.

Manipulation. When closed manipulation is used to reduce a fracture, the patient is given a local or general anesthetic which not only relieves pain but also causes muscle relaxation. The physician then reduces the fracture by pulling on the distal fragment (manual traction) while he (or someone else) applies countertraction to the proximal fragment until the bone fragments *engage* or fall into their normal relationship. The physician may also apply direct pressure over the site of the fracture to correct angulation or lateral displacement of a fragment. Usually when this type of reduction is used, a cast is applied to hold the fragments in the desired position while healing occurs.

Traction. Continuous traction for a period of days or even weeks may be necessary to reduce fractures of the femur, because the large muscles exert a strong pull and draw the bone fragments out of normal alignment so that immediate reduction by manual traction is impossible. Continuous traction may also be used to reduce fractures when there has been very extensive tissue damage and when the physical condition of the patient is such that anesthetics cannot be given. Traction may therefore be used for immobilizing the limb while soft tissue healing takes place, reducing the fracture, and maintaining correct position of fragments during bone healing.

Open reduction. Open reduction may be necessary if closed manipulation or traction fails to reduce a fracture. This may be the procedure of choice in certain fractures such as fracture of the femur, compound fractures, comminuted fractures, fractures involving joints, fractures in which soft tissue is caught between bone fragments, and fractures accompanied by severe blood vessel or nerve injury. Open operation permits the surgeon to view the bone fragments and adjacent injured structures and to arrange the fragments in their proper position. The disadvantages of this method of reduction are that it requires anesthesia and imposes surgery upon a patient who has already suffered from the trauma of the original injury. However, since open reduction permits anatomic approximation, better function and quicker healing usually occur. This is now the treatment of choice for many fractures in adults but not in children.

Immobilization

The purpose of immobilization is to hold the bone fragments in contact with each other until healing takes place. All activity of the part that might cause separation of the fragments is restricted, and the fractured bone is kept in position by immobilizing the entire limb. Usually immobilization includes the joints immediately proximal to and distal to the fractured bone. Bandages, adhesive tape, plaster-of-Paris casts, splints, traction, internal fixation, and bed rest are methods of securing immobilization. Metal pins, screws, plates, and nails all made of stainless steel or Vitallium are used to hold the fragments together when an open reduction is done; a plaster-of-Paris cast is often used to provide extra protection when internal fixation is used. This is especially true in treatment of compound fractures of the lower leg.

General care. Nursing care during the time of immobilization includes prevention of complications and maintenance of general health. The patient whose activity is limited by a fracture usually has digestive and elimination problems. Appetite may be poor, yet the body requirements must be met if repair is to progress normally. The diet should be high in protein, iron, calcium, and vitamins. It should also be high in roughage since constipation is often a real problem which causes inconvenience and discomfort and may interfere with appetite. The patient who is ambulatory and being cared for at home should be encouraged to eat plenty of uncooked green vegetables and fresh fruits. The patient in the hospital should be permitted to have relatives bring such foods to him if the hospital menu is somewhat lacking in uncooked vegetables and fresh fruits.

Thrombosis and embolism and muscle and joint changes, with resultant deformity or limitation of function, are possible complications when a patient is immobilized in the treatment of a fracture. It is a nursing responsibility to see that the patient does deep-breathing exercises and exercises his good limbs by means of muscle setting, resistive exercises, or other exercises depending on his particular circumstances. Because of the complex arrangement of muscle attachments and because of muscle action, the nurse needs specific orders from the surgeon before assisting or encouraging the patient to exercise the involved limb. A safe rule is never, under any circumstances, have the patient move or use the joint either immediately distal to or immediately proximal to the fracture unless there is an order permitting this. For example, if the fracture is in the radius, the wrist and elbow joints should not be moved without an order. However, the shoulder can and should be protected from muscle weakness, muscle shortening, and joint changes by regular motion and exercise. The legs, trunk, and unaffected upper limb should be checked regularly (at least daily) to be certain that the patient is doing some systematic routine exercises.

The patient who must remain in bed for a long period of time in traction or in a cast should be in a bed with a firm mattress, and a fracture board should be placed under the mattress. The patient should, from the beginning of his confinement, pay particular attention to his posture. The "small" of the back can be supported by small pillows or a bath towel or rolled bath blanket. The unaffected foot (or feet) should rest against a footboard at least part of the day. This helps to maintain the foot in the normal walking position, prevents the weight of bedclothes from contributing to foot drop, and provides something firm against which the patient can do resistive foot exercises. The patient should be taught to check the position of his lower limb when at rest. He should "toe in" to prevent external rotation of the hip and pronation of the foot which cause serious difficulty when walking is resumed.

The patient with a fracture who is confined to bed should do full range-of-joint exercises for all unaffected joints daily (see Chapter 4). If he is to eventually use crutches, he should practice push-up exercises or other resistive exercises to strengthen the triceps muscle. These can be done, for example, when the patient in a body cast is turned on his abdomen, the patient in traction and in a back-lying position can straighten his elbows while holding weights on his palms.

The patient's skin should be inspected for pressure areas or signs of other irritation. In caring for patients who are immobilized for a long time, there should be a regular schedule (such as weekly) for cutting the nails and giving special attention to the skin in addition to frequent turning, massage, and cleansing of areas such as the perineum. Urinary output should be checked at intervals since the patient who is immobilized for a time may develop urinary retention and renal calculi.

Patients who have been on bed rest for some time should be mobilized gradually; the change of position from a flat to an upright one causes weakness and dizziness. The patient should be prepared for this and should be closely supervised until he can be safely left alone. A tilt table is useful since it allows the patient to become accustomed to an upright position before actual standing is attempted. The walker is extremely helpful, particularly for elderly patients, since the seat provides a resting place if they become too tired from standing. Often the walker is useful in preparing the patient to use crutches.

Before leaving the hospital, the patient should be relatively self-sufficient in getting in and out of bed and in and out of a chair. If he lives alone, he must be able to manage stairs. When he practices these activities in the hospital, the casters should be removed from the hospital bed to lower it and to make it more stable. A visiting nurse can usually help the patient in his home to adjust to his immediate environment and to supervise his progress. A nursing referral should be sent to the public health nursing agency so that the visiting nurse will know exactly what the patient may or may not do and what his progress was during hospitalization and at discharge.

Healing of fractures

When a bone is broken, the ends of bone do not heal by actual growth of new tissue from the bone itself but by a "soldering together" of the fragments by new tissue that is layed down around and between them.[13] This new tissue starts with the hematoma that forms around the bone ends immediately after injury. The hematoma is not absorbed during healing, as are hematomas that occur elsewhere in the body, but becomes changed into granulation tissue. From the sixth to the tenth day after injury the granulation tissue changes into a tissue called the *callus.* Callus is different from other granulation tissue in that it contains cartilage, calcium and phosphate ions, and osteoblasts. The callus temporarily holds the bone fragments together but will not support weight or withstand much activity. It eventually is replaced by true bone which grows from beneath the periosteum of each fragment to meet and fuse across the defect. The length of time required for a bone to heal depends on its location, blood circulation to the part, and age and general physical condition of the patient. Fractures in young children unite much more quickly than do those in older patients. Fractures of the humerus usually heal within ten to twelve weeks; of the forearm, within eight to ten weeks; of the femur, in six months; of the lower leg, in three months; and of the spine, within six to twelve months. The larger the bone, the longer it usually takes to heal.

Delayed healing or *delayed union* is said to occur when the fracture has not healed within the usual time for the particular bone involved. Delayed healing will occur if the space between the two bones is such that neither the callus nor the bone can bridge the gap, if the callus is broken or torn apart by too much activity, if muscle or fascia is caught between the fragments, if an infection develops, or if there is poor blood supply to the part or marked dietary deficiency. Occasionally delayed union occurs with no obvious cause. Open reduction and more complete immobilization may be necessary.

Nonunion is the term used when healing does not take place even in a much longer time than is usually needed. Congenital conditions and obscure medical disease occasionally account for this, and nonunion may occur in the aged. When this occurs, the patient may have to wear a brace to support the limb; if the fracture is in the lower extremity, crutches may have to be used indefinitely. Surgery may be performed and an attempt made to unite the fragments with a bone graft. Nonunion occurs most often in the middle of the humerus, the neck of the femur in older people, the lower third of the tibia, and the carpal bones.

Plaster casts

Plaster-of-Paris casts have been used for many years and are still widely used in the treatment of fractures. Unless a cast has been applied to the entire trunk, the patient who is treated with a plaster-of-Paris cast can usually move about and carry on most of the activities of daily living. Often he may, for example, return to school or to work and participate in many activities without damage to the site of injury. Use of casts shortens hospitalization, and many patients with simple fractures can be treated in a doctor's office or the outpatient department of a hospital. After a short period of observation, they can be discharged and treatment continued under close medical supervision.

Plaster-of-Paris casts do, however, restrict activities because of their weight and their inflexibility. They also present some potential hazards. A cast can cause complications due to interference with normal physiologic functions and can cause actual physical injury if incorrectly applied and improperly cared for. A cast applied to the arm or shoulder may limit the kind of clothing worn and may interfere with eating, writing, or other uses of the arm. If applied to the leg, a cast may change body alignment, put strain on certain muscle groups, and limit locomotion.

The nurse must not only know how to maintain the effectiveness of the cast, but she must also remember the patient in the cast and understand how he is affected by it. She must help the patient be as independent as possible yet provide assistance as needed. The nurse should help to prevent complications from developing and be alert for early signs of complications which must be reported to the physician promptly.

Application of the cast. Most hospitals have a room set aside for the application of casts which provides the necessary space and contains all the equipment required for this procedure. Some hospitals also have a cart equipped with plaster and other cast materials that can be taken to the bedside for use.

Plaster-of-Paris bandages come in various widths (2 to 8 inches). Each roll is wrapped in waxed paper to prevent sifting of the plaster from the bandage and to prevent deterioration from exposure to moisture. The bandage itself is made of crinoline into which plaster of Paris (gypsum or calcium sulfate) has been rubbed. When water is added, the gypsum assumes its crystalline state and the wet plaster bandage can be molded to fit the shape of a body part or wrapped about a limb. When the water evaporates, the cast becomes firm and is able to withstand considerable stress and strain. The number of layers of plaster used determines the strength of the cast.

After reduction has been accomplished and before the cast is applied, the skin is usually protected with sheet wadding (a thick, nonabsorbent cotton web covered with starch to hold it together), and felt or sponge rubber is used over bony prominences to protect them from pressure. Tubular stockinette, from 2 to 18 inches wide, is used as lining for the cast and is applied so that it will extend over the edge to cover the rough edges of the plaster. The excess stockinette and sheet wadding are usually folded back over the cast after it has been applied and bound down with a final roll of plaster.

If the cast is applied elsewhere than in a special plaster room, the floor and table should be protected from wet plaster. When the doctor is ready to apply the cast, the bandage is placed in a bucket of warm water at 35 to 40° C. (95 to 104° F.) until air bubbling ceases. The bubbles of air rise in the water until water has penetrated all parts of the bandage. When bubbling has ceased, the bandage should be carefully removed so that none of the plaster is lost. It should be held horizontally with an end in the palm of each hand and gently compressed to remove excess water. It should then be quickly handed to the doctor so that it can be used before it begins to set. Only a few bandages should be placed in the water at a time. The bucket containing the water should be lined with a cloth or paper to collect waste plaster. When the procedure has been completed, the cloth or paper containing excess plaster can be removed and discarded into a garbage can and the water emptied into the sink, if there is no loose plaster. Plaster of Paris will clog ordinary plumbing and should never be emptied into ordinary drains.

Care of the cast. Although plaster sets within seven minutes, it does not dry for many hours. Usually it is dry in twenty-four hours, although thick body casts may take several days to dry completely. The cast can be cracked or broken by inadequate support or by unwise handling during this time. A wrinkle in the plaster and indentations caused by the finger tips or from continuous pressure can alter the inner shape of the cast and cause pressure on the body part encased in the plaster.

A fracture board should always be used to provide a firm mattress and prevent uneven weight on the fresh plaster cast. To protect the new cast and ensure its efficiency, the patient should be carefully transferred from the stretcher onto his bed. If he is conscious, he can move onto the bed with the assistance of one nurse while another supports the wet cast with the palms of her hands at the areas of greatest strain—usually at the normal joints. If the patient is asleep or is in a body cast, three or four people should lift him onto the bed. The entire cast and the patient's head and his free leg below the cast must be fully supported.

The wet cast should not lie unsupported on the hard bed because it may become flattened, over bony prominences and weight-bearing areas such as the back of the heel, buttocks, and shoulders, and this can cause pressure. The cast should always be fully supported on a pillow or pillows that are protected with rubber or plastic material to prevent their becoming damp. The patient should be in proper body alignment, and there should not be any break in the support provided by the pillows to cause weakening of the cast. If the patient has a cast on the leg, the foot should extend over the edge of the pillow or the bed to avoid pressure upon the heel.

In order for the cast to dry, there must be provision for evaporation by exposure to circulating air. The cast should not be covered with bed linen until it is dry. Therefore, the bed must be made in such a way that the cast is exposed but the patient kept warm and free from drafts. A hair dryer can be used to provide warm moving air; this is particularly helpful when wet, humid weather delays drying. Heat from radiant lamps is not advocated, because it can cause severe burns beneath the cast. Cradles equipped with electric bulbs are not recommended unless there is also provision for free circulation of air; moisture-laden air becomes trapped under the cradle and delays the drying process. Since the patient easily becomes chilled while the cast is drying, blankets should be used to protect body parts not encased in plaster.

The patient should be turned at least every four hours to ensure uniform drying of the cast, to prevent continuous pressure on any one area while the cast is drying, and to make him more comfortable. He should always be turned on the "good side"; the side of the body with the fracture must always be uppermost when the patient is turned. The cast must be very carefully handled and supported until it is completely dry.

To protect body and long leg casts from becoming soiled or wet, waterproof material should be applied around the perineal area. Continuous dampening will soften the cast and impair its effectivness, and a soiled cast lining will irritate the patient's skin and cause an offensive odor. The area can be covered with plastic material, oiled silk, or waxed paper, which can be anchored with adhesive or cellophane tape and changed as necessary. Shellac and varnish protect the entire cast from staining and soiling but should not be applied until the cast is completely dry. If the cast becomes dirty, it can be cleaned with a damp cloth and an abrasive or scouring powder. Soap and water cannot be used, because their continued use may soften the plaster. Mold will usually form on a damp cast; when this happens the cast is usually thoroughly dried and then reinforced with fresh plaster. Old stockings or stockinette can be used to cover the cast to protect it from soiling and from moisture.

Care of the patient in the cast. After the patient has been carefully transferred into bed and the cast is supported on pillows, the nurse should check the patient's general condition. If he has had an anesthetic, he must be watched carefully until vital signs are normal (see Chapter 13). After reduction and immobilization, he should be observed for signs of *delayed shock* such as sudden faintness, dizziness, pallor, diaphoresis, or change in pulse rate. Medication, if ordered, should be given for *general pain.* Complaints of *pressure* may be relieved by elevating the extremity or changing the patient's position. However, if the patient complains of continuous pressure that is unrelieved by change of position, it should be reported to the physician; it may be possible to relieve pressure by cutting out small edges of the cast, or it may be necessary to bivalve all or part of the cast. Areas of pressure are usually over the instep, the lateral border of the foot, heel, malleoli, iliac crests, and sacrum. Changes in skin color should also be watched carefully since they, too, indicate that there may be pressure constricting circulation.

The skin should be inspected frequently and routinely for signs of *circulatory impairment.* There may be swelling and slow return of color after pressure has been applied to the fingers or the toes below the cast; the skin also may be cold or cyanotic. The patient may complain of tightness of the cast and of numbness or tingling of the fingers or toes. These signs and symptoms should be reported to the doctor immediately so that the cast can be divided to relieve constriction if necessary. Most swelling occurs within the first twenty-four to forty-eight hours. Interference with circulation is usually due to a tight cast or to edema. Occasionally it is due to bruising of a blood vessel during manipulation or surgery.

Compression of a nerve can also occur. The nerve most often affected is the peroneal nerve which is located below the head of the fibula on the lateral side of the leg. Continuous pressure on this superficial nerve by a leg cast results in paralysis, with a loss of the ability to dorsiflex the foot or to extend the toes. The patient's complaint of pressure on the lateral side of the leg or of numbness and tingling in the foot must always be reported to the physician at once since pressure must be relieved immediately; this is often done by bivalving the cast.

The patient in a new wet cast should be warmly covered to prevent *chilling;* blankets can be used for this. Plaster on the skin should be removed with plain water. The skin around and directly under the cast edges should be washed and then massaged with alcohol and cream to prevent skin irritation. (See Figure 137.) The skin should also be inspected for pressure areas and signs of irritation from rough plaster edges. As the patient remains in the cast, his elbows may become irritated from bracing himself to move about in bed. Frequent massage and protective pads help, but probably the best thing, if the patient is able to use one, is to provide him with a Balkan frame and crossbar so that he may lift himself.

If the patient is in a body cast or a long leg cast, the head of the bed should be elevated when a bedpan is used. If the cast is new and still damp, it is better to elevate the head of the bed on shock blocks instead of using the gatch, which will put a strain on the cast and may cause it to crack. A pillow should be placed against the small of the back, and a cotton pad protected with plastic material may be tucked under the sacral area to protect the cast from soiling. The leg in the cast should be supported with pillows so that the patient does not feel insecure in this position. Every effort should be made to simplify this procedure so that the patient will not feel he is a problem to the nurses and hesitate to take enough food and fluids on this account. An overhanging trapeze will permit him to help lift himself as the nurse places the bedpan under him. (See Figure 140.) Side rails also assist the patient to turn and give him protection from falling out of bed.

Many patients are discharged after the cast is dry if there is no evidence of circulatory or nerve impairment. If a cast is applied to the arm, the patient should wear a sling to support the full weight of the cast, and the hand should be supported to prevent wrist drop from de-

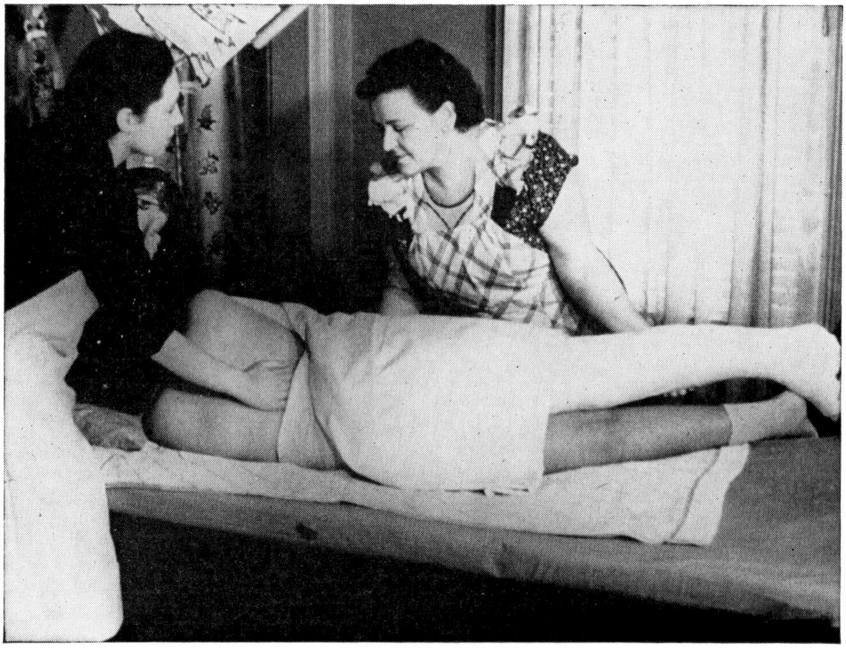

Figure 137

The public health nurse assists a member of a patient's family in home care of the patient in a body cast. (Courtesy Visiting Nurse Association of Brooklyn, Inc., and Clay-Adams, Inc., New York, N. Y.)

veloping. The ends of the sling should be secured with two pins instead of being tied at the back of the neck. If the sling is to be worn for some time, sling ties may be lengthened with bandage or muslin so that they can be crossed in the back and brought around and tied in the front of the body. This helps to prevent forward and downward pull on the neck, which may cause postural defect and fatigue. A member of the patient's family should be taught how to apply the sling correctly.

If a cast is applied to the leg, the patient usually must not bear weight on the cast. If weight-bearing is permitted, the cast is usually fitted with a piece of iron (walking iron) which prevents wear on the plaster. This lengthens the limb and causes an awkward posture, but its use is usually only temporary and the patient progresses to the use of crutches when the cast is removed (see Chapter 19).

Cast removal. The cast is usually removed when roentgenograms show that union is sufficient to allow safe removal. This is often done in the doctor's office or in the hospital outpatient or emergency departments. The cast is bivalved with manual or electric plaster cutters. While the procedure is not painful, the patient may feel some pressure or vibration and is nervous for fear that he may be cut. The skin is usually dry and scaly and should be washed with mild soap and water and lubricated with mineral oil. Since there is usually some stiffness of the joints, the limb should be moved very gently. (See Figure 138.) The patient is usually encouraged to move the limb as much as he is able within limits of pain or stiffness. Exercises for the stiff joint are usually started and muscle-setting exercises continued. After a leg cast is removed, swelling and edema occur for some time when the leg is placed in a dependent

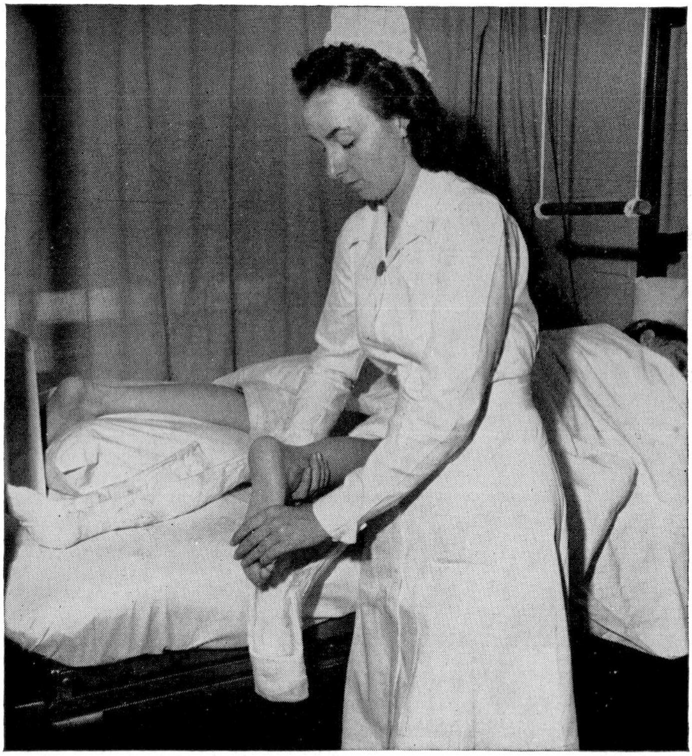

Figure 138

Use of a bivalved cast permits removal of the extremity to give care and exercise. (From Newton, Kathleen: Geriatric Nursing, St. Louis, 1954, The C. V. Mosby Co.)

position. The patient is usually advised by his doctor to sleep with the limb elevated and to elevate it at intervals during the day.

Traction

Continuous traction, or pull, is used to reduce and immobilize fractures, to overcome muscle spasm, and to stretch adhesions and correct certain deformities. Continuous traction may be maintained in several ways, but it always involves pull against bone proximal to the site of pathology (fixed point) or use of countertraction. The fixed point may be established in the bone by means of Kirschner wires or Steinmann pins, or it may be established externally by such means as a Thomas splint. Traction is also achieved by pull from a rope and pulley with weights attached and countertaction provided by the patient's body. The head or foot of the bed is elevated so that the patient's body weight provides pull in one direction while the attached weights exert pull in the opposite direction. Pelvic bands, shoulder straps, ankle straps, and head halters may be used to ensure countertraction by preventing the patient from slipping to the elevated end of the bed. These are likely to be used when a good deal of traction is needed and the patient is light in weight.

Nursing care. Before the nurse attempts to give care to a patient in traction, she must know the nature of the patient's difficulty and what is to be achieved by the use of traction. Any deviation from the basic rules for care of any patient in traction must be approved by the doctor before it is permitted. For example, the patient with arthritis may be permitted to partially release traction by sitting upright for a few moments when the lower limb is being treated, while the patient with a fresh fracture of the femur might do himself harm by doing this.

In order for traction to be effective, the patient must lie on his back. Turning onto the side or sitting up changes body alignment, and the pull (traction) is lost or becomes less effective. The nurse should explain this to the patient and help him to be as comfortable as possible while remaining in the correct position. The patient who must lie flat often feels handicapped and helpless because he cannot readily see what is going on about him; turning the bed to one side sometimes helps this.

The nurse must be certain that the *weights hang free* with no obstruction to interfere with straight, even, continuous pull. Traction should be inspected frequently. For example, when traction is being applied to the lower limb, bedclothes must not be pressing on the rope or against the footplate; the footplate must never be pushing against the foot of the bed or the pulley, since this will completely negate traction. There should be no knots in the rope, since these may become caught in the pulley and interfere with traction; the rope must be long enough so that weights will not be hampered by the pulley as the patient pulls himself up in bed, yet not long enough to rest on the floor if he slips to the foot

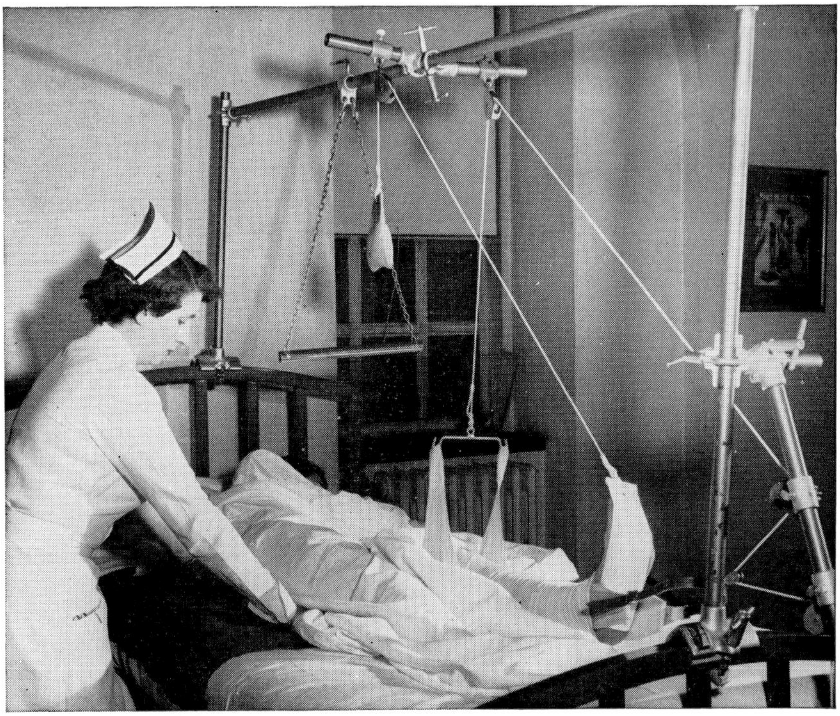

Figure 139

The patient may turn slightly with certain conditions for which Russell traction is used. Note the hammock under the knee, the placement of the four pulleys, and the apparatus used to prevent foot drop.

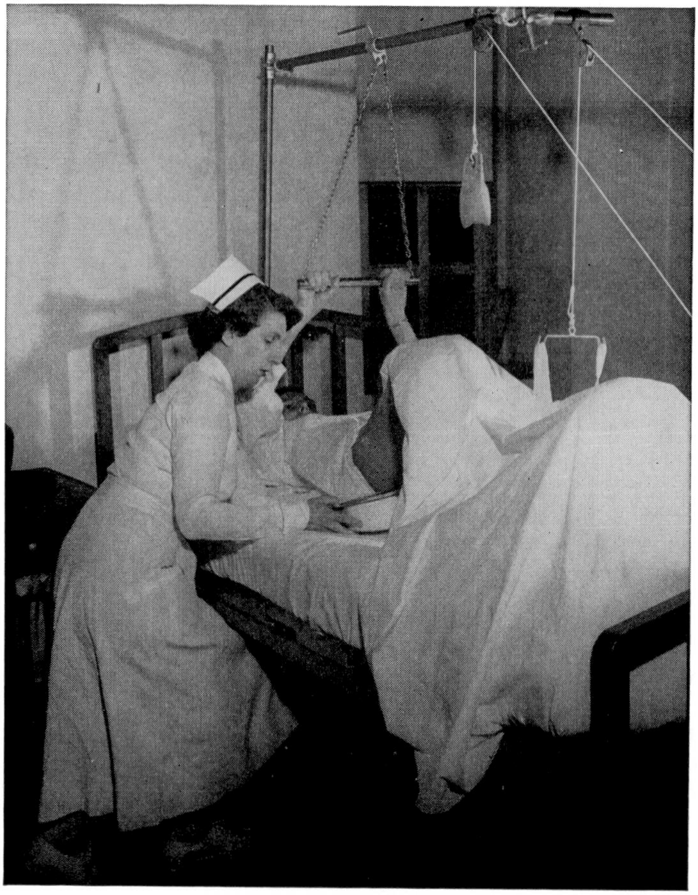

Figure 140

Assisting the patient in Russell traction onto a bedpan. Note the small bedpan, the flexion of the patient's good leg against the bed, the use of the overhead bar, and the nurse's body mechanics.

of the bed; the rope must be strong enough so that it will not break if more weights are added; the weights must be securely fastened so that they will not drop off if the equipment is accidentally touched; and the equipment should be uncovered so that it is not jarred or swung inadvertently. Sandbags are often used for weights and are tied to the rope; when regular scale weights are used, they should be fastened with adhesive tape so that they will not slip off. Jarring the bed and swinging the weights may cause pain and are upsetting to the patient.

An important concept in the care of the patient in traction is that the patient should not suffer from lack of any kind of nursing care because of his immobilization. At first glance it might sometimes appear that good back care, for example, is impossible. This is not true. The patient in traction should, of course, be on a firm bed and should have a Balkan frame or overhead attachment so that he can help to lift himself and take some weight off his back for short periods. He can be moved enough for good back care to be given and for linen to be changed. (See

Figure 139.) This must be accomplished, however, by having the patient raise himself straight up in the bed while care is given and the bed linen slid under him. It is a good practice for a second nurse or an attendant to steady the traction and even increase the pull slightly as the patient carefully and steadily raises himself with assistance. The same procedure is followed when the patient has a bowel movement. A very small, flat bedpan should be used, and the back above the pan should be supported by a small pillow or a bath blanket folded to the correct height. (See Figure 140.)

The patient who is in traction needs the same attention to nutrition, elimination, exercise of noninvolved extremities, prevention of postural defects, and skin care as any other patient who is immobilized. Particular attention must be given to the skin that comes into contact with any traction apparatus. For example, the skin over bony hip prominences may become reddened and painful if a pelvic band is being used, adhesive tape may work downward and straps may rub against the ankle malleolus when skin traction is used on the lower limb, and a Thomas splint may cause injury to the skin of the groin. Skin irritation of this kind must be reported to the doctor, who may alter the amount of weight used or take other action.

Types of traction

Skin traction. Skin traction is achieved by applying wide bands of moleskin adhesive directly to the skin and attaching weights to these. The pull of the weights is transmitted indirectly to the involved bone. *Buck's extension, Bryant's traction,* and *Russell traction* are the three most common forms of skin traction used for injury to the lower extremities. Buck's extension is the simplest and is often used to relieve muscle spasm and to immobilize a limb temporarily, such as the leg and thigh when a hip fracture has been sustained by an elderly person and internal fixation is to be done within a short time. The skin of the leg is shaved and tincture of benzoin is applied for protection. The adhesive is then applied to the lateral and medial aspects of the thigh and leg and is joined to a tape which is attached to a footplate or a spreader to prevent pressure on the toes. This, in turn, is attached to the rope and pulley. Bryant's traction, which is skin traction applied to both lower limbs, can be used to reduce fractures of the femur in children under 6 years of age. Both lower limbs are suspended vertically. This kind of traction is not used for patients over 6 years of age because the countertraction (weight of the trunk) is not sufficient and because the position hampers arterial circulation of the feet.

Russell traction is widely used because it permits the patient to move about in bed somewhat freely and permits bending of the knee joint. This is skin traction in which four pulleys are used and in which the knee is suspended in a hammock or sling. One pulley is attached to the footplate, one to a Balkan frame exactly over the tubercle of the tibia of the affected limb, and two to the crossbar at the foot of the bed. Moleskin adhesive is applied to the leg as in Buck's extension. By means of the pulleys, the actual weight on the line of fracture is double that of the weight placed on the pulley at the foot of the bed (see references and specialized texts for details). (See Figure 141.) Since there is upward pull from the hammock, skin under the popliteal space should be protected with a piece of felt or sponge rubber and should be inspected regularly. Any complaints of pain or discomfort should be reported to the doctor at once; occasionally thrombophlebitis develops from inactivity and from pressure on the popliteal vessels. The patient's heel should just clear the bed so that there is no weight or pressure on the heel. This traction results in slight flexion of the hip; the angle between the thigh and the bed should be approximately 20 degrees. Usually the foot of the bed is elevated to provide countertraction. Russell traction is widely used in treatment of aged persons with fractures since it is com-

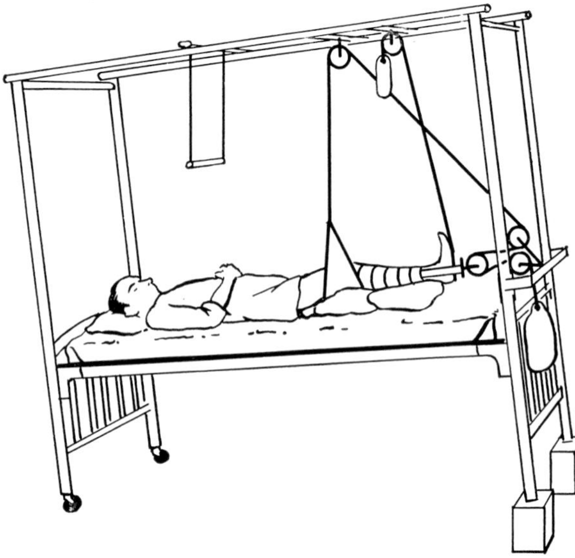

Figure 141

Russell traction. Note that the leg is supported on pillows and the heel extends beyond the pillow.

fortable for most patients; often the patient is permitted to have the head of the bed slightly elevated. Usually a pillow is placed lengthwise under the thigh and a second pillow is placed under the leg.

Skeletal traction. Skeletal traction is applied directly to the bone. Under the strictest of aseptic precautions, a rustless *Steinmann pin* or *Kirschner wire* is inserted directly through the bone fragment distal to the fracture and out through the skin on the opposite side of the limb. A metal spreader is then attached to the wire or pin and then the weights are attached to the spreader. Skeletal traction can be used for fractures of the tibia, femur, humerus, and the skull. Skeletal traction to the skull is achieved by use of *Crutchfield tongs* (see Chapter 34).

Usually the patient goes to the operating room or the fracture room for the insertion of pins or wires. The skin and periosteum are anesthetized with procaine hydrochloride; general anesthesia is not usually used. The ends of the pin or wire are protected with cork, and small sterile dressings are placed around the points of entry and exit. These must be watched for signs of local infection, and care must be taken that they do not become wet or soiled. Usually a cast is also used when Steinmann pins or Kirschner wires are necessary.

Suspension. Suspension is used in conjunction with skin or skeletal traction to permit the patient to move about in bed more freely. The slack caused by the moving is taken up by the suspension so that the line of traction is not changed. The limb no longer rests on the bed and the patient can move more easily, turn partially on his side, and get on and off a bedpan while traction is still maintained. Pressure on the sacrum is often greatly relieved by this form of treatment.

The limb is placed in a canvas hammock provided by a half-ring or a full-ring splint such as a *Thomas* or a *Hodgen splint*. The hammock is made of canvas (muslin towels may be used occasionally) and is lined with sponge rubber or cotton. The ring or half-ring must be protected with oiled silk or other protective material since it fits firmly in the groin. Skin care at the point of pressure has already been mentioned. The end of the splint is attached by a rope to a pulley above the limb; weight at the end of the rope helps the patient lift himself against gravity. The patient in balanced traction or suspension may also be provided with a *Pearson attachment* which permits flexion of the knee. This is attached at the level of the knee and is equipped with a hammock to support the leg. The patient may then, by means of pulleys, exercise his knee joint as desired and prescribed.

Reduction and fixation by operation

When internal fixation is to be used to reduce and immobilize a fracture, the patient is prepared as for other operations (see Chapter 12). However, because bone infection is a serious complication, surgery is delayed and other methods of reduction and immobilization are used if there are lacerations, abraisons, or extensive ecchymosis about the area of the fracture.

When surgery is to be done, the skin is carefully prepared, and the greatest care is taken not to cut the skin or cause even minor abrasions. After the incision is made and reduction is accomplished, the bone fragments may be held in place with steel wire, plates and screws, nails, bolts and screws, or intramedullary nails. These are all made of stainless steel or Vitallium, which are nonirritating metals. A plaster cast may be applied to help prevent muscle pull on the newly reduced fragments if the break is in such a location that there will be strain upon them.

Fractures of the neck of the femur are often treated by *pinning* (internal fixation); no cast is needed when this is done. A variety of nails and pins are used in the treatment of this very common fracture in aged women. This treatment has led to remarkable drop in the death rate from fracture of the femur in aged persons, since immobilization in a body cast and its attendant complications are obviated.

If the patient is placed in a cast following operation, the nursing care is essentially that given any patient in a cast. Immediately following the patient's return from the operating room, he should be watched carefully for signs of shock and hemorrhage. Blood pressure and pulse and respiratory rates should be taken every fifteen minutes until they are stabilized since it may be impossible to detect hemorrhage under a heavy body cast for some time. If bleeding is extensive, however, it will eventually become apparent either as oozing around the edge of the cast or as staining of the cast as blood saturates the damp plaster. Reddened staining on a cast is marked with a pencil, together with a notation of the time, so that its rate of progress can be noted if it continues.

The patient who has had an operation for reduction of a fracture usually has quite severe pain for several days; narcotics for pain and sedatives for sleep are usually ordered.

Local and systemic signs of infection should be watched for. These include pain in the wound, odor, drainage about the cast, and increase in the pulse and respiratory rates and an elevated temperature. Antibiotics are usually given prophylactically prior to surgery and continued postoperatively.

REFERENCES AND SELECTED READINGS*

1 Bruck, Helen: The Drying of Plaster Casts, Am. J. Nursing **46**:400-402, June 1946.
2 *Calderwood, Carmelita: Russell Traction, Am. J. Nursing **43**:464-469, May 1943.
3 *Calderwood, Carmelita: The Patient Comes Out of His Cast, Am. J. Nursing **44**:202-205, March 1944.
4 Cecil, Russell L., and Loeb, Robert F.: A Textbook of Medicine, ed. 10, Philadelphia, 1959, W. B. Saunders Co.
5 Donaldson, John S., and Williams, Mary Edna: Replacement Arthoplasties of the Hip and Nursing Care, Am. J. Nursing **55**:565-567, May 1955.

*References preceded by an asterisk indicate material particularly well suited for student reading.

6 *Hacker, Garnet I.: The Medullary Nail, Am. J. Nursing **50**:104-106, Feb. 1950.
7 Harmer, Bertha, and Henderson, Virginia (revised by): Textbook of the Principles and Practice of Nursing, ed. 5, New York, 1955, The Macmillan Co.
8 Larson, Carroll B., and Gould, Marjorie: Calderwood's Orthopedic Nursing, ed. 4, St. Louis, 1957, The C. V. Mosby Co.
9 *Larson, Carroll B., and Gould, Marjorie L.: Fractures of the Hip and Nursing Care of the Patient With a Fractured Hip, Am. J. Nursing **58**:1558-1563, Nov. 1958.
10 *Mayo, Richard A., and Hughes, Joanne M.: Intramedullary Nailing of Long Bone Fractures and Nursing Care After Intramedullary Nailing, Am. J. Nursing **59**:236-240, Feb. 1959.
11 Miller, Bernice L.: Well-Leg and Well-Hip Splints, Am. J. Nursing **48**:572-576, Sept. 1948.
12 Moore, Moore, Jr.: Ambulation Following Fractures of the Lower Extremity, Am. J. Nursing **53**:174-175, Feb. 1953.
13 Moseley, H. F. (editor): Textbook of Surgery, ed 3, St. Louis, 1959, The C. V. Mosby Co.
14 Newton, Kathleen: Geriatric Nursing ed. 3, St. Louis, 1960, The C. V. Mosby Co.
15 *Wilde, Delphine: Fracture Nursing Problems, Am. J. Nursing **39**:964-967, Sept. 1939.
16 *Wilde, Delphine: Traction and Suspension, Am. J. Nursing **53**:1465-1468, Dec. 1953.

Index

B

G

H

J

K

O

W

X

Y

Z